HANDBUCH
DER EXPERIMENTELLEN
PHARMAKOLOGIE

BEGRÜNDET VON A. HEFFTER

FORTGEFÜHRT VON W. HEUBNER

ERGÄNZUNGSWERK

HERAUSGEGEBEN VON

O. EICHLER   UND   A. FARAH

PROFESSOR DER PHARMAKOLOGIE
AN DER UNIVERSITÄT HEIDELBERG

PROFESSOR DER PHARMAKOLOGIE
AN DER STATE UNIVERSITY OF NEW YORK

DREIZEHNTER BAND

THE ALKALI METAL IONS IN BIOLOGY

BY

H. H. USSING, P. KRUHØFFER, J. HESS THAYSEN AND N. A. THORN

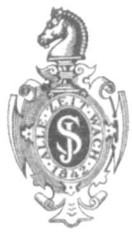

SPRINGER-VERLAG

BERLIN · GÖTTINGEN · HEIDELBERG

1960

THE ALKALI METAL IONS
IN BIOLOGY

I. THE ALKALI METAL IONS
IN ISOLATED SYSTEMS AND TISSUES

BY

HANS H. USSING

II. THE ALKALI METAL IONS
IN THE ORGANISM

BY

P. KRUHØFFER, J. HESS THAYSEN AND N. A. THORN

WITH 47 FIGURES

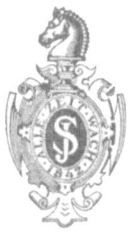

SPRINGER-VERLAG
BERLIN · GÖTTINGEN · HEIDELBERG
1960

ISBN-13: 978-3-642-49248-8   e-ISBN-13: 978-3-642-49246-4
DOI: 10.1007/978-3-642-49246-4

© by Springer-Verlag oHG. Berlin · Göttingen · Heidelberg 1959

Contents

Part I: The alkali metal ions in isolated systems and tissues

By HANS H. USSING

Page

I. General introduction 1

II. Physical and chemical properties of the alkali metal ions 2
    a) Introduction 2
    b) Chemical properties 3
    c) Chemical binding 4
    d) Chelates with low-molecular anions 4
    e) Binding by ion exchange resins 5
    f) Binding by phosphate esters and polyphosphates 6
    g) Binding by nucleic acids 8
    h) Binding by polyvalent acid polysaccharides 8
    i) Binding by proteins 9

III. Role of alkali metal ions in enzymatic processes 10
    a) Introduction 10
    b) Specific effects on enzymatic processes 11
        1. Pyruvic phosphoferase 11
        2. Fructokinase 12
        3. Bacterial hexokinase 13
        4. Phosphofructokinase 13
        5. Acetate-activating enzyme (and "choline acetylase") 14
        6. Phosphotransacetylase 15
        7. Glutathione synthesizing enzyme system 15
        8. Aldehyde dehydrogenase (from yeast) 16
        9. β-galactosidase (from Escherichia coli) 16
      10. Apyrase (brain adenosinetriphosphatase) 17
      11. Bacterial apyrase 17
      12. ATP-ase from crab nerve 17
      13. Myosin ATP-ase 18
      14. Urease 18
    c) Non-specific effects of alkali metal ions 19
    d) Comments 20

IV. Effect of alkali metal ions on mitochondria 21

V. Metabolic effects on tissues and tissue slices 23
    a) Effects on oxygen consumption 24
        1. Brain slices 24
        2. Peripheral nerve 25
        3. Liver slices 25
        4. Muscle 26
        5. Kidney slices 27
        6. Isolated frog skin 27
    b) Effects on glycolysis 28
    c) Effect on acetyl choline synthesis 28
    d) Effect on glycogen synthesis 29
    e) Effects on fatty acid metabolism 31
    f) Effects on cellular accumulation of various substances 31
    g) Morphogenetic effects of lithium 32
        1. The effects of lithium 32
        2. Mechanism of the Li effect 34

VI. Distribution of the alkali metal ions between cells and their surroundings . . 36
    a) General remarks 36
    b) State of potassium in living cells 37
    c) State of Rb and Cs in living cells 43
    d) State of sodium in living cells 44

Page

VII. Active and passive transport of the alkali metal ions 45

A. Characterization and biological role 45
   a) Introduction 45
   b) Passive transport 47
   c) "Simple" passive transport 47
   d) The flux ratio 49
   e) The effect of solvent drag 51
   f) Passive permeability and membrane structure 54
   g) Permeability of intercellular cements 55
   h) Ionic permeability and the development of bioelectric potentials 56
   i) Active transport of the alkali metal ions (The „Sodium pump") 57
   j) Relation of the active transport to metabolism. 60
   k) Quantitative relationship between oxygen consumption and active ion
      transport   61
   l) Temperature dependency of the "sodium pump" 62
   m) Effects of drugs and hormones on active and passive transport 63
      1. Steroid hormones 63
      2. Cardiac glycosides and their aglucones 64
      3. Different Hormones 64
         Acetyl choline p. 64. — Histamine p. 65. — Adrenaline p. 65. — Neuro-
         hypophyseal hormones p. 65.
   n) Role of alkali ion transport in the regulation of the volume of living cells . . 65
   o) Mechanisms proposed for the active transport of alkali metal ions 67
      1. Simple membrane-carrier transport p. 67. — 2. Electron-linked carrier
      transport p. 68. — 3. Propelled carrier transport p. 68. — 4. "Asymme-
      trically collapsing lattice" theories p. 69. — 5. The fluid circuit mecha-
      nisms p. 69. — 6. Pinocytosis p. 69.

B. Transport between cells and their surroundings 70
   a) Erythrocytes 71
      1. Transport of potassium in human erythrocytes 73
      2. Transport of sodium in human erythrocytes. 75
      3. Effect of p_H on the Na transport 76
      4. Effect of temperature 76
      5. Transport of Li in human erythrocytes 77
      6. Transport of Rb in human erythrocytes 77
      7. Transport of Cs in human erythrocytes 77
      8. Evidence for a coupling between active sodium extrusion and potassium
         uptake 77
      9. Relation of the active and passive transports to metabolism 78
     10. Effects of cardiac glucosides on the transport processes 79
     11. Ion transport by red cell "ghosts" 80
     12. Mechanism of the active transport 81
     13. Nature of the diffusion of alkali metal ions through the erythrocyte
         membrane 81
     14. Alkali metal ion transport in other mammalian red cells 82
     15. Transport of K and Na in bird red cells 82
     16. Transport of K and Na in red cells of lower vertebrates 83
   b) Muscle 84
      1. Development of the "sodium pump" concept 85
      2. Net transports of K and Na in muscle 88
      3. The sodium flux across the frog-muscle fibre membrane 89
      4. Energy requirement of the active Na transport in frog muscle 91
      5. The potassium fluxes of frog muscle 93
      6. The potassium fluxes of mammalian muscle 95
      7. Alkali metal ion shifts in relation to muscular activity 95
   c) Peripheral nerve 95
      1. Movements of potassium and sodium in the resting nerve 96
      2. Effect of temperature on cation fluxes in nerve 98
      3. Active transport of Na in cephalopod giant axons 99
      4. Coupling between Na-outflux and K-influx 99
      5. Nature of the passive movement of K through the cephalopod giant axon
         membrane 100
      6. Passive potassium transport during current flow 101

Page

7. Passive transport of Na through the giant fibre membrane 101
8. Potassium and sodium shifts during activity 102
d) Leucocytes 103
e) Brain slices and isolated retina 103
f) Mouse ascites carcinoma cells 105
g) Liver slices 106
h) Kidney cortex slices 106
i) Seminal vesicle mucosa 107
j) Yeast cells 108
k) Ulva lactuca 109
l) Halicystis and Valonia 109
m) Nitellopsis (Characeae) 111
n) Higher plants 111
C. Transport through epithelial membranes 112
a) Introduction 112
b) The amphibian skin 114
1. The active sodium transport of the frog skin and its relation to the skin
potential 114
2. The relation between oxygen consumption and active sodium transport 120
3. The work performed by the active sodium transport mechanism . . . 120
4. The electromotive force of the active sodium transport 122
5. Inhibitors of the active sodium transport 125
6. Stimulants of active sodium transport 126
7. The action of neurohypophyseal hormones upon the transfer of water and
salt across the frog skin 127
8. The relationship between active sodium transport and transport of water
across the skin 128
c) The rumen of ruminants 129
d) The toad urinary bladder 130
e) Intestinal mucosa 131
1. Net transport of sodium 131
2. The dependency of the sodium transport upon different factors 133
3. The unidirectional sodium fluxes 134
4. Intestinal potentials and their relation to active sodium transport . . . 136
5. The transport of potassium across the intestinal wall 138
f) Kidney tubulus 139
g) The Malpighian tubules of insects 140
h) The formation of the endolymph 141
i) Active K transport in the formation of bull seminal plasma 142
j) The gills of Eriocheir sinensis (The "woolhanded crab") 142
VIII. Relation of the alkali metal ions to bioelectric phenomena 144
A. Relation to maintained potentials 144
a) Introduction 144
b) Effect of K on the resting potential of muscle and nerve 144
1. Striated muscle 144
2. Heart muscle 147
3. Smooth muscle 147
4. Nerve 148
c) Dependency of the K effect upon other ion species 150
d) Effect of external Na upon the resting potential of nerve and muscle . . . 150
e) Effects of the non-biological alkali metal ions upon the resting potential . . 151
B. Relation to the electric activity of nerve and muscle 151
a) The "sodium" theory of excitation (HODGKIN-HUXLEY-KATZ) 151
b) The relation of the external Na concentration to the action potential of
single nerve fibres 153
c) Effect of Li upon the action potential of single nerve fibres 154
d) Relation of K to the action potential of single nerve fibres 154
e) The contributions of Na and K to the membrane current in squid axons . 154
f) The applicability and limitations of the sodium theory of electric activity . 160
g) Effect of external Na concentration upon excitation and conduction . . . 162
1. Effects on nerve 162
2. The nerve sheath as a diffusion barrier 162
3. Effects on striated muscle 163

Page

    4. Effects on heart muscle 164
   h) Effect of internal Na concentration on electric activity in muscle 164
   i) Effects of K upon excitation and conduction 165
    1. Nerve 165
    2. Striated muscle 166
    3. Heart muscle 167
 C. Relations to the electric activity of neuromuscular junctions and synapses . . 168
   a) Neuromuscular junctions 168
    1. Effects of Na 169
    2. Effects of potassium 170
   b) The sub-synaptic membrane 170
 D. Relation to the electric activity of electric organs 171
IX. Role of the alkali metal ions in muscular contraction 172
 A. Introduction: Non-living models 172
 B. Effects on skeletal muscle 174
   a) Effects of Na 174
   b) Effects of K 174
    1. Introduction 174
    2. Potassium contracture 175
    3. Effects of K on the mechanical response 177
    4. The Fleckenstein hypothesis 179
 C. Effects on heart muscle 183
   a) Introduction 183
   b) Temperature and ionic effects on the heart 185
   c) Effects on the heart rate (the rhythm) 186
   d) Effects upon the mechanical response of the heart 186
   e) The Hajdu hypothesis 188
    1. The "staircase" phenomenon 188
    2. Potassium ions and the development of tension 189
    3. Potassium ions and contracture 189
    4. Effect of Na upon the staircase 190
    5. Formulation of the hypothesis 190
 D. Effects on smooth muscle 191
   a) Effect of sodium ions 191
    1. Intestinal muscle 191
    2. Uterus muscle 192
   b) Effect of potassium ions 192
    1. Intestinal muscle 192
    2. Uterus muscle 193
    3. Vascular muscle 195

Part: II The alkali metal ions in the organism
By P. KRUHØFFER, J. HESS THAYSEN and N. A. THORN.
 I. Introduction 196
 II. Distribution of alkali metals in body compartments and tissues. By N. A. THORN 198
 A. The sodium and potassium of the extracellular compartment (and some tissues
   built mainly of extracellular components) 198
   a) Blood plasma 198
   b) Lymph 203
   c) Interstitial spaces 204
   d) Tendon 206
   e) Corium 207
   f) Cornea 207
 B. The sodium and potassium of cartilage and bone 208
   a) Cartilage 208
   b) Bone 210
    Amount of sodium in bone p. 210. — Nature of sodium in bone p. 211. —
    "Availability", function of sodium in bone p. 212.
 C. The sodium and potassium of fluids contained in special extracellular cavities . 214
   a) Synovial fluid 214
   b) Cerebrospinal fluid 215
   c) Aqueous humour 216

Page

d) Vitreous humour 217
e) Endolymph, perilymph 217
f) Amniotic fluid 218
g) Transport over placenta 219

D. The sodium and potassium of different tissues mainly composed of cells . . . 219
a) Introduction 219
b) Epidermis, lens 220
c) Muscular tissues 221
d) Blood cells 222
e) Neural tissues 222
f) Glandular tissues 222
g) Miscellaneous 222

E. Distribution of lithium, rubidium and cesium. 223
Distribution of naturally occurring lithium p. 223. — Distribution of lithium
after administration p. 223. — Distribution of naturally occurring rubidium
p. 224. — Distribution of rubidium after administration p. 224. — Distribution of naturally occurring cesium p. 225. — Distribution of cesium after
administration p. 225.

III. Total body contents of sodium and potassium. Total exchangeable sodium and
potassium. By N. A. Thorn. 226

A. Total body contents. 226

B. Total exchangeable sodium and potassium (Na_e, K_e) 227

C. Relation between total body contents and total exchangeable contents . . . 231

D. Relation between isotope dilution data and data from metabolic balance studies 232

E. Relation between Na_e and K_e and serum concentrations 232

IV. Handling of alkali metal ions by the kidney. By P. Kruhøffer 233

A. Introduction 233

B. Processes involved in tubular transport of water and the predominant ions of
plasma; their nature and localization 234
a) The proximal tubules 234
b) The distal tubular system 242
Distal tubular processes concerned with water (and salt) reabsorption
p. 242. — Distal reabsorption of sodium (and secretion of potassium)
p. 251. — Concluding remarks p. 260.

C. Transport of fluid in the nephron as a whole (relationship between glomerular
and tubular factors) 261

D. Physical factors (pressures) affecting sodium (and water) excretion 268
a) Effect of changes in the oncotic pressure of plasma 269
b) Effect of changes in renal arterial pressure 271
c) Effect of increase in ureteral (pelvic) pressure 272
d) Effect of elevation of renal venous pressure 274
e) Effects of pressures acting on the outside of the kidney 276

E. Effects of changes in plasma sodium (and chloride) concentration on sodium
excretion 277

F. "Osmotic diuresis" and sodium (and potassium) excretion 280

G. Interrelationship between urinary acidification and sodium and potassium
excretion 285
a) Potassium excretion as related to sodium excretion 286
b) The effects of primary changes in the acid-base status of the body fluids . . 288
Hyperventilation (respiratory alkalosis) p. 288. — Increased pCO_2
(respiratory acidosis) p. 290. — Effects of non-respiratory ("metabolic")
alkalosis on potassium excretion p. 291. — Potassium excretion in non-respiratory acidosis p. 292.
c) The effects of potassium deficiency and potassium excess 292
Effects of potassium deficiency upon bicarbonate reabsorption p. 293. —
Effects of administration of potassium salts (potassium excess) p. 294.
d) The effects of carbonic anhydrase inhibitors 296

Page

H. Hormonal factors affecting the renal handling of sodium, potassium (and water)   301
   a) Hormones of the adrenal cortex and other steroids   301
      Effects of adrenocortical insufficiency p. 301. — Natural corticosteroids
      p. 304. — Effects of corticoids on renal sodium and potassium excre-
      tions (and renal function in general) p. 316. — Corticoid derivatives
      p. 336. — Licorice extract p. 338 — Progesterone p. 339. — Oestrogens p.
      339. — Androgens p. 340.
   b) Hormones of the adrenal medulla   340
   c) Hormones of the adenohypophysis   340
   d) Neurohypophyseal hormones   342
      Vasopressin (antidiuretic hormone, ADH, β-hypophamine) p. 343. —
      Oxytocin p. 353.
   e) Hormones of the pancreas   354
      Insulin p. 354. — Glucagon p. 354.
   f) Miscellaneous   355
      Renin and hypertensin p. 355. — Serotonin p. 355.

I. Effect of the renal nerves and sympathicomimetic amines on sodium and
   potassium excretion   356
   a) The renal nerves   356
   b) Effects of sympathomimetic amines   359

J. Influence of the central nervous system on body contents and renal excretion
   of sodium (and water)   362

K. Effects of changes in the state of the cardiovascular system on sodium excretion   368
   a) Effects of changes in total blood volume   369
   b) Procedures causing redistribution of the blood volume   372
   c) Influence of posture   375
   d) Sodium retention in circulatory failure (formation of cardiac oedema) . . .   378

L. Effect of exercise on renal sodium excretion   387

M. Diurnal variations in the renal excretion of sodium and potassium   387

N. Diuretic and natriuretic agents   388
   a) Introduction (definitions and types of diureses)   388
   b) Water   389
   c) Osmotic diuretics   390
   d) Salts   391
   e) Acidifying diuretics   393
   f) Mercurial diuretics   395
      The typical response p. 396. — Mechanism of the renal response p. 397. —
      Cellular site of action p. 405. — Factors influencing the diuretic response
      to mercurials p. 406. — Effects of mercurials on urinary potassium excre-
      tion p. 408.
   g) Xanthine diuretics   410
      The typical response p. 411. — The mechanism of xanthine diuresis p. 411.
   h) Diuretics chemically related to xanthines   415
   i) Unsubstituted sulphonamides (carbonic anhydrase inhibitors)   416
   j) Chlorothiazide (and derivatives)   416
   k) Antialdosterones   417

O. The renal excretion of lithium, rubidium and cesium   419
   a) Lithium   419
   b) Rubidium and cesium   422
   c) Note on thallous ions   423

P. Transport of sodium and potassium across the urinary bladder wall   423

V. Handling of alkali metals by exocrine glands other than the kidney. By J. HESS
   THAYSEN   424

A. The duct possessing glands   424
   a) Introduction   424
      The outward transfer of electrolytes p. 427. — The morphological site of
      the outward transport of electrolytes p. 430. — The reabsorption of
      sodium p. 431. — The morphological site of sodium reabsorption p. 434. —
      Glandular sodium and potassium balance during secretion p. 434. —
      Glandular oxygen consumption in relation to electrolyte transport p. 435.

Page

— Factors affecting sodium and potassium excretion by the duct-possessing glands p. 436. — Criticism of the present theory of sodium and potassium secretion p. 438.

b) The sweat glands 438
Type of gland p. 439. — Rate of secretion p. 440. — Skin temperature p. 442. — Duration of secretion p. 442. — Type of stimulus p. 443. — Plasma concentration of Na und K p. 443. — Glandular blood flow p. 443. — Adaptation to salt depletion p. 444. — Adrenal cortical steroids p. 445. — Drugs p. 445. — Individual differences in sweat composition p. 445. — — The secretion of Li, Cs and Rb p. 447. — The effect of prolonged sweating on the homeostasis of water, sodium and potassium p. 447. — Water loss p. 447. — Electrolyte loss p. 448. — Replacements p. 448. — The effect of sweating without replacement of water and salt p. 449. — The effect of sweating with replacement of water but not of salt p. 450. — The effect of sweating with replacement of salt but not of water loss p. 450.

c) The salivary glands 450
Type of gland p. 451. — Rate of secretion p. 452. — Gland temperature p. 454. — Duration of secretion p. 454. — Type of stimulation p. 455. — Glandular blood flow p. 455.—Plasma concentration of Na and K p. 455.— Salt depletion p. 456. — Adrenal cortical steroids p. 457. — The effect of various drugs p. 458. — Individual variations p. 459. — The secretion of Li, Cs and Rb p. 459.

d) The pancreatic gland 460
Rate of secretion p. 461. — Duration of secretion p. 461. — Type of stimulation p. 461. — Plasma concentration of the alkali metals p. 462. — The effect of certain drugs p. 463. — Individual variations p. 463.

e) The lacrymal gland 463
Rate of secretion p. 464. — Duration of secretion p. 464. — Plasma concentration ·p. 464.

B. The glands of the gastrointestinal tract 464
a) The oesophageal glands 464
b) The gastric mucosa 465
Type of gland p. 467. — Rate of secretion p. 468. — Type of stimulus p. 471. — Duration of secretion p. 473. — Plasma concentrations of Na and K (total osmolar concentration) p. 473. — Mucosal blood flow and oxygen supply p. 474. — Gland temperature p. 475. — Salt depletion and adreno-cortical steroids p. 475. — Individual differences p. 477. — The secretion of lithium p. 477. — The alkali metal content of the gastric mucosa p. 477. — Mechanism of alkali metal secretion p. 478.

c) The intestinal mucosa 483
Type of gland p. 483. — Rate of secretion p. 485. — Plasma concentration of the alkali metals (total osmolar concentration of the plasma) p. 485. — The alkali metals in the intestine p. 486. — The mechanism of intestinal secretion p. 486.

C. The liver and the gall bladder 486
a) Hepatic bile 486
Collection of hepatic bile p. 486. — The electrolyte composition of hepatic bile p. 487. — Rate of secretion p. 488. — Plasma concentration of the alkali metals (total osmolar concentration of the plasma) p. 489. — Hepatic blood flow and oxygen supply p. 489. — Temperature p. 490. — The excretion of lithium in the hepatic bile p. 490. — The mechanism of alkali metal excretion in the bile p. 490.

b) Gall bladder bile 492
The electrolyte composition of gall bladder bile p. 492. — The reabsorptive functions of the gall bladder p. 493. — The secretory functions of the gall bladder p. 496.

c) The alkali metals in hepatic tissue 496
D. The mammary gland 497
E. Male organs of reproduction 499
F. Female organs of reproduction 501
G. The glands of the respiratory tract 502

Page

H. Concluding remarks on glandular secretion 503

VI. Intestinal absorption of alkali metal ions. By P. KRUHØFFER and J. HESS THAYSEN 508

A. Introduction 508

B. Resins and intestinal absorption of alkali metal ions 510
   Properties of ion exchange resins p. 510. — The state of charging of resins
   present in the intestinal contents p. 511.

C. Influence of corticoids on intestinal absorption of alkali metal ions 512

D. Use of resin therapy for potassium depletion 514

E. Intestinal lavage as a measure to correct electrolyte imbalances. 514

F. Intestinal absorption as a problem in ureterocolic anastomoses 514

VII. Intakes and general turnovers. By N. A. THORN 516

A. Intakes 516
   a) Contents in food components 516
   b) Normal intakes 516
   c) Diets ensuring low intakes 517

B. Daily turnovers 517

VIII. Effects of excesses and deficits. By N. A. THORN 519

A. Introduction (remarks on homeostasis) 519

B. Effects of sodium loading 520
   a) Acute 520
   b) Chronic 520

C. Effects of potassium loading 521
   a) Acute 521
   b) Chronic 522

D. Effects of lithium loading 523
   Gastrointestinal tract p. 524. — Muscular and nervous systems p. 524. —
   Circulation p. 524. — Kidneys p. 524. — Treatment of lithium intoxication
   p. 525.

E. Effects of rubidium loading 525
   a) Acute 525
   b) Chronic 525

F. Effects of cesium loading 526
   a) Acute 526
   b) Chronic 526
   c) Factors influencing the excretion of cesium 526

G. Sodium depletion 527
   a) Acute 527
   b) Chronic 528

H. Potassium depletion 529
   a) Acute 529
   b) Chronic 531

I. Function of rubidium and cesium in replacement of potassium 533

J. Influence of age on the efficiency of homeostasis 533

IX. Internal shifts and displacements of alkali metal ions. By N. A. THORN 535

A. Mobilization from or deposition in extracellular structures, especially bone . . 535

B. Factors affecting the distribution of alkali metals between cells and extracellular
   fluid 535
   a) Hormones 535
   b) Excesses or deficits — primary changes in p_H 537

Author Index 539

Subject Index 576

The alkali metal ions in isolated systems and tissues

By

Hans H. Ussing

I. General introduction

More than thirty years have passed since the appearance of Höber's treatise[1] on the alkali metal ions in this handbook. Since then the literature on the biological functions and effects of these ions has encreased enormously. The mere bulk of material has forced the authors to abandon the vain attempt to cover all the papers with a bearing on the field. Instead they have tried to choose from the abundance primarily what they feel can be organized into a coherent picture of the biological role of the alkali metal ions.

Thus great emphasis has been placed upon describing physiological events such as secretion, osmotic regulation excitation, conduction, creation of electric, currents etc. in terms of active and passive transports of Na and K. But although a certain degree of understanding of the biological role of the alkali metal ions seems to be emerging from the huge sea of experimental knowledge, one should not conceal the fact that the picture is in many respects incomplete. On the physico-chemical level the details of the processes going on in cell membranes during active transport and excitation are unknown or known only by inference, and the possible role of alkali metal ions in the contraction of muscle is still a matter of argument.

Similarly, if we consider the highest organization level, the intact organism, it often becomes impractical to resolve the functions and effects of alkali metal ions into active transports, passive permeabilities, inhibitions or activations of enzymes etc. The correlations found between the behavior of K and Na in the body fluids and tissues on the one hand and the functional state of the organism as a whole on the other may, however, be considered as physiological laws in their own right. In other words: The correlations found are expressions of the ability of the organism to maintain homeostasis.

In the present book the material is arranged according to increasing levels of organization. Part one treats the functions and effects of the alkali metal ions on the basis of experiments with enzymes, mitochondria, tissue slices and isolated organs, whereas part two is concerned with the behavior and effects of the alkali metal ions in the whole organism, with special emphasis on mammals. This arrangement means that the material is presented as far as possible according to the intentions behind the respective inventigations and the most likely interests of the users of the chapters in question (the authors do not cherish the idea that many will read the book in toto), but cross references will be used to integrate the different chapters.

The delimitation of the subject of this book is obviously rather artificial since the behaviour of the alkali metal ions in the organism is closely interrelated with

---

[1] Höber, R.: Alkali- und Erdalkalimetalle. In: Handbuch der Experimentellen Pharmakologie Bd. III p. 214—275 Berlin: Springer 1927.

that of other body constituents, in particular other electrolytes and the body water. Consequently it has been necessary to discuss some of these relationships in considerable detail.

The pharmacology and physiology of the anions with which the alkali metal ions are associated in the living organisms have been treated thoroughly by EICHLER[2] and his book should be consulted in the reading of the present volume.

II. Physical and chemical properties of the alkali metal ions[3,4,5,6,7,8]

a) Introduction

This is not the place to give a general treatment of the chemistry of the alkali metals. It may, however, be appropriate to bring a condensed account of those of the properties of the alkali metal ions which are generally held to be of special importance for their behaviour in living organisms.

The name alkali metals is used to designate those elements of the first group in the periodic system which follow immediately after the noble gases (compare table 1).

Of the alkali metals one, namely number 87 (francium) exists in nature only as a radioactive decay product of actinium, with a half life of 21 min. The seven artificially prepared isotopes of this element have even shorter half lives. Francium therefore has little biological interest and will not be treated in this volume.

Each of the elements potassium and rubidium has a naturally occurring radioactive isotope. K^{40} decays to Ca^{40} with a half life of 1.2×10^9 year. This isotope constitutes 0.012 % of natural potassium.

Table 1

0	1	2
He 2	Li 3	Be 4
Ne 10	Na 11	Mg 12
Ar 18	K 19	Ca 20
Kr 36	Rb 37	Sr 38
Xe 54	Cs 55	Ba 56
Rn 86	Fr 87	Ra 88

It is interesting to note that most natural Ca has been forwarded in this way. Rb^{87} which decays to Sr^{87} makes up 27.8 % of natural rubidium and has a half life of 6.2×10^{10} years.

Artificial radio-isotopes, useful for tracer work, can be prepared of all the alkali metals except lithium, whose artificial isotopes all have half lives shorter than one second.

For Na two radioactive tracers are commercially available, namely Na^{24} (half life 15.06 hr) and Na^{22} (half life 2.6 years).

[2] EICHLER, O.: Die Pharmakologie anorganischer Anionen. Handbuch der Experimentellen Pharmakologie. Ergänzungswerk, Bd. 10. 1206 pp. Berlin, Göttingen, Heidelberg: Springer 1950 .

[3] EMELEUS, H. J., and J. S. ANDERSON: Modern aspects of inorganic chemistry, 536 pp. New York: Van Nostrand 1938.

[4] HARNED, H. S., and B. B. OWEN: The physical chemistry of electrolytic solutions, 611 pp. New York: Reinhold 1943.

[5] LATIMER, W. M.: The oxidation states of the elements and their potentials in aqueous solution, 392 pp. New York: Prentice-Hall 1952.

[6] FERNELIUS, W. C.: Frontiers in chemistry V, chemical architecture. New York: Interscience 1948.

[7] LEHNINGER, A. L.: Role of metal ions in enzyme systems. Physiol. Rev. 30, 393 (1950).

[8] Nuclear data. United States Department of Commerce. National Bureau of Standards: Circular 499 (1950).

One radioactive tracer has been used for potassium, namely K[42] (half life 12.4 hr). Since for certain types of diffusion and permeability experiments two tracers for the same element are needed, it may be of interest that one more potassium isotope with a suitable half life is known and can possibly be produced if needed (K[45]: half life 22 hr).

Only one rubidium isotope has been used in biological work so far, namely Rb[86] (half life 19.5 days), but other radio-isotopes of this element with suitable half lives are known (Rb[81]: 5 hr; Rb[82]: 6.3 hr).

Finally, three isotopes of caesium are available, namely Cs[131] with half life 9.6 days, Cs[134] with half life 2.3 years and Cs[137], half life 37 years.

b) Chemical properties

The alkali metals very easily give off their valence electron to form the corresponding ions which have a complete noble gas outer shell of electrons. This gives the ions a high degree of stability. Even though the alkali metal ions do form complexes with other ions and molecules, their tendency to do so is generally only slight and definitely less than that of the alkaline earth metals.

With respect to complex formation and also in other respects, Li occupies a position between the alkaline earth ions and the typical alkali metal ions. Thus it is characteristic that both the carbonate and the phosphate of Li are only slightly soluble in water, whereas the corresponding salts of the other alkali metal ions are easily soluble. Most salts of the typical alkali metal ions are highly soluble in water and nearly insoluble in organic solvents. Well-known exceptions from this rule are sodium uranyl acetate and the chloroplatinate, perchlorate, phosphotungstate, and tartrate of potassium, which are all sparingly soluble in water.

A more detailed study of the solubilities of the salts of the different alkali metal ions reveals very close similarities between the K, Rb and Cs salts, whereas the properties of the Na salts are often different from the others. Thus anions which form insoluble or poorly soluble K salts usually form higly soluble Na salts and vice versa. Primarily these differences in solubility seem to be reflexions of differences in the ionic radii of the cations. Table 2 gives values for the radii of the alkali metal ions both in the hydrated and the non-hydrated state.

The non-hydrated radii can be obtained either theoretically from wave-mechanics considerations (PAULING[9A]) or from X-ray studies on crystals, whereas the hydrated radii are computed from diffusion rates in aqueous solution[9B].

Table 2.
Ionic radii of alkali metal ions[9a, 9b]

	Crystal radius, Å	Hydrated radii, Å from mobility
Li	0.60	2.31
Na	0.95	1.78
K	1.33	1.22
Rb	1.48	1.18
Cs	1.69	1.16
NH_4^+	1.48	1.21

It will be noticed that the non-hydrated radius increases with increasing atomic number whereas the reverse is true for the hydrated radius. This state of affairs is due to the fact that the force with which the water dipoles are attracted to the ion by the positive charge of the nucleus decreases as the number of electron shells surrounding it increases.

[9a]. PAULING, L.: The nature of the chemical bond. Cornell Univ. Press, Ithaca. N. Y. 1940.

[9b]. See for instance: KRESSMAN, T. R. E., and J. A. KITCHENER: Cation exchange with a synthetic phenolsulfonate resin. I. Equilibrium with univalent cations. J. chem. Soc. 1949, 1190—1201.

Whereas the non-hydrated radii are physically well defined numbers, the same cannot be said about the "hydrated radii". No method has yet been devised which gives an unambiguous value for the number of "bound" water molecules associated with an ion[9c].

The ability of metal ions to form ionic complexes generally increases with the so-called ionic potential (that is, the ratio of charge to ionic radius). Ions of low potential like Cs, Rb and K show little tendency to form complexes. Na shows an intermediary tendency, and Li a rather pronounced tendency to do so. Thus it may be said that in solution the alkali metal ions form complexes with the solvent (hydration) and that the ability to form such complexes decreases with increasing atomic number. This is true not only for watery solutions, but quite generally for all solvents in which the alkali metal ions dissolve. Thus DAVIES[10] (1950) has pointed out that the rate-limiting step in the diffusion of salts through the water-nitrobenzene interface is the process of replacing the water molecules belonging to the sphere of hydration of the ions by solvation molecules belonging to the non-watery phase.

The force necessary to strip off the water of hydration is considerable. In systems like the living organisms which contain a high percentage of water we therefore mostly have to do wih the fully hydrated forms of these ions, although it is conceivable that during diffusion through lipoid membranes some or all of the molecules of hydration are replaced by other molecular species belonging to the membrane phase.

The ionic diameter is decisive for the rate of free diffusion, but even more so for the penetration through narrow pores. When the pore diameter approaches the dimensions of the dIffusing particles, even small differences in ionic radius may determine whether or not a particular species will be able to penetrate.

c) Chemical binding

Since nearly all salts of these ions are totally dissociated in watery solution it may seem queer that the topic of chemical binding of the alkali metal ions should warrant a discussion of any length. The very conspicuous differences in biological behaviour and biological effect among these ions, notably between Na and K, do, however, suggest that they take a direct part in vitally important processes and thus must be at least temporarily bound to the reacting molecules. Furthermore, according to current thinking, the distinction between the alkali metal ions by the secretory mechanisms of the living organisms requires some kind of specific binding to organic "carrier" molecules.

The word binding is used here in a loose sense to designate partial or total immobilization of one or more ion species. The possibilities for such immobilization are many, for instance inclusion in a molecular cage (clathrate formation) and accumulation in the form of counter ions in polyvalent macromolecules.

d) Chelates with low-molecular anions[11, 12]

The attraction by a single negative charge does not suffice in watery solution to immobilize the alkali metal ions. If, however, two or more negative charges are

---

[9c]. See for instance: Modern aspects of electrochemistry. Ed. J. O. M. BOCKRIS. London: Butterworths 1954.

[10] DAVIES, J. T.: Diffusion of ions at phase boundaries. J. Physiol. Coll. Chem. **54**, 185—204 (1950).

[11] MARTELL, A. E. M., and M. C. CALVIN: The chemistry of the metal chelate compounds. New York: Prentice-Hall 1952.

[12] ROSENBERG, T.: The concept and definition of active transport. Symp. Soc. exp. Biol. 8, 27—41 (1954).

situated sufficiently close together to allow simultaneous interaction with the monovalent ion, its movement may be more or less impeded. Notably if the ion in question can be made to close a 5 or 6-membered ring, a certain stability may arise. Small differences in atomic distances and valence angles may become decisive in determining the stability of the alkali metal ion complex.

Thus, according to SCHWARZENBACH[13, 14, 15] and collaborators, ethylene diamine tetraacetic acid (versene) and several related compounds form complexes with Na but fail to do so with K. β-dicarbonyl compounds such as esters of acetoacetic acid, on the other hand, form K complexes which are more stable than the Na compounds (SIDGWICK and BREWER)[16]. Several of these complexes are more soluble in lipoid solvents than in water. Thus the complexes of K and Na with di-β-naphthol sulphide, which has the alkali metal ion placed in an 8-membered ring, are easily soluble in ethyl ether[17].

In this context it may be pertinent to mention that a guaiacol-containing layer of an organic solvent will preferentially dissolve K from a watery solution containing K and Na. This property of guaiacol to complex with K was made use of by OSTERHOUT[18] in his model experiments designed to explain ion accumulation in living cells.

e) Binding by ion exchange resins[19]

The cation exchange resins are synthetic high polymeres containing an excess of acidic groups which are able to give off their hydrogen ions in exchange for other cations from the bathing solution.

The number of such resins already known is very large and an almost unlimited number can be synthesized. Among the factors which determine the ionic selectivity of the resins the most important ones are 1) the nature of the acidic functional group and 2) the denseness of the structure which is largely determined by the degree of cross linkage.

As regards the first point it is characteristic that the affinity of the alkali ions to strongly acidic groups (sulfonic acid groups etc.) decreases in the order K > > Na > Li, whereas the order is precisely the opposite for the weakly acidic carboxyl, secondary phosphate, and phenol groups. According to BREGMAN[20] this phenomenon can be explained as follows: The electrostatic binding of a monovalent ion is determined primarily by the polarizability of the anionic group and by the ionic potential of the ion[21]. As already mentioned, the ionic potential

[13] SCHWARZENBACH, G., u. H. ACKERMANN: Komplexone. V. Die Äthylendiamin-tetraessigsäure. Helv. chim. Acta 30, 1798—1804 (1947).

[14] SCHWARZENBACH, G., E. KAMPITSCH u. R. STEINER: Komplexone. III. Uramildi-essigsäure und ihr Komplexbildungsvermögen. Helv. chim. Acta 29, 364—370 (1946).

[15] SCHWARZENBACH, G., A. WILLI u. R. O. BACH: Komplexone. IV. Die Acidität und die Erdalkalikomplexe der Anilindiessigsäure und ihrer Substitutionsprodukte. Helv. chim. Acta 30, 1303—1320 (1947).

[16] SIDGWICK, N. V., and F. M. BREWER: Co-ordinated compounds of the alkali metals. II. J. chem. Soc. 127, 2379—2387 (1925).

[17] EVANS, W. J., and S. SMILES: Covalent alkaline derivatives of di-2-hydroxy-1-naphtyl sulphide and of di-2-hydroxy-1-naphtylmethane. J. chem. Soc. 1937, 727.

[18] OSTERHOUT, W. J. V.: Some models of protoplasmic surfaces. Cold Spr. Harb. Symp. quant. Biol. 8, 51—62 (1940).

[19] A series of valuable papers on ion exchange resins anditheir chemical properties is found in: Ion Exchange Resins in Medicine and Biological Research. Editor: R. W. MINER. Ann. N. Y. Acad. Sci. 57, 61—323 (1953).

[20] BREGMAN, J. I., and Y. MURATA: Phosphonous and phosphonic cation-exchange resins. J. Amer. chem. Soc. 74, 1867—1868 (1952).

[21] TEUNISSEN, P. H., u. H. G. BUNGENBERG DE JONG: Negative, nicht amphotere, Bikolloide als hochmolekulare Elektrolyte II. Kolloid.-Beih. 48, 33—92 (1938).

decreases with increasing atomic number. If the negative group is more polarizable than water, then its preference for alkali metal ions is in the order $Li > Na > K$. If the negative group is less polarizable than water the order of preference is reversed because it is now the ionic radius of the hydrated ion which determines the closest approach between the negative and the positive charge. The order of polarizability for some biologically important anionic groups is $PO_4^{---} > COO^- > H_2O > SO_4^{--}$. For the phosphonic resins Nalcite-X-219 BREGMAN[22] found that at acid p_H of the bathing solution the resin showed a slight preference for K relative to Na (1/0.8). When the p_H was shifted to 7.5 the binding capacity for cations increased due to the increased dissociation of the phosphoric acid groups, but now Na was preferred in the ratio 1.5 to 1, calculated on the basis of all the cation bound. That means that the dissociation of the second H leads to a negative group which prefers Na to K in the proportion 2.2 to 1. Also carboxylic[23] and phenolic[23] resins may show a preference for Na relative to K.

The second important factor determining the ionic selectivity is the degree of cross linkage[24]. If we compare the ions K, Na and Li, the selectivity for the first-mentioned ion increases with increasing degree of cross-linkage until a maximum is reached. In very highly cross linked resins, however, the selectivity for K drops off sharply and the resin may even show a higher affinity to Li than to K[25]. Possibly the explanation is that the meshwork making up the resin no longer admits the hydrated ions and the selectivity is determined by the relative sizes of the unhydrated ions. The conditions then are similar to those pertaining in the active layer of a glass electrode where H, and to a much lesser extent also Li and Na are able to move, whereas larger cations like K are excluded.

It will be seen from the foregoing that just by varying the nature of the acidic group and the structure of the resin, its binding properties towards the different alkali metal ions varied over a rather wide range. Presumably, if chelating groups were introduced as acidic functions, the selectivity could be increased even more.

Between a particle of such resins as discussed above and the surrounding fluid a type of equilibrium is established which is quite analogous to the Gibbs-Donnan equilibrium. For the development of the equilibrium it is evidently quite immaterial whether the negative charges inside the system are kept from leaving by a semipermeable membrane or by being part of the polymer. In dilute salt solutions the conditions of the Donnan equilibrium lead to practical exclusion of mobile anions from the interior of the resin. Furthermore, the high concentration of mobile cations inside the resin gives rise to an osmotic suction which brings about a swelling of the resin. The swelling is brought to stop when the tension in the molecular chains has increased to the point where it balances the osmotic pressure. From the foregoing it will be clear that the swelling is greater when the association of the cationic species with the negative charges (the "complex formation") is less and vice versa.

f) Binding by phosphate esters and polyphosphates

In view of the importance of phosphate esters in metabolism, the binding capacity for alkali metal ions of phosphate derivatives warrants special attention.

[22] BREGMAN, J. I.: Cation exchange processes. Ann. N. Y. Acad. Sci. **57**, 125—143 (1953).

[23] GUPTA, S. L., M. BOSE, and S. K. MUKHERJEE: Ion exchange in synthetic resins. J. Physiol. Coll. Chem. **54**, 1098—1109 (1950).

[24] GREGOR, H. P.: Gibbs-Donnan equilibria in ion-exchange resin systems. J. Amer. chem. Soc. **73**, 642—650 (1951).

[25] GREGOR, H. P., and J. I. BREGMAN: Studies on Ion-exchange resins. IV. Selectivity coefficients of various cation exchangers towards univalent cations. J. Coll. Sci. **6**, 323—347 (1951).

Actually, binding by phosphate esters has been claimed by some authors to be the reason for specific accumulation of K over Na in bacteria and in muscle. Although the evidence against such static binding being the main reason for K accumulation in living cells is nearly conclusive (see p. 37), there can be little doubt that in the processes leading to cation accumulation and ionic extrusion phosphate metabolism plays a great part. MELCHIOR[26] estimated the binding of K and Na by ATP from the shifts in the pK values brought about when an alkali ion replaced the non-complexing tetraethylammonium ion in its ATP salts (Bjerrum-Calvin method). Both K and Na form complexes with ATP to an appreciable extent; but no difference in stability of the K and Na salts could be observed.

The binding of alkali metal ions by several biologically important phosphate compounds has been studied by SNELL[27] and by TOSTESON[28], both using a potentiometric method for evaluating the ion binding. The method makes use of the fact that the electric potential which develops across an anion — impermeable, cation — permeable membrane, separating two salts of the same cation, is determined only by the activities of the cation in the two solutions. In order to measure this potential one has of course to design an electrochemical cell where at least one of the contacts between the reversible electrodes and the experimental solution is made with a saturated KCl bridge. The small uncertainty with respect to diffusion potential between saturated KCl and the experimental solutions can usually be disregarded. The following cell can be used[28]:

membrane

$$\text{Hg, Hg}_2\text{Cl}_2 \text{ sat KCl Me}^+\text{Cl}^- \;\Big|\; \text{Me}^+ \text{ A}^{-z} \text{ sat KCl, Hg}_2\text{Cl}_2, \text{Hg}$$
$$(1) \qquad\qquad (2)$$

where Me is the cation under study, and A^{-z} is the anion whose alkali binding is being determined. In this cell, due to its symmetrical construction, the electromotive force is determined by

$$E = \frac{RT}{F} \ln \frac{a_{\text{Me}(1)}}{a_{\text{Me}(2)}}$$

where $a_{\text{Me}(1)}$ and $a_{\text{Me}(2)}$ are the activities of the ion in question in the left hand and right hand compartment, respectively. Knowing the concentrations in the two compartments and the mean activity coefficient of MeCl in the left hand compartment, one can calculate the activity for Me in the right hand compartment. The cell used by SNELL was designed slightly differently but the kind of information obtained was the same.

The following anionic species were studied by SNELL: Glucose-1-phosphate, glucose-6-phosphate, glycerophosphate, fructose-1-6-diphosphate, adenosine triphosphate (ATP), inorganic pyrophosphate. TOSTESON's studies were concerned with the following compounds: Adenosine triphosphate, inosine triphosphate, guanosine triphosphate, uridine triphosphate, cytidine triphosphate, triphosphopyridine nucleotide (TPN), coenzym A, and isethionate ($HOCH_2CH_2SO_3H$).

No significant difference in the activity coefficients of K and Na was found with any of these anions. SNELL found that the activity coefficients for both

[26] MELCHIOR, N. C.: Sodium and potassium complexes of adenosine triphosphate: Equilibrium studies. J. biol. Chem. 208, 615—627 (1954).

[27] SNELL, F. M.: Activity coefficients of some sodium and potassium phosphates in solution, in Electrochemistry in Biology and Medicine, p. 284. Editor: T. SHEDLOWSKY. New York: John Wiley & Sons 1955.

[28] TOSTESON, D.: Potassium and sodium binding by nucleotides. J. cell. comp. Physiol. 50, 199—202 (1957).

these cations varied with concentration in a manner which agreed reasonably well with the behaviour predicted by the Debye-Hückel theory. Only in the case of polymetaphosphate did he find evidence for incomplete dissociation, but K and Na also behaved practically identically in this compound.

This is in agreement with results obtained by VAN WAZER and CAMPANELLA[29]. Through polarographic studies and p_H titration curves in the presence and absence of neutral salts they were led to the conclusion that polyphosphates form weak complexes with alkali metal ions. Li was bound more firmly than K and Na, but much less than the divalent ions. The absence of discrimination between Na and K by polyphosphate was also demonstrated by ANDERSEN and LEHMANN[30]. They found the Na/K ratio to be the same in an ultrafiltrate from the K, Na salt of polyphosphate and in the non-filtrable residue. LAMM and MALMGREN[31], on the other hand have observed a preferential binding of Na by polyphosphate. Possibly small differences in the preparation of the polyphosphate ("hexametaphosphate" prepared according to TAMMANN[32]) are responsible for this discrepancy.

g) Binding by nucleic acids

HAMMARSTEN[33] in his classical study of the properties of thymonucleic acid, found the apparent dissociation constant of dilute solutions of its Na salt to be around 0.2, judging from osmotic pressure and Donnan equilibrium determinations. A comparative study of the K and Na binding was not undertaken, but it was shown that the deviation from normal behaviour of the nucleic acid salts with monovalent ions decreased with increasing diameter of the cation, as is the case with cation exchange resins having phosphate groups as acidic functions. More recently the cation binding by nucleic acids has been studied by VEIS[34].

h) Binding by polyvalent acid polysaccharides

Just like the nucleic acids, the acid polysaccharides (hyaluronic acid, chondroitin sulfuric acid, heparin etc.) have a pronounced ability to bind alkali metal ions (and other ions as well). Thus VEIS[34] (cited after KLOTZ[35]) has demonstrated that arabic acid binds 50 or more moles Na or K per mole (290,000 g) when the concentration of alkali ion is 0.005 molar. At concentrations below one millimole per liter of K and Na the quantity of Na bound is nearly four times the amount if K. At higher concentrations the affinity for the two alkali ions becomes more equal and at about 4 millimole per liter the binding of K exceeds the sodium binding.

The interaction of alkali metal ions and acid polysaccharides in certain enzymatic processes is discussed on p. 19.

[29] WAZER, J. R. VAN, and D. A. CAMPANELLA: Structure and properties of the condensed phosphate. IV. Complex ion formation in polyphosphate solutions. J. Amer. chem. Soc. 72, 655—663 (1950).

[30] ANDERSEN, B., and K. LEHMANN: On the alleged complexity of sodium in polyhexametaphosphate. Acta chem. scand. 6, 613—614 (1952).

[31] LAMM, O., u. H. MALMGREN: Dispersitätsmessungen an einem hochpolymeren Metaphosphat nach TAMMAN. Z. anorg. allg. Chem. 245, 103—128 (1940).

[32] TAMMANN, G.: Beiträge zur Kenntnis der Metaphosphate. J. prakt. Chem. 45, 417—474 (1892).

[33] HAMMARSTEN, E.: Zur Kenntnis der biologischen Bedeutung der Nucleinsäureverbindungen. Biochem. Z. 144, 383 (1924).

[34] VEIS, A.: The interaction of the alkali ions with some linear polyelectrolytes. J. physiol. Chem. 57, 189—194 (1953).

[35] KLOTZ, J. M.: Some metal complex with proteins and other large molecules in "Modern Trends in Physiology and Biochemistry", edited by E. S. G. BARRON. New York: Academic Press 1952.

i) Binding by proteins

Proteins are so numerous and the investigations so relatively few that general rules concerning alkali binding cannot be given.

Some proteins do not bind alkali metal ions to a measurable extent. Thus NORTHROP and KUNITZ[36] concluded from Donnan potential measurements that gelatin does not bind alkali metal ions. This result should be considered in the light of the fact that the effective valence of polyvalent ions decreases as the distance between the charged groups increases (SIMMS[37]). Thus gelatin does not affect the ionic strength of the solution more than an equivalent amount of a divalent ion.

Other proteins, for example serum albumin (SCATCHARD et al.[38]) hemoglobin and hemerythrin[39] also seem unable to bind alkali metal ions.

MIYAMOTO and SCHMIDT[40] did not find any alkali metal binding in casein. More recent studies by CARR and TOPOL[41], using a permselective membrane to estimate the activity coefficient of the cations, revealed a pronounced Na binding by casein at alkaline p_H (8.7). The Na activity in a 0.01 molar NaCl solution was lowered 25 % by 1 % casein. The Na binding was still appreciable at p_H 7, but nil at p_H 5.2. The affinity of casein for the different alkali metal ions was not studied. That proteins may distinguish sharply between the alkali metal ions is born out, for instance, by the studies of GURD et al.[42, 43] on γ-globulin. The solubility of this protein in Na-acetate buffers greatly exceeds that in Li-acetate of the same molarity.

Myosin has a large cation binding capacity. MONTIGEL[44] first observed that K is strongly adsorbed by myosin. However, this binding is not selective in the sense that K is preferred to Na. As shown by ERDÖS[45] the affinity for Na and K is the same. This point is also stressed by SZENT-GYÖRGYI[46] in his well known monograph on muscular contraction. Thus the alkali metal ion binding by myosin cannot explain why K is concentrated more than Na in muscle. Compare, however BAIRD, KARREMAN, MUELLER and SZENT-GYÖRGYI[46a].

[36] NORTHROP, J. H., and M. KUNITZ: Combination of salts and proteins. III. The combination of CuCl$_2$, MgCl$_2$, CaCl$_2$, AlCl$_3$, LaCl$_3$, KCl, AgNO$_3$, and Na$_2$SO$_4$ with gelatin. J. gen. Physiol. **11**, 481—493 (1928).

[37] SIMMS, H. S.: The ionic activity of gelatin. J. gen. Physiol. **11**, 613—628 (1928).

[38] SCATCHARD, G., J. H. SCHEINBERG, and S. H. ARMSTRONG: Physical chemistry of protein solutions. IV. The combination of human serum albumin with chloride ion. J. Amer. chem. Soc. **72**, 535—540 (1950).

[39] BATTLEY, E. H., and J. M. KLOTZ: Interaction of sodium and potassium ions with hemoglobin and with hemerythrin. Biol. Bull. **101**, 205 (1951).

[40] MIYAMOTO, S., and C. L. A. SCHMIDT: Transference and conductivity studies on solutions of certain proteins and amino acids with special reference to the formation of complex ions between the alkaline earth elements and certain protein. J. biol. Chem. **99** 335—358 (1933).

[41] CARR, C. W., and L. TOPOL: The determination of sodium-ion and chloride-ion activities in protein solutions by means of permselective membranes. J. Physiol. Coll. Chem. **54**, 176 to 184 (1950).

[42] GURD, F. R. N.: The specificity of metal-proteins interactions, in "Ion Transport Across Membranes". Editor: H. T. CLARKE. New York: Academic Press 1954.

[43] ONCLEY, J. L., F. H. GORDON, F. R. N. GURD, and R. A. LONTIE: Abstr. 119th Meeting Amer. Chem. Soc. Boston, p. 28 C (April 1951).

[44] MONTIGEL, C.: Myosin and Kalium. Helv. physiol. Pharmacol. Acta **1**, C 47—C 48 (1943).

[45] ERDÖS, T.: The combined action of potassium and sodium on acto-myosin. Hung. Acta Physiol. **1**, 33—34 (1946).

[46] SZENT-GYÖRGYI, A.: Chemistry of muscular contraction, pp. 1—150. New York: Academic Press 1947.

[46a] BAIRD, S. L., G. KARREMAN, H. MUELLER, and A. SZENT-GYÖRGYI: Ionic semipermeability as a bulk property. Proc. Nat. Acad. Sci. USA. **43**, 705—708 (1957).

The affinity of myosin for alkali metal ions can be demonstrated by adding KCl to a salt free solution of myosin. A precipitate is formed already at KCl concentrations as low as 0.025 molar, and this precipitate after washing with alcohol contains no chloride but rather large quantities of K. This phenomenon has been studied in greater detail by BANGA[47]. She found that the five first K ions adsorbed per UW (17,600 g) of myosin are bound rather firmly, forming an electro-neutral myosinate. The latter substance then is able to bind loosely extra potassium. The real isoelectric point of myosin is 5.2, but in the presence of 0.025 molar KCl the myosin will be isoelectric up to p_H 7. The K-binding of myosin strongly depends upon the p_H of the solution. Whereas at p_H 7.5 in 0.1 molar KCl myosin binds 7 equivalents of K per mole, the same amount of myosin under similar conditions binds only 2 equivalents of K at p_H 6.5. Thus it is seen that the cation binding of myosin is exceedingly sensitive to small changes in acidity exactly in the biological range of p_H.

Other structural proteins seem to possess qualitatively similar binding capacities for K and Na (LAJTA[48]).

III. Role of alkali metal ions in enzymatic processes

a) Introduction

It has been recognized for a long time that numerous enzymatic processes show a strong dependency upon the ionic strength of the medium. Since the alkali metal ions do not measurably combine with most proteins it has been the general view until recently that these ions influence enzyme reactions mainly or exclusively via their effect on the ionic strength of the solution. This attitude has not furthered detailed kinetic studies concerning the effects of the individual alkali metal ions

Table 3. *Influence of the alkali metal ions and the ammonium ion on some enzymatic reactions.* a signifies activating effect, 0 no effect, and i inhibitory effect. Double letters indicate a stronger effect. "low" and "high" refer to concentration. For references see text

	Cs	Rb	NH$_4^+$	K	Na	Li
Pyruvic Phosphoferase		aa	aa	aa	low a high i	0
Fructokinase			low a high i	a	0	
Bacterial Hexokinase	i	a	a	a	i	
Phosphofructokinase			a	a	0	
Acetate-activating enzyme		a	a	a	i	i
Phosphotransacetylase			a	a	i	i
Glutathion synthesizing complex				aa		
Yeast aldehyde dehydrogenase	i	a	a	a	low a high i	i
β-galactosidase						
a) lactose	a	a	a	aa	a	(a)
b) o-nitrophenol-D-galactopyranoside				a	aa	
Brain apyrase						a
Bacterial apyrase	a	a	a	a	a	
Crab nerve ATP-ase				high i	a	
Myosine ATP-ase						
+ versene		a	a	a	0	0
+ Ca^{++}		a	a	a	a	a
Urease				i	ii	

[47] BANGA, J.: cit. from [46].
[48] LAJTA, A.: cit. from [46].

on enzymatic processes. Nevertheless several cases of specific activation or inhibition by ions of this group have become known, and in recent years some of the enzyme systems in question have been studied intensively. These studies have led to the realization of the fact that certain enzymes do indeed bind one or a few alkali metal ions in a highly specific way.

Table 3 lists some of the enzyme systems which are known to depend on one or more alkali metal ions. It is indicated for each of these ion species (plus the ammonium ion) whether it activates (a) inhibits (i) or is without effect. (aa) means strong activation and (ii) strong inhibition. The list does not pretend to be complete, but it is hoped that none of the well-established cases is missing. Some systems where the effect is possibly non-specific are included.

At first sight the list gives the impression of a decisive predominance of enzymes engaged in the phosphate metabolism. Such a conclusion should be drawn with some caution, however, until systematic studies of the importance of these ions for other types of enzymes have been carried out. As regards the enzymes of the glycolytic sequence, apart from pyruvic phosphoferase and phospho-fructokinase, none seems to require potassium or other alkali metal ions for activation[49], [50].

b) Specific effects on enzymatic processes

1. Pyruvic phosphoferase

(catalyzes the reaction 2-phosphopyruvate + ADP = pyruvate + ATP). In experiments with yeast, OHLMEYER and OCHOA[51] found that the transfer of phosphate from phosphopyruvic acid to glucose is inhibited by Na and accelerated by K and NH_4. In 1942, BOYER, LARDY and PHILLIPS[52] discovered that the transfer of phosphate from 3-phosphoglycerate to creatine by homogenized muscle could not be carried out unless boiled muscle juice was added. It turned out that K could replace the muscle juice whereas Na was inactive. Further, it was found that K was unnecessary for the phosphate transfer from ATP to creatine. In a subsequent study[53] the same authors demonstrated that the action of K is the result of an accelerating effect on the transfer of phosphate from 2-phospho-pyruvate to ADP. Besides K, Mg^{++} or Mn^{++} were essential for the transfer. NH_4 could replace K in vitro. Ca^{++} was strongly antagonistic to K, and even Na and inorganic phosphate in relatively high concentration were inhibitory to the trans-phosphorylation. In 1945 LARDY and ZIEGLER[54] demonstrated that the reaction catalyzed by pyruvic phosphoferase is reversible and that the synthesis of phospho-pyruvic acid from ATP and pyruvic acid also required K.

The inhibition of the pyruvic phosphoferase of brain homogenates by Na was first demonstrated by UTTER[55].

[49] LARDY, H. A.: The influence of inorganic ions on phosphorylation reactions. In W. D. McELROY and B. GLASS: Phosphorus metabolism I, 477—499. Baltimore: Johns Hopkins Press 1951.

[50] BOYER, P. D.: The role of potassium and related cations in the action of pyruvic phosphoferase and other enzymes. J. Lancet 73, 195—196 (1953).

[51] OHLMEYER, P., u. S. OCHOA: Über die Rolle der Cozymase bei der Phosphatüber-tragung. Biochem. Z. 293, 338—350 (1937).

[52] BOYER, P. D., H. A. LARDY, and P. H. PHILLIPS: The rôle of potassium in muscle phosphorylations. J. biol. Chem. 146, 673—682 (1942).

[53] BOYER, P. D., H. A. LARDY, and P. H. PHILLIPS: Further studies on the role of potassium and other ions in the phosphorylation of the ademylic system. J. biol. Chem. 149, 529—541 (1943).

[54] LARDY, H. A., and J. A. ZIEGLER: The enzymatic synthesis of phosphopyruvate from pyruvate. J. biol. Chem. 159, 343—351 (1945).

[55] UTTER, M. F.: Mechanism of inhibition of anaerobic glycolysis of brain by sodium ions. J. biol. Chem. 185, 499—517 (1950).

KACHMAR and BOYER[56] have studied the kinetics of the potassium activation and calcium inhibition of pyruvic phosphoferase. Only in the presence of one of the ions K, Rb or NH_4 did the enzyme show any appreciable activity. The experiments indicate that although the inhibition shown by Ca^{++} can be in part overcome by additional K, it is not a simple competitive inhibition. In the absence of K, Na was found to possess a real but weak activating capacity, whereas Li gave practically no activation. Both Na and Li counteracted the activation by K, but the nature of this inhibition was not studied.

In the cases of the activating ions K, Rb and NH_4, the "Michaelis constants" for the combination of the activating ion with the enzyme were determined. In all three cases "K_M" was around 0.011 M, meaning that the enzyme was half saturated with K at a concentration in the medium of 11 millimoles K/liter. The "K_M" for the combination of the three cations studied remained relatively constant at different concentrations of phosphopyruvate, just as the K_M for combination of the enzyme with phosphopyruvate seemed to be independent of the concentration of the activating ion. The latter constant was 8.6×10^{-5} M, indicating that the affinity of the protein for phosphopyruvate is greater than its affinity for the activating ion. These data speak for an independent combination of K and phosphopyruvate with the protein.

From kinetic analysis, BOYER et al. deduced that one equivalent of potassium combines with the enzyme for each mole of bound phosphopyruvate. The authors point out that the ions which activate the enzyme have similar hydrated and non-hydrated radii, whereas both Li and Na have larger hydrated and smaller crystal lattice radii. Apparently the configuration of the enzyme at or near the active center is "just right" when a monovalent cation of certain dimensions is associated with it.

The requirement of K by pyruvic phosphoferase is not limited to enzyme of mammalian origin. BOYER[57] found that extracts from 19 different tissues of 11 vertebrates and invertebrates contained pyruvic phosphoferase which was strongly activated by K. The affinity for K in the different preparations varied appreciably, however. The "Michaelis constant" (which is an inverse measure of the affinity) was for example 30—40 times higher for rabbit muscle enzyme than for the enzyme prepared from Anodonta muscle. The properties of the enzyme and its activity in red cells of various species has been studied by SOLVONUK and COLLIER[58].

2. Fructokinase

Fructokinase is the fructose phosphorylating enzyme of muscle and liver. These organs, in contrast to yeast, have separate hexokinases for the phosphorylation of glucose and fructose (CORI and SLEIN[59]). The enzyme catalyses the reaction:

$$\text{fructose} + \text{ATP} \rightarrow \text{fructose-1-phosphate} + \text{ADP}$$

The fructokinase from ox liver has been studied in some detail by HERS[60]. An essential step in the purification procedure is centrifugation at 20,000 g, which

[56] KACHMAR, J. F., and P. D. BOYER: Kinetic analysis of enzyme reactions. II. The potassium activation and calcium inhibition of pyruvic phosphoferase. J. biol. Chem. 200, 669—682 (1953).

[57] BOYER, P. D.: The activation by K and occurrence of pyruvic phosphoferase in different species. J. cell. comp. Physiol. 42, 71—77 (1953).

[58] SOLVONUK, P. F., and H. B. COLLIER: The pyruvic phosphoferase of erythrocytes. I. Properties of the enzyme and its activity in erythrocytes of various species. Canad. J. Biochem. Physiol. 33, 38—45 (1955).

[59] CORI, G. T., and M. W. SLEIN: Gluco- and fructokinase in mammalian tissues. Fed. Proc. 6, 245—246 (1947).

removes all phosphatases and the glucose phosphorylating system. The enzyme is activated by K whereas Na has only little effect. NH_4 which activates at low concentrations is inhibitory at higher concentrations. For activity the enzyme required not only K but also Mg^{++}. This makes it likely that a magnesium complex of ATP is the actual substrate for the enzyme. The affinity of the enzyme for this complex is said to be five times greater in the presence of K than in the presence of Na.

As the concentration of K is increased this ion becomes inhibitory, but the inhibition can be counteracted by the addition of extra Mg^{++} and ATP. HERS advances the following hypothesis to explain the experimental results: The enzyme has two active centers, of which one normally binds K whereas the other binds Mg—ATP:

$$E \big\langle {}^{K}_{MgATP}$$

Excess Mg is inhibitory because it leads to the displacement of K:

$$E \big\langle {}^{MgATP}_{MgATP}$$

Similarly excess of K leads to another inactive complex:

$$E \big\langle {}^{K}_{K}$$

The sodium complex,

$$E \big\langle {}^{Na}_{MgATP} ,$$

is active, but less so than the corresponding potassium complex.

3. Bacterial hexokinase

CLARK and MacLEOD[61] have demonstrated that NH_4, K and Rb stimulate glycolysis in cell free extracts of Lactobacillus arabinosus 8014. Na and Cs counteract in a competitive manner the activation by K, Rb and NH_4. The inhibition of glycolysis by Na and Cs was reflected primarily in an increase in the lag period preceding the initiation of glycolysis. Intermediates like hexosemonophosphate, fructosediphosphate etc., could restore the glycolysis in the absence of the activating cations and would also allow glycolysis in the presence of Na or Cs. Extra ATP, on the other hand, was ineffective. These observations indicate that the alkali metal antagonism is mainly concerned with the conversion of glucose to hexosemonophosphate.

4. Phosphofructokinase

This enzyme catalyses the process fructose-6-phosphate + ATP → fructose-1,6-phosphate + ADP. In 1947 MUNTZ[62] found that K or NH_4 were necessary for

[63] HERS, H. G.: Role du magnésium et du potassium dans la réaction fructokinasique. Biochim. biophys. Acta 8, 424—430 (1952).
[61] CLARK, J. A., and R. A. MacLEOD: Ion antagonism in glycolysis by a cell-free bacterial extract. J. biol. Chem. 211, 531—540 (1954).
[62] MUNTZ, J. A.: The role of potassium and ammonium ions in alcoholic fermentation. J. biol. Chem. 171, 653—665 (1947).

the normal fermentation of glucose by dialyzed yeast maceration juice. In the absence of K or NH_4 glucose is only converted to hexose monophosphates which accumulate, whereas hexose diphosphate undergoes fermentation. This was taken to mean that either of the ions K or NH_4 is necessary for the formation of hexose diphosphate from hexose monophosphate. In this process K does not appear to be antagonized by Na. The concentration of NaCl could be increased up to 0.08 M without impairing the fermentation.

MUNTZ and HURWITZ[63] have studied the phosphofructokinase from rat brain. With samples where all K and NH_4 were replaced by Na by treatment with an ion exchange resin, the reaction rate was slow but not insignificant. The addition of NH_4 more than doubled the reaction rate.

Further purification of the brain phosphofructokinase (MUNTZ, 1953[64]) gave, however, a preparation which could no longer be activated by K but only by NH_4. Possibly the purification procedure brings about a change in the structure of the enzyme, or K excerts its effect on some other reaction which in crude extracts influences the phosphofructokinase activity.

5. Acetate-activating enzyme (and "choline acetylase")

(catalyses the process: acetate + ATP + CoA → acetyl-CoA + AMP + pyrophosphate). In 1943 NACHMANSOHN and MACHADO[65] discovered that cell-free extracts from rat brain contained an enzyme system which acetylates choline under strictly anaerobic conditions. This acetylation derives its energy from the breakdown of ATP. The system was found to require K for activation. According to NACHMANSOHN and JOHN[66] the optimal K concentration was about 0.08 moles per liter. (Compare also NACHMANSOHN, HESTRIN and VORIPAIEFF[67].)

These findings attained increased significance when it was found by KOREY, DE BRAGANZA and NACHMANSOHN[68] that acetyl-CoA was a necessary intermediate in the acetylation of choline. When an enzyme preparation from the head ganglia of the squid was incubated with acetate, ATP, CoA and choline, acetyl choline was formed. This process was activated by K whereas there was some inhibition by Na. This sodium inhibition was, however, rather slight. Concentrations of NaCl up to 100 millimolar had no effect. 200 mmols per liter reduced the synthesis of acetyl choline to 60%, 300 mmolar NaCl reduced the synthesis to 40%, and still higher concentrations practically stopped the reaction. The authors therefore considered the Na inhibition to be non-specific.

The synthesis of acetyl choline from acetate, choline and ATP evidently proceeds by at least two enzymatic steps:

a) acetate + ATP + CoA → acetyl-CoA + AMP + pyrophosphate and
b) acetyl-CoA + choline → acetyl choline + CoA.

[63] MUNTZ, J. A., and J. HURWITZ: The effect of ammonium ions upon isolated reactions of the glycolytic scheme. Arch. Biochem. **32**, 137—149 (1951).

[64] MUNTZ, J. A.: Partial purification and some properties of brain phosphofructokinase. Arch. Biochem. **42**, 435—445 (1953).

[65] NACHMANSOHN, D., and A. L. MACHADO: Formation of acetylcholin. A new enzyme: "choline acetylase". J. Neurophysiol. **6**, 397—403 (1943).

[66] NACHMANSOHN, D., and H. M. JOHN: Studies on choline acetylase. 1. Effect of amino acids on the dialysed enzyme inhibition by α-keto acids. J. biol. Chem. **158**, 157—171 (1945).

[67] NACHMANSOHN, D., S. HESTRIN, and H. VORIPAIEFF: Enzymatic synthesis of a compopund with acetyl choline-like biological activity. J. biol. Chem. **180**, 875—877 (1949).

[68] KOREY, S. R., B. DE BRAGANZA, and D. NACHMANSOHN: Choline acetylase. V. Esterifications and Transacetylations. J. biol. Chem. **189**, 705—715 (1951).

The action of alkali metal ions on process b) has not been investigated. Recently, however, v. KORFF and collaborators[69, 70, 71] have prepared from heart muscle an enzyme which catalyses reaction a). This system is strongly stimulated by K, Rb and NH_4, whereas Na and Li act as potent inhibitors. K and Na do not, however, behave like true antagonists towards this enzyme. K will stimulate in the presence of Na, but the sodium inhibition cannot be overcome by an excess of potassium. Maximum activation by K, Rb and NH_4 is obtained with 50 milliequivalents per liter. 50% inhibition is reached at a Na concentration of 20 meq/l.

It is well known that acetyl coenzyme A is now regarded as one of the key substances in the intermediary metabolism. One of its most important functions is to be the acetyl-donor in the reaction with oxaloacetate, a reaction which is catalysed by the condensing enzyme of OCHOA and coworkers[72]. If the acetate-activating enzyme is coupled with the condensing enzyme to give a system which synthesizes citrate from acetic acid and oxaloacetate, the citrate formation is increased by K and decreased by Na.

When comparing the observations of NACHMANSOHN and his group on "choline acetylase" with those of v. KORFF on the acetate activating enzyme, it appears surprising that the former workers find Na to be a weak inhibitor, whereas v. KORFF finds Na-inhibition to be very powerful. It should be remembered, however, that the high tolerance to Na was found in a preparation from squid ganglia, whereas the strong inhibition by Na occurred with an enzyme from mammalian muscle. Since the salt concentration in the blood of the squid is some 5 times higher than that of mammalian blood, it is perhaps not surprising that the squid enzyme is adapted to tolerate a higher Na-concentration than is the mammalian enzyme. In any case, there seems no reason to doubt that the potassium requirement of the choline acetylase system is due to the step involving the acetate activating enzyme.

6. Phosphotransacetylase

(catalyses the process acetylphosphate + CoA → acetyl-CoA + inorganic phosphate). STADTMAN[73] has prepared from Clostridium kluyveri an enzyme which he called phosphotransacetylase and which catalyses the process given above.

The purified enzyme shows obligatory requirements for K or NH_4. It is inhibited by Na and Li. Furthermore, it is inhibited non-competitively by inorganic phosphate, barbiturate, citrate and pyrophosphate. Therefore one cannot use buffers containing these anions in studies with this enzyme.

7. Glutathione synthesizing enzyme system[74, 75, 76]

The system by which glutamic acid, cysteine and glycine are coupled at the expense of chemical energy from ATP to form glutathione, is activated to some extent by K.

[69] BEINERT, H., D. E. GREEN, P. HELE, H. HIFT, R. W. v. KORFF, and C. V. RAMAKRISHNAN: The acetate activating enzyme system of heart muscle. J. biol. Chem. 203, 35—45 (1953).

[70] v. KORFF, R. W.: The effects of alkali metal ions on the acetate activating enzyme system. J. biol. Chem. 203, 265—271 (1953).

[71] v. KORFF, R. W.: The effect of alkali metal ions on acetate activation by an enzyme from heart muscle. J. Lancet 73, 196—197 (1953).

[72] STERN, J. R., B. SHAPIRO, E. R. STADTMAN, and S. OCHOA: Enzymatic synthesis of citric acid. III. Reversibility and mechanism. J. biol. Chem. 193, 703—720 (1951).

[73] STADTMAN, E. R.: The purification and properties of phosphotransacetylase. J. biol. Chem. 196, 527—524 (1952).

[74] JOHNSTON, R. B., and K. BLOCH: Enzymatic synthesis of glutathione. J. biol. Chem. 188, 221—240 (1951).

[75] SNOKE, E. J., and K. BLOCH: Formation and utilization of γ-glutamyl cysteine in glutathione synthesis. J. biol. Chem. 199, 407—414 (1952).

Omission of KCl (0.01 molar) from the reaction mixture (pigeon liver extract + + Mg^{++} + ATP + the three aminoacids) reduced the reaction rate by about 50%. According to SNOKE and BLOCH[75], γ-glutamylcysteine is formed first. Then this compound reacts with glycine. For both reactions ATP is necessary. The reaction: γ-glutamyl-cysteine + glycine → glutathione shows at least the same dependency on K as does the overall reaction. Systematic studies of the effects of the different alkali metal ions are lacking. It might be tempting to relate this K effect to the K dependence of the acetate activating enzyme. It has been shown, however, that acetyl glycine is not an intermediate. Possibly the reaction goes via an amino acid-coenzyme A compound, whose formation may show a similar K-sensitivity to that of the acetate activating enzyme.

8. Aldehyde dehydrogenase (from yeast)

(catalyses the process: $R-CHO + DPN + H_2O \rightarrow R-COOH + DPNH_2$). BLACK[77] prepared from yeast an aldehyde dehydrogenase which catalyses the oxidation of several aldehydes. The enzyme can use either DPN or TPN as coenzyme. Inside the cell this system probably collaborates with additional factors to form acetyl-CoA from acetaldehyde. The isolated enzyme, however, forms acetic acid. K and cysteine are essential for the enzyme's activity. Rb and NH$_4$ can be substituted for K. Li, Na and Cs inhibit the reaction in the presence of K. In the absence of any of the strongly activating ions, Na shows some activation of its own at low concentrations, but becomes inhibitory at higher concentrations. Apparently this is the only case of a dehydrogenase which requires an inorganic ion as cofactor.

9. β-galactosidase (from Escherichia coli)

COHN and MONOD[78] prepared from E. coli a β-galactosidase which showed a rather remarkable dependence upon the alkali metal ions. Depending upon the concentration of other cations, a given species such as for instance Na, could act either as an inhibitor or as an activator for the enzyme. These effects evidently are the results of the competition between the monovalent cations. In order to account for the findings, the authors assume two factors to be essential for the action of a given species, namely 1) its affinity for the enzyme and 2) its activance, i. e. the activity of the enzyme when saturated with the ion in question.

For the hydrolysis of lactose, K shows the highest "activance" while Na is only weakly active. Nevertheless Na has a much higher affinity for the enzyme than have the other monovalent cations, including K.

The affinities for the enzyme of the different alkali metal ions (including NH$_4$) decrease in the order Na > K > Cs > Li > Rb > NH$_4$.

The apparent "Michaelis" constant for combination of the alkali metal ions with the enzyme protein was for K: 3×10^{-3} M, for Rb: 2×10^{-2} M and for NH$_4$: 4×10^{-2} M.

Technical difficulties made it impossible to determine the constant accurately for Na, but it must be very low.

The "activance" (with lactose as the substrate) falls off in a way which is entirely different from the sequence of the affinities: K > Rb > NH$_4$ > Cs > > Na > Li. When o-nitrophenol-β-D-galactopyranoside is used as the substrate,

[76] BLOCH, K.: The synthesis of glutathione in isolated liver. J. biol. Chem. 179, 1245—1254 (1949).
[77] BLACK, S.: Yeast aldehyde dehydrogenase. Arch. Biochem. and Biophys. 34, 86—97 (1951).
[78] COHN, M., and J. MONOD: Purification et propriétés de la galactosidase (lactase) d'Escherichia coli. Biochim. biophys. Acta 7, 153—174 (1951).

the "activance" of Na, surprisingly enough, is higher than that of K. Thus it seems that the slight differences in atomic distances arising in the active center of the enzyme when one alkali metal ion replaces another at the cationic site may adjust the enzyme so as to prefer another substrate.

10. Apyrase (brain adenosinetriphosphatase)

It has been known for some time that Na inhibits glycolysis in tissue homogenates. Thus RACKER and KRIMSKY[79] found Na to inhibit the glycolysis of mouse brain homogenates and LE PAGE[80] reported similar findings for tumor homogenates.

The phenomenon of Na inhibition was studied in more detail by UTTER[55] who used homogenates of nervous tissue of the cotton rat. According to this study the observed effect of Na involves two enzymes, namely pyruvic phosphoferase which is inhibited, and apyrase which is stimulated by Na. The effect of Na upon pyruvic transphosphorylase has been discussed above.

The reason why stimulation of apyrase leads to a reduction of glycolysis is that ATP is necessary for the initial phosphorylation of the hexoses. Na stimulates both the splitting off of the first and the second phosphate from ATP, but the mechanism for the splitting off of the second phosphate may be due to the action of a myokinase.

Stimulation of apyrase by Na can be detected at a concentration as low as 0.003 molar. Since glycolysis was appreciably inhibited only above this concentration of Na, it seems likely that the activation of apyrase is the main reason for the sodium-induced inhibition of glycolysis.

Na exerts its stimulatory effect on apyrase only in the presence of magnesium ions. The sodium-activation is evident even in the presence of K, but no data are available to show whether there is any inhibition of the sodium effect by an excess of potassium ions.

The brain apyrase seems to be largely adsorbed to the particulate matter of the homogenate (MEYERHOF and WILSON[81]). This explains why the inhibition of glycolysis by Na is more pronounced with homogenates than with centrifuged extracts.

11. Bacterial apyrase

According to CLARK and MACLEOD[61] the cell-free extract of Lactobacillus arabinosus contains an apyrase which is stimulated by NH_4, K, Rb, Na and Cs, whereas it is inhibited by Mn^{++}. All the alkali metal ions activate to about the same extent. The inhibitory effect of Mn^{++} is remarkable because this ion promotes the apyrase activity of brain extract (UTTER[55]).

12. ATP-ase from crab nerve

SKOU[82] has studied an adenosinetriphosphatase which is associated with the microsome fraction of crab nerve. The presence of Mg^{++} is an obligatory require-

[79] RACKER, E., and I. KRIMSKY: Effect of nicotinic acid amide and sodium on glycolysis and oxygen uptake in brain homogenates. J. biol. Chem. 161, 453—461 (1945).
[80] LE PAGE, G. A.: Glycolysis in tumor homogenates. J. biol. Chem. 176, 1009—1020 (1948).
[81] MEYERHOF, O., and J. R. WILSON: The rate of turnover of hexosediphosphate in brain preparations. Arch. Biochem. 14, 71—82 (1947).
[82] SKOU, J. C.: The influence of some cations on adenosinetriphosphatase from peripheral nerves. Biochim. biophys. Acta 23, 394—401 (1957).

ment for the activity of this enzyme. In the presence of Mg^{++}, Na^+ activates strongly. The activity increases rapidly with increasing Na concentration.

K cannot replace Na but if Na and Mg^{++} are present, addition of K gives an augmentation of the reaction rate. Potassium ions in high concentration inhibit that part of the activity which is due to Na. In a medium containing K, Na, Ca^{++} and Mg^{++} in concengrations roughly equal to those of crab axoplasma, either an increase in Na concentration or a decrease in K concentration will lead to a stimulation of the enzyme activity.

13. Myosin ATP-ase

It is well known that part of the ATP-ase activity of muscle is associated with the protein, myosin, which is also an integral part of the contractile mechanism. The property of reacting with actin and that of splitting ATP seem to reside in the same molecule. It is, however, possible by treatment with proteolytic enzymes like trypsin or chymotrypsin (see GERGELY et al.[83]) to obtain preparations which have lost the capacity for forming a superprecipitate with actin but which retain the ATP-ase activity. The behaviour of the ATP-ase toward inorganic ions seems, however, to be the same before and after treatment with the proteolytic enzymes.

The myosin ATP-ase is strongly activated by K with an optimum concentration around 0.2 molar[84]. Na, on the other hand, has little effect when added alone. When Na and K are added together, Na acts as an inhibitor at concentrations which produce no effect when it is present alone. Conversely, if Na is present, the concentration of K necessary to attain optimum activity is higher than without Na[85]:

It has long been known that ATP-ase is activated by Ca^{++}, but, surprisingly enough, the chelating agent ethylenediamine tetraacetate (versene) which binds Ca^{++} is also a powerful activator of myosine ATP-ase[86]. In the presence of this agent there is virtually no activity when Li or Na are added, but a very high activity with K, Rb or NH_4[87]. In the presence of 0.005 molar $CaCl_2$ all the alkali metal ions seem to have the same effect[88].

Mg^{++} is an activator of myosin ATP-ase at low K concentrations and an inhibitor at high K concentrations.

14. Urease

As early as in 1913, ARMSTRONG and ARMSTRONG[89] found that, with potassium phosphate buffers, the activity of urease first increases and then decreases again with increasing concentrations of potassium ions. Furthermore it was found that for equivalent concentrations, Na-phosphates caused a greater inhibition than did K phosphates. These experiments were performed with impure preparations of

[83] GERGELY, J., M. A. GOUVEA, and D. KARIBIAN: Fragmentation of myosin by chymotrypsin. J. biol. Chem. **212**, 165—177 (1955).

[84] BOWEN, W. J., and T. D. KERWIN: A study of the effects of ethyldiaminetetraacetic acid on myosin adenosinetriphosphatase. J. biol. Chem. **211**, 237—247 (1954).

[85] MOMMAERTS, W. F. H. M., and I. GREEN: Adenosinetriphosphatase systems of muscle. J. biol. Chem. **208**, 833—843 (1954).

[86] FRIESS, E. T.: The effect of chelating agent on myosin ATPase. Arch. Biochem. Biophys. **51**, 17—23 (1954).

[87] KIELLY, W. W., H. M. KALCKAR, and L. B. BRADLEY: The hydrolysis of purine and pyrimidine nucleoside triphosphates by myosin. J. biol. Chem. **219**, 95—101 (1956).

[88] HASSELBACH, W.: Conversion of actomyosin-adenosinetriphosphatase into L-myosin-adenosinetriphosphatase activators and the resulting effects. Z. Naturforsch. **7b**, 163—174 (1952).

[89] ARMSTRONG, E. F., and H. E. ARMSTRONG: Studies on the processes operative in solutions and on enzyme action; the nature of enzymes and of their action as hydrolytic agents. Proc. roy. Soc. B. **86**, 561—586 (1913).

urease. More recently, however, FASMAN and NIEMAN[90] have studied the kinetics of the splitting of urea by urease in the presence of sodium and potassium ions. The kinetic analysis indicates that phosphate ions activate, whereas K and Na inhibit urease. Na was found to be a more powerful inhibitor than K.

c) Non-specific effects of alkali metal ions

Besides those listed above, several enzymes are known whose action is profoundly influenced by the concentration of alkali metal ions. Thus, according to NACHMANSOHN[91] the cholinesterase from the electric ray (Torpedo) is nearly inactive after dialysis, but is reactivated by K and Na if the salt concentration is higher than 0.1 molar. Cholinesterases of different origin seem to have rather different sensitivities towards the alkali metal ions[92, 93, 94], but it appears that K and Na always have qualitatively as well as quantitatively identical effects.

Even certain plant esterases are very powerfully activated by alkali metal ions, for example the *pectinesterases*. As early as 1925 KOPACZEWSKI[95] stated that a neutral mixture of purified pectin and dialyzed enzyme from alfalfa showed no activity except in the presence of alkali or alkaline earth salts. This finding was verified and extended by LINEWEAVER and BALLOU[96]. Their kinetic studies of the process led to the conclusion that the action of the cations is primarily one of deinhibition. K and Na have essentially the same effect which is about ten times weaker than that of the alkaline earth metal ions. The enzyme is markedly inhibited (at slightly acid p_H) by the carboxyl groups of pectic acid which is formed by the enzyme reaction. The cations prevent inhibition by complexing with the carboxyls. The cations do not affect the enzyme-substrate dissociation constant.

The action of NaCl on the degradation of hyaluronic acid catalyzed by *hyaluronidase* seems also to be one of deinhibition (compare the reviews by MEYER[97] and by MEYER and RAPOPORT[98]). The enzyme[99] is strongly activated by NaCl, the optimum concentration being around 0.1 molar. The effect of NaCl does, however, show a pronounced dependence upon the source of the substrate[100]. Thus the degradation of hyaluronate from umbilical cord was 20 times faster in

[90] FASMAN, G. D., and C. NIEMANN: A reinvestigation of the kinetics of the *urease*-catalysed hydrolysis of urea. I. The activity of urease in the presence of sodium and potassium phosphate. J. Amer. chem. Soc. **73**, 1646—1650 (1951).

[91] NACHMANSOHN, D.: Action of ions on choline esterase. Nature (Lond.) **145**, 513—514 (1940).

[92] GLICK, D.: Effect of sodium and potassium ions on choline esterase. Nature (Lond.) **148**, 662 (1941).

[93] MENDEL, B., D. MUNDELL, and F. STRELITZ: Cholinesterase and electrolytes. Nature (Lond.) **144**, 479—480 (1939).

[94] ALLES, G. A., and R. C. HAWES: Cholinesterases in the blood of man. J. biol. Chem. **133**, 375—390 (1940).

[95] KOPACZEWSKI, M. W.: Sur la coagulation de la pectine. Bull. Soc. Chim. biol. **7**, 419—428 (1925).

[96] LINEWEAVER, H., and G. A. BALLOU: The effect of cations on the activity of alfalfa pectinesterase (pectase). Arch. Biochem. **6**, 373—387 (1945).

[97] MEYER, K.: Biological significance of hyaluronic acid and hyaluronidase. Physiol. Rev. **27**, 335—359 (1947).

[98] MEYER, K., and M. M. RAPPORT: Hyaluronidases. Advanc. Enzymol. **13**, 199—236 (1952).

[99] MADINAVEITIA, J., and T. H. H. QUIBELL: Diffusing factors. 9. The effect of salts on the action of testicular extracts on the viscosity of vitreous humour preparations. Biochem. J. **35**, 456—460 (1941).

[100] HADIDAN, Z., and N. W. PIRIE: The preparation and some properties of hyaluronic acid from human umbilical cord. Biochem. J. **42**, 260—265 (1948).

the presence of 0.15 molar NaCl than when the salt was absent, whereas the splitting of material from synovial fluid proceeded at a rate, in salt-free solution, which was about $^2/_3$ of that in 0.15 molar NaCl. Further studies in MEYER's laboratory led to the conclusion that NaCl counteracts inhibition of the enzyme by certain inhibitors like heparin or chondroitin sulfate. These findings are related to the studies of McCLEAN[100 a] on the inhibitory action of heparin and chondroitin sulfate on the in vitro decapsulation of streptococci by hyaluronidase. It was found that a series of acid polysaccharides inhibit, whereas two neutral polysaccharides were without effect on the action of hyaluronidase. The ability of polyvalent ions like uronic acids to combine with alkali metal ions has been discussed in a previous chapter. It was pointed out that the affinity for different alkali metal ions may differ appreciably among these polyvalent acids. Unfortunately no material is at hand concerning the relative effects on the hyaluronidase reaction of the different alkali metal ions.

d) Comments

From the foregoing it appears that enzymes often are influenced differently by the various species of alkali metal ions. Usually K, Rb (and NH_4) have essentially the same effect which is opposed more or less markedly by Na and Li. The effect of Cs usually comes closer to that of the K = group than to that of the Na = group, in agreement with the fact that K, Rb and Cs are rather similar with respect to ionic diameter etc. In the cases where the kinetic study has been carried far enough to draw reasonably safe conclusions (pyruvic transphosphorylase, fructokinase, β-galactosidase) it appears, however, that the "antagonism" between the K group and the Na group of alkali metal ions is not a true antagonism in the sense that the two groups have opposite effects on the enzymatic processes. Rather it seems that the action of K and Na is of qualitatively the same nature, but that one ion has a much stronger effect than the other. The approach, most clearly formulated by COHN and MONOD, which distinguishes between the "activance" (see p. 16) and the affinity of an activating ion seems to offer a satisfactory basis for future work. The predominance of K — activated over Na — activated enzymes raises the question whether K is *per se* better suited as activator for enzymes than is Na. If that were the case it would help explaining why all living cells must maintain a high concentration of K. It should be remembered, however, that all the enzymes which are activated by K seem to be intracellular. If for any reason (see for instance BOYLE and CONWAY[101]) potassium ions tend to accumulate in the cells, their enzyme systems would have had to adapt to the K = rich environment in the course of phylogenetic development. In this context it is worth remembering that the β-galactosidase of E. coli is activated by K more than by Na towards the natural substrate lactose, whereas Na is a better activator when the synthetic substrate o-nitrophenol-β-D-galacto-pyranoside is used. Similarly, the acetate activating enzyme of the squid seems to be only little inhibited by Na whereas the corresponding enzyme from mammalian muscle is strongly inhibited by this ion, in agreement with the fact that the Na concentration is likely to be much higher in the tissues of the squid than in those of the mammal.

It is evident from the foregoing discussion that several enzymes are able to bind alkali metal ions quite strongly and specifically. Such binding must be

---

[100a] McCLEAN, D.: Studies on diffusing factors. 2. Methods of assay of hyaluronidase and their correlation with skin diffusing activity. Biochem. J. **37**, 169—177 (1943).

[101] BOYLE, P. J., and E. J. CONWAY: Potassium accumulation in muscle and associated changes. J. Physiol. **100**, 1—63 (1941).

assumed both when an ion species acts as activator and when it is inhibitory. Apart from the interest which the enzymologist takes in such specific binding of one or more of the alkali metal ions, this binding is also of great interest for purely chemical reasons. In a previous chapter it was stated that most proteins do not show any measurable tendency to bind alkali metal ions. The consequence of this seems to be that the alkali metal ion-binding enzymes must possess prosthetic groups or molecular structures which are not typical of proteins in general.

On the other hand, binding of alkali metal ions is exhibited by many natural and artificial polyvalent anions (see chapter II). It is interesting to speculate that alkali metal ion activation or inhibition is more common among enzymes connected with phosphate metabolism than among other enzymes, because they have a dense population of negative charges belonging to phosphate and phosphate esters in the vicinity of the active center. At present our knowledge is too limited to prove or disprove this hypothesis.

It goes without saying that the elucidation of the mechanisms by which enzymes bind alkali metal ions might also bring clues to the intriguing problems connected with active transport of alkali metal ions (see chapter VII).

IV. Effect of alkali metal ions on mitochondria

Whereas some enzymes, for instance those responsible for glycolysis, are present mainly in dissolved form in the cytoplasm, several important enzyme systems are confined almost exclusively to the particulate or insoluble fraction of the cells. As far as metabolism is concerned, the mitochondria or "large granules" deserve particular interest because they seem to contain most of the enzymes responsible for the oxidative metabolism. Thus cytochrome oxidase, succinoxidase, the enzymes involved in the KREBS-tricarboxylic acid cycle and the system responsible for the oxidation of fatty acids to acetoacetate are present in the mitochondria (for references see for instance KENNEDY and LEHNINGER[102]).

The effects of ions in general and of alkali metal ions in particular upon the enzymatic processes catalyzed by mitochondria differ profoundly from the effects elicited in systems containing the same enzymes in solution. The reason for this seems to lie in the organization of the mitochondria. CLAUDE, in 1946[103], pointed out that the function of the mitochondria was very sensitive to the osmotic pressure of the suspension medium. As a matter of fact the mitochondria behave towards osmotic changes as if they were surrounded by a semipermeable membrane, and electron microscopic studies have provided strong support for the idea that such mitochondrium membranes do in fact exist[104, 105, 106].

---

[102] KENNEDY, E. P., and A. L. LEHNINGER: Oxidation of fatty acids and tricarboxylic acids cycle intermediates by isolated rat liver mitochondria. J. biol. Chem. 179, 957—972 (1949).

[103] CLAUDE, A.: Fractionation of mammalian liver cells by differential centrifugation I, problem, method, and preparation of extract, II experimental procedures and results. J. exp. Biol. Med. 84, 51—89 (1946).

[104] SJÖSTRAND, F. S., and V. HANZON: Membrane structures of cytoplasma and mitochondria in exocrine cells of mouse pancreas as revealed by high resolution electron microscopy. Exp. Cell. Res. 7, 393—414 (1954).

[105] PALADE, A. E.: The fine structure of mitochondria. Anat. Rec. 114, 427—451 (1952).

[106] BEAMS, H. W., T. N. TAHMISIAN, R. L. DEVINE, and L. E. ROTH: Phasecontrast and electron microscope studies on the nebenkem, a mitochondrial body in the spermatids of the grasshopper. Biol. Bull. 107, 47—56 (1954).

Modern methods for the isolation of functional mitochondria, like those of HOGEBOOM, SCHNEIDER and PALLADE[107], are based on the protection of the particles against osmotic damage by the use of sucrose solutions of a suitable tonicity. Thus, the effects of alkali metal ions on mitochondria must be considered from two aspects: 1) to what extent do solutions containing these ions as major or minor constituents protect mitochondria against osmotic damage, and 2) how do these ions influence the processes going on in the mitochondria.

Both problems are further complicated by the fact that the mitochondria possess the ability to concentrate certain ionic species, under some conditions K^{108} and sometimes Na^{109}. Thus an analysis of the suspension medium may give a distorted picture of the true ionic concentrations at the site of the enzyme reactions.

Tracer experiments[108, 109, 110] have shown that both K and Na exchange at a high rate across the mitochondrion membrane, although a minor fraction of the mito-chondrion K may be confined, under certain conditions like low temperature and low oxygen tension, in an unexchangable form within the particles. Consider-ing the relative ease with which these ions penetrate into the particles it is perhaps not surprising that solutions of the non-penetrating sucrose are preferable to those containing alkali chlorides for the preparation of mitochondria. Sucrose will remain in the outside medium irrespective of the metabolic state in the mitochondria whereas the maintenance of a given alkali metal ion concentration must depend upon metabolicaly driven active transport mechanisms (see chap-ter VII). According to POTTER and RECKNAGEL[111], maximum oxygen uptake and maximum sensitivity to dinitrophenol pertain at a tonicity of 0.25 molar sucrose. A 0.154 molar solution of KCl, isotonic with the sucrose solution men-tioned, could not replace it.

DE DUVE and collaborators[112] have shown that the acid phosphatase of rat liver mitochondria will leak out if the particles are suspended in distilled water. The leakage is slowed down, but is not fully inhibited, by 0.15 molar NaCl. Even 0.44 molar NaCl does not stop the loss of phosphatase, whereas 0.25 molar sucrose, both in the absence and presence of NaCl, blocks the leakage effectively.

A point of great interest is that a typical substrate for the phosphatase, for example glycerophosphate, is not attacked by intact mitochondria. This shows that not only does the membrane keep the enzyme from leaking, but it also stops the diffusion of the substrate into the particles.

In the case of some enzyme systems the alkali metal ions in appropriate concentration do give sufficient protection against osmotic damage to mito-chondria. One example is provided by the fatty acid oxidation complex. It was

[107] HOGEBOOM, G. H., W. C. SCHNEIDER, and G. E. PALLADE: Cytochemical studies of mammalian tissues I. Isolation of intact mitochondria from rat liver, some biochemical properties of mitochondria and submicroscopic particulate material. J. biol. Chem. 172, 619—636 (1948).

[108] STANBURY, S. W., and G. H. MUDGE: Potassium metabolism of liver mitochondria. Proc. Soc. exp. Biol. (N. Y.) 82, 675—681 (1953).

[109] BARTLAY, W., and R. E. DAVIES: Secretary activity of mitochondria. Biochem. J. 52, XX (1952).

[110] SPECTOR, W. G.: Electrolyte flux in isolated mitochondria. Proc. roy. Soc. Ser. B, Biol. Sci. Lond. 141, 268—279 (1953).

[111] POTTER, V. R., and R. O. RECKNAGEL: The regulation of the rate of oxidation in rat liver mitochondria, in "A Symposium on Phosphorous Metabolism", Vol. I, p. 377—391. Baltimore: Johns Hopkins Press 1951.

[112] DUVE, C. DE, J. BERTHET, L. BERTHET, and F. APPELMANS: Permeability of mito-chondria. Nature (Lond.) 167, 389—390 (1951).

first shown by POTTER[113] that the addition of K promoted the oxidation of fatty acids by rat liver homogenate suspended in distilled water. Later, LEHNINGER and KENNEDY[114] pointed out that the fatty acid oxidase activity of the liver homogenates was bound to the mitochondria. The material showed no activity when suspended with ATP, Mg^{++} and dilute phosphate buffer. When saline was used in stead of distilled water as suspending medium, the preparations were highly active. KCl, LiCl and sucrose solutions were equally effective. Low-molecular substances like glycerol, acetamide and ethylene glycol were without effect. The authors concluded that the beneficial effect of alkali metal ions was solely due to their contributions to the osmotic pressure of the medium (compare also KENNEDY and LEHNINGER[102]).

PRESSMAN and LARDY[115, 49], also studied the effect of the different alkali ions upon the respiration of rat liver mitochondria in the presence of Krebs cycle intermediates. They found that K, Rb and Cs gave higher rates of respiration than did Na and Li. These authors also made the highly interesting observation that the addition of microsomes or a heat-stable, acetone-soluble extract of microsomes to the mitochondria greatly increased the sensitivity of the latter to added K.

V. Metabolic effects on tissues and tissue slices

We have seen that some factor, presumably the existence of the selective membrane, makes the enzymes of mitochondria and the corresponding free enzymes respond differently to the alkali metal ions. As one would expect, it becomes even more difficult to explain the effects of the alkali metal ions upon whole cells and tissues in terms of effects on individual enzymes. In the first place, most cells — and animal cells in particular — are damaged if the osmotic pressure of the medium is varied beyond certain limits. Since sodium ion is the major cation of most biological fluids, it often seems to play the role of an inert, but osmotically active particle. In this role Na can be partly or totally replaced by other ions, organic as well as inorganic. Furthermore, hydrophilic organic non-electrolytes like the sugars may take the place of most of the ions in the medium with at least some of the vital functions retained. But even if certain cell types can for a time carry on their functions in a medium practically free of alkali metal ions, this does not mean that these ions are necessarily non-essential for the enzymatic processes. Rather it is an expression of the fact that most cells have the ability to retain at least part of their internal ionic composition with great tenacity. The study of ion effects on the metabolism is therefore intimately correlated with the problems of ionic permeability and active ion transport. These problems are discussed in chapter VII.

Another point which should be born in mind is that isolated tissues and tissue slices consist of more or less severely damaged cells. The damage may be slight so that the cells might recover if returned to the organism as a transplant. Or, the damage may be irreversible, so that what are studied are stages on the way to total death. These facts constitute a warning against taking effects found with tissue slices as direct evidence for similar effects in the intact organism. Rather the study of isolated tissues indicates reaction patterns of which only some may

---

[113] POTTER, V. R.: The assay of animal tissues for respiratory enzymes IV. Cell structure in relation to fatty acid oxidation. J. biol. Chem. **163**, 437—446 (1946).

[114] LEHNINGER, A. L., and E. P. KENNEDY: The requirements of the fatty acids oxidase complex of rat liver. J. biol. chem. **173**, 753—771 (1948).

[115] PRESSMAN, B. C., and H. A. LARDY: Influence of potassium and other alkali cations on respiration of mitochondria. J. biol. Chem. **197**, 547—556 (1952).

be realisable with the same cells in situ. On the other hand it is possible to vary the conditions in the incubation media to such extremes as to reveal reactions which are barely discernible as long as the cells are subject to the homeostasis of a whole organism.

For some of the uses that have been made of isolated tissues it has been essential to reduce as much as possible the importance of the cell membranes as a diffusion barrier to metabolites. No doubt the well-known Krebs Ringer-Phosphate fulfills the requirements for a medium allowing maximum oxygen uptake by many tissues. But, being calcium-free, it changes the membrane properties profoundly, so that ionic effects measured in this medium cannot be expected to be valid for cells in a balanced medium.

As it will appear from the following the gaps in our present knowledge are many. The experimental material concerning the metabolic effects of Li, Rb and Cs is deplorably inadequate. The data also bear out the fact that a certain ionic composition of the medium may well be beneficial for one cellular function and inhibitory for another. There is no such thing as an optimum medium which maximizes all cellular functions. Rather, by choosing the proper medium one can exaggerate one or another of the functions. The different functions are therefore discussed separately below.

a) Effects on oxygen consumption

1. Brain slices

It was first shown by ASHFORD and DIXON[116] that the addition of potassium ions to the incubation medium increases the oxygen consumption of brain slices. The phenomenon was studied in greater detail by DICKENS and GREVILLE[117]. They found that the addition of 0.1 molar KCl to the Tyrode solution in which the brain slices were incubated led to an increased respiration whether the substrate was glucose, fructose, lactate or pyruvate. Rb and Cs had the same effect as K, whereas Li and Na had only little effect. The divalent ions Ca^{++} and Mg^{++} depressed the oxygen consumption. In the presence of a balanced medium containing Ca^{++}, K and Na, the respiration was low and steady. When Ca was left out, the respiration became high and not very steady, and if Na was the only cation, the respiration was initially high, but fell off rapidly.

K stimulates respiration in concentrations as low as those encountered in mammalian serum[119]. The latter authors found the optimum concentration of K for the respiration of Guinea pig brain slices to be 0.04 molar. K does not stimulate except in the presence of at least 0.02 M. NaCl.

The antagonism observed by DICKENS and GREVILLE[117] between Ca^{++}, which depresses, and K which stimulates respiration, has been verified by CANZANELLI et al.[118]. In a medium fully balanced as to inorganic ions the respiration was found to be the same as in a solution containing Na as the only cation. These authors assume Ca^{++} to depress respiration solely by antagonizing the stimulatory effect of K.

---

[116] ASHFORD, C. A., and K. C. DIXON: The effect of potassium on the glucolysis of brain tissue with reference to the Pasteur effect. Biochem. J. 29, 157—168 (1935).

[117] DICKENS, F., and G. D. GREVILLE: The metabolism of normal and tumor tissue. XIII Neutral salt effects. Biochem. J. 29, 1468—1483 (1935).

[118] CANZANELLI, A., G. ROGERS, and D. RAPPORT: Effects of inorganic ions on the respiration of brain cortex. Amer. J. Physiol. 135, 309—315 (1941).

[119] LIPSETT, M. N., and F. CRESCITELLI: Effects of increased potassium concentration on metabolism of rat cerebral cortical slices. Arch. Biochem. 28, 329—337 (1950).

Li was found to stimulate respiration in concentrations greater than 0.01 molar.

As mentioned above the KCl = induced stimulation of respiration can be brought about with glucose, fructose, lactate and pyruvate as substrates. However, no stimulation could be noticed with succinate, L-glutamate or ketoglutarate. As a matter of fact, the last three substances mentioned, as well as citrate, inhibited the stimulation in the presence of glucose. Malonate in a concentration of 10^{-3} moles/liter depressed the K = stimulated oxygen consumption down to the level of non-stimulated metabolism.

The mechanism underlying the K-effect on the metabolism is not quite clear. TERNER, EGGLESTON and KREBS[120] have shown that brain slices cannot maintain normal K concentration unless both glucose and glutamate are added to the medium. They further point out that effects similar to those given by high potassium (increased glycolysis and increased oxygen consumption) are also elicited by the addition of L-glutamate to the medium. They therefore conclude: "The effects produced by potassium and glutamate have presumably a common root: both substances raise the potassium concentration in the tissue slice". However, this hypothesis does not explain the fact that glutamate reduced the stimulation of oxygen consumption brought about by high K in the medium containing glucose[121].

2. Peripheral nerve

According to CHANG, SHAFFER and GERARD[122], high K concentrations depress the oxygen consumption of frog nerve. Maximum depression, about 50% of the normal respiration, was obtained when K made up about 50% of the total cation. K-free solutions gave the same respiration rate as normal Ringer. A stimulating effect of excess Na could not be demonstrated with certainty. The depressant action which K exerts upon frog nerve respiration does not show any simple correlation with the other physiological effects of K.

The effect of the K concentration upon the respiration of crab nerve has been studied by SHANES and HOPKINS[123]. The oxygen consumption showed a pronouced maximum when the K concentration in the medium was around 30 mM. Thus between zero and 10 mM. K the respiration was constant and equalled about 100 mm³/g wet weight/hr. As 30 mM K concentration was increased towards 100mM, the respiration dropped to about 50 mm³/g/hr.

3. Liver slices

According to AEBI[124], K markedly increases the respiration of liver slices of guinea pig. Optimum conditions for respiration of the slices are obtained with a medium containing Na, Ca⁺⁺ and Mg⁺⁺ in concentrations equal to those found in serum but having a concentration of K twice that of serum. The respiration is not related in a simple way to the K content of the slices, however. In many cases a high oxygen consumption goes with high cellular K (and a low degree

[120] TERNER, C., L. V. EGGLETON, and H. A. KREBS: The rôle of glutamic acid in the transport of potassium in brain and retina. Biochem. J. 47, 139—149 (1950).

[121] WEIL-MALHERBE, H.: Observations on tissue glycolysis. Biochem. J. 32, 2257—2275 (1938).

[122] CHANG, T. H., M. SHAFFER, and R. W. GERARD: The influence of electrolytes on respiration in nerve. Amer. J. Physiol. 111, 681—696 (1935).

[123] SHANES, A. M., and H. S. HOPKINS: Effect of potassium on resting potential and respiration of crab nerve. J. Neurophysiol. 11, 331—342 (1948).

[124] AEBI, H.: Kationenmilieu und Gewebsatmung. Helv. physiol. pharmacol. Acta 8, 525—543 (1950).

of swelling) but sometimes the opposite is more nearly true[125]. Nevertheless, the importance of a high intracellular K concentration is made clear by the fact that slices kept under optimal conditions with ample oxygen supply, a balanced salt medium, and substrate, show no swelling, maintain a normal intracellular K concentration, and keep their oxygen consumption going at a constant rate for several hours. Thus high cellular K is a measure of the viability of the preparation, but does not necessarily give maximum oxygen consumption.

4. Muscle

When isolated frog muscle is placed in an isotonic sugar solution it becomes non-irritable. At the same time there is an enormous increase in oxygen consumption[126] and an increased loss of phosphoric acid. The respiration rate can be normalized by the addition of a small amount of isotonic NaCl to the medium, whereas KCl is without effect[127]. FENN, also found that the salt-free sugar solution induced a slight contracture and an increased lactic acid formation. According to CHANG et al. the increased O_2 consumption is mainly due to the contracture. In any event FENN found it possible to control the oxygen consumption by the K/Ca^{++} ratio, both in the presence of sugar and with NaCl as the osmotically active component. K causes a rise while Ca^{++} causes a fall in the metabolic rate. However, these effects are not likely to play any great role in the intact organism since, presumably, the concentration changes necessary in the extracellular fluid are beyond the physiological range.

The effect of increased K concentration on the respiration of frog muscle was studied in greater detail by HEGNAUER et al.[128]. The oxygen consumption increased as much as tenfold in the first hour after the K concentration of the medium had been raised to 25 mM. Also the heat production is stimulated strongly by increased K in the medium[139]. According to SOLANDT[129,130] the increase in heat production sets in at an outside K concentration which does not elicit any measurable contracture. KEYNES and MAISEL[131] confirm this view, finding no signs of contracture in muscles subjected to 10 mM potassium, at which concentration the oxygen consumption was significantly increased.

The effect of the ionic composition of the medium on the oxygen consumption of minced pigeon breast muscle has been studied by KLEINZELLER[132]. The optimum K concentration was 0.385 M for a medium containing 0.02 M phosphate buffer and 0.0425 M NaCl, but no Ca^{++} and Mg^{++}. The optimum K concentration was, however, much lower, namely 0.0034 M, when a trace of Mg^{++} (0.00085 M) was added to the medium. The optimum Mg^{++} concentration depends, on the other hand, upon the concentration of K, and may vary between 0.0085 and 0.01M.

[125] AEBI, H.: Zusammenhänge zwischen Atmung, Quellung und Elektrolytgehalt überlebender Gewebsschnitte. Helv. physiol. pharmacol. Acta 10, 184—206 (1952).

[126] EMBDEN, G., and H. LANGE: Muskelatmung und Sarkoplasma. Z. physiol. Chem. 125, 258—282 (1923).

[127] FENN, W. O.: The oxygen comsumption of muscles made non-irritable by sugar solutions. Amer. J. Physiol. 97, 635—647 (1931).

[128] HEGNAUER, A. H., W. O. FENN, and D. M. COBB: The cause of the rise in oxygen consumption of frog muscles in excess of potassium. J. cell. comp. Physiol. 4, 505—526 (1934).

[129] SOLANDT, D. Y.: The effect of potassium on the excitability and resting metabolism of frog's muscle. J. Physiol. 86, 162—170 (1936).

[130] SMITH, C. G., and D. Y. SOLANDT: The relation of contracture to the increment in the resting heat production of muscle under the influence of potassium. J. Physiol. 93, 305 to 311 (1938).

[131] KEYNES, R. D., and G. W. MAISEL: Energy requirement for sodium ion extrusion from a frog muscle. Proc. roy. Soc. B 142, 383—392 (1954).

[132] KLEINZELLER, A.: The effect of electrolytes on the respiration of pigeon breast muscle. Biochem. J. 34, 1241—1244 (1940).

Mg^{++} and K can partly, but not completely, replace each other. This recalls the fact that certain enzymes like pyruvic transphosphorylase and fructokinase require both K and Mg^{++}. No doubt the muscle fibre membranes of minced muscle are severely damaged, especially in a Ca^{++}-free medium and direct ionic effects on enzymes are more likely to show up here than in most cellular systems.

In the course of a study of glycogen synthesis by rat heart slices, STADIE et al.[133] measured the oxygen consumption as a function of the NaCl concentration of the medium, the osmotic pressure being maintained constant by proper addition of inert sugars. The respiration showed a positive correlation with the Na concentration, whereas, surprisingly enough, the opposite was true with respect to glycogen formation.

5. Kidney slices

In the course of their study of the paraamino hippurate uptake by kidney slices, TAGGART, SILVERMAN and TRAYNER[134] also measured the oxygen consumption at various K/Na ratios in the medium. The outcome of one of these experimental series is shown in table 4.

Table 4. *Influence of cellular electrolyte composition on the respiration and p-aminohippurate accumulation in rabbit kidney slices*
By leaching in 0.15 M NaCl the K concentration in the slices are reduced from 78.7 mMoles/kg to 31.7 mMoles/kg[134]

K concentration in			Na + K in slices mMoles/kg	Resp. q_{O_2}	PAH Slices/medium
Slices	medium				
final mMoles/kg	initial mMoles/l	final mMoles/l			
29.5	0	0.8	134	0.91	2.6
45.3	2	0.8	135	1.02	6.9
60.1	5	2.8	137	1.10	10.1
66.3	10	6.9	139	1.04	9.6
77.0	30	25.9	136	0.93	8.9
98.0	60	53.9	136	0.79	7.0

It is seen that maximum oxygen consumption was obtained at a final K concentration in the medium of 2.8 meq/liter. This outer concentration allowed the slices to maintain a K concentration of 60.1 meq/liter. The tissue concentration of K turned out to be of greater importance than the potassium concentration of the bathing solution in supporting the metabolic functions of the slices. The cellular K level itself is, however, the result of the metabolically-driven active transport of Na out of, and possibly also transport of K into the cells (see p. 57). Li in concentrations ranging from 10—100 meq./liter has no significant effect upon the respiration although it depresses the PAH transport[134].

6. Isolated frog skin

The isolated frog skin possesses a powerful mechanism for active sodium transport (see p. 114), which is also responsible for the maintenance of the observed potential difference across the skin when it is in contact with Ringer on both

[133] STADIE, W. C., N. HAUGAARD, and M. PERLMUTTER: The synthesis of glycogen by rat heart slices. J. biol. Chem. **171**, 419—429 (1947).
[134] TAGGART, J. V., L. SILVERMAN, and E. M. TRAYNER: Influence of renal electrolyte composition on the tubular excretion of P-aminohippurate. Amer. J. Physiol. **173**, 345—350 (1953).

sides (the inside being between 10 and 160 mV positive relative to the outside solution). If this potential difference is short-circuited by a suitable "voltage clamp" system, the active sodium transport gives rise to a maintained electric current. The strength of this current is a direct measure of the rate of active transport (compare p. 118). If the outside and inside solutions are contained in closed systems during the short-circuting, the oxygen consumption can be measured simultaneously with the measurement the rate of of active sodium transport. Using this procedure, ZERAHN has demonstrated that the oxygen consumption is some 50% higher when the outside medium is Ringer than when the sodium of the solution is replaced by an inert ion like choline or magnesium. Furthermore it was shown that the extra oxygen consumption associated with replacement of the inert ion with Na is proportional to of the rate of active sodium transport. If the active transport is increased by addition to the inside solution of antidiuretic hormone (which presumably acts by increasing the pore size of some layer presenting a passive resistance to ion flow (p. 127) the oxygen consumption goes up in proportion to the rate of current flow. Thus the resistance determines the current flow and the current flow in turn determines the oxygen consumption. We have here a clear case of the active ion transport being the pace setting reaction determining the level of a sizable fraction of the oxygen consumption.

b) Effects on glycolysis

The glycolysis of *brain slices* is profoundly affected by the K concentration of the incubation fluid. Thus, ASHFORD and DIXON[116] found that addition of potassium salts to glycolysing brain slices increases the aerobic and decreases anaerobic glycolysis. The effect is not shown by the corresponding Na^+ salts. Very high K concentrations (0.5 M) depressed both aerobic and anaerobic glycolysis. This, however, may have been partly an osmotic effect, since no attempt was made to keep the tonicity of the medium constant.

The inhibition of anaerobic glycolysis by KCl was irreversible. Probably anaerobiosis is detrimental to the cells. ASHFORD has pointed out that damage to the tissue diminishes the glycolysis. The findings of ASHFORD and DIXON have been verified and extended by DICKENS and GREVILLE[117].

The glycolysis of *tumor tissue* (Flexner-Jobling tar carcinoma and Jensen sarcoma) also depends upon the K concentration. For instance, the addition to the saline medium of KCl to give a concentration of 0.0025 M, increase the glycolysis of Jensen sarcoma by about 70% as compared with the lactive acid formation in a potassium-free medium[135, 136]. This potassium stimulation was observed during anaerobic conditions. Evidently, the tumor tissue is less sensitive to oxygen lack than is brain tissue.

c) Effect on acetyl choline synthesis

MANN, TENNENBAUM and QUASTEL[137] discovered that brain slices will synthesize much more acetyl choline if potassium ions are added to the saline or bicarbonate-Locke medium containing a suitable substrate. 0.027 M K gave

[135] LASNITZKI, A., and O. ROSENTHAL: Über den Einfluß der Kationen auf das Gärvermögen der Tumorzelle I. Biochem. Z. 207, 120—140 (1929).

[136] LASNITZKI, A.: Über den Einfluß der Kationen auf das Gärvermögen der Tumorzelle III. Weitere Untersuchungen über die Wirkung des Kaliums. Biochem. Z. 264, 285—291 (1933).

[137] MANN, P. J. G., M. TENNENBAUM, and J. H. QUASTEL: Acetylcholine metabolism in the central nervous system. The effects of potassium and other cations on acetylcholine liberation. Biochem. J. 33, 822—835 (1939).

maximum augmentation of the synthesis. High potassium concentrations inhibit the acetyl choline formation. Rb and to a smaller extent Cs gave effects similar to those given by K, whereas NH_4 inhibited the synthesis. The divalent ions Ca^{++} and Mg^{++} counteracted the acceleration given by K. The same authors also found that the addition of acetyl choline to the medium depresses the synthesis, if K is also present. From this and other observations they argued that potassium ions influence the rate of synthesis by making the cell membrane more permeable. Therefore, acetyl choline escapes from the cells, and the equilibrium is displaced in the direction of synthesis. Extra acetyl choline added to the medium would reduce the rate of escape and thus depress the rate of acetyl choline formation. However, McLENNAN and ELLIOT[138], who have studied the process more recently, were unable to find any depression of the acetyl choline formation by addition of extra acetyl choline.

The same authors[139] found that the synthesis of acetyl choline in brain extracts is strongly dependent upon the ATP concentration below about 2 mmoles/liter. Since respiring brain slices contain about 30 mmoles/liter of acid labile phosphate (mostly ATP), it seems unlikely that the level of ATP is rate = limiting for the synthesis in the slices. Thus the effect of K on the rate of synthesis could very well be related to some process going on in the cell membrane.

Whether or not high K ion concentrations increase the permeability of brain slices to acetyl choline, is may be pertinent to recall the fact that the acetate activating enzyme which is involved in the acetyl choline synthesis is strongly activated by K and inhibited by Na (compare p. 14). This may be at least a contributing factor in the augmentation of the synthesis by high K concentrations in the medium.

d) Effect on glycogen synthesis

It was first observed by HASTINGS and BUCHANAN[140] that a medium rich in K promotes the synthesis of glycogen from glucose by rat liver slices. The phenomenon was studied in more detail by BUCHANAN, HASTINGS and NESBETT[141]. More glycogen was synthesized from glucose added to a medium rich in K (optimum K-concentration 145 mmoles/liter) than when the medium was ordinary Ringer. Ca^{++} and Mg^{++} also increased glycogen formation. (It should be recalled that Ca^{++} depressed respiration!)

Succinate reduced the glycogen formation. If succinate and phosphate were given simultaneously the synthesis fell to zero. Since both succinate and phosphate form nearly insoluble Ca^{++} salts, the effect may be one of calcium deprivation.

The formation of glycogen with pyruvate as the substrate is also favoured by high K concentration. BUCHANAN, HASTINGS and NESBETT[141] made the striking observation that the formation of carbohydrate from pyruvate will proceed independently of the K concentration in the medium. If, however, K is absent, non-glycogen carbohydrate piles up, whereas in the presence of K a large fraction of the carbohydrate is made into glycogen. Ca^{++} is necessary for both reactions. Na seems to stimulate carbohydrate synthesis, but also favours glycogenolysis.

---

[138] McLENNAN, H., and K. A. C. ELLIOTT: Factors affecting synthesis of acethylcholine by brain slices. Amer. J. Physiol. **163**, 605—613 (1950).

[139] McLENNAN, H., and K. A. C. ELLIOTT: Adenosine triphosphate concentration and the synthesis of acetylcholine by brain preparations. Arch. Biochem. **36**, 89—96 (1952).

[140] HASTINGS, A. B., and J. M. BUCHANAN: The role of intracellular cations in liver glycogen formation in vitro. Proc. nat. Acad. Sci. (Wash.) **28**, 478—482 (1942).

[141] BUCHANAN, J. M., A. B. HASTINGS, and F. B. NESBETT: The effect of the ionic environment on the synthesis of glycogen from glucose in rat liver slices. J. biol. Chem. **180**, 435—445 (1949).

Since phosphorylation of the pyruvate must be the first step in carbohydrate synthesis from this substance, one might have thought that the K-sensitive pyruvic transphosphorylase was responsible for the K requirement of the carbohydrate synthesis. However, HASTINGS et al.[142, 143, 144] were able to demonstrate that the total amount of carbohydrate formed by rat liver slices from pyruvate was the same with a K/Na ratio of 110/0 and 5/105 in the medium. This finding seems to rule out the pyruvic transphosphorylase reaction as the step responsible for the K-sensitivity of the slices.

With glucose as the substrate, the rat liver slices form more glycogen and also accumulate much more non-glycogen carbohydrate in a medium rich in K than in one of low potassium concentration. Low K and high Na concentrations lead to lower glucose uptake and lower glycogen formation (Fig. 1). The above authors favour the idea that potassium ions somehow facilitate the formation of glucose 6-phosphate. An alternative hypothesis would be that K somehow facilitates the transport of glucose into the cells.

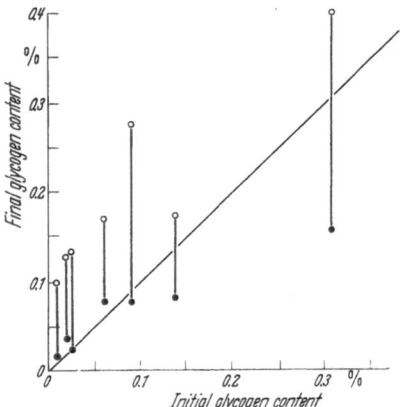

Fig. 1. Final glycogen concentration in rat liver slices plotted against initial glycogen concentration. Medium contains glucose and is rich either in potassium (○) or sodium (●). Points of net glycogen break down fall below the line, points of net accumulation above the line (after HASTINGS and BUCHANAN[140])

The ability of *human placenta* slices to form glycogen also depends on the K concentration in the medium[145]. No net formation of glycogen could be observed in a medium containing 140 mM Na and 5 mM Mg^{++} per liter. Optimum synthesis was obtained when the medium contained 50 mM K, 80 mM Na and 10 mM Mg^{++} per liter. At higher concentrations K became inhibitory to the synthesis.

The glycogen formation by isolated *rat diaphragm* is, on the other hand, only slightly sensitive to the K concentration of the medium[146]. K concentrations up to 75% of the total cation failed to influence the rate of synthesis. At still higher K concentrations the synthesis was inhibited. If the glycogen synthesis is stimulated by insulin, potassium ions become inhibitory to glycogen formation. Maximum synthesis is then obtained in the complete absence of K from the medium. This does not mean, however, that there is no K left in the fibres. It has bee shown by KAMMINGA, WILLEBRANDS, GROEN and BLICKMAN[147] that rat diaphragm, in contrast to most tissues, does not lose its potassium in a saline

[142] HASTINGS, A. B., A. K. SOLOMON, C. B. ANFINSEN, R. G. GOULD, and J. M. ROSENBERG: Incorporation of isotopic carbondioxide in rabbit liver glycogen in vitro. J. biol. Chem. 177, 717—731 (1949).

[143] BUCHANAN, J. M., A. B. HASTINGS, and F. B. NESBETT: The effect of the ionic environment on the synthesis of glycogen and total carbohydrate from pyruvate in liver slices. J. biol. Chem. 180, 447—455 (1949).

[144] HASTINGS, A. B., C. T. TENG, F. B. NESBETT, and F. M. SINEX: Studies on carbohydrate metabolism in rat liver slices. J. biol. Chem. 194, 69—81 (1952).

[145] VILLEE, C. A.: The metabolism of human placenta in vitro. J. biol. Chem. 205, 113 to 123 (1953).

[146] STADIE, W. C., and J. A. ZAPP JR.: The effect of insulin upon the synthesis of glycogen by rat diaphragm in vitro. J. biol. Chem. 170, 55—65 (1947).

[147] KAMMINGA, C. E., A. F. WILLEBRANDS, J. GROEN, and J. R. BLICKMAN: Effect of insulin on the potassium and inorganic phosphate content of the medium in experiments with isolated rat diaphragms. Science 111, 30—31 (1950).

medium. KREBS et al.[120] take this as evidence that the glycogen formation always requires a high cellular K concentration, but that high external potassium concentration is required only by tissues which, like placenta and liver slices, cannot otherwise keep up the normal cellular potassium level.

This hypothesis may not cover the whole truth, however: STADIE, HAUGAARD and PERLMUTTER[133] found that rat heart slices will form only very little glycogen in a NaCl medium. With K as the cation the synthesis is still smaller or does not occur at all. It turned out that isosmotic solutions, containing no ions at all, or very low concentrations of inorganic ions, were most favourable for glycogen formation from glucose. Isosmolarity could be obtained with sorbitol, L-arabinose, and mannose, none of which are glycogenic. Smaller molecules, like urea and creatinine were ineffective. It is extremely unlikely that sliced heart muscle would be able to withstand incubation in an ion-free solution without loss of potassium. Tentatively one might offer the hypothesis that inert molecules such as sorbitol protect the cells of the slices against osmotic swelling, thereby preserving their ability to form glycogen.

As mentioned above, maximum O_2 consumption does not coincide with maximum glycogen formation. On the contrary, respiration increases with increasing NaCl concentration.

e) Effects on fatty acid metabolism

GEYER et al.[148, 149] have studied the influence of Na, K and Li upon the fatty acid metabolism of liver and kidney slices from the rat. The metabolism of the C^{14} labelled octanoic acid-1-C^{14} was studied in media where Na was partly replaced by K and Li. Both of these ions greatly increased the octanoate consumption by liver slices and the main product of octanoate breakdown was found to be acetoacetate. If an all-Na buffer system was used, the ratio of radio-acetoacetate to $C^{14}O_2$ was below one, whereas the ratio was above three when K or Li were present.

K, but not Li caused an increase in the octanoate metabolism of kidney.

The preponderance of acetoacetate formation relative to oxidation to CO_2 observed in the presence of K and Li might indicate that the tricarboxylic acid cycle cannot under the circumstances cope with the amount of active acetyl groups (probably acetyl-CoA, made available by the breakdown of octanoate).

f) Effects on cellular accumulation of various substances

While themselves subject to cellular accumulation [(i. e. K and Rb) or extrusion (Na)] the alkali metal ions also influence the cellular accumulation of other substances. Isolated kidney tubules and kidney slices have proved particularly well suited for the study of these phenomena. The method of FORSTER and TAGGART[150] for the isolation of individual renal tubules of the flounder has been used by PUCK, WASSERMAN and FISHMAN[151] to study the effects of inorganic ions upon the phenol red accumulation. Their results may be summarized as follows: If the incubation medium is relatively low in K and high in Ca^{++}, accumulation of

---

[148] GEYER, R. P., M. F. MEADOWS, L. D. MARSHALL, and M. S. GONGAWARE: The influence of sodium, potassium, and lithium on fatty acid metabolism. J. biol. Chem. **205**, 81—85 (1953).

[149] GEYER, R. P., E. J. BOWIE, and J. C. BATES: Effect of pyruvate on octanoate metabolism as influenced by potassium and lithium. J. biol. Chem. **203**, 625—628 (1953).

[150] FORSTER, R. P., and J. V. TAGGART: Use of isolated renal tubules for the examination of metabolic processes associated with active cellular transport. J. cell. comp. Physiol. **36**, 251—270 (1950).

[151] PUCK, T. T., K. WASSERMAN, and A. P. FISHMAN: Some effects of inorganic ions on the active transport of phenol red by isolated kidney tubules of the flounder. J. cell. comp. Physiol. **40**, 73—88 (1952).

phenol red is limited to the lumen of the tubules and none is visible in the tubule cells. If, on the other hand, the K concentration is high and Ca^{++} is absent, the dye accumulates in the cells while little or none appears in the lumen. In the absence of Ca^{++}, the rate of accumulation is directly proportional to the concentration of K in the medium. These observations led to the conclusion that the transport of phenol red into the tubular lumen proceeds in two steps, the first of which is stimulated by K whereas the other requires Ca^{++} (see also WASSERMAN, BECKER and FISHMAN[152]).

Kidney slices, those of the rabbit for instance, will concentrate p-aminohippurate (PAH). This process also depends on the ionic composition of the medium. In a preliminary study of this phenomenon CROSS and TAGGART[153] came to the conclusion that the optimum composition of the medium for PAH accumulation was 110 meq K per liter. Later it turned out, however, that the decisive factor is the K concentration of the tissue and not the concentration in the medium[134]. Depending on the efficiency of the active ion transport going on in the tissue, optimum K concentration within the cells may be attained at widely different concentrations in the bathing fluid (compare chapter VII B.). Maximum accumulation is obtained when the cellular K/Na ratio is similar to that prevailing in the intact kidney cells. The experiment given in table 4 shows that the intracellular concentration of K giving maximum PAH transport coincides with that giving maximum respiration.

Li in concentrations ranging from 10—60 meq per liter depressed PAH accumulation by as much as 40% without significantly affecting the respiration. Tissue analyses failed to reveal any significant displacement of Na or K by Li.

Rat kidney cortex slices and to a lesser extent also slices of kidney medulla and liver have the ability to concentrate inorganic sulfate[154]. The accumulated sulfate is lost during cooling to room temperature but is regained at 37 degrees C. If the total osmotic pressure of the medium is kept constant by the addition of the necessary amount of sugar, while the concentrations of K and Na are varied, it turns out that the degree of sulfate accumulation is a function of the concentrations of both Na and K. Maximum accumulation in the slice (about 18 times the concentration in the medium) is obtained with 0.04 M potassium and no sodium in the bathing fluid. With increasing Na concentration, the sulfate accumulation decreases, but the optimum concentration of K remains the same. The medium concentration of about 0.04 M K just suffices to restore the tissue level of K to that prevailing in freshly cut slices.

g) Morphogenetic effects of lithium

1. The effects of lithium

Since the discovery by HERBST[155, 156] that small amounts of lithium added to the medium result in an abnormal development in sea urchin embryos, the

[152] WASSERMAN, K., E. L. BECKER, and A. P. FISHMAN: Transport of phenol red in the flounder renal tubule. J. cell. comp. Physiol. **42**, 385—393 (1953).

[153] CROSS, R. J., and J. V. TAGGART: Renal tubular transport: Accumulation of P-aminohippurate by rabbit kidney slices. Amer. J. Physiol. **161**, 181—190 (1950).

[154] DEYRUP, I. J., and H. H. USSING: Accumulation of sulfate labelled with S^{35} by rat tissue in vitro. J. gen. Physiol. **38**, 599—612 (1955).

[155] HERBST, C.: Experimentelle Untersuchungen über den Einfluß der veränderten chemischen Zusammensetzung des umgebenden Mediums auf die Entwicklung der Tiere. I. Z. wiss. Zool. **55**, 446—518 (1893).

[156] HERBST, C.: Experimentelle Untersuchungen über den Einfluß der veränderten chemischen Zusammensetzung des umgebenden Mediums auf die Entwicklung der Tiere, II. Mitt. Zool. Stat. Neapel **11**, 136—220 (1895).

morphogenetic effects of the lithium ion have been studied extensively. An interesting discussion of the literature up to 1942 is found in NEEDHAM's book[157]. For references to papers which have occurred since then see for instance the reviews by RUNNSTRÖM and GUSTAFSON[158] and RAVEN[159].

What has made the lithium effect especially attractive to workers in the field of chemical embryology is the fact that it is so strictly limited to certain phases of the development. Once the embryo has passed a certain stage the effect of Li declines rapidly. In Limnaea embryos, for instance, the period of maximum sensitivity is limited to a short time towards the end of the four-cell stage, although a secondary peak of sensitivity appears at the 24 cell stage. The Li effect is also organ-specific, or, rather, it concerns some organs much more than others. In the sea urchin embryo in the presence of Li, the mesenchymatic and entodermal organs develop at the expense of the ectodermal organs, resulting often in the abnormality called extragastrulation. In most sea urchin species $20-30$ mM Li in the sea water suffices to bring about the effect, which is characterized by retardation of development, a shift of the mesenchymering towards the animal pole, and enlargement of the entodermal region, followed by extragastrulation.

In the fresh water snail, Limnaea stagnalis, Li treatment also leads to extragastrulation[160, 161, 162]. Moreover it brings about head malformations like synophthalmia, cyclopia, anophthalmia etc. If the medium is tap water, 0.01% LiCl gives a maximum number of malformations in the embryo. If, however, the medium is distilled water, as little as 2.16×10^{-5} molar LiCl suffices to give a large number of head malformations.

Contrary to what has been found in sea urchins, K does not antagonize Li in Limnaea, but even intensifies the morphogenetic effects.

In the newt, Triton alpestris[163], the main primary effect of Li is a suppression of the formation of the notochord. Since, however, this organ is essential for the development of the neural tube, Li treatment leads to more or less complete suppression of the central nervous system. The development of other tissues is remarkably normal. In order to bring about the disappearance of the notochord, the developing egg has to be treated with LiCl in concentrations of 1/400 to 1/600 in 24 hr or 1/200 to 1/300 in about 6 hr.

The late effects of Li treatment in this species depend on the time of Li application because the head organizer and the tail organizer differ very appreciably in their sensitivities to Li. Thus at an early stage of development the head organizer is very sensitive and the tail organizer quite insensitive to Li. Later on the reverse is true. The Li effect on frog larvae (Rana fusca) resembles those described for Triton (Lallier).

[157] NEEDHAM, J.: Biochemistry and morphogenesis. 785 pp. Cambridge: University Press 1942.
[158] RUNNSTRÖM, J., and T. GUSTAFSON: Developmental physiology. Ann. Rev. Physiol. 13, 57—74 (1951).
[159] RAVEN, C. P.: Lithium as a tool in the analysis of morphogenesis in Limnaea stagnalis. Experientia (Basel) 8, 252—257 (1952).
[160] RAVEN, C. P.: Effects of monovalent cations on the eggs of Limnaea. Pubbl. Staz. Zool. Napoli 28, 136—169 (1956).
[161] RAVEN, C. P.: The influence of lithium upon the development of the pond snail, Limnaea stagnalis L. Proc. Ned. Akad. Wetensch. 45, 856—860 (1942).
[162] RAVEN, C. P.: Morphogenesis in Limnaea stagnalis and its disturbance by lithium. J. exp. Zool. 121, 1—78 (1952).
[163] LEHMANN, F. E.: Mesodermisierung des präsumptiven Chordamaterials durch Einwirkung von Lithiumchlorid auf die Gastrula von Triton alpestris. Arch. Entwickl.-mech. Org. 136, 112—146 (1937).

2. Mechanism of the Li effect

Some workers (CHILD[164], for instance) consider the Li effect on sea urchin larvae to be rather unspecific and comparable to that produced by azide or crowding. However, no uniformly accepted explanation has so far been offered of the Li effect on embryos. Undoubtedly, progress in this field would be furthered by chemical or spectrographic Li analyses of the species studied. It is a surprising fact that in no case known to the present author has the Li effect been correlated to the Li content of the organism in question, although we know from RANZI and FALKENHEIM's[165] spectrographic measurements on the ash of Li-treated sea urchin larvae that Li can be taken up by the embryo. The early workers like HERBST and SPEK[166] interpreted the Li development in sea urchin larvae in terms of an effect on the vegetative part of the egg. MACARTHUR[167] and RUNNSTRÖM[168] emphasized the effect on the animal part of the larva. As far as the sea urchins and the snail Limnaea is concerned, the Li effect is now being looked upon as a depression of a "gradient field" with maximum at the animal pole of the egg. The Swedish school (RUNNSTRÖM, LINDAHL[168, 169], HÖRSTADIUS[170] etc.) in particular have made very thorough studies of the cytochemical and metabolic effects on the different parts of the egg of sea urchins by the treatment. Only the main features can be given here.

RUNNSTRÖM[171] discovered that Li in concentrations which are too low to influence the development can be made active by simultaneous application of an atmosphere of CO, containing 5% of oxygen. Cyanide poisoning (LINDAHL[169]) has a similar effect. The Li effect is countered by pyocyanin, thiocyante, iodide and other "animalizing" agents. According to LINDAHL[172] and LINDAHL and ÖHMAN[173], the respiration of the sea urchin gastrula is composed of two parts. One which is concerned with the combustion of fat remains constant, whereas the other which is due to the burning of carbohydrate is steadily increasing. Only the latter one can be inhibited by Li. Both the metabolic and the morphogenetic effects of Li can be antagonized by K. The Li effect is accentuated by partial anaerobia, by organic acids and by 4,6-dinitro-o-cresole. Even in frog larvae Li reduces respiration. After treatment with 9% LiCl for three hours the cytochrome system seems to be unaffected, whereas the dehydrogenase activity is 25%

[164] CHILD, C. M.: Exogastrulation by sodium azide and other inhibiting conditions in strongylocentrotus purpuratus. J. exp. Zool. 107, 1—38 (1948).

[165] RANZI, S., and M. FALKENHEIM: Ricerche sulle basi fisiologische nell'embrione degli Echinodermi. Pubbl. Staz. zool. Napoli 16, 436—458 (1937).

[166] SPEK, J.: Differenzen im Quallungszustand der Plasmakolloide als eine Ursache der Gastrula-Invagination, sowie der Einstülpungen und Faltungen von Zellplatten überhaupt. Kolloidchem. Beih. 9, 259—399 (1918).

[167] MACARTHUR, J. W.: An experimental study and a physiological interpretation of exogastrulation and related modifications in Echinoderm embryos. Biol. Bull. 46, 60—87 (1924).

[168] RUNNSTRÖM, J.: Zur experimentellen Analyse der Wirkung des Lithiums auf den Seeigelkeim. Acta zool. (Stockh.) 9, 365—424 (1928).

[169] LINDAHL, P. E.: Neue Beiträge zur physiologischen Grundlage der Vegetativisierung des Seeigelkeimes durch Lithiumionen. Arch. Entwickl. Mech. Org. 140, 168—194 (1940).

[170] HÖRSTADIUS, S.: Über die zeitliche Determination im Keim von Paracentrotus lividus, Lk. Arch. Entwickl.-Mech. Org. 135, 1—39 (1937).

[171] RUNNSTRÖM, J.: Kurze Mitteilung zur Physiologie der Determination des Seeigelkeimes. Arch. Entwickl.-Mech. Org. 129, 442—444 (1933).

[172] LINDAHL, P. E.: Zur Kenntnis der physiologischen Grundlagen der Determination im Seeigelkeim. Acta zool. (Stockh.) 17, 179—365 (1936).

[173] LINDAHL, P. E., and L. O. ÖHMAN: Weitere Studien über Stoffwechsel und Determination im Seeigelkeim. Biol. Zbl. 58, 179—218 (1938).

inhibited. Moreover the sedimentable ribonucleic acid is reduced to half its normal value (LALLIER[174]).

The effects of Li upon Limnaea stagnalis larvae shows similarities to that on sea urchins, but there are also distinctive differences. Contrary to what has been found in sea urchins, K does not antagonize Li but even intensifies the morphogenetic effects of this ion as it does in amphibia. Low oxygen tension does not increase the Li effect and under anaerobic conditions the characteristic head malformations do not appear at all.

The interference by Li with respiratory enzymes in sea urchin eggs has given rise to the hypothesis that metabolic changes are the cause of the morphogenetic effects. Most workers now think, however, that both respiratory inhibition and developmental derangements are secondary to structural changes in the cytoplasm. RUNNSTRÖM 1928 first described the Li effect on the cytoplasm of sea urchin eggs as a coarsening of the cytoplasmatic structure. It can be seen in cases where the inhibition of the oxidative metabolism is not apparent (LINDAHL[169]). The physical state of the cells of larvae which have been treated with Li in sea water differs profoundly from that of controls which have developed in pure sea water. Isolated epithelial cells of normal larvae after stretching with microneedles quickly become spherical again. The Li treated cells under similar conditions remain distorted and spindle-shaped (RUNNSTRÖM[175]).

In the Limnae larvae Li treatment makes the cytoplasm more dense and more easily stainable and the cytoplasmic vacuoles are reduced in size. In the decapsulated egg of Limnaea, low concentrations of LiCl induce an increase in overall viscosity. Moreover Li has an effect upon the consistency and adhesiveness of the vitelline membrane and the egg cortex similar to that of Ca ions. RAVEN has proposed that Li acts by interfering with the displacement of substances, maybe ribonucleic acid, from the vegetative towards the animal cells of the embryo.

According to RANZI and CITTERIO[176] substances which vegetalize the sea urchin embryo (Li, Mg, valine, leucine, NaN_3 and thiourea) induce an increase in viscosity in fibrillar protein solutions (for instance actomyosine, protein from amphibian eggs etc.). The vegetalizing substances thus seem to stabilize protein particles. Animalizing substances on the other hand (thiocyanate, NaI, methylen blue, lysine lactate, maleinate, iodobenzoate, glucose at a concentration of 0.03 molar), and the agents inducing the formation of notochord in amphibians (urea, high p_H), induce a decrease in viscosity of fibrillar protein solutions. Protein particles so treated become less resistant to the *demolishing* action of urea. The stabilizing action on the protein particles exerted by lithium chloride or magnesium chloride cannot be reversed by ATP. It is interesting that lithium and magnesium show similar effects, since Li in its general chemical behaviour shows similarities to the alkaline earth ions.

The foregoing discussion takes it for granted that the Li effect on developing eggs is concerned with some cellular change in the developing egg. Some of the most drastic Li-effects are, however, seen in the extracellular coatings, notably the hyaline layer. Thus Li softens this layer in Arbacia and Echinarchinus eggs

---

[174] LALLIER, R.: Chlorure de lithium et biochimie du développement embryonnaire. C. R. Acad. Sci. (Paris) **235**, 98—100 (1952).

[175] RUNNSTRÖM, J.: An analysis of the action of lithium on sea urchin development. Biol. Bull. **68**, 378—384 (1935).

[176] RANZI, S., and P. CITTERIO: Sul meccanismo di azione degli ioni che inducono cambiamenti nella precoce determinazione embrionale. Pubbl. Staz. Zool. Napoli **25**, 201—240 (1954).

to the extent that the individual cells of the blastula can be picked off with a micro needle. Since the hyaline layer serves as a support for the cells during gastrulation, its dispersion is likely to lead to extragastrulation (CHAMBERS[177], MOORE and BURT[178]).

VI. Distribution
of the alkali metal ions between cells and theirs surroundings

a) General remarks

It is a very old observation that the potassium of living organisms is largely confined to the cells[179], very little being present in the extracellular phase, whereas the opposite is true with respect to sodium. This rule for the distribution of the two ion species holds true in the case of nearly all living cells, microorganisms, plant cells and animal cells alike.

In assigning a certain potassium- or sodium-concentration to a cell we are making the usually unjustified assumption that the element in question is uniformly distributed over the cell. Actually, all cells are heterogenous systems and there is no a priori reason why the ionic concentrations in mitochondria, nuclei, vacuoles and cytoplasm should be the same. In most cases it is, however, almost impossible to obtain trustworthy analyses of the different "organelles" making up a cell.

The giant cells of the marine algae Halicystis and Valonia offer unique opportunities to analyse the vacuolar sap as distinguished from the cytoplasm (see VII Bl.), but here the latter forms a thin layer surrounding the vacuole and so far has not been analyzed for cations.

The Characeans also have giant cells, several centimeters long and often one millimeter in diameter. The careful work of COLLANDER[180, 181] has shown that these algae will concentrate in the sap practically all cations to which they are exposed. At all concentrations, however, K is concentrated relatively much more than Na. Although the cytoplasm of these cells makes up only a small fraction (of the order of a few per cent) of the total cell contents, HOLM-JENSEN, KROGH and WARTIO-VAARA[182] succeeded in separating cytoplasm and sap of the characean Tolypellopsis (now Nitellopsis) by careful centrifugation and analyzed both fractions for K and Na. There seemed to be little difference between the concentrations of these ions in sap and cytoplasm. The same conclusion was reached by MACROBBIE and DAINTY, who estimated the abundance of the two ions in sap and cytoplasm from the kinetics of the exchange of radioactive Na and K between the cells and the soaking medium (see VII Bm). The important implication of these observations is that the high concentration of K in the cytoplasm of these cells must be due to free potassium ions and not to potassium preferentially bound by cytoplasmic constituents, considering that the K of the sap (which is a dilute solution of inorganic ions) shows an equally large K accumulation.

---

[177] CHAMBERS, R.: The relation of extraneous coats to the organization and permeability of cellular membranes. Cold Spr. Harb. Symp. quant. Biol. 8, 144—153 (1940).

[178] MOORE, A. R., and A. S. BURT: On the locus and nature of the forces causing gastrulation in the embryos of Dendraster excentricus. Amer. J. exp. Zool. 82, 159—171 (1939).

[179] MACOLLUM, A. B.: On the distribution of potassium in animal and vegetable cells. J. Physiol. 32, 95—128 (1905).

[180] COLLANDER, R.: Der Zellsaft der Characeen. Protoplasma 25, 201—210 (1936).

[181] COLLANDER, R.: Permeabilitätsstudien an Characeen III. Die Aufnahme und Abgabe von Kationen. Protoplasma 33, 215—257 (1939).

[182] HOLM-JENSEN, I., A. KROGH, and V. WARTIOVAARA: Some experiments on the exchange of potassium and sodium between single cells of Characeae and the bathing fluid. Acta Bot. Fenn. 36, 3—22 (1944).

It should not be inferred, however, that vacuoles necessarily have an ionic composition similar to that of the cytoplasm. The contractile vacuole of amoebae seems mainly to serve the purpose of osmotic regulation, removing the excess water taken up by diffusion through the surface of the animal (compare KIT-CHING[183]). Obviously, then, its content of inorganic ions must be quite low. With respect to the mitochondria, their concentration of K and Na, while in the intact cells is unknown. Isolated mitochondria seem, however, to be able to concentrate alkali ions preferentially. Thus under the conditions used by DAVIES et al.[184, 185], kidney mitochondria showed a preference for Na whereas STANBURY and MUDGE[108] found kidney cortex mitochondria to concentrate K. What makes the mitochondria prefer one or the other of the two alkali metal ions has not so far been explained satisfactorily.

b) State of potassium in living cells

The nature of the forces maintaining the intracellular potassium at a high and relatively constant level has been the subject of much speculation in the past, and even today no general agreement has been achieved. The hypotheses advanced to explain the phenomenon are based on four principally different concepts. 1) The cell membrane is impermeable to potassium. This hypothesis now has only historical interest. 2) The potassium ions are free in the cell interior but are kept from leaving the cell by the electric potential difference between the cell and its surroundings (Donnan equilibrium). This situation seems to be approached in several cell types. The Donnan distribution of potassium ions clearly demands that sodium which is normally present in abundance outside the cells is somehow kept from entering. For a long time all cells were though to be impermeable to sodium, but most workers now assume that there is a sodium pump extruding sodium from the cells just as fast as it enters (these problems are discussed in detail in chapter VII).

3) The potassium ions are chemically bound by or adsorbed to non-diffusible cell constituents. Although some workers believe in such binding, definite proof is lacking and so far no cell constituent present in sufficient amount has been found to bind potassium selectively (compare chapter II, c—i).

4) The potassium ions are supposed to be free in the cell interior but are transported actively inward through the cell membrane. There is mounting evidence that active potassium transport inward does take place in certain cell types, but rigorous proof is made difficult by the fact that many cells are so leaky to potassium that this ion will become Donnan-distributed no matter whether it is being transported actively into the cells or not. Certain cell types like the erythrocyte give practically conclusive proof of active potassium transport inward. The problems of active transport are discussed in chapter VII.

The idea that some or all cellular K is in some way "bound" has been expressed frequently, and there are indeed facts which speak in favour of the idea that some potassium is bound or immobilized somehow in some cells. In cases where the potassium concentration of the cells is the one predicted for Donnan distribution between cells and surroundings (see VII B b) it seems at least likely that most of the K is "free". However, the calculation of the equilibrium concentration for potassium requires knowledge of the membrane potential, or, alternatively, an

[183] KITCHING, J. A.: Osmoregulation and ionic regulation in animals without kidneys. Symp. Soc. exp. Biol. 8, 63—75 (1954).
[184] BARTLEY, W., and R. E. DAVIES: Active transport of ions by subcellular particles. Biochem. J. 57, 37—49 (1954).
[185] BARTLEY, W., R. E. DAVIES, and H. A. KREBS: Active transport in animal tissues and subcellular particles. Proc. roy. Soc. B 142, 187—196 (1954).

estimate of the concentration ratio cell/surroundings of one or more ionic species which are manifestly easily diffusible, not actively transported and not adsorbed by cell constituents. The techniques of measuring membrane potentials by intracellular microelectrodes have made great strides forward in recent years; but many cell types remain for which nothing is known about the membrane potential.

Unfortunately, much of the work done concerning the ability of cells to concentrate potassium has been performed with systems for which the membrane potential is unknown. Thus, ROBERTS et al.[186, 187] have suggested that the high potassium concentration in Eschericia coli is due to binding by hexose phosphates. There is, however, no evidence that such a specific affinity for K exists among hexose phosphates. On the other hand, the presence of non-diffusible phosphate esters in the cell interior requires a certain amount of counter ions. Whether the membrane potential of the bacteria suffices to bring about electrochemical equilibrium between cellular and extracellular potassium is unknown. As pointed out by MITCHELL[188], however, the interior of some bacteria, for instance Staphylococcus aureus, must be rather strongly negative since the basic amino acid lysine which shows every sign of behaving largely passively in the system is concentrated as much as 196 times in the cells relative to the medium (GALE[189]).

CONWAY et al. from studies of extracellular and intracellular p_H and K concentration of yeast have found a striking disagreement between the data obtained and those expected in case of an equilibrium of the Donnan type. They prefer, however, to explain the findings in terms of an active transport of K into, and H ions out of the cells (see VII Bj.).

Many plant physiologists consider the high K concentration of the protoplasm of higher plants to be due to chemical binding (compare ARISZ[190], EPSTEIN[191]). Direct evidence for this view is lacking since the potential difference between protoplasm and cell sap as well as that between protoplasm and extracellular fluid is unknown. According to STEWARD and MILLAR[192], extracts from artichoke tissue culture contain a protein or peptide which forms a Cs-complex. The complex is stable in methyl alcohol; whether or not it is stable in the presence of water was not tested, however.

The behaviour of K in red cells in general can be explained satisfactorily on the bases of an active transport inward (coupled with an active Na transport outward) located in the membrane, counteracting the passive diffusion processes (see p. 71). There are, however, observations which do not fit into that picture. As is well known (see p. 72) red cells lose K at low temperatures and when the glycolysis is inhibited by NaF. PONDER[193] found, however, that if NaF is used to poison red cells at 4°, some 20—40% of the K show a rate of leakage from the

[186] ROBERTS, R. B., I. Z. ROBERTS, and D. B. COWIE: Potassium metabolism in escherichia coli II. Metabolism in the presence of carbohydrates and their metabolic derivatives. J. cell. comp. Physiol. **34**, 259—291 (1949).

[187] ROBERTS, R. B., and I. Z. ROBERTS: Potassium metabolism in escherichia coli, III. Interrelationship of potassium and phosphorous metabolism. J. cell. comp. Physiol. **36**, 15—39 (1950).

[188] MITCHELL, P.: Transport of phosphate through an osmotic barrier. Symp. Soc. exp. Biol. 8, 254—261 (1954).

[189] GALE, E. F.: The accumulation of amino-acids within staphylococcal cells. Symp. Soc. exp. Biol. 8, 242—253 (1954).

[190] ARISZ, W. H.: Significance of the symplasm theory for transport across the root. Protoplasma **46**, 5—62 (1956).

[191] EPSTEIN, E.: Absorption of ions by plant roots. In: Electrolytes in biological systems. Ed.: A. M. SHANES. Amer. Physiol. Soc. 101—111. Washington, D. C. 1955.

[192] STEWARD, F. C., and F. K. MILLAR: Salt accumulation in plants: A reconsideration of the role of growth and metabolism. Symp. Soc. exp. Biol. 8, 367—406 (1954).

cells very much smaller than the rest. He interprets this finding as indicating that a fraction of cellular K is immobilized by forces related to the orderly arrangement of materials in the cell surface and the interior. In kidney slices, according to MUDGE, all potassium is exchangeable in an atmosphere of oxygen. If, however, the gas phase over the incubation medium is nitrogen, 45% of the K is non-exchangeable against K^{42}. STANBURY and MUDGE[108], also studied the exchangeability of liver mitochondria and found the exchange rate to be dependent on the metabolic activity. At zero degrees mitochondrial potassium does not exchange with that of the suspension medium. Similarly, HARRIS[194, 195] has found that frog muscle, kept in potassium phosphate at zero degrees, will not exchange a certain fraction of its K with radioactive K in the medium. Low temperatures also bring about non-exchangeability of part of the potassium in mammalian muscle[199]. Thus, whereas there is general agreement that all K of mammalian muscle is totally exchangeable at body temperature (NOONAN et al.[196], CREESE[197, 198], GOURLY et al.[199]), an appreciable fraction of rat sartorius and extensor digitorum becomes nearly inexchangeable at 20° C, and, according to HASHISH[200], nearly half the K of rat diaphragm exchanges at a very low rate indeed at one degree C.

The non-uniformity of cellular potassium was especially clearly brought in experiments where frog sartorius muscles were equilibrated with K^{42}-containing Ringer for several hours, whereupon their contents of K was leached out in successive lots of distilled water (HARRIS and STEINBACH[201, 202]). It then turned out that even after 12 hr loading with radioactive potassium the labelling was not uniform as indicated by the fact that the specific activity of radio-K in the successive washings was continuously falling. Thus the potassium which was more easily leached out had been more completely equilibrated with the K of the surrounding medium than had the less readily extracted K.

The degree of equilibration which is reached depends on the time of soaking, the temperature and the potassium concentration in the solution. Thus, if soaked in a modified Ringer containing one millimolar potassium for 24 hr most of the fibre potassium had reached only some 40% equilibration. If the K concentration of the soaking medium is higher, the degree of equilibration reached within the same period of time is also higher. A muscle which had been soaked in 12 mM K-Ringer for 18 hr showed about 80% equilibration in the first H_2O washing and even after repeated washings with distilled water, K of a specific activity of 66% of that of the medium could be extracted. The higher degree of equilibration

[193] PONDER, E.: Anomalous features of the loss of K from human red cells. J. gen. Physiol. **34**, 359—372 (1951).

[194] HARRIS, E. J.: The exchangeability of the potassium of frog muscle, studied in phosphate media. J. Physiol. **117**, 278—288 (1952).

[195] HARRIS, E. J.: The exchange of frog muscle potassium. J. Physiol. **120**, 246—253 (1953).

[196] NOONAN, T. R., W. O. FENN, and L. HAEGE: The distribution of injected radioactive potassium in rats. Amer. J. Physiol. **132**, 474—488 (1941).

[197] CREESE, R.: Exchangeability of muscle potassium. J. Physiol. **115**, 23P (1951).

[198] CREESE, R.: Measurement of cation fluxes in rat diaphragm. Proc. roy. Soc. B **142**, 497—513 (1954).

[199] GOURLEY, D. R. H., and H. JONAS: Potassium turnover in rat skeletal muscle in vitro. Fed. Proc. **13**, 59 (1954).

[200] HASHISH, S. E. E.: The effects of low temperatures and heparin on potassium exchangeability in rat diaphragm. Acta physiol. scand. **43**, 189—199 (1958).

[201] HARRIS, E. J., and H. B. STEINBACH: Interchangeable Na and K in frog muscle. J. Physiol. **131**, 20—21 (1956).

[202] HARRIS, E. J., and H. B. STEINBACH: The extraction of ions from muscle by water and sugar solution with a study of the degree of exchange with tracer of the sodium and potassium in the extracts. J. Physiol. **133**, 385—401 (1956).

achieved at high outside K concentrations may be associated with the increased metabolic rate pertaining in such a medium (see V a4.). It is worth mentioning that the dimensions of the frog sartorius muscle are such that the establishment of diffusion equilibrium in the interspaces between the fibres with the potassium of the medium takes only minutes (compare chapter VII). The slow equilibration with medium potassium therefore must be associated with the structure of the fibres. Clearly, the treatment with distilled water is non-physiological, killing the fibres and making them give off their electrolytes, but the fact that the specific activity of K is not the same throughout the muscle after many hours of soaking in K[42]-containing solutions is evidence of a heterogeneity of cellular potassium which existed in the living muscle.

The non-uniform exchange of fibre potassium is explained by the above authors as being due to the fact that "much of the internal movement in the muscle takes place between adsorption sites in the cellular material rather than by random diffusion". The kind of kinetics involved thus would be related to the "single file diffusion" proposed by HODGKIN and KEYNES (p. 51) for the passive movement of K through the nerve fibre membrane, but in muscle that kind of movement would involve a sizable fraction of the muscle mass. It is obvious, however, that incomplete mixing of fibre potassium could also be related to a compartmentalization of cellular potassium.

The question as to whether or not potassium is uniformly distributed in the muscle fibre is an old one. MACOLLUM[179] performed histochemical studies on different types of muscle fibres and concluded that the potassium was located in the A-bands. The localization was based on in situ precipitation of K with cobaltonitrite reagent. BUREAU[203], using a similar technique also found the potassium of frog muscle fibres mainly located in the A-bands, but claimed that the slightest contraction caused even distribution of the potassium. DEUCHER[204] also confirmed MACOLLUM's finding of the concentration of potassium in the A-discs. The cobaltonitrite precipitation procedure was criticized by GERSH[205]. GERSH studied the K distribution in frozen-dried frog muscle and came to the conclusion that potassium was evenly distributed in the fibres. The problem has been reviewed by DUBUISSON[206] and by STEINBACH[207]. DUBUISSON comes to the conclusion that as much as 98% of the fibre potassium is localized in the anisotropic bands. The potassium he assumes to be held there as counter-ion for protein-bound organic phosphates like ATP and creatine phosphate. STEINBACH also concluded that the histochemical evidence of MACOLLUM and others must indicate a heterogeneity of K distribution in the intact fibre. Whereas alternating zones of potassium-rich and potassium-poor character may exist in striated muscle, the methods used were probably never good enough to indicate whether the potassium-rich zones were really the anisotropic bands. The recent discovery by HUXLEY[208] that it is the isotropic and not the anisotropic bands which contract, invites a reexamination of

[203] BUREAU, V.: Recherches sur la répartition du potassium dans les cellules et sur les déplacements qu'il subit au cours des phénomènes d'excitation. Arch. int. Physiol. **39**, 311 to 328 (1934).

[204] DEUCHER, F.: Topochemische Untersuchungen über Glycogen-, Kalium- und Aschegehalt in Warmblüterherzen. Z. mikrosk. Anat. **49**, 401—424 (1941).

[205] GERSH, I.: Improved histochemical methods for chloride, phosphate-carbonate, and potassium applied to skeletal muscle. Anat. Rec. **70**, 311—329 (1937/38).

[206] DUBUISSON, M.: Sur la répartition des ions dans le muscle strié. Arch. int. Physiol. **52**, 439—463 (1942).

[207] STEINBACH, H. B.: Intracellular inorganic ions and muscle action. Ann. N. Y. Acad. Sci. **47**, 849—874 (1946-47).

[208] HUXLEY, A. F.: Muscle structure and theories of contraction. Progress in Biophysics **7**, 255—318 (1957).

the problem. Obviously one would want to find the actomyosin, the adenosine triphosphate, and the creatine phosphate together with their counter-ions in the zones which perform the contraction, and this type of wishful thinking may have induced previous workers to identify the potassium-rich zones by the anisotropic bands which for a long time were thought to be the seats of contractility. If the organic phosphates are indeed located in certain bands, it is a simple physical necessity that the counter-ions be found in the same zones. Actually, micro-incineration gives a pattern of ash which corresponds to the striation of the fibres (Scott and Packer[209]). Unfortunately studies of the sodium distribution in the fibres seem not to have been performed. Thus we do not know whether the zones that are rich in potassium are also rich in sodium or whether it is the other way around. Since the phosphate esters and the actomyosin do not seem to discriminate significantly between potassium and sodium (p. 9) it is quite possible that the two alkali metal ions are both concentrated in certain zones. This would imply that the activity of potassium might very well be the same in the isotropic and the anisotropic bands. This assumption would be in agreement with the fact that the membrane potential which presumably is a function of the potassium concentration ratio across the fibre membrane (see p. 144) seems to be the same everywhere on a given fibre. In certain muscle fibres, at least (crab, insects), the striation is coarse enough so that it is possible to decide with certainty whether it is punctured in an A- or an I-band.

If we attempt on the basis of the evidence available to form a picture of the state of potassium in striated muscle it may be summarized as follows: Some complexing takes place between actomyosin and potassium and some potassium also complexes with ATP and other organic phosphates. These complexes, however, are of a very loose nature and there is no indication that a discrimination in favor of potassium relative to sodium takes place as the result of this complex formation, although we must admit that the structures of intact muscle may show a higher power of discrimination than do the isolated parts. The binding of K by ATP and other known muscle constituents is mainly of electrostatic nature and the potassium must be easily exchangeable. Therefore this binding cannot explain the low exchangeability which under certain experimental conditions is exhibited by muscle potassium. Spatial factors are probably responsible for this finding. Either the fibre interior is compartmentalized, the different compartments having different K permeabilities, or, the access for potassium to certain parts of the fibre is through narrow pores or through a lattice of fixed charges where neighbouring cations have difficulty passing each other. It is probably futile to speculate as to which anatomical entities could be acting as compartments governing the potassium exchange. It may be pertinent, however, to mention that according to Huxley[208] electric stimulation can only reach the mucle fibre via certain points in the vicinity of the Z-membranes. Thus it would seem that certain ionic species can move more easily here. It has already been mentioned that under certain conditions mitochondrial potassium shows a very low exchange rate. The fraction of muscle potassium which can be localized in the mitochondria probably amounts to only a few per cent, however, and the major irregularities in the K exchange kinetics must be ascribed to other structures.

The fact that the isolated actomyosin-ATP system does not discriminate between K and Na as for as the capacity for contraction is concerned, seems to make it unlikely that gross differences in potassium/sodium binding ratio should exist within the muscle fibre. However, it would be rash to identify the ionic

[209] Scott, G. H., and D. M. Packer: An electron microscope study of magnesium and calcium in striated muscle. Anat. Rec. 74, 31—43 (1939).

requirements of the contractile substance of intact muscle fibre with those of the isolated systems. As a matter of fact, there are workers who prefer to think of the muscle fibre as a kind of ion exchange resin with a specifically high affinity for K and a very low affinity for sodium (LING[210, 211], SHAW and SIMON[212, 213]). These hypotheses will be discussed below in connection with the state of sodium in the cells.

From the foregoing it will appear that part of the cellular potassium can under certain conditions behave as if it were more or less trapped or bound inside the cells. The trapping seems, however, to be related to states of low temperature or low metabolic activity whereas during normal conditions all cellular K is exchangeable and tends towards forming a single "pool".

There are, indeed, certain facts which are hard to reconcile with the presence of large amounts of bound K in the cells. In the first place, if osmotic equilibrium is assumed between cells and tissue fluids, calculations show that at least in muscle K has to be free and osmotically active (compare HILL and KUPALOV[214]). Secondly, impedance measurements at different frequencies on cell suspensions make it possible to calculate the resistance of the membranes and the cell interior separately[215]. The conductivity of the protoplasm of most cells turns out to be quite high, so high indeed that the cellular K practically has to be free with a mobility that does not differ very much from its mobility in free solution.

Even more direct evidence for this view has been obtained by HODGKIN and KEYNES[216]. They labelled the K of a short length of the axis cylinder of a cuttlefish giant nerve fibre with K^{42}. Then a longitudinal current of known strength was passed through the fibre for a certain time. The distribution of radioactivity was then determined in the fibre, and from this data the mobility of K in the axis cylinder was calculated. It appeared that the internal K exists mainly as free ions and that chemical binding does not occur to any significant extent. Similar experiments with frog sartorius muscle (HARRIS[217]) showed that even here the mobility of K was from $80-100\%$ of that in free solution.

It will appear from the foregoing that chemical binding plays a minor role in explaining the high potassium level in most of the systems where sufficient data are at hand. Furthermore it has already been pointed out that the negative potential of most cells allows these to have a high potassium concentration in electrochemical equilibrium with the surroundings. But this is a qualitative statement. Accurate measurements under a variety of conditions show that the K concentrations are not always in accord with the electric potential. Such findings by themselves do not invalidate the view that the K concentration is a function of the potential. If the cells go through cycles of activity and recovery, the distribution of ions like K and H may well lag behind due to the limited rates

[210] LING, G.: The role of phosphorus in the maintenance of the resting potential and selective ionic accumulation in frog muscle cells. In Phosphorus Metabolism, Vol. II, edited by W. D. McELROY and B. GLASS. 748—795. Baltimore: Johns Hopkins Press 1952.

[211] LING, G.: Muscle electrolytes. Amer. phys. Med. 34, 89—101 (1955).

[212] SHAW, F. H., and S. E. SIMON: The nature of the sodium and potassium balance in nerve and muscle cells. Aust. J. exp. Biol. med. Sci. 33, 153—178 (1955).

[213] SHAW, F. H., S. SIMON, and B. M. JOHNSTONE: The non-correlation of bioelectric potentials with ionic gradients. J. gen. Physiol. 40, 1—17 (1957).

[214] HILL, A. V., and P. S. KUPALOV: The vapour pressure of muscle. Proc. roy. Soc. B 106, 445—477 (1930).

[215] For references see R. HÖBER: Physical chemistry of cells and tissues, p. 281. London: Churchill 1945.

[216] HODGKIN, A. L., and R. D. KEYNES: The mobility and diffusion coefficient of potassium in giant axons from Sepia. J. Physiol. 119, 513—528 (1953).

[217] HARRIS, E. J.: Iontophoresis along frog muscle. J. Physiol. 124, 248—253 (1954).

of diffusion through the living membranes. But cases are known where apparently the potassium ions of the cells are never in electrochemical equilibrium with those outside.

Let us for example consider erythrocytes. As it is well known, these cells are extremely permeable to small anions like Cl and HCO_3. Assuming that the chloride ions are not subject to active transport into or out of the red cells, and that chloride ions are not bound by other components of the cells, the potential across the membrane must be

$$E = \frac{RT}{F} \ln \frac{[Cl_i]}{[Cl_0]}$$

Inserting proper values in this equation, one gets a potential difference of 5 to 10 mV across the membrane, the inside being negative relative to the medium. In order that the cellular potassium ions be maintained at a concentration which is, say, 40 times the plasma value, the potential difference would have to be nearly 100 mV. It is readily seen that even if a fraction of 20—40% of the cellular K were "immobile" (compare PONDER[193]) it still is impossible to account for all the red cell K. It must therefore be assumed that there is an active transport of K through the red cell membrane (just as there must be an active transport of Na ions outward). It has also been mentioned above that the accumulation of K in the yeast cells during fermentation does not represent an approach to electrochemical equilibrium since H ions are excreted while K ions are taken up.

The more detailed discussion of the active transport processes will be postponed until after the treatment of the diffusion of the alkali metal ions through membranes. For the present problem — the state of cellular potassium — the concept of active transport of potassium ions means that we can accept three apparently contradictory observations: Cellular potassium is largely free; it exchanges more or less readily with extracellular K; and it is not in electrochemical equilibrium with the extracellular K. At present it is not known whether active K transport is a property of only certain cell types like red cells, or whether it is a general cellular mechanism which is working faster in some cells than in others.

c) State of Rb and Cs in living cells

The behaviour of Rb and Cs in living cells has been reviewed recently by RELMAN[218]. By and large the ions of these two elements distribute themselves between cells and surroundings in a way similar to potassium. Tracer experiments have shown that muscle, erythrocytes, and several other tissues of different mammals including man create concentration ratios tissue/plasma for these two ions equal to or higher than those existing for potassium[219, 220, 221]. In rat skeletal muscle[222] the order of preference is cesium > rubidium > potassium. This

[218] RELMAN, A. S.: The physiological behaviour of rubidium and cesium in relation to that of potassium. Yale J. Biol. Med. **29**, 248—262 (1956).

[219] KILPATRIC, R., H. E. RENSCHLER, D. S. MUNRO, and G. M. WILSON: A comparison of the distribution of K^{42} and Rb^{86} in rabbit and man. J. Physiol. **133**, 194—201 (1956).

[220] LOVE, W. D., R. B. ROMNEY, and G. E. BURCH: A comparison of the distribution of potassium and exchangeable rubidium in the organs of the dog, using rubidium[86]. Circulat. Res. **2**, 112—122 (1954).

[221] TYOR, M. P., and J. S. ELDRIDGE: A comparison of the metabolism of rubidium[86] and potassium[42] following simultaneous injection into man. Amer. J. med. Sci. **232**, 186—193 (1956).

[222] HOOD, S. L., and C. L. COMAR: Metabolism of cesium[137] in rats and farm animals. Arch. Biochem. **45**, 423—433 (1953).

behaviour, as pointed out by RELMAN[223], is incompatible with Donnan distribution, which demands that the concentration ratios cell/medium be the same for all three ion species. The results would be understandable either in terms of active transport of all three species into the muscle fibre or in terms of preferential adsorption inside the fibres. A systematic study of the behaviour of Rb and Cs in different cell types would be likely to shed light also upon the state of potassium in the cells.

d) State of sodium in living cells

The state of sodium in living cells has not been studied very extensively. SOLOMON and associates have given evidence that a small fraction of the sodium of red cells shows exchange kinetics which are definitely different from the bulk of cell sodium (see p. 77). According to HARRIS and STEINBACH[201, 202] there is within the isolated frog sartorius a small fraction of sodium which is practically non-exchangeable against sodium from the outside medium. When the muscles had had occasion to exchange sodium with bicarbonate Ringer containing Na^{24}, most of the Na which could be extracted with H_2O showed a uniform specific activity, not differing much from that of the presoaking medium. However, some sodium remained in the residue which was only slightly radioactive. This non-exchanging sodium seemed to be associated with the connective tissue rather than with the muscle fibres.

As it will be discussed in detail in chapter VII, p. 57, the low concentrations of sodium in most cells is assumed to be due to active transport of this ion in the outward direction.

The only alternative to the sodium pump theory which has been seriously considered in recent years is the "fixed charge" hypothesis of LING[210, 211]. According to this hypothesis the fibre membrane is not responsible for the ion distribution, which is determined solely by the structure of the bulk phase of the fibre. The latter is supposed to have fixed negative charges corresponding in number to the intracellular cations. Due to its smaller hydrated diameter, K is supposed to be able to approach the negative charges more closely than can the bigger Na ions. As a result of this K is selectively accumulated.

Metabolic work is required, not to expel Na, but to maintain the intracellular structure so as to prefer K for Na. [The latter part of the hypothesis is made necessary by the fact that none of the major muscle constituents (myosin, lactomyosin, phosphate esters etc.) show any preference for K relative to Na.]

In spite of its apparent simplicity, the fixed charge hypothesis presents many serious difficulties, some of which have been discussed on p. 42. The existence of the fibre membrane as the seat of the major fibre resistance and the electric potential difference is well established. The longitudinal mobility of fibre K corresponds to that of K in free solution[217]. K has to be thermodynamically active to give the osmotic equivalent necessary to explain osmotic equilibrium of muscle fibres. Li ions which are larger than Na ions, attain a steady state distribution ratio fibre/medium which is higher than that for Na.

Perhaps the strongest argument against the fixed charge theory is an indirect one, namely that active Na transport can be demonstrated beyond doubt in a large number of cell types and tissues (see p. 112). Thus the reabsorption of Na in kidney and intestine, frog skin, large intestine, toad urinary bladder, rumen of ruminants etc. and in gills of fresh water animals like eriocheir, cannot take place

---

[223] RELMAN, A. S., A. T. LAMBIE, A. M. ROY, and B. A. BURROWS: The nature of the cation accumulation by muscle cells: the displacement of potassium by rubidium and cesium. Res. Proc. 4, 150 (1956).

without active Na transport; the ion distribution between red cells and their surroundings must also require active extrusion of Na since the interior of red cells has neither the rigid structure nor the number of fixed charges required by the fixed charge theory.

One of LING's main reasons for advancing his hypothesis apparently is the notion that the exchange rate for muscle fibre Na would require an unreasonable expenditure of energy in case it were due to leakage of Na into, and active transport of Na out of the fibres. Of particular interest is LING's finding that frog muscles maintain for hours their normal K/Na ratio when poisoned with 0.5 Mm monoiodo-acetate in pure N_2 at 0° C. Under these conditions both glycolysis and respiration are blocked and the only energy available is represented by creatine phosphate and ATP. From experiments with Na^{24} LING estimated that the Na exchange was higher than could be accounted for by the decline in energy-rich phosphates, assuming that there were a passive diffusion of Na into the fibres and an active transport outward. As it will be further discussed below, however, CAREY and CONWAY (p. 91) have presented evidence that some of the apparently intracellular Na is actually located in a "third compartment" which is not truly intracellular, but possibly is identical with the sarcolemma. A similar extracellular compartment has been proposed by HARRIS p. 94. Should such a third compartment exist as indeed it seems, and if part of its Na exchanges at about the same rate as the intracellular Na, the estimate of the active transport rate and thus the energy expenditure must become too high.

LING's arguments for his hypothesis thus are not quite as compelling as they seemed at first. For a penetrating analysis and criticism of the "fixed charge" hypothesis, see CONWAY [224]. Recently, SHAW and SIMON [212] have argued in favour of LING's hypothesis. Working on toad muscles (Bufo marinus) they notice that even in dead muscles, the K concentration might be several times that of the Ringer used as soaking medium. Later the situation reversed, so that the K level of the dead muscle became lower than that of Ringer.

Although very interesting, these observations neither prove nor disprove LING's hypothesis. They emphasize, however, what has been pointed out already (see p. 41) that cells in general and muscle fibres in particular cannot always be treated as bagsful of a homogenous solution. The exchange kinetics of K in frog muscle and several other cells (see p. 41) suggests that under certain conditions, at least, there is some kind of compartmentalization or preferential binding of part of the cellular K. At present, the weight of evidence seems to be for a dual nature of cellular K, a minor fraction of it being bound or constrained in its movements, whereas the bulk of the cellular K is "free" and is being kept there by the action of the sodium pump, which may or may not act also as a K pump.

VII. Active and passive transport of the alkali metal ions[225—235]

A. Characterization and biological role

a) Introduction

The mechanisms by which the alkali metal ions pass through living membranes are of supreme importance in the physiological function of these ions. Such

[224] CONWAY, E. J.: Membrane equilibrium in skeletal muscle and the active transport of sodium, p. 73—114. In: Metabolic aspects of transport across membranes. Ed.: Q. R. MURPHY. Madison: University of Wisconsin Press 1957.

[225] HÖBER, R.: Physikalische Chemie der Zelle und der Gewebe, 6th ed. Leipzig: W. Engelmann 1926.

diverse phenomena as glandular secretion, intestinal and tubular absorption of salt solutions, nervous activity, and bioelectric potentials are all intimately related to the movements of sodium and potassium ions across cell membranes. The mechanisms by which these ions pass through the cell surfaces have not been explained in detail, but a classification of considerable usefulness can be based upon the distinction between active and passive transport. The reason for the usefulness of the concept of active transport is that it is related, often in a stoichiometrical way, to the expenditure of metabolic work. A survey of the pertinent literature will reveal that there is a certain ambiguity in the use of the term active transport. It is, however, common to most definitions that active transport must be performed at the expense of work done by the cell whose membrane is being traversed by the substance in question. In the following, active transport is defined as a transfer which cannot be accounted for by physical forces. According to this definition transport of an ion taking place due to a difference in electric potential across the membrane is no more active than is transport brought about by a differences in concentration or activity coefficient. Neither would it be appropriate to consider as active a transfer resulting from solvent drag, i. e. the force exerted upon a solute by the flow of solvent through pores in the membrane. It is implicit in the above considerations that active transport must be due to chemical processes in which the ion in question is taking part. It must be stressed, however, that our present knowledge does not allow a distinction between transport brought about by chemical reactions directly involving the ion in question and transport caused by mechanical events within the membrane phase (contraction of fibrils etc.), granted that the latter process has acquired specificity from such ionic properties as size or polarizability. As a matter of fact it is hardly justified to distinguish between chemical and physical specificity on the molecular level. We shall return later to some of the hypotheses advanced to explain active transport of the alkali metal ions. It should be pointed out here, however, that the concept of active transport has turned out to be of considerable operational value, notwithstanding our ignorance of its detailed mechanism.

[225] KROGH, A.: The active and passive exchanges of inorganic ions through the surfaces of living cells and through living membranes generally. Croonian Lecture, Proc. roy. Soc. B 133, 140—200 (1946).

[227] ROSENBERG, T.: On accumulation and active transport in biological systems. I. Thermodynamical considerations. Acta chem. scand. 2, 14—133 (1948).

[228] USSING, H. H.: Transport of ions across cellular membranes. Physiol. Rev. 29, 127 to 155 (1949).

Many important papers bearing upon the problem of defining active transport are found in the following publications:

[229] Symposia of the society for experimental biology VIII: Active transport and secretion, 516 pp. Cambridge University Press 1954.

[230] CLARKE, H. T.: Ion transport across membranes. 298 pp. New York, N. Y.: Academic Press 1954.

[231] Electrolytes in biological systems. Ed.: A. M. SHANES. 243 pp. American Physiological Soc. 1955.

[232] Metabolic aspects of transport across cell membranes. 379 pp. Ed.: Q. R. MURPHY. Madison: The University of Wisconsin Press 1957.

[233] USSING, H. H.: Some aspects of the application of tracers in permeability studies. Advanc. Enzymol. 13, 21—65 (1952).

[234] KOEFOED-JOHNSEN, V., and H. H. USSING: The contributions of diffusion and flow to the passage of D_2O through living membranes. Acta physiol. scand. 28, 60—76 (1953).

[235] ANDERSEN, B., and H. H. USSING: Solvent drag on non-electrolytes during osmotic flow through isolated toad skin and its response to antidiuretic hormone. Acta physiol. scand. 39, 228—239 (1957).

b) Passive transport

Passive transport is often loosely referred to as diffusion. Strictly speaking, however, diffusion is a propagation due to thermal movements and does not include movement under the influence of an electric field or a solvent drag force. The property of allowing passive transport of an ion species will be referred to as passive permeability to that species. It has become increasingly clear during recent years that not only the active transport but also the passive transport of alkali metal ions is often highly specific. The major portion of most cell surfaces seems to be practically impermeable to ions, and among the "patches" which are permeable to alkali metal ions two kinds can often be distinguished: one which is accessible for Na and Li, but little permeable to K and Rb (and Cs), and another kind which admits K, Rb and sometimes Cs, but not Na and Li. No satisfactory analogy to this peculiarity has been found among non-living systems, although ion-exchanger resin membranes may show preference for one or the other of the alkali ions. Thus in certain cells showing the phenomenon of impulse conduction, the permeabilities to K and to Na depend strongly, but in different ways, upon the membrane potential, a dependency quite out of proportion to what one would expect for an inanimate membrane. Finally, the study by means of tracers of the permeation kinetics of certain cell membranes has revealed that the permeation of these ions is sometimes subject to peculiar restraints, probably arising from the binding of these ions to membrane elements.

c) "Simple" passive transport

From the foregoing it will be apparent that the only safe way of demonstrating active transport is to exclude the possibility that the transport in question is of passive nature. For this reason alone, knowledge of the laws governing passive transport is desirable. But in itself passive transport of Na and K is of enormous physiological importance. It therefore seems warranted to give a brief account of some of the expressions which are useful in the description of passive permeability of living membranes to ions.

Even if one assumes the existence of a steady state, the description of passive transport of ions is made difficult by the fact that the ions are acted upon simultaneously by diffusion force, electric force, and possibly solvent drag force. These forces may vary in an unknown way along the path of transport, just as the resistance to the movement is an unknown function of the path. The attempts to circumvent these difficulties must obviously be based upon simplifying assumptions. The most commonly used approximation has been to disregard the effects of solvent drag. Doing this one can make reasonably safe predictions of the *direction* of passive transport, which will always be from the higher to the lower electrochemical potential. The electrochemical potential of the j'th ion is defined by the equation:

$$\bar{\mu}_j = R\,T \ln a_j + zF\,\psi + J \,, \tag{1}$$

where R is the gas constant, T the absolute temperature, F, Faradays number, a_j the chemical activity of the ion, z, its charge, ψ, the electrical potential and J a constant which may be considered the electrochemical potential of the ion in a standard system where it is present at zero potential and unit activity. The j'th ion is in equilibrium with respect to a given membrane when

$$\bar{\mu}_{j\,(0)} = \bar{\mu}_{j\,(i)} \tag{2}$$

where subscripts (0) and (i) denote "outside" and "inside" solutions, respectively. This can also be written

$$R\,T \ln a_{j\,(i)} + zF\,\psi_{(i)} = R\,T \ln a_{j\,(0)} + zF\,\psi_{(0)}$$

or, by rearrangement

$$\frac{RT}{zF} \cdot \ln \frac{a_{j(i)}}{a_{j(0)}} = \psi_{(i)} - \psi_{(0)} = E \qquad (3)$$

where E is the electric potential difference between the inside and outside solutions. If concentrations are substituted for activities in this equation, it is the well-known Nernst equation.

The above considerations provide information only about the direction of passive transport of the ion in question, but do not say anything with respect to the rate of this transport. In order to obtain such information it would be necessary to solve the differential equation for the movements of an ionic species under the simultaneous effects of diffusion and electric force. The equation may be written:

$$M_j = -z_j u_j c_j \left[\frac{d \ln c_j}{dx} + z_j F \frac{d\psi}{dx} \right] \qquad (4)$$

where M_j is the flux across unit area (that is, the amount crossing unit area in unit time), u_j is the mobility of the ion and c_j its concentration (both are functions of x, the distance in the membrane phase from the side of origin in the direction normal to the membrane), $-RT \dfrac{d \ln c_j}{dx}$ (5) is the diffusion force and $-zF \dfrac{d\psi}{dx}$ (6) the electric force acting upon one mole of the ion in the x direction.

In order to solve this equation it is necessary to make further assumptions which are not very well justified. Nevertheless the solutions obtained can often be used to make tolerably good predictions of diffusion rates. One solution in particular which was first derived by GOLDMAN[236] has found considerable use. The assumptions made are that the mobility, u_j, is a constant throughout the membrane and that the electric potential changes linearly across the membrane (in other words: the electric field is constant). These assumptions lead to the following equation:

$$M_j = \frac{z_j^2 u_j F E}{x_0} \cdot \frac{c_{j(i)} - c_{j(0)} \exp\left[-z_j F E/RT\right]}{1 - \exp\left[-z_j F E/RT\right]} \qquad (7)$$

where x_0 is the thickness of the membrane, $c_{j\,(i)}$ is the concentration of the ion in the inside solution and $c_{j\,(0)}$ is its concentration in the outside solution.

This equation gives qualitative but usually not quantitative agreement with experiments on biological systems. Model experiments performed by TEORELL[237] upon artificial membranes with many fixed charges have shown that often the electric potential gradient is far from being linear. TEORELL[237, 238, 239, 240] in his treatments of the problem therefore has preferred to consider the concentration gradient as being linear. The original papers should be consulted for details of this approach. A related treatment which, however, is based upon the assumption of no fixed charges in the membrane phase has been worked out by LINDERHOLM[241].

[236] GOLDMAN, D. E.: Potential, impedance and rectification in membranes. J. gen. Physiol. **27**, 37—60 (1944).

[237] TEORELL, T.: Zur quantitativen Behandlung der Membranpermeabilität. Z. Elektrochem. **55**, 460—469 (1951).

[238] TEORELL, T.: Membrane electrophoresis in relation to bio-electrical polarization effects. Arch. Sci. Physiol. **3**, 205—219 (1949).

[239] TEORELL, T.: Transport processes and electrical phenomena in ionic membranes. Progr. Biophys. biophysical Chem. **3**, 305—369 (1953).

[240] TEORELL, T.: Transport phenomena in membranes. Disc. Faraday Soc. **21**, 9—26 (1956).

[241] LINDERHOLM, H.: Active transport of ions through frog skin with special reference to the action of certain diuretics. Acta physiol. scand. **27**, suppl. 97, 1—144 (1952).

The treatments so far discussed have in common that the mobility, u_j, as well as the area available for diffusion, is assumed to be non-variant with x. Even for a single cell membrane these assumptions may be grossly in error and they are hardly ever justified in the treatment of transcellular transports (across epithelial membranes, etc.), although they may lead to predictions which are qualitatively correct (compare LINDERHOLM [241]).

d) The flux ratio

Evidently, the precise prediction of permeation rates through living membranes requires detailed information about the structure of the membrane, information which at present is out of our reach. Despite this it is, however, possible to ascertain whether or not the ionic species in question moves passively and without combining with other moving particles through a living membrane. The reason is that there exists a function of the permeability to such uncombined and passive ions which depends solely upon the electrochemical potential difference across the membrane and it is independent of the variations along the path of diffusion of such variables as potential, concentration, activity coefficient, mobility etc. This function is the flux ratio, that is: the ratio between the unidirectional fluxes of the ion in the inward and outward directions. These flux-values can be determined simultaneously or separately by suitable tracer experiments (see USSING [242]).

If we denote by M_{in} the flux in the inward direction and by M_{out} the flux in the outward direction, we have [242]:

$$R T \ln (M_{in}/M_{out}) = \bar{\mu}_{j\,(0)} - \bar{\mu}_{j\,(i)} \ . \tag{8}$$

The equation is implicit in EYRING's theory of rate processes [243]. Equations of the same form can be immediately obtained from the Goldman equation and from those derived by TEORELL and LINDERHOLM, but it is much more generally applicable since it is not based upon the specific assumptions made in the derivation of these equations.

The above equation can also be written:

$$M_{in}/M_{out} = (a_{j\,(0)}/a_{j\,(i)}) \exp (z F E/R T) \tag{9}$$

where $a_{j\,(0)}$ and $a_{j\,(i)}$ are the activities of the ion in the inside and outside solutions, respectively.

As already mentioned, this equation holds for ions which move in the uncombined state through a membrane where they are not subject to solvent drag. It is immaterial whether or not the ions are temporarily bound by fixed charges in the membrane. Binding to moving particles, however, upsets the relationship given by the equation. Experiments with living membranes have shown that the flux ratio equation holds well in several cases of passive ion transport. Spectacular exceptions have been found, however, indicating strong interaction with other moving particles even in cases where there was every reason to consider the transport strictly passive.

In a purely formal way the deviations from "normal passive behaviour" can be divided in two classes characterized by the relationships

a) $|R T \ln (M_{in}/M_{out})| < |\bar{\mu}_0 - \bar{\mu}_i|$,

b) $|R T \ln (M_{in}/M_{out})| > |\bar{\mu}_0 - \bar{\mu}_i|$.

---

[242] USSING, H. H.: The distinction by means of tracers between active transport and diffusion. Acta physiol. scand. 19, 43—56 (1949).

[243] For references, see: FRANK H. JOHNSON, HENRY EYRING, and MILTON J. POLISSAR: The kinetic basis of molecular biology, 874 pp. New York: John Wiley and Sons 1954.

Case a) is met with rather frequently in passive transport of ions. A good example is the exchange of potassium ions across the membrane of duck erythrocytes[244] (see p. 82). Despite a steep electrochemical gradient in the direction inside-out, K moves in and out at about the same rate, and the rate of this exchange is rather enhanced when in the simultaneous absence of oxygen and presence of fluoride, the energy sources for active transport are abolished. This process of "uphill" transport of one ion coupled with the concomitant "downhill" transport of another ion of the same species obviously can only be observed by the use of isotopic tracers. The phenomenon has been termed "exchange diffusion" (USSING[245]). Exchange diffusion of sodium ions seems to be very pronounced in kidney mitochondria. Isolated mitochondria maintain a sodium concentration which may be much higher than that of the suspension medium and they obviously possess an active sodium transport which is responsible for the concentration difference[246]. However, the sodium of the mitochondria exchanges with that of the medium at such a rate that it would be energetically impossible to consider the outflux of Na as a measure of "leakage" and the influx as a measure of active uptake. It has also turned out that, under certain circumstances, part of the Na-exchange with the medium of muscle must be due to exchange-diffusion (see KEYNES[247, 248], also p. 92). As a matter of fact the phenomenon was first proposed to account for part of the rather high exchange of Na in isolated frog sartorius muscle (USSING[249], LEVI and USSING[250]). The phenomenon may be explained as follows: The cell membrane is little permeable to free sodium ions. It contains, however, "carrier" molecules (probably negatively charged) which can combine with Na to form a complex, and this complex — in contrast to the carrier itself — is able to cross the membrane from one boundary to the other. It is easy to see that if the "carrier" can use no other "return freight" than Na and cannot pass the membrane except when loaded with Na, the flux of Na catalyzed by the carrier must be the same in both directions. Neither a difference in concentration nor in electric potential can affect this one-to-one relationship if the system works ideally. Any real system of this type is, however, likely to show some "leakiness". Thus the carrier may be able to cross the membrane unloaded and it may show some affinity towards other ionic species than Na. According to CROGHAN[251], the brine shrimp, Artemia salina, exchanges its Na rapidly with that of the surrounding water, but if offered potassium instead, this ion will exchange freely against the Na of the animal. The sodium exchange shows every sign of being largely exchange diffusion since the whole metabolism of the animal would not suffice to excrete against a concentration gradient the huge amounts of Na which

[244] TOSTESON, D.: Sodium and potassium transport in red blood cells, in: ABRAHAM M. SHANES: Electrolytes in biological systems. American Physiological Soc. Washington D. C. 1955.

[245] USSING, H. H.: The use of tracers in the study of active ion transport across animal membranes. Cold Spr. Harbor Symp. quant. Biol. **13**, 193—200 (1948).

[246] DAVIES, R. E.: Relations between active transport and metabolism in some isolated tissues and mitochondria. Symp. Soc. exp. Biol. 8, 453—475 (1954).

[247] KEYNES, R. D., and R. H. ADRIAN: The ionic selectivity of nerve and muscle membranes. Farady Soc. Disc., **1956**, No. 21, 265—271.

[248] SWAN, R. C., and R. D. KEYNES: Sodium efflux from amphibian muscle. Abstr. comm. 20. International Physiological Congress, p. 869—870. Brussels 1956.

[249] USSING, H. H.: Interpretation of the exchange of radiosodium in isolated muscle. Nature (Lond.) **160**, 262—263 (1947).

[250] LEVI, H., and H. H. USSING: The exchange of sodium and chloride ions across the fibre membrane of the isolated fibre membrane of isolated frog sartorius Acta physiol. scand. **16**, 232—249 (1948).

[251] CROGHAN, P. C.: The osmotic and ionic regulation in Artemia Salina (L). J. exp. Biol. **35**, 219—233 (1958).

judging from the tracer experiments are constantly entering from the highly concentrated salt solution. But in this case the exchange system does not discriminate between Na and K.

With respect to the foregoing discussion of the mechanism of exchange diffusion, it should be emphasized that the carrier need not be an independent molecule. A side-chain belonging to some membrane constituent, having certain degrees of freedom to move within the membrane phase, would have the same effect. No cell constituent which can with any certainty be identified with a carrier has ever been isolated, and it is wise at the present state of our knowledge to consider the carrier concept mainly as a mental help. It assists us in understanding that it is no violation of the second law of thermodynamics that there is a fast flow of, say, Na uphill as long as there is an equally large flow going downhill. Thermodynamically the work involved is nil. The true molecular bases of exchange diffusion may be rather different from the picture outlined here.

In almost all cases so far studied the deviations from the flux equation belonging to class b) (p. 49) have turned out to be due to active transport. The flux ratio is an expression of the "onesidedness" of the transport and if the onesidedness is more pronounced than predicted from the electrochemical potential difference, there is every reason to suspect active transport whether the transport is uphill or downhill. One spectacular exception from this interpretation has been reported, however. According to HODGKIN and KEYNES[252] giant decapod axons which have been poisoned with dinitrophenol to inhibit active transport will slowly lose potassium. During this leakage the flux ratio is determined by a function of the form

$$RT \ln(M_{in}/M_{out}) = n(\bar{\mu}_0 - \bar{\mu}_i)$$

where n has a value between 2 and 3. This means that either the potassium exchange is of type b), or potassium must during its passage through the membrane behave as if it had three positive charges. According to HODGKIN and KEYNES this peculiar behaviour of the potassium ion can be explained if it is assumed that the paths which the potassium ions must follow have 2 to 3 sites in succession, all of which must be occupied by potassium ions, and that, further, it is impossible for two potassium ions to pass each other within the membrane phase. Given these restrictions, all potassium ions in a row must move as one unit if they are to move at all. By statistical considerations HODGKIN and KEYNES have demonstrated that such "single file" movement must lead to the above-mentioned relationship. One additional possibility of explaining the deviation from the predicted flux ratio might be worth mentioning. If, during its leakage out, the potassium ions pass through a pore through which there is a net flow of water, the solvent drag (see below) might substantially change the ionic fluxes. Even in this case the potassium ions would be moving more or less in single file, but the coupling between their movements would be due to hydrostatic rather than electric force.

e) The effect of solvent drag

If ions pass a membrane by way of pores through which there is a flow of solvent, those moving "downstream" will be speeded up and those going "upstream" will be slowed down. If the pores were large, so that interference with the walls were of minor importance, it would be natural to ascribe to the solution in the pores a certain velocity. This is the device used by ONSAGER[253, 254], who in

[252] HODGKIN, A. L., and R. D. KEYNES: The potassium permeability of a giant nerve fibre. J. Physiol. **128**, 61—88 (1955).

[253] ONSAGER, L.: Theories and problems of liquid diffusion. Ann. N. Y. Acad. Sci. **46**, 241—265 (1945).

his treatment also takes into account the co-diffusion terms arising from inter-action with other diffusing molecules. In biological membranes, however, the pores, if present, must be very small, and the ions passing through them are impeded in their movements by interaction with the pore wall. At least it is a fact that the permeability coefficient for water is generally several orders of magnitude larger than those for inorganic ions and organic molecules of similar size. Therefore it is advantageous to consider the effect of the solvent flow as a force acting upon solute molecules which are relatively stationary with respect to the membrane phase[233, 234, 235].

The force, acting upon one mole of water in the direction of flow, may be put equal to $-dP/dx$, i. e. the hydrostatic pressure gradient. If g'_w is the friction exerted upon one mole of water, moving in the membrane at unit velocity, the linear rate of flow must be $-(dP/dx)(1/g'_w)$. The force, arising from solvent drag upon one mole of solute of the j' species then is: $-(dP/dx)(G_j/g'_w)$, where G_j is the friction between one mole of solute and water at unit velocity. This frictional coefficient, G_j, is assumed to be the same in the pore as outside, since it is only concerned with the interaction between solute and solvent. Thus G_j can be derived from the free diffusion coefficient, D_j, of the j'th species: $G_j = RT/D_j$.

The flux, M_j, across unit area normal to the direction of flow is assumed to be proportional to the force per mole, to the concentration of the diffusing species to the fraction, A, of the unit area which is available to diffusion of the species in question. The flux is further assumed to be proportional to the mobility of the ion in the membrane, u_j. Thus we get:

$$M_j = -A u_j c_j \left(RT \frac{d \ln c_j}{dx} + RT\, d \ln f/dx + z_j F \frac{d\psi}{dx} + \frac{dP}{dx} \cdot \frac{G_j}{g'_w} \right). \qquad (10)$$

A, u_j, c_j, ψ, P and g'_w are all unknown functions of x. In the expression for the flux ratio, however, most of the unknowns cancel (compare p. 49) and we obtain (discarding the subscript)

$$\ln(M_{in}/M_{out}) = \ln(a_0/a_i) + (zF/RT)(\psi_0 - \psi_i) + \frac{G}{RT} \int_0^{x_0} \frac{1}{g'_w} \left(\frac{dP}{dx} \right) dx ,$$

or

$$\ln(M_{in}/M_{out}) = \ln(a_0/a_i) + \frac{zF}{RT}(\psi_0 - \psi_i) + \frac{1}{D} \int_0^{x_0} \frac{1}{g'_w} \left(\frac{dP}{dx} \right) dx . \qquad (11)$$

The linear rate of flow, $\dfrac{dP}{dx} \cdot \dfrac{1}{g'_w}$, may vary in an unknown way with x. But the volume-rate must be the same for all values of x since water is non compressible. If the volume rate of flow is called Δ_w, we have:

$$\Delta_w = A \cdot \frac{1}{g'_w} \left(\frac{dP}{dx} \right)$$

where, as mentioned above, A is the fraction of unit area available for flow. By rearrangement we get:

$$\frac{\Delta_w}{A} = \frac{1}{g'_w} \left(\frac{dP}{dx} \right).$$

---

[254] Compare also J. G. KIRKWOOD: Transport of ions through biological membrane form the standpoint of irreversible thermodynamics. In: Ion transport across membranes. H. T. CLARKE ed. New York, N. Y.: Academic Press 1954.

Introducing this expression in eq. (11), we finally obtain

$$\ln\left(M_{in}/M_{out}\right) = \ln\frac{a_0}{a_i} + \frac{zF}{RT}\left(\psi_0 - \psi_i\right) + \frac{\varDelta_w}{D}\int_0^{x_0}\frac{1}{A}\,dx\,. \qquad (12)$$

The activity as used here means the absolute activity, including the effect of pressure on the activity cofficient. The integral occurring in the last term of this expression cannot be evaluated directly. It will be noticed, however, that it is independent of the nature of the ionic species in question. It is also the same for non-charged molecules as long as they are not actively transported. Since all the parameters in the above expression with the exception of the integral are accessible to measurement, it can serve the evaluation of the integral, using a passive test substance. As such, a non-charged molecule can be used with advantage, as its movements are not influenced by the potential. If an estimate of the drag effect exerted upon an ion is desired, it is advantageous to use as test substance an uncharged hydrophilic substance of about the same molecular size as the ion in question. In order to determine the influx and outflux of the test substance simultaneously, the test molecules should be available in two differently labelled forms. Thus ANDERSEN and USSING[235] used thiourea labelled with C^{14} and S^{35} and acetamide labelled in positions 1 and 2 with C^{14} to study the solvent drag created by osmotic water flow through the isolated toad skin. An equally good estimate was, however, obtained by using heavy water (D_2O) to measure influx, and volume measurements to measure the difference between influx and outflux of water (KOEFOED-JOHNSEN and USSING[234]).

The above equation states that the drag effect is inversely related to the diffusion coefficient of the ion in question. In other words: the solvent drag increases with increasing apparent ionic diameter.

Model studies[257] on a positive ion exchanger resin membrane have shown that the flux ratios for both Na and Cl are given with satisfactory accuracy by eq. (12) under a variety of conditions when sodium chloride is the only salt present in the system. More experiments are desirable to demonstrate its general applicability.

In the above treatment, the water flow is supposed to be due to a hydrostatic pressure gradient, dP/dx. Such a gradient might arise due to a difference in hydrostatic pressure between inside and outside solution. The result would, however, be exactly the same if the water flow were due to a difference in osmotic pressure[256, 233, 255, 235, 258, 259]. Also electroosmosis and water movements associated with active transport of solutes may result in drag effects which can be treated along the line indicated above. In conclusion it should be stressed that although solvent drag may play a role in organs where sizable differences in osmotic pressure

[255] USSING, H. H.: General principles and theories of membrane transport, in: Metabolic aspects of transport across cell membranes. Q. R. MURPHY ed. The University of Wisconsin Press, Madison 1957. p. 39—56.

[256] JACOBS, M. H.: The measurement of cell permeability with particular reference to the erythrocyte, in: Modern trends in physiology and biochemistry, ed. E. S. GUZMAN. BARRON. New York: Academic press 1952.

[257] MEARES, P., and H. H. USSING: The fluxes of sodium and chloride ions across a cation-exchange resin membrane. Part 1. — Effect of a concentration gradient. Trans. Faraday Soc. 55, 142—155 (1959).

[258] PAPPENHEIMER, J. R., E. M. RENKIN, and L. M. BORRERO: Filtration, diffusion and molecular sieving through periferal capillary membranes. Amer. J. Physiol. 167, 13—46 (1951).

[259] GARBY, L.: Studies on transfer of matter across membranes with special reference to the isolated human amniotic membrane and the exchange of amniotic fluid. Acta physiol. scand. 40, Suppl. 137, 84 (1957). ·

exist, present experience indicates that the solvent drag term can usually
disregarded in the first approximation when the object is to distinguish pass
from active transport.

f) Passive permeability and membrane structure

The extent to which solvent drag influences the movements of ions in liv
systems is still largely unknown. As already mentioned, the solvent drag depe
upon the existence of a porous membrane-structure, and the demonstration o
pronounced drag effect upon a suitable test substance can, in fact, be used
demonstrate the existence of "pores", that is a continuous water phase, throug
membrane. The work of PAPPENHEIMER and coworkers has demonstrated bey
reasonable doubt the existence of such "pores" in capillary walls, and pores m
also play an important role in the transfer of water and solutes through the ski
amphibia and through the gastric mucosa (SOLOMON et al.[260]). In all these ca
there is, however, the theoretical possibility that the water-filled channels
constituted by the interspaces between epithelial cells. As far as cell membra
go, the drag effect has been demonstrated beyond doubt in certain aquatic e
(ZEUTHEN and PRESCOTT[261]) and has been found to vary widely between spec
indicating pore sizes from little more than that of a water molecule to such t
might allow even protein molecules to pass through.

It should be stressed that the pore dimensions calculated from such
periments should be used with the utmost caution since they are, at best, eo
valent diameters, based upon the assumptions of cylindrical shape and lami
flow. Such values thus cannot be used to estimate whether or not a given io
species will be able to penetrate the membrane. As mentioned in chapter II. p
precise or even remotely correct figures for the diameters of ions in solution can
be given, since the mobility and thus the self diffusion constant of ions depend
the effect of the charge upon the solvent as well as on the ionic diameter. Th
for the time being, the absolute permeabilities of biological membranes to i
is of largely empirical nature and is awaiting a unifying theory. (For an interest
although unconventional approach, see MULLINS[262].)

Any theory of passive permeability to ions must take into account that cert
cell membranes, for instance those of nerve and "fast" muscle fibres, possess
property of changing, often within milliseconds, from a predominately K perme
to a predominately Na permeable state and back again. These changes seem
have nothing to do with active transport. At any time during the process the i
concerned are flowing down their electrochemical potential gradient. The class
view, favoured since the time of BERNSTEIN, that the cell membranes have p
large enough to permit potassium ions to pass, but too small to let thro
sodium ions, fails to account for the sodium-slectivity which sets in and ap
disappears during the conducted impulse of muscle and nerve. A maintai
sodium-selectivity seems to be characteristic of the outward-facing cell membr
of the frog skin epithelium and possibly of several other epithelia. The inw
facing cell membranes of these epithelium cells are, on the other hand,
dominately potassium permeable, like the membrane of resting muscle and ne
fibres.

[260] DURBIN, R. P., H. FRANK, and A. K. SOLOMON: Water flow through gastric muc
J. gen. Physiol. **39**, 535—551 (1956).
[261] PRESCOTT, D. M., and E. ZEUTHEN: Comparison of water diffusion and water filtra
across cell surfaces. Acta physiol. scand. **28**, 77—94 (1953).
[262] MULLINS, L. J.: In: Molecular structure and functional activity of nerve cells. A
Inst. Biol. Sci. Washington 1956.

The type of membrane characteristic of the conducted impulses in nerve and muscle is not the only membrane type capable of sudden changes in ionic permeability. A rather different type is found in the motor end plates of muscle and the subsynaptic membrane of neurons. This type of membrane, when acted upon by acetyl-choline, suddenly changes from a state where it is permeable to K and Cl but not to Na into one where it is highly permeable to all small ions, including sodium. It would be tempting to look for the same type of mechanism in gland cells which are stimulated by acetyl-choline like, for instance, salivary and sweat glands. At least for the salivary glands it is known that stimulation leads to potassium loss and sodium gain by the gland cells.

g) Permeability of intercellular cements

Ordinarily it is assumed that the cell membrane proper is the structure which impedes the diffusion of ions whereas they move relatively freely in the interspaces. In many cases it is undoubtedly true that the interstices offer little more resistance to, say K or Na, than to water. The studies of the isotopic exchange kinetics of alkali metal ions in different tissues have given values for the diffusion in the interspaces as a by-product. For frog-sartorius, HARRIS and BURN[263] estimate the diffusion coefficient of Na to be $2.9 \cdot 10^{-6} \, cm^2/sec$. The diffusion coefficient of K could not be calculated accurately because the exchange of this ion across the cell membranes goes on at a rate not very different from the exchange between interspaces and bathing solution. The diffusion coefficient for K seemed, however, to be somewhat larger than that for sodium.

In other cases the diffusion resistance of the interspaces is much higher, however. Thus in the extracellular space of sympathetic ganglia of different mammals, the rate of diffusion of sodium has been estimated at only 1/50 of that in free solution (HARRIS and MCLENNAN[264]).

Obviously the intercellular substances (hyaluronic acid, etc.) may impede the diffusion of inorganic ions pronouncedly.

Ordinarily the mobility of potassium is higher than that of sodium in the interspaces, as it is in free solution. There may be exceptions from this rule, however. Thus it has been claimed by CATCHPOLE, JOSEPH and ENGEL[265], that, judging from liquid junction potentials, the mobility of potassium relative to sodium was only 0.7 in the symphyseal connective tissue of pregnant guinea-pigs whereas, during extreme relaxation induced by hormone treatment, the ratio of 1.3 was found between the mobility of potassium and that of sodium. In water the ratio is 1.5. Thus it seems that the more dense packing of the negative charges of the ground substance favours the diffusion of sodium relative to potassium.

As it has been pointed out in chapter II, the relative affinities of potassium and sodium may differ appreciably in polyelectrolytes. There is, however, no simple relationship between the affinity of the polyelectrolyte to an ion and the ability of that ion to diffuse within the polyelectrolyte.

Extended studies of the relative mobilities of the two alkali metal ions in different types of ground substance material would be highly desirable. They may also shed light upon the means available to cells to make the membranes relatively potassium or sodium selective.

---

[263] HARRIS, E. J., and G. P. BURN: The transfer of sodium and potassium ions between muscle and the surrounding medium. Trans. Faraday Soc. 45, 508—528 (1949).

[264] HARRIS, E. J., and H. MCLENNAN: Cation exchanges in sympathetic ganglia. J. Physiol. 121, 629—637 (1953).

[265] CATCHPOLE, H. R., N. R. JOSEPH, and M. B. ENGEL: Electrochemical state of symphyseal connective tissue under hormonal stimulation. Amer. J. Physiol. 167, 774 (Soc. Proc. 1951).

h) Ionic permeability and the development of bioelectric potentials

In the above treatment of the permeability, the potential difference was considered an independent variable, but, of course, the equations mentioned can equally well be used to calculate the potential difference from concentration and flux data, that is: treating the potential as a dependent variable. Before the advent of isotopic tracers, flux data were not available, and information about membrane permeability to ions had to be obtained by indirect means. The method of choice often was study of the dependence of the membrane potential upon the ionic composition of the bathing solutions.

This line of research, among whose pioneers we may mention NERNST and MICHAELIS, has been developed in part at least on the basis of work with artificial porous membranes (collodium, ion exchange resins) and is still in rapid progress. Although the equations obtained are mostly derived for simplified systems, i. e. membranes of uniform thickness and uniform properties throughout, several of them are useful for the approximate calculation of bioelectric potentials. For recent discussions of the merits of the different treatments, see HARRIS[266], TEORELL[240], MEYER and SIEVERS[267], SCATCHARD[268], SOLLNER[269], and others [270a], [270b].

Of particular importance is the Nernst equation (29) which is valid when the membrane is permeable only to one of the ionic species present. The validity of the relation furthermore is restricted to cases with no electric current flow. For the general cases of current flow and/or net transport of more than one ionic species no generally valid treatment can be given, unless simplifying assumptions are introduced. As already mentioned, GOLDMAN[236] has given a solution to the general diffusion equation making the assumption that electric potential gradient is linear. From the GOLDMAN equation[236] HODGKIN and KATZ[271] have derived an expression for the potential difference, E, which is used repeatedly in the following. It takes into account only the contributions to the potential of monovalent ions.

$$E = \frac{RT}{F} \ln \frac{P_{Cl}(Cl)_i + P_{Na}(Na)_0 + P_K(K)_0 + \cdots}{P_{Cl}(Cl)_0 + P_{Na}(Na)_i + P_K(K)_i + \cdots}. \tag{13}$$

P_{Cl}, P_{Na} and P_K are the permeability constants for Cl, Na and K, respectively. Subscript i refers to concentrations in the inside, subscript 0 to concentrations in the outside solution. If other monovalent ions than Cl, Na and K are present, the appropriate terms should be added.

This equation makes it possible to estimate the membrane potential from the concentrations of all permeating ionic species present, and a permeability constant assigned to each species. It is interesting that SOLLNER and collaborators[269], [272],

[266] HARRIS, E. J.: Transport and accumulation in biological systems, 291 pp. London: Butterworth's scientific publications 1956.

[267] MEYER, K. H., and J. F. SIEVERS: La permenbilité des membranes. I. Théorie de la perm8nbilité ionique. Helv. chim. Acta 19, 649—664 (1936).

[268] SCATCHARD, G.: Transport of ions across charged membranes. In: Ion transport across membranes, ed. HANS T. CLARKE. New York: Academic Press 1954.

[269] SOLLNER, K.: Electrochemical studies with model membranes. In: Ion transport across membranes, ed. HANS T. CLARKE. New York: Academic Press 1954.

[270a] Several papers in: Electrochemistry in biology and medicine THEODORE SHEDLOVSKY. 369 pp. New York: John Wiley and Sons 1955.

[270b] Several papers in: Discuss. Faraday Soc. 21, (1956).

[271] HODGKIN, A. L., and B. KATZ: The effect of sodium ions on the electrical activity of the giant axon of the squid. J. Physiol. 108, 37—77 (1949).

[272] SOLLNER, K., S. DRAY, E. GRIM, and R. NEIHOF: Membranes of high electrochemical activity in studies of biological interest. In: Electrochemistry in biology and medicine. Ed. THEODORE SHEDLOVSKY, JOHN WILEY and Sons, New York (1955) p. 65—90.

working on collodion membranes, have obtained essentially the same equation. Other expressions may, however, give equally good or better agreement with experimental findings. TEORELL[239, 240], LINDERHOLM[241], MEYER[267, 273], in particular the TEORELL and MEYER-SIEVERS treatments seem to give satisfactory results with membranes having a high density of fixed charges.

Since BERNSTEIN[621] in 1902 advanced the idea that the resting potentials of muscle and nerve were diffusion potentials (see p. 144) arising from the potassium selectivity of the fibre membrane, this membrane theory of bioelectric potentials has had many advocates and although the original idea has undergone modifications, the basic concept of the biopotentials being diffusion potentials is now better founded than ever. Thus the membrane potentials of nerve and muscle, both in rest and during activity, have been found to behave as if they were determined solely by the concentration gradients and permeabilities of a small number of inorganic ionic species, among which K and Na play a decisive role.

Perhaps one might have expected that the active transport of these same ions would have offset the potentials one way or the other. It seems, however, that the active transport processes, although being necessary for the maintenance of the cellular ionic composition and thus ultimately for the potential development, do not otherwise contribute to the membrane potential. This is understandable if the active ion transport is walays a "forced exchange" of one ion, say sodium, against another, for example potassium or hydrogen ion with the same charge. Recent work suggests that even when we are dealing with a net active transport of sodium across epithelial membranes giving rise to a maintained membrane potential across the epithelium the active step itself is not electrogenic. Rather the active mechanism is again an electroneutral ion pump, keeping the cellular sodium low and the cellular potassium high. The implication is that the potential across an epithelium can be described as the sum of one diffusion potential across the outward facing cellmembrane and another across the inward facing membrane, each potential being determined by the passive ionic permeabilities of the membrane in question and the concentration gradients across it. But all the potentials would run down unless they were maintained by the active ion transport. It should be pointed out, however, that much work remains before it can be said with certainty that active ion transport is never electrogenic. The detailed discussion of the role of K and Na in the development of bioelectric potentials is given in chapter VII Ah.

i) Active transport of the alkali metal ions
(The "Sodium pump")

It is now becoming commonly accepted that most if not all animal cells are capable of active sodium transport. Recent observations from different quarters indicate that active sodium transport is also of great importance in some plant cells (yeast, Halicystis, Ulva, Nitella). Originally it was the characteristic distribution of the alkali metal ions between muscle fibres and their surroundings which inspired the idea of a "sodium pump" which would extrude the sodium ions as fast as they entered (DEAN[274], KROGH[226]). But against the "pump" hypothesis it was argued that the ionic distribution of the living cells might just as well be a static and not a dynamic phenomenon. If so the cytoplasm would possess specific binding sites preferring K and excluding Na (compare chapter VI). The hypotheses

[273] MEYER, K. H., and P. BERNFELD: The potentiometric analysis of membrane structure and its application to living animal membranes. J. gen. Physiol. **29**, 353—378 (1946).
[274] DEAN, R. B.: Theories of electrolyte equilibrium in muscle. Biol. Symp. **3**, 331—348 (1941).

of this type, although not very likely, are difficult to rule out entirely because it is so difficult to measure intracellular ionic activities with any accuracy. The idea of the active sodium transport as the factor responsible for the cellular ionic pattern thus probably would not have been so readily accepted were it not for the fact that numerous cases are known where cells perform a net transport of sodium under such conditions that there can be no question about the active nature of the process. Thus the capacity for active sodium transport has to be accepted anyway and it then seems simpler to consider the same mechanism as being responsible for the cellular rejection of sodium and preference for potassium. Membranes which show a manifest active transport of sodium are the skin of amphibia, toad urinary bladder, toad and frog large intestine, guinea pig caecum, rumen epithelium of the ruminants etc. Moreover a large and increasing body of evidence points to active sodium-transport in tubular reabsorption of sodium and in the formation of other glandular excertions (sweat, saliva etc.).

As we shall see later there are, indeed, a sufficient number of similarities between the mechanisms performing the net sodium transports and those which seem responsible for the maintenance of the cellular K/Na ratio to support the hypothesis of their being closely related if not identical.

But although all available evidence makes it necessary to accept the existence of a "sodium pump", active transport of sodium alone cannot always account for the K/Na ratios observed in all cells. It is true that the cellular potential is often sufficiently negative relative to the surroundings to account for the high cellular potassium level. In other words: cellular and extracellular potassium ions are often close to electrochemical equilibrium. But this is by no means always the case. Erythrocytes of most mammalian species have a potassium concentration many (often about 40) times higher than that of plasma, and there is every reason to believe that the potential difference between cell interior and plasma is only a few millivolts. Thus the potassium accumulation as well as the sodium depletion must be assumed to be due to active transport. Actually the outward transport of Na and the inward transport of K show such interdependence that it seems natural to consider the potassium ion as the "return freight" for the active sodium transport (see p. 77). There is also good evidence that the active extrusion of Na from nerve and muscle is mainly such a forced exchange of Na against K. Whether it is justified quite generally to consider the "sodium pump" as a coupled sodium-potassium pump is still an open question. Such a mechanism would explain the alkali ion distribution in many cells better than the pure sodium pump hypothesis. Notably, it would explain the fact that the cellular potassium concentration quite often is higher than demanded by electrochemical equilibrium with the surroundings. A coupled Na-K pump would also help explain why the steady state concentration ratio for K is usually different from Rb and Cs ions. Thus these three ions might have a different affinity for the ion pump, or they might leak out again from the cells at unequal rates.

There are cases of cellular ion transport where transport of K does not seem to be coupled with that of Na. In yeast, for example, in the absence of Na there is a forced exchange of K against H (see p. 108). In general the capacity of plant cells to accumulate K normally, even when grown in sodium-free media, points to the existence of one or more alternative partners for potassium other than Na.

When we consider transcellular transport of sodium it seems at first sight as if potassium is usually not acting as partner. Thus sodium is transported inward through the frog skin without any potassium being transported *actively* from the inside solution to that bathing the outside of the skin. Nevertheless potassium ions in the inside bathing solution are absolutely necessary for the sodium transport. Recent work suggests that K is, in fact, the active exchange partner for sodium in the frog skin, but potassium moves in a closed circuit, being "pumped" into the epithelium cells from the inside bathing solution and returning again to the latter by passive transport. Fig. 2 shows how the operation of an active sodium-potassium exchange can be operated so as to bring about a net transport from the outside in of sodium and chloride ions. It is seen that the net transport is due to the fact that the epithelium cell is polar in the sense that the membrane facing outward is selectively (but passively) permeable to Na (and Cl) whereas that facing inward is passively permeable to K and Cl but not to Na. Furthermore only the inward-facing membrane possesses the ion-pump. For comparison is shown a nonpolar cell (for instance a muscle cell) having the capacity for active ion transport as well as the passive permeabilities evenly distributed over its surface. The same elements which in the muscle cell serve only for the maintenance of the internal ionic composition, in addition, accomplish a net salt transport in the epithelial cell. Clearly, by a proper distribution of the passive permeabilities, but with the very same active mechanism, the epithelial cell would have been transporting potassium chloride in the outward direction instead of sodium chloride inward. If like the muscle cell the epithelium cell had retained the ion pump on both faces, more complicated ion transport patterns would ensue, even to the extent of having sodium and potassium being subject to net transport in the same direction as shown in Fig. 2c. These hypothetical cases are mentioned because they have an important bearing upon our interpretation of the active transports across epithelial membranes which have been described. Thus

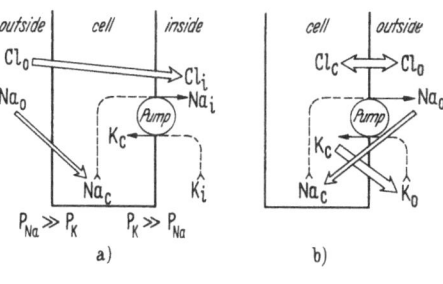

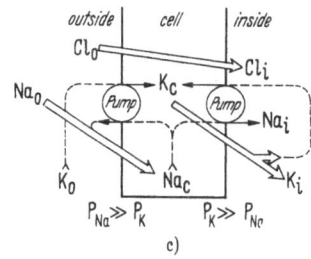

Fig. 2. Tentative representation of ionic fluxes across the cell membranes of different cell types, a) represents an asymmetric cell, viz. an epithelial cell, b) represents a symmetrical cell with the same permeability and the same "pump" mechanism at all cell borders, viz. a muscle cell, c) represents a cell with an equally distributed "pump" mechanism but with different permeabilities at different borders. Oblique arrows designate passive diffusion. The "pump" effects a one-to-one exchange of K for Na

in the malpighian tubule of insects there is an active excretion of K whereas Na seems to behave passively. In vertebrate kidney tubules both the reabsorption of Na and the excretion of K seem to be of an active nature, the gills of crabs actively take up both K and Na, etc. But the above discussion of the potentialities of an epithelium with a sodium-potassium pump and proper passive permeabilities has taught us that the determination of which ion or ions are subject to net transport does not tell us unambiguously which ions are originally transported actively. Further studies are needed before it can be said whether the hypothesis of an ubiquitous sodium/potassium pump is tenable. In some cases, at least, the hydrogen ion rather than the potassium ion may serve as partner for sodium. Thus the tubular acidification of the urine in vertebrates seems to depend upon a forced exchange of sodium against hydrogen ions.

From a pharmacological viewpoint it is important to realize that the effect of any agent upon the net transport of an ion may be due to changes either in the passive or the active elements usually governing its transcellular transfer.

j) Relation of the active transport to metabolism[275-286]

The active transport of the alkali metal ions, like all active transports, requires metabolic energy. For convenience we shall in the following speak of the energy requirements of the "sodium pump" although in all probability K is also actively transported in the opposite direction. The justification for focussing the interest mainly upon the sodium ion lies in the fact that in most cells by far the greater part of the work performed is done upon the sodium ion, the cellular potassium ion being close to electrochemical equilibrium with that of the surroundings.

In most animal cells and tissues the active cation transport depends for its energy supply upon oxidative metabolism, that is, they cannot continue the transport for an extended period of time without oxygen supply. This is the case with brain, retina, nerve, kidney, mammalian muscle, frog skin, toad and frog large intestine, toad urinary bladder etc. In some cases an active transport at strongly reduced rate will continue for hours in the absence of oxygen, evidently energized by glycolysis (toad urinary bladder?).

The seminal vesicle mucosa of the guinea-pig is an example of a tissue which will support its active ion transport on the basis of oxidative metabolism under aerobic conditions but is able to utilize glycolysis to maintain normal cellular concentration of K and Na in the absence of oxygen. Finally there are cells like mammalian erythrocytes which depend exclusively upon glycolysis for their active ion transport.

In cells depending on oxidative metabolism, dinitrophenol is usually a powerful inhibitor of the active transport, whereas this poison has little effect upon the ion transport of erythrocytes, which do not respire, and frog muscle, which apparently is able to provide sufficient energy for the ion transport by glycolysis. Such observations have made several investigators suspect that energy rich phosphate bonds were utilized in the active transport of the alkali metal ions and the hypothesis has recently been strengthened considerably by the finding that decapod giant axons which had stopped extruding sodium after their store of energy-rich phosphates had run down, started up the sodium transport again on

[275] FLINK, E. B., A. B. HASTINGS, and J. K. LOWRY: Changes in potassium and sodium concentration in liver slices accompanying incubation in vitro. Amer J. Physiol. **163**, 598—604 (1950).

[276] MUDGE, G. H.: Studies on potassium accumulation by rabbit kidney slices; effect of metabolic activity. Amer. J. Physiol. **165**, 113—127 (1951).

[277] WHITTAM, R., and R. E. DAVIES: Active transport of water, sodium, potassium and α-oxyglutarate by kidney-cortex slices. Biochem. J. **55**, 880—888 (1953).

[278] CALKINS, E., I. M. TAYLOR, and A. B. HASTINGS: Potassium exchange in the isolated rat diaphragm; effect of anoxia and cold. Amer. J. Physiol. **177**, 211—218 (1954).

[279] HODGKIN, A. L., and R. D. KEYNES: Active transport of cations in giant axons from Sepia and Loligo. J. Physiol. **128**, 28—60 (1955).

[280] ZERAHN, K.: Oxygen consumption and active sodium transport in the isolated and short-circuited frog skin. Acta physiol. scand. **36**, 300—318 (1956).

[281] ANDERSEN, B., and H. H. USSING: Unpublished.

[282] BREUER, H. J., and R. WHITTAM: Ion movements in seminal vesicle mucosa. J. Physiol. **135**, 213—225 (1957).

[283] TOSTESON, D. C., and J. S. ROBERTSON: Potassium transport in duck red cells. J. cell. comp. Physiol. **47**, 147—166 (1956).

[284] MAIZELS, M.: Cation transport in chicken erythrocytes. J. Physiol. **125**, 263—277 (1954).

[285] KEYNES, R. D., and G. W. MAISEL: The energy requirement for sodium extrusion from a frog muscle. Proc. roy. Soc. B **142**, 383—392 (1954).

[286] CALDWELL, P. C., and R. D. KEYNES: The utilization of phosphate bond energy for sodium extrusion from giant axons. J. Physiol. **137**, 12P—13P (1957).

injection of ATP into the fibre. It may also be mentioned that human erythrocytes which are washed free of glucose show a parallel drop in ATP content and active potassium transport (DUNHAM [287]).

k) Quantitative relationship between oxygen consumption and active ion transport

Precise simultaneous determinations of oxygen consumption and active sodium transport have only been obtained for a few tissues. ZERAHN [280, 288] found that for each sodium ion transported actively through the isolated frog skin there was an extra oxygen consumption of 1/16 to 1/20 molecule of oxygen (see p. 120). In other words: for each electron passing through the cytochrome system there was an active transport of 4—5 sodium ions. Similar results were obtained by LEAF and RENSHAW [289, 290]. In a later study ZERAHN [291] showed that the extra oxygen consumption associated with the transport of a sodium ion was independent within wide limits of the transport *work* performed. Thus the Na/O ratio was the same whether the transport took place against a concentration gradient, against an electric potential gradient or between solutions of the same composition and at the same potential. This means that there is a stoichiometric relationship between sodium transport and metabolic rate. An analogous relationship was discovered by LUNDEGARDH [292] for the ion uptake by plant roots where the oxygen consumption increases in proportion to the rate of ion uptake. LUNDEGARDH named this reaction "Anionenatmung", assuming that one electron was carried through the cytochrome system in exchange for each anion taken up.

LUNDGARDH's observations have recently been reinterpreted by CHANCE and WILLIAMS [293] who consider the increase in oxygen consumption as being brought about as follows: The addition of a salt whose anion is capable of being absorbed, induced an active salt transport into the root. This active transport takes place at the expense of ATP or other high-energy phosphates. The ADP formed will then diffuse to the mitochondria and as its concentration is rate limiting, it will activate the respiratory chain. The important implication of this is that it is not the oxygen consumption which determines the rate of active transport, but rather the drain on the ATP caused by the active transport which sets the rate of oxygen consumption. The correctness of the consideration that it is the sodium transport that sets the metabolism as far as the frog skin is concerned is born out by the following experiment: An isolated frog skin is placed between modified "Ringer" solutions having in stead of chloride a non penetrating anion. In this system sodium ion can only move from the outside to the inside solution to an extent governed by the resistance of an external circuit. Thus, by adjusting the resistance in this circuit the rate of active transport can be set at any desired value[294].

[287] DUNHAM, E. T.: Parallel decay of ATP and active cation fluxes in starved human erythrocytes (in preparation).

[288] ZERAHN, K.: Oxygen consumption and active transport of sodium in the isolated, short-circuited frog skin. Nature (Lond.) 177, 937—938 (1956).

[289] LEAF, A., and A. RENSHAW: A test of the redox hypothesis of active ion transport. Nature (Lond.) 178, 156—157 (1956).

[290] LEAF, A., and A. RENSHAW: Ion transport and respiration of isolated frog skin. Biochem. J. 65, 82—90 (1957).

[291] ZERAHN, K.: Oxygen consumption and active sodium transport in isolated amphibian skin under varying experimental conditions. Diss. Copenhagen 1958.

[292] For references, see H. LUNDEGARDH: Anion respiration. Symp. Soc. exp. Biol. 8, 262—296 (1954).

[293] CHANCE, B., and G. R. WILLIAMS: The respiratory chain and oxidative phosphorylation. Advanc. Enzymol. 17, 65—134 (1956).

[294] ANDERSEN, B.: In preparation.

As one would predict from the foregoing, the adjustment of the resist
actually determined the rate of oxygen consumption. The situation is not u
that of mucsular contraction where it is the drain on ATP arising from the con
tions which determines how much oxygen is to be used.

Reliable figures for the oxygen consumption in relation to ion transpor
also available for the isolated gills of the wool-handed crab, Eriocheir sine
KOCH[295] found that for each μmol of oxygen consumed, the gill would tak
12.3 μmols of sodium. Thus here roughly 3 sodiums are transported per elec

For frog muscle KEYNES and MAISEL[285] found that the ratio of sodium
transported to oxygen molecules used was from 2—5.7, whereas for nerve HOD
and KEYNES[296] found one sodium to be transported outward for each equiv
of oxygen consumed.

Due to the experimental difficulties involved the figures for muscle and r
fibres are not as accurate as those for the epithelial membranes and it can ther
not be stated with certainty that the stoichiometric efficiency is less for the cel
than for transcellular transport. It should further be born in mind that in ce
organs there may be drains upon the ATP system other than those associated
active sodium (and potassium) transport.

The realization that active ion transport is stoichiometrically related tc
expenditure of energy has rather important implications with respect to cal
tions of the energy requirements of glands. If we consider an organ like the ki
it is well known that practically all the sodium chloride ultrafiltered in the gl
ruli is reabsorbed in the tubuli, no matter whether the urine ultimately form
concentrated or dilute. One would therefore predict that the transport
would be determined largely by the filtration rate whereas the composition o
urine would be immaterial.

For glands like the sublingualis where the primary secretion does not see
undergo any modification by reabsorption of sodium, the minimum er
requirements must be determined simply by the number of ions excreted.]
there is some reason to believe, both the sodium and the chloride ion are su
to active transport, the energy requirements might be considerably higher th
the secretion were formed by the activity of the sodium pump alone.

1) Temperature dependency of the "sodium pump"

As one might expect, the rate of active transport of sodium increases marl
with temperature, as long as it does not lead to damage of the tissue. Ta
shows the temperature coefficient, Q_{10}, for the active sodium transport
number of tissues. The highest values were found for sodium extrusion ir
isolated Sepia axon[279] (3.2 for the interval 10—20 degrees C.). For frog sart
muscle between 0 and 20° it will be noticed that the estimation of the tempera
coefficient from the isotopic exchange rate gives much lower figures [1.5 (
and USSING[250]), 1.7 (HARRIS[297])] than does the net extrusion rate 2.5 (S1
BACH[298]). This may indicate that the isotopic exchange measures a mixtu
exchange diffusion of sodium having a relatively low temperature coefficient
active transport of this ion. The net extrusion, on the other hand, measures

[295] KOCH, H.: Cited by K. ZERAHN. Diss. Copenhagen 1958.

[296] HODGKIN, A. L., and R. D. KEYNES: Movement of cations during recovery in r
Symp. Soc. exp. Biol. 8, 423—437 (1954).

[297] HARRIS, E. J.: The transfer of sodium and potassium between muscle and the surr
ing medium. Trans. Faraday Soc. 46, 872—882 (1950).

[298] STEINBACH, H. B.: The regulation of sodium and potassium in muscle fibres. S
Soc. exp. Biol. 8, 432—452 (1954).

active transport, thus yielding the higher temperature coefficient. The relatively low Q_{10} for sodium exchange in rat muscle[299] might be explained along the same line. The participation of exchange diffusion cannot be ruled out in erythrocytes[300] and crab nerves[301], either. It is a fact, however, that the isolated amphibian skin (several species of frog and toad) has also a Q_{10} around 2. Here there can be no question of exchange diffusion since the parameter measured was the net current output of the short-circuited skin, a quantity which is equal to the net sodium transport. Thus it might be concluded that the sodium pump of Sepia and that of frog skin (and several other tissues) differ in principle as indicated by the difference in temperature dependency. It should be remembered, however, that in Sepia nerve the sodium ions passes

Table 5. *Q_{10} for sodium transport in different tissues*

organ	quantity measured	Temp. range °C	Q_{10}	Ref.
Frog muscle .	outflux	1—20	1.5	250
Frog muscle .	outflux		1.7	297
Frog muscle .	net transport	4—22	2.8	298
Sepia axon . .	outflux	9—19	3.4	279
Rat muscle .	outflux	0—20	1.5	299
Frog skin . .	net transport	10—20	1.75	291
Toad skin . .	net transport		1.6	291

only one cell membrane whereas in the frog skin it passes at least two. Thus the rate limiting step in the two systems need not be the same even if the "ion pumps" were identical.

In all events the temperature coefficients of all the sodium transports shown in the table are much larger than that for free diffusion which is ca. 1.3 and thus are compatible with the idea that they describe the properties of one or more chemical processes. On the other hand, as pointed out by DANIELLI[302], it is not possible from the magnitude of the temperature coefficient to decide whether it is due to a chemical process or a diffusion process. If the activation energy of diffusion is large (meaning that there is a high energy barrier to be overcome by the thermal movements) the temperature coefficient will also be high.

m) Effects of drugs and hormones on active and passive transport

There is mounting evidence that several hormones and drugs owe their effects to their ability to alter the passive and active transport of ions (mainly Na and K) through cell membranes. The detailed analysis of these effects in terms of specific changes in permeability constants and active transport rates so far has been carried out only in a few cases (acetyl choline on end-plates, neurohypophyseal hormones on amphibian skin, see below). As, however, the proper methods for such studies now exist or are being developed, rapid progress in the field can be anticipated.

1. Steroid hormones

The profound effects of the steroid hormones, notably those of the adrenal cortex, upon the handling of Na and K in the organism has long been recognized (see part II). Even the sex hormones (estradiol, progesteron etc.) may exert

[299] McLENNAN, H.: Physical and chemical factors affecting potassium movements in mammalian muscle. Biochem. biophys. Acta **22**, 30—37 (1956).

[300] SOLOMON, A. K.: The permeability of the human erythrocyte to sodium and potassium. J. gen. Physiol. **36**, 57—110 (1952).

[301] SHANES, A. M.: Effect of temperature on potassium liberation during nerve activity. Fed. Proc. **13**, 134 (1954).

[302] DANIELLI, J. F.: In H. DAVSON and J. F. DANIELLI, The permeability of natural membranes, 361 pp. Cambridge: University Press 1943.

some (or all) of their effects via their abilities to change the electrolyte pattern of cells (compare IX D a 2). Despite the great interest in these hormones, a satisfactory analysis in terms of effects on active and passive transports has hardly been carried through. According to a hypothesis advanced by GLYNN (see VII B a 10) the steroid hormones are transformed metabolically to substances related to the cardiac aglucones before they become physiologically active.

2. Cardiac glycosides and their aglucones

Among the drugs which effect the "cation pump" the cardiac glycosides and their aglucones have attracted particular interest by recent years because they seem to have a direct inhibitory effect on the active transport mechanism. So far the effect has been observed in red cells (p. 79) heart muscle (p. 189) skeletal muscle (see JOHNSON[303]), giant nerve fibre (KEYNES[304]) mouse ascites tumor cells (see p. 106) and frog skin epithelium (see p. 126). Furthermore there is indirect evidence that it also inhibits the active sodium reabsorption in kidney proximal tubule of Necturus (SOLOMON[305], personal information). The fact that these drugs inhibit the cation pump of such diverse cells and tissues constitutes a strong indirect evidence that in essence we are dealing with the same active transport mechanism in all the cells in question. In particular it is worthy of note that the regulation of the cellular cation-level for instance in red cells and the transcellular sodium transport across epithelia (frog skin and kidney tubule) make use of the same type of cation-pump.

In the details of the inhibition pattern there are interesting differences between the different cell-types. Thus in red cells, not only the active fluxes of Na and K are inhibited, but also a sizable fraction of the passive diffusion fluxes. In the ascites tumor cell the active transport outward and the passive leakage inward of sodium ions are inhibited, and to the same extent. In striated muscle although the active transports are inhibited, the passive permeability to potassium must remain high as evidenced by the fact that the membrane potential is unaffected by the drugs.

In heart muscle the drugs induce a loss of potassium which indicates that the passive permeability to potassium is not greatly impeded. In the frog skin, the glycoside G-strophanthin inhibits strongly the net sodium transport, and at the same time the epithelium cells start leaking potassium towards the chorium side. Thus the passive diffusion of K cannot have been inhibited.

It thus seems that the common feature of these drug effects is the stoppage of the cation pump. The passive transports are sometimes inhibited and sometimes not. It would be tempting to interpret these findings in the way that passive diffusion can either take place through pores (potassium in muscle and frog skin) in which case the heart poisons have no effect, or by way of a "passive" or "ideling" carrier system using carriers similar or identical to those functioning in the active transport system. Only in the latter case would the heart poisons have an effect.

3. Different Hormones

Acetyl choline. In motor end-plates and in the subsynaptic membrane of nerve cells, acetyl choline brings about a pronounced increase in passive permeability to all small ions including Na and K (see p. 168). It now seems that even in

---

[303] JOHNSON, J. A.: Influence of ouabain, strophanthidin and dihydrostrophantidin on sodium and potassium transport in frog sartorii. Amer. J. Physiol. **187**, 328—332 (1956).
[304] KEYNES, R. D.: Personal communication.
[305] SOLOMON, A. K.: Personal communication.

the case of the heart muscle, the acetyl choline effect can best be explained in terms of an increase in passive permeability, but here it is mainly or solely the permeability to potassium ions which is increased (BURGEN and TERROUX[306], see also WEIDMANN[307, 308] and BROOKS, HOFFMAN, SUCKLING and ORIAS[309]). In the parotis gland, acetyl choline induces loss of K and gain of Na which very well could be interpreted in terms of an increased passive permeability of the cell membrane to both alkali metal ions (part II, chapter).

According to NACHMANSOHN[310] and associates acetyl choline plays a role in bringing about the increased sodium permeability associated with the rising phase of the spike in.

Histamine. Histamine gives rise to the release of K from isolated intestinal muscle[311, 312]. The detailed mechanism of this effect is not known.

Adrenaline. In certain cases adrenaline seems to decrease permeability. Thus it partly inhibits the loss of K from isolated skeletal muscle to the soaking medium[313] (Tyrode-solution). In the isolated frog skin adrenaline brings about a large increase in passive sodium permeability. The effect may be mainly or solely concerned with the mucus gland cells which are stimulated to secretion by adrenaline. In the parotis gland the effect of adrenaline and acetyl choline are very similar. Thus, by inference, adrenaline may increase the permeability of the gland cells to sodium and well as to potassium.

Neurohypophyseal hormones. These hormones bring about an increase in pore-size in some layer of the amphibian skin. This leads to an increased water permeability as well as to an increase in active sodium transport (compare p. 126). It is still an open question whether or not the effects of these hormones on other organs (kidney, uterus muscle etc.) can be explained along the same lines.

n) Role of alkali ion transport in the regulation of the volume of living cells

It is readily seen that the capacity of actively transporting ions must be a factor of great importance for the osmotic regulation of the individual cell as well as for the organism as a whole. It has been known for some years that the hydration of several isolated tissues depends upon the cellular respiration (STERN et al.[314])

[306] BURGEN, A. S. V., and K. G. TERROUX: On the negative inotropic effect in the cat's auricle. J. Physiol. **120,** 449—464 (1953).

[307] WEIDMANN, S.: Elektrophysiologie der Herzmuskelfaser, 100 pp. Bern, Stuttgart: Huber 1956.

[308] WEIDMANN, S.: Electrophysiology of the heart, 20' International Physiological Congress, p. 239—244, Brussels 1956.

[309] BROOKS, C. McC., B. F. HOFFMAN, E. E. SUCKLING, and O. ORIAS: Excitability of the Heart. New York: Grune and Stratton 1955.

[310] WILSON, I. B., and D. NACHMANSOHN: The generation of bioelectric potentials. In: Transport across Membranes (H. T. CLARKE and D. NACHMANSOHN, eds.). New York: Academic Press 1954.

[311] PARROT, J. L., J. THOUVENOT, and S. LONGUEVALLE: Libération de potassium par l'histamine, étude sur le jéjuno-iléon isole du cobaye. C. R. Soc. Biol. (Paris) **146,** 359—362 (1952).

[312] PARROT, J. L., J. THOUVENOT, and S. LONGUEVALLE: Libération de potassium par les organes isolés du cobaye, action de l' histamine et de l'un de ses antagonistes de synthèse. J. Physiol. (Paris) **45,** 215—218 (1953).

[313] GOFFART, M., and W. L. M. PERRY: The action of adrenaline on the rate of loss of potassium ions from unfatigued striated muscle. J. Physiol. **112,** 95—101 (1951).

[314] STERN, J. R., L. V. EGGLESTON, R. HEMS, and H. A. KREBS: Accumulation of glutamic acid in isolated brain tissue. Biochem. J. **44,** 410—418 (1949).

and that metabolic inhibitors bring about swelling of the tissues (OPIE[315], ROBIN-SON[316], AEBI[317]). This phenomenon was first interpreted as indicating that the cells were normally hypertonic relative to the extracellular fluid and that the swelling was opposed by an active transport of water energized by the cell metabolism (see for instance ROBINSON[316]). This view was, however, contested by MUDGE[318] who pointed out that since the depression of the metabolism by appropriate inhibitors is associated with an uptake of not only water but of a corresponding amount of inorganic ions as well, the depression of metabolism must lead to an isosmotic increase in cellular hydration.

The close relationship between water and electrolyte shifts is becoming increasingly apparent. Several groups of workers were able to demonstrate that the electrolyte shifts as well as the volume increase produced by metabolic inhibitors were reversed more or less completely when the tissue was incubated in a medium free of inhibitor and generally favourable for the metabolism (TERNER, EGGLESTON and KREBS[120], MUDGE[318], ROBINSON[316], DEYRUP[319], WHITTAM and DAVIES[277]).

The idea that the cells were normally hypertonic became even less tenable when CONWAY[224] was able to demonstrate that the contents of tissues rapidly frozen in liquid air and disintegrated in the frozen state were isotonic with the extracellular fluid. It was used as an argument for tissue hypertonicity that the sum of Na and K of many tissues is higher than the sum of these ions in blood plasma, but as pointed out by MUDGE[320], the presence of polyvalent anions in tissues actually demands that the cellular cation concentration is higher than that of the extracellular fluid in order that osmotic equilibrium be established.

Careful studies on slices of guinea pig kidney cortex, rat liver and rat cerebral cortex (LEAF[321]) have revealed that the swelling associated with metabolic inhibition was indeed associated with the uptake of sodium and chloride ions to such an extent that the overall result was the transfer of a solution isotonic with the medium. More sodium was always taken up than potassium lost, the difference being equal to the uptake of chloride ions. Leaf points out that the phenomenon can be considered a simple consequence of the stoppage of the sodium pump. Reestablishment of the metabolic activity will result in extrusion of sodium and chloride with reduction of the cell volume. A similar hypothesis has been advanced independently by WILSON[322]. As stated by the above authors the sodium pump is supposed to pump only sodium. If, as there now is some reason to believe, the sodium pump is moving Na and K in opposite directions, the problem of volume control becomes somewhat more involved. A class-room example of this is the depen-

[315] OPIE, E. L.: The movement of water in tissues removed from the body and its relation to movement of water during life. J. exp. Med. 89, 185—208 (1949).

[316] ROBINSON, J. R.: Osmoregulation in surviving slices from the kidneys of adult rats. Proc. roy. Soc. B 137, 378—402 (1950).

[317] AEBI, H.: Elektrolyt-Akkumulierung und Osmoregulation in Gewebeschnitten. Helv. physiol. Acta 11, 96—121 (1953).

[318] MUDGE, G. H.: Electrolyte and water metabolism of rabbit kidney slices. Effect of metabolic inhibitors. Amer. J. Physiol. 167, 206—223 (1951).

[319] DEYRUP, I. J.: Reversal of fluid uptake by rat kidney slices immersed in isosmotic solutions in vitro. Amer. J. Physiol. 175, 349—352 (1955).

[320] MUDGE, G. H.: Electrolyte metabolism of rabbit-kidney slices. Studies with radioactive potassium and sodium. Amer. J. Physiol. 173, 511—522 (1953).

[321] LEAF, A.: On the mechanism of fluid exchange of tissues in vitro. Biochem. J. 62, 241—248 (1956).

[322] WILSON, T. H.: Ionic permeability and osmotic swelling of cells. Science 120, 104—105 (1954).

dence of the osmotic resistance of erythrocytes upon their Na—K-pump [323,324,325]. As it will be discussed in greater detail below (p. 71), the erythrocytes of humans and many other mammals, although being highly permeable to chloride ions and other small anions, exhibit only a slight passive permeability to K and Na. Nevertheless, the leakiness to these ions would in the long run lead to loss of the cellular K and gain of Na, were it not for the activity of the "cation-pump". Inhibition of the glycolytic metabolism either by metabolic poisons, by cooling or by withdrawal of glucose from the substrate stops the ion pump and the ionic distribution drifts towards equilibrium. The normal ion distribution with high K and low Na in the cells is usually reestablished when conditions are provided for a normal glycosis. It is obvious, however, that during stoppage of the metabolic ion pumping, the osmotic equilibrium of the cells must be disturbed. Given enough time, K and Na as well as Cl and HCO_3 must be considered diffusible and since the colloid osmotic pressure of the cells is larger than that of the plasma, the cells must in the long run swell, and ultimately cytolyze. The rate at which this happens depends upon the composition of the cells, the ionic composition of the medium and on the membrane permeabilities to K and to Na. In the normally metabolizing cell in normal plasma the cell volume must be determined by three parameters: The pumping rate of the Na—K-pump, the passive leaking in rate of Na, and the passive leaking-out rate of K. Since these three processes seem to make use of independent pathways, we can thus, at least in theory, influence the cell volume by influencing any one of them.

This viewpoint can probably be extended to many other cell types. The relative magnitudes of the cation pumping and the passive leaks to K and Na may be among the main tools used by the organisms to regulate cell volumes. Thus, when the rat uterus starts increasing in size under the effect of estradiol (see p .194), the initial effect is an augmentation of the cellular K and Cl, whereas the growth in protein and phosphate content lags behind a day or more. Such a swelling with increased K, Cl content of the cells might result for example from an inhibition of the passive diffusion out of the cells of K with retained pumping rate and a normal Na leak.

o) Mechanisms proposed for the active transport of alkali metal ions

Although great progress has been made in recent years towards characterizing the active transport of K and Na and its relation to metabolism and to bioelectric potentials, the mechanism of transport has remained unknown. A number of hypotheses have however been advanced to explain the phenomenon, and it may be appropriate to give a short account of some of these hypotheses together with the evidence which speaks for or against each of them.

1. Simple membrane-carrier transport (OSTERHOUT[18]). The ionic species which is transported is supposed to form a "complex" with a membrane constituent. Due to some metabolic process the concentration of the carrier is kept lower at one membrane boundary than at the other, thus creating a diffusion gradient for the complex in the direction of transport. At the boundary where the complex-forming molecule is metabolically removed, there is a release of the ion in question, whereas, at the boundary where the complex-former is created, the transported ion is being "trapped". The complex-former may be a metabolite (ROSENBERG[227]) or an integral part of the membrane (USSING[245]).

[323] MATTHIES, H.: Über Stoffwechselleistungen von roten Blutkörperchen. Naunyn-Schmiedeberg's Arch. exp. Path. Pharmak. **221**, 497—505 (1954).

[324] TEITEL, P.: Favorable effect of insulin on the osmotic resistance of stored erythrocytes. Rep. Roumanian Soc. Physiol. June 27, 1957.

[325] TOSTESON, D. C.: In preparation.

In the case of the alkali metal ions the requirements to a proper carrier mole-cule are very exacting. Thus in human red cells the active inward transport mechanism of K must have a preference for this ion exceeding that for Na by a factor of at least 100. Conversely the outward transport of Na in red cells, muscle and nerve fibres must have an equally large preference for Na relative to K. The same is the case for the active transport of Na through frog skin and presumably many other epithelial membranes. As it will appear from chapter II, none of the known binders of K and Na show the required specificity. The likelihood of a coupling between the transport of Na in one direction and of K in the other, makes it look as if the hypothetical carrier is transformed at one boundary from a K-binder into a Na-binder whereas at the other boundary the reverse reaction takes place. The fact that ATP, at least in the case of the giant squid axon, has been shown to energize the active sodium-potassium exchange, might suggest that ATP itself is the prostetic group of the compound which acts as membrane-carrier. Since ATP in the free state does not discriminate measurably between K and Na, the specificity necessary might arise from the combination of ATP with, say, an enzyme-like protein. At least it is a fact that certain enzymes distinguish rather sharply between Na and K (see p. 10). The hypothesis outlined here is, however, so far without experimental proof.

2. Electron-linked carrier transport (LUNDEGARDH[292], CONWAY[326]). The fact that electrons can be shuttled along chains of electron carriers, giving rise to a definite, albeit small separation of the hydrogen ion and the hydroxyl formed in the cellular oxydation of hydrogen atoms, has inspired several workers to assume that chains of electron carriers are operative in active transport of ions. The possible applicability in acid secretion is immediately apparent, and LUNDEGARDH has devised a hypothetical scheme whereby electron transport could be exploited in anion transport in plant roots. This is not the place to discuss the merits and drawbacks of these models. It is evident that specific active transport of, for instance Na in the presence of K or vice versa cannot be the result of "simple" electron transport. CONWAY has proposed an intricate combination of electron transport and transport by membrane carrier. The implication is, however, that there exists a one-to-one relationship between the number of, say, Na ions trans-ported and the number of electrons carried from substrate to oxygen. However, the experiments by ZERAHN and by LEAF on isolated frog skins and toad urinary bladder have shown conclusively that more than one Na ion is transported for each equivalent of oxygen used (see p. 120). Also it is difficult to explain that in certain cases active Na transport can take place at the expense of ATP (squid nerve?) and that in many organs active transport is abolished by dinitrophenol poisoning (known to inhibit the formation of ATP) even though the oxygen consumption is augmented.

3. Propelled carrier transport (DANIELLI[327], GOLDACRE[328]). The hypotheses of this group assume that a complex between a membrane constituent and the transported ion is drawn through the membrane by the contraction of a con-tractile fibre. Such a mechanism might explain that ions and molecules, having themselves a low diffusion coefficient can be actively transported at a high rate.

---

[326] CONWAY, E. J.: The biochemistry of gastric acid secretion. 185 pp. Springfield, Ill.: Thomas 1953.

[327] DANIELLI, J. F.: Morphological and molecular aspects of active transport. Symp. Soc. exp. Biol. 8, 502—516 (1954).

[328] GOLDACRE, R. J., and I. J. LORCH: Folding and unfolding or protein molecules in relation to cytoplasmic streaming, amoeboid movement and osmotic work. Nature (Lond.) **166**, 497—500 (1950).

For the time being it seems that our knowledge about membrane structure and requirements for diffusion within it is too meagre to make the assumption of propelled transport imperative. In several cases it seems that the work necessary to overcome the internal resistance of the membrane must be rather limited since the electrochemical potential level to which ions can be lifted by active transport approaches the theoretical maximum (ZERAHN[280]). An interesting implication of the hypothetical propelled active transport is that accumulation on one side of the membrane may arise without chemical destruction of the binding sites.

In essence the hypothesis assumes that some macromolecule is alternating between an extended and a coiled state. The process of uncoiling involves breaking of bonds, thus releasing affinities which can be satisfied by the adsorption of molecules or ions. When the macromolecule is recoiled, the original bonds are reformed and the adsorbed ions are released.

4. "Asymmetrically collapsing lattice" theories. The proposal by BOWYER of a "onesidedly collapsing lattice" as being the operative in active transport exemplifies a group of hypotheses which assume the active transport to be brought about by a kind of "peristaltic wave" through the molecular lattice enclosing the substance to be transported (see [327]). Specificity would arise from mesh dimensions and possibly specific binding sites within the meshwork. Models of this type picture the active transport as a true mechanical ion pump. Although at the first sight the existence of an apparently fixed stoichiometric relationship between the oxygen used and the number of, say, sodium ions transported speaks in favour of the carrier hypotheses, a mechanical pump might have a more or less constant "stroke", transporting a relatively fixed number of ions. Conceptually the lattice specifically enclosing certain ionic species may be considered the negative image of a membrane carrier and on the molecular level the difference tends to vanish.

5. The fluid circuit mechanisms. The prototype of the fluid circuit mechanisms was proposed by INGRAHAM, PETERS and VISSCHER[329] to explain salt uptake in the gut. The net transport of salt was supposed to arise from the one way transport of a salt solution through a set of relatively large pores, and a transport in the opposite direction of more or less pure water through a set of narrow pores. As originally proposed the reason for the flow of solutions is left unexplained, but the authors pointed out that electroosmosis might be of importance as driving force. It is evident that it is hard to design a fluid circuit system with sufficient specificity to separate K and Na and other closely related pairs of substances. Thus, although solvent drag may play a role in intestinal transport, it is hard to assume that it is the principal force in salt transport in the gut or in other salt transporting organs. To operate the pumping of solvent through living membranes forces other than electroosmosis and simple osmosis may be invoked. Thus FRANCK and MAYER[330] have pointed out that if a substance goes through a polymerization-depolymetrization cycle within the cell or membrane, and granted that the two oppositely directed processes are spatially separated, an osmotic pressure gradient can be maintained which may be used for moving water or solutes. These authors also calculate the efficiency of such a solute circuit pump.

6. Pinocytosis. Pinocytosis consists in the uptake by cells of minute droplets of environmental fluid. The phenomenon is seen in unicellular organisms and some epithelial cells, especially as a response to high concentrations of proteins and salts.

---

[329] INGRAHAM, R. C., H. C. PETERS, and M. B. VISSCHER: On the movement of materials across living membranes against concentration gradients. J. phys. Chem. 42, 141—150 (1938).
[330] FRANCK, J., and J. E. MAYER: An osmotic diffusion pump. Arch. Biochem. 14, 297—313 (1947).

It is easily seen that the first step must lack specificity entirely. Thus the strict discrimination between closely related inorganic ions shown by most animal cells must rest upon another principle. In cells which do possess pinocytosis the phenomenon may influence the electrolyte balance, but it remains uncertain whether the pinocytosis suffices quantitatively to account for any appreciable fraction of the ionic exchange.

It is, however, conceptionally possible to visualize a gradual transition from the uptake of microscopic droplets via submicroscopic ones until the situation is reached which could more rationally be described by a mechanical molecular pump like the one called "one-sidedly collapsing lattice". No matter how the transport of small elements of solution is pictured, it remains hard to explain the coupled exchange of Na against K which seems characteristic of a large number of animal cells (p. 58).

B. Transport between cells and their surroundings

The importance of active transport for the distribution of K and Na between cells and their surroundings has been studied most extensively in three rather specialized cell types, viz. nerve- and muscle-fibres and erythrocytes. The evidence for the existence of a coupled Na—K-pump in these structures is quite convincing and will be given in detail below. For most other cell types the picture is not quite as clear. It seems that most cells must possess an active extrusion of Na in order to keep down the cellular concentration of this ion, but since the cell interior in practically all cells studied is distinctly negative relative to the medium, the high cellular K concentration might well be the result of the potential difference (a kind of Donnan distribution, compare chapter VI.b on the state of K in living cells). Nevertheless several pieces of evidence do point to the possibility that the coupled Na—K-pump is widely distributed among animal cells. It is, however, by no means certain that there is in general a one-to-one coupling between active transport of Na and of K. Thus in the acidification of the urine in the kidney tubules it seems as if hydrogen ions can be used as a substitute for K in the active exchange against Na (see part II).

In evaluating the experiments with isolated cells and tissues it must be remembered that almost any kind of cell damage is known to lead to a loss of K and a more or less equivalent uptake of Na. This phenomenon is often seen in cases of reversible traumata within the body (see part II). In particular, however, removal of tissues from an animal usually leads to the above mentioned electrolyte shift. Thus many freshly isolated tissues and tissue slices are decidedly abnormal with respect to their Ka and Na concentrations. In some tissues the damage seems practically irreparable. Thus KREBS et al.[331] found that slices of guinea pig liver and pigeon liver as well as pigeon gizzard and pigeon pancreas were unable to maintain normal K—Na-distribution with any combination of substrates. In several tissues, however, more or less complete recovery can take place, especially if proper substrates are offered. With respect to the beneficial effect of added substrates cells vary widely. Some types like striated muscle normally have an ample supply of glycogen and are, on the other hand, rather impermeable to several substrates which consequently are of minor value. Other tissues like brain and kidney combine a rapid ion-exchange with a very limited store of "fuel", and in such tissues substrates, notably members of the tricarboxylic acid cycle, often accelerate the ion transport.

---

[331] KREBS, H. A., L. V. EGGLESTON, and C. TERNER: In vitro measurements of the turnover rate of potassium in brain and retina. Biochem. J. 48, 530—537 (1951).

It is not uncommon that tissues which cannot restore the cellular electrolytes to normal in physiological saline, will do so if a higher than normal K concentration is offered in the medium. Thus rat liver slices require as much as 34 mM K in the medium to maintain the normal cellular level of this ion (see below).

It is worth remembering that certain tissues like epithelia and glandular tissue are composed of asymmetrical cells which, while maintaining their internal electrolyte composition, perform active transport of certain ions from one boundary to the other (see p. 112). Thus the bathing fluid and also often the electric potential are normally different at the two faces of the cell. When such tissues are studied in isolation, for instance in the form of tissue slices, their electric asymmetry is short-circuited by the medium and both faces are now in contact with identical solutions. Thus their electrolyte balance may be severely offset. Actually, the fact that certain glandular and epithelial tissues can maintain practically normal electrolyte composition in isolation and in the form of slices calls for an explanation, the most likely one being that the one of the cellular faces (probably the normal blood side) is much more permeable than the other to water and diffusible ions, so that osmotic and ionic equilibrium is always maintained with respect to this side. The electrical and chemical "short-circuiting" does, however, put a severe strain upon the metabolic machinery which "attempts" to maintain the physiological asymmetry with respect to potential and ion distribution (see p. 120).

a) Erythrocytes

Introduction. Until relatively recently it was generally held that erythrocytes were impermeable to the alkali metal ions, and to practically all other cations with the exception of the hydrogen and ammonium ions. It was also believed that the erythrocytes, especially the non-nucleated ones of the mammals, were essentially dead, and the impermeability to cations thus was the necessary and sufficient condition for maintaining at the same time a cation composition which was different from that of the plasma and a high permeability to small anions like Cl and HCO_3. Among the first to demonstrate that K can be lost and regained by erythrocytes were HENRIQUES and ØRSKOV[332] who showed that lead injected into the blood of rabbits made the erythrocytes loose K, and that K was regained by the red cells as the lead ions disappeared from the circulation.

It was, however, the introduction of radioactive tracers in the study of cell permeability which made it clear that a constant although not very rapid exchange of cations is going on across the red cell surface. Thus COHN and COHN[333] showed that the Na of dog red cells exchanged with Na^{24} injected into the blood stream, and MULLINS, FENN, NOONAN and HAEGE[334] as well as HAHN and HEVESY[335] found the same to be true in the case of rabbit red cells. The exchangeability of K in the rabbit red cells was first demonstrated by HEVESY and HAHN[336].

[332] HENRIQUES, V., and S. L. ØRSKOV: Untersuchungen über die Schwankungen des Kationengehaltes der roten Blutkörperchen II. Änderung des Kaliumgehaltes der Blutkörperchen bei Bleivergiftung. Skand. Arch. Physiol. 74, 78—85 (1936).

[333] COHN, W. E., and E. T. COHN: Permeability of red corpuscles of the dog to sodium-ion. Proc. Soc. exp. Biol. (N. Y.) 41, 445—449 (1939).

[334] MULLINS, L. J., W. O. FENN, T. R. NOONAN, and L. HAEGE: Permeability of erythrocytes to radioactive potassium. Amer. J. Physiol. 135, 93—101 (1941).

[335] HAHN, L., and G. HEVESY: Rate of penetration of ions into erythrocytes. Acta physiol. scand. 3, 193—223 (1942).

[336] HEVESY, G., and L. HAHN: Exchange of cellular potassium. Kgl. danske Vidensk. selsk. Biol. Medd. 16, 1—27 (1941).

At about the same time it was found by DANOWSKI[337] and by HARRIS[338] that red cells would lose K and gain Na when stored in the cold but that this process could be reversed if the cells were incubated at 37° with glucose. Also mono-iodoacetic acid poisoning led to a reversible loss of K and gain of Na.

In the years that have passed since these discoveries the cation transports across the red cell membrane have been studied vigorously by several groups. Valuable reviews and discussions of the pertinent literature have been written by SHEPPARD[339], PARPART and HOFFMAN[340], SOLOMON[300], MAIZELS[341], HARRIS[342], TOSTESON[244] and GLYNN[343]. Red cells of various species have turned out to handle the alkali metal ions in rather different ways. In some species, like for instance the dog, the red cells have a cation composition which is not very different from that of the plasma; that is: the dominating cation is Na and the K concentration is only a few mM/l. In this species the dominating process in the cation transport across the membrane seems to be ordinary ("simple") diffusion. In most species, however, K is the predominant internal ion whereas the Na concentration is quite low. Present information speaks strongly in favour of active transport inward of K as well as active transport outward of Na as being responsible for this distribution of the cations. One alternative hypothesis, namely that the cell contains sufficient specific binding sites for K and at the same time a structure such that Na ions would enter in low concentrations only, is not tenable. As well known, the red cells behave like almost ideal osmometers, and calculations show that all K has to be free in order to give the internal osmotic pressure required. As a matter of fact, there is no indication that any of the major components of red cells (notably hemoglobin) bind potassium (compare p. 9).

At one time it was proposed that the red cells possessed one active transport mechanism only, namely one expelling Na (MAIZELS[344]). If such were the case, K would have to be kept from leaving by an electric potential difference, arising as a consequence of the active Na transport. A direct measurement of the intra-cellular potential of red cells has not been performed as yet. From the equilibrium distribution ratio of chloride ions between red cells and the medium it is, however, possible to estimate the potential (HODGKIN[345,346]). If the ratio of cell to plasma chloride concentrations (per kg water) is 0.8 and it is assumed that the activity coefficient for chloride is the same on both sides of the membrane, the potential difference works out to be $(RT/F) \log_e 0.8 = -6 \, \text{mV}$, the cell interior being negative relative to the medium. This small potential can by no means account for the potassium concentration ratio cell/medium of about 35 in normal human cells.

[337] DANOWSKI, T. S.: The transfer of potassium across the human blood cell membrane. J. biol. Chem. 139, 693—705 (1941).

[338] HARRIS, E. J.: The influence of metabolism of human erythrocytes on their potassium content. J. biol. Chem. 141, 579—595 (1941).

[339] SHEPPARD, C. W.: New developments in potassium and cell physiology: 1940—1950. Science 114, 85—91 (1951).

[340] PARPART, A. K., and J. F. HOFFMAN: Ion permeability of the red cell. In: Ion transport across membranes, pp. 69—74. Ed. by H. T. CLARKE. New York: Acad. Press. 1954.

[341] MAIZELS, M.: Active cation transport in erythrocytes. Symp. Soc. exper. Biol. 8, 202—227 (1954).

[342] HARRIS, E. J.: Linkage of sodium- and potassium-active transport in human erythrocytes. Symp. Soc. exp. Biol. 8, 228—241 (1954).

[343] GLYNN, I. M.: The ionic permeability of the red cell membrane. Progr. in Biophysics 8, 241—307 (1957).

[344] MAIZELS, M.: Cation control in human erythrocytes. J. Physiol. 108, 247—263 (1949).

[345] HODGKIN, A. L.: The ionic basis of electrical activity in nerve and muscle. Biol. Rev. Cambridge Phil. Soc. 26, 339—409 (1957).

[346] DAVSON, H.: A textbook of general physiology, pp. 659. Blakiston: Churchill 1951.

Thus both K and Na have to be transported actively in red cells of the species having high K content.

Under normal conditions red cells are neither gaining nor losing cation. The situation is thus characterized by the fact that the active uptake of K is balanced by an equally large loss, just as the Na extrusion is countered by an inward transport of the same amount of Na.

The hypothesis has been advanced (SOLOMON[300]) that both the "uphill" transports, that is K in and Na out, and the "downhill" transports (K out and Na in) are due to specific carrier systems. A simpler hypothesis (HARRIS[342]), is that the "downhill" processes are due to simple diffusion, whereas the "uphill" transports are performed by a single carrier system which transports Na actively in the outward direction and K or H^+ actively in the inward direction. In a summary way one may visualize the active transport as being brought about by the fact that the membrane carrier can exist in two forms one with a high affinity for K and another with a high affinity for Na. The "Na-modification" is formed by a reaction taking place at the inner boundary of the membrane. When this modification — loaded with Na — arrives at the outer boundary it is changed into the "K-modification" and has to release its Na and take up K. When the "K-modification" reaches the inner boundary the cycle is completed by the re-formation of the "Na-modification" and the release of K. The arguments for assuming one system pumping both Na and K rather than two independent pumps will be discussed below. The way in which this cycle is "geared" to the metabolism is not known in detail, but it is known that it can be driven, and in the mammalian red cell is solely driven, by glycolysis, compare MAIZELS[347, 341]. As the glycolysis scheme contains fewer elements and is generally much simpler than respiration, the red cell system must be considered favourable as an object for studying the relation between active cation transport and metabolism (see p. 60), and much promising work has been done in this field.

The study of the relationship between metabolic energy and transport work has led to the interesting finding that, in duck red cells, TOSTESON and ROBERTSON[283] but not in mammalian cells, the K ion exhibits rapid exchange diffusion (see p. 50), that is: the influx of K derives all or most of the necessary energy for overcoming the concentration difference from the simultaneous outflux of the same ionic species and not from the metabolism (see below).

1. Transport of potassium in human erythrocytes

Human red cells have a K concentration of about 140 mM/kg cell water, whereas the Na concentration is 15 mM/kg water. When suspended in blood plasma the intracellular K is exchanging with the extracellular K at a rate which is approximately 1.6 mM/hr per (liter blood cells) at 37°. A more recent, and probably more accurate figure for the steady state flux of K at 37° is 2.1 mM/hr per liter blood (STREETEN and SOLOMON[348]). [It should be noticed that in most papers dealing with erythrocytes the exchange rates and flux values are expressed per liter red cells rather than per unit area of membrane (RAKER et al.[349], SHEPPARD and MARTIN[350], SOLOMON[300]).] It is an interesting fact that the steady

[347] MAIZELS, M.: Factors in the active transport of cations. J. Physiol. 112, 59—83 (1951).
[348] STREETEN, D. H. P., and A. K. SOLOMON: The effect of ACTH and adrenal steroids on K transport in human erythrocytes. J. gen. Physiol. 37, 643—661 (1954).
[349] RAKER, J. W., I. M. TAYLOR, J. M. WELLER, and A. B. HASTINGS: Rate of potassium exchange of the human erythrocyte. J. gen. Physiol. 33, 691—702 (1950).
[350] SHEPPARD, C. W., and W. R. MARTIN: Cation exchange between cells and plasma of mammalian blood. J. gen. Physiol. 33, 703—722 (1950).

state in- and outflux of K are smaller than the Na fluxes which under similar conditions are 3.0 mM/l cells per hour (SHEPPARD, MARTIN and BEYL[351], SOLOMON[300]).

It has been shown that if the K concentration of the medium is varied, the influx of K exhibits saturation kinetics (see Fig. 3). It is seen that at very low outside K concentrations, the K influx increases violently with increasing K

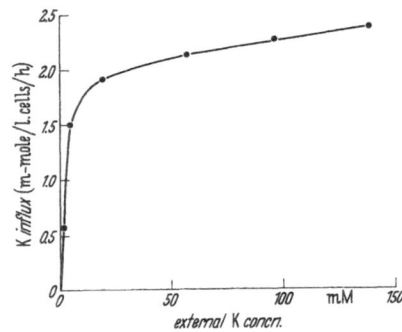

concentraton but that when the K concentration approaches the normal physiological level of 4 mM the rate of increase is strongly reduced and was for some years assumed to be nearly non-variant with respect to the K concentration.

According to TOSTESON, compare also STREETEN et al.[348] and GLYNN[343], however, the K influx shows a significant increase with outside K concentration over the range from 4 mM to 140 mM. The shape of the curve can be explained in the light of the hypothesis (HARRIS[342], TOSTESON[244]) that the influx of K is due to two independent processes: 1) An active trans-

Fig. 3. Dependence of K. influx upon external K concentration in human red cells (after GLYNN[351a])

port process which is carrier-limited and reaches its maximum (saturation) rate at about 4 mM K in the plasma, and 2) a process of passive diffusion which is proportional to the outside K concentration.

Following the treatment of TOSTESON[244] which is also closely related to that used by HARRIS[342] we can write:

$$^0M_K = {}^0k_K \, [K]_c \qquad (14)$$

where ^0M_K is the K outflux, ^0k_K the outward rate constant for K transport, and $[K]_c$ is the cellular K concentration, and

$$^iM_K = {}^i_aM_K + {}^i_dk_K \, [K]_m \qquad (15)$$

where ^iM_K is the influx, $^i_dk_K$ is the inward rate constant for K diffusion, $^i_aM_K$ the active transport flux of K, and $[K]_m$ the K concentration in the medium.

For a passively diffusing ion we have, however (USSING[242]), that the flux ratio (influx/outflux) is independent of the membrane structure and equal to $(c_i/c_0) \exp(EzF/RT)$, where E is the electric potential difference across the membrane. If chloride ions are supposed to be in equilibrium in the red cells, we have

$$[Cl]_c/[Cl]_m = \exp(EzF/RT) \, , \qquad (16)$$

thus by substitution of (16) into (15), we obtain

$$^iM_K = {}^i_aM_K + {}^0k_K \, [K]_c \cdot [[Cl]_m/[Cl]_c] \, . \qquad (17)$$

The K exchange (and thus presumably the outflux) is roughly proportional to the intracellular K conc. (SHEPPARD, MARTIN and BEYL[351], see also RAKER[349] et al.) Since, however, it is impossible to lower the cellular K conc. without changing the system, no safe conclusions can be drawn from these observations.

[351] SHEPPARD, C. W., W. R. MARTIN, and G. BEYL: Cation exchange between cells and plasma of mammalian blood. II. Sodium and potassium exchange in the sheep, dog, cow and man. J. gen. Physiol. **34**, 411—429 (1951).

[351a] GLYNN, I. M.: The action of cardiac glycosides on sodium and potassium movements in human red cells. J. Physiol. 1957, 148—173.

Introducing the appropriate figures from his own and other published experiments, TOSTESON finds that the K influx (in millimoles/liter red cells) can be expressed by the equation

$$^iM_K = 1.9 + 0.017 \, [K]_m \, , \tag{18}$$

whereas the outflux is

$$^0M_K = 0.014 \, [K]_c \, . \tag{19}$$

These figures apply to red cell systems at p_H 7.4 and with an adequate supply of glucose. Under such conditions influx and outflux of K are about equal at all but the very lowest medium concentrations of K. During prolonged exposures to high K, the cells do, however, show a net uptake of this ion. When the medium K concentration is 130 mM the cells hemolyze in 24 hours. From the rate of net gain of K, TOSTESON calculates an inward rate constant of K diffusion of 0.018, in good agreement with the value of 0.017 given above.

In the absence of glucose the potassium influx is strongly reduced, and it is characteristic that the reduction concerns only the "saturable" part of the influx (the active transport) whereas the linear fraction retains its slope (GLYNN[352]).

2. Transport of sodium in human erythrocytes

The influx of Na into the red cells according to HARRIS[342] seems to be proportional to the Na concentration between 150 and 75 mM/l, if osmotic equilibrium is maintained by the addition of an appropriate non-penetrating substance like choline chloride or sugar.

According to SOLOMON (1952) the sodium influx can be described by the equation

$$^iM_{Na} = 0.72 + 0.19 \, [Na]_m \, . \tag{20}$$

Since, however, the low Na concentrations were brought about by replacing Na by sugar, the cells must have lost Cl and gained OH (DAVSON[353], compare also HARRIS[342], TOSTESON[244]). Now, as we have seen, the Cl concentration ratio defines the potential difference across the membrane as well as the cellular p_H, and both of these factors are bound to influence the sodium flux. Thus the relationship found by SOLOMON between influx and medium concentration of Na does not speak against the assumption that Na enters the cell by simple diffusion, assisted by the small potential difference, and that the influx can be described by the equation:

$$^iM_{Na} = {}^ik_{Na} \, [Na]_m \, , \tag{21}$$

in analogy with the outflux of K which was also taken to be due to diffusion.

TOSTESON gives the value of 0.020 for $^ik_{Na}$, thus the Na influx is

$$^iM_{Na} = 0.020 \, [Na]_m \, . \tag{22}$$

From the rate constant for inward diffusion, $^ik_{Na}$, the rate constant for outward diffusion, $^0_d k_{Na}$, can be determined by the equation:

$$^0_d k_{Na} = {}^ik_{Na} \, ([Cl]_c / [Cl]_m) \tag{23}$$

in analogy with the procedure used to relate the outward and inward diffusion constants for K.

[352] GLYNN, I. M.: Sodium and potassium movements in human red cells. J. Physiol. **134**, 278—310 (1956).
[353] DAVSON, H.: Studies on the permeability of erythrocytes. VI. The effect of reducing the salt content of the medium surrounding the cell. Biochem. J. **33**, 389—401 (1939).

The outflux of Na, however, differs from the influx of K in being roughly proportional to the concentration in the solution of origin (HARRIS and MAIZELS[354]). One can thus write

$$^0M_{Na} = {^0k_{Na}} \ [Na]_c \ . \tag{24}$$

Of this flux a certain fraction arises from simple diffusion, namely [from eq. (23)]

$$_d^0M_{Na} = {^ik_{Na}} \ ([Cl]_c/[Cl]_m) \ [Na]_c \ . \tag{25}$$

The remaining and usually by far the larger part of the Na outflux then must be due to active transport. Thus:

$$_a^0M_{Na} = {_a^0k_{Na}} \ [Na]_c = {^0M_{Na}} - {_d^0M_{Na}} \ . \tag{26}$$

The linear relationship between active transport of Na and cellular Na concentration must be accepted with some reserve since the preparation of cells with a higher than normal Na content implies the treatment with metabolic poisons, lack of glucose or low temperature. It seems to be safe to say, however, that the sodium active transport system is not saturated even at the highest cellular Na concentrations tested, whereas the K active transport system (carrying K inward) is saturated at an outside K concentration of a few mM/l.

On the basis of the available evidence it cannot be excluded that part of the Na exchange is due to exchange diffusion.

3. Effect of p_H on the Na transport

According to HARRIS and MAIZELS[355] both influx and outflux of Na are independent of p_H between p_H 7 and 7.5. Below this region, both decrease, notably the outflux, and the cells gain Na. Above p_H 7.5, both influx and outflux increase, but the influx more so than the outflux, and again the cellular Na increases. As a consequence of these conditions the cellular Na concentration is at a minimum at about neutral solution. The active transport component of the outflux seems to have its maximum about p_H 7.4.

4. Effect of temperature

Like the inward and outward transports of K, the Na transports have high apparent activation energies. Thus for Na influx the values range about 20,000 cal/mole, whereas for outflux the value is about 15,000 cal/mole (RAKER et al.[349], SHEPPARD et al.[350], SOLOMON[300]). The fact that the apparent activation energies for both influx and outflux are so high has been taken as indication that the influx as well as outflux are due to active processes and not to diffusion, but as already discussed under the transport of K high apparent activation energies can also be found for passive processes.

As it can be seen from the numerical values of the apparent activation energies, low temperature ought to lead to a decrease in cellular Na. It is well known, however, that the opposite is the case. The cells gain Na and loose K at low temperatures. Obviously, then, the activation energy for outflux must be greater than that for influx. This only goes to show that the technical difficulties in evaluating the apparent activation energies are considerable.

---

[354] HARRIS, E. J., and M. MAIZELS: Distribution of ions in suspensions of human erythrocytes. J. Physiol. 118, 40—53 (1952).

[355] HARRIS, E. J., and M. MAIZELS: The permeability of human erythrocytes to sodium. J. Physiol. 113, 506—524 (1951).

Perhaps the most serious difficulty is that all cellular Na does not exchange with the same rate (see SHEPPARD[350], SOLOMON[300], GOLD and SOLOMON[356]). It is clear that this fact makes the determination of the Na fluxes somewhat arbitrary until the nature and location of the small slowly exchanging Na fraction has been cleared up. At present one can only say that both the passive diffusion and the active transport of Na through the red cell membrane have high temperature coefficient, but that that for the active transport is the higher one.

5. Transport of Li, in human erythrocytes

Li is found in human blood in very low concentration. According to BERT-RAND[357] one l human blood contains 19 micrograms of Li, of which 15 are found in the plasma and 4 in the corpuscles. Calculated on the water phase of the plasma this gives approximately 30 micrograms per liter against 16 micrograms per liter red cell water phase. The concentration ratio (cell water/plasma water) of two may be taken to mean that Li is being expelled by the cells, but less effectively than Na. This is in accord with the fact that cells swell appreciably when Li replaces two thirds of the extracellular Na (SOLOMON[300]). About 2.23 meq Li enters one liter cells per hour from a solution containing 95 meq. Li/liter. This gives a rate constant for Li influx which is slightly lower than that for Na. Similar results have been obtained by MAIZELS[341]. The reason for the swelling of the cells evidently is that active transport in the outward direction of Li is rather ineffective (HARRIS and MAIZELS[355]). The active transport mechanism is probably identical with that transporting Na but conclusive evidence for this hypothesis is still lacking. Li does not compete for influx with the K transport system. Li influx undoubtedly is due to simple diffusion.

6. Transport of Rb in human erythrocytes

As in most other biological systems, Rb behaves in the red cell almost like K. According to SOLOMON[300] Rb competes on equal terms with K for transport in the carrier-limited active transport system (see also LOVE and BURCH[358]). Neither is its passive diffusion constant for transport out of the cells significantly different from that of potassium.

7. Transport of Cs in human erythrocytes

Cs penetrates very slowly indeed into the red cells. Apparently it enters via the same carrier system as K and Rb (LOVE and BURCH[358], SOLOMON[300], TOSTESON and DUNHAM[359]), but the affinity for the system seems to be only 1/5 of that of K. The outflux of Cs presumably is due to diffusion only. The rate constant for outflux is about 60% of that of K.

8. Evidence for a coupling between active sodium extrusion and potassium uptake

The hypothesis (HARRIS[342], compare also GLYNN[360]) that the Na and K active transports are coupled and probably mediated by a single carrier system derives

---

[356] GOLD, G. L., and A. K. SOLOMON: The transport of sodium into human erythrocytes in vivo. J. gen. Physiol. **38**, 389—404 (1955).

[357] BERTRAND, D.: Sur la repartition du lithium du sang entre le plasma et les globules. Bull. Soc. Chim. biol. **33**, 827—828 (1951).

[358] LOVE, W. D., and G. E. BURCH: Chloride exchange between human erythrocytes and plasma studied with Cl[36]. Proc. Soc. exp. Biol. (N. Y.) **82**, 131—133 (1953).

[359] TOSTESON, D. C., and E. T. DUNHAM: Effect of sickling on sodium and cesium transport. Fed. Proc. **13**, 523 (1954).

[360] GLYNN, I. M.: Linked sodium and potassium movements in human red cells. J. Physiol. **126**, 35 P (1954).

support from several observations. 1) The K influx is high in cells which are expelling Na at a high rate (MAIZELS[347], PONDER[361]). 2) The active Na-outflux is very much reduced when the K concentration of the medium is below a certain level (ca. 1 mmolar) (HARRIS and MAIZELS[354], SOLOMON[300]). Finally 3) the active extrusion of Na and the uptake of K seem to depend on the same metabolic factors (compare MAIZELS[347], MAIZELS[341]).

The fact remains, however, that the apparent active transport rate for Na is always larger than that for K. HARRIS gives 3/2 as the ratio between the active fluxes of Na and K. Thus for each time the hypothetical carrier transports out 3 Na ions, it must return with two potassium ions and, maybe, with one hydrogen ion. It is possible, however, that part of the Na-exchange is due to exchange-diffusion. If so, the true active Na transport might still equal the active transport of K.

Although the coupling between Na and K active transport cannot be considered as proven beyond doubt, its existence seems very likely, the more so since a coupled active K—Na exchange is indicated in several other cell types such as muscle (STEINBACH[362]), nerve (HODGKIN and KEYNES[363]) and frog skin (KOEFOED-JOHNSEN and USSING[364]).

9. Relation of the active and passive transports to metabolism

As is well known mammalian red cells have an extremely low respiration rate whereas they glycolyze at an appreciable rate. One liter of cells at $37°$ and p_H 7.5 metabolize 1.5 mM glucose to lactic acid in one hour (RAKER et al.[349]). It is therefore not surprising that changing the gas composition from O_2 to N_2 does not effect the rate of action transport of K and Na (RAKER et al.[349], SOLOMON[300], TOSTESON[244]).

The cation transport can be energized by glucose, mannose and fructose, but not by pyruvate and lactate (MAIZELS[347]). Removal of glucose from the medium reduces K influx without appreciably changing the outflux in normal cells (GLYNN) and in cells from patients with sickle cell anemia (TOSTESON, CARLSEN and DUNHAM[365]). It is thus apparent that the active ion transport of red cells is associated with glycolysis. This view is also supported by work with metabolic inhibitors.

Thus iodoacetate and fluoride ions[366, 367, 368, 369, 370, 371, 372] both of which inhibit glycolysis are also powerful inhibitors of active cation transport in red

[361] PONDER, E.: Accumulation of potassium by human red cells. J. gen. Physiol. **33**, 745—757 (1950).

[362] STEINBACH, H. B.: On the sodium and potassium balance of isolated frog muscles. Proc. nat. Acad. Sci. (Wash.) **38**, 451—455 (1952).

[363] HODGKIN, A. L., and R. D. KEYNES: Sodium extrusion and potassium absorption in Sepia axons. J. Physiol. **120**, 46 P (1953).

[364] KOEFOED-JOHNSON, V., and H. H. USSING: The nature of the frog skin potential. Acta physiol. scand. (1958) **42**, 298—308 (1958).

[365] TOSTESON, D. C., E. CARLSEN, and E. T. DUNHAM: The effect of sickling on ion transport. 1. Effekt of sickling on potassium transport. J. gen. Physiol. **39**, 31—53 (1956).

[366] LOVE, W. D., J. A. CRONVICK, and G. E. BURCH: Mechanisms controlling cation concentrations in the human cell. Evidence from the effect of iodoacetate on Na and K exchange rates of the erythrocytes. J. clin. Invest. **34**, 61—66 (1955).

[367] GREEN, J. W., and A. K. PARPART: The effect of metabolic poisons on potassium loss from rabbit red cells. J. cell. comp. Physiol. **42**, 191—202 (1953).

[368] DUNKER, E., and H. PASSOW: Verteilung von Anionen und Kationen bei Fluorid-vergiftung menschlicher Erythrocyten. Pflügers Arch. ges. Physiol. **252**, 542—550 (1950).

[369] WILBRANDT, W.: Die Abhängigkeit der Ionenpermeabilität der Erythrocyten vom glycolytischen Stoffwechsel. Pflügers Arch. ges. Physiol. **243**, 519—539 (1940).

[370] FLYNN, F., and M. MAIZELS: Cation control in human erythrocytes. J. Physiol. **110**, 301—318 (1949).

cells. The effect of these two agents is complex, however. In low concentration they inhibit glycolysis and active ion transport. Higher concentrations also change the diffusion characteristics of the membrane so that the passive diffusion of Na and notably K is augmented.

Thus when human cells are suspended in 30 mmolar fluoride they will shrink due to a loss of K without concomitant uptake of Na (WILBRANDT[373], DUNKER and PASSOW[368]). Similar observations were made on rabbit cells by DAVSON[374].

Metabolic poisons which do not inhibit glycolysis seem to be without effect on active ion transport in red cells. Thus cyanide, 2—4-dinitrophenol, malonate azide and carbon monoxide fail to affect the reaccumulation of K and extrusion of Na in cells which have been depleted of K and have gained Na during storage in the cold (MAIZELS[347]). Inhibitors of carbonic anhydrase also are without effect on the active transport.

LINDVIG, GREIG and PETERSON[375] have found that acetylcholine in a concentration of 10^{-2} M decreases the influx of Na and K in red cells and delays hemolysis in isotonic $NaHCO_3$ solution. Other esters (like, for instance, triacetin) which are split by erythrocyte cholinesterase have the same effect (GREIG and HOLLAND[376]). Acetyl choline also gives rise to a small net gain of K in cells suspended in $NaHCO_3$ and in NaCl. PARPART and HOFFMANN[340] have pointed out, however, that the effect of acetylcholine may be due to the reduction of cellular p_H produced by the splitting of this compound. The relation of acetyl choline and acetyl cholinesterase to the active transport of cations in red cells thus remains uncertain.

Many lytic agents (alcohols, dyes, etc.) bring about K loss and Na gain prior to hemolysis (PONDER[377, 378, 379, 380]).

10. Effects of cardiac glucosides on the transport processes

SCHATZMANN[381] was the first to observe the powerful inhibitory effect of cardiac glucosides (Strophanthin etc.) and their aglucones (Strophanthidin, Digitoxigenin) upon the expulsion of sodium and reaccumulation of potassium in red cells which had previously been exposed to storage in the cold. Since then the

[371] TAYLOR, I. M., J. M. WELLER, and A. B. HASTINGS: Effect of cholinesterase and choline acetylase inhibitors on the potassium concentration gradient and potassium exchaneg of human erythrocytes. Amer. J. Physiol. 168, 658—665 (1952).

[372] ECKEL, R. E.: Effect of fluoride on potassium permeability in human erythrocytes in vitro. Amer. J. Physiol. 179, 632 (1954).

[373] WILBRANDT, W.: A relation between the permeability of the red cell and its metabolism. Trans. Faraday Soc. 33, 956—959 (1937).

[374] DAVSON, H.: The effect of some metabolic poisons on the permeability of the rabbit erythrocyte to potassium. J. cell. comp. Physiol. 18, 173—185 (1941).

[375] LINDVIG, P. E., M. E. GREIG, and S. W. PETERSON: Studies on Permeability. V. The effect of acetylcholine and physostigmin on the permeability of human erythrocytes to sodium and potassium. Arch. Biochem. 30, 241—250 (1951).

[376] GREIG, M. E., and W. C. HOLLAND: Studies on permeability of erythrocytes. IV. Effect of certain choline and non-choline esters on permeability of dog erythrocytes. Amer. J. Physiol. 164, 423—427 (1951).

[377] PONDER, E.: The prolytic loss of K from human red cells. J. gen. Physiol. 30, 235—246 (1947).

[378] PONDER, E.: Prolytic ion exchanges produced in human red cells by methanol, ethanol, guaiacol and resorcinol. J. gen. Physiol. 30, 479—491 (1947).

[379] PONDER, E.: K—Na exchange accompanying the prolytic loss of K from human red cells. J. gen. Physiol. 30, 379—387 (1947).

[380] PONDER, E.: The permiability of human red cells to cations after treatment with resorcinol, n-butyl alcohol, and similar lysins. J. gen Physiol. 32, 53—62 (1949).

[381] SCHATZMANN, H. J.: Herzglykoside als Hemmstoffe für den aktiven Kalium- und Natriumtransport durch die Erythrocytenmembran. Helv. physiol. Acta 11, 346—354 (1953).

phenomenon has been studied extensively [382], [383], [384], [385], [386], [387], [388] and results similar to those of SCHATZMANN have been obtained with a series of different cardiac glucosides.

Since the glucosides prevent the active transport of K and Na, they might seem to be specific inhibitors of the ion transport itself or of the energizing mechanism. With respect to the latter possibility it has been demonstrated that they do not inhibit glycolysis (SCHATZMANN [382]) and do not interfere with the formation of ATP (WHITTAM [389]). Thus it would seem that they must act upon the reaction by which ATP is utilized in the active transport process. There are, however, certain facts which are hard to reconcile with this hypothesis. Thus, according to GLYNN [384], [385] digitoxin and scillaren inhibit the passive sodium and potassium fluxes as well as the active ones. He therefore concludes that these drugs interfere with the carrier mechanisms, the implication being that closely related carrier molecules are responsible for all the K and Na fluxes through the membrane, no matter whether the transport is passive or active.

Certainly, there seems to be no reason why carrier molecules which are "idling" should not catalyze a certain passive flow of ions. The passive cation-permeability of red cells would then be in principle different from, say, the passive potassium permeability of muscle cells where the permeability seems associated with "pores". This might be the reason why the heart poisons hit the active cation transport in heart muscle and striated muscle, but do not prevent the passive loss by these cells of potassium.

The strong effect of the heart poisons upon erythrocytes is in striking contrast to the feeble action of adrenal steroids upon these cells (STREETEN and SOLOMON [390], SCHATZMANN [382], GLYNN [385]). The latter author advances the hypothesis that in organs where the mineralocorticoids do act (kidney, tubule, sweat glands, etc.) they do so by being converted into substances related to the cardiac aglucones.

11. Ion transport by red cell "ghosts"

Red cells which have been lysed and have lost most of their hemoglobin by exposure to hypotonic solution are still capable of active transport of K (and Na) when returned under suitable conditions to normal shape in blood-isotonic solution (STRAUB [391], GÁRDOS [392]). Thus, the membrane of the cells possesses the

[382] SCHATZMANN, H. J.: Die Wirkung von Desoxycorticosteron auf den aktiven Kationenaustausch an Rattenblutzellen. Experientia (Basel) 10, 189—190 (1954).

[383] JOYCE, C. R. B., and M. WEATHERALL: Cardiac glycosides and the potassium exchange of human erythrocytes. J. Physiol. 127, 33 P (1955).

[384] GLYNN, I. M.: The action of cardiac glycosides on red cells. J. Physiol. 128, 56—57 P (1955).

[385] GLYNN, I. M.: The action of cardiac glycosides on sodium and potassium movements in human red cells. J. Physiol. 136, 148—173 (1957).

[386] KAHN JR., J. B., and G. H. ACHESON: Effects of cardiac glucosides and other lactones and of certain other compounds on cation transfer in human erythrocytes. J. Pharmacol. 115, 305—318 (1955).

[387] HARRIS, E. J., and T. A. J. PRANKERD: The rate of sodium extrusion from human erythrocytes. J. Physiol. 121, 470—486 (1953).

[388] SOLOMON, A. K., T. J. GILL, and G. L. GOLD: Effect of cardiac glycosides on potassium transport in human red cells. Fed. Proc. 15, 174 (1956).

[389] WHITTAM, R. in: GLYNN, J. M.: The ionic permeability of the red cell membrane. Progress in Biophysics, 8, 241—307 (1957).

[390] STREETEN, D. H. P., and A. K. SOLOMON: The effect of ACTH and adrenal steroids on potassium transport in human erythrocytes. J. gen. Physiol. 37, 643—661 (1954).

[391] STRAUB, F. B.: Über die Akkumulation der Kaliumionen durch menschliche Blutkörperchen. Acta physiol. Hung. 4, 235—240 (1954).

[392] GÁRDOS, G.: Akkumulation der Kaliumionen durch menschliche Blutkörperchen. Acta physiol. Hung. 6, 191—199 (1954).

remarkable property of being able to close the "holes" through which the hemo-globin escapes during the lysis.

During the lysis not only hemoglobin but also coenzymes, substrates etc. can pass in and out through the cell membrane. Thus it is a necessary condition for reconstitution of the active transport of cations that the appropriate diffusible cell constituents are included in the hemolysis fluid.

The reconstituted cells are able to accumulate potassium at the expense of glycolysis just like ordinary red cells. Such "ghosts" whose content of co-factors and substrates can be varied within wide limits provide an excellent object for the study of the relation between metabolism and active transport. Thus STRAUB demonstrated that if the formation by the metabolism of ATP was inhibited there was no active cation transport. GÁRDOS actually demonstrated that if suitable amounts of ATP were introduced into the cells during the permeable period, the cells accumulate K in the absence of substrate.

12. Mechanism of the active transport

Based on his studies of the effect of metabolic inhibitors MAIZELS[341] made the suggestion that the ion transport in red cells is somehow associated with the consumption of energy-rich phosphate bonds. He also pointed out that under normal conditions the active ion transport requires a minimum of somewhat less than 10% of the energy released by glycolysis. If, however, we consider the stoichiometry of the situation, it appears that the fraction of the metabolism concerned with ion transport must be quite large, as the following calculation may show.

For one liter cells in one hour at $37°$ and p_H 7.5 we have:

glucose glycolyzed:	1.5 mmoles
active Na transport:	3.0 mmoles
active K transport:	2.0 mmoles

Each glucose molecule is split into two molecules of lactic acid, with a net yield of two energy-rich phosphate bonds. 1.5 mmoles glucose thus yields 3 mmoles ATP. Now, if ATP or some other energy-rich phosphate participates in the transport process there must be at least one energy-rich phosphate bond split for each cycle of the carrier system. If the carrier binds only one cation and if, further, K and Na are transported by independent carriers there will be a consumption of 5 moles of ATP per hour against a resynthesis of only three. This situation obviously is not tenable. If, however, the transports of K and Na are geared together, so that for each cycle of the carrier system one Na is expelled and one K (or sometimes perhaps one hydrogen ion) is transported in, the production of ATP would just suffice to keep up with the consumption.

The nature of the membrane carrier or carriers involved is at present quite uncertain. A lipoid material which will take K and Na into ether solution and which thus must form complexes with alkali metal ions has been prepared from red cells by KIRSCHNER (personal comm.). Similar observations have been made by SOLOMON (personal comm.). Possibly these materials are related to the carriers.

13. Nature of the diffusion of alkali metal ions through the erythrocyte membrane

One of the surprising features of the diffusion components of the ionic fluxes through the human red cell membrane is that the rate constants for Na diffusion is larger than that for diffusion of K (see p. 82). This fact has been taken by, for instance, HARRIS[310] (compare however HARRIS and PANKERD [392a]) to mean that even the passive diffusion is due to specific carrier molecules in the membrane.

Although attractive, this argument is not quite compulsive, however, since, as pointed out by TOSTESON, such selectivity could also be shown by resins having a specific affinity for Na.

14. Alkali metal ion transport in other mammalian red cells

Table 6 shows the cation distribution as well as the flux values for K and Na of a number of mammals. Some of them like, for instance, the rabbit red cell, show great similarity to that of man.

The red cells of beef and dog are representative of a type which has Na as the major intracellular ion. According to FRAZIER et al.[393] the K influx into dog red cells is roughly proportional to the medium K concentration in accord witht he theory of passive diffusion where there is no K accumulation. TOSTESON calculates an inward rate constant for diffusion of K in dog cells $^ik_K = 0.016$ as compared with $^ik_{Na} = 0.093$ which he calculated from the data of SHEPPARD et al.[351]. Thus the diffusion of Na is nearly 6 times as fast as the diffusion of K through the dog cell membrane. Active ion transport is absent in these cells.

Table 6. *Sodium and potassium concentrations and exchange rates in different mammalian red blood cells*

Species	Cellular conc. (mMoles/l red cells)		Exchange rate (mMoles/hr/l red cells)		Ref.
	K	Na	K	Na	
Man	95	10	1.7	1.5—3	351, 300
Pig	108	12			393a
Rat	90—100	13	7.2		393a, 334
Rabbit	90—100	17	4.5		393a, 334
Cow	25	80	1	11	351
Dog	6—10	110	0.1—0.8	13	351
Cat	6—12	95—110	5.4	13	393a, 334b

15. Transport of K and Na in bird red cells

Although the nucleated red cells of birds show a cation distribution which is very similar to that of man, there seems to be gross differences in the transport mechanisms. Quite possibly different species of birds show dissimilarities just like those in mammals, but until now only a few species have been studied.

MAIZELS[347] states that the net accumulation of K and the extrusion of Na in hen red cells is energized by respiration rather than by glycolysis. Thus the active ion transport is inhibited by cyanide, CO_2, dinitrophenol etc., and lactate can substitute for glucose as energy source.

The transport of K in duck red cells has been studied by TOSTESON and ROBERTSON[283]. They found that re-accumulation of K in cells which had lost this ion in a K free and glucose-free medium, could take place both aerobically and anaerobically from a medium containing 10 mM K per liter. The restoration of high cellular K was, however, faster in N_2 than in O_2. Thus in ducks at least both respiration and glycolysis can support net accumulation.

The detailed study of the penetration kinetics of K revealed several anomalous features. When incubated at 37° in a medium containing 140 mM Na and 5 mM K per liter with glucose as the substrate and 5% CO_2 in O_2 as the gas phase, the

[392a] HARRIS, E. J., and T. H. J. PANKERD: Diffusion and permeation of cations in human and dog erythrocytes. J. Gen. Physiol. **41**, 197—218 (1958).

[393] FRAZIER, H. S., A. SICULAR, and A. K. SOLOMON: Potassium uptake by the dog erythrocyte. J. gen. Physiol. **37**, 631—641 (1954).

[393a] KERR, S. E.: Studies of the inorganic compounds of blood. J. biol. Chem. **117**, 227—235 (1937).

approach to isotopic equilibrium indicated at least two intracellular K phases. If the gas phase were 5% CO_2 in nitrogen all cellular K behaved as one phase.

The steady state exchange of K was higher in nitrogen than in oxygen and strongly enough the K flux was stimulated by fluoride, an agent which did not induce any net loss of K in a concentration which depressed glycolysis. The K influx shows saturation kinetics. Notably when the gas phase is nitrogen, the K influx (and outflux) are almost independent of outside K concentration when the latter is above 10 mM/kg H_2O. In this respect the system resembles that of active K transport in human red cells. If, however, the energetics of the system is considered, it becomes apparent that exchange diffusion and not active transport is responsible for the larger part of the K flux. TOSTESON and ROBERTSON [283] calculate that if the influx of K were due to active transport and the outflux to diffusion, the K transport alone would require 56 cal/l red cells per hour in nitrogen. Under the same conditions there was an energy release by glycolysis of 89 cal/hr. Thus there would be very little energy left for Na transport.

In fluoride-poisoned cells inward active transport and outward diffusion are still less able to account for the K exchange. In 30 mM NaF the energy required for K transport was 78 cal/l red cells per hour, whereas the glycolysis would yield less than 50 cal per hour per liter red cells.

If we accept the view that, during active transport, each cycle of the carrier mechanism is energized by, say, one energy-rich phosphate bond (or any other definite reaction in the glycolytic cycle like for instance the transfer of an electron or a hydrogen atom) the inadequacy of the concept of "active transport in/diffusion out" becomes even more striking.

During the fluoride poisoning experiment discussed the glycolysis gave rise to 0.4 mmole lactate per hour and liter red cells, whereas the K influx was 66 mmole/hr per liter cells. Thus for each mole of ATP formed there would be a transport of $66/0.4 = 165$ moles of K. Since the idea of a carrier transporting 165 K ions per revolution is quite unreasonable the major part of the K exchange must be due to exchange-diffusion which is a process by which the potential energy lost by an ion going "downhill" the electrochemical potential gradient can be used for carrying another ion "uphill".

It is interesting that although both NaF and iodoacetate inhibit glycolysis, exchange diffusion of K is stimulated by NaF and inhibited by iodoacetate.

From this and other inhibitor experiments, TOSTESON and JOHNSON[393b, 393c] conclude that the exchange diffusion of K depends upon the concentration of some organic phosphate compound, and they draw attention to the suggestive fact that phytic acid (hexa phosphomesoinositol) is present in large amounts in bird red cells in contrast to mammalian cells.

16. Transport of K and Na in red cells of lower vertebrates

According to MAIZELS[341] cation transport in the gras snake cells resembles that in the hen cells in being based on respiration. The transport is unaffected by Ca. In a number of other forms: African tortoise, snapping turtle and in various

---

[393b] TOSTESON, D. C., and J. JOHNSON: The coupling of potassium transport with metabolism in duck red cells. I. The effects of sodium fluoride and other metabolic inhibitors. J. cell. comp. Physiol. 50, 169—183 (1957).

[393c] TOSTESON, D. C., and J. JOHNSON: The coupling of potassium transport with metabolism in duck red cells. II. The effect of adenosine and other substrates. J. cell. comp. Physiol. 50, 185—197 (1957).

teleosts and elasmobranchs the alkali metal ion transport apparently is also dependent upon respiration, but these cells will invariably lose K and gain Na unless Ca ions are present.

b) Muscle

References to the recent literature about this topic are found in reviews by HARRIS[394], CONWAY[395], MANERY[396] and WILDE[397]. For the earlier literature, see the articles by FENN[398, 399], KROGH[226], CONWAY[400], USSING[228] and HODGKIN[345].

Muscle fibres share with most other cells the property of having a continuous exchange of Na as well as of K with the surrounding medium. But besides these resting exchanges the muscle, like other excitable tissues such as nerve and electric organs, exhibit grossly increased K and Na shifts during activity. The electrical manifestations of activity are associated with a net loss of K and a net gain of Na (compare p. 151), but during recovery, the ionic composition of the fibres is reconstituted. The active transport of sodium (and perhaps also K) which brings the muscle electrolyte composition back to normal is usually so efficient that the fluctuations of muscle K and Na arising from activity are barely noticible. Under special conditions they may be of physiological importance, however. Thus, in an isolated frog's heart which is not working, the activity of the ion pump leads to a condition where the muscle potassium concentration becomes too high (and the sodium concentration possibly too low) for optimum contraction. Consequently, when the heart is induced to start working, the first contractions are decidedly submaximal, but as K is lost (and Na gained) due to the ionic "leakiness" during the contractions, the mechanical response is improved (the "staircase phenomenon", see p. 189). Similar phenomena are exhibited by uterus muscle, see p. 194.

Most experiments concerning the ion transports across the muscle fibre membrane have been performed with frog muscle (especially sartorius), but it should be stressed that with respect to ion transport, the frog muscle probably should not be considered typical. Thus its capacity to maintain normal ion composition is independent of the presence of oxygen, indicating that glycolysis and possibly other types of anaerobic processes suffice to energize the transport. In contrast to this, mammalian muscle depends on respiration for its active ion transport. At least it is a fact that mammalian muscle, both in the isolated state and in situ, will leak potassium and gain sodium when the oxygen supply is cut off (see p. 88). If the oxygen-lack is not extended over too long a period, these "ischaemic" cationshifts are reversible. As a rule, during the period of oxygen lack the uptake of Na exceeds the loss of K, and as a consequence of this, more Na has to be extruded than K taken up during recovery. Offhand it thus would seem that a sodium pump would be better suited than a coupled Na—K pump to bring about normal ionic distribution. Since, however, the fibres of most muscle cells are highly permeable to K and have a K concentration which is not far from Donnan equilibrium with the surroundings, it makes no great difference whether

[394] HARRIS, E. J.: Transport through biological membranes. Ann. Rev. Physiol. **19,** 13—40 (1957).

[395] CONWAY, E. J.: Nature and significance of concentration relations of potassium and sodium ions in skeletal muscle. Physiol. Rev. **37,** 84—132 (1957).

[396] MANERY, J. F.: Water and electrolyte metabolism. Physiol. Rev. **34,** 334—417 (1954).

[397] WILDE, W. S.: Transport through biological membranes. Ann. Rev. Physiol. **17,** 17—36 (1955).

[398] FENN, W. O.: Electrolytes in muscle. Physiol. Rev. **16,** 450—487 (1936).

[399] FENN, W. O.: The role of potassium in physiological processes. Physiol. Rev. **20,** 377—415 (1940).

[400] CONWAY, E. J.: Exchanges of K, Na and H ions between cell and environment. Irish J. med. Sci. **262,** 593—609 (1947).

we think of the pump as a "pure" sodium pump or a Na—K pump. Some evidence is at hand that in frog muscle at least the latter case is realized (see p. 87).

Estimates of the rate of the active sodium transport process have been obtained in two ways. One is based on the rate at which sodium is extruded and potassium taken up from a suitable test solution by muscles which have been induced to take up sodium and lose potassium by soaking in a potassium-free medium. This method obviously yields minimum values for the rate, since it measures the difference between the sodium extruded and that leaking in during the experimental period.

The sodium outflux, as measured with tracer sodium, ought to give a better measure of the amount actively transported; but, as it will be discussed below, the experimental determination of the sodium flux from the fibres presents certain difficulties, particularly because there can be doubt as to which part of the fibre sodium is truly intracellular.

Also it seems that, under certain conditions at least, part of the exchange of fibre sodium with sodium of the bathing fluid is due to exchange-diffusion rather than passive diffusion inward and active transport outward.

By and large the ion shifts in muscle can be treated satisfactorily on the basis of the membrane theory, i. e. that the active and passive ion movements are associated with the cell membrane whereas the alkali ions, both sodium and potassium, are free and unimpeded in the interior of the fibre. The evidence for this view has been reviewed in chapter VI.

It will be recalled, however, that the simple membrane concept fails to account for certain observation. Thus, although most of the fibre potassium of muscle exchanges readily with the surroundings, it is often possible to demonstrate a small fraction of less readily exchangeable K. The phenomenon depends strongly on the temperature, so that at zero degrees centrigrade an appreciable part of the K is immobilized. This means that either there are groups which under suitable conditions can bind potassium, or, perhaps more likely, there is a compartmentalization of the fibre K which becomes manifest in the exchange pattern only when one or more of the compartments are closed off from the rest of the fibre. Evidently, the interior of a muscle fibre is so highly organized that some caution is warranted when data from tracer experiments are to be translated into values for active and passive transports.

1. Development of the "sodium pump" concept

The K permeability of muscle was first demonstrated in 1916 by MEIGS and ATWOOD[401] who found that muscles kept in solutions with a great excess of potassium would swell and take up KCl. Later it was found by FENN and COBB[402,403] that isolated frog sartorii lose K and gain Na when placed in ordinary Ringer solution with a K concentration of 2 mM/l; but as it was later found to be the case for many other tissues, a maintenance concentration of outside potassium could be found at which K was neither lost nor gained. This maintenance concentration depends strongly upon the p_H of the medium. Thus FENN and COBB found that at p_H 7.2 the equilibrium concentration was 4.8 mM/l, whereas at p_H 5.6 an outside concentration of 11.8 mM/l was required. Similar results were obtained by MOND

[401] MEIGS, E. B., and W. G. ATWOOD: The reactions of striated muscle to potassium chloride solutions. Amer. J. Physiol. **40**, 30—42 (1916).

[402] FENN, W. O., and D. M. COBB: Evidence for a potassium shift from plasma to muscles in response to an increased carbon dioxide tension. Amer. J. Physiol. **112**, 41—55 (1934).

[403] FENN, W. O., and D. M. COBB: Electrolyte changes in muscle during activity. Amer. J. Physiol. **115**, 345—355 (1936).

and NETTER[404-406] (see also NETTER[407]) on perfused frog muscle. Due, presumably, to the low concentration of H+ ions and their slow penetration which is a consequence hereof, the ionic equilibria mentioned above take many hours to develop.

For some years it was the general opinion that K and H were the only ions which were able to penetrate into the muscle fibres. FENN[408, 409], however, showed that as K is lost from muscles in the intact body due to fatigue, sodium enters instead. Also low potassium diets given to rats (HEPPEL[410, 411], MILLER and DARROW[412]) leads to a partial exchange of muscle K against Na, presumably due to low potassium concentration in the blood plasma.

The reversibility of this process of K-loss and Na-uptake by muscle was also established. Thus STEINBACH[413] observed the phenomenon in frog sartorii which had been depleted of K by soaking in a K-free medium. Placed in a medium containing 10 mM K per liter, these muscles could regain K and expel Na if they had not been allowed to lose more than half their initial K content. At about the same time MILLER and DARROW[412] showed that low-K animals (rats) corrected their muscle electrolyte composition on injection of KCl, and FENN[399] pointed out that the K—Na exchange going on during muscular activity was reversed in the recovery period.

An uptake of Na by frog sartorius muscles incubated in Ringer solution was also observed by BOYLE and CONWAY[101]. At the time, however, these authors believed that the Na uptake was irreversible and that normal fibres were impermeable to Na and quite permeable to K, Cl and other ions with a hydrated diameter smaller than that of Na. As a matter of fact, it was later shown by CAREY and CONWAY[414] that this initial uptake of Na exhibited by excised muscles is largely inhibited if frog's plasma is used as soaking medium. (Possibly this beneficial effect of plasma is related to its content of bicarbonate since, according to CREESE[415], isolated rat diaphragms lose K to bicarbonate-free Krebs-saline but regain it when bicarbonate is added.) Based upon the thesis of the impermeability of muscle to Na, BOYLE and CONWAY[101] developed a set of equations which very satisfactorily describe the volume changes and the K and Cl concentrations in the muscle as a function of the composition of the medium. The Boyle-Conway

[404] MOND, R., u. H. NETTER: Über die Regulation des Natriums durch den Muskel. Pfllügers Arch. ges. Physiol. **230**, 42—69 (1932).

[405] MOND, R., u. K. AMSON: Über die Ionenpermeabilität des quergestreiften Muskels. Pflügers Arch. ges. Physiol. **220**, 69—81 (1928).

[406] MOND, R., u. H. NETTER: Ändert sich die Ionenpermeabilität des Muskels während seiner Tätigkeit? Pflügers Arch. ges. Physiol. **224**, 702—709 (1930).

[407] NETTER, H.: Die Stellung des Kaliums im Elektrolytsystem des Muskels. Pflügers Arch. ges. Physiol. **234**, 680—695 (1934).

[408] FENN, W. O.: Factors affecting the loss of potassium from stimulated muscles. Amer. J. Physiol. **124**, 213—229 (1938).

[409] FENN, W. O., D. M. COBB, J. F. MANERY, and W. R. BLOOR: Electrolyte changes in cat muscle during stimulation. Amer. J. Physiol. **121**, 595—608 (1938).

[410] HEPPEL, L. A.: The electrolytes of muscle and liver in potassium depleted rats. Amer. J. Physiol. **127**, 385—392 (1939).

[411] HEPPEL, L. A.: The diffusion of radioactive sodium into the muscles of potassium-deprived rats. Amer. J. Physiol. **128**, 449—454 (1940).

[412] MILLER, H. C., and D. C. DARROW: Relation of muscle electrolyte to alterations in serum potassium and the toxic effects of injected potassium chloride. Amer. J. Physiol. **130**, 747—758 (1940).

[413] STEINBACH, H. B.: Sodium and potassium in frog muscle. J. biol. Chem. **133**, 695—701 (1940).

[414] CAREY, M. J., and E. J. CONWAY: Comparison of various media for immersing frog Sartorii at room temperature and evidence for the regional distribution of fibre Na+. J. Physiol. **125**, 232—250 (1954).

[415] CREESE, R.: Bicarbonate ion and muscle potassium. Biochem. J. **50**, XVIII (1952).

treatment has been of great importance for the development of modern electrolyte physiology because it related quantities which could be tested experimentally, but as it will appear from the foregoing, even at the time of its appearance, the evidence against the thesis of sodium impermeability was quite heavy. As a matter of fact, Na seems to penetrate into muscle quite rapidly. This became apparent when HEPPEL[411] showed that the muscle-fibre Na of low-K rats would equilibrate with injected Na[24] within one hour. Even in the isolated frog sartorius the fibre Na exchanges rapidly with the Na of the soaking medium as evidenced by tracer experiments (LEVI and USSING[250], HARRIS and BURN[264, 416]).

Since BERNSTEIN advanced his theory of the origin of the injury potential (see p. 144) the K-permeability of muscle fibres has been accepted by most workers, as it did not seem to present any theoretical difficulties. The membrane potential would have a magnitude sufficient to keep K from leaving the fibre. The same condition was required by the Boyle-Conway hypothesis which describes a muscle in its medium as a sort of double Donnan equilibrium system where the non-penetrating cation Na is in high concentration outside and non-penetrating anions like proteins and phosphate esters in high concentration inside, thus forcing the penetrating ions K, Cl etc. to take on a distribution which make for electro-neutrality on both sides of the membrane. Even in this system, therefore, the K permeability might be quite high (as a matter of fact it might be infinitely high!) without introducing theoretical difficulties. The realization that the sodium ion was also able to pass through the membrane gave rise to a serious problem, however. Both the concentration gradient and the potential gradient would tend to drag Na into the fibre. In order to explain that the level of muscle Na remains low despite the unquestionable sodium permeability, DEAN[274] proposed a "sodium pump", that is an active transport mechanism expelling Na at the same rate as it enters. A similar scheme was proposed by KROGH[226]. Such a mechanism would result in the maintenance of a more or less constant electrolyte distribution between fibre and surroundings as long as the amount of non-diffusible anion inside the membrane was conserved.

This sodium pump or active sodium transport concept seemed to give an explanation of the electrolyte composition of muscle which was satisfactory in most respects, and it has been used in most recent discussions of ionic regulation in muscle. The Ling "fixed charge hypothesis" has been discussed on p. 42.

Recently KEYNES[417] has proposed that in frog muscle at least the sodium pump is using potassium as partner in a forced exchange process, so that, like in red cells and nerve, we have in reality a sodium-potassium pump. KEYNES bases his assumption up on the observation that the sodium outflux in frog muscle is reduced in K-free media and increased in media rich in potassium ions. In this context it may be pertinent that, as shown by STEINBACH[298] the net extrusion of Na and the uptake of K by Na-rich frog muscles depends strongly upon the K concentration of the recovery medium. At a medium concentration of 20 mM K per liter, the rate of Na extrusion is optimal. STEINBACH offered the provisional explanation of these findings that the inward diffusion of K becomes the limiting factor in the exchange process, but obviously the result could equally well be due to some form of coupling between active Na transport outward and K transport inward.

---

[416] See also E. J. HARRIS: The exchange of frog muscle potassium. J. Physiol. **120**, 246—253 (1953).

[417] KEYNES, R. D.: The ionic fluxes in frog muscle. Proc. roy. Soc. B. **142**, 359—382 (1954).

Although, thermodynamically, nothing seems to be gained by the active pumping of K (this ion being at approximately the same electrochemical potential at both sides of the membrane) the process might serve to speed up the K transfer. There is some evidence that muscle fibres are only sparingly permeable to hydrogen ions. Thus in crab muscle, measurements with intracellular glass electrodes have indicated that hydrogen ions are present at a concentration decidedly lower than demanded by the Donnan equilibrium[418]. Evidently, metabolic processes consume hydrogen ions faster than they can diffuse in from the surroundings under the influence of the membrane potential. Now, if in the active transport of sodium, hydrogen ions and not potassium ions were used as exchange partners for sodium, the cell interior would receive so many hydrogen ions that one would expect it to become more and not less acid than calculated for Donnan distribution. More experiments are needed, however, before it can be said with certainty that the sodium pump of frog muscle is in reality a sodium-potassium pump.

2. Net transports of K and Na in muscle

It has already been mentioned that soaking in a K-free Ringer forces muscle to give up some of its K and take up Na. Such muscles have been used extensively, notably by STEINBACH[298], to study the extrusion of Na and uptake of K. This sodium extrusion is independent of the sodium concentration of the medium and also independent of the internal Na concentration as long as the latter is high. At low cellular Na concentrations there is a strong positive correlation between internal Na concentration and the rate of expulsion of this ion. However, the rate of extrusion of Na depends very much on the composition of the medium[419].

According to STEINBACH, the Q_{10} of the Na extrusion process as measured by this recovery method is quite high (more than 3.0 compare p. 62).

The uniqueness of the sodium ion in the active transport process is clearly illustrated by the fact that although frog muscle can exchange a sizable fraction of its K against choline ions when placed in "choline Ringer", such muscles cannot rid themselves of the choline ion and cannot regain K when returned to cholinefree recovery media.

In contrast to nerve, frog muscle can maintain its cation composition under anaerobic conditions. Thus Dean showed that frog muscle would not lose its K in oxygenfree medium. Neither would monoiodoacetate poisoning alone give rise to potassium loss. However, oxygen lack combined with monoiodoacetate poisoning led to a rapid loss of potassium as rigor set in. This may be interpreted as meaning that the energy stored in the form of creatine-phosphate and ATP is applicable for maintaining normal K/Na ratio in the muscle fibres. In the ligth of this hypothesis it is perhaps not so surprising that the Na outflux as measured with Na24 is only little affected by metabolic poisons like dinitrophenol cyanide and monoiodoacetate (KEYNES and MAISEL[285]) see below.

Mammalian muscle seems to depend much more on oxydative metabolism for maintaining its ionic composition. Already in 1935 BAETJER[420] observed that K was lost from leg muscle of cat when the oxygen supply was reduced by 80%. The isolated rat diaphragm loses K both with and without the addition of monoiodoacetate when incubated anaerobically at 37°, although, under aerobic

[418] CALDWELL, P. C.: An investigation of the intracellular p_H of crab muscle fibres by means of micro-glass and micro-tungsten electrodes. J. Physiol. **126**, 169—180 (1954).

[419] DESMEDT, J. E.: Electrical activity and intracellular sodium concentration in frog muscle. J. Physiol. **121**, 191—205 (1953).

[420] BAETJER, A. M.: The diffusion of potassium from resting skeletal muscles following a reduction in the blood supply. Amer. J. Physiol. **112**, 139—146 (1935).

conditions, constant K content of the tissue could be maintained for at least 4 hs (CALKINS, TAYLOR and HASTINGS[278]). Incidentally, the anaerobic potassium loss in mammalian muscle may start a vicious circle since an increase in extra-cellular K stimulates its oxygen consumption.

3. *The sodium flux across the frog-muscle fibre membrane*

When isolated frog muscles are kept in Ringer containing Na^{24}, all muscle Na will exchange with that of the medium in the matter of a few hours as evidenced by the fact that the specific activity of muscle Na and medium Na become equal.

Brought back into an inactive medium, such Na^{24}-containing muscles lose their radioactivity by exchange of muscle Na against Na from the medium. As shown by LEVI and USSING[250] and HARRIS and BURN[264], see also KEYNES[417] and JOHNSON[421] the time course of this exchange can usually be described quite satisfactorily as being determined by two rate constants. The fast component of exchange was ascribed to the exchange of extracellular Na and the slow component to the exchange of fibre Na. It can easily be seen from the Fig. 4 that the intercept of the straight line representing the slow component (plotted in a semilogarithmic coordinate system) on the ordinate, gives a measure of the total a mount of fibre Na in the muscle. Under the assumption that the remaining Na of the muscle is present in the form of extracellular fluid of a composition not differing much from Ringer, one can calculate the fibre volume and the fibre concentration of Na. The slope of the slow exchange com-

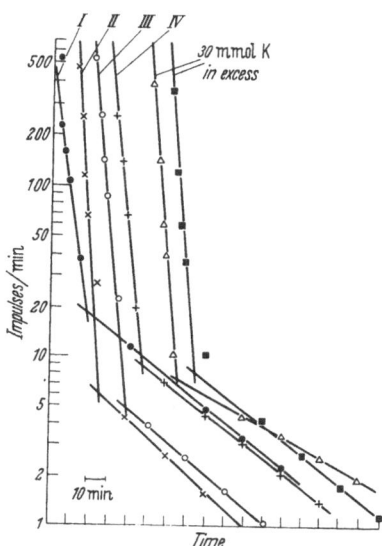

Fig. 4. Wash-out curve for Na^{24} from isolated frog sartorius (from LEVI and USSING[250])

ponent gives the rate at which this fibre Na exchanges, so that the amount exchanging per unit time and volume can be obtained. The calculation of the Na flux (that is the amount passing unit area of membrane per unit time) can be obtained, assuming the fibre to be cylinders of uniform diameter. Table 7 gives values found by different workers for intracellular Na concentration and Na flux values, calcu-

Table 7.
Resting sodium fluxes in frog muscle (10^{-12} Moles/cm² sec)

Muscle	Na conc. mMoles/kg water	Na_{in}	Na_{out}	Ref.
Sartorius	25		14	250
Sartorius	22	13	16	422
Sartorius	15		5—10	422a
Abdominal muscle.	15		5	422a

lated on the assumption that the volume to surface ratio of the fibres is 0.002 cm.

It should be realized, however, that the simple exchange kinetics with only two exponentials is not seen under all circumstances. Thus HARRIS[297] demonstrated that the slow phase of the washout of Na^{24} in frog sartorius would usually

---

[421] JOHNSON, J. A.: Kinetics of release of radioactive sodium, sulfate and sucrose from the frog sartorius muscle. Amer. J. Physiol. 181, 263—268 (1955).

resolve in two if followed over several hours. The same has been found by KEY-NES[422a] to be the case for the small cylindrical muscle extensor longus digit. IV. According to HARRIS only the slower on of the two slow components describes the exchange of truly intracellular Na, whereas the other one is due to the exchange of Na which is adsorbed to the fibres. Other factors may contribute to the occurrence of a third exponential in the Na washout.

In the first place all fibres are not of equal diameter: a given flux will exhaust the activity sooner in the thin fibres than in the thicker ones[422 a].

Secondly the fibres may have different physiological properties. Thus the "slow fibres" have a lower membrane potential than fast fibres (KUFFLER and VAUGHAN WILLIAMS[423]). Possibly, the two kinds of fibres have different Na flux.

Thirdly the exchange properties of the fibres may change during prolonged washouts. A gradual reduction in the Na flux might show up in the washout curve in a way simulating the contribution of a third compartment. The existence of an amount of Na adsorbed to the fibres is perhaps the most important factor in giving the third exponential.

Thus Ling's finding that a considerable exchange of apparent fibre Na continues under conditions where there seems to be no energy available for active transport (see above p. 45) might be understood if there is a fraction of the muscle Na which is extracellular in the sense that it is outside the membrane where the active transport takes place, but which is exchanging much more slowly than the rest of the extracellular Na. In this context it is of interest that JOHNSON[421] found both sulfate and sucrose to show a washout kinetics with a fast and a slow exponential. From the intercept on the ordinate of the washout curve for these two substances, JOHNSON estimated that a volume of the muscle amounting to $3\% \pm 1\%$ of the total gave off its sucrose and sulfate much more slowly than the rest of the interspaces. Possibly the region which is responsible for the slow phase of sulphate and sucrose exchange is also responsible for the intermediary phase of Na exchange.

CAREY and CONWAY[414] also came to the conclusion that a sizable fraction of the fibre Na and some K is located in a region, possibly the sarcolemma, outside the general body of the fibres. Actually, of the 24 meq Na in one kg muscle, 14 are supposed to be located in the interspaces, 8 in the "special region" (sarcolemma?) and only 2 in the fibres.

They base this view mainly upon two pieces of evidence: 1) the exchange of muscle K (measured with K^{42}) shows a rapid phase, apparently stemming from a K space which contains more K than the interspaces, but which is much smaller than the total fibre volume. The K content of this space seems to vary in proportion to the external K concentration. 2) Most of the apparent fibre Na is lost rapidly to a glucose solution containing KCl, but more slowly to a pure glucose solution. CAREY and CONWAY interpret this latter observation as meaning that if potassium ions are available they can replace Na in the "special zone" and thus facilitate the Na washout.

CAREY and CONWAY's interpretation of their data is not, however, quite convincing. The fact that part of the fibre K exchanged faster than the rest might mean that there is a heterogeneity of the intracellular K; and the fact

---

[422] For a mathematical treatment of such complications, see: R. CREESE, M. W. NEIL and G. STEPHENSON: Effect of cell variation on potassium exchange of muscle. Trans. Faraday Soc. **52**, 1022—1032 (1956).

[422a] KEYNES, R. D.: Ph. D. Thesis, University Library, Cambridge.

[423] KUFFLER, S. W., and E. M. VAUGHAN WILLIAMS: Smallnervejunctional potentials. The distribution of small motor nerves to frog skeletal muscle, and the membrane characteristics of the fibres they innervate. J. Physiol. **121**, 289—317 (1953).

that most of the apparent fibre Na is lost faster to a sucrose solution if K is present in the medium could equally well be due to a potassium requirement of the sodium pump. As a matter of fact KEYNES [417] has shown that the Na outflux from the fibres of sartorius and toe muscle of frog is 50%—100% higher in Ringer than in K-free Ringer and higher still in Ringer containing 10 mM K./l. It has already been mentioned that KEYNES takes these results to mean that the "sodium pump" is really a coupled active transport of Na outward and K inward.

4. Energy requirement of the active Na transport in frog muscle

Any attempt to estimate the energy requirement of the steady state active transport outward of Na in muscle rests on the assumption of the correctness of the membrane theory. In order to estimate the electrochemical potential difference which the work of the "sodium pump" has to overcome, one must further assume that the activity coefficient to be applied for intracellular Na is the same as that for extracellular Na, and that the membrane potential measured by micropuncture gives a true measure of the electric potential of the phase containing the intracellular Na. Also one must know the intracellular Na-concentration.

As it will have appeared from the foregoing, the estimation of all three parameters (activity coefficient, electric potential and intracellular concentration) is subject to some uncertainty. However, the successful application which HODGKIN and coworkers have made of these parameters in describing the action potential of nerve and muscle (see p. 151) lends some support to the belief that they are essentially trustworthy. This implies that we shall consider potassium binding within the fibre as being of at most secondary importance. Also we shall for the moment assume, in contrast to CAREY and CONWAY [414, 424], that Na adsorbed in the sarcolemma or elsewhere accounts for only a minor fraction of the "intracellular Na".

In order to estimate the secretory work performed one must know also the rate of steady state transport. The simplest assumption obviously is to identify the rate of active transport with the Na-outflux as estimated with tracer-Na.

The first attempt to compare the Na-outflux and the metabolism in frog muscle was made by LEVI and USSING [250]. If the amount of Na leaving the fibres contained in one kg muscle in one hour is called Q, the minimum work expenditure per hour and kg is

$$W = Q \left(\bar{\mu}_{Na_{(0)}} - \bar{\mu}_{Na_{(i)}} \right), \tag{27}$$

$\bar{\mu}_{Na_{(0)}} - \bar{\mu}_{Na_{(i)}}$ can also be written: $R T \ln (c_{Na_{(0)}}/c_{Na_{(i)}}) + EF$, where E is the membrane potential.

Since it is usually inconvenient to measure the membrane potential during the isotope experiment one can either use an average value for membrane potentials measured in other experiments or else one can use the concentration ratio of cellular to external K as a measure of the membrane potential [although this latter estimate is likely to be too high (see p. 145)]. Using the latter approach, the equation for the electrochemical potential difference overcome by the transport of Na becomes

$$R T \left(\ln c_{Na(0)} - \ln c_{Na(i)} + \ln c_{K(i)} - \ln c_{K(0)} \right)$$

or

$$R T \ln \frac{c_{Na(0)} \cdot c_{K(i)}}{c_{Na(i)} \cdot c_{K(0)}}$$

[424] CONWAY, E. J.: Some aspects of ion transport through membranes. Symp. Soc. exp. Biol. 8, 297—324 (1954).

and we have that the work performed is

$$W = QRT \ln \frac{c_{Na(0)} \cdot c_{K(i)}}{c_{Na(i)} \cdot c_{K(0)}} \, . \tag{28}$$

LEVI and USSING estimated the transport work performed on the Na ion to be about 50 cal/hr/kg muscle. Simultaneous determinations of the O_2 consumption were not performed, but from figures in the literature it was estimated that some 30 % of the energy made available by the resting metabolism was use for the active Na-transport. HARRIS[297] estimated the caloric efficiency of the Na-transport at 20 %.

Recently KEYNES and MAISEL have reinvestigated the problem, parallel measurements being made of oxygen consumption and outflux of Na in frog sartorius muscle. They find values for the secretory work which are of the same order of magnitude as those found by LEVI and USSING. The oxygen consumption which varied between 34 and 194 mm^3/g, was, however, appreciably higher than the estimate used by USSING and LEVI. As a consequence of this, the minimum fraction of the metabolism used for Na extrusion turned out to be from 6—16 %, with an average of 10 %. HODGKIN and KEYNES also found the Na extrusion in 200 μ Sepia axons to have a caloric efficiency of about 10 %[296].

The "coulomb efficiency", i. e. the number of equivalents transported per mole of oxygen is quite high, varying between 2.0 and 5.7 with an average of 4.1. This means that in case one Na is transported per electron transferred to oxygen (compare CONWAY's hypothesis p. 68), every single electron transfer should result in the transfer of one Na, even granted that the variation in the coulomb efficiency is due to experimental error and not to true variations in the coulomb efficiency. It is worthy of note, however, that the high value of 5.7 for the coulomb efficiency was found as an average for two experiments performed in ordinary Ringer, whereas the low values were found in experiments where the K concentration of the bathing solution was either 0 or 10 mM/l. Now, it is a well known fact that high K increases the metabolism (see p. 26) possibly by giving rise to contracture, although it seems that the increase in O_2-consumption sets in before contracture is manifest (SOLANDT[129]). Thus in the high-K experiments the coulomb efficiency might have been low due to this extra oxygen consumption. In experiments with K-free Ringeres, the coulomb efficiency must also have been unduly low, due to the fact that, as shown by HODGKIN and KEYNES, lack of K inhibits the extrusion of Na in muscle. Thus it seems that under optimum conditions (that is: in Ringer) nearly 1.5 equivalents of Na are transported per electron transferred to O_2, even if all the electrons were involved in the process. The direct involvement of electron transfer in the Na extrusion is made even more unlikely by the fact that frog muscle is able to retain its cation composition under anaerobic conditions (see above p. 88), and that, indeed, frog muscle poisoned with monoiodoacetate in a N_2 atmosphere (DEAN[274]) will not start losing K rapidly until rigor sets in. It seems then that energy sources other than glycolysis and respiration can keep the Na transport going.

The possibility of a certain contribution of exchange-diffusion (see p. 50) in the Na exchange in isolated frog muscle cannot be excluded, however, and obviously the exchange accounted for by exchange diffusion does not require any metabolic work apart from that necessary to maintain the membrane structure. It will be recalled that the major part of the K exchange in duck red cells is due to exchange diffusion and other well established cases are discussed on p. 50. The possibility of some non energy-consuming exchange of intracellular Na plus the possibility that part of what we measure as Na-flux through the fibre membrane may come from exchange of Na adsorbed to the surface of the fibres should warn us not to take the values for caloric efficiency and coulomb efficiency given above as more than rough estimates.

5. The potassium fluxes of frog muscle

In the above treatment of the Na flux, use was made of the fact that radiosodium washes out of the muscle with a time course which can be resolved into two exponentials. Due to the high Na concentration in the interspaces and the relative high diffusion rate of Na in the interspaces, the chance of back diffusion of washed out radio-Na into other fibres is very small compared to the chance that the radio-Na shall reach the soaking medium. In the case of potassium the situation is different. The K concentration in the interspaces is quite low, so that even a moderate flux of K across the fibre membrane would tend to raise the specific activity of the interspace K sufficiently to give a very significant back diffusion of activity into the fibres. These problems have been mathematically treated by HARRIS and BURN [224] for the case of a flat sheet of muscle tissue and by KEYNES [417] for the case of a cylindrical muscle.

HARRIS and BURN [264] conclude that in the case of the sartorius muscle the exchange of K across the fibre membrane proceeds at a rate which is about the same as that at which interspace potassium exchanges with the K of the soaking solution. Under such conditions, the time course for the loss of radioactive K from the muscle does not give unambiguously a value for the flux across the fibre membrane. In order to obtain the flux, one must assume some figure for the diffusion constant for potassium in the interspaces.

Assuming that the diffusion constant for K is some 25% higher than that for Na in the interspaces (like it is in free diffusion) HARRIS and BURN estimate the interspace K diffusion constant at 3×10^{-6} cm² sec⁻¹. Taking all muscle fibres to have a diameter of 80 μ they arrive at a K flux across the fibre membrane of 0.0068 μeq [5] cm⁻² hr⁻¹, when the medium is ordinary Ringer. The flux is proportional to the outside K concentration up to 12 mM.

It is of interest that an increased Ca concentration does not affect the potassium flux.

It has already been mentioned that isolated frog muscle loses K constantly when placed in ordinary Ringer. This fact obviously is disturbing in studies of the steady state potassium exchange. In one series of experiments HARRIS [194] circumvented this difficulty by using a potassium phosphate medium which was 0.1 M with respect to phosphate and contained 140—150 meq/l of K (p_H 6.8 to 6.9). In this medium the muscle maintains a constant volume and a constant K concentration. Experiments performed at 18°C showed that practically all fibre K exchanges in a simple exponential manner. At 0°, however, not only is the exchange slower, but some 20% of the potassium is much less readily exchanged than the rest. HARRIS takes this to mean that part of the fibre K is only slightly ionized at low temperatures. Increasing the temperature, accordingly, would have a dual effect: increasing the membrane permeability to K and increasing the ratio of free to bound K. He draws attention to the fact that the membrane potential increases more with increasing temperature than can be accounted for by the increase in T in the Nernst equation

$$E = \frac{RT}{F} \ln (K_i/K_0) \,. \tag{29}$$

Later HARRIS [416] found that frog muscle can be maintained for many hours without loss of K in a modified Ringer solution where part of the Cl has been substituted by bicarbonate (30 mM), just like, according to Creese[415] bicarbonate favours the K retention in rat muscle.

Using such modified Ringers, Harris found that frog sartorii exchanged their K with a time course which could be resolved in two exponentials. One has a time constant of about 20 min and involved only a small fraction of the muscle K (1—5%). The other has a time constant of 2—16 hr. But usually this exchange only concerned part of the fibre K (from 20—100%). The non-exchangeable fraction seemed to be larger at 0° than at room temperature. Increasing the external K concentration also seemed to lower the non-exchangeable fraction.

Carey and Conway[414] using frog plasma or sulfate Ringer to minimize the net loss of potassium also found that there are two distinct phases in the exchange of frog sartorius muscle potassium. The rapid component which seems to involve 3—4% of the muscle K has a half time of 8 min at room temperature. Carey and Conway, as mentioned above, assume that this rapidly exchanging K is located in a special region which may possibly be identical with the sarcolemma.

Table 8. *Potassium fluxes in extensor longus dig. IV muscle of the frog*[417]

K conc. mMoles/l myoplasm	influx 10^{-12} Moles/cm²sec	outflux 10^{-12} Moles/cm²sec
81.5	5.0	6.1
91.0	4.0	4.2
90.0	3.8	4.9
86.3	4.5	5.4
82.5	4.8	4.7
98.0	2.7	4.2

All experiments concerned with the potassium exchange in frog sartoriusmuscle suffered from the uncertainty arising from back diffusion of radioactive ions into the fibres from the interspaces. Notably, if all fibre K does not exchange at the same rate, the equation derived by Harris and Burn[264] is not to be applied safely. It is obvious that the errors arising from such diffusion effects can be greatly reduced by using smaller muscles where the average path travelled from the fibres to the soaking solution can be made short. This principle has been applied by Keynes[425, 417] see also Abbott[426], using a toe muscle, extensor longus dig. V., from the frog (R. esc. and temp.). According to Keynes, radioactive K disappeared from an activated muscle, washed in inactive Ringer, according to a single exponential when plotted against time. The K concentration of the muscles was determined by activation analysis. Influx was determined in another series of experiments from the rate of entry of K⁴² during immersion in radioactive Ringer.

Table 8 shows some of the figures found. It is seen that the influx is slightly less than the outflux which is understandable since the fibres were slowly losing K. All the K that did exchange, exchanged at the same rate. Keynes states that if non-exchangeable K does exist in this muscle, it must amount to less than 20% of the total. The K fluxes are seen to increase with increasing K concentration in the bathing fluid, like it was found by Harris and Burn[264].

Abbott[426] has also used the frog toe muscle to measure the rate of K exchange in Ringer. Abbott's figures for the rate of K exchange were roughly of the order of one fifth of those obtained by Keynes. Apparently there must have been a difference between the frogs used by the two investigators.

The temperature coefficient of K fluxes in sartorius muscle was found by Keynes[417] to be 1.5. Harris and Burn[264] and Harris[416] have obtained the same value.

[425] Keynes, R. D.: The role of electrolytes in excitable tissues. Instituto de Biofisica, Universidade do Brasil. Rio de Janeiro 1951.
[426] Abbott, R.: Potassium exchange in frog muscle. J. Physiol. **117**, 24P (1952).

6. The potassium fluxes of mammalian muscle

When kept in modified Krebs Ringer, containing 25—30 mM/l of bicarbonate (but not in bicarbonate-free Krebs Ringer) isolated rat diaphragm will maintain a high and constant K concentration for many hours CREESE[198, 415], CALKINS, TAYLOR and HASTINGS[278]) under aerobic conditions at 37°C. All K of the diaphragm is exchangeable and exchanges at the same rate (CREESE[197]). CALKINS et al. find that on an average 1.6% of the K of the tissue exchanges per minute. This corresponds to a potassium influx of 0.89 μM/g wet weight/min and an outflux of 0.91 μM/g wet weight/min. The dimensions of the fibres have not been measured in the studies mentioned, so that the flux cannot be expressed as amount per unit area and unit time.

Both anoxia and cold bring about a net loss of K. There is, however, the difference between the effects of these two factors that cold primarily inhibits the influx of K and changes the outflux only little, whereas anoxia primarily leads to an increased outflux of K. The fact that anoxia does not immediately hit the influx of K is taken by CALKINS et al. to indicate that the tissue potassium concentration is not maintained primarily by a "potassium pump".

7. Alkali metal ion shifts in relation to muscular activity

The increased potassium loss and the gain of sodium by muscle associated with contraction has been mentioned above.

Since these phenomena seem so intimately associated with the mechanical manifestations of muscle, they are discussed in chapter IX, in connection with the effect of the alkali ions upon muscular contraction. Notably the loss of potassium associated with the contraction of heart muscle (frog and turtle) has been studied in recent years (see p. 189 and 182).

c) Peripheral nerve

Valuable reviews have been prepared by HODGKIN[427], SHANES[428], KEYNES[425], and HODGKIN and KEYNES[296] Numerical values for the concentrations of K and Na in nerve are found in Table 9. The figures are given as milliequivalents per liter of fibre water. The most reliable figures are probably for cephalopod giant nerves. For these, however, the analyses are mostly made on extruded axoplasm and not on the whole fibre.

Nearly all work on ion transport in nerve fibres has been performed on isolated nerves. This is particularly worthy of note because, as first shown by STEIN-BACH and SPIEGELMAN[429], isolated ner-

Table 9. *Estimated intracellular concentrations of sodium and potassium in nerve fibres (mMoles/l axoplasm)*

Na	K	animal	Ref.
—	342	Carcinus maenas	[438]
47	340	Loligo forbesi	[431]
54	379	Loligo pealii	[439]
77	267	Sepia officinalis	[279]
42	135	Toad	[428]
28	123	Cat	[428a]

ves when in contact with a solution having the same K and Na concentration as the blood plasma are often losing K and gaining Na. The steady state pertaining as long as the nerves are intact thus is easily upset by the process of isolation.

[427] HODGKIN, A. L.: Ionic movements and electrical activity in giant nerve fibres. Proc. roy. Soc. B 148, 1—37 (1957).

[428] SHANES, A. M.: Factors governing ion transfer in nerve. In: Electrolytes in biological systems. Amer. Physiol. Soc. Wash. D. C. 1955, 157—175.

[428a] KRNJEVIC, K.: The ion distribution in cat nerves. J. Physiol. 128, 473—488 (1955).

[429] STEINBACH, H. B., and S. SPIEGELMAN: The sodium and potassium balance in squid nerve axoplasm. J. cell. comp. Physiol. 22, 187—196 (1943).

The technique of isolation and the general treatment of the isolated fibres are probably of great importance for the maintenance of more or less normal K and Na values in the fibre. Thus HODGKIN and KEYNES [279] in recent work on Sepia and Loligo axons find good maintenance of fibre K and even net recovery of K from the medium, whereas in earlier work (KEYNES [430], KEYNES and LEWIS [431]) the fibres always showed net loss of K and net gain of Na.

There seem, also, to be considerable species differences as to the ability to maintain constant electrolyte composition of the nerve fibres outside the body. Thus SHANES and BERMAN [432] have pointed out that toad myelinated nerve fibres can be soaked in Ringer for more than 24 hr without losing any of their K, whereas frog nerve fibres, judging from the falling K/Na ratio, deteriorate in a matter of hours after desheathing. This is particularly important because the transport of ions across the fibre membrane cannot be studied very well in the presence of the sheath. As discussed on p. 162 the sheath represents an important diffusion barreer to many substances, and it has been shown (SHANES [433, 434]) that the Na exchange rate between the frog ischiadicus and the soaking medium is solely determined by the sheath.

1. Movements of potassium and sodium in the resting nerve

From the foregoing it will be apparent that isolated nerves usually exhibit slow net changes in their content of the alkali metal ions, so that K is lost for instance to solutions with low K concentrations whereas it is taken up from K-rich media. The movements of Na are usually a mirror image of the movements of K, but under several experimental conditions a certain independence of the shifts of the two ion species can be demonstrated, see for instance SHANES [428]. The detailed analysis of such shifts has been made possible mainly by the use of tracers.

Determinations of the K and Na fluxes through nerve membranes have been performed by ROTHENBERG [436], KEYNES [437], SHANES [435], HODGKIN and KEYNES [296].

Table 10 shows representative values for the K and Na fluxes found in different nerve fibre preparations. The interpretation of these data depends of course upon the ideas we have concerning the state of the alkali metal ions within the fibre. These problems have been discussed elsewhere in this book (p. 36). In so far as a definite conclusion can be drawn at the present stage of our knowledge, by far the greater part of the fibre K, at least of the giant fibres of Sepia, must be "free" in the sense that its mobility under the influence of a longitudinal electrical field

[430] KEYNES, R. D.: The ionic movements during nervous activity. J. Physiol. **114**, 119—150 (1951).

[431] KEYNES, R. D., and P. R. LEWIS: The sodium and potassium content of cephalopod nerve fibres. J. Physiol. **114**, 151—182 (1951).

[432] SHANES, A. M., and M. D. BERMAN: Penetration of the desheathed toad sciatic nerve by ions and molecules. II. Kinetics. J. cell. comp. Physiol. **45**, 199—240 (1955).

[433] SHANES, A. M.: Effect of sheath removal on the sciatic of the toad, Bufo marinus. J. cell. comp. Physiol. **43**, 87—98 (1954).

[434] SHANES, A. M.: Sodium exchange through the epineurium of the bullfrog sciatic. J. cell. comp. Physiol. **43**, 99—105 (1954).

[435] SHANES, A. M.: The ultraviolet spectra and neurophysiological effects of "veratrine" alkaloids. J. Pharmacol. exp. Ther. **105**, 216—231 (1952).

[436] ROTHENBERG, M. A.: Studies on permeability in relation to nerve function. Biochem. biophys. Acta **4**, 96—114 (1950).

[437] KEYNES, R. D.: The leakage of radioactive potassium from stimulated nerve. J. Physiol. **113**, 99—114 (1951).

[438] KEYNES, R. D., and P. R. LEWIS: The resting exchange of radioactive potassium in crab nerve. J. Physiol. **113**, 73—98 (1951).

[439] SHANES, A. M., and M. D. BERMAN: Kinetics of ion movement in the squid giant nerve. J. gen. Physiol. **39**, 279—300 (1955).

is the same as would be expected for free K ions (Hodgkin and Keynes[216]). This would be in keeping with the fact that the axoplasm of these fibres forms a nearly homogeneous gel which can be squeezed out. On the other hand it is quite conceivable that the cortical protoplasmic layer which is left behind when the axoplasm is squeezed out contains some K with a different mobility.

Calculations show (see p. 148, compare also Hodgkin[345]) that the ratio of inside to outside K in nerve fibres is not very far from the ratio predicted from the potential difference across the membrane. The fact that the concentration ratio is usually somewhat larger than expected from the potential could be explained by the fact that the isolated fibres were slowly deteriorating; thus no true equilibrium

Table 10. *Fluxes of Na and K in resting and stimulated single nerve fibres*
(10^{-12} Moles/cm^2 sec)

	resting		stimulated 100 imp/sec		animal	Ref.
	influx	outflux	influx	outflux		
Na	32	39			Sepia officinalis	279
K	31	28				
Na	61	31	1050	700	Loligo forbesi	430
K	16.7	55	55	530		

would be established. Furthermore the activity coefficient for cellular K might be slightly less than the one to be applied for medium-K; finally some of the fibre-K might be contained in certain compartments such as mitochondria, granules etc., and thus not taking immediate part in the establishment of the potential.

Thus it was for several years the common notion that although an active transport process would be necessary to expel the Na which leaked in, the distribution of K was the necessary consequence of the potential difference created by the Na transport (Hodgkin[456], Ussing[228]). Although the idea that K was actively transported inward had its proponents (see for instance Shanes[428]), it could be argued that since the work necessary to transfer K from the outside to the inside solutions was practically nil, no purpose could be served by an active K transport. The situation was changed, however, when Hodgkin and Keynes[279] presented evidence that in the cephalopod giant axon at least, active Na transport in the outward direction is coupled to an active K transport inward. As is the case in red cells, it seems that the ratio of actively transported Na to actively transported K is higher than one (see below). The active K transport then would be incidental to the Na active transport, but the mechanism might serve the purpose of bringing the cellular K to a concentration which was somewhat higher than the equilibrium potential, while at the same time depleting the fibre of Na. The evidence for this hypothesis will be discussed below in connection with the detailed description of the ion transport through the cephalopod giant axon membrane.

It still remains to be found out whether a similar mechanism is also responsible for the maintenance of K/Na ratio of other nerve fibres. According to this theory we have to consider in the resting nerve fibre three processes: 1) Passive diffusion of Na (responsible for the influx of Na and a small fraction of the Na outflux). 2) Passive diffusion of K, which must be responsible for a sizable fraction of K-influx as well as of K-outflux. And 3) active transport of Na in the outward direction coupled with active transport of K in the inward direction. This mechanism is responsible for practically the whole of the Na outflux and a fraction of the K influx.

The active transport mechanism must of course cope not only with the small amount of Na leakage in and K leakage out taking place in the resting nerve, but also with the often much larger ion shifts resulting from nervous activity. The active Na—K transport thus can be considered the charging device, creating the concentration gradients necessary for electrical activity. It might be worth stressing that the process of forcibly exchanging one Na for one K does not in itself contribute to the resting potential; it arises from the fact that the membrane is much more premeable to K than to Na in the resting state. In cells like erythrocytes where the passive permeabilities to K are low, the active K/Na exchange does not seem to give rise to any appreciable potential. This view is in contrast to the hypothesis discussed for instance by GRUNDFEST that the active transport process ("the sodium pump") gives a contribution to the potential over and above that defined by the ion distribution and the passive ion permeabilities.

It should be mentioned that some workers still believe that K and Na are actively transported in nerve by independent mechanisms. Thus this view is taken by SHANES[428] in his recent review.

In the nerve fibres so far studied oxidative metabolism is supplying the energy for the active cation transport. This can be seen from the depressing effect of anaerobic conditions[432] or cyanide poisoning upon the active fluxes of Na and K in cephalopod nerve[296] (although SHANES[428] claims that in toad nerve anaerobiosis as well as metabolic poisons affect only the active transport of K in the inward direction, but not the transport of Na in the outward direction).

Furthermore there is ample evidence that anoxia leads to a net loss of K and a net gain of Na, and that return to oxygen after a period of anoxia reverses the ionic movements[440, 441, 442, 443, 444, 445].

Although anaerobic processes like, for instance, glycolysis, cannot serve to maintain normal K and Na concentrations in nerve, it seems that enough energy can be drawn from such processes to delay the cation leakage, since fluoride and iodoacetate accelerate the anoxic ion shifts.

The active cation transport of nerve is highly sensitive to dinitrophenol (HODGKIN and KEYNES[279]). It thus seems that it is the formation of energy rich phosphates and not oxidative metabolism as such which is required by the ion transport mechanism. Actually injected ATP can support active sodium extrusion in the giant fibre of Loligo.

2. Effect of temperature on cation fluxes in nerve

According to SHANES[446] the resting loss of K from Loligo nerve is about three times higher at 6° C than at 24 degrees. This obviously may be due to the fact that the active inward transport of K is inhibited at low temperatures (see above p. 62). But also the K loss during stimulation is greater at low temperatures

[440] BISHOP, G. H.: Action of nerve depressants on potential. J. cell. comp. Physiol. 1, 177—194 (1932).

[441] FENN, W. O., and R. GERSHMAN: The loss of potassium from frog nerves in anoxia and other conditions. J. gen. Physiol. 33, 195—204 (1950).

[442] HARREVELD, A. VAN: Asphysial potassium loss of mammalian nerve. J. cell. comp. Physiol. 38, 199—206 (1951).

[443] GERARD, R. W.: The response of nerve to oxygen lack. Amer. J. Physiol. 92, 498—541 (1930).

[444] SHANES, A. M.: Potassium retention in crab nerve. J. gen. Physiol. 33, 643—649 (1950).

[445] SHANES, A. M., and D. E. S. BROWN: The effect of metabolic inhibitors on the resting potential of frog nerve. J. cell. comp. Physiol. 19, 1—13 (1942).

[446] SHANES, A. M.: Effect of temperature on potassium liberation during nerve activity. Amer. J. Physiol. 177, 377—382 (1954).

than at room temperature. This conclusion has also been reached by Hodgkin and Huxley[447] from their mathematical analysis of the spike.

Even the leg nerves of the crab, Libinia emarginata, showed increased resting and activity loss of K when the temperature was lowered, whereas the reabsorption of K was decreased Shanes[444].

Hodgkin and Keynes[279] found that potassium influx in Sepia axons (which is assumed to be largely active transport) had a Q_{10} of 3.3. The passive processes, namely K outflux and Na influx, are much less sensitive to temperature. Thus Q_{10} for K outflux is 1.1 and that for Na influx 1.4.

3. Active transport of Na in cephalopod giant axons

Recent work by Hodgkin and Keynes[279] working on axons from Loligo and Sepia has contributed greatly to the characterisation of the active ion transport processes in cephalopod giant axons.

Metabolic poisons such as dinitrophenol, cyanide or azide and also low temperature (1° C) depress the outflux of Na to a small fraction of the control value. The effect is particularly apparent in fibres which are recovering after a period of activity where the fibres had carried 10,000—40,000 impulses. Evidently the active transport mechanism is stimulated by a period of electric activity or possibly by the increase in cellular Na and the drop in K associated with activity.

It is significant that the metabolic depressants mentioned do not inhibit the sodium influx which is a "downhill" movement and most certainly due to passive diffusion. Thus the effect of these agents cannot be a general decrease in Na permeability.

Neither do dinitrophenol and cyanide have any appreciable effect on the resting and action potentials. This shows that the active Na transport *per se* has no effect on the membrane potential. In itself this observation indicates that the active Na transport must consist in a forced exchange of one positive ion against another. The potential difference is a function of the ion distribution resulting from the active transport and the passive diffusion characteristics of the membrane.

4. Coupling between Na-outflux and K-influx

The same agents which inhibit active Na transport also greatly reduce the uptake of K from sea water (containing 10.4 mM K per liter). The uptake of K from potassium rich solutions (52 mM) is not affected. These observations can be taken to mean that K can enter the cells by two paths, one of which depends upon the same metabolic factors as does the active Na transport.

The concept of an active K transport inward coupled with the active Na extrusion gains further support from the fact that the decrease in K influx brought about by dinitrophenol poisoning is nearly equal to the decrease in Na outflux. Furthermore the Na outflux drops to about one third when K is removed from the medium. This reduction in the active Na transport is immediate in contrast to the inhibitions brought about by metabolic poisons. The fact that some Na extrusion remains in K free solution seems to indicate that the coupling between active Na transport and active K transport is not a rigid one. Also the experiments show that the active Na flux exceeds the active K flux. The extra sodium flux over the active K flux must be associated with the transfer of some other cation in the opposite direction, or with an anion in the same direction; but nothing is known

---

[447] Hodgkin, A. L., and A. F. Huxley: A quantitative description of membrane current and its application to conduction and excitation in nerve. J. Physiol. 117, 500—544 (1952).

about this reaction-partner. When sodium ions are extruded into a K- and Na-free solution (sucrose or Choline chloride substituting for NaCl) Na obviously must be accompanied by some anion, but its nature is unknown. The fact that metabolic poisons (for instance dinitrophenol) inhibit the outflux to Na-free solutions may be taken as evidence that even this "downhill" transport of Na is an active transport. Possibly it is activated by the small amounts of K which are steadily leaking out and which may be present in significant amounts at the sites of active transport. Part of the K would thus be recirculated to the fibre interior while an amount of Na over and above that diffusing out passively would be extruded.

5. Nature of the passive movement of K through the cephalopod giant axon membrane

As mentioned earlier (p. 49), for ions diffusing independently the following relationship is valid [242, 448, 449]:

$$M_{in}/M_{out} = \frac{c_0}{c_i} e^{zFE/RT}$$

where M_{in} and M_{out} are the influx and outflux, c_i and c_0 are the inside and outside concentrations of the ion in question, E is the potential difference across the membrane $(E_0 - E_i)$, z is the change of the ion; F is Faraday's number, R is the gas constant and T is the absolute temperature. It will be recalled that the application of this relationship gave a satisfactory description of the passive K movements in human red cells.

Early work by KEYNES [437] on cephalopod nerve fibres gave flux ratios (M_{in}/M_{out}) which were in reasonably good agreement with the ratio calculated from the resting potential (E) and the K concentrations in the medium and the fibres according to the equation mentioned. Thus the simple diffusion of K through the resting fibre membrane seemed well established. When, however, HODGKIN and KEYNES [252] made a study of the K transport in fibres poisoned with dinitrophenol (which stops the active transport components of the ion fluxes) it turned out that the remaining K fluxes did no longer obey the laws for independent passive diffusion. Nevertheless there could be not doubt that the K movements were passive. Thus the net movement was always downhill the electrochemical potential gradient and influx was equal to outflux at a potential which corresponded to the calculated equilibrium potential for the potassium ion. One therefore had to conclude that the agreement between experiment and theory for free diffusion in the non-poisoned fibres of KEYNES [430] was fortuitous, the influx of K being apparently composed of an active transport-component as discussed above and a passive flux-component which, however, must be due to a type of penetration which is not free diffusion. The type of potassium diffusion exhibited by the dinitrophenol poisoned fibre is characterized by the fact that the flux ratio varied with the driving electrochemical potential as if K had a positive charge of about 2—3 in stead of one. Thus the ratio of influx to outflux changed by a factor of 2400 as the electrochemical potential for the K ion was altered from —50 to + 30 mV. If K ions had been moving independently, an electrochemical potential change of that magnitude would have changed the flux ratio only by a factor of 24. Other observations also support the assumption that the potassium ions were not moving independently. Thus the influx at constant membrane potential was not proportional to the K concentration of the medium, but increased more steeply.

[448] TEORELL, T.: Membrane electrophoresis in relation to bio-electrical polarization effects. Arch. Sci. Physiol. **3**, 205—219 (1949).
[449] HODGKIN, A. L., and A. F. HUXLEY: Currents carried by sodium and potassium ions through the membrane of the giant axons of Loligo. J. Physiol. **116**, 449—472 (1952)

HODGKIN and KEYNES[252] concluded that some kind of interaction must exist between potassium ions while crossing the membrane, and that a satisfactory kinetic picture would ensue if the potassium ions were constrained to move in "single file" (without being able to pass each other) in the membrane phase. It is clear that if K has to pass the membrane along a path having, say, 3 sites in series each of which is always occupied by a K, the three of them have to move simultaneously if they are to move at all. It is therefore not surprising that K behaves as if it had a charge higher than one.

HODGKIN and KEYNES showed by statistical considerations and also by model experiments with a mechanical model that movement in single file leads to the type of relationship between flux ratio and electrochemical potential difference which was found in their experiments on cephalopod nerve.

6. Passive potassium transport during current flow

The strong dependence of the membrane potential of nerve upon the K concentration of the medium is generally taken to show that the membrane is much more permeable to K than to other ion species (except Rb which in nearly all respects behaves like K). These questions are discussed on p. 148. A point of particular interest here is that the K selectivity which is already very pronounced when the fibre is allowed to develop its normal membrane potential, is still more conspicuous when the fibre is more or less completely depolarized. This increased K selectivity is primarily due to a rise in K permeability resulting from depolarization. In the squid nerve, a depolarization by 10—50 mV caused by an applied electro-motive force, gives rise to a large outward-directed current for a considerable period of time. This current may be nearly 100 times that caused by an equally large hyperpolarization (COLE and CURTIS[450]), HODGKIN and HUXLEY[451] using Sepia axons compared the membrane current during voltage clamp (compare p. 154) with the potassium outflux measured with K^{42}, and were able to demonstrate that over a wide range of cathodal currents, the quantity of K leaving the depolarized section of the axon and the amount of electric current passing through the same section were identical. Thus in the more or less depolarized fibre the passive K permeability far exceeds the permeability to all other species.

7. Passive transport of Na through the giant fibre membrane

Passive diffusion of Na through the nerve fibre membrane has two entirely different aspects namely 1) the very high but transient Na-permeability during the spike and 2) the resting, very low Na influx into the fibre (see Table 11).

The first problem is discussed elsewhere (p. 154). It should be noted here, however, that accor ding to the mathematical analysis of HODGKIN and HUXLEY[447] Na movements during the period of activity is governed by the laws for the independent movement of singly charged positive ions. This does not exclude the participation of a membrane carrier, but the

Table 11. Net movements of Na and K in stimulated unmyelinated nerve fibres $(10^{-12}$ Moles/cm² impulse)

Na entry	K loss	animal	Ref.
	2.4	Carcinus maenas	437
3.8	3.6	Sepia officinalis	431
3.5	3.0	Loligo forbesi	431
	3.1	Loligo pealii	446

[450] COLE, K. S., and H. J. CURTIS: Membrane potential of the squid giant axon during current flow. J. gen. Physiol. 24, 551—563 (1941).

[451] HODGKIN, A. L., and A. F. HUXLEY: Movement of radioactive potassium and membrane current in a giant axon. J. Physiol. 121, 403—414 (1953).

latter must then be without net charge and combine with just one Na and, furthermore, the carrier must be present in excess, so that it is the Na concentration which is rate-limiting.

Thus there is no indication of exchange diffusion or single file diffusion of Na during the spike. Neither is there any evidence for these diffusion "anomalies" with respect to the Na influx in the resting fibre. The contribution of exchange diffusion in the resting Na exchange between fibre and medium is made unlikely by the fact that the outflux is unaffected by substitution of choline for Na in the medium (KEYNES[437]). On the basis of the material at hand one cannot say whether or not "single file" diffusion of Na takes place in the resting fibre.

8. Potassium and sodium shifts during activity

It has been known for some time (COWAN[452], YOUNG[453], ARNETT and WILDE[454]) that nerve fibres, both non-myelinated and myelinated, lose K to the medium when stimulated to fatigue. HODGKIN and HUXLEY[455], using an indirect method, were able to demonstrate that the isolated fibre from the shore crab Carcinus maenas gives off an amount of K during stimulation which is roughly proportional to the number of impulses conducted and that the fibres regained the K lost within a few minutes when the stimulation ceased. The estimation of the movements of K out of and into the fibre depended on the assumption that the membrane conductance is mainly determined by the K concentration in the outside solution (compare HODGKIN[456]). The axons were immersed in oil and therefore surrounded by a very small volume of solution. When the fibres were stimulated, the membrane conductance rose but returned to normal with a half time of a few minutes. From the volume of adhering medium and the effects on membrane conductivity of known concentrations of K, the K leakage associated with activity could be estimated. The average value for K loss was 1.7×10^{-12} mol per impulse per cm^2 of fibre membrane. K was regained by the resting fibre at a rate of about 3×10^{-10} mole cm^{-2} sec^{-1} from a medium where the K concentration was three times the normal value.

A fibre with a diameter of $30\,\mu$ loses about $1/100,000$ of its K per impulse.

By direct chemical analysis SHANES[457, 435] found that frog nerve loses less than $1/100,000$ of its K per impulse, whereas spider crab nerve loses at least 25 times as much. Thus, as might be expected, the non-myelinated nerves lose relatively more K than the myelinated fibres during the passing of an impulse.

The loss of K and the gain of Na in stimulated nerve is intimately correlated with the process of conduction. This and related problems are discussed on p. 151 and the following pages in connection with Hodgkin's theory of the ionic basis for electrical activity in nerve. According to this theory there is during the rising part of the action potential a short period of enormously increased permeability to Na, followed by a period of increased permeability to K. Neither the inflow of Na leading to the reversal of the potential, or the outflow of K associated with the return of the potential to the resting level show any sign of active transport.

[452] COWAN, S. L.: The action of potassium and other ions on the injury potential and action current in Maia nerve. Proc. roy. Soc. B 115, 216—260 (1934).

[453] YOUNG, A. C.: The effect of stimulation on the potassium content of limulus leg nerve. J. Neurophysiol. 1, 4—6 (1938).

[454] ARNETT, V., and W. S. WILDE: Potassium and water changes in excised nerve on stimulation. J. Neurophysiol. 4, 572—577 (1941).

[455] HODGKIN, A. L., and A. F. HUXLEY: Potassium leakage from an active nerve fibre. J. Physiol. 106, 341—367 (1947).

[456] HODGKIN, A. L.: The effect of potassium on the surface membrane of an isolated axon. J. Physiol. 106, 319—340 (1947).

[457] SHANES, A. M.: Factors in nerve functioning. Fed. Proc. 10, 611—621 (1951).

Both seem to be diffusion processes down the electrochemical potential gradient. The sequence of permeability changes giving rise to the spike has been deduced from indirect evidence, which, however, seems quite convincing.

Table 11 shows examples of the net loss of K and net gain of Na per impulse for isolated nerve fibres of different species. These net changes arise due to the sequence of permeability changes which are discussed in chapter VII. Actually there is good quantitative agreement between the ion shifts calculated form the electrical measurements and those found experimentally.

Since the movements Na and K during activity are strictly passive, both influx and outflux of these ions must exhibit an average increase during activity. This is indeed the case. Table 10 shows example of the exchange of Na as well as of K are enormously increased over and above the resting values when the fibre is stimulated at a rate of 100 impulses per sec.

d) Leucocytes

With respect to their handling of sodium and potassium, leucocytes differ markedly from erythrocytes. Thus, whereas the latter exchange K and Na only slowly, leucocytes (rabbit) exchange more than 90% of their Na within 75 min[458].

Since the cellular Na concentration is about half that of the medium, there can be little doubt that Na is actively extruded. Table 12 gives the concentrations of Cl, Na and K in the cellwater and in the physiological saline with which they have been allowed to equilibrate (temperature: 37°, glucose as substrate).

It is readily seen that the product of K and Cl in the cells is more than ten times the corresponding product for the medium. Thus the system is far from Donnan distribution of these two ions and either K or Cl must be actively transported into (or bound in) the cells. It may be taken as evidence for the active inward transport of K that this ion is concentrated in leucocytes (horse) when glucose is added to the medium and is given up again to the solution as the glucose concentration falls due to utilisation[459].

Table 12. *Intracellular concentrations of some ions in leucocytes equilibrated with physiological saline*[458]

	meq/l		
	Cl	Na	K
Medium . .	145	169	4.8
Cells. . . .	93	80	106

Mechanical agitation[460] also makes leucocytes lose potassium. In two hours at 37° rabbit cells which were shaken, lost almost all their K, whereas the controls showed only little loss.

e) Brain slices and isolated retina

Slices of guinea pig brain lose about 40% of their K within a few minutes of being suspended in bicarbonate saline or homologous serum, but normal K concentration is restored in the course of about half an hour under aerobic conditions with glucose and L-glutamate as substrates (KREBS et al.[331]). Isolated retina shows a similar behaviour. Tracer experiments indicate a very fast exchange of the cellular K in these tissues. Since it is known that nerve cells, just like the

[458] WILSON, D. L., and J. F. MANERY: The permeability of rabbit leucocytes to sodium, potassium and chloride. J. cell. comp. Physiol. **34**, 493—519 (1949).

[459] PULVER, R., and F. VERZAR: Kalium- und Kohlenhydratstoffwechsel der Leukocyten. Helv. chim. Acta **24**, 272—277 (1941).

[460] HEMPLING, H. G.: Potassium loss in rabbit leucocytes in response to mechanical agitation. J. cell. comp. Physiol. **40**, 161—164 (1952).

axons, are strongly negative relative to the surroundings, the cellular K may not be far from electrochemical equilibrium with that of the medium and the steady state K exchange cannot be used to evaluate the metabolic work involved in the cation transport. The rapid recovery of the K lost initially indicates, however, that brain and retina possess a very powerful cation transport system. The transport system seems not to be wholly dependent upon oxidative metabolism. Thus DIXON [461] found that brain slices did nor lose K to the bathing fluid in the presence of glucose whereas the absence of the substrate or poisoning with fluoride led to potassium leakage.

Whether the cation transport of nerve cells is a pure sodium pump or a Na-K exchange pump cannot be decided at present. There is, however, some evidence

Table 13. *Changes in water and electrolytes of rat retina assuming inulin space = extracellular space* [463]

		units per gram dry weight				meq/l			
		H_2O ml	Na meq	K meq	Cl meq	[Na]	[K]	[Cl]	[K]×[Cl]
Medium						143.7	3.6	126	454
Retina	Initial level	3.40	.131	.439	.082	38.5	129	24.1	3110
	10' in basic medium	3.05	.094	.423	.071	30.8	139	23.3	3240
	60' in basic medium	2.95	.085	.439	.060	28.8	149	20.4	3030
	10', 5 mM glutamate	3.87	.262	.358	.141	67.7	92.5	36.5	3370
	60', 5 mM glutamate	4.80	.265	.529	.124	55.2	110.2	25.9	2850
	10', 5 mM glutamine	3.17	.106	.414	.073	33.5	131	23.0	3020
		3.65	.087	.446	.057	23.8	122	15.6	1905

that the active transport of Na alone cannot explain the ionic composition of rat retina. AMES and HASTINGS [462], also AMES [463] have made a careful study of this tissue under a variety of conditions. The intercellular space was measured with inulin, and analyses were made for K, Na and Cl concentrations, and total water content on fresh tissues and on tissues which had been exposed to a medium closely resembling cerebrospinal fluid. In some cases glutamate or glutamine, both of which are concentrated by the tissue, were added.

The figures in table 13 are calculated from data given by AMES [463].

It is readily seen that the cells are capable of reaccumulating K and extruding Na. Moreover it is apparent that both glutamate and glutamine are taken up, whereby the cell volume increases, probably due to simple osmotic water uptake. What is of special interest, however, is the feature shown in the last column, namely, that the product of the concentrations of cellular K and Cl far exceeds the corresponding product for the medium. Of course, this might be an artifact due to an inability of inulin to reach all of the intercellular space, but the discrepancy is rather too large for that explanation. AMES and HASTINGS propose as

---

[461] DIXON, K. C.: Anaerobic leakage of potassium from brain. Biochem. J. **44**, 187—190 (1949).

[462] AMES, A., and A. B. HASTINGS: Studies of water and electrolytes in nervous tissue. I. Rabbit retina: Methods and interpretation of data. J. Neurophysiol. **19**, 201—212 (1956).

[463] AMES, A.: Studies on water and electrolytes in nervous tissue. II. Effect of glutamate and glutamine. J. Neurophysiol. **19**, 213—223 (1956).

an alternative hypothesis that some of the cellular chloride is "bound", or, less likely, that the tissue contains damaged cells, rich in chloride. Still another possibility is, however, worth considering, viz. that there is nothing abnormal with the chloride distribution, but that the potassium ion is present in a concentration higher than demanded by the Gibbs-Donnan equilibrium. This possibility would seem to be in accord with recent findings in peripheral nerve (p. 97) where, presumably, K is being pumped in at approximately the same rate at which Na is being pumped out. Compare also Eccles et al. p. 171.

f) Mouse ascites carcinoma cells

Extensive studies on the electrolyte and amino acid transport have been carried out by CHRISTENSEN and associates[464, 465, 466] using the Ehrlich mouse ascites carcinoma cell. The latter is a variant of the Ehrlich breast carcinoma of the mouse which, when inoculated intraperitoneally into mice will multiply rapidly as single cells in free suspension. Such a cell population shows an average electrolyte composition of 134 meq K, 50 meq Na and 64 meq Cl per liter, and possesses a pronounced tendency to concentrate amino acids, e. g. glycine. This property is, however, strongly inhibited if the K level of the medium is raised. A similar inhibition also exists in the cases of rat diaphragm and erythrocytes. Conversely, a high level of glycine in the medium, while bringing about accumulation of the amino acid, causes a loss of K with sodium replacement. Another indication of some link between amino acid and alkali metal ion transport lies in the fact agents which are known to stimulate amino acid accumulation cause cellular loss of potassium (and chloride) with a concomitant uptake of Na.

Foremost among substances having these effects stands pyridoxal and 4-nitrosalicylaldehyde, but also indoleacetate and phenylacetate are active. CHRISTENSEN proposes that there may be a common reactant or reaction in the two transport processes, or, alternatively, that the substances in question may transform amino acid-leaky areas of the cell membrane into potassium-leaky areas. The latter hypothesis implies that the cellular potassium level is normally maintained higher than the equilibrium level by active transport.

According to MAIZELS, REMINGTON and TRUSCOE[467, 468, 469], the active extrusion of sodium by these cells is strongly depressed in potassium-free medium. This is in accord with the idea that even here, we have a coupled Na-K pump. HEMPLING[470] however, has found that glucose enhances the accumulation of K by cells which have been kept at low temperature for 24 hr whereas sodium extrusion is uninfluenced by glucose addition. He therefore feels that, under

[464] CHRISTENSEN, H. N.: Mode of transport of amino acids in tocells. In Amino acid metabolism ed. WILLIAMS D. MCELROY and BENTLEY GLASS, p. 63—106. Baltimore: The Johns Hopkins Press 1955.

[465] CHRISTENSEN, H. N., and T. R. RIGGS: Concentrative uptake of amino acids by the Ehrlich mouse ascites carcinoma cell. J. biol. Chem. **194**, 57—68 (1952).

[466] CHRISTENSEN, H. N., T. R. RIGGS, and B. A. COYNE: Effects of pyridoxal and indoleacetate on cell uptake of amino acids and potassium. J. biol. Chem. **209**, 413—427 (1954).

[467] MAIZELS, M., M. REMINGTON, and R. TRUSCOE: The effects of certain physical factors and of the cardiac glycosides on sodium transfer by mouse ascites tumor cells. J. Physiol. **140**, 61—79 (1958).

[468] MAIZELS, M., M. REMINGTON, and R. TRUSCOE: Metabolism and sodium transfer of mouse ascites tumor cells. J. Physiol. **140**, 80—93 (1958).

[469] MAIZELS, M., M. REMINGTON, and R. TRUSCOE: Data for the calculation of the rate coefficients of sodium transfer by mouse ascites tumor cells. J. Physiol. **140**, 48—60 (1958).

[470] HEMPLING, H. G.: Potassium and sodium movements in the Ehrlich mouse ascites tumor cell. J. gen. Physiol. **41**, 565—583 (1958).

certain conditions at least, the K transport can be dissociated from the active Na transport.

As one would expect, if the sodium transport is a Na-K exchange in media poor in K, sodium ion leaks into the cell faster than it is expelled, and the cells swell. Addition of K to the medium make the cells excrete the sodium, and they shrink to attain normal volume. If the metabolism is inhibited, there may be a temporary shrinkage, apparently because K (accompanied by some diffusible anion) diffuses out faster than sodium diffuses in, but once electrochemical equilibrium with respect to potassium is attained, swelling sets in, because Na is still far from equilibrium and continues to diffuse in.

Oddly enough the temperature coefficient for sodium influx is higher than that for outflux, although only the latter represents the active transport. The Q_{10}'s vary between 2.4 and 3.4. HEMPLING[470] has found much lower Q_{10} for the sodium transport viz. 1.2—1.6. On the other hand he found extremely high temperature coefficients for K exchange: about 5. Apparently, the sodium extrusion is proportional to the cellular sodium concentration, since the extrusion appears as a first order process.

It seems that both respiration and glycolysis can energize the cation pump. Iodoacetate even in concentrations which leave respiration unaffected, depresses the ion transport in cells depleted of substrate. If now, in addition, cyanide is added the active ion transport is still further inhibited.

Cardiac glycosides (Digitoxin and Strophantin G) inhibit both outflux in of influx sodium to about the same extent.

g) Liver slices[275]

Rat liver slices, when incubated in bicarbonate Ringer, show an initial loss of K of considerable magnitude. This loss reaches its maximum about 15 min after slicing. Then the partial recovery sets in and within one hour a cellular K level is reached which is about 80% of the normal. The difference is made up by Na. Metabolic inhibitors like fluoride, as well as anaerobiosis for any length of time, increase the initial K-loss and inhibit the recovery.

h) Kidney cortex slices

According to TERNER et al.[120] and KREBS et al.,[331] kidney cortex slices can recover the K lost initially if the medium contains L-glutamate and glucose or ketoglutatate. MUDGE[318, 276] using kidney cortex slices from rabbits found that agents which decrease the oxygen consumption (anoxia, cyanide) also prevent reaccumulation of K and extrusion of Na. 2,4-dinitrophenol and related compounds inhibit K uptake at concentrations which are known to depress the cellular pool of energy-rich phosphate bonds. Thus it is probably ATP etc. and not the respiration per se which is essential for the ion transport. Compounds like azide, Hg, Cu, theopylline and Benemid depress the cation transport at concentrations significantly lower than those required to depress oxygen consumption. Inhibitors of alkaline phosphatase, cholinesterase and carbonic anhydrase were without effect (see however DAVIES and GALSTON[471]). The sum of the tissue concentrations of K and Na remained practically constant, but anoxia and several metabolic inhibitors increased the water content of the tissue. According to WITTHAM and

---

[471] DAVIES, R. E., and A. W. GALSTON: Rapid rate of turnover of potassium ions in kidney slices. Nature (Lond.) **168**, 700 (1951).

DAVIES[277], Guinea-pig kidney cortex slices in Krebs bicarbonate saline with ketoglutarate (10 mM) as substrate, when incubated at 0°, lose most of their K (and ketoglutarate) and gain Na until the concentrations are almost equal in cells and medium. Anaerobic incubation at 37° has a similar effect. Even in the absence of any energy supply to drive the ion transport the cells retain a small but distinct excess of K over and above that of the medium, and the cell sodium is correspondingly lower than required by full concentration equilibration. This phenomenon may be due to preferential binding of K by certain cell constituents or there may be certain compartments in the cells which are closing themselves off more or less completely under adverse conditions. Thus MUDGE[320] has demonstrated that during anaerobiosis about 8 meq K per kg of rabbit kidney cortex is non exchangeable, and a similar fraction is found aerobically at 2°. The cellular sodium does not show this phenomenon.

Even the aerobic K exchange at 37 degrees indicates that the cellular potassium is multiphasic, in that part of the K exchanges much more slowly than the rest. It is interesting that DPN greatly decreases the slow component of the K exchange. It would be tempting then to consider the slow exchange a measure of the active part of the K transport. Such a view is dangerous, however. Poisoning of the phosphate metabolism might very well influence the passive permeability of the cell to potassium ions. Furthermore it is known from puncture experiments with micro electrodes that the interior of the cells in the kidney cortex is negative relative to the blood. Thus the cell potassium may not be far from electrochemical equilibrium with that of their surroundings. It is clear that the rate of exchange between inside and outside K in near-equilibrium need bear no direct relationship to the active transport. At least we can say with certainty that a passive exchange of unknown magnitude must be superimposed upon the, possibly, active part of the K exchange. Since the sodium extrusion from the tissue is taking place uphill against the electrochemical gradient, one might expect to find a better measure of the active ion transport in the behaviour of this ion. Unfortunately the data for Na exchange are subject to the uncertainty associated with the distinction between intracellular and extracellular sodium pools. On the whole, the tracer exchange experiments are extremely difficult to interpret when obtained with a tissue composed of grossly different cells.

i) Seminal vesicle mucosa

The mucosa of the seminal vesicle of the guinea-pig can be separated cleanly from the underlying tissue. This preparation has been used by BREUER and WHITTAM[282] for a study of the conditions for the maintenance of its ionic composition. High K and low Na concentration could be maintained both aerobically and anaerobically when the tissue was kept at 37° in Krebs phosphate or bicarbonate saline solution. The addition of glutamate, aspartate, glutamine or fructose to the medium resulted in higher K and lower Na concentration than obtained with glucose alone. Thus it may be postulated that the cells of this tissue also possess active Na extrusion, possibly in the form of the coupled Na-K-pump. Since the secretion from this gland contains only traces of K and Na, the ion shifts probably take place across the serosal membrane of the cells rather than across that facing the lumen. Tracer experiments indicate that all the cellular K is exchangeable. The concentration gradients of the two alkali metal ions are reduced by DNP poisoning under aerobic conditions and by fluoride in the absence of oxygen. Thus the ion pump can be energized by the aerobic as well as by the anaerobic metabolism.

j) Yeast cells

Yeast cells possess mechanisms for active accumulation of K as well as for the active extrusion of Na. The potassium transport was discovered first (PULVER and VERZAR[472, 473], ROTHSTEIN and ENNS[474], CONWAY and O'MALLEY[475]). If yeast is fermenting in the presence of KCl (0.1—0.2 molar), potassium ions are taken up and hydrogen ions excreted so that the medium becomes strongly acidic. In unbuffered solution, the p_H may become as low as 1.4. This active K-H exchange has been described in detail in a series of important papers by CONWAY and associates[476, 477, 478].

The process is inhibited by azide (0.05 M), and also dinitrophenol is inhibitory towards the ion transport, although it hardly affects the fermentation. Since the

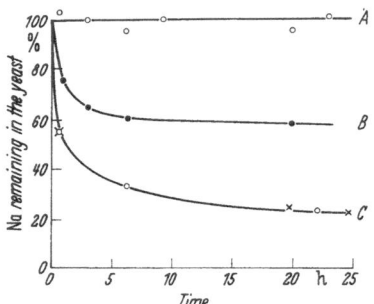

Fig. 5. Rate of Na excretion from yeast into different media, viz. (A) 0.1 M NaCl, (B) tap water, and (C) 0.1 M NaCl + 0.1 M KCl (x) or 0.1 M KCl (o) (after CONWAY, RYAN and CARTON[479])

potential of the cell interior is not known it could, of course, be postulated that it is sufficiently negative to account for the uptake of K in a purely passive way. The active transport would then be a simultaneous transport of hydrogen ions outward and hydroxyl ions inward (the cell interior becomes rather strongly alkaline during the process). For the time being it seems simpler to accept the idea of an active K-H exchange. Besides this mechanism the cells do, however, possess an active sodium extrusion mechanism which seems rather closely related to that of animal cells. CONWAY, RYAN and CARTON [479] discovered that yeast which has been enriched in Na by fermenting for 2 hr in 0.2 M sodium

citrate +5% glucose, after washing and resuspension was able to extrude an appreciable fraction of the Na even against a concentration gradient. The efficiency of the sodium extrusion was greatly enhanced if potassium ions were present in the medium (see Fig. 5). The active transport process led to the replacement of most of the cellular Na by K. In the absence of substrate in the medium, the active sodium extrusion is inhibited by anoxia and cyanide, but Na can be extruded anaerobically if the yeast ferments a 5% glucose solution.

CONWAY[480] points out a number of similarities but also some differences between the cation transport of yeast and of animal cells. One important point

[472] PULVER, R., and F. VERZAR: Connection between carbohydrate and potassium metabolism in the yeast cell. Nature (Lond.) **145**, 823—824 (1940).

[473] PULVER, R., and F. VERZAR: Der Zusammenhang von Kalium- und Kohlehydrat-Stoffwechsel bei der Hefe. Helv. chim. Acta **23**, 1087—1100 (1940).

[474] ROTHSTEIN, A., and L. H. ENNS: The relationship of potassium to carbohydrate metabolism in baker's yeast. J. cell. comp. Physiol. **28**, 231—252 (1946).

[475] CONWAY, E. J., and E. O'MALLEY: The nature of cation exchanges during yeast fermentation with formation of 0.02 n-H ion. Biochem. J. **40**, 59—67 (1946).

[476] CONWAY, E. J., and M. DOWNEY: p_H values of yeast cell. Biochem. J. **47**, 355—360(1950).

[477] CONWAY, E. J., and T. G. BRADY: Biological production of acid and alkali. I. Quantitative relations of succinic acid and carbonic acids to the potassium and hydrogen ion exchange in fermenting yeast. Biochem. J. **47**, 360—369 (1950).

[478] CONWAY, E. J., T. G. BRADY, and E. CARTON: Biological production of acid and alkali. II. A redox theory for the process in yeast with application to the production of gastric acidity. Biochem. J. **47**, 369—374 (1950).

[479] CONWAY, E. J., H. RYAN, and E. CARTON: Active transport of sodium ions from the yeast cell. Biochem. J. **58**, 158—167 (1954).

[480] CONWAY, E. J.: Evidence for a redox pump in the active transport of cations. Int. rev. cytol. **4**, 377—396 (1955).

in common is the great specificity towards Na of the extrusion mechanism. Thus although both K and Na may be present in the cells, no detectable amount of K is excreted under condition of rapid Na transport. The only cation which can compete with Na for the active transport mechanism is Li. With respect to Li transport most animal cells are rather less effective than yeast (compare Schou [480a]). An important difference from the animal Na transport system is the insensitivity of the yeast Na transport to dinitrophenol poisoning. Whether that means that the active transport of Na in yeast is independent of the availability of ATP is not clear. Conway prefers to think that the Na transport ion yeast is directly linked to the electron transport cennected with metabolic oxydation-reduction processes.

A complicating factor in evaluating transport experiments with yeast is the likelihood of separate compartments within the yeast cell. Thus some of the intracellular ions may be contained in vacuole-like structures.

k) Ulva lactuca

The transport of K and Na in fronds of the green alga Ulva lactuca has been studied by Scott and Hayward [481, 482, 483, 484, 485]. The cells of this plant have a rather small vacuole and the cytoplasm represents a relatively large fraction of the individual cell. Thus the transports described may relate to the ionic composition of the cytoplasm proper. Under normal conditions the cellular K level of this organism is about 310 mM/l and the Na level 190 mM/l cell water. Darkness (which probably means lack of substrate) and a number of metabolic inhibitors such as 4,6-dinitro-o-cresol and phenylurethane make the cells lose K and gain Na. Iodoacetate enhances the ion shift in the dark but has little effect during illumination, probably because enough energy can be supplied via photosynthesis even with the glycolytic path cut off. Since the kinetics of potassium loss differs from that of the sodium gain, for instance during dinitro-o-cresol poisoning the above authors assume the transport mechanism for K and Na to be independent. It should be remembered, however, that if the cells, like most plant and animal cells, have the cell interior negative relative to the surroundings, part (or all) of the K shift may be passive and one should not expect the movements of Ka and Na to be mirror images of each other, even if the ion pump were a coupled Na-K-mechanism.

l) Halicystis and Valonia

For references to the older litteratire see Blinks [486] and Osterhout [18].

[480a] Schou, M.: Biology and pharmacology of the lithium ion. Pharmacol. Rev. 9, 17—58 (1957).

[481] Scott, G. T., and H. R. Hayward: Metabolic factors influencing the sodium and potassium distribution in Ulva lactuca. J. gen. Physiol. 36, 659—671 (1953).

[482] Scott, G. T., and H. R. Hayward: The influence of iodoacetate on the sodium and potassium content of Ulva lactuca and the prevention of its influence by light. Science 117, 719—721 (1953).

[483] Scott, G. T., and H. R. Hayward: The influence of temperature and illumination on the exchange of potassium ion in Ulva lactuca. Biochim. Acta 12, 401—404 (1953).

[484] Scott, G. T., and H. R. Hayward: Evidence for the presence of separate mechanisms regulating potassium and sodium distribution in Ulva lactuca. J. gen. Physiol. 37, 601—620 (1954).

[485] Scott, G. T., and H. R. Hayward: Sodium and potassium regulation in Ulva lactuca and Valonia macrophysa. In: Electrolyte in Biological Systems, ed.: A. M. Shanes, p. 35—64. Amer. Physiol. Soc. Washington, D. C. 1955.

[486] Blinks, L. R.: The relations of bioelectric phenomena to ionic permeability and to metabolism in large plant cells. Cold Spr. Harb. Symp. quant. Biol. 8, 204—215 (1940).

The coenocytic marine algae Halicystis and Valonia offer unique opportunities for the study of ion transport across cell membranes. These nearly spherical algae which attain a diameter of the order of one cm, in a sense are unicellular since the thin layer of cytoplasm surrounding the central vacuole is not divided up in individual cells although it contains many nuclei. Thus substances passing from the outside to the vacuole pass only two cell membranes, viz. that facing outward and the tonoplast surrounding the vacuole. Furthermore, these cells can be impaled and samples taken from the vacuole without ill effects to the cell. Actually the sap can be replaced by, for instance, sea water so that the concentration difference between the two sides of the cytoplasm is abolished. Most

Table 14. *Ionic composition of the cell sap and the potential of some giant algal cells*

	Composition of cell sap (mM)			PD(mV) outside zero	Ref.
	Na	K	Cl		
Halicystis ovalis . . .	257	337	543	—80	487, 487a
Valonia macrophysa .	140	500	615	+10	487b

species of both genui maintain a high K level in the vacuole (H. Osterhoutii does not concentrate K), but whereas the sap of for instance H. ovalis is some 80 mV negative relative to the sea water[487], the sap of Valonia macrophysa is some 8 mV positive.

Representative values for the ionic composition of the sap of V. macrophysa and H. ovalis are given in Table 14. It should be mentioned that it was the ionic composition of the sap of Valonia which inspired Osterhout's classical model experiments on ion accumulation.

The high K concentration of the Valonia-sap and the positive sign of the potential makes it apparent that K enters the sap due to active transport. Since the sap is a dilute solution of inorganic ions, there is no question of K binding to macromolecules. It can, however, be demonstrated that the cell also possesses the ability to transport Na actively. Thus Valonia can be induced to lose K and gain Na by cooling to 2—5 degrees or by poisoning with phenyl urethane. When the cells are returned to optimal conditions, Na is again extruded and K taken up. Iodoacetate poisoning in the dark also leads to K loss and Na gain, but this effect is inhibited by light.

Active sodium transport has also been demonstrated in Halicystis ovalis (BLOUNT[488]). A simple calculation, based upon the concentrations and the potential actually measured, using equation 9, p. 49, indicates that in the steady state neither the sodium ion nor the chloride ion of the sap are in electrochemical equilibrium with the surrounding sea water: Sodium must be under the influence of an active transport in the outward direction, whereas chloride ions must be transported inward. The potassium ion of the sap, on the other hand, although its concentration there is much higher than in the sea water, is close to electrochemical equilibrium with the latter.

[487] BROOKS, S. C.: Composition of the cell sap of Halicystis ovalis. (Lyng) Areschoug. Proc. Soc. exp. Biol. (N. Y.) **27**, 409—412 (1929—1930).
[487a] HOLLENBERG, G. J.: Some physical and chemical properties of the cell sap Halicystis Ovalis. J. gen. Physiol. **15**, 651—653 (1931).
[487b] JACQUES, A. G.: The kinestics of penetration 1 and 11. J. gen. Physiol. **22**, 147—164, 501—520 (1938).
[488] BLOUNT, R. W.: A quantitative analysis of active ion transport in the single celled alga Halicystis ovalis. Diss. Univ. of California, Los Angeles 1958.

In order to determine the contribution of the active Na transport to the eletric potential, BLOUNT has applied the "short-circuiting" technique to impaled Halicystis cells. It should be mentioned, that already 1930 BLINKS showed that partly short-circuited Halicystis cells would generate electric current for several days. The short-circuited method is described in detail in connection with the active sodium transport of the frog skin (p. 116). Suffice it here to mention that the principle is to use solutions of identical composition in the vacuole and in the surrounding medium and at the same time connecting vacuole and outside medium through a short-circuit of zero effective resistance. The current generated by the cell under such conditions must consist exclusively of actively transported ions and can be compared with the amounts of the different ionic species actually transferred. The measurement of ion transports can be made with tracers. The experiments showed that the cell is able to transport Na actively and specifically in the outward direction, but it also turned out that there was an "extra" current not accounted for by the active sodium transport. This current was identified beyond reasonable doubt with the active transport of chloride into the vacuole.

The active Na transport, but not the chloride transport, was strongly inhibited by dinitrophenol.

The fact that the K ion of the sap is in electro-chemical equilibrium with that of the bathing fluid in the steady state does not necessarily mean that we are dealing with a "pure" sodium pump. If both the plasma membrane and the vacuole membrane are easily permeable to K it will attain electrochemical equilibrium no matter whether it participates in the sodium transport or not. Additional experiments are needed to test this point.

m) Nitellopsis (Characeae)

The large cells of this fresh water and brackish water form belonging to the Characeans can be punctured with microelectrodes and the potential difference between sap and surroundings measured. It is also relatively easy to obtain sufficient sap for chemical analysis. From such measurements in connection with measurements of ionic fluxes with isotopes MACROBBIE and DAINTY[489, 490] concluded that sodium ions, although being able to exchange between sap and medium were always present in the former at a much lower electrochemical potential than in the latter whereas the opposite was true for chloride. Potassium, on the other hand, was present in the sap at the concentration predicted from the magnitude of the (negative) potential difference between sap and medium. Thus, as in the case for Halicystis ovalis, the cells must possess an active transport of sodium in the outward direction and an active chloride transport inward.

n) Higher plants

Although the accumulation of inorganic cations by tissues of higher plants has been studied extensively (for references see for instance LUNDEGARDH[292], STEWARD[192], SUTCLIFFE[491], SCOTT RUSSEL[492], EPSTEIN[191]) such studies have in

[489] MACROBBIE, E. A. C.: Studies in diffusion and permeability in biological systems. Diss. Univ. Edinburgh 1957.
[490] MACROBBIE, E. A. C., and J. DAINTY: Ion transport in Nitellopsis obtusa. J. Gen. Physiol. 42, 335—358 (1958).
[491] SUTCLIFFE, J. F.: Cation absorption by non-growing plant cells. Symp. Soc. exp. Biol. 8, 325—342 (1954).
[492] SCOTT RUSSEL, R.: The relationship between metabolism and the accumulation of ions by plants. Symp. Soc. exp. Biol. 8, 343—366 (1954).

general not been correlated with measurements of the membrane potentials, and it cannot therefore be said with certainty whether the potassium accumulation in the cell sap is due to Donnan distribution or whether it requires an active transport of this ion. LUNDEGÅRDH[493] (see also [494]) has shown that the bleeding sap from barley roots is negative relative to the culture medium and it is thus possible that the cation uptake is secondary to the active uptake by the roots of anions.

C. Transport through epithelial membranes

a) Introduction

The physiological role of the transport of alkali metal ions across epithelial membranes is great, especially if we take into account that all glands must be considered as being derived from epithelial tissues. Several epithelia, especially such that can be obtained in the form of reasonably large flat sheets are well suited for the study of diffusion and active transport. They often constitute systems where massive transport of ions is going on under conditions where both the concentrations and the activity coefficients for the ions in question can be determined in the bathing solutions and where, furthermore, the potential drop across the membrane is easily accessible. Thus the parameters necessary to distinguish between active and passive transport (compare p. 49) can be obtained with better accuracy than in the cases where we are concerned with the transport into and out of cells. It must be admitted, however, that this advantage is gained at the expense of the complication that the transported ions must pass at least two cell boundaries to get across even the simplest epithelium, one cell layer thick.

As it will appear from the following, there is mounting evidence that the transport into and out of cells is brought about by mechanisms which do not in principle differ from those responsible for the transport across epithelial membranes. All epithelia seem, however, to consist of asymmetrical cells, one membrane having properties grossly different from those of the other. Any net transport brought about by such a membrane must be considered the resultant of the processes going on at the two boundaries.

In some membranes, like the endothelium[495] of the blood vessels, the intercellular diffusion is probably of considerable importance. In many other epithelia (skin, urinary bladder etc.) the intercellular "leakage" can probably be neglected as evidenced by the high electrical resistance and diffusion resistance of these structures.

Although the epithelial membranes serve extremely diverse purposes in the organisms, it seems possible to discern a few distinct patterns according to which they treat the alkali metal ions. Thus, for instance, the amphibian skin, the urinary bladder of the toad, the rumen epithelium of the ruminants, the large intestine epithelium of the toad, the bull frog and the guinea pig perform an active transport of sodium from the morphological outside to the morphological inside (see below). It is highly likely that the same type of transport is also found in the tubule cells of the kidney. This active sodium transport gives rise to an electric potential difference, making the "blood side" positive relative to the morphological outside.

[493] LUNDEGÅRDH, H.: Ionenkonzentration und Ionenaustausch in der Grenzfläche Protoplasma: Lösung. Biochem. Z. **298**, 51—73 (1938).

[494] SCHUFFELEN, A. C., and R. LOOSJES: The importance of the ion activity of the medium and the root potential for the cation-absorption by the plant. Proc. Acad. Sci. Amsterdam **49**, 80—86 (1946).

[495] See for instance: B. W. ZWEIFACH: The structural basis of permeability and other functions of blood capillaries. Cold Spr. Harb. Symp. quant. Biol. **8**, 216—223 (1940).

This potential difference in turn is solely or mainly providing the force, dragging in the anions, primarily chloride. The mechanism seems almost specific to sodium, Li being the only ion which to some extent can substitute for Na.

This pattern of behaviour has been most carefully studied in the isolated frog skin, but it seems to be surprisingly similar in all the tissues mentioned. As discussed above (p. 57) it is entirely possible that the active net transport of Na is due to the activity of a Na—K pump. (In the frog skin, at least, the sodium pump requires a certain minimum amount of potassium ions in the inside bathing solution.) If so, the reason why the skin pumps sodium one-sidedly and not potassium lies in the fact that the outward facing membrane is impermeable to potassium ions while passively permeable to sodium ions. The same Na—K pump, combined with suitable passive ion permeabilities would make the epithelium transport sodium, potassium or both actively. An example of simultaneous active transport of K and Na in opposite directions is found in the part of the distal kidney tubule where K (and H) are excreted while Na is reabsorbed. Whether the active uptake of Na and K in the gills of crustaceans (wollhanded crab, shore crab etc., see p. 142) is due to the same type of ion pump or whether there is another type which does not distinguish between the two ions is not entirely clear.

There are, however, epithelial cells whose ion transport pattern is not dominated by any kind of sodium pump. A good example is the gastric mucosa. Although accurate measurements do show a weak active sodium transport from the mucosal to the serosal side, this transport is far too small to affect the potential development[496]. This modest active cation transport may be related to the cation regulation of the cells which like other cells keep potassium high and sodium low. The potential across the epithelium is primarily determined by the active transport of chloride ions in the direction serosa mucosa (HOGBEN[497]). Active chloride transport is also characteristic of the skin gland cells of the frog skin which are normally resting, but can be stimulated by adrenaline[498] or by nervous stimulation. This active chloride transport is largely responsible for the characteristic secretion potential.

Thus active sodium transport may be characteristic of cells which perform a transport of sodium and chloride into the organism, whereas the type that secrete ions may be dominated by the active chloride transport. In this context it may be worth mentioning that according to LUNDBERG's (see part II) electro-physiological studies of the parotid gland, the primary secretion formed in the acini seems to be associated with an active chloride transport. The primary secretion would then be dependent of the active chloride transport whereas the modification of the secretion taking place during the flow of the primary secretion through the ducts, according to the hypothesis advanced by HESS THAYSEN (see part II) depends on an active sodium ion reabsorption.

It is tempting to identify the sodium transporting element of the frog skin etc. with the sodium reabsorbing mechanism of kidney tubules. One may stretch the comparison still further and propose that the same element is operative in the production of many glandular secretions. Thus according to HESS THAYSEN both the sweat and the saliva from the parotid gland are elaborated by reabsorption of Na and certain other substances, notably water from a presecretion during its

---

[496] HOGBEN, C. A. M.: In preparation.

[497] HOGBEN, C. A. M.: Active transport of chloride by isolated frog gastric epithelium. Origin of the gastric mucosal potential. Amer. J. Physiol. 180, 641—649 (1955).

[498] KOEFOED-JOHNSEN, V., H. H. USSING, and K. ZERAHN: The origin of the short-circuitcurrent in the adrenaline stimulated frog skin. Acta physiol. scand. 27, 38—48 (1952).

flow through the ducts. However, much work has still to be done before it can be decided whether or not such a generalisation is justified. Even if we limit our discussion to the organs where the active sodium transport of the abovementioned type is manifestly demonstrated, it must be said to play a great role biologically.

The following examples of active and passive transport of alkali metal ions through epithelia are not meant to cover completely the cases where these ions are known to undergo net transfer. The tissues discussed are some for which sufficient data are available to warrant a meaningful evaluation of the contributions of passive and active transports to the overall transfer.

b) The amphibian skin

1. The active sodium transport of the frog skin and its relation to the skin potential

The early literature concerning the frog skin potential has been reviewed by DEAN and GATTY[499]. Reviews which also comprise the recent developments concerning active ion transport and potential are those by LINDERHOLM[241], HUF[500] and USSING[501, 502].

More than a hundred years ago DU BOIS REYMOND[503] observed that the isolated frog skin maintains an electric potential between its inside and outside. The phenomenon was studied in more detail by GALEOTTI[504, 505]. He made the interesting observation that the potential can only be maintained in the presence of Na or Li ions. In order to explain this phenomenon he assumed that the skin were more permeable for sodium and lithium in the direction outside-in than in the direction inside-out. As it turned out he was not far from the truth, but at the time his hypothesis was not well received since it seemed to violate the second law of thermodynamics. In the following years the frog skin potential was made the subject of many studies. Various views were expressed concerning the origin of the skin potential. Thus as late as 1946, MEYER and BERNFELD[273] proposed that the potential arose from the fact that the hydrogen ions diffuse faster from the cells to the inside bathing solution than do the bicarbonate ions, so that the formation of metabolic carbon dioxide would be the real source of the potential. Other explanations, see ORBELI[506], UHLENBROCK[507], HASHIDA[508], MOTOKAWA[509, 510, 511],

[499] DEAN, R. B., and O. GATTY: The bioelectrical properties of frog skin. Trans. Faraday Soc. 33, 1040—1046 (1937).

[500] HUF, E. G.: Ion transport and ion exchange in frog skin. In: Electrolytes in Biological Systems. Ed. A. M. SHANES. Amer. Physiol. Soc. Washington D. C. 1955.

[501] USSING, H. H.: Transport through biological membranes. Ann. Rev. Physiol. 15, 1—20 (1953).

[502] USSING, H. H.: Ion transport across biological membranes. In: Ion transport across membranes, p. 3—22. Ed. H. T. CLARKE. New York Academic Press 1954.

[503] DU BOIS REYMOND, E.: Untersuchungen über tierische Elektricität. Berlin 1848.

[504] GALEOTTI, G.: Concerning the EMF which is generated at the surface of animal membranes on contact with different electrolytes. Z. physic. Chem. 49, 542—562 (1904).

[505] GALEOTTI, G.: Ricerche di elettrofisiologia secondo i criteri dell'elettrochimica. Z. allg. Physiol. 6, 99—118 (1907).

[506] ORBELI, L. A.: Die Abhängigkeit der elektromotorischen Wirkungen der Froschhaut von den Eigenschaften der Ableitungsflüssigkeiten. Z. Biol. 54, 329—386 (1910).

[507] UHLENBROCK, P.: Über bioelektrische Ströme an der Froschhaut. Z. Biol. 82, 225 bis 243 (1925).

[508] HASHIDA, K.: Untersuchungen über das elektromotorische Verhalten der Froschhaut. I. Die Abhängigkeit des elektromotorischen Verhaltens der Froschhaut von den ableitenden Flüssigkeiten. J. Biochem. 1, 21—67 (1922).

[509] MOTOKAWA, K.: Studien über die EMK der toten Froschhaut vom kolloidchemischen Standpunkt. I. Mitteilung: Über die Bedeutung der Kolloidzustandsänderungen der Haut für die Entstehung der EMK. Jap. J. med. Sci., Biophysics 3, 69—93 (1935—1936).

GREVEN[512] and LUND and coworkers[513]. In the meantime another characteristic property of the frog skin attracted the interest of physiologists. In 1935 HUF[514] found that the isolated surviving frog skin, when in contact with Ringer solution on both sides, would transport chloride ions from the outside to the inside. Although he did not analyze for sodium, HUF assumed the process to be an active transport of NaCl in the inward direction. Shortly afterwards, KROGH[515], in 1937, demonstrated that chloride-depleted frogs are able to take up salt through the skin from solutions as dilute with respect to NaCl as 10^{-5} molar. KROGH[516] further demonstrated that sodium is indeed taken up through the skin and that neither potassium nor calcium can replace sodium in this process. That even the isolated frog skin with Ringer on both sides will transport sodium appeared from the fact that radioactive sodium passes faster inward than outward through this preparation (KATZIN[517]). As a matter of fact, when the inside solution is Ringer and the outside solution is varied with respect to its sodium chloride concentration, the influx of sodium is always larger than the outflux, as long as the concentration of sodium in the outside solution is no more dilute than about one millimolar (see Fig. 6). It is seen that both the influx and the outflux of sodium increase with increasing outside Na concentration in a way which suggests that the transfer of sodium approaches asymptotically

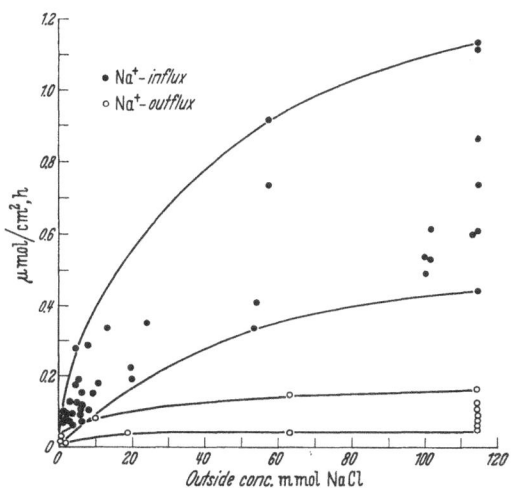

Fig. 6. Na influx (●) and Na outflux (○) through the isolated frog skin as functions of outside NaCl-concentration (from USSING[518])

a limiting rate (USSING[245, 518]). In all the experiments on which the figure was based, there was a potential difference between the solutions such that the solution bathing the inside of the skin was positive relative to the outside. This clearly indicates that the transfer of sodium must be an active process since it takes place against a concentration gradient as well as against an electric potential

[510] MOTOKAWA, K.: Studien über die EMK der toten Froschhaut vom kolloidchemischen Standpunkt. II. Mitteilung: Über den zeitlichen Verlauf der EMK der toten Froschhaut und den Zusammenhang der Potentialdifferenz mit anderen kolloidchemischen Eigenschaften. Jap. J. med. Sci., Biophysics 3, 95—116 (1935—1936).

[511] MOTOKAWA, K.: Thermodynamische Studien über Epithelströme. I. Mitteilung: Die Temperaturabhängigkeit der Ruheströmung der Froschhaut und die Kritik der Membrantheorie. Jap. J. Med. Sci. Biophysics 5, 95—124 (1938).

[512] GREVEN, K.: Ein Beitrag zum Problem des Ruhestroms der Froschhaut. Pflügers Arch. ges. Physiol. 244, 365—405 (1941).

[513] LUND, E. J.: Bioelectric fields and growth, 391 pp. Austin: Univ. of Texas Press 1947.

[514] HUF, E.: Versuche über den Zusammenhang zwischen Stoffwechsel, Potentialbildung und Funktion der Froschhaut. Pflügers Arch. ges. Physiol. 235, 655—673 (1935).

[515] KROGH, A.: Osmotic regulation in the frog (R. esculenta) by active absorption of chloride ions. Skand. Arch. Physiol. 76, 60—74 (1937).

[516] KROGH, A.: The active absorption of ions in some freshwater animals. Z. vergl. Physiol. 25, 335—350 (1938).

[517] KATZIN, L. J.: The use of radioactive tracers in the determination of irreciprocal permeability of biological membranes. Biol. Bull. 79, 342 (1940).

[518] USSING, H. H.: The active ion transport through the isolated frog skin in the light of tracer studies. Acta physiol. scand. 17, 1—37 (1949).

gradient. Later work showed that the transfer of chloride ions across the skin could be explained as being the consequence of the electrochemical potential gradient for this ion. The electric potential difference was usually of such a magnitude that the electrochemical potential of the chloride ion was higher in the outside than in the inside medium, and the flux ratio for chloride ions as determined by tracers turned out to be of the same magnitude as that calculated for a passively diffusing monovalent negatively charged ion (KOEFOED-JOHNSEN, LEVI and USSING[519]).

The sodium influx usually was considerably higher than the chloride influx. Thus sodium and chloride are not transferred in equal amounts in the form of, say, minute droplets or a continuous stream of sodium chloride solution. Furthermore, factors which favour a high potential difference, for instance a high p_H of the internal solution, also increase the influx of sodium. On the basis of these observations the hypothesis was advanced that the potential difference across the skin is maintained at its actual level by the active transport of sodium ions from the outside to the inside solution, and that the transport of chloride takes place due to the potential created by the active sodium transport (USSING[518]).

If identical solutions are placed on both sides of the skin and if the active sodium transport is blocked by metabolic poisons like cyanide, the potential will drop to zero. If, however, the outside solution is more dilute with respect to NaCl than is the inside solution, the potential difference reverses its sign, the outside solution becoming positive due to the fact that the dead skin is more permeable to sodium than to chloride (AMBERSON[519a]). Thus, to state the hypothesis clearly, the potential should be considered as the resultant of the passive diffusion of all ion species present plus the unique contribution of the active inward transport of the sodium ion. In order to prove the correctness of this hypothesis one therefore has to demonstrate that no ionic species except the actively transported sodium ion contributes measureably to the electric asymmetry of the skin. The rela-

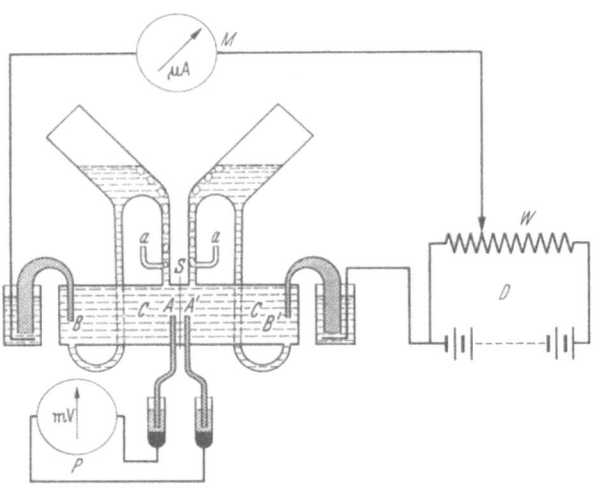

Fig. 7. Diagram used for the determination of short-circuit current and Na fluxes through an isolated membrane. The membrane, S, separates the two chambers, C. Two agar-Ringer bridges, A and A', connect the bathing solutions with calomel electrodes. The potential difference across the skin is measured by the valve potentiometer, P. By mean of the potential divider, W, a variable current can be passed through the skin via the agar-bridges, B and B'. The current passing the circuit is read on the microammeter. M. The bathing solutions are aerated and mixed by air from the inlets, a (from USSING and ZERAHN[520])

[519] KOEFOED-JOHNSEN, V., H. LEVI, and H. H. USSING: The mode of passage of chloride ions through the isolated frog skin. Acta physiol. scand. 25, 150—163 (1952).

[519a] AMBERSON, W. R.: On the mechanism of the production of electromotive forces in living tissues. Cold Spr. Harb. Symp. quant. Biol. 4, 53—62 (1936).

[520] USSING, H. H., and K. ZERAHN: Active transport of sodium as the source of electric current in the short-circuited isolated frog skin. Acta physiol. scand. 23, 110—127 (1951).

tionship between active sodium transport and the output of electric energy by the frog skin can be studied by the "short circuiting" technique. It was shown already in 1933 by FRANCIS[521] that a frog skin which is partially shortcircuited will generate electric energy for many hours. The shortcircuiting technique was improved by STAPP[522] and LUND and STAPP[523] who used large lead-leadchloride electrodes to make the electric contacts with the outside and inside bathing solutions. None of the authors mentioned related the currents drawn from the skin to ionic movements. From LUND and STAPP's figures it could be calculated, however, that the skin of Rana cathespiana shortcircuited through an outer resistance of 87.5 ohms per square centimeter gives a maximum current of 0.059 coulombs/cm²/hr. Considerably higher current densities can be obtained, however, if a complete shortcircuit is brought about. The shortcircuiting device developed by USSING[523a] and ZERAHN[524] is shown diagramatically in Fig. 7. The skin, S, is shown separating the Ringer solutions in two celluloid or lucite chambers. Two Ringer-agar bridges, A, and A^1, open on either side in the immediate vicinity of the skin. The outer ends of these bridges make contact with saturated KCl-calomel electrodes. The potential difference between the latter is read on the tube potentiometer P.

Another pair of Ringer-agar bridges, B and B^1, make contact with the bathing solutions, as far as possible from the skin. The outer ends of these bridges dip into beakers with saturated KCl. Spirals of silver wire immersed in these beakers serve as electrodes in the shortcircuit. The shortcircuit is completed by the microammeter, M, and the voltage supply consisting of a battery, D, and a voltage divider, W, connected in series with the silver electrodes. During operation the applied EMF is adjusted by the voltage divider so that the potential drop across the skin as read on the potentiometer, P, is maintained at zero. (In principle this arrangement is electrically similar to the voltage clamp system as developed by HODGKIN and associates for the study of the ionic currents through the nerve fibre during activity.) When there is no potential difference between the inside and outside of the skin, it is by definition shortcircuited. The current generated by the skin now passes through an outer circuit of zero effective resistance and can be read on the microammeter.

The transport rate of sodium across the skin is so low that the chemical demonstration of the exact transport/current relationship would meet with great difficulties. The tracer method, on the other hand, allows us to determine the transport rate with very good accuracy, the net Na transport being the difference between the influx and outflux of this ion. In early experiments both influx and outflux were determined with Na²⁴ in parallel experiments. The most accurate results are however obtained with the double labeling technique, influx being determined with Na²² and outflux with Na²⁴ in the same experiment. As it will be seen from Table 15, the shortcircuit current arises solely from the active transport of sodium. Both the sodium influx, the sodium outflux and the electric current are expressed as millicoulombs/cm²/hr. It is seen that the sodium influx is slightly

[521] FRANCIS, W. L.: Output of electrical energy by frog-skin. Nature (Lond.) 131, 805 (1933).

[522] STAPP, P.: Efficiency of electrical energy production by surviving frog skin, measured by iodine coulometer. Proc. Soc. exp. Biol. (N. Y.) 46, 382—384 (1941).

[523] LUND, E. J., and P. STAPP: Use of the iodine coulometer in the measurement of bioelectrical energy and the efficiency of the bioelectrical process. In: Bioelectric Fields and Growth, by E. J. LUND. p. 235—254. Austin: Univ. Texas Press 1947.

[523a] USSING, H. H.: The relation between active ion transport and bioelectric phenomena. Publicaçoes do instituto de Biofisica. Rio de Janeiro 1955.

[524] ZERAHN, K.: Studies on the active transport of lithium in the isolated frog skin. Acta physiol. scand. 33, 347—358 (1955).

larger than the corresponding current and that the outflux is only a small fraction of the influx. Δ_{Na} which is the difference between sodium in- and outflux represents the net sodium current, i. e. the net rate of active sodium transport. It is seen that this quantity is identical with the current measured electrically. There is only one notable exception from this rule: the adrenaline stimulated skin gives a current which is larger than the net Na transport. All other drugs so far tested have failed to disturb the identity between active sodium transport and the short-circuit current. The number of agents tested is already very large. A few examples are shown in Table 16. It will be noticed that though Cu^{++} ions in the concentration of 10^{-5} molar in the outside solution has no effect on the sodium transport and the current, such a treatment induces an increase in the skin potential which may in the course of one hour reach a level some 60 mV higher than its value before Cu was added. This is in accord with the hypothesis (Ussing[242]) that Cu ions increase the potential by changing the skin surface so that it becomes very poorly permeable

Table 15. *Short-circuit current and sodium flux values for a number of short-circuited frog skins (Rana temporaria)* (Ringer's solution on both sides)

	μamps/cm^2			
	Na in	Na out	Δ Na	Current
I	20.1	2.4	17.7	17.8
II	11.1	1.5	9.6	9.9
III	40.1	0.89	39.2	38.6
IV	62.5	2.2	60.3	56.8
V	47.9	2.5	45.4	44.3

to anions. Adrenaline has two different effects, one is to increase strongly the sodium influx and outflux, especially the latter. The other effect disturbs the identity between sodium net flux and electric current. It has been shown that this is due to activation by adrenaline of an active transport of chloride ions in the outward direction. This transport is most probably performed by the skin glands which are normally dormant. Neurohypophyseal hormones (antidiuretic hormone etc.) which in the intact skin bring about a rather large increase in potential seem to augment sodium influx, sodium outflux and electric current to the same degree. The rule of equality of current and active sodium transport thus still holds. We shall revert to the nature of the effect of the neurohypophyseal hormones later. The last example is the effect of adding 5% CO_2 to the air or oxygen used for mixing the bathing solutions. It is seen that both current and sodium influx are strongly inhibited so that the net sodium flux becomes practically nil. In general the active sodium transport depends strongly upon the p_H of the inside bathing solution. Maximum active sodium transport is achieved at about 8.5, whereas at p_H 5.7 the transport is almost totally inhibited (compare also Schoffeniels[525]).

The transport mechanism is highly specific to sodium, lithium being the only cation so far studied which can substitute to some extent. In this context it may be remembered, however, that the frog skin is practically impermeable to divalent ions like magnesium and calcium. Even the monovalent choline ion does not seem to penetrate[526]. Only small monovalent ions would have any chance to be transported. The behaviour of the potassium ion in the frog skin is particularly interesting. Under all experimental conditions so far tested the skin will actively transport sodium and not potassium. Even if the skin is placed in contact with modified Ringer solution where, on a molar basis, 35% of the sodium is replaced by potassium, the shortcircuit current is still equal to the net rate of sodium transport.

[525] Schoffeniels, E.: Influence du p_H sur le transport actif de sodium à travers la peau de grenouille. Arch. int. Physiol. **63**, 513—530 (1955).
[526] Kirschner, L. B.: On the mechanism of active sodium transport across the frog skin. J. cell. comp. Physiol. **45**, 61—87 (1955).

Table 16. *Influence of a number of agents upon sodium-flux and total current values, as obtained on totally shorted frog skins* [523a]

Group a comprises results from influx-experiments, group b results from outflux-experiments. Each experiment is represented by a control period and one or two periods following the application of the agent in question. Duration of periods generally one hour. In experiments a 3 and b 3 the first period after application of adrenaline lasted only 30 minutes. These periods may not represent steady states. The following dosages were used. $CuSO_4$, aq: 0.2 mg, added to outside solution. Adrenaline: 50 μl $1^o/_{oo}$ adrenaline hydrochloride, added to inside solution. Neurohypophyseal extract: The equivalent of 1 mg dry gland, added to inside solution.

a			b		
	mCoul. cm^{-2}h^{-1}			mCoul. cm^{-2}h^{-1}	
Exp. No.	Na	Short circuit current	Exp. No.	Na	Short circuit current
1. Control	99	86	1. Control . , . . .	10.9	176
Cu^{++} outside	91	87	Cu^{++} outside	8.6	165
Cu^{++} outside	99	89	Cu^{++} outside	10.5	139
2. Control	57	49	2. Control	13.5	112
Adrenaline	87	76	Adrenaline	41.0	126
Adrenaline	111	88			
3. Control	47	92	3. Control	1.2	153
Adrenaline	129	140	Adrenaline	67.0	174
Adrenaline	115	101	Adrenaline	58,0	126
4. Control	105	100	4. Control	5.6	124
Neurohypophyseal extract	168	158	Neurohypophyseal extract	8.5	164
				9.5	164
5. Control	126	118	5. Control	1.6	77
Neurohypophyseal extract	246	232	Neurohypophyseal extract	3.1	129
				5.4	164
6. 5% CO_2 + 95% O_2	4.5	0	6. 5% CO_2 + 95% O_2	5.5	0
5% CO_2 + 95% O_2	3.8	0	5% CO_2 + 95% O_2	6.1	0
Atmospheric air . . .	165	150	Atmospheric air . . .	8.3	161
Atmospheric air . . .	173	163	Atmospheric air . . .	15.3	158

Table 17. *Effect of partial replacement of Na^+ by K^+*

	K/Na × 100 in solution	Influx μeq Na/hr/cm^2	Outflux μeq Na/hr/cm^2	Δ Na μeq/hr/cm^2	Na current μamp/cm^2	Total current μamp/cm^2
I	35.0	1.89	0.08	1.8	48.4	41.2
	35.0	1.34	0.12	1.2	32.9	33.6
II	35.0	0.83	0.05	0.77	20.7	22.5
	35.0	0.88	0.05	0.83	22.1	22.0
	35.0	0.79	0.06	0.72	19.4	20.4
III	35.0	0.58	0.15	0.43	11.6	12.1
	35.0	0.76	0.15	0.61	16.3	16.6
	35.0	0.76	0.13	0.63	16.9	17.3

The contribution to the total current of active transport of potassium thus remains nil (compare Table 17). This does not mean, however, that the potassium ion does not play a role in the development of the electric potential and the shortcircuit current in the frog skin. The effect of the potassium concentration on the potential is discussed on p. 123.

The active sodium transport depends strongly upon the potassium concentration of the inside bathing solution and drops to a very low value if potassium-free bathing solutions are used (compare HUF et al.[527, 528, 500], USSING[529]).

That lithium can to some extent substitute for Na was indicated by the early work of GALEOTTI[504] and has been clearly born out in studies carried out by ZERAHN[525]. He showed that when both Li and Na are present in the outside bathing solution, they contribute to the shortcircuit current in proportion to their molar fractions. Nevertheless Li cannot fully replace sodium in the transport system. If lithium ions comprise more than 20% of the total cation there is a pronounced inhibition of the transport of sodium as well as of lithium. This is indicated by a drop in the shortcircuit current. This phenomenon is accompanied by an accumulation of Li in the skin epithelium. Calculations show that the Li concentration in the epithelium becomes 5 to 10 times higher than in the bathing solution. Thus it seems that the cells can take up lithium and sodium equally well but are unable to expel lithium towards the inside solution as fast as they can sodium. This excess intake of lithium ultimately inhibits the sodium transport mechanism or it may possibly derange the cellular metabolism.

2. The relation between oxygen consumption and active sodium transport

The short-circuiting technique is well suited for determining the amount of oxygen consumed per equivalent of sodium transported. According to ZERAHN[280, 288] for each equivalent of sodium transported by the shortcircuited frog skin with Ringer on both sides, on an average 0.74 equivalents of oxygen, (that is 0.185 moles O_2) are consumed. Similar figures have been obtained by LEAF and RENSHAW[289, 290]. This finding is important because certain hypotheses advanced to explain active ion transport make the assumption that one cation is transported for each electron being transferred to oxygen. The experiments of ZERAHN and LEAF seem to rule out this possibility. Actually, the efficiency of the sodium transport mechanism must be such that the true sodium to oxygen ratio is even higher, considering that the frog skin contains other cells than the sodium-transporting epithelial cells and that even these cells must require energy for other purposes than sodium transport. According to ZERAHN, in the absence of Na in the outside bathing solution (Na being replaced by an inert nonpenetrating ion like magnesium) the oxygen consumption is depressed relative to that of a skin in contact with Ringer. If only the extra oxygen consumption observed in the presence of sodium is considered to be a measure of the part of the metabolism concerned with the active transport, between 4 and 5 sodium ions are transported for each equivalent of oxygen consumed (i. e. roughly 20 Na for each molecule of oxygen). This line of reasoning is confirmed by the fact that the extra oxygen consumption is proportional to the rate of active sodium transport over a wide range of sodium transport rates. In the absence of oxygen the sodium transport drops off rapidly but is usually not reduced to zero even one or two hours of oxygen lack. The residual may be energized by glycolysis since, according to LEAF and RENSHAW[530], the lactic acid production is increased under such circumstances.

3. The work performed by the active sodium transport mechanism

We shall consider the general case of a skin transporting sodium from a lower outside concentration to a higher inside concentration against an electric potential

---

[527] HUF, E. G., and J. WILLS: Influence of some inorganic cations on active salt and water uptake by isolated frog skin. Amer. J. Physiol. 167, 255—260 (1951).

[528] HUF, E. G., and J. WILLS: The relationship of sodium uptake, potassium rejection, and skin potential in isolated frog skin. J. gen. Physiol. 36, 473—487 (1953).

[529] USSING, H. H.: Active transport of inorganic ions. Symp. Soc. exp. Biol. 8, 407—422 (1954).

[530] LEAF, A., and A. RENSHAW: The anaerobic active ion transport by isolated frog skin. Biochem. J. 65, 90—93 (1957).

difference. The work performed necessary to accomplish the transport of one equivalent of sodium may be broken down into three components:

a) the work required to overcome the concentration gradient:

$$w_i = RT \ln (c_i/c_0) \, ,$$

b) the work required to overcome the potential gradient:

$$w_2 = FE \, ,$$

c) the work required to overcome the internal sodiumresistance of the skin:

$$w_3 = RT \ln (M_{in}/M_{out}) \, ,$$

where M_{in} is the influx, and M_{out} is the outflux of sodium (compare USSING[242], ZERAHN[280]).

The total work (per mole Na) thus is

$$W = w_1 + w_2 + w_3 = RT \ln (c_i/c_0) + FE + RT \ln (M_{in}/M_{out}) \qquad (30)$$

or

$$W = F [(RT/F) \ln (c_i/c_0) + E + (RT/F) \ln (M_{in}/M_{out})] \, . \qquad (31)$$

Using ordinary logarithms this equation becomes

$$W = F [0.058 \log (c_i/c_0) + E + 0.058 \log (M_{in}/M_{out})] \, ,$$

which gives the work in joules. Since one joule is equal to 0.239 calories, we obtain

$$W = 0.239 \times 96{,}500 \, [0.058 \log (c_i/c_0) + E + 0.058 \log (M_{in}/M_{out})] \, . \qquad (32)$$

If we want to know the apparent driving force of the active sodium transport, E_{Na}, we can divide through by Faraday's number in eq[(32)].

$$E_{Na} = W/F = 0.058 \log (c_i/c_0) + E + 0.058 \log (M_{in}/M_{out}) \, . \qquad (32a)$$

E_{Na} is the total active transport potential for sodium. In the case of the short-circuited frog skin with Ringer on both sides, E_{Na} becomes equal to 0.058 $\log (M_{in}/M_{out})$ (compare USSING and ZERAHN[520]). The work performed under these conditions is equal to

$$W = 1.340 \log (M_{in}/M_{out}) \qquad (33)$$

calories.

From ZERAHN's figures it can be seen that one square centimeter of frog skin consumes in the order of one microequivalent of oxygen per hour per square centimeter. One equivalent of oxygen corresponds to 25,000 calories. Thus we have that one square centimeter of frog skin has an energy output of 25,000 times 10^{-6} calories per hour per square centimeter. Taking the active transport rate of sodium to be 1.25 microequivalents per hour per square centimeter and putting the flux ratio for sodium, M_{in}/M_{out}, equal to 30 we find that the electric work performed, according to eq.[(33)], is 2.5 times 10^{-3} calories. Thus the gross efficiency of the "pump" is 10%. If, however, only the extra oxygen consumption (see above) is taken to be concerned with the sodium transport, so that between 4 and 5 sodium ions are transported for each equivalent of oxygen consumed, the efficiency of the sodium pump seems to be as high as 40 to 50%. Similar values are obtained even if the sodium transport is taking place against a concentration- or potential gradient (see ZERAHN).

4. The electromotive force of the active sodium transport

As mentioned above, equation[32a] can serve to give an estimate of the active sodium transport potential. Cases of particular interest arise when M_{in} is made equal to M_{out} or in other words if there is no net transport of sodium. This situation

Table 18. *The maximum driving force of the sodium transport mechanism in isolated frog skin estimated by different methods*

Max force, E_{Na} mV	Method of estimation	Ref.
Ca. 120	Potential making M_{in} and M_{out} equal when $C_0 = C_i$	520
122	Short-circuited skin, $E_{Na} = (RT/F) \ln (M_{in}/M_{out})$	520
136	Potential measured for C_i/C_0 making $M_{in} = M_{out}$	531
152	Max. potential observed with impermeable anion (increased inside K conc, 5 mM)	364

can be achieved by applying a counter-EMF making the inside solution sufficiently positive relative to the outside or by lowering the outside sodium concentration by substituting for sodium a nonpenetrating inert ion like Mg^{++} or the choline ion. Finally one can substitute for chloride a non-penetrating anion like sulfate. In this case no net salt transport can take place and the influx and outflux of cations must become equal. Table 18 gives examples of the estimates of E_{Na} which have been obtained by the different methods mentioned. It is evident that higher driving potentials are obtained when no current is being drawn than during current flow.

It ought to be stressed that the active transport potential as defined here is the effective active transport potential. It includes the effects of sodium leaks in the membrane or membranes through which Na is transported. LINDERHOLM [531,532] has attempted to determine the true value of the driving force. In order to do so he has to make a number of assumptions, which are not accessible to experimental verification. LINDERHOLM's equation as well as another interesting kinetic treatment of the sodium transport in the frog skin given by KIRSCHNER [526] are both based on the assumption that sodium ions in a concentration equal to that of the outside bathing solution can react immediately with the hypothetical carrier system which performs the transport. LINDERHOLM claims that the sodium ions do not go through the epithelial cells of the skin but between them to reach the basement membrane where the active transport is supposed to take place.

In support of his view LINDERHOLM draws attention to the study by OTTOSON, SJÖSTRAND, STENSTRÖM and SWAETICHIN [533] who claim that when the frog skin is pierced with a microelectrode only one potential jump is seen which is located at the level of the basement membrane. Recent work by HOSHIKO and ENGBAEK [534,535] has

[531] LINDERHOLM, H.: On the behavior of the "Sodium Pump" in frog skin at various concentrations of Na ions in the solution on the epithelial side. Acta physiol. scand. 31, 36—61 (1954).

[532] LINDERHOLM, H.: The electrical potential across isolated frog skins and its dependence on the permeability of the skins to chloride ions. Acta physiol. scand. 28, 211—217 (1953).

[533] OTTOSON, D., F. SJÖSTRAND, S. STENSTRÖM, and G. SWAETICHIN: Microelectrode studies on the EMF of the frog skin related to electron microscopy of the dermoepidermal junction. Acta physiol. scand. 29, Suppl. 106, p. 611—624 (1953).

[534] HOSHIKO, T., and LISE ENGBAEK: Microelectrode study of the frog skin potential. Abstr. Comm. XXth International Physiological Congress. p. 443. Brussels 1956.

[535] ENGBAEK, L., and T. HOSHIKO: Electrical potential gradients through frog skin. Acta physiol. scand. 39, 348—355 (1957).

shown, however, that two or sometimes three distinct potential levels can always
be discerned when the frog skin is pierced by a microelectrode. Thus the overall
skin potential is the sum of two or three potential steps. The nature of the skin
potential is especially clearly brought out when the skin is studied in contact
with salt solution having as their only anion a non-penetrating one like sulfate.
Under such conditions the outward facing side of the skin behaves like an almost
ideal sodium electrode over a wide range of concentrations (1—120 mM Na/l)
whereas the inward facing side of the skin behaves like a potassium electrode[536, 364].
The skin potential thus seems to be the sum of the sodium diffusion potential
determined by (RT/F ln (Na_0/Na_c) and the potassium diffusion potential (RT/F)

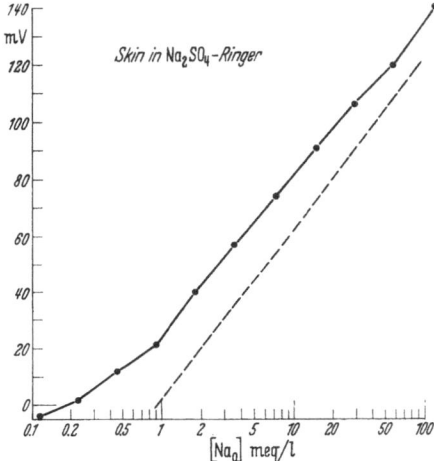

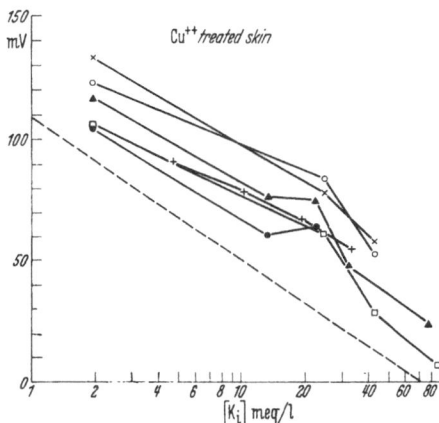

Fig. 8. Dependence of potential difference across the isolated frog skin upon the outside Na concentration. The use of sulfate prevents short-circuiting by anion permeation (from KOEFOED-JOHNSEN and USSING[364])

Fig. 9. Dependence of potential difference across the isolated frog skin upon inside K concentration. Short-circuiting effect of chloride ion is diminished by treating the skin with 10 M^{-5} Cu++ (from KOEFOED-JOHNSEN and USSING[364])

ln (K_c/K_i), where the concentrations marked with subscript o refer to the outside
bathing solution, those marked c to the cellular phase and those marked i to the
inside bathing solution. It should be realized, however, that we have at present
no direct way of determining the concentration of ions in the cell interior. Skins
in which the chloride permeability has been strongly reduced by treatment of
the outside surface with 10^{-5} molar copper sulfate also show a potential which
seems to be largely composed of a sodium diffusion potential at the outer border
and a potassium diffusion potential at the inner border of the skin epithelium.
Fig. 8 shows the skin potential as the function of log Na_0. The Na of the outside
sodium sulfate solution was replaced stepwise with the non-penetrating magnesium
ion.

Similar results are obtained if other non-penetrating ions like choline, arginine
or even potassium ions are replacing Na. The dotted line indicates the slope valid
for an ideal Na electrode (that is 60 millivolts for a ten times change in Na concentration). Fig. 9 shows the response of the skin potential to changes in the potassium
concentration at the inner border of the skin. It is immaterial whether or not the
potassium concentration is changed on both sides or on the inside only. In this

[536] KOEFOED-JOHNSEN, V., and H. H. USSING: Nature of the frog skin potential. Abstr.
Comm XXth International Physiological Congress. p. 511—512. Brussels 1956.

case the skin has been made nearly impermeable to chloride by copper-treatment.

From these and other observations a hypothesis can be deduced which describes the magnitude of the skin potential under a wide variety of conditions. 1) The active transport mechanism, which is located at the inner border of the epithelial cells, maintains a low sodium and high potassium concentration in the cells, but does not otherwise contribute to the membrane potential. 2) The inner border of the epithelial cells is highly permeable to potassium ions and practically impermeable to free sodium ions. Sodium thus crosses this membrane almost exclusively via the active transport mechanism. 3) The outward-facing cell membrane is highly permeable to sodium ions but practically impermeable to potassium ions. Despite the specificity of the sodium permeability of this membrane it is of a strictly passive nature like the sodium permeability of the nerve fibre during the rising part of the spike.

Fig. 10 shows in diagrammatic form the essential elements of this hypothesis. It will appear from the figure that for the idealized skin the driving force for the system is

$$E_{\mathrm{Na}} = (RT/F)\, [\ln (\mathrm{Na}_0/\mathrm{Na}_c) + \ln (\mathrm{K}_c/\mathrm{K}_i)] \quad (34)$$

This presupposes that the outer membrane is absolutely tight for K and the inner one for free Na. This undoubtedly is an oversimplification. Even during shortcircuiting of strongly transporting skins there is an outflux of Na of the order of one per cent of the current or more, and although this Na leakage might conceivably take place via the "sodium pump" system and not by passive diffusion through the inner cell boundary, there is always a chemically demonstrable leakage of K through the outer border.

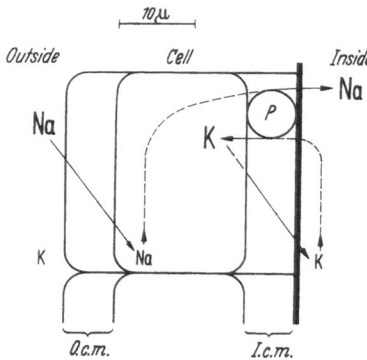

Fig. 10. Diagrammatic representation of movements of cations across the outer (O. c. m.) and inner (I. c. m.) cell membrane of an epithelial cell. The oblique arrows designate passive though highly specific diffusion. P is a "pump" mechanism with a one-to-one exchange of K for Na. The size and the level of the chemical symbols indicate the concentration levels of the cations (from KOEFOED-JOHNSEN and USSING[244])

The skin P.D. measured across the skin is always smaller than E_{Na} on account of the shorting effect of diffusible anions. Formally it could be approximated by the Hodgkin-Huxley-Goldman equation (see p. 56, eq. (13)).

It will appear from eq.[34] that high cellular K concentration and low cellular Na concentration must be characteristic of a high electromotive force of the system. When the skin is short-circuited, the current is determined by this EMF, by the resistance to Na diffusion in the outward facing cell membrane and in cytoplasm of the epithelial cells themselves, and by the resistance to K of the inward facing boundary of the epithelium. Undoubtedly one should also introduce a term for the Na resistance of the connective tissue; this term, however, is likely to be small.

If the sodium pump (or the Na/K-pump) cannot keep pace with the loss of potassium and the gain of sodium by the epithelium the electromotive force of the system would gradually drop until a new steady state is reached. According to this hypothesis it ought to be possible to charge the skin battery treating the skin inside with a high potassium, low sodium solution for some time. As a matter of fact this conclusion seems to be correct.

The question may be raised whether the sodium pump is a sodium-potassium exchange mechnism or whether the partner in the forced exchange process against sodium is really the hydrogen ion. In the latter case hydrogen ions would be carried into the cells to the extent sodium is extruded towards the inside solution. If the inwardfacing membrane were highly permeable to hydrogen ions, the diffusion of these would create a diffusion potential which in turn would determine the level of potassium in the cells. This latter assumption would imply a high H permeability of the inward facing membrane. As a matter of fact, MEYER and BERNFELD have claimed that this membrane behaves towards hydrogen ion concentration changes almost like a glass electrode, indicating a high selectivity towards hydrogen ions. It seems, however, that the effect of hydrogen ions on this boundary is not simply that of an ion penetrating with relative ease. Thus, the sodium pump is inhibited strongly by a lowering of the p_H. A detailed study of the effect of p_H on sodium transport and on sodium resistance of frog skin has been performed by SCHOFFENIELS[524]. For the time being it is impossible with certainty to distinguish between the possibilities that the partner in the forced exchange of sodium is potassium (MACROBBIE and USING [536a]) or that it is the hydrogen ion. The former possibility seems, however, to be the more promising one.

5. Inhibitors of the active sodium transport

It has already been mentioned that lack of oxygen reduces the sodium transport very much indeed, and so do all inhibitors interfering with oxidative metabolism such as cyanide. The inhibitory effect of dinitrophenol has already been mentioned. It probably acts by uncoupling phosphorylation from oxidation. Dinitrophenol poisoning is associated with a loss of potassium from the cells of the skin. According to LINDERHOLM, compare also HUF[537] other poisons like the xanthines reduce the sodium movement without inducing any potassium loss. Higher concentrations of the xanthines also lead to a loss of potassium as well to complete inhibition of the sodium transport (compare also LEVINSKY and SAWYER[538]).

The skin potential and thus presumably also the active sodium transport is strongly depressed by monoiodo- and monobromo-acetate (HUF[537], FRANCIS and GATTY[539], BORGHGRAEFF[540]). This may be taken as evidence that the glycolytic cycle is of importance in the frog skin metabolism. Even monofluoracetate depresses the transport, indicating the involvement of the citric acid cycle. The effects of other inhibitors are shown in Table 19. In several cases the nature of the effect is obscure. Thus, although a number of carbonic anhydrase inhibitors have a decisive inhibitory effect on the sodium transport, carbonic anhydrase has not so far been demonstrated in the skin. Anti-cholinesterases like tetraethylpyrophosphate and eserin when applied from the inside are powerful inhibitors of the active sodium transport[542, 543]. The most striking feature is that although such poisoning stops the current and the active sodium transport, the

---

[536a] MACROBBIE, E. A. C., and H. H. USSING: in prep.

[537] HUF, E. G., N. S. DOSS, and J. P. WILLS: Effects of metabolic inhibitors and drugs on ion transport and oxygen consumption in isolated frog skin. J. gen. Physiol. **41**, 397—417 (1957).

[538] LEVINSKY, N. G., and W. H. SAWYER: Relation of metabolism of frog skin to cellular integrity and electrolyte transfer. J. gen. Physiol. **36**, 607—615 (1953).

[539] FRANCIS, W. L., and O. GATTY: The effect of iodoacetate on the electrical potential and on the oxygen uptake of frog skin. J. exp. Biol. **15**, 132—142 (1938).

[540] BORGHGRAEFF, R.: In preparation.

[541] NEDERGAARD, S., and H. H. USSING: Acta physiol. scand. (in press).

[542] KIRSCHNER, L. B.: Effect of cholinesterase inhibitors and atropine on active sodium transport across frog skin. Nature (Lond.) **172**, 348—349 (1953).

[543] FUHRMAN, F. A.: Inhibition of active sodium transport in the isolated frog skin. Amer. J. Physiol. **171**, 266—278 (1952).

Table 19. *Agents inhibiting sodium transport in amphibian skin*

Group	Substance	Dose giving at least 50% inhibition M/l	Applied on	Remark	Ref.
Metabolic inhibitors	cyanide	$3 \cdot 10^{-5}$	inside	Rana pipiens	[537]
	fluoroacetate	$1 \cdot 10^{-3}$	inside	Rana pipiens	[537]
	azide	$1 \cdot 10^{-3}$	inside	Rana pipiens	[537]
	diethylmalonate	$1 \cdot 10^{-3}$	inside	Rana pipiens	[537]
	iodoacetate	$1 \cdot 10^{-3}$	inside		[539] [537]
	2,4 dinitrophenol	$5 \cdot 10^{-5}$	inside outside both sides	Rana pipiens Rana temps.	[543] [537] [538]
	arsenite	$1 \cdot 10^{-4}$	inside	Rana pipiens	[537]
	fluoride	$1 \cdot 10^{-2}$	inside	Rana pipiens	[537]
Cholinesterase inhibitors	(TEP) tetraethylpyrophos- phate eserin	$6 \cdot 10^{-3}$ $>1 \cdot 10^{-2}$	inside outside	Rana esc. Rana temp. Rana temp.	[547]
Sulfonamides	p-toluenesulfonamide sulfanilamide	$1.8 \cdot 10^{-3}$ $2 \cdot 10^{-3}$	inside inside	Rana temp.	[543]
Narcotics	CO_2	5%	both sides	Rana temp.	[520]
Cardiac glucosides	g-strophanthin	$1 \cdot 10^{-6}$	inside	Rana temp.	[544]

skin does not die, as evidenced by the fact that the skin resistance goes up whereas in dead skins it drops to nearly zero.

G-strophantin in concentrations as low as 10^{-6} molar strongly inhibits the active sodium transport[544] when added to the inside bathing solution. Added from the outside it has no effect. The drug also induces a violent drop in cellular potassium in the skin, as much as 60% being lost in three hours. The loss takes place exclusively towards the inside bathing solution.

An effect which superficially resembles that of strophantin is exerted by a toxin from a diniflagellate. The toxin drastically reduces the skin potential (ABBOT and BALLANTINE[545]). Also the membrane potential of muscle and nerve is depressed by this agent. Since, however, the toxin can induce a reversal of sign of the frog skin P.D. even if it is in contact with Ringer on both sides, a mere inhibition of the sodium pump cannot be the explanation, If, however, the passive Na—permeability of the inward-facing membrane of the epithelium cells were increased strongly and selectively, a reversal of potential might ensue. A greatly increased passive sodium permeability would also explain the depolarizing effect in nerve and muscle.

6. Stimulants of active sodium transport

It is characteristic of the isolated amphibian skin that addition of substrates are normally without effect on the rate of active transport. The active transport can, however, be augmented considerably by a number of agents (see table 20). The substances listed all under proper conditions give rise to an increase in sodium

---

[544] KOEFOED-JOHNSEN, V.: The effect of g-strophanthin (ouabain) on the active transport of sodium through the isolated frog skin. Acta physiol. scand. **42**, Suppl. 145, 87—88 (1957).

[545] ABBOT, B. C., and D. BALLANTINE: The toxin from Gymnodinium veneficum Ballantine. J. Mar. Biol. U. K. **36**, 169—189 (1957).

Table 20. *Agents stimulating active sodium transport in amphibian skin*
Only agents capable of giving at least 25% increase in sodium current in short-circuited skins
are listed

Group	Substance	Dose	Applied on	Remark	Ref.
Neurohypo-physeal hormones	vasopressin oxytocin	0.1—4.0 I.U./25 ml 0.1—2.0 I.U./25 ml	inside inside	Rana esc., Rana temp. R. pipiens, Bufo bufo Bufo bufo Rana	546 546 520
Oxidants	permanganate bromine periodate	$3 \cdot 10^{-4}$ M/l $1 \cdot 10^{-3}$ M/l $5 \cdot 10$ M/l	inside inside inside	R. temp. Bufo bufo R. temp. Bufo bufo R. temp. Bufo bufo	541
Reductants	BAL	$3 \cdot 10^{-4}$ M/l	inside	Rana temp.	541
Heavy metals	Ag^+	$1 \cdot 10^{-4}$ M/l	inside	Rana temp. Bufo bufo	541
Alkaloids	atropine curares	$0.3—9 \cdot 10^{-4}$ M/l $0.1—1.3 \cdot 10^{-4}$ M/l	outside outside	Rana esc. not R. temp. R. esc.	547
Diuretics	mersalyl aminophylline	10^{-4} $2 \cdot 10^{-3}$	inside inside	Rana temp. Rana temp.	531, 537 531, 537 538

transport by short-circuited skins of at least 25%. The mode of action of the neurohypophyseal hormones[546] has been partly cleared up and will be discussed below. With Ringer on both sides of the skin the neurohypophyseal hormones increase the rate of sodium transport but not the apparent driving force, E_{Na}. By contrast, agents like permanganate, BAL and silver ions[541] increase both the sodium current and the apparent driving potential. Since the experiments are performed under conditions of short-circuiting where there is no net flow of anions, the substance in question must act either by facilitating the diffusion of potassium through the inward facing membrane of the stratum germinativum cells or by stimulating the sodium pump for instance by releasing carrier molecules in the membrane. Most of them are so powerful cell poisons that they are most unlikely to act inside the cells. None of them stimulated the sodium transport if added to the outside solution. The alkaloids atropin, tubocurarin, histamine and pilocarpine[547], on the other hand, are powerful stimulants of the active sodium transport when added from the outside but do not stimulate when added from the inside. Possibly they facilitate the diffusion of sodium through the outward facing membrane of the epithelium cells. It is a peculiar fact that the atropin effect cannot be elicited in R. temporaria although it is pronounced in R. esculenta and Bufo bufo.

7. *The action of neurohypophyseal hormones upon the transfer of water and salt across the frog skin*

It is a well known fact that the neurohypophyseal hormones induce an increased uptake of water through the skin of amphibians. This effect has been

[546] FUHRMAN, F. A., and H. H. USSING: A characteristic response of the isolated frog skin potential to neurohypophyseal principles and its relation to the transport of sodium and water. J. cell. comp. Physiol. 38, 109—130 (1951).
[547] KIRSCHNER, L. B.: The effect of atropine and the curares on the active transport of sodium by the skin of Rana esculenta. J. cell. comp. Physiol. 45, 89—102 (1955).

studied under the name of the BRUNN[548] reaction or the water balance reaction. The pertinent literature has been discussed by HELLER[549], JØRGENSEN[550] and SAWYER[551]. All three authors agree that the neurohypophyseal hormones increase the rate of water uptake through the skin besides depressing the renal excretion of water. With respect to the mechanism, SAWYER[551] assumed it to be due to increased permeability whereas CAPRARO et al.[552] preferred to think of it as an increase in active water transport. The phenomenon can be seen not only in intact animals but also in the isolated skin of toads (NOVELLI[553]) and frogs (FUHRMAN and USSING[546], SAWYER[551]). It has been mentioned above that the neurohypophyseal hormones also increase the active transport of sodium. The most reasonable explanation of these phenomena is that the hormones increase the pore size of some layer in the skin. The following facts speak in favor of an effect on the pore size: 1) The hormones increase the rate of active sodium transport without affecting the driving force, E_{Na}. Thus the effect must consist in a drop in the resistance to the flow of sodium ions rather than a stimulation of the metabolic mechanism behind the sodium transport. 2) They increase the water permeability in a way which indicates an increase in pore size (compare KOEFOED-JOHNSEN and USSING[364]). 3) They increase the permeability of the skin to inert hydrophilic substances like thiourea and acetamide. 4) They increase the solvent drag upon uncharged molecules during osmosis (ANDERSEN and USSING[235]). 5) They make possible the stimulation of the active sodium transport by added glucose, indicating a breakdown of a barrier for the diffusion into the cells of this substance. 6) It permits the rapid poisoning of the skin by noxious substances like monoiodoacetate or fluoracetate, which otherwise take a long time to exert their effects.

In so far as a small fraction of the water transfer in the presence of an osomotic gradient, and the total water transfer in the absence of a gradient, is associated with the active sodium transport one may say that the hormones stimulate active water transport, but what these hormones do in all cases is simply to lower the resistance to water flow and to the flow of sodium ions.

8. The relationship between active sodium transport and transport of water across the skin

As early as 1890, REID[554] demonstrated a small net transfer of water in the inward direction across the skin in the absence of a hydrostatic or osmotic pressure difference. The phenomenon has been studied by, for instance, MAXWELL[555],

[548] BRUNN, F.: Beitrag zur Kenntnis der Wirkung von Hypophysenextrakten auf den Wasserhaushalt des Frosches. Z. ges. exp. Med. 25, 170—175 (1921).

[549] HELLER, H.: The effect of neurohypophysiol extracts on the water balance of lower vertebrates. Biol. Rev. 20, 147—158 (1945).

[550] JØRGENSEN, C. B.: The amphibian water economy with special regard to the effect of neurohypophyseal extracts. Acta physiol. scand. 22, Suppl. 78, 79 pp. (1950).

[551] SAWYER, W. H.: Effect of posterior pituitary extract on permeability of frog skin to water. Amer. J. Physiol. 164, 44—48 (1951).

[552] CAPRARO, V., and G. BERNINI: Mechanism of action of extracts of the posthypophysis on water transport through the skin of the frog. Nature (Lond.) 169, 454 (1952).

[553] NOVELLI, A.: Lobulo posterior de hipófisis e imbibición de los batracios. II. Mecanismo de su acción, Rev. Soc. argent. Biol. 12, 163—170 (1936).

[554] REID, E. W.: Report on experiments upon "Absorption without Osmosis". Brit. med. J. 1892 I, 323—326.

[555] MAXWELL, S. S.: On the absorption of water by the skin of the frog. Amer. J. Physiol. 32, 286—294 (1913).

Wertheimer[556], Huf[557] and Capraro[552]. With Ringer on both sides, the net transfer of water across the frog skin is of the order of $1-5$ mg cm^{-2} hr^{-1}. Huf[500] found the net inward transport of about one mg water per cm^2 per hour.

Cyanide inhibits the transfer of water as well as of salt. The water transfer seems to be strictly associated with the active sodium transport. Thus if the salt solution bathing the outside of the skin is replaced by Ringer-isotonic sugar solution there is no net transfer of water (Krogh[515]). If dilute Ringer or water is used as an outside solution so that an osmotic gradient is present across the skin, water transfers of considerably larger magnitude are obtained. In the presence of an osmotic gradient there seems to be very little dependence of the water transfer upon the active transport of sodium.

Possibly, the water transfer associated with the active sodium transport, even in the absence of an osmotic gradient should be considered as the resultant of the drag exerted on the water by the net movement of sodium and (or) chloride ions. In a sense, then, this water flow may be considered as being due to electro-osmosis.

c) The rumen of ruminants

The transport of sodium and potassium across the rumen of the ruminates seems to follow a pattern very similar to that described for the isolated frog skin. The first evidence for active salt transport in the rumen mucosa was provided

Table 21. *Net ion shifts in the goat rumen* (Ref. [558])

Time hr.		Na mM	K+ mM	HPO$_4$$^{--}$ mM	Cl− mM
0	Introduced 150 ml	169	0	31	86
4.5	Removed 39 ml	156	trace	36	77
22	Pouch emptied 45 ml	152	27	70	28
Introduced (mMoles)		24	0	4.65	12.9
Removed again (mMoles)		12.9	1.2	4.55	4.3

by Sperber and Hydén[558]. They studied the absorption of salt solutions from the posterior ventral blind sack of the rumen of the goat with intact blood supply. Table 21 shows results from a typical experiment. It is seen that if sodium chloride solution is introduced, the chloride concentration steadily decreases with time. The sodium concentration shows a considerably smaller reduction with time and potassium which was originally absent accumulates in the rumen to give a final concentration after 22 hs of 27 mmoles per liter. If we consider the amounts of the different ions transferred it is seen that 11.1 millimoles of sodium are absorbed, chloride is absorbed to a somewhat lesser extent, namely 3.6 millimoles, whereas 1.2 millimoles of potassium appear in the rumen contents. The phosphate transfer is practically nil. Sperber and Hydén conclude that chloride must pass through the rumen wall as the result of an active process, and that the same was probably true for sodium. Potassium also passes through against a concentration gradient,

[556] Wertheimer, E.: Weitere Studien über die Permeabilität lebender Membranen. V. Mitteilung. Über die Kräfte, die die Wasserbewegung durch eine lebende Membran bedingen. Pflügers Arch. ges. Physiol. **201**, 591—602 (1923).

[557] Huf, E. G.: Die Reproduzierbarkeit des Reidschen Versuchs. Pflügers Arch. ges. Physiol. **238**, 97—102 (1937).

[558] Sperber, I., and S. Hydén: Transport of chloride through the rumen mucosa. Nature (Lond.) **169**, 587 (1952).

but in the opposite direction. PARTHASARATHY and PHILLIPSON[559] confirmed the observation that chloride is taken up against a concentration gradient. Later, however, DOBSON and PHILLIPSON[560] using the washed reticulo-rumen sack of the sheep in situ, demonstrated that the net flux of chloride ions across the epithelium took place always in the direction dictated by the electrochemical potential difference for the chloride ion. The electric potential difference across the rumen epithelium varied between 25.4 and 44.0 mV, the blood side positive relative to the lumen side. Changing the chloride concentration in the rumen sack, they found that the transport could always be accounted for as the resultant of the combined effects of the potential and concentration gradient. The sodium transport, however, according to DOBSON[561] took place always against the electrochemical potential, that is Na^+ was always being transferred from the lumen to the blood side. In 8 periods where the concentration ratio of Na across the rumen epithelium was near unity, net uptakes of 0.25—0.48 milliequivalents per minute were observed. This corresponds to 1.0 milliequivalents per minute per kg wet weight of epithelium. Thus the chloride transport is passive whereas the sodium transport is active and can be — and probably is — the source of the electric potential difference. The transfer of potassium into the lumen of the rumen sack, observed by SPERBER and HYDÉN, might very well be due to the electrical potential difference. Quite recently, DOBSON and PHELLIPSON[562] have observed that if solutions, having a high potassium and low sodium concentration, are placed in the rumen, small net movements of chloride take plate into the rumen contents against the electrochemical potential of this ion. DUBSON assumes that this small active transport of chloride into the lumen corresponds to the active chloride excretion by the frog skin glands which is elicited by stimulation with adrenalin.

d) The toad urinary bladder

LEAF[563] has demonstrated that the urinary bladder of the toad (Bufo bufo), when in contact with Ringer solution on both sides maintaines a potential (the lumen side negative) of similar magnitude as that of the isolated frog skin. If short-circuited (see under the frog skin) the toad bladder gives rise to a steady electric current from the mucosal to theserosal surface. In 226 experiments it was on an average $0.00850\ \mu Eq/cm^2/min$. The net sodium transport during the same periods was $0.00847\ \mu Eq/cm^2/min$. Thus the active sodium transport was responsible for the total short circuit current. Addition of neurohypophyseal extract to the serosal side gives a powerful increase in both sodium transport and current, the equality of the two quantities being maintained.

Adrenaline had no effect on the sodium fluxes and neither did it effect the short circuit current. This may be taken as evidence that the adrenaline effect on the frog skin is mainly associated with the skin glands which are lacking in the urinary bladder.

[559] PARTHASARATHY, D., and A. T. PHILLIPSON: The movement of potassium, sodium, chloride and water across the rumen epithelium of sheep. J. Physiol. **121**, 452—469 (1953).

[560] DOBSON, A., and A. T. PHILLIPSON: The forces moving chloride ions through rumen epithelium. J. Physiol. **125**, 26 P—27 P (1954).

[561] DOBSON, A.: The forces moving sodium ions through rumen epithelium. J. Physiol. **128**, 39 P—40 P (1955).

[562] DOBSON, A., and A. T. PHILLIPSON: The movements of ions across the reticulo-rumen sack. Abstr. Comm. XXth int. Physiol. Congress. Brussels 1956.

[563] LEAF, A.: Ion transport by the isolated bladder of the toad. Resumes dez Communications 3ème Congrès International de Biochemie, p. 107. Brussels 1955.

e) Intestinal mucosa

1. Net transport of sodium

It has been recognized for a long time that the transfer of sodium ions across the intestinal wall involves the participation of active transport. Thus HEIDEN-HAIN[564] concluded from experiments on the resorption of sodium chloride solutions in dog small intestine that the transport does not strictly follow the diffusion laws. The sodium chloride resorption is brought about by the combined effects of a physical and a physiological driving force. The latter force, according to HEIDEN-HAIN, could be inhibited by sodium fluoride in the infusion fluid. HÖBER[565] first contested this view, and claimed that the resorption of salts depended upon their diffusibility. Thus the factors governing salt resorption would be physical and the cells would play no particular role. Furthermore, HÖBER assumed that only lipoid soluble salts could be resorbed intracellularly, whereas lipoid non-soluble salts diffused solely between the mucosal cells. The work of WALLACE and CUSHNY[566] and KATZENELLENBOGEN[567] was not in agreement with HÖBER's view, however. HÖBER[568] later accepted HEIDENHAIN's original view that the resorption of salt does not depend solely upon the physical factors but was aided by a special "Triebkraft". In the small intestine hypertonic sodium chloride solutions usually undergo dilution whereas hypotonic solutions are concentrated by the absorption of water, so that, finally, an almost isotonic sodium chloride solution is reabsorbed. Such experiments thus do not show with certainty whether it is sodium, chloride or the sodium chloride solution as such which is being actively transported. Methodologically it was therefore a great step forward when KATZENELLEN-BOGEN[567] introduced the technique of mixing the NaCl solution with a substance like mannitol which is not easily absorbed in the intestine. The mannitol by its osmotic effect stops the flow of water from the intestine to the blood without stopping the absorption of Na and Cl. With this technique he demonstrated that sodium chloride could be absorbed against a concentration gradient in the dog small intestine. Mannitol can be replaced by magnesium chloride or sodium sulfate (COBET[569]). The ability to transport NaCl against the concentration gradient is more pronounced in the large intestine than in the small intestine (GOLDSCHMIDT and DAYTON[570]).

The above mentioned technique of studying the uptake of NaCl against the concentration gradient in the presence of an osmotically active substance which is not, or only slowly, absorbed, has been applied with great success by VISSCHER and collaborators.

According to INGRAHAM and VISSCHER[571], chloride can be absorbed from mixtures of KCl and K_2SO_4, just as well as from mixtures of NaCl and Na_2SO_4. In

[564] HEIDENHAIN, R.: Neue Versuche über die Aufsaugung im Dünndarm. Arch. ges. Physiol. **56**, 579—631 (1894).

[565] HÖBER, R.: Über Resorption im Dünndarm. Arch. ges. Physiol. **74**, 246—271 (1899).

[566] WALLACE, G. B., and A. R. CUSHNY: Über Darmresorption und die salinischen Abführmittel. Arch. ges. Physiol. **77**, 202—209 (1899).

[567] KATZENELLENBOGEN, M.: Der Einfluß der Diffusibilität und der Lipoidlöslichkeit auf die Geschwindigkeit der Darmresorption. Arch. ges. Physiol. **114**, 522—534 (1906).

[568] HÖBER, R.: Physikalische Chemie der Zellen und Gewebe. 5. Aufl., 906 pp. Leipzig: Engelmann 1924.

[569] COBET, R.: Über die Resorption von Magnesiumsulfatlösungen im Dünndarm und die Wirkungsweise der salinischen Abführmittel. Arch. ges. Physiol. **150**, 325—360 (1913).

[570] GOLDSCHMIDT, S., and A. B. DAYTON: Studies in the mechanism of absorption from the intestine III: the colon: the osmotic pressure equilibrium between the intestinal contents and the blood. Amer. J. Physiol. **48**, 440—449 (1919).

fact potassium was absorbed somewhat faster than sodium. They therefore concluded that sodium does not play any specific role for the transport of chloride. It
should be remembered, however, that if NaCl and KCl of equal tonicity are being
absorbed, the potassium gradient from intestine to blood must always be much
steeper than the sodium gradient, since, in the blood, the Na concentration is high
and the potassium concentration is low. Another factor which must be born in
mind is that even if sodium-free solutions are introduced into the intestine, sodium
must always be present during the absorption since it is secreted continuously into
the intestine by the intestinal glands. Furthermore Na diffuses through the
intestinal wall into the intestine contents. This can be demonstrated by introducing
sodium chloride-free media into the intestine and analyzing after a suitable period
of time (HÖBER[565], COBET[569], KNAFFL-LENZ and NOGAKI[572], RABINOWITCH[573],
BURNS and VISSCHER[574], MacDOUGAL and VERZAR[575], DENNIS[576], VISSCHER
and coll.[577], VISSCHER, ROEPKE and LIFSON[580] and GOLDSCHMIDT and DAYTON[570]).
In their experiments with dog small intestine INGRAHAM and VISSCHER[578] usually
found that the chloride resorption exceeded the net absorption of sodium. This
finding has been verified by BUDOLFSEN[579]. This fact might speak in favour of the
chloride transport being independent of the active sodium transport, but it
should be remembered that whereas sodium and chloride ions have usually been
given in equivalent concentrations in the infusate, the two ions are not present in
identical concentrations, in the lymph and the blood, roughly one third of the
anion of the blood plasma being bicarbonate, whereas Na makes up nearly all of
the cation. Consequently, the chloride diffusion gradient toward the blood is
steeper than the sodium gradient. Clearly then, during resorption experiments,
chloride in the intestine will exchange against bicarbonate ions from the blood
(compare INGRAHAM and VISSCHER[578], VISSCHER, ROEPKE and LIFSON[580], BUCHER,
ANDERSON and ROBINSON[581]). It is obvious that without knowledge of the electric
potential difference across the intestine under the specific conditions of the experiments it is impossible to judge whether chloride is being actively transported

[571] INGRAHAM, R. C., and M. B. VISSCHER: The influence of various poisons on the
movement of chloride against concentration gradients from intestine to plasma. Amer. J.
Physiol. **114**, 681—687 (1935/36).
[572] KNAFFL-LENZ, E., and S. NOGAKI: Über die Resorption aus ausgeschalteten Darm-
schlingen. Naunyn-Schmiedebergs Arch. exp. Path. Pharmak. **105**, 109—123 (1925).
[573] RABINOWITCH, J.: Factors influencing the absorption of water and chlorides from
the intestine. Amer. J. Physiol. **82**, 279—289 (1927).
[574] BURNS, H. S., and M. B. VISSCHER: The influence of various anions of the lyotropic
series upon the sodium and chloride content of fluid in the intestine. Amer. J. Physiol. **110**,
490—498 (1934—35).
[575] MacDOUGAL, E. J., and F. VERZAR: Die Resorption von Wasser aus Kochsalz- und
Zuckerlösungen. Arch. ges. Physiol. **236**, 321—328 (1935).
[576] DENNIS, C.: Injury to the ileal mucosa by contact with distilled water. Amer. J.
Physiol. **129**, 171—175 (1940).
[577] VISSCHER, M. B., R. H. VARCO, C. W. CARR, R. B. DEAN, and D. ERICSON: Sodium
ion movement between the intestinal lumen and the blood. Amer. J. Physiol. 141, 488—505
(1944).
[578] INGRAHAM, R. C., and M. B. VISSCHER: Further studies on intestinal absorption
with the performance of osmotic work. Amer. J. Physiol. **121**, 771—785 (1938).
[579] BUDOLFSEN, S. E.: Sammenlignende Undersøgelser over Resorptionen i Tyktarmen
og den distale Del af Tyndtarmen (with an English summary), 173 pp. Diss. 1952, Aarhus,
Denmark.
[580] VISSCHER, M. B., R. R. ROEPKE, and N. LIFSON: Osmotic and electrolyte concentration relationships during the absorption of autogenous serum from ileal segments. Amer.
J. Physiol. **144**, 457—463 (1945).
[581] BUCHER, G. R., C. E. ANDERSON, and C. S. ROBINSON: Chemical changes produced
in isotonic solutions of sodium sulfate and sodium chloride by the small intestine of dog.
Amer. J. Physiol. **163**, 1—13 (1950).

or whether its transfer is due to the combined effects of the concentration and potential gradients. Furthermore, with an organ like the intestine where gross net transfers of water can take place, the effect of solvent drag cannot be neglected. Recent work indicates that in the small intestine of the rat both Cl and Na are being actively absorbed (see p. 137). In the large intestine of the toad and the frog as well as in the coecum of the guinea-pig, the active sodium transport dominates the picture and there is no indication of active chloride transport (see p. 137).

It is well established that the uptake of sodium does not depend critically on the chloride concentration. Thus sodium is rapidly taken up from solutions of NaCl, NaBr, Na I, Na-acetate. The rate does depend on the nature of the anion, however. Thus Na is absorbed faster from isotonic NaCl than from isotonic solutions of Na_2SO_4 (although the Na concentration is higher in the latter solution)[582]. Unfortunately, in none of these experiments was the electric potential measured; thus a rigorous treatment of the material is not possible. As a general rule one can say that in the duodenum and the jejunum, Na^+, Cl^+ and water move roughly in the direction of their concentration gradients. Apparently the permeability here is so large that the purely physical factors dominate over the active transport processes. In the ileum the passive permeability is apparently less and the active transport of Na becomes of more importance. In the colon the transport rates are low, but under proper conditions the active transport of sodium and chloride make themselves manifest by the establishment of a concentration which is lower than in the blood. This statement as far as the absolute rates of transfer go, must be taken with some reserve. One can, of course, compare sections of intestine of equal length, but what matters in the absorption process is the area of exposed epithelium, which, due to the development of villi and folds in the gut can only be estimated with a low degree of accuracy.

Besides the existence of a transport of NaCl "uphill" one other factor has often been mentioned as being indicative of active transport, namely that the transport is not proportional to the concentration in the intestine. Thus, according to RABINOWITCH, the NaCl uptake increases with the concentration in the infusate to reach an about constant level around isotonic solution. At still higher concentrations, about 1.5% NaCl, the amount absorbed per unit time actually decreases. Similar results were obtained by MACDOUGAL and VERZAR[575] in experiments with rat jejunum (see also DENNIS and VISSCHER[583], experiments in the ileum of dogs). Also BUDOLFSEN[579] experiments on dogs. A "saturation" type of transport kinetics is, however, no proof of active transport.

2. The dependency of the sodium transport upon different factors

As long as the p_H of the infusion fluid remains within physiological limits, it does not seem to influence the sodium transport. Thus BUDOLFSEN found the absorbed amount of Na and Cl in dog small intestine and large intestine to be the same whether the p_H was 6.0, 7.0 or 8.3. According to the same author, K depresses the Na transport markedly in the small intestine of the dog, whereas little effect is seen on the sodium transport in the large intestine. The Cl transport is unaffected by potassium. BUDOLFSEN assumes this above mentioned reduction of the Na absorption by potassium ions to be due to a specific interference by K with the

[582] VISSCHER, M. B., E. S. FETCHER, C. W. CARR, H. P. GREGOR, M. S. BUSHEY, and D. E. BARBER: Isotopic tracer studies on the movement of water and ions between intestinal lumen and the blood. Amer. J. Physiol. 142, 550—575 (1944).

[583] DENNIS, C., and M. B. VISSCHER: Studies on the rates of absorption of water and salts from the ileum of the dog. Amer. J. Physiol. 131, 402—408 (1940).

sodium transport mechanism. A simpler explanation is that concomitant with absorption of NaCl from a mixture of NaCl and KCl solutions in the small intestine, there is an exchange of K from the intestine against Na from the blood. Due to the steeper K gradient towards the blood, more potassium than Na would leave the intestine, even if the two ionic species diffused at the same rate. This explanation would be in bearing with the notion that in the small intestine the physical forces dominate over the active transport force in determining the direction of movement for Na. It should be mentioned, however, that addition of KCl to a glucose solution reduces its rate of reabsorption in the small intestine, although no effect is seen in the large intestine. This unquestionably speaks in favor of a specific effect of K upon the processes in the mucosa unless the transport of sugar in some way depends upon the sodium transport. No such coupling has so far been demonstrated with certainty, but it is known that the transport of isotonic NaCl solution through isolated loops of small intestine of rats is only possible in the presence of glucose in the intestinal contents (FISHER[584], SMYTH and TAYLOR[585]). It speaks in favour of some coupling between Na transport and active glucose transport in the small intestine that both phenomena are inhibited by phlorhizin. The fact that this glycoside acts much more strongly on glucose absorption than on sodium chloride absorption is not unexpected since, as mentioned above, the merely physical forces dominate in the NaCl resorption in the small intestine, whereas the glucose transport is largely of active nature. In the large intestine K does not interfere with Na resorption and here also phlorhizin is without effect, possibly because the membrane is impermeable to the glycoside. Many toxic substances have been studied with respect to their ability to influence the sodium chloride absorption in the gut. Most of the poisons studied show a highly unspecific effect. Thus, according to INGRAHAM and VISSCHER, mercury chloride, arsenic, NaF, and HCN all make the intestinal wall permeable to sulfate ions. It is therefore not surprising that the same poisons make it impossible for the intestinal epithelium to perform transport against the concentration gradient of NaCl.

3. The unidirectional sodium fluxes

VISSCHER and collaborators were the first to use isotopes in an extensive study of the absorption kinetics of inorganic substances from the intestine. They prepared chronic Thiry-Vella loops from different sections of the gut of dogs. Solutions containing Na-salts labelled with Na^{24} were introduced, and after a suitable time the volume changes and the changes in Na concentration and Na^{24} activity were determined. From these measurements the Na fluxes into and out of the gut could be calculated. The figures shown in Table 22 are extracted from the paper by VISSCHER et al.[577]. In all experiments shown in the table the solution placed in the loop was isotonic with the blood and consisted of equal parts, on an osmolar basis, of NaCl and Na_2SO_4. It will be seen that in agreement with what has been said already, the fluxes are highest in the jejunum, lower in the ileum and lowest in the colon. More interesting, however, than the absolute amount transferred are the flux ratios — that is the ratio of the Na-flux out of the gut to the sodium flux into the gut. For the jejunum this figure is close to one, it seems higher in the ileum and has arisen to about 3 for the colon. Thus the "one-sidedness" of the sodium transport is definitely more pronounced in the large intestine,

[584] FISHER, R. B.: The absorption of water and of some small solute molecules from the isolated small intestine of the rat. J. Physiol. 130, 655—664 (1955).

[585] SMYTH, D. H., and C. B. TAYLOR: The inhibition of water transport in the vitro intestinal preparation. J. Physiol. 128, 81 P—82 P (1955).

although the net transfers are smaller. This result is in full agreement with the one obtained on the basis of the ability of the different sections of the gut to deplete the intestinal contents of Na ions.

VISSCHER et al. also studied the net transfer and total exchange of water across the dog gut, using heavy water as a tracer. Table 23 shows the mean rates of water movement between gut loops and blood. It further gives the flux ratios found, and those calculated according to "classical osmotic theory". The experiments are divided into three groups, according to whether the NaCl solution introduced into the intestinal loop was hypotonic, nearly isotonic or hypertonic to the blood. Ileal loops of dogs about 10 cm long were used. The water

Table 22. *Na-flux into and out of intestinal loops of the dog.* Solutions in intestine: 50% of isotonic NaCl and isotonic Na_2SO_4. (Figures extracted from VISSCHER et al.[577])

	meq/min			Flux ratio Na out/Na into
	Na out	Na into	Na net	
Jejunum	0.459	0.382	0.077	1.20
	0.323	0.373	—0.050	0.87
	0.580	0.538	0.042	1.08
Ileum	0.157	0.138	0.019	1.14
	0.209	0.129	0.080	1.62
	0.259	0.176	0.083	1.47
Colon	0.099	0.031	0.068	3.19
	0.153	0.056	0.097	2.73
	0.083	0.025	0.058	3.22

transfers are given as cm³ per loop per ten minutes. Since the effective area cannot be measured, the results cannot be expressed as ml per unit area. R_{out} is the rate at which water leaves the intestinal contents as measured by the disappearance rate of the heavy water, R_{net} is the net disappearance rate. The sign is positive if more water leaves than enters the gut and negative if the reverse is true. $R_{net, calc}$ is the

Table 23. *Mean rates of water movement between gut loops and blood*
Observed rates compared with rates predicted from osmotic theory (ml/10 min). (Ref. [582])

Na Cl Solution in gut	R_{out} obs	R_{into} obs	R_{out}/R_{into} obs	R_{into} calc	R_{out}/R_{into} calc
Hypotonic . .	21.2	11.0	1.93	21.15	1.002
Isotonic . . .	11.1	9.5	1.17	11.11	0.999
Hypertonic .	7.4	12.1	0.61	7.47	0.991

disappearance rate calculated under the assumption that the rates of transfer out of and into the gut are proportional to the water vapour tensions of the gut contents and of the blood, respectively. In other words, the calculation is based upon the classical assumption that osmosis arises as the difference between the amount of solvent diffusing in one direction and the amount diffusing in the opposite direction, and that diffusion is proportional to the water activities in the two bathing solutions. The flux ratio is derived on the same assumption. It is seen that the flux ratio found differs greatly from that calculated. VISSCHER et al. interpreted these results as indicating that the water exchange in the gut is due mainly to active transport processes. As a matter of fact it is still a matter of doubt whether active water transport does take place. Thus there is a significant resorption of water (and salt) from isotonic solutions. But it is also apparent that the osmotic pressure of the gut contents is of greater importance than the active water transport as evidenced by the fact the direction of net water flow is reversed when hypertonic solutions are introduced.

In a recent study of the sodium, chloride and water absorption by the small intestines of the rat CURRAN and SOLOMON[586] found no evidence for active water transport. FISHER[584], however, working with isolated small intestine of the rat found that the rate of water absorption was unaffected by rather large differences in osmotic pressure gradient and therefore concluded that water was actively transported.

As discussed on p. 51, the so called "simple osmotic theory" is not valid if osmotic flow takes place through pores, in which case it is the laws of laminar flow and not those of diffusion which dominate the picture. Osmosis through a porous membrane will always show a larger flux ratio than that predicted from "classical theory". Thus the results of VISSCHER et al. as far as water is concerned can be satisfactorily explained as arising from osmosis through a porous membrane, superimposed upon a small but significant active water transport. The situation seems to be quite similar to that pertaining in the isolated amphibian skin. VISSCHER and collaborators' experiments therefore cannot be taken as evidence for his ingenious fluid circuit theory which is discussed on p. 69.

There are, however, several observations indicating an intimate relationship between water movements and salt resorption in the gut. Thus the water flux, as measured with D_2O is more than twice as big when the solution in the gut is one third isotonic than when it is hypertonic. Possibly the epithelium cells swell when the intestinal contents is hypotonic and this might in a purely mechanical way increase the pore size and the water permeability. It is known that the mucosa swells strongly when distilled water is introduced into the gut (DENNIS)[576].

4. Intestinal potentials and their relation to active sodium transport

In all the papers on intestinal sodium resorption so far discussed observations on the electrical potential difference between intestinal contents and the blood are lacking. It is indeed a peculiar fact that, whereas the gastric potentials have been studied to a considerable extent, the potentials across the intestine have attracted only little attention. Some information can be obtained from a paper by NISTLER[587]. He studied the potential between an arbitrary point at the stomach of the frog and points along the intestine, as well as points in the interior of the gastro-intestinal tract. The material suggested that the potential differences larger than a few millivolts across the wall of the organ existed only in the stomach and in the large intestine. The potential drop across the small intestine was negligible. This last-mentioned observation is in good agreement with the view that the small intestine is highly permeable to ions like Na and Cl, and thus unsuited for the maintenance of a potential difference of any magnitude. Both NISTLER's observation of a significant potential in the large intestine and the finding by VISSCHER and collaborators of a more pronounced "onesidedness" of the sodium transport in the large intestine of the dog indicate that this organ would be the place to look for a well developed active sodium transport system. As a matter of fact it can be shown that in the large intestine of toad[588] and frog and in the isolated mucosa from the coecum of the guinea pig, there is an easily demonstrable potential difference between the lumen and the blood side, the latter being positive relative to the former. This electric asymmetry arises mainly as the result of the

---

[586] CURRAN, P. F., and A. K. SOLOMON: Ion and water fluxes in the ileum of rats. J. gen. Physiol. **41**, 143—168 (1958).

[587] NISTLER, L.: Mikro-Elektr. Untersuchungen im Verdauungskanal. Diss. Mähr.-Ostrau: Jul. Kittls Nachf. 1932.

[588] COOPERSTEIN, I. L., D. CHALFIN, and C. A. M. HOGBEN: Ionic transfer across the isolated large bullfrog large intestine. Fed. Proc. **16**, 24 (1957).

active transport of sodium ions (USSING and ANDERSEN[589]). This can be demonstrated with the short-circuiting technique. The mucosa of the large intestine of the toad can be rather easily stripped off and when placed as a membrane in the flux apparatus (see p. 116) can maintain a potential difference of considerable magnitude, as much as 60 mV, for hours. During short-circuiting this organ will give electric current for many hours and the flux-analysis, using Na^{22} for determining influx and Na^{24} for determining outflux, demonstrates that all the current comes from active sodium transport (see Table 24).

The net sodium transport Δ_{Na} is seen to be almost identical with the electric current generated by the mucosa. Recent studies on the isolated large intestine of the bullfrog have shown that even here the active transport of sodium ions must be responsible for the electric potential and for practically all the electric current generated by the intestine during short-circuiting. Similar results have been obtained with the stripped-off mucosa of the guinea-pig coecum. Thus

Table 24. *Sodium flux values and short-circuit current for 3 isolated toad large intestines*[589]
Both sides Ringer. p_H 8.3

	$\mu amps/cm^2$				p.d.(mV) before shorting
	Na in	Na out	Δ Na	current	
I	47	21	26	31	37
	44	24	20	24	
II	34	9	25	23	16
III	37	16	21	20	30

in these three large intestinal preparations studied, the active sodium transport is by far the more important active transport process in so far as the establishment of the electric potential is concerned. With the stripped coecum preparations potentials ranging from 6 to 20 mV were observed. A few cursory observations indicate that similar potential values are found in vivo when Ringer solutions is being absorbed in the guinea-pig coecum. Systematic studies of the relationship between potential and ionic composition of the intestinal contents during salt absorption are, however, urgently needed. The toad and frog large intestine preparation in many respects behaves like the isolated frog skin. Thus traces of Cu in the lumen side increases the potential, probably by impeding the diffusion of chloride ion Neurohypophyseal hormones applied to the serosal side of stripped toad large intestine increase very markedly the potential and, presumably, the active Na transport. The transport of sodium in the intestinal preparations is strongly dependent on aerobic metabolism and is inhibited by DNP.

In the small intestine potentials of only a few millivolts are encountered. To some extent this is due to the large permeability to ions of this part of the intestinal tract. Recent work by CURRAN and SOLOMON[586] indicates, however, that a contributing factor to the lack of a sizable potential is the active absorption of chloride ions. Thus the transport potentials of the Na^+ and the Cl^- ions nearly neutralize each other. Working with loops of small intestine of the rat, these authors found the intestinal lumen to be as much as 18 mV positive relative to the external medium when the sodium chloride concentration in the loop was low (25 mM/l), whereas the lumen became slightly negative when the salt concentration was 163 mM/l. The flux ratios measured with isotopes indicated active transport of both ionic species, and it was clear that they were transported by independent mechanisms. The water absorption going on simultaneously with the transport of ions could be accounted for by osmosis. In the isolated small intestine of the bull

[589] USSING, H. H., and B. ANDERSEN: The relation between solvent drag and active transport of ions. Proc. Third int. Congress of Biochem., p. 434—440. Brussels 1955.

frog[589a] there is no evidence for active sodium transport, whereas there is a weak, but significant active chloride transport, giving rise, under proper conditions, to a potential difference of a few millivolts.

5. The transport of potassium across the intestinal wall

The absorption of potassium in the intestine has not been studied very extensively. The early work by HÖBER, WALLACE and CUSHNY, KATZENELLENBOGEN indicated that potassium passes readily through the intestinal wall in both directions. According to INGRAHAM and VISSCHER[590], potassium is resorbed faster than sodium in the dog small intestine. This result was based upon the observation that K disappeared faster from isotonic mixtures of KCl and K_2SO_4 than did sodium from the corresponding mixtures of its chloride and sulfate. BUDOLFSEN found that NaCl and KCl are resorbed at the same rate as estimated from the disappearance rate of chloride from the small intestine of the dog. However, the analyses for the alkali metal ions showed that K disappeared much faster than did Na from mixtures of NaCl and KCl. As it has already been pointed out, the gradient for potassium in the direction gut — blood is much steeper than the Na-gradient, when equimolar solutions of the two alkali metal ions are being used. Thus the permeability coefficient for the two alkali ions may very well be about the same. The problem should, however, be reinvestigated with tracers and with simultaneous measurement of the intestinal potential. According to BUDOLFSEN[579] Na and K are resorbed at the same rate in the large intestine, when isotonic solutions of the chlorides of the two ions are applied. Again, if calculated on the basis of the permeability constants it will probably turn out that the large intestine is more permeable to sodium than to potassium. This was to be predicted in case the active sodium transport mechanism were of the same type as that of the frog skin. Whether or not there is an active uptake of K in the gut is unknown. The low potassium concentration in the blood would under normal circumstances lead to a potassium diffusion gradient in the direction intestine-blood, so that an active transport of this ion would not seem necessary. In studying dogs with surgically prepared Thiry-Vella loops, DENNIS and WOOD[591] found that adrenalectomy decreases the rate of resorption of both sodium and potassium, but effect on potassium was less marked than that upon sodium. The most striking effect on the intestinal absorption of adrenalectomy is, however, the failure of the ability of the intestine to absorb water.

When saline is introduced into the colon of humans, the K concentration increases to about 30 mM per liter as sodium, chloride and water are absorbed[592], and it is well known that the feces are normally almost devoid of Na whereas K is always present (see part II). Thus it is apparent that the active cation transport of the large intestine exhibits a strong preference for sodium relative to potassium. We know (see above, p. 137) that the active sodium transport of the colon gives rise to a potential difference between lumen and blood, which would tend to bring about a movement of potassium from blood to lumen. Unfortunately, the material at hand does not indicate whether the potential difference is large enough to account for the high K concentration of the colon contents. If so, the situation

[589a] HOGBEN, C. A. M.: Personal communication.

[590] INGRAHAM, R. C., and M. B. VISSCHER: The production of chloride-free solutions by the action of the intestinal epithelium. Amer. J. Physiol. 114, 676—680 (1935/36).

[591] DENNIS, C., and E. H. WOOD: Intestinal absorption in the adrenalectomized dog. Amer. J. Physiol. 129, 182—190 (1940).

[592] DARROW, D. C.: Some aspects of ion exchange in clinical medicine. In: Metabolic aspects of transport across cell membranes. p. 23—38. Ed. Q. R. MURPHY. Madison the University for Wisconsin press 1957.

would be very similar to that exhibited by the isolated frog skin where the active transport of sodium inward creates a potential difference which drags in chloride and to a lesser extent "pushes" potassium ions outward.

In addition to the effect of the electric potential there might, of course, be active potassium transport in the outward direction, possibly in the form of a coupled Na/K pump.

f) Kidney tubulus

The transport of sodium and potassium in kidney is discussed in part II. The regulation of the cellular concentration of these ions has already been considered (p. 106). It may, however, be appropriate to consider briefly the handling of sodium and potassium in the kidney tubules as a case of net transport through an epithelial membrane. The generally accepted view is that sodium (and chloride) are reabsorbed in the proximal as well as in the distal tubules (for references, see part II). Furthermore, in a special section of the distal tubule there is a sodium reabsorption which takes place in exchange for an excretion of potassium and (or) hydrogen ions. Recent studies [593, 593a, 593b] have shown that the lumen in both proximal and distal tubules of the rat are strongly negative relative to the peritoneal fluid. For the proximal tubule the P. D. ranged from $19-39$ mV whereas the potential difference assumed to originate in the distal tubule ranged from $34-70$ mV. Thus, qualitatively, it can be stated that the sodium transport is active, whereas chloride may be carried along by the electric potential difference. In the case of the proximal tubules where the reabsorption seems to take place as an almost isotonic solution, the movement of sodium must be against the electro-chemical potential gradient, whereas the movement of chloride must be "down-hill". Although the conditions in the distal tubules are less well established, the likelihood is that even here an active sodium transport of the type found in the frog skin would suffice to account for the electrolyte shifts. In the case of the special zone where K is excreted in exchange for sodium, there is at least the theoretical possibility that the potassium transport is largely passive, the negative potential strongly favouring the transfer of K from the blood to the lumen. At present it is impossible to say if the potential is large enough to explain the potassium transport. It has been shown that frog skins having a low permeability to chloride and thus developing a high electric potential exhibit a marked net transfer of potassium ions from the inside to the outside solution (LEVI and USSING[250], HUF[528]). If, however, the active sodium transport of the epithelium cells should turn out to be a Na—K pump, one might say that a discussion of the problem as to whether the potassium transport in the kidney is passive or active is of mostly academical interest. In cases where the urine is being acidified there is also the problem whether or not the ion (in case the hydrogen ion) exchanging against Na is transported by an independent active mechanism, by a coupled Na—H pump, or by the elctric potential difference. The latter certainly has the right sign, but since p_H values of the urine as low as 4.6 may be encountered, passive excretion of hydrogen ions would require the lumen to be as much as 180 mV negative relative to the blood.

Apparently K and hydrogen ions compete in this particular region as exchange partners for sodium. If the supply of accessible hydrogen ions from the carbonic

[593] SOLOMON, S.: Transtubular potential differences of rat kidney. J. cell. comp. Physiol. 49, 351—365 (1957).

[593a] SOLOMON, A. K.: Ion and water transport in single protimal tubules of the necturus kidney. In: The Method of Isotopic Tracers Applied to the study of Active Ion Transport. I Colloque de Biologie de Saclay 1958, 196 pp. Pergamon Press. Londen.

[593b] GIEBISCH, G.: Electrial potential measurements on single nephrons of nectures J. cell. comp. Physiol. 51 221—239 (1958).

acid system is reduced by the application of carbonic acid anhydrase inhibitors, there is a drop in hydrogen ion and an increase in potassium excretion.

g) The Malpighian tubules of insects

As shown by RAMSAY[594, 595, 596, 597, 598] the formation of urine in the malpighian tubules of insects must involve an active transport of potassium ions from the haemolymph to the lumen of the tubules. The transfer of sodium ions, on the other hand, could be considered a passive process in most species, judging from the fact that the electrochemical potential gradient for this ion is downhill from haemolymph to urine. Table 25 gives a compilation of the results obtained in different species. In this context it should be recalled that inorganic ions usually make up only a minor fraction of the osmotically active matter of insect blood, the major fraction being made up of amino acids. Also the sodium to potassium ratio of

Table 25. *The calculated equilibrium potential for Na and K across the wall of Malpighian tubules of different insects as compared with the observed potential differences*[594]

Insect	$\frac{C_{urine}}{C_{blood}}$ (Na)	$\frac{C_{urine}}{C_{blood}}$ (K)	calculated equilibrium p.d. (mV)		found p.d. (mV) ψ urine- ψ blood
			for Na ψ urine- ψ blood	for K ψ urine- ψ blood	
Locusta	0.81	6.2	+ 5	—46	—16
Dixippus	0.40	8.8	+23	—55	+21
Pieris	0.70	6.0	+ 9	—45	+28
Tenebrio	0.24	6.4	+36	—47	+45
Dytiscus	0.31	31.1	+29	—86	+22
Rhodnius	0.75	17.7	+ 7	—72	—35
Aedes (distilled water adapted)	0.28	29.3	+32	—85	+21

insect haemolymph differs markedly from species to species[599], sodium being the major ion in carnivorius insects, whereas K dominates in the herbivorius species. But despite these differences the active nature of the potassium transport seems a common feature in all species. The lumen is always positive relative to the haemolymph, the potassium concentration is always higher in the urine than in the haemolymph, and the sodium concentration is generally less. On the face of it then we may postulate that the potassium transport is active, whereas the sodium transport may take place by passive diffusion. The fact that the cells of the tubules in all species were decidedly negative (24—47 mV) relative to the haemolymph seems, however, to demand some mechanism like an active sodium extrusion to keep the cells from swelling due to the uptake of Na. Thus like it was the case with the cells forming the endolymph in the vertebrate ear, we may postulate the existence of the sodium-potassium pump at both the inward-facing and the outward-facing cell membrane, the net flow of potassium resulting from a relatively greater leakiness to K of the luminal border of the tubule cells.

[594] RAMSAY, J. A.: Active transport of potassium by the Malpighian tubules of insects. J. exp. Biol. **30**, 358—369 (1953).

[595] RAMSAY, J. A.: Osmotic regulation in mosquito larvae. J. exp. Biol. **27**, 145—157 (1950).

[596] RAMSAY, J. A.: Osmotic regulation in mosquito larvae: the role of the Malpighian tubules. J. exp. Biol. **28**, 62—73 (1951).

[597] RAMSAY, J. A.: The excretion of sodium and potassium by the Malpighian tubules of Rhodnius. J. exp. Biol. **29**, 110—126 (1952).

[598] RAMSAY, J. A.: Exchanges of sodium and potassium in mosquito larvae. J. exp. Biol. **30**, 79—89 (1953).

[599] BONÉ, G.-J.: Le rapport sodium/potassium dans le liquide coelomique des insectes. I. Ses relations avec le régime alimentaire. Ann. Soc. zool. Belg. **75**, 123—132 (1944).

In considering the physiological role of the potassium excretion in the tubules it should be remembered that the ions excreted into the Malpighian tubules are not necessarily lost by the organism since these organs empty into the rectum where a sizible reabsorption may take place. Thus in the moscito Aedes sodium ions as well as potassium ions are reabsorbed by the rectum. Active absorption of both alkali metal ions can also take place from the surrounding water through the "anal gills" (see below p. 143).

h) The formation of the endolymph

Whereas the perilymph of the inner ear of the vertebrates has a composition not very different from a blood ultrafiltrate (see part II), the endolymph is characterized by a high K and a low Na concentration (SMITH, WU and LOWREY[600], see Table 26). This clearly indicates the participation of an active transport mechanism involved in the formation of the endolymph. Further proof comes from the existence of a marked potential difference between endolymph and perilymph, the former being some 50 mV positive relative to the latter (BEZEKY[601]). Thus, the sodium ion in the endolymph is not far from electrochemical equilibrium with that of the perilymph.

Table 26. *Ionic concentrations and potentials of endolymph and perilymph*[600, 601]

	mM/l		potential (mV)
	K	Na	
Endolymph	140	15	—50
Perilymph	6	150	0

The potassium ion, on the other hand, must be transported uphill against the electrical potential as well as against the concentration gradient.

The chloride ion is also not in equilibrium, but this does not mean that it has to be transported actively during the formation of the endolymph, since its electrochemical potential gradient from perilymph to endolymph is downhill. It can be inferred, however, that there is a considerable resistance to chloride in the cells separating perilymph and endolymph. If we were to characterize these cells, we should say that they were freely permeable to Na, sparingly permeable to Cl and performing an active transport of K from perilymph to endolymph.

The apparent near-equilibrium between sodium in the endolymph and in the perilymph is possibly fortuitous. Inside the Reissner membrane and the organ of Corti the potential is about 80 mV negative relative to the perilymph and 130 mV negative relative to the endolymph. Without an active extrusion of Na towards both sides the cells would be flooded with sodium ions. Thus it is possible that these cells possess a sodium-potassium exchange pump at both the boundary facing the endolymph and that facing the perilymph, and that the net transport of K is the resultant of a greater passive K permeability of the side facing the endolymph. The cell membrane towards the perilymph must, however, possess some passive permeability to potassium ions, judging from the fact that increasing the potassium concentration of the perilymph by a factor of six suppresses the electrical responses of the cochlea to sound (TASAKI and FERNANDEZ[602]).

[600] SMITH, C. A., M. WU, and O. H. LOWRY: The electrolytes of the Endolymph and Perilymph. Science 116, 529 (1952).

[601] BEZEKY, G. V.: Resting potentials, inside the cochlear partition. J. Acoust. Soc. Amer. 24, 72—76 (1952).

[602] TASAKI, I., and C. FERNANDEZ: Modification of cochlear microphonics and action potentials by KCl solution and by direct currents. J. Neurophysiol. 15, 497—512 (1952).

i) Active K transport in the formation of bull seminal plasma

Bull seminal plasma has a higher K concentration (43.9 mM) than the blood plasma, whereas both the sodium concentration (112.3) and particularly the Cl concentration (49.3) are lower than expected for a blood plasma ultrafiltrate[603]. This strongly suggests a process of active K transport[282], but more detailed information is needed to confirm this hypothesis. In particular the potential in the different parts of the sexual tract should be measured. It is known that most of the seminal plasma originates in the seminal vesicles, the urethral glands and in the ampullary glands. In the guinea-pig the secretion of the seminal vesicles has a very low concentration of alkali metal ions, but species difference may exist with respect to the composition of this secretion.

j) The gills of Eriocheir sinensis (The "woolhanded crab")

It was first discovered by KROGH[604] that the "woolhanded crab", Eriocheir sinensis, which most of its life lives in fresh water, is capable of taking up both sodium and potassium ions even from dilute solutions of these ions. The uptake is performed by the epithelium of the gills. More recently this ion transport has been studied by KOCH and collaborators[605, 606, 607, 608, 609, 610, 611].

KOCH and EVANS assume that Na and K are taken up by independent mechanisms, but conclusive proof of this is still lacking. It is clear, however, that potassium ions do not exert any competitive inhibition upon the uptake of sodium ions. Li, on the other hand, inhibits both the uptake of Na and of K. Curiously enough, Li itself is absorbed from dilute solutions of LiCl, although, when added to sodium chloride solutions in concentrations sufficient to inhibit Na transport, the Li transport is also inhibited. Unfortunately the uptake experiments have not been combined with measurements of the electric potential. It is therefore not possible to say to what extent the uptake of alkali metal ions is secondary to active transport of chloride.

Eriocheir can, however, take up Na from solutions as dilute as 0.2 mmolar. The blood concentration of this ion is 200—300 mmolar. Thus it would take a

[603] LORD ROTHSCHILD, and H. BARNES: Constituents of bull seminal plasma. J. exp. Biol. 31, 561—572 (1954).

[604] KROGH, A.: Osmotic regulation in aquatic animals. 242 pp. Cambridge University Press 1939.

[605] KOCH, H. J.: Cholinesterase and active transport of sodium chloride through the isolated gills of the crab, Eriocheir sinensis (M. Edw.). In: Recent developments in cell physiology. Ed. J. A. KITCHING. London: Butterworths scientific publications 1954.

[606] KOCH, H. J.: L'intervention de cholinestérases dans l'absorption et transport actif de matières minérales par les branchies du crabe, Eriocheir sinensis M. Edw. Arch. int. Physiol. 62, 136 (1954).

[607] KOCH, H. J., J. EVANS, and E. SCHICKS: Inhibition a l'aide de colorants basiques du transport actif de matières minérales par les branchies isolées du crabe, Eriocheir sinensis M. Edw. Arch. int. Physiol. 61, 476—484 (1953).

[608] KOCH, H. J., J. EVANS, and E. SCHICKS: The active absorption of ions by the isolated gills of the crab Eriocheir sinensis. Meded. Vlaamse Acad. Kl. Wet. 16, nr. 5, 1—16 (1954).

[609] KOCH, H. J.: On the influence of lithium on the uptake of sodium and potassium by the crab Eriocheir sinensis (M. Edw.). Meded. Vlaamse Acad. Kl. Wet. 18, nr. 6, pp. 1—10 (1956).

[610] KOCH, H. J., and J. EVANS: On the absorption of sodium from dilute solutions by the crab Eriocheir sinensis (M. Edw.). Meded. Vlaamse Acad. Kl. Wet. 18, nr. 7, pp. 1—15 (1956).

[611] KOCH, H. J., and J. EVANS: Influence of a basic dye, thionine, on the absorption of sodium by the crab Eriocheir sinensis (M. Edw.). Meded. Vlaamse Acad. Kl. Wet. 18, nr. 8, pp. 1—11 (1956).

potential difference of more than 180 mV to account for the sodium uptake as a passive process. The sensitivity of the sodium uptake to specific inhibitors of the anticholinesterase type (Eserin, tubocurarine, diisopropylfluorophosphate, tetra-ethylfluorophosphate, thionin, etc.) also point to the active nature of the sodium transport (compare the effects of these drugs on the sodium transport of frog skin, p. 126). If so, we have here the interesting case of an active transport of K and Na in the same direction. This cannot, however, be taken as evidence that the underlying mechanism is different from the sodium-potassium exchange pump. It is entirely possible that the gill epithelium cells are provided with the transporting units both at the outward-facing and the inward-facing boundary. Thus K would be pumped into the cells and Na would be extruded from the cells in both directions.

Now, let us further assume that, like the frog skin epithelium cells, those of the gill are passively permeable only to sodium at the outward facing boundary and to potassium only at the boundary facing inward. It is then clear that a net transport inward of both ionic species would result. In this context it may be worth mentioning that certain crustaceans like the brackish water shrimp Palaemonetes varians are able to take up sodium chloride through the gills when living in fresh water, whereas it excretes salt by the same route when kept in sea water[612]. It would be tempting to assume that again the sodium-potassium pump is operative at both boundaries of the gill epithelium cell and that the adapation from life in fresh water to life in the sea consists "merely" in changing the passive permeabilities of the two cell membranes so that the one facing outward becomes potassium permeable and that facing inward sodium permeable.

Active uptake of potassium as well as sodium seems to be rather widespread among arthropods. (For reviews, see KROGH[604], BEADLE[613], ROBERTSON[614].) Thus the common shore crab, Carcinus maenas takes up Na as well as K through the gills (WEBB[615]). HOLM-JENSEN[616], using radioactive isotopes, found indications of active uptake of K as well as of Na from the medium in the cladoceran, Daphnia magna. Heavy metals (Hg, Cu, Pb) strongly inhibited the uptake, but not the loss of the two alkali metal ions. The mosquito larvae which absorbe salt through special organs, the anal papillae (KOCH and KROGH[618]) are capable of absorbing both K and Na against steep concentration gradients (RAMSEY[598], TREHERNE[619,620], KOCH[617]). A similar although less efficient transport of K as well as Na is found in the larva of the beetle, Helodes. Here, however, part of the transport takes place in the gut.

[612] PANIKKAR, N. K.: Osmoregulation in some palaemonid prawns. J. Mar. Biol. Ass. U. K. 25, 317—359 (1941—43).
[613] BEADLE, L. C.: Comparative physiology: Osmotic and ionic regulation in aquatic animals. Ann. Rev. Physiol. 19, 329—358 (1957).
[614] ROBERTSON, J. D.: Osmotic and ionic regulation in aquatic invertebrates, p. 229—246. In: Recent Advances in Invertebrate Physiology. Univ. Oregon Publ. 1957.
[615] WEBB, D. A.: Ionic regulation in Carcinus maenas. Proc. roy. Soc. B 129, 107—136 (1940).
[616] HOLM-JENSEN, I.: Osmotic regulation in Daphnia magna under physiological conditions and in the presence of heavy metals. Kgl. Danske Vidensk. Selsk. Biol. Medd. 20, 1—64 (1948).
[617] KOCH, H. J.: The absorption of chloride ions by the anal papillae of Diptera larvae. J. exp. Biol. 15, 152—160 (1938).
[618] KOCH, H. J., and A. KROGH: La fonction des papilles anales des larves de Diptères. Ann. Soc. Sci. Brux. 56, 459—461 (1936).
[619] TREHERNE, J. E.: The exchange of labelled sodium in the larva of Aedes aegypti. J. exp. Biol. 31, 386—401 (1954).
[620] TREHERNE, J. E.: Osmotic regulation in the larvae Helodes (Coleoptera: Helodidae). Trans. roy. entomol. Soc. London 105, 117—130 (1954).

VIII. Relation
of the alkali metal ions to bioelectric phenomena
A. Relation to maintained potentials
a) Introduction

Active ion transports, passive ion transports and potential development are intricately interwoven. It has been pointed out above that whereever the active transport of some ionic species sets up a concentration gradient, an electric potential defference is likely to occur. The magnitude and sign of this potential is, however, a function of the passive permeabilities of the membranes concerned (see p. 56). Thus erythrocytes have a high internal K and low Na, but only a small potential difference between the interior and the medium (p. 72) whereas muscle cells often come cose to the maximum potential obtainable if the membrane were selectively permeable to K.

The relationship between active ion transport and potential development across epithelial membranes has been discussed. Since the relationship between active sodium transport and potential development has been studied in greatest detail for the isolated frog skin, this organ was used as example, but it is likely that several other epithelia follow the same pattern.

The electrophysiological approach has, however, been primarily concerned with the function of nerve and muscle. A discussion of the role of the alkali metal ions for the potential development in these cell types is therefore warranted.

b) Effect of K on the resting potential of muscle and nerve

1. Striated muscle

Ever since BERNSTEIN[621] developed his membrane theory of biopotentials it has been recognized that the external K concentration is one of the major factors determining the magnitude of the muscle- (and nerve-) resting or injury potential[623, 624]. As it is well known this theory which was developed on the basis of W. OSTWALD's[622] work on semipermeable membranes, assumed that the membrane potential is a diffusion potential, arising as a consequence of the diffusion of K ions out of the muscle. Under the assumption that the fibre membrane is impermeable to all ions present except K, the diffusion potential becomes:

$$E = (RT/F) \ln ([K_i]/K_0) \qquad \text{(eq 29, p. 93)}$$

where E is the potential difference across the membrane, R is the gas constant, T the absolute temperature, F Faraday's number, and $[K_i]$ and $[K_0]$ the inside and outside K concentrations (strictly speaking activities), respectively. Expressed in ordinary logarithms and taking the temperature to be $22°C$, the expression for the membrane potential is (E being expressed in millivolts):

$$E = 59 \log ([K_i]/[K_0]) . \qquad (35)$$

[621] BERNSTEIN, J.: Untersuchungen zur Thermodynamik der biologischen Ströme. Pflügers Arch. ges. Physiol. **92**, 521—562 (1902).

[622] OSTWALD, W.: Elektrische Eigenschaften halbdurchlässiger Scheidewände. Z. physiol. Chem. **6**, 71—82 (1890).

[623] HÖBER, R.: Über den Einfluß der Salze auf den Ruhestrom des Froschmuskels. Pflügers Arch. ges. Physiol. **106**, 599—635 (1905).

[624] HÖBER, R., M. ANDERSH, J. HÖBER, and B. NEBEL: The influence of organic electrolytes and non-electrolytes upon the membrane potentials of muscle and nerve. J. cell. comp. Physiol. **13**, 195—218 (1939).

In its derivation this is clearly an approximation since ions other than K must certainly penetrate the membrane, if only slowly. The experimental testing of the theory has met with difficulties which have not as yet been fully overcome. The most important one is concerned with the value to be used for $[K_i]$. As already mentioned it is the chemical activity and not the concentration which should be applied. Thus the proper measuring device would be a reversible K electrode. But since such a device of practical applicability does not exist we have to use the chemically determined concentration together with an estimate of the activity coefficient. But this brings us back to the much disputed problem as to what fraction of the cellular K can be considered "free" (see p. 37).

If the true $[K_i]$ is unknown, the above equation may be written:

$$E = E_s - 59 \log (1/[K_0]) , \qquad (36)$$

where E_s is the resting potential measured at an arbitrary standard outside K concentration. Thus a partial check of the validity of the BERNSTEIN hypothesis can be obtained without knowledge of the concentration of free K in the fibres.

HEGENAUER, FENN and COBB[128] found that the injury potential of the frog sartorius varied in the way to be predicted from eq. (36) at outside K concentrations higher than 20 mg-%. As $[K_0]$ was lowered towards zero, however, the relationship broke down and the potential approached a maximum of about 60 millivolts. The value for E_s, that is the injury potential with 24 mg-% K in the outside medium was surprisingly small. Taking all fibre K to be free, and applying eq. (36), HEGNAUER et al. concluded that the potential ought to be as high as 73 mV when in fact they found only 41.6 mV. They suggested that the discrepancy be due to the technique used for measuring the injury potential. One end of the muscle was soaked in a modified Ringer solutions with varied K concentration, whereas the other end was depolarized by dipping in saturated KCl. The potential difference was measured between the two soaking solutions, using KCl bridges to eliminate diffusion potentials. The procedure has at least one serious source of error, namely that the injury potential is more or less short-circuited via the interspaces of the muscle which provide an open electric lead between the two soaking solutions.

It was therefore a great step forward when LING and GERARD[625, 626] developed the technique of using capillary microelectrodes introduced through the cell surface for measuring the normal membrane potential of muscle fibres. When tip diameters well under one μ were used the cell damage seemed to be negligible and highly constant and reproducible values were obtained. In the frog sartorius fibres the membrane potential averaged 78.4 mV when the muscle was in contact with ordinary Ringer. In a more recent study, the resting potential of frog muscle fibres was found to be from 90—95 mV, whereas the value predicted from the potassium concentration of the fibre was 102 mV (ADRIAN[627]).

Still, the potassium-diffusion potential concept may be upheld if the activity of the intracellular K is assumed to be lower than that of extracellular K, in other words if some of the cellular K is more or less firmly "bound" to cell constituents. But even if such is the case, equation[36] which relates the membrane potential to the K concentration of the outside solution should still be valid.

[625] LING, G., and R. W. GERARD: The normal membrane potential of frog sartorius fibres. J. cell. comp. Physiol. 34, 383—396 (1949).

[626] LING, G., and R. W. GERARD: External potassium and the membrane potential of single muscle fibres. Nature (Lond.) 165, 113—114 (1950).

[627] ADRIAN, R. H.: The effect of internal and external potassium concentration on the membrane potential of frog muscle. J. Physiol. 133, 631—658 (1956).

This equation states that if $[K_i]$ remains constant the membrane potential should decrease by 59 mV for each time $[K_0]$ is increased by a factor of ten. As shown in Fig. 11 it is clear that the expected dependency of the potential upon the outside K concentration was not found in LING and GERARD's (1950) studies on the frog sartorius fibres. Between 2.5 millimolar and 100 millimolar in the bathing solution (the sum of the molar concentrations of K and Na being maintained), the membrane potential decreases in a linear way with log $[K_0]$. But the decrease for a tenfold increase in K concentration is only 47.6 mV against the expected 59 mV. The average slope for 8 different curves was -44 mV ± 9.5 mV

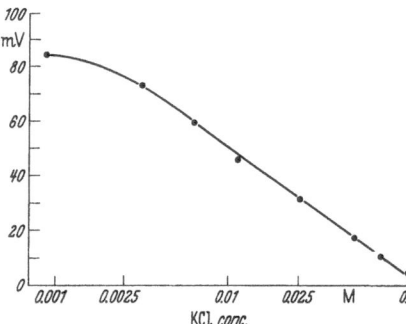

Fig. 11. The potential difference across the cell membrane of a single muscle fibre as a function of the external K concentration (after LING and GERARD [636])

for log $([K_i]/[K_0]) = 1$. Similar values for the slope have been obtained by previous workers (see STEINBACH[628], OSTERHOUT and HARRIS[629]), but internal shorting could not be excluded in those cases.

It is evident that the experiments are not in accord with the Bernstein hypothesis. In other words: the muscle fibre does not behave as an ideal potassium electrode. This, as a matter of fact is not so surprising. As early as in 1905 HÖBER pointed out that not only the K concentration, but also the nature and concentrations of the anions influenced the injury potential. Later BOYLE and CONWAY[101] demonstrated that the isolated frog sartorius is relatively permeably to small anions like Cl and HCO_3 and that, consequently, the potential is not a simple potassium diffusion potential. Rather, if due time is allowed for equilibration, the small anions as well as the potassium ion becomes Donnan distributed between fibre and surroundings. In case of equilibrium the Nernst equation gives the relationship between potassium concentrations and membrane potential no matter whether the BERNSTEIN hypothesis or the BOYLE-CONWAY hypothesis of Donnan distribution is correct. Until diffusion equilibrium is attained, however, the potential is determined by an equation of a different type[236], and the potential becomes a function of the concentration gradients and permeability constants for all diffusible ions present.

As mentioned above HODGKIN and KATZ[271] have derived from the constant field theory of GOLDMAN[236] the following approximate equation for the resting potential, taking into account only the major ions involved:

$$E = \frac{RT}{F} \cdot \ln \frac{P_{Cl}(Cl)_i + P_{Na}(Na)_0 + P_K(K)_0 \ldots}{P_{Cl}(Cl)_0 + P_{Na}(Na)_i + P_K(K)_i \ldots} \qquad \text{(eq 13, p. 56)}$$

where P_K, P_{Na} and P_{Cl} are the permeability constants for the individual ions.

HODGKIN and HOROWICZ[630] have recently shown that when the ionic milieu is varied, the membrane potential is usually closer to the chloride equilibrium potential than to the potassium potential which means that the membrane is

[628] STEINBACH, H. B.: Electrolyte balance of animal cells. Cold Spr. Harb. Symp. quant. Biol. 8, 242—254 (1940).

[629] OSTERHOUT, W. J. V., and E. S. HARRIS: The concentration effect in Nitella. J. gen. Physiol. 12, 761—781 (1929).

[630] HODGKIN, A. L., and P. HOROWICZ: Effects of K and Cl on the membrane potential of isolated muscle fibres. J. Physiol. 137, 30 P (1957).

more permeable to Cl than to K. This is in striking contrast to nerve (see below) where in the resting state, the membrane is more permeable to K than to all anions, including chloride.

The fact remains, however, that even in the steady state potassium seems to be present in muscle somewhat over and above the calculated equilibrium concentration. This could be due to some binding or adsorption of K in the fibre. In addition it should be remembered that if the active transport mechanism, removing sodium from the fibre, is in reality a sodium/potassium exchange pump, the potassium concentration of the fibre would be constantly somewhat above that predicted from the membrane potential.

In evaluating experiments where the ionic composition is being changed suddenly, it might not be correct to ignore totally the drag effect of water being transferred osmotically across the membrane. In this context it may be pertinent that EDWARDS and HARRIS[631] have observed the movement of Na^{24} out of the frog sartorius to be faster when water is being osmotically withdrawn than when it is going in. Although the above authors explain their results in a different way, solvent drag might have been involved. Similar experiments seem not to have been performed with potassium.

2. Heart muscle

Using the internal micro-electrode technique, BURGEN and TERROUX[632] have studied the dependency of the resting potential of the cat auricle upon the K concentration of the medium. The mean value of the potential was found to be 60.4 mV when the medium was Tyrode solution. When the external K concentration was increased, the resting potential decreased inversely with the logarithm of the K concentration ion just as it is the case with nerve and striated muscle. The shift for a tenfold change in K concentration was only 38 mV. For an ideal K electrode at 37° centigrade the slope should have been 61.5 mV, but the discrepancy is probably to be explained by a certain leakiness to other ion species (compare p. 146). The shortcoming of the simple K-electrode concept is also apparent from the fact that with the concentration ratio of $K_i/K_0 = 26/1$ the potential ought to have been 87 mV, whereas the value actually found was only some 70% of that. In the case of the Purkinje fibre of the kid, DRAPER and WEIDMANN[633] found a resting potential which, calculated on the basis of the K concentration, was 87% of theory.

3. Smooth muscle

Smooth muscle differs rather markedly from striated muscle in its electric properties. Thus the membrane potential of fibres of the taenia coli, measured with an internal microelectrode, depends on the degree of stretch (in contrast to striated muscle). At the in situ length the fibres have a membrane potential of about 60 mV, whereas, when stretched to a degree where no movement could be seen, the potential had dropped to 45 mV (BÜLBRING[634]). The relation between

---

[631] EDWARDS, C., and E. J. HARRIS: Do tracers measure fluxes? Nature (Lond.) 175, 262 (1955).

[632] BURGEN, A. S. V., and K. G. TERROUX: The membrane resting and action potentials of the cat auricle. J. Physiol. 119, 139—152 (1953).

[633] DRAPER, M. H., and S. WEIDMANN: Cardiac resting and action potentials recorded with an intracellular electrode. J. Physiol. 115, 74—94 (1951).

[634] BÜLBRING, E.: Membrane potentials of smooth muscle fibres of the Taenia Coli of the guinea-pig. J. Physiol. 125, 302—315 (1954).

resting potential and the logarithm of the external K concentration is linear for concentrations greater than 20 mM/l with a slope of 33 mV for a tenfold change in K concentration[635].

4. Nerve

The resting potential of nerve behaves very much like that of muscle towards variations in the K concentration of the bathing fluid. It should be pointed out at the outset, however, that the response of nerves to changes in K concentration is in many cases very much delayed due to the low permeability of the epineurium to inorganic ions (see p. 162). With single fibres and desheathed nerves, however, the typical responses to changing K concentration are readily obtained. Thus even before the invention of intracellular microelectrodes, curves like those established for muscle (see Fig. 11) had been found valid for different types of nerve. For instance such curves have been found for the squid giant nerve by STEINBACH[636], for crustacean nerve by COWAN[452] and SHANES and HOPKINS[123], and for myelinated nerve by FENG and LIU[637].

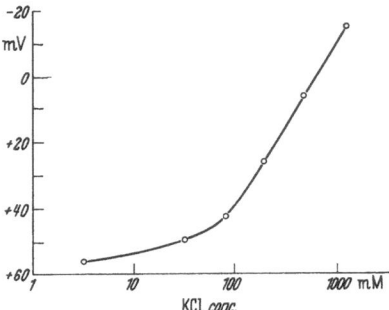

Fig. 12. Resting potential of squid giant axon as a function of external K concentration (after CURTIS and COLE[638])

It is now generally recognized, however, that the classical method of measuring the resting potential between an intact portion and a damaged portion of the nerve does not give reliable values for the resting potential. Satisfactory results can be obtained with intracellular electrodes introduced sufficiently far through the cut end of the fibre (CURTIS and COLE[638]), micro-electrodes of the LING-GERARD type introduced transversely, or by applying special methods to reduce to zero the external short-circuiting between the electrodes (HUXLEY and STÄMPFLI[639], STÄMPFLI[640]).

The first nerve preparation to be carefully studied with intracellular electrodes was the giant axon of the squid. CURTIS and COLE (1942) found the resting potential of this preparation to vary between 46 and 59 mV. When the outside K concentration was varied, the slope of the potential — log $[K_0]$ curve was about 50 mV for a tenfold change in K concentration at high K-levels. In the biological range of K concentrations the potential showed only a slight dependency upon changes in K concentration (see Fig. 12).

It can be predicted from eq. (13) or eq. (29) that when the outside K concentration reaches a level higher than the effective inside K concentration, the resting potential should change sign so that the inside of the fibre becomes positive

[635] HOLMAN, MOLLIE E.: The effect of changes in potassium chloride concentration on the membrane potential, electric activity and tension of intestinal muscle. J. Physiol. **137**, 77 P (1957).

[636] STEINBACH, H. B.: Chemical and concentration potentials in the giant fibres of squid nerves. J. cell. comp. Physiol. **15**, 373—386 (1940).

[637] FENG, T. B., and Y. M. LIU: The concentration-effect relationship in the depolarization of amphibian nerve by potassium and other agents. J. cell. comp. Physiol. **34**, 33—42 (1949).

[638] CURTIS, H. J., and K. S. COLE: Membrane resting and action potentials from the squid giant axon. J. cell. comp. Physiol. **19**, 135—144 (1942).

[639] HUXLEY, A. F., and R. STÄMPFLI: Direct determination of membrane resting potential and action potential in single myelinated nerve fibres. J. Physiol. **112**, 476—495 (1951).

[640] STÄMPFLI, R.: Nouvelle méthode pour enregistrer le potentiel d'action d'un seul étranglement de Ranvier et sa modification par un brusque changement de la concentration du milieu extérieur. J. Physiol. (Paris) **48**, 710—714 (1956).

relative to the outside medium. This prediction, as a matter of fact, can be shown to be correct both in nerve and in muscle. Thus in the squid axon the potential reversed sign by about 15 mV when isotonic KCl was used as bathing solution. Observations of this sort emphasize the view that the so called "depolarization" which is obtained when potassium chloride solutions are applied to muscle, nerve and other living cells can in no way be considered as a simple annihilation of the membrane potential. Even though, as we shall see later (p. 158), a lowering of the membrane potential tends to change the selectivity of the membrane, the reversal of the membrane potential at high K concentration implies that K must diffuse through the membrane much faster than does Cl. Thus the situation is entirely different from that pertaining when a micro-electrode containing, say, three molar KCl is introduced through the membrane into the cytoplasm. We then can assume that K and Cl show the same mobility at the boundary between cytoplasm and electrode. If the structure of the cytoplasma should happen to be such that this condition of equal mobility for K and Cl is notfulfilled, the absolute value of the potential would be in error even though the electrode would register changes in potential faithfully. There is for the time being no absolute proof that the true values of the intracellular potentials are measured correctly, but it is generally assumed that the error is not appreciable.

A tentative estimate of the liquid junction potential sea-water/axoplasm can be obtained by making the assumption (CURTIS and COLE[638]) that the anions are monovalent and have a mobility sufficient to give the axoplasm its measured value of 28 ohm, cm. In this way CURTIS and COLE obtained a value of 6 mV for the junction potential between isotonic KCl and axoplasm (KCl being positive). Using a similar approach HODGKIN and KATZ calculated a junction potential between sea water and axoplasm of 14 mV (the latter becoming negative relative to the former).

Squid fibres, like most isolated tissue and cell preparations cannot be maintained in a steady state with respect to ionic composition in a medium having the potassium concentration of the blood. They tend to gain Na and Cl and to lose K. Therefore the transfer of charge associated with the movements of Na and Cl have to be taken into account in calculating the membrane potential.

If proper values are chosen for the permeability constants of K, Na and Cl, eq. (13) gives the dependency of the membrane potential upon the potassium concentration in a very satisfyctory way. Thus, if $P_K : P_{Na} : P_{Cl} = 1 : 0.04 : 0.45$ in the physiological range and equal to $1 : 0.025 : 0.3$ at high K concentrations, a curve is obtained which is nearly identical to that given in Fig. 12. Also the resting potential of the Lologo axon is given satisfactorily by this equation.

The dependency of the resting potential of single myelinated nerve fibres (from Rana escuelenta) upon the outside K concentration has been studied by HUXLEY and STÄMPFLI[641]. The potential was measured between two nodes one of which was "depolarized" with isotonic (117 mM) KCl solution. The short-circuiting between the electrodes was reduced by an interposed oil seal and the residual shorting compensated by a special electrode arrangement. While this method is not likely to give the true value for the resting potential, it must be assumed to give a faithful picture of the (potential/$[K_0]$) relationship which indeed turned out to be practically identical to that found with internal electrodes in the squid axon.

[641] HUXLEY, A. F., and R. STÄMPFLI: Effect of potassium and sodium on resting and action potentials of single myelinated nerve fibres. J. Physiol. 112, 496—508 (1951).

c) Dependency of the K effect upon other ion species

According to HÖBER[623] (see also HÖBER and STROHE[642]) the potential change arising from an increase in K concentration is delayed or fully abolished when a frog nerve is first treated with isotonic solution of $CaCl_2$, $SrCl_2$ or $BaCl_2$. Similar results have been obtained by GUTTMAN[643] in the case of the spider crab nerve. STEINBACH, SPIEGELMAN and KAWATA[644], however, found that excess Ca has practically no effect upon the depression of the injury potential of the giant squid nerve, exposed to increased K concentrations. In view of the importance of the perineurium as a diffusion barrier, some of the effects of earth alkali ions observed on whole nerves may conceivably have been due to effects on this structure rather than upon the fibres themselves. A reinvestigation of these relationships with modern methods is therefore needed.

d) Effect of external Na upon the resting potential of nerve and muscle

When the Na of the solution bathing a nerve fibre is replaced by an inert, non-penetrating ion like choline the resting potential increases slightly or remains constant (HODGKIN and KATZ[271], HUXLEY and STÄMPFLI[641]). The same is the case with frog muscle (NASTUK and HODGKIN[645]). In the range from 8—150 mM Na (substitution of NaCl by isosmotic sucrose) DRAPER and WEIDMAN[633] did not find any consistent change in resting potential in Purkinje fibres of the kid and in the "false tendon" of the dog.

These results are in agreement with the view that the resting potential is determined by the relative rates of diffusion of the major penetrating ions K, Cl and Na. Inspection of eq. (13) shows that the replacement of Na by an ion with a lower permeability constant will tend to increase the resting potential. It is also natural that Li which has a larger hydrated diameter than Na will act like choline when it is used to replace Na in the bathing solution. Thus HUXLEY and STÄMPFLI[641] found that in the frog myelinated fibre ordinary Ringer gave a resting potential which was 3 mV lower than a Ringer in which NaCl was replaced by LiCl.

It is clear that these considerations cannot apply to the nerve fibre in the intact organism. If Na were constantly diffusing in and K leaking out, the ionic unequilibrium of the fibre would soon come to an and. Therefore active transport of Na and possibly K must restore the diffusion losses (see p. 97). This implies, however, that many of the statements which can be made concerning the resting potential of isolated nerves are valid for such preparations only.

In the case of the giant axon of the squid the resting potential is slightly increased by dilution of the medium with isotonic sucrose solution, whereas hypertonic sodium-rich solutions did not affect the resting potential or reduced it slightly (HODGKIN and KATZ[271]).

Nevertheless Na-rich solutions may have special effects upon the fibres. Thus LUNDBERG[646] found that treatment of the frog spinal roots with NaCl at

[642] HÖBER, R., and H. STROHE: Über den Einfluß von Salzen auf die elektrotonischen Ströme, die Erregbarkeit und das Ruhepotential der Nerven. Pflügers Arch. ges. Physiol. 222, 71—88 (1929).

[643] GUTTMAN, R.: Stabilization of spider crab nerve membranes by alkaline earths, as manifested in resting potential measurements. J. gen. Physiol. 23, 343—364 (1940).

[644] STEINBACH, H. B., S. SPIEGELMAN, and N. KAWATA: The effects of potassium and calcium on the electrical properties of squid axons. J. cell. comp. Physiol. 24, 147—154 (1944).

[645] NASTUK, W. L., and A. L. HODGKIN: The electrical activity of single muscle fibres. J. cell. comp. Physiol. 35, 39—73 (1950).

[646] LUNDBERG, A.: On the ability of some cations to inhibit the potassium depolarization of frog nerve fibres. Acta physiol. scand. 22, 365—375 (1951).

2—3 times the concentration of Ringer decreases very much both the depolarization obtained with a subsequent application of isotonic KCl and the rate at which maximum depolarization was obtained. Most osmotically active substance could not duplicate this effect of Na ions, but tetraethyl ammonium chloride was even more effective than Na. Since the experiments were not performed with isolated fibres the significance of this observation is not entirely clear.

e) Effects of the non-biological alkali metal ions upon the resting potential

The effects of the ions Li, Rb and Cs upon the resting potential of muscle and nerve is in general agreement with the diffusion potential concept. Their rates of penetration seem to be determined by their apparent hydrated diameters (see p. 3). Thus the change in resting potential brought about by equivalent concentrations of the alkali chlorides falls off in the order K > Rb > Ca > Na > Li (HÖBER[623], HÖBER et al.[624]). For frog nerve the order is the same (NETTER[647], VAN HÉUVERSWYN[648]), whereas with the unmyelinated nerve of the spider crab the order is Rb > K > Na > Li (WILBRANDT[649]).

B. Relation to the electric activity of nerve and muscle

a) The "sodium" theory of excitation (HODGKIN-HUXLEY-KATZ)

For many years it was generally assumed (compare BERNSTEIN[621], HÖBER[623], EBBECKE[650, 651], LILLIE[652]) that the active state and the associated action potential of nerve and muscle arose as the consequence of a sudden breakdown of the K selectivity of the membrane, so that Na, Cl etc. could move through freely. The situation was compared with that existing in an injured portion or a cut end of the fibre. The word depolarization has therefore been used rather indiscriminately to characterize the situation during the passage of an impulse and that pertaining when the fibre was in contact with, say, isotonic KCl.

There can be no doubt that a sudden increase in membrane permeability takes place during the active state. Thus COLE and CURTIS[653] found that the resistance of the fibre membrane of the squid axon drops from 100,000 ohms/cm^2 in the resting state to 500 ohms/cm^2 during the passage of an impulse. But that the classical theory nevertheless had to be wrong became clear when it was realized that the action potential of the squid giant axon — when measured correctly between an external and an internal electrode — exceeded the resting potential by some 50 mV (HODGKIN and HUXLEY[654], CURTIS and COLE[638]).

[647] NETTER, H.: Über den Ruhestrom der Nerven und die Ionenpermeabilität seiner Hüllen. Pflügers Arch. ges. Physiol. 218, 310—330 (1928).

[648] HEUVERSWYN, J. VAN: Etude de la perméabilité du nerf sciatique de la grenouille au sodium, au potassium et au chlore par la mesure des potentiels de concentration. Arch. int. Physiol. 43, 316—326 (1936).

[649] WILBRANDT, W.: The effect of organic ions on the membrane potential of nerves. J. gen. Physiol. 20, 519—541 (1937).

[650] EBBECKE, U.: Membranänderung und Nervenerregung. Pflügers Arch. ges. Physiol. 195, 555—587 (1922).

[651] EBBECKE, U.: Membranänderung und Nervenerregung. II. Mitteilung. Über das Nervenschwirren bei Reizung sensibler Nerven. Pflügers Arch. ges. Physiol. 197, 482—499 (1922).

[652] LILLIE, R. S.: Protoplasmic action and nervous action. Chicago University Press 1923.

[653] COLE, K. S., and H. J. CURTIS: Electric impedance of the squid giant axon during activity. J. gen. Physiol. 22, 649—670 (1939).

[654] HODGKIN, A. L., and A. F. HUXLEY: Action potentials recorded from inside a nerve fibre. Nature (Lond.) 144, 710—711 (1939).

This means that during the spike the potential difference across the nerve membrane changes sign, the inside becoming positive instead of negative towards the outside medium (Fig. 13).

Several attempts were made to explain this "overshoot" of the potential. Thus COLE and CURTIS pointed out that the phenomenon could be explained in terms of a membrane inductance. This explanation which is formally quite satisfactory suffers, however, from the weakness that no molecular interpretation of the inductance element in membrane permeability could be given. Other explanations, proposed, for instance, by HODGKIN and HUXLEY[655], HÖBER[656] and GRUNDFEST[657] were equally unsatisfactory in operating with assumptions which were hardly accessible to experimental verification. A much more fruitful hypothesis was advanced by HODGKIN and KATZ[271]. Their main assumptions

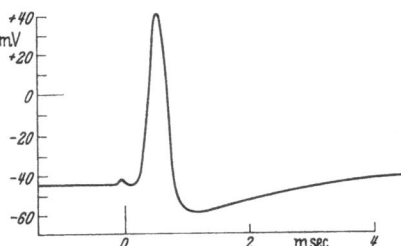

were the following: In the resting state the fibre membrane is readily permeable to K (and also to Cl) ions whereas the permeability to Na is extremely low. The resting potential is determined by the distribution and relative permeabilities of the penetrating ions K and Cl. The hypothesis assumes, however, that during activity the membrane acquires a transient high permeability for Na, many times higher than that for K and Cl.

Fig. 13. Action potential of giant axon (after HODGKIN and HUXLEY[655])

If the outside medium has a higher Na concentration than the interior of the fibre, the preferential Na permeability clearly should lead to a reversal of the sign of the potential. With a fibre whose internal Na concentration is one tenth of that of the medium the reversed potential might be as great as 60 mV.

In order for the potential to return to normal it is further required that there exist in the membrane a mechanism which reduces the Na permeability so that it becomes once again largely K-selective.

According to current views the impulse is normally set off by a critical lowering of the membrane potential (for the squid axon at 20° a depolarization of about 15 mV). The HODGKIN-KATZ hypothesis now implies that a lowering (depolarization) of the membrane potential has two effects: 1) A rapid, transient increase in Na permeability and 2) a delayed, but maintained increase in potassium permeability. Both effects are assumed to be reversible in the sense that repolarization restores the permeabilities to their original values (compare HODGKIN[345, 427]).

This hypothesis has turned out to explain a wide variety of observations and may now be considered a rather well established theory. The theory in its present form does not imply any explanation of the transition from K selectivity to Na selectivity and back again. Certain aspects of the permeability changes will be discussed in more detail below (p. 154). The above short account of the "sodium" theory is intended to serve as an introduction to the discussion of the effects of alkali metal ions upon the action potential and nerve conduction.

[655] HODGKIN, A. L., and A. F. HUXLEY: Resting and action potentials in single nerve fibres. J. Physiol. 104, 176—195 (1945).

[656] HÖBER, R.: The membrane theory. Ann. N. Y. Acad. Sci. 47, 381—394 (1946—47).

[657] GRUNDFEST, H.: Bioelectric potentials in the nervous system and in muscle. Ann. Rev. Physiol. 9, 477—506 (1947).

b) The relation of the external Na concentration to the action potential of single nerve fibres

The relation between action potential and external sodium concentration has been studied by HODGKIN and KATZ for the giant axon of the squid and by HUXLEY and STÄMPFLI for single myelinated nerve fibres of the frog (Rana esculenta). If it is assumed that, during the initial part of the active state the membrane becomes much more permeable to Na than to all other ions, HODGKIN and KATZ[271] pointed out that the potential at the peak of the spike should be given by

$$E = 58\,\text{mV} \times \log_{10} \frac{\text{Na } (inside)}{\text{Na } (outside)}$$

where E is the potential of the outside solution minus that of the axoplasm. Na(inside) and Na(outside) are sodium concentrations or, more strictly, Na activities, in the axoplasm and external solution. Since the intracellular Na activity is usually not known with sufficient accuracy, the hypothesis can be put to test by studying the change in potential, ΔE, brought about by a given change in external Na concentration:

$$\Delta E_a = E_{a\,(test)} - E_{a\,(Ringer)} = 58\,\text{mV} \times \log_{10} \frac{\text{Na } (Ringer)}{\text{Na } (test)}\,.$$

As a matter of fact this equation describes the behaviour of the spike height at varying Na concentrations remarkably well (see Fig. 14). The equation predicts that the spike height should be a linear function of the logarithm to the Na concentration which, indeed, it is. In the experiments of HUXLEY and STÄMPFLI[641] the isotonicity of the bathing solution was maintained by substituting choline for Na. Choline is also a satisfactory substitute for Na in squid nerve (HODGKIN, HUXLEY and KATZ[658]). If isotonicity is obtained by adding appropriate amounts of dextrose, deviations from the theory occur at low Na concentrations (HODGKIN and KATZ)[271].

The "sodium" hypothesis predicts that the rise in action potential should be determined by the rate at which the membrane capacity is discharged by entry of Na. In their experiments with the squid axon HODGKIN and KATZ found the rate of rise of the action potential to be roughly proportional to the external Na concentration. It is interesting that the falling phase

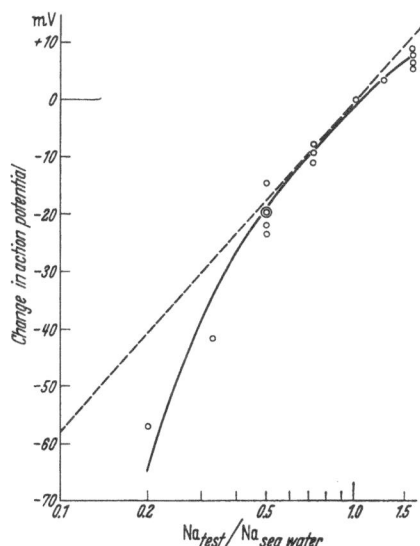

Fig. 14. Change in action potential of the squid giant axon as a function of the change in external Na concentration (after HODGKIN and KATZ[270])

of the action potential, during which the fibre is supposed to be very little permeable to Na is much less affected by the external Na concentration than is the rising phase.

[658] HODGKIN, A. L., A. F. HUXLEY, and B. KATZ: Ionic currents underlying activity in the giant axon of the squid. Arch. Sci. Physiol. **3**, 129—150 (1949).

c) Effect of Li upon the action potential of single nerve fibres

As regards the effect upon action potential, Li seems to behave exactly like Na (HODGKIN and KATZ, HUXLEY and STÄMPFLI).

d) Relation of K to the action potential of single nerve fibres

Fig. 15 shows the spike height of the squid fibre action potential as a function of outside K concentration. It will be seen that a perfectly normal action potential can be obtained even in the absence of K in the solution bathing the nerve fibre. As the K concentration is increased, the spike height remains practically the same until the K concentration is about 1.5 times that of sea water (which is used as standard medium for experiments with squid axons). The fibre ceased to conduct at a K concentration between 2.5 and 6 times that of sea water. No sudden cessation of the action potential was observed. Even after 3 min immersion in isotonic KCl solution the action potential returned to normal height when sea water replaced the KCl solution. Essentially identical results were obtained by HODGKIN and KATZ[271]. Comparing outside media with no potassium, with 10 mM (equal to sea water) and with 20 mM K they noticed a decrease with increasing K in action potential from 88.5 mV to 75.5 mV, whereas the resting potential decreased from 49—42 mV.

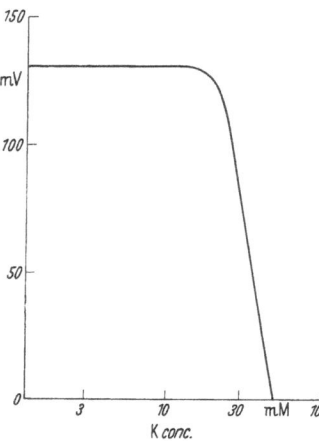

Fig. 15. Spike height in millivolts of squid giant axon as a function of external potassium concentration (after CURTIS and COLE[636])

The frog myelinated fibre action potential is affected by the outside K concentration in very much the same way as that of the squid axon (HUXLEY and STÄMPFLI[641]).

e) The contributions of Na and K to the membrane current in squid axons

The sodium theory for the development of the action potential (see above) has been further developed by HODGKIN and HUXLEY[449, 659, 660, 447] to account quantitatively for the electric and ionic events in the squid giant axon. The rigorous treatment of the theory was made possible by the "voltage clamp" procedure (HODGKIN, HUXLEY and KATZ[661]). In short the principle of this very elegant method is the following: A pair of long silver wire electrodes are inserted longitudinally inside the fibre. One internal electrode is used for recording the potential inside the fibre. Through the other one current can be passed across a well defined section of the fibre membrane to the surrounding medium. A pair of guard electrodes placed on either side of the section of fibre under study prevent propagation within that region by making the potential and the membrane current the same over a considerable distance. A feedback amplifier adjusts the membrane current in such a way that the potential difference across the membrane can be kept constant at any desired level. Furthermore the setup is arranged so that the

[659] HODGKIN, A. L., and A. F. HUXLEY: The components of membrane conductance in the giant axon of Loligo. J. Physiol. **116**, 473—496 (1952).

[660] HODGKIN, A. L., and A. F. HUXLEY: The dual effect of membrane potential on sodium conductance in the giant axon of Loligo. J. Physiol. **116**, 497—506 (1952).

[661] HODGKIN, A. L., A. F. HUXLEY, and B. KATZ: Measurement of current-voltage relations in the membrane of the giant axon of Loligo. J. Physiol. **116**, 424—448 (1952).

potential level can be suddenly displaced upward or downward for a preset period of time upon which it returns to the starting value. As the result of this applied single "square wave" of potential, electric current passes through the membrane and the time course of the current flow can be recorded. With this device it is possible to study the dependency of the current upon the magnitude of the applied potential and upon the ionic composition of the bathing fluid.

For the study of the ionic permeability changes this arrangement has great advantages. Thus by holding the potential constant one eliminates the effect of the membrane capacitance except for a quick pulse in connection with the displacement of the potential, and this contribution can easily be calculated from the well known expression: $I = C\dfrac{dV}{dt}$, where I is the current, C the capacity and $\dfrac{dV}{dt}$ the rate of change of the potential. The lack of propagation eliminates disturbing currents from neighboring points which would otherwise have been in a different phase of ionic permeability. Finally, the voltage clamp eliminates the all-or-non response.

Under practically all conditions the current obtained with this setup differs from the one which would have been obtained if the current was passing through an ohmic resistance. The most striking features are shown by records of the membrane current when the membrane potential is suddenly lowered from its resting value by some ten mV or more. Following the quick outward pulse through the membrane capacity, there is an initial current in the inward direction. This ingoing current obviously corresponds to the rising phase of the action potential which would have appeared in the absence of the "voltage clamp". Thus according to the "sodium theory" this inward phase of the current on the voltage clamp records would be carried by sodium ions, moving passively under the influence of concentration and potential differences. If the voltage clamp is maintained for a

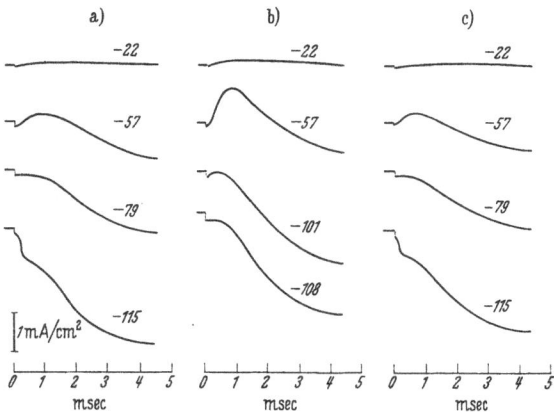

Fig. 16. Time course of membrane current associated with a sudden depolarisation in a squid giant axon under voltage clamp. The figure on each curve gives the potential displacement in mV. Inward current is shown upwards. a, axon in modified sea water (30% Na ad 70 %choline), b, axon in sea water, c, after replacing sea water with 30% Na and 70% choline (after HODGKIN and HUXLEY[44])

sufficient period of time, there is a reversal of the direction of current, corresponding to the falling part of the action potential. According to the theory the potassium permeability should dominate in this period. One can predict that if the sodium ions in the outside medium are replaced by non-penetrating choline ions, the ingoing component of the membrane current following a depolarization of the membrane should disappear. This, as a matter of fact, is the case. The record of the current under such conditions shows a hump in the outward direction, conceivable due to diffusion of Na out of the fibre. Fig. 16 shows the effect of the sodium concentration and the degree of depolarization on the time course of the ionic current. (The curves are corrected for the initial contribution of current passing the membrane capacitance.) The numbers show the displacement of the membrane potential in mV. The tracings in column a and c refer to experiments where the medium was sea water with 70% of its Na replaced by choline ion. Column b comprises tracings from experiments with the fibre in pure sea water. It is seen that depolarization of 22 mV give rise to very little current (when corrected for the capacity current). 43 mV depolarization, however, elicits the positive surge of current, and the peak is definitely higher with high sodium than with low. With increasing displacement of the membrane potential the positive surge diminishes and in the low-Na system it has entirely vanished around 79 mV displacement. In the case of sea water, however, 108 mV displacement of the membrane potential is required to extinguish the positive phase of the current. These results are easily explainable in terms of the "sodium hypothesis". If the current is carried solely by sodium ions, it will be directed inward as long as the electrochemical potential of the sodium ion is higher outside than inside the fibre. The concentration difference between the outside and the inside media give rise to a "sodium potential", E_{Na}, which, according to the Nernst equation, is:

$$E_{Na} = \frac{RT}{F} \ln \frac{[Na]_i}{[Na]_o} .$$

This potential will tend to drive sodium inward unless it is opposed by an electric potential of equal or larger size. If Na_0 is the sodium activity in sea water and Na_0' the sodium concentration in modified sea water with reduced sodium, we can deduce from the above equation that the difference between the corresponding sodium potentials E_{Na}' and E_{Na} is given by:

$$E_{Na}' - E_{Na} = \frac{RT}{F} \left(\ln \frac{[Na]_i}{[Na]_o} - \ln \frac{[Na]_i}{[Na]_o} \right) = \frac{RT}{F} \ln \frac{[Na]_o}{[Na]_o'} . \tag{37}$$

The displacements of the membrane potential making influx and outflux of sodium equal (and thus just extinguishing the positive inflexion of the current curve) are called $V_{Na} = E_{Na} - E_r$ and $V_{Na}' = E_{Na}' - E_r'$, where E_r and E_r' are the values of the resting potential in sea water and in the test solution, respectively. We thus have

$$(V_{Na}' - V_{Na}) + (E_r' - E_r) = \frac{RT}{F} \ln \frac{[Na]_o}{[Na]_o'} . \tag{38}$$

It is seen that the theory can be tested without knowledge of the actual Na concentration inside the fibre, although it must be considered constant. As it will be seen from Table 27 the agreement between theory and experiment must be considered very satisfactory indeed. It is thus well established that the current during the initial part of the voltage clamp is carried by sodium ions, and by this ionic species only. The delayed outward current associated with prolonged depolarization, on the other hand, is little affected by replacing sodium ions with choline ions. The proof that the outward current following the inward directed phase is mainly due to potassium is mostly indirect. In the first place it is highly

Table 27. *Observed and theoretical changes in sodium potential in giant axons of Loligo when the external sodium concentration is lowered* [449]

$\frac{(Na)_o'}{(Na)_o}$	VNa mV	V'Na mV	$E_{Na}'-E_{Na}$ mV	Sodium shift obs	Potential (mV) theo.
0.3	—105	—78	+3	30	28.9
0.1	— 96	—45	+4	55	55.3
0.1	—100	—48	+4	56	55.6
0.1	— 95	—45	+4	54	55.6

suggestive that the outward current associated with prolonged depolarization is the same current that causes the falling phase of the spike and as mentioned on p. 102 the amount of potassium given off per impulse from the stimulated nerve is of the right magnitude to explain the repolarization.

By making a few simple assumptions HODGKIN and HUXLEY succeeded in separating the ionic currents into a sodium current and a potassium current. The assumptions are the following:

1) The time course of the potassium current is the same in the presence of low sodium solution and in sea water, if the potential during the voltage clamp is the same.

2) The time course of the sodium current is similar in the two cases, even if the amplitude and sometimes the direction of the sodium current is different.

3) $\frac{dI_K}{dt} = 0$ initially for a period of about one-third of that taken by I_{Na} to reach its maximum.

Using these assumptions it is now possible to resolve the voltage clamp current into a sodium component and a potassium component (see Fig. 17).[662] Assuming further that both the sodium current and the potassium current are determined solely by the electrochemical potential gradient for the ion in question and the conductance of the membrane for that ion, it can be easily shown that the conductance changes are identical for the fibre in sea water and in sodium-free choline sea water. In the resting state the fibre has a potassium conductance of about 0.5 mmho/cm². The sodium conductance is much less, perhaps 0.01 mmho/cm². If, by applying the voltage clamp, the potential difference across the membrane is increased (that is the inside of the fibre is made more negative) both the potassium conductance and the sodium conductance fall and remain less than they are in the resting state, as long as the voltage clamp is maintained. If, however, the membrane potential is reduced to zero, he sodium conductance starts rising and within one or two milliseconds reaches a value around 15 mmho/cm², whereupon it decays to a low value along an exponential curve with a time constant of about one millisecond. The potassium conductance does not change notably at first but rises along an S-shaped curve; having reached a peak level about equal to that of sodium, the potassium conductance again drops and reaches a constant level about 20 mmho/cm². This level is maintained as

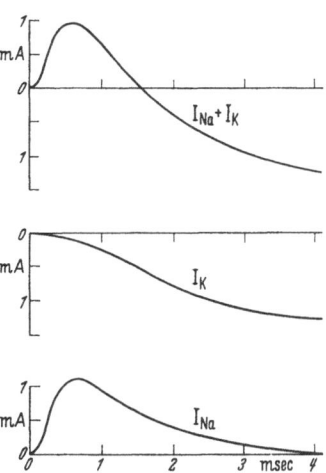

Fig. 17. Separation of ionic currents through the membrane of a giant axon into currents carried by Na and K. Resting potential lowered by 56 mV. Upper curve, axon in sea water, middle curve, axon in modified sea water (10% Na and 90% choline), lower curve, difference between upper and middle curve. Inward currents are shown upwards (after HODGKIN and HUXLEY[662])

long as the membrane potential is clamped at zero. When the membrane potential is brought back to its original value, the sodium permeability of the membrane thus is characterized by a fast formation of a permeability element and a somewhat slower decay or inactivation of this element. Both the rate of formation and the rate of inactivation of the sodium permeable membrane element increase with increasing depolarization.

[662] HUXLEY, A. F.: Electrical processes in nerve conduction. In: Ion transport across membranes, p. 23—34. Ed.: HANS T. CLARKE. New York: Acad. Press. 1954.

Small changes in the membrane potential give rise to large alterations in the ability of the membrane to give the characteristic increase in sodium conductance. The inactivation process also is very sensitive to the potential level. Thus a steady depolarization of 10 mV reduces the sodium current associated with a subsequent depolarization of 45 mV by about 60%, whereas a steady rise in potential enhances the power of the membrane to become permeable to sodium. The inactivation, if allowed to proceed for a sufficient period of time, makes the fibre refractory. In other words: it cannot undergo the increase in sodium conductance if suddenly depolarized. At high potentials, however, the inactivation is rapidly reversed.

Also the potassium permeability depends strongly upon the membrane potential, but as with sodium, the permeability element takes some time to form and to disappear. Following a period of depolarization the potassium conductance will remain high for a short time, thus assisting the inactivation process in holding the fibre in an unexcitable state.

As long as the chemical nature of the membrane processes is unknown it is clearly impossible to deduce the behaviour of the membrane from first principles. Instead, HODGKIN and HUXLEY have developed empirically a set of differential equations which describe the voltage clamp currents very closely. It then turned out that the parameters which were found to govern the voltage clamp system could also be used to describe the spike of the non-propagated impulse and even of the propagated impulse. The original paper must be consulted for the details of the treatment. The success of this treatment to predict correctly the behaviour of the fibre under the most varied conditions speaks strongly in favour of the belief that the three major processes going on in the fibre membrane during conductions are indeed the formation of a sodium conducting element, the inactivation of this element and the formation of a potassium permeability element. It is a striking fact that the sodium permeable element seems to be entirely inaccessible for potassium just as the potassium permeable element cannot be passed by sodium. It is worth emphasizing that the "setting" of the rate constants determining the permeability for the two alkali metal ions is determined by the displacement of the potential and is independent of the outside sodium concentration. On the other hand it is highly sensitive to the concentration of bivalent cations like Ca and Mg[664], as one would expect from the well known effects on the excitability of these ions.

A few apparent shortcomings of the theory call for comment. The first one is that the membrane potential and the apparent equilibrium potential for potassium do not obey the Nernst equation if the external K concentration is less than about 20 mM (HODGKIN and HUXLEY, HODGKIN and KEYNES[252]). According to FRANKENHAEUSER and HODGKIN[663] (compare, however, SHANES[665, 435, 666]) the explanation is that there is a narrow space immediately outside the excitable membrane where, temporarily, the K concentration may be different from that of the external medium. The fibre behaves as if a single impulse increased the external K concentration by about 1.6 Mm at 18°. The excess K then disappeared exponentially with a time constant of 30—100 msec. The diffusion barrier has a

[663] FRANKENHAEUSER, B., and A. L. HODGKIN: The after-effects of impulses in the giant nerve fibres of Loligo. J. Physiol. 131, 341—376 (1956).

[664] WEIDMANN, S.: Effects of calcium ions and local anaestetics on electrical properties of Purkinje fibres. J. Physiol. 129, 568—582 (1955).

[665] SHANES, A. M.: Potassium movements in relation to nerve activity. J. gen. Physiol. 34, 795—807 (1951).

[666] SHANES, A. M., H. GRUNDFEST, and W. FREYGANG: Low level impedance changes following the spike in the squid giant axon before and after treatment with "veratrine" alkaloids. J. gen. Physiol. 37, 39—51 (1954).

resistance of about 4 ohms/cm² and is quite unselective. The space in question is probably located beneath the Schwann cells.

GRUNDFEST[667] and collaborators have argued against the HODGKIN-HUXLEY theory that the membrane potential is not dependent upon the intracellular potassium concentration. They base this statement upon experiments in which they have injected KCl, K glutamate or K aspartate into the squid fibre. Notably the K salts of the non-penetrating aspartate and glutamate ions ought to have produced an increase in the membrane potential. It might be argued of course, that the injection damages the membrane sufficiently to offset the increase in potential, but the problem certainly invites further study. It is to be hoped that the improved micro-injection technique developed by HODGKIN and KEYNES will help solve the problem. The latter authors have studied the sodium outflux from fibres micro-injected with readioactive sodium. The sodium outflux turned out to be proportional to the internal Na concentration. Thus the active transport mechanism for sodium seems to be undamaged by the injection procedure. The injected Na reduced the overshoot of the spike by the amount predicted by the Hodgkin-Huxley theory. Thus, as far as sodium is concerned, the micro-injection results do not give rise to doubt about the theory.

It is an old idea that the fibre membrane goes through a state of increased permeability during activity. The feature in the Hodgkin theory which clashed most against conventional physiological thinking was perhaps that, at least for a short period of time, the sodium permeability exceeds the permeability to K by a factor of at least 30. For years it has been a dogma that cell membranes must always be more permeable to K than to Na, because the hydrated potassium ion is smaller than the hydrated sodium ion and thus is able to pass through smaller pores than the latter.

As a matter of fact there are several exceptions to the rule that cells are more permeable to K than to Na. In erythrocytes of certain species the reverse is true (see p. 82) even though the K and Na permeabilities are of the same order of magnitude. The outward facing side of the frog skin epithelium is highly permeable to Na and Li, but very little permeable to K and other cations (see p. 123). Thus structures similar to the kind which serve the sodium permeability during conduction in nerve may be in permanent function in other cell types.

With respect to the chemical nature of the structures in the nerve fibre membrane accounting for the specific sodium and potassium permeabilities very little can be said at the present time. The fact that the sodium permeability is still high when the potassium permeability is developing seems to rule out the otherwise rather tempting possibility that it is the same type of membrane structure which serves as vehicle for both ionic species in succession.

No matter what theory concerning their nature is put forward, it must account for two striking facts, namely the ionic specificity and the sensitivity to the membrane potential.

With respect to the first point, it seems that the sodium permeable element of sepia nerve is accessible only to sodium and lithium ions. The potassium permeable element, on the other hand, allows K, Rb, Cs and NH_3^+ to pass through. Judging from their ability to reduce the membrane potential Rb seems to pass through somewhat faster than K, whereas Cs seems to diffuse through much less readily. The fact that there is an increased influx of Ca during nerve activity might

────────

[667] GRUNDFEST, H.: The nature of the electrochemical potentials of bioelectric tissues. In: Electrochemistry in biology and medicine. p. 141—166. Ed. T. SHEDLOVSKY. New York: John Wiley and Sons 1955.

tentatively be taken as indicating that Ca can use either the sodium "path" or the potassium "path". It is tempting to assume that it is the competition between Ca and, say, sodium ions for the sodium paths which is responsible for the effect of Ca upon nervous activity.

In any event Ca profoundly changes the dependency between the membrane potential and the parameters governing the sodium conductance (FRANKEN-HAEUSER and HODGKIN[663], WEIDMANN[664]).

According to HODGKIN and HUXLEY, the sensitivity of the sodium and potassium permeabilities of the nerve fibre to the membrane potential indicates that the underlying structures are charged molecules or dipoles whose orientation is determined by the electric field. One possibility which they mention is that bridges of sodium or potassium specific sites are formed across the membrane by a lowering of the potential. This hypothesis has found some support in the "single file" phenomenon characteristic of potassium diffusion through the membrane (see p. 51). In any case the binding sites involved must have high chemical specificity to exclude one or the other of the two principal alkali ions. In this respect the alkali ion permeable structures resemble those responsible for the active transport of the same ions. But all available evidence indicates that the ionic movements during activity is always down an electrochemical potential gradient and that no active transport is involved. The active transport process is concerned only with the recharging of the fibre during recovery.

f) The applicability and limitations of the sodium theory of electric activity

It will appear from the foregoing the essential elements involved in the electric activity are common to the non-myelinated squid nerve fibre and the myelinated fibre of the frog. The question may therefore be asked: are we able to describe the conducted impulse in other excitable cells and tissues in terms of the sequence of permeability changes which has turned out to work so successfully in the description of the events in squid nerve. At the present time it seems justified to say that the essential elements of the mechanism must be operational in most excitable animal tissues, nerve fibres, striated muscle fibres and heart muscle fibres alike, but that the rates of the processes involved in different tissues vary widely and certain details of the mechanism may even be different in principle from one tissue to the other. The question of the applicability of the "sodium theory" upon the mammalian motoneuron in situ has been studied by ECCLES and collaborators[668, 669, 670].

The technique applied was to alter the internal ionic milieu of the axon by electrophoretic injection via one channel of "double-barrelled" microelectrode, the other one being used for potential recordings. With this method it was possible to demonstrate that the mammalian motoneuron behaved in most respects as would be predicted from the sodium theory of nervous activity. There are, however, differences which may be of importance functionally. It will be recalled that in the giant axon the increased K permeability following the initial surge of Na permeability seems to be an immediate consequence of the potential drop. With the motoneuron the high potassium permeability must be caused by the increased

---

[668] COOMBS, J. S., J. C. ECCLES, and P. FATT: The electrical properties of the motoneurone membrane. J. Physiol. **130**, 291—325 (1955).

[669] COOMBS, J. S., J. C. ECCLES, and P. FATT: The specific ionic conductances and the ionic movements across the motoneuronal membrane that produce the inhibitory post-synaptic potentials. J. Physiol. **130**, 326—373 (1955).

[670] ECCLES, J. C.: The physiology of nerve cells. 270 pp. Baltimore: Johns Hopkins Press 1957. London: Oxford Univ. Press 1957.

sodium concentration, since a lowering of the potential does not in itself bring about an increased potassium conductance. Like in the giant axon, the sodium pump seems to be coupled with the pumping inward of potassium. At least judging from the concentrations and the electric potential, the potassium ion is present in the fibre at a concentration decisively above the equilibrium concentration. In this context it should also be mentioned that the motoneurons show a pronounced after-hyperpolarization. This apparently is due to the increased K permeability relative to that for other ionic species. This state of affairs obviously will tend to bring the membrane potential closer to the equilibrium potential of the K ion which is above the normal resting potential of the fibre. In certain types of neurons like the crustacean stretch receptor cell, the hyperpolarization is absent, apparently because the potassium ion is already in Donnan equilibrium with the surrounding medium[671, 672].

With the spectacular exception of crab muscle (see below), the sodium theory seems also applicable to striated muscle and heart muscle (BRADY and WOODBURY[673]). In the latter the action potential is, however, greatly prolonged which may be due to the fact that the period of increased permeability to K, following the initial surge of sodium current, is lacking in heart muscle (see p. 167). A similar phenomenon can be elicited even in squid nerve if tetraethylammonium ions are injected into the axon (TASAKI and HAGIWARA[674]). FATT and KATZ found that crustacean muscles which had been treated with tetrabutylammonium ions gave greatly prolonged action potentials in the total absence of monovalent cations in the medium. Thus, either the membrane current must be carried by an anion, or the membrane must become temporarily permeable to one of the divalent cations. It has been known for some time that tetraethylammonium ions can restore excitability to B and C fibres of frog nerve which have been blocked by treatment with sodium-free solutions (LORENTE DE NÓ[675]). Recently it has been found that even the excitability of the A-fibres can be restored in the absence of sodium if the fibres are treated with guanidinium ions and certain quaternary ammonium compounds (LORENTE DE NÓ et al.[676, 677]). Whether the organic cations can actually substitute for sodium in the excitation process is still an open question. In general it seems, however, that we can safely use the sodium theory as the basis for our discussion of the effects of sodium and potassium upon excitation and conduction in excitable tissues, but it should be born in mind that there is a group of fast electrophysiological events which are of an entirely different nature: The non-conducted potential changes elicited by neurohormones (acetylcholine etc.) in motor endplates, subsynaptic membranes and electric organs. These phenomena will be treated on p. 168 and the following pages.

[671] EYZAGUIRRE, C., and S. W. KUFFLER: Processes of excitation in the dendrites and in the soma of single isolated sensory nerve cells of the lobster and crayfish. J. gen. Physiol. **39**, 87—119 (1956).

[672] EYZAGUIRRE, C., and S. W. KUFFLER: Further study of soma dendrite and axon excitation in single neurons. J. gen. Physiol. **39**, 121—153 (1956).

[673] BRADY, A. J., and J. W. WOODBURY: Effects of sodium and potassium on repolarization in frog ventricular fibres. Ann. N. Y. Acad. Sci. **65**, 687—692 (1957).

[674] TASAKI, I., and S. HAGIWARA: Demonstration of two stable potential states in the squid giant axon under tetraethylammonium chloride. J. gen. Physiol. **40**, 859—885 (1957).

[675] LORENTE DE NÓ, R.: On the effect of certain quaternary ammonium ions upon frog nerve. J. cell. comp. Physiol. 33. Suppl. (1949).

[676] LORENTE DE NÓ, R., F. VIDAL, and L. M. H. LARRAMENDI: Restoration of sodium-deficient frog nerve fibres by onium ions. Nature (Lond.) **179**, 737—738 (1957).

[677] LARRAMENDI, L. M. H., R. LORENTE DE NÓ, and F. VIDAL: Restoration of sodium deficient frog nerve fibres by an isotonic solution of guanidinium chloride. Nature (Lond.) **178**, 316—317 (1956).

g) Effect of external Na concentration upon excitation and conduction

1. Effects on nerve

It is a well established fact that nerve fibres become inexcitible when the Na concentration of the medium is less than some 10% of that of the ordinary Ringer solution, isotonicity being maintained with glucose or sucrose. This has been demonstrated in the case of Loligo giant axon (WEBB and YOUNG[678], HODGKIN and KATZ[271]), Sepia giant axon (KEYNES[430]), Carcinus nerve (KATZ[679]), frog medulated nerve (KATO[680], ERLANGER and BLAIR[681], LORENTE DE NÓ[682], FENG and LIU[683], HUXLEY and STÄMPFLI[641]). In most cases the conduction block also occurs when the Na ion of the outside medium is replaced by an inert non-penetrating cation like choline. Among the alkali metal ions only Li can replace Na with the excitability retained. As demonstrated by LORENTE DE NÓ[675], however, tetraethylammonium ions and to a lesser extent certain other quaternary ammonium compounds can maintain excitability in the B and C fibres but not the A fibre of frog nerve. Whereas this is of great theoretical interest, there is, however, no reason to believe that quaternary ammonium ions are present in the tissue fluids in sufficient amounts to play the role of "Na substitute" in any of the animal species so far studied. It has been known for some time that the blood of insects, notably of herbivorous species, contains very little Na and rather large K concentration (for references, see HOYLE[684]). The work of HOYLE has shown, however, that the space between the nerve sheath and the fibres has an ionic composition which is entirely different from that of the blood or hemolymph, being for one thing, much poorer in K. While, to the author's knowledge, the Na concentration inside the nerve sheath has not been measured, it is at least conceivable that these nerves also depend for their function upon the presence of Na.

2. The nerve sheath as a diffusion barrier

Even in animal forms where the blood concentration of Na is high (that is most of the animal kingdom) the nerve sheaths play a great role as diffusion barriers. Thus, the slow penetration of Na through the sheath must be considered the reason why frog nerve trunks can conduct for a long time in media free of Na. This was already observed by OVERTON[685], and the phenomenon was used by LORENTE DE NÓ[686, 687, 688] as evidence that extracellular Na is unimportant for

[678] WEBB, D. A., and J. Z. YOUNG: Electrolyte content and action potential of the giant nerve fibres of Loligo. J. Physiol. **98**, 299—313 (1940).

[679] KATZ, B.: The effect of electrolyte deficiency on the rate of conduction in a single nerve fibre. J. Physiol. **106**, 411—417 (1947).

[680] KATO, G.: On the excitation, conduction, and narcotisation of single nerve fibres. Cold Spr. Harb. Symp. quant. Biol. **4**, 202—213 (1936).

[681] ERLANGER, J., and E. A. BLAIR: The action of isotonic, salt-free solutions on conduction in medullated nerve fibres. Amer. J. Physiol. **124**, 341—359 (1938).

[682] LORENTE DE NÓ. R.: A study of nerve physiology. In: Studies Rockefeller Inst. Med. Res. **131** and **132**. New York (1947).

[683] FENG, T. P., and Y. M. LIU: The connective tissue sheath of the nerve as effective diffusion barrier. J. cell. comp. Physiol. **34**, 1—16 (1949).

[684] HOYLE, G.: Potassium ions and insect nerve muscle. J. exp. Biol. **30**, 121—135 (1953).

[685] OVERTON, E.: Beiträge zur allgemeinen Muskel- und Nervenphysiologie. II. Mitteilung. Über die Unentbehrlichkeit von Natrium- (oder Lithium)-Ionen für den Kontraktionsact des Muskels. Pflügers Arch. ges. Physiol. **92**, 346—386 (1902).

[686] LORENTE DE NÓ, R.: Equilibria of frog nerve with different external concentrations of sodium ions. J. gen. Physiol. **35**, 145—182 (1952).

[687] LORENTE DE NÓ, R.: The ineffectiveness of the connective tissue sheath of nerve as a diffusion barrier. J. cell. comp. Physiol. **35**, 195—240 (1950).

[688] LORENTE DE NÓ, R.: Observations on the properties of the epineurium of frog nerve. Cold Spr. Harb. Symp. quant. Biol. **17**, 299—315 (1952).

nerve conduction, whereas intracellular Na is involved in metabolic processes of importance for the function of nerve, see also LORENTE DE NÓ[682, 687, 686], CALLEGO[689]. A key point in LORENTE DE Nó's argument was that the removal of the sheath damages the nerve so that results obtained with desheathed nerves would lead to erroneous results.

However, in 1951 CRESCITELLI and GEISSMANN[690] found 1) that in the first place desheathing does not materially damage the nerve since resheathed nerves behave like normal ones, and that 2) the sheath acts as an effective barrier against a number of substances. Similar results were obtained by FENG and LIU[691] (Compare also RASHBASS and RUSHTON[692], LUNDBERG[646], CRESCITELLI[693]). Still more conclusive are the experiments performed by KRNJEVIC[694] on perfused frog sciatic nerve. In this preparation a Na-free solution blocks conduction reversibly within 6—7 min, whereas isotonic KCl blocks reversibly in one minute. Thus, when the sheath is bypassed via the vascular system, Na is as necessary for conduction in intact nerve as it is in isolated fibres. The rate at which the lack of Na in the bathing solution makes itself felt seems to be a simple function of the rate at which Na can diffuse away from the surface of the fibre.

3. Effects on striated muscle

From the classical work of OVERTON[685] it was known that muscle became non-excitable when the Na concentration of the bathing fluid contained less than 10% of that of Ringer. In recent times the phenomenon has been studied by NASTUK and HODGKIN[645]. The dependency of the muscle fibre action potential (of Rana temporaria) upon the external Na concentration turned out to be remarkably similar to that of nerve fibres. Thus there is every reason to believe that the sodium theory of conduction and excitation is also valid for muscle (see HODGKIN[345]).

It should be pointed out, however, that the nervelike type of conduction is only typical of the "fast" muscle fibres. The system of "slow" fibres, discovered by KUFFLER and VAUGHAN WILLIAMS[423], is unable to propagate an impulse. These fibres have numerous end-plates and the stimulation of these gives rise to local depolarization and maintained contraction in the depolarized region.

In crustacean muscle the action potential is abolished when sugar is substituted for NaCl. But if choline or tetraethylammonium ions replace Na, stimulation can be achieved and, as a matter of fact, the spike height is increased. Spikes as high as 90 mV (in choline-Ringer) or even 110 mV (in tetramethylammonium-Ringer) are obtained as compared with 60—70 mV in Na-Ringer (FATT and KATZ[695]). These observations are undoubtedly related to the finding of LORENTE DE Nó that certain quaternary ammonium ions can substitute for Na in the conduction of B and C fibres in frog nerve.

[689] CALLEGO, A.: Loss and recovery of excitability by normal and by degenerating nerves deprived of sodium. J. gen. Physiol. **35**, 129—144 (1952).

[690] CRESCITELLI, F., and T. A. GEISMANN: Certain effects of antihistamines and related compounds of frog nerve fibres. Amer. J. Physiol. **164**, 509—519 (1951).

[691] FENG, T. P., and Y. M. LIU: Chinese J. Physiol. **17**, 207 (1950).

[692] RASHBASS, C., and W. A. H. RUSHTON: The relation of structure to the spread of excitation in the frog's sciatic trunk. J. Physiol. **110**, 110—135 (1949).

[693] CRESCITELLI, F.: Nerve sheath as a barrier to the action of certain substances. Amer. J. Physiol. **166**, 229—240 (1951).

[694] KRNJEVIC, K.: Some observations on perfused frog sciatic nerves. J. Physiol. **123**, 338—356 (1954).

[695] FATT, P., and B. KATZ: Conduction of impulses in crustacean muscle fibres. J. Physiol. **115**, 45 P (1951).

Thus it seems that the conduction in excitable tissues is not strictly associated with external Na. If, however, the mechanism underlying the development of an action potential requires, say 10 meq/l external fluid, of the participating ion, it would seem as if in most species, the mechanism will have to depend on Na.

4. Effects on heart muscle

In most respects the effect of the Na concentration on excitation and conduction of heart tissue resembles the one exerted by this ion upon striated muscle. That is: Reduction of the Na concentration of the Ringer or Tyrode solution used as outside medium results in a decrease in action potential. In the Purkinje fibre of the kid DRAPER and WEIDMANN[633] found the membrane reversal to vary with the logarithm of the extracellular Na concentration, in agreement with the sodium theory (compare p. 151). Qualitatively similar results have been obtained by CRANEFIELD, EYSTER and GILSON[696] in the case of the heart of the snapping turtle (Chelydra serpentina), and by BRADY and WOODBURY[673] on the frog ventricle.

The production of conducted action potentials required a Na concentration in the medium of at least 10—20% of the normal.

As it is the case with other conducting tissues, the rate of rise of the action potential is a decisive factor as regards the rate of conduction and as such of considerable interest. Besides that, however, the maximum rate of rise of the action potential, according to the Hodgkin theory of electric activity is a measure of the inward sodium current: The driving force for the transfer of Na is made up of the potential difference and the concentration gradient. If the potential at the point of maximum rise is kept constant, the rate of rise in current must be a direct measure of the Na permeability. This line of reasoning was used by WEIDMANN[697] to study the relationship between the "resting" potential of Purkinje fibres, artificially clamped at series of values (compare p. 154) and the Na permeability during activity following the clamping period. It was found that the calculated Na permeability was at a maximum when the membrane potential had been clamped at 90 mV or higher before stimulation, and that it fell off along an S-shaped curve as the clamp potential was lowered. In agreement with the ideas of HODGKIN and HUXLEY this phenomenon was explained as follows: The diffusion of Na into the fibres during the spike, although it is not active transport, depends upon the availability of a membrane carrier which acts as a "ferry boat" for Na. The availability of the carrier at the surface of the membrane, for some reason not yet understood, depends upon the membrane potential as it is immediately before stimulation. If a potential of more than 90 mV has been acting on the membrane, the amount of carrier is at a maximum, whence at a clamp potential of some 50 mV nearly all carrier is temporarily inactivated. Reactivation is, however, a very rapid process, taking place with a time constant of a few milliseconds on applying a clamp potential of sufficient magnitude.

h) Effect of internal Na concentration on electric activity in muscle

In the experiments of NASTUK and HODGKIN[645] the Na concentration of the soaking medium was varied, whereas the fibre Na concentration was supposedly constant. It has been shown by DESMEDT[419], however, that the sodium theory

    [696] CRANEFIELD, P. F., J. A. E. EYSTER, and W. E. GILSON: Effect of reduction of external sodium chloride on the injury potentials of cardiac muscle. Amer. J. Physiol. **166**, 269—272 (1951).

    [697] WEIDMANN, S.: The effect of the cardiac membrane potential on the rapid availability of the sodium-carrying system. J. Physiol. **127**, 213—224 (1955).

of the action potential (see p. 151) does also predict satisfactorily the magnitude of the action potential of muscle when the concentration of fibre Na is varied. An increased level of fibre Na can be obtained by soaking the muscle in K free Ringer, whereas lower than normal Na levels are obtained in modified Ringers with increased K-concentration (compare FENN and COBB[698], STEINBACH[413], BOYLE and CONWAY[101]; for a further discussion of the K-Na exchange in muscle, see p. 88).

The muscles (frog sartorii) were soaked for 10—68 hr at 2—3°C. Control experiments showed that the interspace volume did not vary significantly as a function of the soaking time. The Na content of the individual muscles could therefore be expressed in terms of concentration in the fibre water, assuming uniform distribution in the fibre (see, however, CONWAY[395]).

The results fit well the equation

$$E_a = 58 \log_{10} (Na_i)/(Na_0) \,,$$

where E_a is the active membrane potential and Na_i and Na_0 are the fibre and outside Na concentrations.

i) Effects of K upon excitation and conduction

1. Nerve

Since an increase in external K concentration imposes a lowering of the membrane potential upon the fibre, it is quite understandable that the application of solutions of high K concentration can stimulate nerve fibres to activity.

But also the magnitude of the action potential depends upon the K concentration (see below) so that it is depressed as the outside K concentration increases. In the squid axon, for example, the action potential is reduced to zero at about 6 times the K concentration of sea water (CURTIS and COLE). If solutions of high K concentration remain in contact with the fibres it therefore leads to block of conduction. Application of excess K to a nerve fibre thus initially tends to give rise to excitation, followed by block of conduction. It is understandable that early studies of the effects of potassium-rich solution on nerve gave rather a complex picture.

For whole nerves the situation is further complicated by the fact that the sheath slows down that diffusion of ions appreciably (compare p. 162). Thus a frog sciatic nerve bathed in Ringer solution containing four times the normal K concentration takes about 30 min to develop a noticeable reduction in the height and rate of rise of the action potential (see for instance ROSENBERG and KITAYAMA[699]). With single frog myelinated fibres, on the other hand, HERTZ[700] found an immediate reduction of the amplitude of the action potential on immersing the fibre in Ringer containing 6—10 times the normal K concentration. According to HUXLEY and STÄMPFLI[641] the depolarization due to increased K concentration takes place in less than one minute. The depressant action of K on nerve activity should always be born in mind in experiments with nerves. Thus COWAN[452] pointed out that the reversible inexitability which is characteristic

---

[698] FENN, W. O., and D. M. COBB: The potassium equilibrium in muscle. J. gen. Physiol. **17**, 629—656 (1934).

[699] ROSENBERG, H., and K. KITAYAMA: Untersuchungen über Nervenaktionsströme. III. Das Verhalten der Negativitätswelle bei Überschuß von Kalium- und Calciumionen. Pflügers Arch. ges. Physiol. **223**, 602—618 (1930).

[700] HERTZ, H.: Relation between fibre diameter and action potential of single nerve fibres. J. Physiol. **104**, 1 P—2 P (1945).

of freshly dissected crab nerve is due to K which has leaked out of the fibres and accumulated at their surface.

According to what has been said above, the stimulatory effect of K ions is usually transitory and is often seen when high K concentration are suddenly established at the fibre surface. Thus CICARDO[701] elicited contractions of the gastrocnemius muscle by injecting KCl into the sciatic nerve. HODGKIN and HUXLEY[655] obtained a transient volley of impulses when a drop of isotonic KCl was placed on the squid axon. Also in mammalian nerve (cat) excess K gives rise to "spontaneous" discharges (LEHMANN[702]).

With respect to its stimulatory effect, K is antagonized by Ca^{++}. If the Ca^{++} concentration of the solution in contact with a frog nerve fibre is lowered by washing with NaCl solution, activity can be maintained with four times the normal K concentration. When the fibre is brought to discharge spontaneously by treatment with sodium citrate, the addition of low concentrations of K will produce an initial increase in discharge frequency, followed by a secondary decline. Conversely, excess Ca^{++} can abolish the stimulatory effect of potassium ions (see for instance BROWN and MacINTOSH[703], CALMA and WRIGHT[704]). For a more detailed account of the stimulatory effects of K ions, see BRINK, BRONK and LARRABEE[705], also GOFFART and BACQ[706]).

The threshold of electric stimulation is in general first lowered and then increased by K ions in moderate concentrations, whereas larger amounts of K cause inexcitability.

For the understanding of the role which K plays in the nerve fibre it is important to realize that the block of conduction brought about by increased K concentration can be relieved by anodal polarization (WORONZOW[707], LORENTO DE N6[682]). Obviously, in the region of the anode the potential drop across the fibre must be increased, and a polarization of sufficient magnitude to counter the lowering of the potential induced by the increased K concentration evidently restores the capacity of the fibre to conduct. This made it likely that the effects of K upon excitability is of a largely indirect nature via its effect upon the membrane potential. This view has been fully substantiated by the later developments. This is also in agreement with the fact that nerves can be stimulated in the total absence of K in the external medium.

2. Striated muscle

The effect of external potassium upon the membrane potential and the threshold of single frog muscle fibres has been studied by JENERICK and GERARD[708].

[701] CICARDO, V. H.: Rev. Soc. Argent. Biol. 14, 12 (1939).

[702] LEHMANN, J. E.: The effect of changes in p_H on the action of mammalian A nerve fibers. Amer. J. Physiol. 118, 600—612 (1937).

[703] BROWN, G. L., and F. C. MacINTOSH: Discharges in nerve fibres produced by potassium ions. J. Physiol. 96, 10 P—11 P (1939).

[704] CALMA, I., and S. WRIGHT: Effects of intrathecal injection of KCl and other solutions in cats. Excitatory action of K ions on posterior nerve root fibres. J. Physiol. 106, 211—235 (1947).

[705] BRINK, F., D. W. BRONK, and M. G. LARRABEE: Chemical excitation of nerve. Ann. N. Y. Acad. Sci. 57, 457—485 (1946).

[706] GOFFART, M., and Z. M. BACQ: Les sensibilisateurs au potassium. Ergebn. Physiol. 47, 555—617 (1952).

[707] WORONZOW, D. S.: Über die Einwirkung des konstanten Stromes auf den mit Wasser, Zuckerlösung, Alkali- und Erdalkalichloridlösungen behandelten Nerven. Pflügers Arch. ges. Physiol. 203, 300—318 (1924).

[708] JENERICK, H. P., and R. W. GERARD: Membrane potential and threshold of single muscle fibres. J. cell. comp. Physiol. 42, 79—102 (1953).

The threshold for electrical stimulation decreases in a linear fashion with log $[K_0]$. The potassium concentration seems to act almost exclusively by setting the membrane potential (compare Fig. 18). The critical potential for propagated impulses is 57 mV in summer and 52 mV in winter. If the membrane potential is suddenly displaced below this value a propagated impulse ensues. If the membrane potential is maintained below threshold but above 30 mV, local responses can be elicited but there is no action potential. Below 30 mV no response is seen.

3. Heart muscle

As in the case of other excitable tissues, K only (or mainly) influences the action potential via its effect upon the resting potential. WEIDMANN[709], [710] found, on the false tendon of calf and sheep hearts, that increasing the K concentration of the Tyrode solution fivefold would reduce the resting potential from 92—54 mV. After that the preparation did not respond to electric stimula-

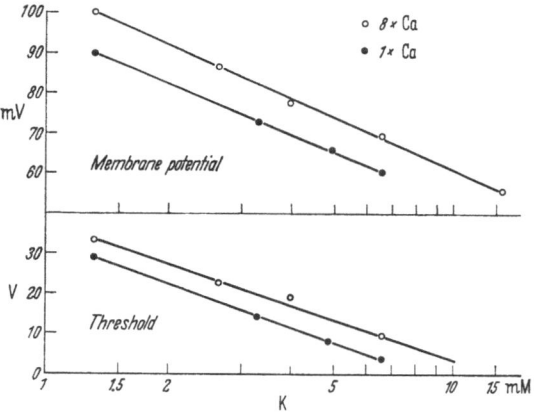

Fig. 18. Membrane potential and threshold of single frog muscle fibres as a function of external K and Ca concentrations. Normal Ca concentration 1.3 mM (after JENERICK and GERARD[708])

tion. If, however, the fibre was repolarized electrically to 92 mV by a voltage clamp procedure, a perfectly normal action potential with a normal rise and a normal overshoot was obtained on stimulation. Even prolonged depolarization by K did not damage the fibres to any extent.

Heart muscle differs from nerve and skeletal muscle in that repolarization is a relatively slow process. This probably is due to the fact that depolarization does not cause any marked increase in K permeability of heart muscle as opposed to the other two cell types. Possibly the repolarization is due to an increased rate of active sodium extrusion.

In the pace maker regions the membrane potential gradually decreases until, at a value around 60 mV, the fall becomes rapidly steeper and continues into the upstroke of an action potential. K ions influence the pacemaker by determining the value of the potential to which the membrane can repolarize after the action potential.

BAMMER and ROTHSCHUH[711] have studied the effect of outside K upon the conduction rate in the frog ventricle strip preparation. The rate of conduction in this preparation in Ringer solution is between 7 and 15 cm/sec. As the K concentration of the solution is increased the rate of conduction increases to reach a plateau around 20 mg-% K. When the concentration is raised still further, there is a drop in conduction rate and around 30 mg-% K there is a complete block of conduction. These results are easily understood in the light of present day ideas

---

[709] WEIDMANN, S.: Elektrophysiologie der Herzmuskelfaser. 100 pp. Bern, Stuttgart: Huber 1956.

[710] WEIDMANN, S.: Rectifier properties of purkinje fibers. Amer. J. Physiol. **183**, 671 (1955).

[711] BAMMER, H., u. K. E. ROTHSCHUH: Über die Erregungsleitung im Froschherzstreifen unter der Wirkung von Kalium-Ionen und anderen herzmuskeleigenen Substanzen. Z. exp. Med. **119**, 402—414 (1952).

about excitable tissues: As the K concentration is increased, a lowering of the membrane potential is brought about which brings the system closer to the state (the critical potential) where activity sets in. If the depolarization is carried further, there is, however, as we have seen in the foregoing, a reduction in the amount of Na-carrier. As a consequence of this the Na current during the spike is decreased and the rate of conduction is slowed down; finally conduction is altogether stopped.

The simultaneous action of K ions and acetyl choline upon the frog ventricle strip preparation has been studied by BAMMER[712]. The increase in conduction rate which is seen at moderate increases in K concentration is accentuated by acetyl choline. On the other hand, the conduction block which is seen with, say, 36.4 mg-% K is obtained much faster in the presence of AcCH (10^{-4} parts) than in the absence of the drug.

Bammer assumes that acetyl choline influences the K effect by changing the membrane permeability to Na. In this context it is of interest that acetyl choline is without effect upon the membrane potential of resting heart muscle (ROTH-SCHUH[713]), whereas it accentuates the action potential of the working frog heart.

C. Relations to the electric activity of neuromuscular junctions and synapses

a) Neuromuscular junctions

For years it was a matter of dispute whether the transfer of the impulse from nerve endings to muscle fibre was mediated electrically or by acetyl choline. (For references, see for instance NACHMANSOHN et al.[714, 715], BULLOCK[716], ECCLES and MacFARLANE[717], KUFFLER[718].) Recent work, especially by CASTILLO and KATZ[719, 720, 721, 722, 723, 724] has, however, helped greatly to clarify the situation. It now seems clear that the arrival of an impulse at the nerve endings brings about the release of a number of discrete "packets" or "droplets" of acetyl

[712] BAMMER, H.: Der Einfluß von Acetylcholin auf die dromotope Kaliumwirkung am Froschherzstreifen. Pflügers Arch. ges. Physiol. **255**, 476—484 (1952).

[713] ROTHSCHUH, K. E.: Elektrophysiologie des Herzens. Darstellung, Kritik, Probleme. Verlag Dr. O. Steinkopff, Darmstadt. Germany (1952).

[714] NACHMANSOHN, D., and I. B. WILSON: The enzymic hydrolysis and synthesis of acetylcholine. Advanc. Enzymol. **12**, 259—339 (1951).

[715] NACHMANSOHN, D.: Metabolism and function of the nerve cell. Harvey Lect. **49**, 57—99 (1953—54).

[716] BULLOCK, T. H.: Conduction and transmission of nerve impulses. Ann. Rev. Physiol. **13**, 261—280 (1951).

[717] ECCLES, J. C., and W. V. MacFARLANE: Actions of anticholinesterases on endplate potential of frog muscle. J. Neurophysiol. **12**, 59—80 (1949).

[718] KUFFLER, S. W.: Transmitter mechanism at the nerve-muscle junction. Arch. Sci. Physiol. **3**, 585—599 (1949).

[719] CASTILLO, J. DEL, and B. KATZ: The failure of local-circuit transmission at the nerve-muscle junction. J. Physiol. **123**, 7 P—8 P (1954).

[720] CASTILLO, J. DEL, and B. KATZ: The effect of magnesium on the activity of motor nerve endings. J. Physiol. **124**, 553—559 (1954).

[721] CASTILLO, J. DEL, and B. KATZ: Quantal components of the end-plate potential. J. Physiol. **124**, 560—573 (1954).

[722] CASTILLO, J. DEL, and B. KATZ: Statistical factors involved in neuromuscular facilitation and depression. J. Physiol. **124**, 574—385 (1954).

[723] CASTILLO, J. DEL, and B. KATZ: Changes in end-plate activity produced by pre-synaptic polarization. J. Physiol. **124**, 586—604 (1954).

[724] CASTILLO, J. DEL, and B. KATZ: The membrane change produced by the neuromuscular transmitter. J. Physiol. **125**, 546—565 (1954).

choline (a few thousand molecules in each). Acetyl choline then acts upon the specially developed part of the muscle fibre membrane beneath the nerve endings, creating an enormous unspecific increase in permeability to all small inorganic ions, including sodium, with the result that the membrane potential drops toward zero. Due to the cholinesterase present in this region the effect rapidly decays. The ensuing current pulse in turn may trigger the conducted impulse in the "normal" fibre membrane. It is beyond the scope of the present book to present the evidence for this theory. It is pertinent, however, to discuss the effects of Na and K on the two structures involved, namely 1) the specially developed muscle fibre membrane at the "end plate", and 2) the nerve endings.

1. Effects of Na

Already in 1895, LOCKE[725] observed that Na was necessary (as well as K, Ca and Mg) for the normal neuromuscular transmission. Later it was found that muscles which were bathed in a solution where NaCl was replaced by sucrose became refractory to acetyl choline as well as to electrical stimulation. The conclusions which could be drawn from these early observations concerning the role of Na in the transmission were limited by the fact that the end plate process could not be studied independent of the mechanical response. Lately, however, the role of Na for the and plate potential has been largely explained by FATT and KATZ and FATT[726, 727, 728, 729, 730]. Using micro electrodes which were introduced into the frog muscle fibre at the site of the end plate, they found that the end plate potential (which means the diminution of the membrane potential associated with a stimulation of the end plate) was reduced and the nerve transmission blocked when the Na concentration of the external solution was lowered below a critical level (osmotic equilibrium being maintained by the addition of glucose).

Even in Na-free solution, the end plate region of the fibre responds to acetyl choline in concentrations between 10^{-7} and 10^{-3}, showing a typical depolarization. The latter is, however, much smaller than normal and it increases as the sodium concentration of the medium is raised. These and other observations led to the conclusion (FATT and KATZ), mentioned above, that the effect of acetyl choline is the production of a large nonselective increase in ionic permeability amounting to an effective short-circuit of the end plate.

The importance of Na for the magnitude of the end plate potential becomes clear when it is considered that before stimulation the end plate region of the muscle fibre is very little permeable to Na, but quite permeable to K and Cl. Thus the latter two ions are normally close to their equilibrium potential, whereas sodium is very far from quilibrium. The transfer of electric charge associated with the increase in permeability is therefore primarily due to the passive flow of sodium ions. Thus, when the external Na concentration is lowered to $1/4$ of that of Ringer, the end plate potential falls to sub-threshold values, and even

[725] LOCKE, F. S.: Notiz über den Einfluß physiologischer Kochsalzlösung auf die elektrische Erregbarkeit von Muskel und Nerv. Zbl. Physiol. 8, 166 (1894).

[726] FATT, P., and B. KATZ: Membrane potentials at the motor end-plate. J. Physiol. 111, 46 P—47 P (1950).

[727] FATT, P.: The electromotive action of acetylcholine at the motor end-plate. J. Physiol. 111, 408—422 (1950).

[728] FATT, P., and B. KATZ: The effect of sodium ions on neuromuscular transmission. J. Physiol. 118, 73—87 (1952).

[729] FATT, P., and B. KATZ: An analysis of the end-plate potential. Recorded with an intra-cellular electrode. J. Physiol. 115, 320—370 (1951).

[730] FATT, P., and B. KATZ: Spontaneous subthreshold activity at motor nerve endings. J. Physiol. 117, 109—128 (1952).

in the non-curarized fibre neuromuscular block ensues. This level of Na is slightly higher than the one which leads to failing conduction in nerve and muscle. The end plate potential increases in a regular way with increasing Na concentration both in untreated and in curarized fibres, the main difference being that the absolute value of the end plate potential is lower in the presence of curare, and that the dependency upon the Na concentration is more pronounced in the presence of this drug. The use of curare very much facilitates the determination of the dependency between Na concentration and e.p.p., because the electric disturbances arising from the action potential of the muscle fibre are eliminated due to the reduction of the e.p.p. to sub-threshold values.

Besides the immediate effect on the end plate potential, Na is also of importance for the release of acetyl choline from the nerve endings. This is understandable because this release seems to be closely correlated to the magnitude of the action potential. The release of acetyl choline "packets" also depends on the concentrations of the divalent cations, Ca stimulating and Mg inhibiting the process.

2. Effects of potassium

The resting potential, as measured with an internal electrode, across the frog muscle end-plate membrane, is the same as elsewhere along the fibre (FATT and KATZ[729]). At 20°C the average value is 90 mV. This value is unaffected by curarine. It depends, however, on the external K concentration in exactly the same way as does the resting potential across the muscle membrane proper (compare p. 146).

Local application of K (or Rb) to the end plate may stimulate it to activity. This was first shown by BUCHTHAL and LINDHARD[731, 732] who found that the lizzard muscle fibre will give a twitch-like contraction on application of as little as $10^4 \mu$g of K. The concentration in which the K was applied was 25—30 mM per liter, that is about 10 times its concentration in Ringer. Similar observations were made by KUFFLER[733] on the frog sartorius. The two species differ, however, in that the lizzard muscle fibre does not respond to K in similar or even 10 times higher amounts when applied to the fibre outside the end plate region, whereas the frog fibre responds equally well to K in the end-plate free parts where AcCh is ineffective.

Thus, for example, according to WALKER and LAPORTE[734] small increases of the K concentration in the fluid surrounding the fibres first facilicate and then depress neuromuscular transmission. During the period of depression a response is followed by a prolonged reduction of responsiveness.

b) The sub-synaptic membrane

The patches of the dendrites and soma of a nerve cell which make immediate contact with the endings of other neurons seem to possess properties very similar

---

[731] BUCHTHAL, F., and J. LINDHARD: Transmission of impulses from nerve to muscle fibre. Acta physiol. scand. 4, 136—148 (1942).

[732] BUCHTHAL, F.: Interaction entre l'acétylcholine, l'adénosine triphosphate et les phénomènes électriques dans la transmission neuro-musculaire. Arch. Sci. Physiol. 3, 603 to 608 (1949).

[733] KUFFLER, S. W.: Specific excitability of the endplate region in normal and denervated muscle. J. Neurophysiol. 6, 99—110 (1943).

[734] WALKER, S. M., and Y. LAPORTE: Effects of potassium on the endplate potential and neuromuscular transmission in the curarized semitendinosus of the frog. Neurophysiol. 10, 79—85 (1947).

to those of the motor end plate. According to ECCLES and collaborators[735, 736] this sub-synaptic membrane when stimulated by the transmitter substance, most likely acetyl choline, responds by becoming highly permeable not only to K, but to Cl and Na as well. As a result of this the membrane potential falls and triggers a conducted impulse in the excitable portion of the soma membrane which covers by far the larger part of the nerve cell and the impulse thus travels down the axon. The unspecific high permeability of the sub-synaptic membrane rapidly decays due to the splitting of the acetyl choline by cholinesterase. The release of acetyl choline just like in the neuromuscular junction, takes place in the form of minute droplets from the nerve endings. The release of these droplets can be inhibited in a highly specific way by botulinus toxin.

Many synapses receive both stimulatory and inhibitory impulses. They arrive through different fibres and probably the transmitter substances are different. Even at the inhibitory nerve endings the transmitter substance acts by increasing the ion permeability of the sub-synaptic membrane, but only the permeabilities to K and Cl are greatly augmented whereas the membrane remains practically tight to Na. This increase in K and Cl permeability has the effect of locking the membrane potential at a value intermediate between the equilibrium potentials of the above mentioned two ions. If the neuron is already close to the Donnan distribution of K and Cl, no potential change will take place. If K is present in the neuron at a concentration above equilibrium (due to the activity of the ion pump) the potential may be slightly increased. The increased permeability now tends to lock the potential in the vicinity of the permeable area and will swamp out any tendency to lower the potential to the critical value for a conducted impulse which might arise due to the arrival of stimuli to the stimulatory synapses.

D. Relation to the electric activity of electric organs

The literature on the physiology of electric organs of fishes has been reviewed recently by KEYNES[737, 738], and by GRUNDFEST[739]. Their papers should be consulted for further references. Organs which on stimulation are able to deliver strong electric chocks are found in certain groups of fishes which are not at all closely related. Thus it is apparent that the development of such organs has taken place independently several times in the course of phyllogenetic evolution. Apparently the processes exploited in creating the very high voltages (as much as 600 V in Electrophorus 50 V in Torpedo) and high current strenghts (1 amp. in Electrophorus to several amp. in Torpedo) seen in electric fishes are nothing but appropriate arrangements in series and in parallel of elementary mechanisms which we are already familiar with from motor end plates, muscle and nerve fibres and gland cells.

In all electrical fishes the electric organ is composed of disk-shaped cells (electroplaxes, electroplaques, electroplates) having one innervated and one non-innervated surface. They are arranged in such a fashion that all innervated

[735] COOMBS, J. S., J. C. ECCLES, and P. FATT: Excitatory synaptic action in motoneurones. J. Physiol. **130**, 374—395 (1955).

[736] COOMBS, J. S., J. C. ECCLES, and P. FATT: The inhibitory suppression of reflex discharges from motoneurones. J. Physiol. **130**, 396—413 (1955).

[737] KEYNES, R. D.: Electric organs in the Physiology of Fishes (M. E. BROWN, ed.) New York: Academic Press 1956.

[738] KEYNES, R. D.: The generation of electricity by fishes. Endeavour **15**, 215—222 (1956).

[739] GRUNDFEST, H.: The mechanisms of discharge of the electric organs in relation to general and comparative electrophysiology. Progress in Biophysics **7**, 1—86 (1957).

(References [740] and [741] have been deleted).

surfaces face in the same direction. The non-innervated surfaces are quite insensitive to both chemical and electrical stimulation and presumably have a constant
ionic permability. The innervated face, on the other hand, under influence of the
transmitter from the nerve endings, undergoes reactions which in Torpedo and
other rays seems virtually identical with those of a motor endplate (see p. 168)
where as in Electrophorus it is more similar to those of a whole muscle fibre or
a nerve axon. A detailed analysis of the reaction in Malapterurus has not been
carried out so far. The nervous control of the electric organs permit them to
fire all electroplaques of an electric organ simultaneously and so the action
potentials of the individual cells (of the order of 100 mV each) add up to give
the full voltage of up to several hundred volts.

IX. Role of the alkali metal ions in muscular contraction

A. Introduction: Non-living models

It is a well established fact that the alkali metal ions Na and K are of great
importance for the mechanical response of muscular tissues. The exact roles
played by these two ions in muscular contraction are, however, not fully understood. One line of attack on the problem has been concerned with model systems
containing among their essential elements the proteins actin and myosin. As is
well known, suitably prepared actomyosin fibres will respond to the addition of
adenosine triphosphate (ATP) with a contraction.

Although the precise role of ATP in muscle contraction is not quite clear
(for references see NEEDHAM[742], FEIGEN[743], MOMMAERTS[744], WEBER and PORT-
ZEHL[745]), many workers are confident that the ATP response of actomyosin fibres
must be related to contraction of living muscle. For this reason various workers,
notably SZENT-GYÖRGYI and his school have studied the relationship of inorganic
ions to the muscle proteins. We cannot at this place present a detailed account
of the delicate interplay between actin, myosin and inorganic ions which this
work has brought to light. The reader is referred to the monographs by SZENT-
GYÖRGYI[46, 746, 747]. We shall, however, consider some of the salient facts having
to do with the role of the alkali metal ions in particular which this work has
revealed. As already mentioned (p. 9), myosin binds K and Na to an appreciable
extent. It has often been claimed that the K binding capacity of myosin speaks
in favor of a particular role of K in muscle-contraction, but it should be remembered
that the affinity of myosin is the same for K and Na (compare SZENT-GYÖRGYI[46]
p. 7). If anything, Na seems to be bound slightly stronger than is K. Thus with
respect to the reactions of muscle proteins, the two alkali metal ions are interchangeable. The adsorption of ATP by actomyosin depends on the simultaneous
adsorption of K (or Na); but the effect of the monovalent cation in turn depends
on the previous adsorption of bivalent cation, and all these reactions are highly
p_H-dependent.

[742] NEEDHAM, D. M.: Adenosine triphosphate and the structural proteins in relation to
muscle contraction. Advanc. Enzymol. **13**, 151—197 (1952).
[743] FEIGEN, G. A.: Muscle. Ann. Rev. Physiol. **18**, 89—120 (1956).
[744] MOMMAERTS, W. F. H. M.: The biochemistry of muscle. Ann. Rev. Biochem. **23**,
381—404 (1954).
[745] WEBER, H. H., and H. PORTZEHL: The transference of the muscle energy in the
contraction cycle. Progress in Biophysics. **4**, 60—111 (1954).
[746] SZENT-GYÖRGYI, A.: Chemical Physiology of Contraction in Body and Heart Muscle.
Academic Press, N. Y. 1953.
[747] SZENT-GYÖRGYI, A. G.: Structural and functional aspects of myosin. Advanc. Biochem.
16, 313—360 (1955).

Among the types of actomyosin fibre whose properties come closest to those of living muscle are those prepared by HAYASHI and ROSENBLUETH[748] from compressed surface films of actomyosin. Such fibres are capable of repeated contractions and elongations. The conditions of shortening are presence of ATP and a low concentration of KCl, whereas for elongation is needed a high concentration of KCl or NaCl, with or without the presence of ATP. Also the glycerol-extracted fibre bundles, prepared according to SZENT-GYÖRGYI[749], give ATP induced contractions which are reversed with suitably high KCl concentrations. These fibres, though inexcitable electrically, develop tensions comparable with those given by normal fibres (see also WEBER and WEBER[750] and WEBER[751]). Definite points of similarity thus can be found between actomyosin fibres, glycerol treated muscle fibres and living fibres. On the other hand, the actomyosin fibers exhibit features which are closely related to those of synthetic long-chain poly-electrolytes like polyvinyl alcohol-polyacrylic acid fibres which, according to KUHN and HAGARTAY[752] distend in alkaline medium and contract when the alkali is neutralized. In this context it may be worth mentioning that myosin contains a greater proportion of charged and polar groups than most other proteins (BAILEY[753]). It is thus not difficult to imagine that the distribution of charges along the actomyosin fibre must influence its length.

From the foregoing it would appear likely that the concentration of mono-valent cation (which is largely K) in muscle fibres is a major factor in determining the contractibility.

As a matter of fact, HAJDU and SZENT-GYÖRGYI[754] have found that the increase in contraction strength in the course of the first few contractions after standstill shown by an isolated frog's heart (staircase phenomenon) is associated with and is probably caused by a loss of fibre potassium. Thus during standstill the heart takes up more potassium than is compatible with maximum contractibility. For each contraction, however, a small amount of K is lost, so that the ratio of monovalent to divalent cations approaches that associated with maximum contractibility. A more detailed discussion of the hypothesis is given on p. 188.

The very fact that the resting heart muscle takes up excess K which is given off again in graded amounts during each contraction emphasizes the importance of a structure which is found in living, but not in artificial fibres: the cell membrane. This structure is also the seat of the electric responses (the action potential) and the conduction of impulses seen in many, though not all, muscle fibres. The electric activity of muscle fibres shows such striking similarities to those of nerve that there can be no doubt about the virtual identity of the phenomena. Recent work, especially with the giant axons of cephalopods, has gone a long way towards elucidating the nature of the electrical activity. The phenomena of resting and action potentials have been treated in chapter VIII whereas the active uptake

[748] HAYASHI, T., and R. ROSENBLUETH: Contraction-elongation cycle of loaded surface-spread actomyosin fibers. J. cell. comp. Physiol. **40**, 495—506 (1952).

[749] SZENT-GYÖRGYI, A.: Free-energy relations and contraction of actomyosin. Biol. Bull. **96**, 140—161 (1949).

[750] WEBER, A., and H. H. WEBER: Zur Thermodynamik der ATP-Kontraktion am Fasermodell. Z. Naturforsch. **5b**, 124—125 (1950).

[751] WEBER, A.: Muscular contraction and a contraction model. Biochem. biophys. Acta **7**, 214—224 (1951).

[752] KUHN, W., and B. HAGARTAY: Muscle-similar work performance of synthetic polymers. Z. Elektrochem. **55**, 490—505 (1951).

[753] BAILEY, K.: Tropomyosin: a new asymmetric protein component of the muscle fibril. Biochem. J. **43**, 271—279 (1948).

[754] HAJDU, S., and A. SZENT-GYÖRGYI: Action of DOC and serum on the frog heart. Amer. J. Physiol. **168**, 159—170 (1952).

and diffusion of ions is discussed in chapter VII. Previously it was generally assumed that a clear line of distinction could be drawn between on the one hand the membrane processes which lead to excitation and, on the other hand, the cont actile processes in the interior of the fibre. The processes at the surface thus wererthought only to trigger events in the interior. Recent work, especially by SANDOW's group in New York and HILL's group in London, has changed this view. It is now clear that the duration of the contraction is determined by processes occurring at the fibre surface (HILL and MACPHERSON[755], SANDOW and KAHN[756]). Some workers go even further than that. Thus Fleckenstein advocates the idea that electric events associated with the exchange of K against Na at the fibre surface provides the energy for the contraction process. But whether or not one is willing to accept this bold idea, it is clear that it is not possible to treat the effects of alkali metal ions on the mechanical response of muscle without considering the processes at the fibre surface. In this chapter, however, electrical responses will be considered only in so far as they are directly related to the contraction, whereas the detailed discussion of them is found in chapter VIII.

B. Effects on skeletal muscle

a) Effects of Na

Since the classical work of OVERTON[685, 757] it has been known that muscles are paralyzed in the absence of sodium ions, even if the osmotic pressure of the medium is maintained at the normal level by the addition of an indifferent non-electrolyte like sucrose. The paralysis is fully reversible with suitable concentrations of Na in the medium. The nature of the anion is immaterial. Of the cations only Li can to some extent replace Na. The Na concentration at which paralysis is complete varies from one species to another. Frog muscle loses its excitability around 12 mM Na/liter whereas rat diaphragm is made totally unresponsive already at 20 mM Na/liter[758].

In recent years the role of Na in muscle has been studied intensively and it has turned out that this ion is of decisive importance in the processes of transmission (see p. 169) and conduction in nerve (p. 162) as well as in the muscle fibre itself (see p. 163). There is, however, no safe information as to the role of Na in the contraction process.

b) Effects of K

1. Introduction

It is well known that a moderate increase in the K concentration of the medium may enhance the mechanical response of skeletal muscle. For a discussion of the older literature see FENN[399]. Higher K concentrations, however, paralyze

---

[755] HILL, A. V., and L. MACPHERSON: The effect of nitrate, iodide and bromide on the duration of the active state in skeletal muscle. Proc. roy. Soc. B **143**, 81—102 (1954).

[756] SANDOW, A., and A. J. KAHN: The immediate effects of potassium on responses of skeletal muscle. J. cell. comp. Physiol. **40**, 89—114 (1952).

[757] OVERTON, E.: Beiträge zur allgemeinen Muskel- und Nervenphysiologie. III. Studien über die Wirkung der Alkali- und Erdalkalisalze auf Skeletmuskeln und Nerven. Pflügers Arch. ges. Physiol. **105**, 176—290 (1904).

[758] TAUGNER, R., G. SIEBERT, and U. GOTTSTEIN: Kontrakturen des Warmblütermuskels bei Hypoglykämie und Hypoxie. Pflügers Arch. ges. Physiol. **257**, 454—463 (1953).

the muscles. Thus OVERTON[757], using the isolated nerve muscle preparation of frog, found that about 10 mM K/liter Ringer solution sufficed to give total paralysis. Similar concentrations of K also paralyze mammalian muscle. Still higher K concentrations give rise to potassium-contracture. As we shall see later this phenomenon is not equally apparent in all types of muscle.

These different effects of K are of a complex nature, K being involved in impulse conduction as well as in transmission and directly in the contraction process. The effect of K upon conduction in nerve and muscle is discussed in chapter VIII, p. 165 whereas the effects on transmission are discussed on p. 170.

2. Potassium contracture

Potassium contracture can be brought about in skeletal muscle as well as in smooth and heart muscle. The older literature on the subject has been discussed by GASSER[759] more recent discussions giving a wealth of information are found in FLECKENSTEIN monograph[760] and in RIESSER[761] Muskelpharmalogie. A contracture is a prolonged, reversible, not conducted contraction of a muscle (GASSER[759], KUFFLER[762]). Muscles which are so fatigued that they do not respond to nervous stimulation nevertheless can respond to KCl treatment with large contractures (KUFFLER[762]). Even iodoacetic acid treated muscles show this response (SANDOW[763]).

Contractures can be brought about by a number of agents all of which have in common that they lower the muscle membrane potential. When the latter reaches a certain low level, contracture ensues. 0.6 % KCl applied to a frog muscle gives a pronounced contracture. Below 0.3 % KCl no visible signs of contracture can be found. 0.2—0.3 % KCl normally elicit propagated impulses. Contracture rather than contraction is brought about if the depolarization is not allowed to be followed by a return of the potential to a non-critical level.

During contracture there is increased breakdown of phosphocreatin as well as increased glycolysis and oxygen consumption (HEGENAUER, FENN and COBB[128], NACHMANSOHN, WAJZER and MARNAY[764]). Heat production is also increased (SOLANDT[130]). An excess of K reduces the contracture, but it is impossible to inhibit totally the K-contracture by excess K (HARDT and FLECKENSTEIN[765]). Prolonged treatment with high concentrations of KCl leads to paralysis of the muscle. This paralysis is, however, fully reversible on washing with solutions low in K.

It is clear that K is an excellent agent for bringing about a maintained depolarization (see chapter VIII). Due to the relatively high permeability of the fibre membrane to this ion, its concentration in the outside medium to a first

---

[759] GASSER, H. S.: Contractures of skeletal muscle. Physiol. Rev. **10**, 35—109 (1930).

[760] FLECKENSTEIN, A.: Der Kalium-Natrium-Austausch als Energieprinzip in Muskel und Nerv. 157 pp. Springer-Verlag 1955.

[761] RIESSER, O.: Muskelpharmakologie und ihre Anwendung in der Therapie der Muskelkrankheiten. 232 pp. Bern 1949.

[762] KUFFLER, S. W.: The relation of electric potential changes to contracture in skeletal muscle. J. Neurophysiol.. **9**, 367—377 (1946).

[763] SANDOW, A.: Contracture responses of skeletal muscle. Amer. J. Phys. Med. **34**, 145—160 (1955).

[764] NACHMANSOHN, D., J. WAJZER, and A. MARNAY: Action de la pilocarpine sur la formation d'acide lactique et sur la décomposition du phosphogène dans le muscle de grenouille isolé et en repos. C. R. Soc. Biol. (Paris) **121**, 139—141 (1936).

[765] HARDT, A., and A. FLECKENSTEIN: Liberation of K from frog muscle by action of contraction-stimulating substances and inhibition of liberation by contraction-inhibiting local anaesthetics. Naunyn-Schmiedebergs Arch. exp. Path. Pharmak. **207**, 39—54 (1948).

approximation determines the membrane potential. It was noticed already by BETHE and FRANKE[766] that K seems to act directly upon the fibres and not "upon the receptive substance of Langley". Sartorius muscles showed just as pronounced a contracture in the nerve-free ends as in the middle. These authors also found that K-contractures can be elicited even during propanol narcosis and when the muscle is made unresponsive by replacing the NaCl in the medium by isotonic sucrose. Evidently the conduction system of nerve and muscle, as well as the end plates, are of secondary or no importance for the phenomenon of K-contracture.

The effect of other ion species upon the K-contracture was studied by GELL-HORN[767]. The phenomenon is enhanced by monovalent cations, notably Rb and NH_4, whereas the earth alkali ions are inhibitory. Among the anions notably SCN and I enhance the K-effect. Hypertonic solutions are inhibitory whereas hypotonic solutions sensitize the muscle to contracture. In the physiological range (p_H 6.1—7.7) the tendency towards K-concentracture increases with increasing p_H. When ions like Rb and SCN enhance the K-contracture, it may be considered as a simple addition of effects, since these latter ions themselves give contracture in sufficient doses. In other cases the synergism is of a more involved nature. Thus, in 1939 SZENT-GYÖRGYI, BACQ and GOFFART[768] noticed that a contracting muscle gives off a substance which when applied to a veratrinized muscle gives rise to contracture. The substance responsible for this humoral transmission of contraction was found to be the potassium ion. Based upon this observation BACQ[769, 770, 771] advanced the hypothesis that veratrine, thiocyanate and several other drugs act by sensitizing nerve, muscle and other organs to potassium. An extensive literature has occurred centring around this concept. In a recent review GOFFART and BACQ[772] conclude that "the group of sensitizers to potassium does not constitute a homogeneous class although the K-ion is involved in all cases". Since, as was mentioned above, any lowering of the membrane potential below the critical level may bring about contracture, it seems doubtful whether it is justified to place potassium in the center of the picture. Some of the so-called sensitizers to potassium are, however, interesting in that they are not in themselves depolarizing agents. Thus veratrine has no effect upon the resting potential of muscle and no effect on the end-plates. It does, however, increase enormously the negative after-potential following the muscle spike, and if the after-potential attains a critical value, repetitive contractions followed by contracture will be the result (KUFF-LER[773]). According to KUFFLER it is characteristic of the veratrinized muscle that its sensitivity to acetyl-choline and potassium is only insignificantly altered.

[766] BETHE, A., and F. FRANKE: Versuche über die Kalikontraktur. Biochem. Z. **156**, 190—200 (1925).

[767] GELLHORN, E.: Zur Kenntnis der Kaliumcontraktur am quergestreiften und glatten Muskel. II. Zur Permeabilität der Muskulatur. Pflügers Arch. ges. Physiol. **219**, 761—788 (1928).

[768] SZENT-GYÖRGYI, A., Z. M. BACQ, and M. GOFFART: A humoral transmission of muscular contraction in the presence of veratrine. Nature (Lond.) **143**, 522 (1939).

[769] BACQ, Z. M.: Sensitisation of skeletal muscle to potassium by veratrine. C. R. Soc. Biol. (Paris) **130**, 1369—1371 (1939).

[770] BACQ, Z. M.: Les sensibilisateurs au potassium. Bull. Acad. Méd. Belg. **12**, 255—275 (1947).

[771] BACQ, Z. M.: Effects of ions and veratrine substances. Arch. int. Pharmacodyn. **63**, 59—87 (1939).

[772] GOFFART, M., and Z. M. BACQ: Les sensibilisateurs au potassium. Ergebn. Physiol. **47**, 555—617 (1952).

[773] KUFFLER, S. W.: Action of veratrine on nerve-muscle preparations. J. Neurophysiol. **8**, 113—122 (1945).

Until recently it was assumed that contractions of the type characterized as contracture were largely artefacts, notably in vertebrate muscle. The whole outlook has changed now after the discovery that all skeletal muscles (of frogs, at least) are composed of two entirely different types of fibres, called twitch fibres and slow fibres, respectively (KUFFLER and VAUGHAN WILLIAMS [423, 774]). The slow fibres differ from the twitch fibres in having a lower membrane potential, around 60 mV, in contrast to the 90 to 95 mV of the twitch fibres. Moreover, they are differently innervated. The twitch fibres' nerve supply consists of nerve fibres with a conduction velocity of 8—40 m/sec, whereas the slow fibres are innervated by small nerve fibres conducting at a rate of 2—8 m/sec. It has been shown that it is only the slow fibres which respond to immersion in solutions of acetyl choline and KCl with a prolonged contracture. Much of the previous work on contracture undoubtedly needs reconsideration in the light of these facts.

It should be mentioned that a contracture-like response is also typical of various motor-responses in many invertebrates (KATZ [775]).

A discussion of FLECKENSTEIN's hypothesis of muscle contraction which to a large extent is based on studies on K-contracture will be given below (p. 179). Other aspects of the contracture problem will be mentioned in connection with the treatment of the different types of muscle tissue.

3. Effects of K on the mechanical response

In much of the early work on this problem no sharp distinction was made between effects on the contractibility and effects upon the excitability of the muscles (for a critical review see FENN [399]). The work of BAETJER [776] and BROWN and v. EULER [777] did, however, indicate strongly that there was a direct effect of K on the muscle fibres, although some of the effects seen might have been exerted upon the motor end-plates. BAETJER made intra-arterial injections of KCl in cats during periods of direct and indirect stimulation. This led to an increase in the height of the recorded muscle contractions. Since the effect was also seen upon direct stimulation of curarized muscles, she attributed it to an action upon the muscle substance itself. BROWN and v. EULER studied the after-effects of tetanus on cat muscle. It had previously been shown (ROSENBLUETH and MORRISON [778]) that a tetanus of suitable duration is followed by an increase of long duration in the twitch tension. BROWN and v. EULER now showed that the potentiation could be observed even in denervated muscle and in muscle completely paralysed by curarine. Thus the effect must be entirely independent of the neuro-muscular transmission apparatus. It turned out that the observed effects could be imitated by close arterial injections of KCl. Similar results were obtained by FENG et al. [779]. WALKER [780] found a definite potentiation by K of the peak tension of the triceps

---

[774] KUFFLER, S. W., and E. M. V. WILLIAMS: Properties of the "slow" skeletal muscle fibres of the frog. J. Physiol. **121**, 318—340 (1953).

[775] KATZ, B.: Neuro-muscular transmission in invertebrates. Biol. Rev. (Cambridge) **24**, 1—20 (1949).

[776] BAETJER, A. M.: The effect of potassium (and calcium) on the contractions of mammalian skeletal muscle. Amer. J. Physiol. **112**, 147—151 (1935).

[777] BROWN, G. L., and U. S. VON EULER: The after-effects of a tetanus on mammalian muscle. J. Physiol. **93**, 39—60 (1938).

[778] ROSENBLUETH, A., and R. S. MORISON: Curarization, fatigue and Wedensky inhibition. Amer. J. Physiol. **119**, 236—256 (1937).

[779] FENG, T. P., L. Y. LEE, C. W. MENG, and S. C. WANG: After-effects of tetanisation on neuromuscular transmission in cat. Chinese J. Physiol. **13**, 79—108 (1938).

[780] WALKER, S. M.: The response of the triceps surae of normal, adrenalectomized, desoxycorticosterone acetate-treated and KCl-treated rats to direct and indirect, single and repetitive stimulation. Amer. J. Physiol. **149**, 7—23 (1947).

surae of the rat on direct stimulation, although a still more pronounced potentiation was obtained on indirect stimulation. The latter effect was, however, partly due to repetitive impulses.

The mechanical response does not seem to be a simple function of the potassium level in the muscle or in the surrounding fluid. This appears, for instance, from the fact that in curarized rat muscles, stimulated directly, the peak tension and the rising time were the same for muscles from normal and adrenalectomized animals (WALKER), although the K level of the latter is elevated as compared to the controls (compare HARRISON and DARROW[781]). The muscles of the adrenalectomized animals did, however, show a marked decrease in tetanic tension after some time's exercise. This fatigue could not be attributed to neuromuscular failure and thus must reside in the muscle itself.

The detailed evaluation of experiments of the types so far discussed suffers from the disadvantage that no records were made of the variations of potassium concentration with time in the tissue fluids and in the muscles. It is therefore impossible to say with certainty which effects are due to cellular and which to extracellular potassium concentration. The work of SANDOW and KAHN[756] therefore represents an important step forward towards an understanding of the effects of the potassium ion on contraction. These workers studied the influence of enhanced concentrations of K on the latent period, the twitch tension and the action potential of isometric contractions of frog sartorius muscle. In order to circumvent the complications arising from conduction, stimulation was effected by the transverse massive electrode method (BROWN and SICHEL[782]). Square wave pulses of sufficient strength to give maximum direct stimulation were used. The general approach was to compare the time course of the electrical and mechanical parameters with that of the average K concentration in the extracellular space of the muscle. As it is well known (compare p. 86) isolated frog muscle loses K to normal Ringer. The K concentration of the bathing fluid has to be increased to the so-called maintenance concentration (around 8 mM/l), before the loss of K is reversed. SANDOW and KAHN assume that those effects which are obtained before the intercellular concentration of K has reached the maintenance level must be due to K-effects on the fibre membrane, whereas effects which are not seen before the fibre-K has commenced to increase again *may* be due to intracellular processes. Their results may briefly be summarized as follows: In all K-enriched media the mechanical parameters (twitch tension and depth of latency relaxation) first increase and then decrease. In solutions containing more than maintenance concentration of K, the decline of the mechanical parameters is quite violent, ending in total paralysis. The action potential spike decreases with time in all K-enriched solutions. Most of these effects are seen before the maintenance concentration is reached and thus must be due to effects on the membrane phase. Only the violent secondary depression of the mechanical parameters is typical of above-maintenance K-concentrations. A point of crucial interest is that potassium ions acting upon the fibre membrane will cause a diminution of the action potential and, at the same time a potentiation of the mechanical response. This observation seems to set apart the membrane processes responsible for the action potential and those governing contraction. The same conclusion can be drawn from the fact that the kinetics of depolarization by K is entirely different from

[781] HARRISON, H. E., and D. C. DARROW: Distribution of body-water and -electrolytes in adrenal insufficiency. J. clin. Invest. 17, 77—85 (1938).

[782] BROWN, D. E. S., and F. J. M. SICHEL: The isometric contraction of isolated muscle fibers. J. cell. comp. Physiol. 8, 315—328 (1936).

that of the changes in the mechanical parameters (MANDEL[783], SANDOW and MANDEL[784]). Thus the elcetrical and the mechanical parameters are quite uncorrelated in the course of the responses to K. This has led these authors to believe that K acts upon two different membrane structures, one of which is responsible for the conduction of the impulse in the longitudinal direction and for the recorded electrical manifestations, whereas the other membrane structure is associated with events which pass inward, leading to the activation of the contractile material. The two membrane structures are, however, assumed to be interdependent in so far as it is the depolarization occurring during the rising phase of the spike which triggers the inward directed activation of the contractile element of the fibres.

The function of K in membrane depolarization is quite well understood and is discussed elsewhere (p. 144). With respect to the mechanical activation process, SANDOW and KAHN[756] (see also SANDOW[785]) have advanced the hypothesis that excitation leads to a release of Ca from the surface of the cells into the interior and that this Ca in turn induces the fibrils to contract. The enhancement of contraction by extra K is then assumed to be due to a positive correlation between outside K concentration and the amount of Ca released into the interior of the cell. It will be seen that this hypothesis is a special case of HEILBRUNN's general theory[786] of stimulation according to which any stimulating agent brings about a release of Ca into the cytoplasma, whereupon the Ca brings about a change in the physical state of the cytoplasma. It is known that treatment with potassium ions can bring about a release of Ca from the cortical region into the cell interior of different eggs (CHURNEY and MOSER[787], MAZIA[788]) but it has not been shown for muscle. The hypothesis that Ca is the chemical mediator of activation in muscle presents the difficulty that, as pointed out by HILL[789, 790], diffusion is far too slow a process to account for the rapid development of full activity in a twitch. The Ca hypothesis of activation must therefore be accepted only with reluctance, and the role of K in the process of activation and contraction cannot be considered as finally settled. A recent development which will have to be taken into account is observation by HUXLEY[791, 792] that electric stimulation through an external micro electrode seems to reach the contractile elements only through points near the Z-membrane in the isotropic substance.

4. The Fleckenstein hypothesis

As mentioned above, FLECKENSTEIN and collaborators have developed the hypothesis that the contraction process derives its energy directly from the K/Na

[783] MANDEL, H.: Masters Thesis. Deptmt. Biol. Washington Square College of Arts and Science, New York Univ. 1951.

[784] SANDOW, A., and H. MANDEL: Effects of potassium and rubidium on the resting potential of muscle. J. cell. comp. Physiol. 38, 271—291 (1951).

[785] SANDOW, A.: Excitation-contraction coupling in muscular response. Yale J. Biol. Med. 25, 176—201 (1952).

[786] HEILBRUNN, L. V.: An outline of General Physiology. Philadelphia: W. B. Saunders Co. 1943.

[787] CHURNEY, L., and F. MOSER: The effect of excess potassium on the cortex of the fertilized egg of arbacia punctulata. Physiol. Zool. 13, 212—217 (1940).

[788] MAZIA, D.: The release of calcium in the arbacia eggs on fertilization. J. cell. comp. Physiol. 10, 291—304 (1937).

[789] HILL, A. V.: Abrupt transition from rest to activity in muscle. Proc. roy. Soc. B 136, 399—420 (1949).

[790] HILL, A. V.: Time required for diffusion and its relation to processes in muscle. Proc. roy. Soc. B 135, 446—453 (1948).

[791] HUXLEY, A. F., and R. E. TAYLOR: Function of Krause's membrane. Nature (Lond.) 176, 1068 (1955).

[792] HUXLEY, A. F., and R. E. TAYLOR: Activation of a single sarcomere. J. Physiol. 130, 49 P—50 P (1955).

exchange which takes place in conjunction with contraction. There are several observations which are hard to reconcile with this hypothesis. But whether or not it is correct, the experimental evidence on which it is based is of considerable interest.

FLECKENSTEIN assumes that it is the distension of the muscle fibres which requires metabolic work, whereas contraction represents a return to a statistically more likely state of the protein chains. This view is closely related to Bethe's hypothesis[793]. The Fleckenstein hypothesis goes a step further and assumes that the distension of the fibres is the immediate result of the membrane potential. (It does not, however, specify in which way the potential difference across the fibre membrane might influence the distribution of charges upon the molecules of the contractile elements. This is a definite weakness in the formulation of the hypothesis.) If, for the sake of argument, we accept this assumption and if at the same time we remember that the membrane potential is mainly determined by the ratio of internal to external K, it appears that the muscle must contract if the internal K is lost in exchange for Na coming from the external medium. Conversely, if we consider a hypothetical, maximally contracted fibre, it is clear that as Na is extruded and replaced by K, the potential must go up and the fibre must distend again. The ultimate source of contraction energy thus would be the active transport process by which Na is extruded and K is taken up (compare chapter VII). On the other hand, the release of the stored energy in the form of a contraction would normally be the immediate result of the passive cation exchange taking place during the state of excitation (see chapter VIII).

It would be outside the scope of this book to discuss the crucial point of the hypothesis, namely whether or not a potential difference across the membrane can be assumed to influence the equilibrium length of protein chains in the cell interior. It is, however, pertinent to discuss two points, namely 1) would the energy associated with cation exchange suffice to bring about the contraction, and 2) is there a sufficiently close correlation between potential difference and height of contraction to justify the assumption of a causal relationship between them.

FLECKENSTEIN[794] concludes that the concentration work represented by the store of K in the fibres amounts to about 0.15 cal/g, whereas the uneven distribution of Na between fibres and surroundings accounts for an additional 0.06 cal/g muscle. The deviations from equilibrium distribution of the two cations thus represents a total of about 0.21 cal/g as compared with 0.23 cal/g as creatin phosphate and 0.09 cal/g of ATP. Thus the "cation storage battery" contains enough energy for many contractions (granted that it can be exploited) and compares favorably with the acknowledged energy stores of creatine phosphate and adenosine triphosphate.

From a formal point of view this calculation of the energy store may seem faulty because the contributions of the membrane potential to the total free energy of the ions has not been taken into account. Thus the transfer of K takes place between two phases where, thanks to the potential difference, the electrochemical potential for this ion is the same. Such a transfer does not require any work in case it takes place in a reversible way. On the other hand, the transfer of Na from the inside to the outside represents not only concentration work but also electrical work since it takes place against the electric field. Nevertheless the

    [793] BETHE, A.: Die Dauerverkürzung der Muskeln. Pflügers Arch. ges. Physiol. **142**, 291—336 (1911).
    [794] FLECKENSTEIN, A.: Über den primären Energiespeicher der Muskelkontraktion. Pflügers Arch. ges. Physiol. **250**, 643—666 (1947).

overall result (Na + K stored energy) is correct if the only process to be considered is a K—Na exchange. If this is the case the net transfer of charge is nil and the potential effect may be disregarded to a first approximation. With respect to the active transport of ions across the muscle fibre membrane the reader is referred to chapter VII, p. 84. As far as the problem of muscle contraction in relation to ionic distribution is concerned we must conclude that there is in the muscle a sufficient store of energy to drive the muscle for many contractions.

The second point to be considered is the close correlation between potential and the degree of contraction postulated by the Fleckenstein hypothesis. The parallelism between membrane potential and the degree of contraction is particularly conspicuous in the K-contracture of the rectus abdominis of the frog, Rana esculenta (FLECKENSTEIN and HER-TEL[795]). In the experiment depicted in Fig. 19, curve II shows the degree of contracture in per cent of the maximum K-contracture as a function of the K-concentration in the bath. The K-concentration was varied by gradual substitution of K for Na. Curve I is the ideal potential difference across the fibre membrane calculated on the assumption that the p. d. is equal to $(RT/F$ (ln $(K_i/K_0))$. The correlation between potential and contracture is obvious, but not striking. If, however, a similar experiment is performed with a muscle which had been penetrated with oxalate-Ringer so that the calcium ion concentration had been reduced practically to zero, a curve like III is obtained. It thus appears that in the absence of Ca there is the theoretical relationship

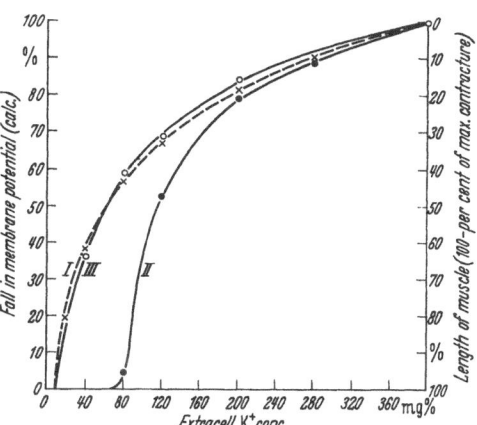

Fig. 19. Dependence of contracture of frog m. rectus abdominis upon external K concentration. Curve *I* gives the calculated fall in membrane potential. Curve *II* and *III* give the change in contracture as a function of external K concentration. Curve *II* is obtained with 20 mg-% CaCl₂ in the bathing solution and curve *III* with oxalate added to remove the Ca (after FLECKENSTEIN and HERTEL[795])

between K-concentration and the degree of contraction. The function of Ca seems to be that of counteracting the depolarizing effect of K. FLECKENSTEIN, WAGNER and GÖGGEL[796] found that both the depolarizing effect (as estimated from the injury potential) and the contracture promoting effect of 0.765% KCl are depressed progressively and to about the same extent by increasing concentrations of CaCl₂.

As we now know (see p. 177) the mechanical response of the rectus muscle is due almost exclusively to the "slow muscle fibres" which make up the major fraction of this muscle. In the case of the "twich" muscle fibres which dominate in, say, the sartorius muscle of the frog, the contraction is usually maximal. According to the FLECKENSTEIN hypothesis this is to be expected because on stimulation the potential is not only reduced to zero but even temporarily reversed

[795] FLECKENSTEIN, A., and H. HERTEL: Über die Zustandsänderungen des contractilen Systems in Abhängigkeit vom extracellulären Kalium und Natrium. Pflügers Arch. ges. Physiol. **250**, 577—597 (1947).

[796] FLECKENSTEIN, A., E. WAGNER, and K. H. GÖGGEL: Relationship between muscle length and membrane potential. Mode of action of local anaesthetics which abolish contractures. Pflügers Arch. ges. Physiol. **253**, 38—54 (1950).

(overshoot, see p. 152). According to the FLECKENSTEIN hypothesis it is, however, necessary that for each contraction there is a K/Na exchange which is at least equivalent to the amount of mechanical work performed. Acording to FLECKEN-STEIN, HILLE and ADAM[797] the K given off to the venous blood does not account for more than 5—10% of the work performed by a muscle. The estimation of the true K/Na exchange in a working muscle is difficult, however. During the contraction the blood stream is temporarily stopped and part of the K released during the contraction may have been reabsorbed by the fibres before it has the chance to be carried away by the blood.

A more satisfactory estimate of the amount of K released during muscular contraction has been obtained by O'BRIEN and WILDE[798] and WILDE and O'BRIEN[799] in the case of the isolated heart of the turtle. The heart was first equilibrated with a solution containing K^{42}. It was then perfused through the coronary artery with a solution containing another radio-isotope (I^{131}, P^{32}) but no K^{42}. The effluent was collected as drops upon a rotating filterpaper. Thus during each contraction cycle, 200 samples were taken, which described the time course of the release of cellular K from the heart muscle fibres. The isotopes I^{131} or P^{32} served as indicators of the volume of the drops so that the amount of K^{42} given off could be expressed in terms of concentration in each individual drop.

The experiments showed that about 1/400 of the total K of the heart was released per systole, or 0.25 μM K per systole per g heart muscle. If a K/Na exchange of this magnitude could be exploited with 100% efficiency it would yield 30—40 gcm of muscular work which is of the order of the normal work output by the heart. It should be pointed out, however, that this estimate of the K/Na exchange is likely to be too high since the exchange of intracellular against extracellular K is included in the figure. It thus remains a question whether or not the cation exchange associated with muscular contraction is of sufficient magnitude to account for the mechanical work performed.

The Fleckenstein hypothesis has been criticized, for instance by SANDOW[785] on the ground that the tension developed does not bear any fixed relation to the size of the action potential (compare SANDOW[763], v. BRÜCKE[800], BREITOFF[801], ROSENBLUETH et al.[802]). This, however, would be to demand a constant efficiency of the contraction mechanism, a requirement which does not seem to be implicit in the hypothesis. A more serious problem is provided by the time relationships of the different events during the contraction. There seems to be a definite time lag between the spike and the development of tension. Furthermore, as we have seen above, actomyosin fibres which in many respects resemble muscle fibres in their reactions, are quite insensitive to the K/Na ratio in the immersion fluid.

[797] FLECKENSTEIN, A., H. HILLE, and W. E. ADAM: Aufhebung der Kontraktur-Wirkung depolarisierender Katelektrotonica durch Repolarisation in Anelektrotonus, die Anode als Antagonist von Acetylcholin, Cholin, Nicotin, Coniin, Veratrin, Kalium- und Rubidium-Salzen usw. Pflügers Arch. ges. Physiol. **253**, 264—282 (1951).

[798] O'BRIEN, J. M., and W. S. WILDE: Rapid serial recording of concentrations in the blood circulation and in perfusion systems: The effluogram. Science **116**, 193—194 (1952).

[799] WILDE, W. S., and J. M. O'BRIEN: Abst. XIX Internat. Congr. Physiol. p. 889. Montreal 1953.

[800] v. BRÜCKE, E. TH.: Über die Beziehungen zwischen Aktionsstrom und Zuckung des Muskels im Verlaufe der Ermüdung. Pflügers Arch. ges. Physiol. **124**, 215—244 (1908).

[801] BREITOFF, J.: Über die Verhältnisse zwischen elektrischem und mechanischem Effekt des Skeletmuskels. Z. Biol. **82**, 119—125 (1925).

[802] ROSENBLUETH, A., J. H. WILLE, and H. HOAGLAND: The slow components of the electrogram of striated muscle. Amer. J. Physiol. **133**, 724—735 (1941).

Certain observations on the development of tension in isolated frog muscle fibres rendered non-conducting by the application of $10-12$ mM K are also hard to reconcile with the Fleckenstein hypothesis. Thus STEN-KNUDSEN[803] found that such fibres when stimulated by a transversal alternating field, developed tension which increased along an S-shaped curve with increasing field strength. At about 4 V/cm the tension reached its maximum which was $95-100\%$ of the tetanus tension. At all field strengths above $1-1.5$ V/cm the membrane potential remained constant at about 45 mV. Thus it is the magnitude of the transversal field and not the membrane potential which determines the strength of contraction.

C. Effects on heart muscle

a) Introduction

The heart consists of several cell types and tissues with different sensitivities to the composition of the bathing fluid. Taking this into consideration and considering that the different manifestations of the heart activity (rythmicity, conductivity, excitability, contractibility) are not influenced in the same way by physiologically active agents, one should not be surprised if the effects of the alkali metal ions on the heart become quite involved. Considerable simplification is obtained if we focus our interest upon the individual cell types and the individual manifestations of activity. Ultimately, of course, it must be the object of physiologists to combine the information concerning the individual reactions to an integrated picture of the heart action, but this stage has not as yet been reached. In this chapter we shall be mainly concerned with the effects of alkali metal ions upon the contraction process, whereas conduction and excitability have been treated in chapter VIII in connection with the corresponding phenomena in other cell types. First, however, it may be appropriate to consider briefly the gross effects of K and Na upon the heart.

Since RINGER's classical studies[804, 805, 806] it has been recognized that the function of the heart depends upon a delicate balance of the cations Na, K, and Ca in the medium. The relationship between K and Ca is often described as one of antagonism, K favouring the diastole whereas a relative excess of Ca prolongs the systole, increases the tone and, in sufficient concentration, brings about a systolic contracture. In pure NaCl solution the contractions become increasingly weaker and ultimately stop entirely. The sodium ions have at least two functions. Firstly, they provide together with the chloride ions the necessary osmotic pressure. In that function NaCl can be replaced by numerous osmotically active substances like sugars, choline chloride etc. But secondly, Na has a specific function. Thus a heart in Na-free Ringer stops after a short while.

As mentioned above, the various cell types of the heart have different sensitivities to the ionic environment. Thus the sinus automatism is much more resistant to changes in the concentration of the critical ions than is the ventricle automatism (SAKAI[807]). Numerous observations indicate that the sinus and atrium are much

[803] STEN-KNUDSEN, O.: Mechanical response and membrane potential during transverse stimulation to frog muscle. Acta physiol. scand. 42, suppl. 145 (1957).

[804] RINGER, S.: Concerning the influence exerted by each of the constituents of the blood on the contraction of the ventricle. J. Physiol. 3, 380—393 (1882).

[805] RINGER, S.: A third contribution regarding the influence of the inorganic constituents of the blood in the ventricular contraction. J. Physiol. 4, 222—225 (1883).

[806] RINGER, S.: On the mutual antagonism between lime and potash salts in toxic doses. J. Physiol. 5, 247—254 (1884—1885).

[807] SAKAI, T.: Über die Wechselwirkung der Na-, K- und Ca-Ionen am Froschherzen. Z. Biol. 64, 505—548 (1914).

less affected by an increased K concentration than is the ventricle (BOEHM[808], MATHISON[809], MARTIN[810, 811]). The frequency of the spontaneous contractions of the frog's heart increases on a lowering of the concentration of NaCl (to 0.1%) or of KCl (to 0.005%). It is also increased by raising the concentration of $CaCl_2$ (to 0.0325%), whereas the frequency of the sinus is reduced by lack of Na or excess of Ca (SAKAI[807], DALY and CLARK[812]).

The concept of ionic antagonism, especially between K and Ca, has played a great role in studies on the heart function, but it has long been known that the antagonism is by no means complete and certainly not of the type of mutual competitive inhibition. Thus K and Ca only to a very limited extent act as antagonists as regards their effects on the conduction of impulses. Just like in nerve and striated muscle conduction is strongly influenced by the K concentration, whereas lack of Ca will cause complete arrest of the movements of the heart, without producing significant changes in the electric responses. According to DALY and CLARK[812] this suggests that although excess of K and lack of Ca give rise to similar mechanical responses, yet K acts primarily by interfering with conduction whereas lack of Ca abolishes the normal mechanical response.

It is interesting to note that although the heart muscle (like other muscles) has a high K- and a low Na-content (see part II) there is no antagonism between Na and K as far the heart function is concerned. Thus reduction of the concentration in the medium of any one of these ions (the osmotic pressure being maintained constant by proper addition of inert solute) leads to a rise in the systolic tone. A similar response is given by excess Ca.

As already mentioned, excess K increases the duration of the diastole and finally brings the heart to a complete stop. In the mammalian heart a plasma concentration of 0.07—0.08% K usually suffices to bring about a complete stopage of the heart function. But smaller doses of K ordinarily lead to an acceleration of the rhythm. This has been observed both in the case of the isolated frog's heart (HALD[813], BOEHM[808], CLARK[814], SAKAI[807]) and in the mammalian heart (HALD[813], HERING[815]).

An interesting example of the complexity of the ionic effects on the heart is the phenomenon of "K-contracture". Already RINGER[804] observed that a frog's heart which has been stopped in diastole by KCl, will contract after a while and remain in a state of contracture. If a frog's heart is washed free of K with K-free Ringer solution, it will for a while show a tendency towards Ca-contracture. But when all extracellular K has been washed out, the tendency towards contracture vanishes and the heart passes into diastolic stoppage. If, now, excess

[808] BOEHM, R.: Über das Verhalten des isolierten Froschherzens bei reiner Salzdiät. Naunyn-Schmiedebergs Arch. exp. Path. Pharmak. 75, 230—316 (1914).

[809] MATHISON, G. C.: The effect of potassium salts upon the circulation and their action on plain muscle. J. Physiol. 42, 471—494 (1911).

[810] MARTIN, E. G.: An experimental study of the rhythmic activity of isolated strips of the heart muscle. Amer. J. Physiol. 11, 103—138 (1904).

[811] MARTIN, E. G.: A study of the relations of the inorganic salts of the blood to the contraction of heart muscle and skeletal muscle. Amer. J. Physiol. 16, 191—220 (1906).

[812] DE BURGH DALY, I, and A. J. CLARK: The action of ions upon the frog's heart. Amer. J. Physiol. 54, 367—383 (1921).

[813] HALD, P. T.: Die Wirkung der Kalisalze auf die Kreislauforgane. Naunyn-Schmiedebergs Arch. exp. Path. Pharmak. 53, 227—259 (1905).

[814] CLARK, A. J.: The action of ions and lipoids upon the frog's heart. J. Physiol. 47, 66—107 (1913/14).

[815] HERING, H. E.: Über erregende Wirkungen des Kaliums auf das Säugetierherz. Arch. ges. Physiol. 161, 544—554 (1915).

KCl is added, a typical contracture is achieved. According to Kolm and Pick[816] the contracture of the ventricle is brought about even when the KCl is only applied to the sinus or the atrium (compare also Hald[813], Beccari[817]). Thus it seems that it is the impulse set off by K in the sinus which induces contracture in the ventricle when the latter is in a state of contracture-readiness. It is, however, possible to bring about a true K-contracture in the isolated frog ventricle if the K-concentration is increased suddenly (compare p. 189).

Another peculiar response of the isolated frog's heart is the "potassium paradox" of Zwaardemaker[818]: A heart maintained for some time in K-free Ringer will stop in diastole when it is perfused with ordinary Ringer. This response is accentuated by atropine and acetyl choline (Meyler[819]).

It is well known that the heart normally shows an all-or-non reaction to stimuli. It has been demonstrated, however, (Zwikster and Boyd[820]) that, after soaking in modified Ringer with 0.2—0.4% KCl, the heart of the turtle or the bull frog shows perfectly graded mechanical responses to graded electric stimuli. The response is located at the cathode and must be considered as a galvanic contracture. The graded response seems to be associated with an uptake of K by the fibres. The normal type of response returns when the extra K taken up has been given off again during soaking for some time in normal Ringer.

b) Temperature and ionic effects on the heart

A peculiar interdependence seems to exist between the effects of temperature and the effects of ions upon the function of the isolated heart. In general the effect of a relative increase in K concentration can be compensated by an increase in temperature. The phenomenon has been observed in the case of the ventricle of a snail (Bachrach et al.[821]), the dorsal blood vessel (equivalent to the heart) of a cricket (Bergerard and Reinberg[822] the frog's heart (J. J. and J. P. Bouckaert and Noyons[823], Reinberg[824], turtle's heart (Martin[810]) and rabbit's heart (Reinberg[824]). For example, a decrease in temperature increases the tone of the vertebrate ventricle, and the same effect can be obtained by an increase in K-concentration. Similarly, the inhibition of the automatism of the heart is observed at a higher temperature when the K-concentration of the medium is high than when it is low (Reinberg[824]). Not only the effects of cations like K.

[816] Kolm, R., and E. P. Pick: Über die Bedeutung des Kaliums für die Selbststeuerung des Herzens. Pflügers Arch. ges. Physiol. 185, 235—247 (1920).

[817] Beccari, L.: Azione del potassio e degli omologhi rubidio e cesio sul cuore. Arch. scienz. biol. 1, 22—36 (1919).

[818] Zwaardemaker, H.: Le paradoxe radio-physiologique. C. R. Soc. Biol. (Paris) 84, 704—706 (1921).

[819] Meyler, F. L.: Sur l'action de l'acétylcholine, de l'atropine et du potassium sur le coeur de la grenouille. Arch. int. Physiol. 61, 323—329 (1953).

[820] Zwikster, G. H., and T. E. Boyd: Reversible loss of the all or none response in the cold blooded hearts treated with excess potassium. Amer. J. Physiol. 61, 560—567 (1935).

[821] Bachrach, E., and N. Guillot: Effect of ions on thermal optimum for physiological function. C. R. Acad. Sci. (Paris) 212, 929—932 (1941).

[822] Bergerard, J., and A. Reinberg: Combined action of cations and temperature on the dorsal vessel of the cricket. C. R. Soc. Biol. (Paris) 141, 1083—1085 (1947).

[823] Bouckaert, J. J., J. P. Bouckaert, and A. K. Noyons: Rapport entre les effets des ions potassium et calcium et le coefficient de température du coeur de grenouille. Arch. int. Physiol. 19, 160—182 (1922).

[824] Reinberg, A.: Etude de la compensation des effects de la température et des cations sur le fonctionnement de coeurs isolé. Arch. Sci. Physiol. 6, 247—271 (1952).

but also the effects of anions (I, Br, SO_4, PO_4) depend on the temperature[825], Thus the augmentation of the contractions of the snail's heart by iodide can be compensated by an increase in temperature, whereas the augmentation brought about by the other anions mentioned can be countered by a lowering of the temperature. It follows that the dependency of the K effects upon the temperature is only an aspect of a more general rule that the effect of ions depend very much upon the temperature.

c) Effects on the heart rate (the rhythm)

As already mentioned, Na deficient solutions slow the spontaneous rhythm of the heart (DALY and CLARK[812], compare also DRAPER and WEIDMANN[633]). The latter authors found that with Na concentrations in the region of 20% of normal, spontaneous activity ceased, but conduction and excitability remained unchanged.

As long as the concentrations are not too different from normal, the rate of the heart beat is not much affected by changes in the ionic environment. SPEALMAN[826] found that, in the case of the guinea pig heart right atrium, the Na concentration in the medium could be varied from $100-160$ mM/l without change in the rate. At higher concentrations there was a reduction in the rate. K could be varied from $2-4$ mN/l without effect, but both at higher and at lower K concentrations there was a reduction in the rate of the heart beat.

d) Effects upon the mechanical response of the heart

Some authors have held that irritability and contractility are closely related phenomena in the sense that an increase in irritability is always associated with an increase in the force of contraction, and vice versa (see for instance LEWIS and DRURY[827], LEWIS[828], WIGGERS[829]). There is, however, mounting evidence that the two phenomena can often be dissociated completely in heart muscle (see GARB[830], SALTER and RUNELS[831]), just as it could in striated muscle (see above). A separate discussion of the effects of the alkali metal ions on the mechanical response of heart muscle is therefore warranted. According to SALTER and RUNELS[831] the frog's heart ventricle contracts maximally when the K concentration of the bathing medium is 4.8 mM/l. Higher and lower K concentrations cause a sharp reduction in contractility. The position of this maximum is independent of the Ca concentration as long as it remains within the physiological range (Fig. 20). Thus there is no true antagonism between K and Ca ions with respect to contractility. The maximum contraction attained at the K optimum (and at any other K concentration) shows, however, a strong positive correlation to the Ca concentration. In the guinea pig right atrium preparation there was an

[825] BACHRACH, E., and A. REINBERG: Etude de la compensation des effets dus aux variations de la température et des anions sur le fonctionnement du ventricule isolé d'escargot. Arch. int. Physiol. **61**, 185—199 (1953).

[826] SPEALMAN, C. R.: The action of ions on the mammalian heart. Amer. J. Physiol. **136**, 332—339 (1942).

[827] LEWIS, T., and A. N. DRURY: Engelmann's evidence for the independence of excitability and contractility in heart muscle. J. Physiol. **55**, XII—XIII (1921).

[828] LEWIS, T.: The law of cardiac muscle with special reference to conduction in the mammalian heart. Quart. J. Med. **14**, 339—351 (1920—21).

[829] WIGGERS, C. J.: Physiology in healt and disease. Philadelphia: Lee 1944, p. 56.

[830] GARB, S.: Separability of contractile force and irritability in mammalian heart muscle. Amer. J. Physiol. **164**, 234—237 (1951).

[831] SALTER, W. T., and E. A. RUNELS: A nomogram for cardiac contractility involving calcium, potassium and digitalis-like drugs. Amer. J. Physiol. **165**, 520—526 (1951).

optimum for the amplitude of the K contraction of 4 mM/l. For Na there was a broad maximum between 140 and 160 mM/l. Outside this range the amplitude of the contraction was progressively diminished. Ca increased the amplitude up to 4 mM/l. At higher concentrations of Ca the contraction height becomes increasingly less (SPEALMAN[826]).

In the case of the cat papillary muscle the K concentration of the medium seemed without effect upon the contractility in the concentration range from 2.15—10.15 mM/l (GREEN, GIARMAN and SALTER[832]). Above this concentration K lowers the contractility. As it was the case with the frog's heart, Ca is not truly antagonistic to K, but increases the contractility irrespective of the level of K in the medium.

The strength of the spontaneous contractions of the turtle heart (Emys orbicularis) is diminished by excess K, whereas acetyl choline has no effect. The K effect upon the atria is even more pronounced and the atria are also depressed by acetyl choline (DELVAUX[833]). Both atria and ventricle aresentisized towards K by CN and urethane ((DELVAUX[834]).

Low Na concentrations in the medium seem in general to be beneficial for optimum contractility. Thus McDOWAL and ZAYAT[835] demonstrated that the strength of the contractions of the stimulated rat ventricle is a function of the frequency. 40 contractions per minute gives a contraction height which is only half that obtained with 4 contractions per minute. If, however, the Na concentration of the bath is reduced to about half that of the Ringer solution (NaCl being replaced by a suitable amount of glucose) there is hardly any reduction of the contraction height with increased rate of stimulation. The experiment is taken to mean that during contractions the rat ventricle takes up Na faster than it can get rid of it. If the outside Na concentration is now lowered, the extrusion of Na is made easier and the uptake is presumable less. The optimum Na content of the fibres can thus be maintained even at a high rate of

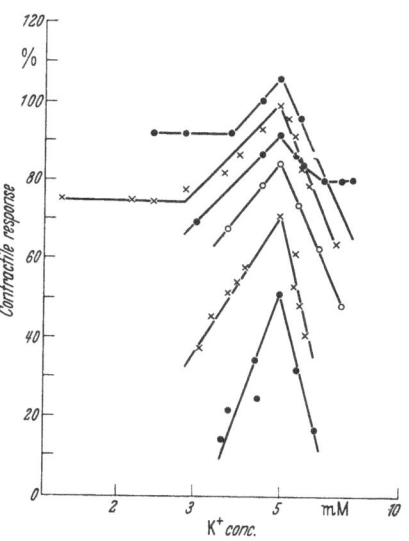

Fig. 20. Dependence of contractility of the frog heart upon external K and Ca concentrations. From top to bottom the Ca concentrations are 125, 100, 66, 50 and 25 per cent of the physiological concentration, respectively (after SALTER and RUNELS[831])

stimulation. To the reviewers knowledeg similar studies with K are lacking. Thus we do not know whether even the mammalian heart depends upon a certain low sum of K and Na on the fibres for maximum contractility, or whether it is only Na which is deleterious to contractility.

[832] GREEN, J. P., N. J. GIARMAN, and W. T. SALTER: Combined effects of calcium and potassium on contractility and excitability of the mammalian myocardium. Amer. J. Physiol. **171**, 174—177 (1952).

[833] DELVAUX, P.: A propos de l'intervention réciproque de l'acétylcholine et du potassium dans le mécanisme de la cardio-inhibition vagale. Arch. int. Physiol. **61**, 26—30 (1953).

[834] DELVAUX, P.: Influence de la respiration tissulaire sur la sensibilité au potassium du ventricle isolé de la tortue. Arch. int. Physiol. **61**, 387—390 (1953).

[835] McDOWAL, R. J. S., and A. F. ZAYAT: Sodium chloride and cardiac muscle. J. Physiol. **120**, 13 P (1953).

Under anoxic conditions the right ventricle of the rat heart is rapidly depressed and is unable to recover even when oxygen is returned as long as the medium is normal Krebs' solution. If the concentration of NaCl is lowered to 0.4—0.5%, however, recovery ensues (McDOWAL and ZAYAT [836]). Thus again, it seems that low fibre-Na is essential for contractility and that the proper Na-level in the fibre can either be maintained by aerobic extrusion of Na or by an outer medium having a low Na-concentration. The fact that sodium-deficient solution increase the force of contraction has also been pointed out by CLARK and DALY [812], see also CLARK [814]).

Both the twitch tension and the potassium contracture tension of heart muscle strips (frog) are determined by the quotient Ca/Na^2 so that the tension increases with increasing values of the quotient [837]. These authors explain this behaviour by assuming 1) that the activator for the contraction is the calcium complex of a substance which is located in the fibre surface and that 2) Na competes with Ca for the anionic binding site responsible for the complex formation. (It will be recalled that even in the case of the striated muscle there are indications that Ca somehow is involved in the activation process.) The cometition is strictly between Ca and Na. Not even Li seems to form an inactive complex with the activator.

The sodium-calcium antagonism is not only concerned with binding sites on the surface of the fibres, however. In low-Na media calcium is rapidly taken up by the cells, bit is extruded again in the presence of high-Na media. Thus there seems to be a cellular store of Ca whose magnitude varies inversely with the sodium concentration of the medium. It can, however, also be increased by omission of K from the Ringer solution. When the store of cellular Ca is low, the strength of contraction is weak, whereas high Ca in the fibres is associated with forceful contractions.

e) The HAJDU hypothesis

1. The "staircase" phenomenon

An interesting attempt has been made by HAJDU [838] to give an integrated interpretation of the effects of alkali metal ions upon the mechanical response of the heart. The hypothesis is based upon a study of the so-called staircase phenomenon which was first described by BOWDITCH [839]. The name staircase relates to the first contractions of a frog's heart after a stoppage. These contractions increase gradually in strength, thus forming a staircase leading up to the relatively constant contractions of the regularly beating heart. This peculiar behaviour of the heart was made the object of a careful study by HAJDU and SZENT-GYÖRGYI [754, 840]. It was found that the staircase phenomenon (recorded isometrically) was abolished by low temperature and by low K concentration in the medium. The preliminary hypothesis was then advanced that each contraction, following a stoppage, lowered the amount of fibre-K a little, and that the lowered concentration of K in the fibres was favorable for contraction. It was further found that serum as well as digitalis glucosides and desoxycortico-

[836] McDOWAL, R. J. S., and A. F. ZAYAT: Sodium chloride and anoxic cardiac muscle. J. Physiol. 117, 75 P—76 P (1952).
[837] NIEDERGERKE, R., H. C. LÜTTGAU, and E. J. HARRIS: Calcium and the contraction of the heart. Nature (Lond.) 79, 1066—1069 (1957).
[838] HAJDU, S.: Mechanism of staircase and contracture in ventricular muscle. Amer. J. Physiol. 174, 371—380 (1953).
[839] BOWDITCH, H. P.: Über die Eigentümlichkeiten der Reizbarkeit, welche die Muskelfasern des Herzens zeigen. Leipzig, Arbeit. Physiol. Anst. 1871, 139—176 (1952).
[840] HAJDU, S., and A. SZENT-GYÖRGYI: Action of digitalis glucosides on isolated frog heart. Amer. J. Physiol. 168, 171—176 (1952).

sterone (DOC) counteracted the staircase phenomenon. HAJDU and SZENT-GYÖRGYI[754, 840] therefore suggested that these agents must somehow bring about the same ionic state in the fibre as do a series of contractions. Later, HAJDU[838] undertook a thorough study of the ionic balance of the heart in relation to the development of tension in the isometrically contracting frog ventricle. Maximal electric stimulation was used throughout.

2. Potassium ions and the development of tension

Fig. 21 (HAJDU[838]) shows in schematic form the relationship between the tension developed and the amount of internal K lost by the heart (expressed in

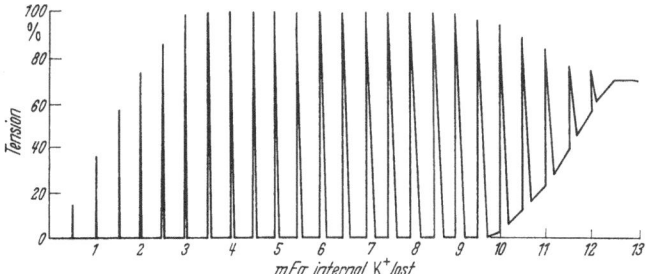

Fig. 21. Diagrammatic representation of height and shape of contractions of frog heart and contracture (rise of base line) as a function of loss of internal K (after HAJDU[838])

meq per kg heart). It is seen that the tension goes up as the fibre K decreases (staircase!) to reach a maximum after the loss of 3 meq of potassium per kg heart. If the loss of K is driven further, the maximal tension remains constant over a wide range of concentrations, but the relaxation time increases. When about 9 meq K have been lost, the tension no longer returns to zero after each contraction, and as the K content of the heart is reduced still further, the heart goes into contracture. The range of intracellular K levels which provide the material for this figure was brought about by different means. K-losses up to 3 meq can be achieved by stimulating at the maximum rate (about 45 contractions/min). Greater losses of K were induced by digitalis (1—5 μg/ml) desoxycorticosterone or progesterone (50—150 μg/ml). These drugs all act in a similar way, preventing

the entry of K into the fibres and thus preserving the favourable conditions for maximal contractions.

3. Potassium ions and contracture

From Fig. 22 it would appear that contracture is only observed when the heart has suffered a considerable loss of K. Actually, however, contracture can be brought about at any internal K level by a sudden lowering of the membrane potential, and since the membrane potential

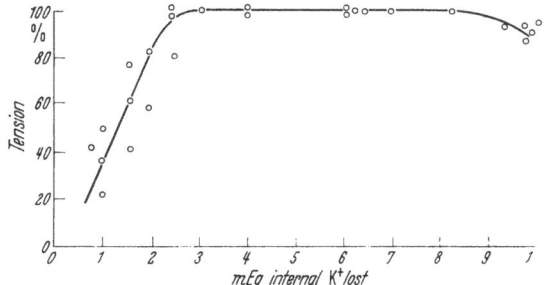

Fig. 22. Dependence of tension developed by frog heart upon loss of internal potassium (after HAJDU[838])

is a function of the outside K concentration (see p. 146), contracture can be elicited by a sudden increase in the external K-concentration. Thus, when the external K concentration is increased suddenly over and above a critical level (which is determined primarily by the internal K concentration) a contracture ensues which will persist until sufficient K has entered the fibres to make them no longer contracture-prone.

From this discussion it is apparent that K in the fibres and K outside the fibres have opposite effects with respect to the development of contracture. The observations of HAJDU and SZENT-GYÖRGYI go a long way towards reconciling the conflicting statements made by previous authors concerning the effects of K upon the heart function (see above).

4. Effect of Na upon the staircase

HAJDU was able to demonstrate that the effects of K upon the staircase was not at all specific. Thus the staircase could be abolished by a lowering of the Na-concentration of the medium, in so far as a non-penetrating cation was used to replace Na (for instance Li or choline ion). Similar results were obtained when part of the NaCl of the Ringer solution was replaced by an isosmotic amount of glucose or mannose. When the sodium concentration of the medium was lowered to 72.6 mM/liter, the heart reached the verge of contracture. At still lower Na concentrations contracture actually occurred.

5. Formulation of the hypothesis

From the experiments mentioned in the foregoing HAJDU concluded that the tension developed in the heart is determined by the sum of potassium and sodium ions in the fibres. Determination of the fibre volume with inuline under different

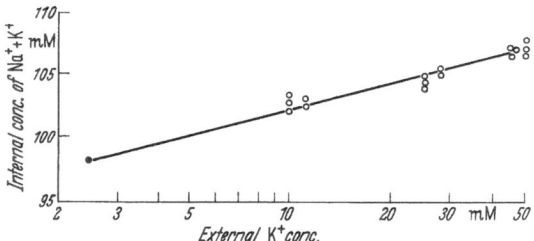

Fig. 23. Correlation between internal Na + K concentration and external K concentration necessary to produce contracture. ● indicates the mean of nine measurements (after HAJDU [838])

experimental conditions showed that what really matters is not the *concentration* of (K + Na) in the fibres but rather the *amount* of alkali metal ion (that is the number of equivalents) in the fibres. (It is perhaps doubtful whether the volume determinations are accurate enough to justify this distinction.) Fig. 23 (HAJDU [838]) shows the level of external K, sufficing to bring about contracture at different levels of internal (K + Na).

In order to explain his findings, HAJDU makes the following two assumptions: Firstly, when the alkali metal ion concentration in the fibres is high, the actomyosin system remains dissociated even during stimulation. According to SZENT-GYÖRGYI [841, 746] this is exactly what one would expect from experiments with the isolated actomyosin system. As the cellular K (and/or Na) is lowered, association takes place and the contractions become increasingly vigorous until finally the actomyosin remains in the contracted state even in the absence of a stimulus.

Secondly, HAJDU assumes that the resting potential exerts a "static action" on the actomyosin which results in a dissociation in a milieu which would otherwise favour association. HAJDU further assumes the hydrogen ion to be the vehicle for the effect exerted by the membrane potential. If a Donnan distribution of hydrogen and potassium ions takes place in the heart muscle, it is obvious that a highly negative potential level inside the fibre would lead to a relative accumula-

[841] SZENT-GYÖRGYI, A.: Chemistry of muscular contraction. Academic Press, N. Y. 1951.

tion of hydrogen ions as well as potassium ions, whereas depolarization would lead to a loss of these ions. Depolarization thus could bring about association (that is contraction) by increasing the cellular p_H. Actual determinations of the fibre p_H were not performed. Recent studies by CALDWELL[418] of the intracellular p_H in crab muscle fibres with a micro-glass electrode seem, however, to throw some doubt upon the validity of HAJDU's argument. CALDWELL found that the intracellular p_H of the 600 μ fibres of the crab Carcinus maenas was about 6.9 against 7.06 in the medium. A value of this magnitude was observed whether the potential was high (50—59 mV) or low (0—9 mV). Thus in the case of the Carcinus muscle the Donnan distribution of hydrogen ions does not apply.

An explanation of the staircase phenomenon differing somewhat from that of HAJDU has been presented by MOULIN and WILBRANDT[842]. They assume that calcium is being lost from the heart during the quiescent period and that Ca like Na moves into the fibres during activity. Thus it would be the gain of Ca and not the loss of K which was responsible for the improved contractility associated with the first contractions. A rather fast exchange of K and Ca has previously been demonstrated by KROGH, LINDBERG and SCHMIDT-NIELSEN[843].

NIEDERGERKE[844], however, has presented evidence that the effects of changes in external K and Ca are too fast to involve equilibration with the internal electrolyte content. He therefore advocates the view that the strength of contraction is determined by the concentration of calcium in a superficially located region of the heart cells. Until more material is forthcoming we therefore cannot consider HAJDU's explanation of the effect of the potential upon muscular contraction as final (compare also FEIGEN[743]).

D. Effects on smooth muscle

a) Effect of sodium ions

1. Intestinal muscle

According to MAGEE and REID[845], lowering of the concentration of NaCl below 0.6% (osmotic pressure being maintained by addition of appropriate amounts of glucose) reduces the size of the contractions in the isolated intestine of the rabbit and ultimately almost abolishes them. The low Na concentration has little or no effect on the frequency. STREETEN[846] found that guinea-pig and human intestines were even more sensitive to a reduction in the NaCl level than was the rabbit gut. Clinical observations have indicated a close correlation between low plasma chloride (and presumably low Na-concentration) and paralytic ileus (LEVY and NORA[847, 848], STREETEN[846], and MARRIOTT[849]) has pointed out that in salt-depleted

---

[842] MOULIN, M., and W. WILBRANDT: Die Wirkung von Kalium und Calcium auf das Treppenphänomen am Froschherzen. Experientia (Basel) **11**, 72—73 (1955).

[843] KROGH, A., A. L. LINDBERG, and B. SCHMIDT-NIELSEN: The exchange of ions between cells and extracellular fluids. II. The exchange of potassium and calcium between the frog heart muscle and the bathing fluid. Acta physiol. scand. **7**, 221—237 (1944).

[844] NIEDERGERKE, R.: The "Staircase" Phenomenon and the action of calcium on the heart. J. Physiol. **134**, 569—583 (1956).

[845] MAGEE, H. E., and C. REID: Studies on the movements of the alimentary canal I. The effects of electrolytes on the rhythmical contractions of the isolated mammalian intestine. J. Physiol. **63**, 97—106 (1927).

[846] STREETEN, D. H. P.: Effects of sodium and chloride lack of intestinal motility and their significance in paralytic ileus. Surg. Gynec. Obstet. **91**, 421—434 (1950).

[847] LEVY, M., and G. NORA: Occlusion intestinale paralytique post-opératoire tardive; inefficacité du chlorure de Sodium administré par voie buccale; insuffisance des quantités de NaCl administrées dans les veines dans la phase post-opératoire. Arch. Mal Appar. dig. **25**, 190—193 (1935).

subjects water absorption is delayed due to gastrointestinal atonia. STREETEN and VAUGHAN WILLIAMS[850] have studied the effect of NaCl depletion upon the rate of intestinal fluid propulsion in the dog. NaCl-depletion was brought about by intraperitoneal infusions of 4.5% dextrose solution, containing appropriate amounts of K, Ca, Mg and PO_4, the infusates being withdrawn two to four hours later. This treatment caused initially a rise in the rate of intestinal propulsion, but soon followed a marked reduction, and ultimately total paralysis of propulsion. In some cases the intestinal loops became completely toneless. It is of interest that the skin elasticity was also markedly impaired, indicating loss of tone in the plain muscle of the skin. The paralysis of propulsion could be reversed within one minute by the injection intracardially of hypertonic NaCl. STREETEN and VAUGHAN WILLIAMS believe that the reduced blood NaCl induces a loss of potassium from the fibres which is supposed to be the ultimate cause of the paralysis (see below, under K).

2. Uterus muscle

Isolated uterus which has been made insensitive to histamine by large doses of this drug regains its sensitivity by treatment with Krebs Ringer solution in which half the NaCl is replaced by sucrose (McDOWAL and SOLIMAN[851]). These authors suggest that in normal Krebs solution the smooth uterus muscle gains Na during contraction, and that this Na is responsible for the insensitivity. Lowering the Na concentration of the bathing fluid makes it easier for the fibres to rid themselves of the excess Na. It is interesting that a low level of NaCl which is highly inhibitory for one type of plain muscle (intestine, skin) seems definitely beneficial for another (uterus). It is worth mentioning, however, that also isolated mammalian heart muscle shows an increased strength of contraction when the Na concentration of the bath is half that of ordinary Krebs solution (sucrose being used to maintain isotonia).

b) Effect of potassium ions

1. Intestinal muscle

The effect of K upon smooth muscle is of a complex nature just as it was the case with skeletal muscle. K-deficiency in the medium increases the tone and the rate of contraction, whereas excess K has no effect on tone but decreases both the rate and the amplitude of the contractions (MAGEE and REID[845], SOLLMAN, VAN OETTINGEN and ISHIKAWA[852, 853], WHITEHEAD[854]). Given in doses of, say, one mg KCl per ml bathing solution, the potassium ion first brings about contraction

[848] LEVY, M., and G. NORA: Le diagnostic de l'occlusion intestinale paralytique postopératoire: le rôle du laboratoire. Arch. Mal. Appar. dig. **35**, 67—73 (1946).

[849] MARRIOTT, H. L.: Water and salt depletion. Brit. med. J. **1947** I, 285—290.

[850] STREETEN, D. H. P., and E. M. VAUGHAN WILLIAMS: Loss of cellular potassium as a cause of intestinal paralysis in dogs. J. Physiol. **118**, 149—170 (1952).

[851] McDOWALL, R. J. S., and A. A. I. SOLIMAN: Sodium chloride and the response of mooth muscle. J. Physiol. **122**, 42 P (1953).

[852] SOLLMAN, T., W. F. VAN OETTINGEN, and Y. ISHIKAWA: The efficiency of bicarbonate and phosphate buffers for experimentation with excised organs. Amer. J. Physiol. **85**, 118 to 128 (1928).

[853] SOLLMAN, T., W. F. VAN OETTINGEN, and Y. ISHIKAWA: The effects of phosphate buffers on intestinal movements, and their interrelation with calcium. Amer. J. Physiol. **87**, 293—304 (1928).

[854] WHITEHEAD, R. W.: Responses of excised intestines to alterations of electrolyte concentrations (Na, Ca, K). Amer. J. Physiol. **89**, 253—265 (1929).

and then inhibits the fresh gut of rabbit and guinea-pig (AMBACHE[855]). The effect was interpreted as being due to a release of acetyl choline from nerve-endings in the gut (AMBACHE[855]).

EMMELIN and FELDBERG[856] (compare also MERCIER and MERCIER[857]), however presented good evidence that the K effects the intestinal muscle directly. Thus benadryl ($1/10^6$) is a much more powerful antagonist of acetylcholine than of K. In experiments where the gut had been treated with benadryl and the drug washed out again, the sensitivity to K returned long before that to acetylcholine. BROWN and FELDBERG also draw attention to the analogous case of the K stimulation of denervated sympathetic ganglia which do not contain acetyl-choline (BROWN and FELDBERG[858]). PLOTKA[859] came to the conclusion that the effect of K is a double one. In small doses it sensitizes to acetyl-choline, whereas larger doses stimulate. This view is supported by HAZARD and CORNEC[860].

There is some evidence that the contractions of the *intestinal muscle* depend critically upon its potassium content. Thus WEBSTER, HENRIKSON and CURRIE[861] found that a K-deficient diet produced, in rats, a condition resembling paralytic ileus, and led to a reduction in the strength and frequency of the contractions in the dog intestine. Clinical considerations led DARROW[862] to the conclusion that paralytic ileus might be caused by low plasma K. It was shown by STREETEN and VAUGHAN WILLIAMS[850], however, that the intestine of NaCl-depleted dogs may become completely toneless at a time when the plasma K level is actually increased. These authors therefore conclude that the paralysis of the intestine is due to a loss of fibre K. This assumption is supported by the finding that contracting intestinal segments in vitro lost more K when immersed in NaCl-deficient Tyrode than in normal Tyrode solution. It has also been shown by WINTER, HOFF and DSO[863] that desoxycorticosterone administration to rats (which lowers the fibre K level) resulted in lowered gastro-intestinal motility.

2. Uterus muscle

A moderate increase in K concentration in the medium usually leads to contraction of uterus muscle (MATHISON[809]). This type of reaction seems to be common to all smooth muscles. The sensitivity to pituitary extract is also increased by excess K. Thus VAN DYKE and HASTINGS[864] found that without exception the uterus of the guinea-pig showed a more vigorous response to pituitrin when the

---

[855] AMBACHE, N.: Interaction of drugs and the effect of cooling on the isolated mammalian intestine. J. Physiol. **104**, 266—287 (1946).

[856] EMMELIN, N., and W. FELDBERG: The smooth muscle contracting effects of various substances supposed to act on nervous structures in the intestinal wall. J. Physiol. **106**, 482—502 (1947).

[857] MERCIER, F., and J. MERCIER: Remarques à propos de l'action du camphosulfonate racémique de potassium sur l'intestine isolé. C. R. Soc. Biol. (Paris) **141**, 502—505 (1947).

[858] BROWN, G. L., and W. FELDBERG: The action of potassium on the superior cervical ganglion of the rat. J. Physiol. **86**, 290—305 (1936).

[859] PLOTKA, C.: Potassium et intestin isolé. C. R. Soc. Biol. (Paris) **141**, 1026—1029 (1947).

[860] HAZARD, R., and A. CORNEC: Action du potassium sur l'intestin isolé de rat et sur sa réactivité à l'acétylcholine. C. R. Soc. Biol. (Paris) **146**, 896—897 (1952).

[861] WEBSTER, D. R., W. H. HENRIKSON, and D. J. CURRIE: The effect of potassium deficiency on intestinal motility and gastric secretion. Ann. Surg. **132**, 779—785 (1950).

[862] DARROW, D. C.: Role of potassium in clinical disturbances of body water and electrolyte. New Engl. J. Med. **242**, 978—983 (1950).

[863] WINTER, H. A., H. E. HOFF, and L. DSO: Effects of potassium deficiency upon gastrointestinal motility. Fed. Proc. **8**, 169 (1949).

[864] DYKE, H. B. VAN, and A. B. HASTINGS: The response of smooth muscle in different ionic environments. Amer. J. Physiol. **83**, 563—577 (1928).

K-concentration of the bathing fluid was raised from 6.2 to 9.3 mM/liter (see, however, TUROLT[865]).

It was mentioned above that the contractility of intestinal muscle depends upon a proper concentration of intracellular K. The same is the case for uterus muscle. It is a well known fact (for references see REYNOLDS[866], ROBERTS and SZEGO[867]) that during the estrus cycle the uterus undergoes reversible changes in electrolyte content as well as in its ability to contract and develop tension. In the estrogen dominated state the water content and the electrolyte content per uterus are increased and so is the contractibility. Some of the gain in water and electrolyte is due to extracellular edema, probably arising from an increased capillary permeability. But a considerable fraction of the water and electrolyte is taken up by the cells. Already TALBOT, LOWRY and ASTWOOD[868] showed that a large retention of cellular K (and phosphate) is induced in uteri of immature rats after the administration of a single dose of estradiol. It is very interesting that the uptake of K preceeds that of phosphate. Possibly KCl is accumulated in the initial phase of the reaction. ROBERTS and SZEGO[867] believe that the sterol hormones primarily influence the permeability of the muscle fibre membranes.

Table 28. *Intracellular ion concentrations* (mM/1 intracellular water)

	Na	K	K + Na	Ratio (K/Na)
Estrogen treated	30	158	188	5.3
Estrogen withdrawn	32	126	158	3.9
Progesterone	45	132	177	2.9

The water and electrolyte retention goes back during the progesterone-dominated part of the cycle, and at the same time the contractility is diminished. CSAPO[869] has demonstrated that progesterone depresses the isometric tension developed in the isolated rabbit uteri. A recent study by HORVATH[870] shows the drastic changes taking place in rabbit uterus muscle electrolytes under the influence of the ovarian hormones (see Table 28).

Castrated females or infantile females were used. One group was treated with daily injections of estrogens for some ten days, the second group was treated the same way, but left untreated for an additional 3—4 days. The last group also received the estrogen treatment initially, but progesteron was given for 3—4 days after the estrogen treatment was discontinued. The figures for the electrolyte concentration were calculated on the basis of intracellular water, the extracellular water space having been estimated from the inulin space.

Closely related to the intracellular K-concentration is the "stair-case" phenomena. The tension of uterus muscle increases with increasing frequency of stimulation (positive staircase) in estrogen dominated uterus muscle, whereas the progesteron treated castrate uteri show negative staircases (that is decreasing

[865] TUROLT, M.: Umkehr der Adrenalinwirkung auf den überlebenden Uterus durch Ionenverschiebung. Arch. Gynäk. **115**, 600—611 (1922).

[866] REYNOLDS, S. R. M.: Determinants of uterine growth and activity. Physiol. Rev. **31**, 244—273 (1951).

[867] ROBERTS, S., and C. M. SZEGO: Steroid interaction in metabolism of reproductive target organs. Physiol. Rev. **33**, 593—629 (1953).

[868] TALBOT, N. B., O. H. LOWRY, and E. B. ASTWOOD: Influence of estrogen on the electrolyte pattern of the immature rat uterus. J. biol. Chem. **132**, 1—9 (1940).

[869] CSAPO, A.: Dependence of isometric tension and isotonic shortening of uterine muscle on temperature and on strength of stimulation. Amer. J. Physiol. **177**, 348—354 (1954).

[870] HORVATH, B.: Ovarian hormones and the ionic balance of uterine muscle. Proc. nat. Acad. Sci. (Wash.) **40**, 515—523 (1954).

tension with increasing rate of stimulation) (CSAPO and CORNER[871]). CSAPO[872] thinks that these observations can be explained by assuming that estrogen dominated uterus contains too much K for the development of maximum tension. As the rate of stimulation is increased, more K is lost than can be recovered during relaxation and the muscle approaches conditions for maximum contractility. This is essentially the same explanation as that advanced by HAJDU and SZENT-GYÖRGYI to explain the staircase of the frog's heart. The "estrogen withdrawal" and progestron uteri, on the other hand have already too little K for maximum contractions, and as the K is lost due to the increased rate of contractions, the lack of intracellular K makes itself felt in the form of a falling tension. It thus becomes an important question where in the sequence of events leading to contraction the K/Na ratio of intracellular electrolyte is of such great importance. According to CSAPO[873] strong electrical chocks will induce contractions even in uterus muscles which are totally depolarized by KCl (124 mM/l). Thus it is possible to activate the contractile element directly. Chocks of similar strength also activate uteri placed in ordinary tyrode, and under such conditions the stair-case phenomena are not seen, although they are very apparent with moderate stimuli. CSAPO therefore believes that the stair-cases are related to activation rather than to the process of contraction. This would explain that less tension is developed when cellular K/Na ratio is low than when it is high despite the fact that for the contractility of actomyosin Na can fully replace K.

3. Vascular muscle

It is well known (for references see GOFFART and BACQ[706], HAZARD and QUINQUAUD[874]) that injections of KCl in the blood circulation of mammals gives rise to an increase in blood pressure. This effect is, however, only partly due to the direct effect on the vascular muscle. HAZARD and QUINQUAUD have demonstrated that a sudden rise in the plasma concentration of K leads to a release of adrenaline from the adrenals and this is the major cause of the rise in blood pressure. Even in adrenalectomized dogs, however, the injection of KCl produces an increase in blood-pressure and this effect seems to be of muscular origin.

[871] CSAPO, A., and G. W. CORNER: Antagonistic effects of estrogen and progesterone on staircase phenomenon in uterine muscle. Endocrinol. 51, 378—385 (1952).

[872] CSAPO, A.: Potassium and myometrial function. J. Lancet 73, 250—251 (1953).

[873] CSAPO, A.: A link between "models" and living muscle. Nature (Lond.) 173, 1019 to 1021 (1954).

[874] HAZARD, R., and A. QUINQUAUD: L'ion potassium vasoconstricteur. J. Physiol. (Paris) 44, 259—262 (1952).

The alkali metal ions in the organism

By

P. W. Kruhøffer, J. Hess Thaysen and N. A. Thorn

I. Introduction

While part I of this book has mainly been devoted to considerations on the biology of alkali metal ions at the cellular and subcellular level, part II has been written with the intention to consider the relation of these ions to the body as a whole or to parts of the body at a higher level of organization.

Part II then deals with the distribution of the alkali metals in the body (Chapter II), and with the total body contents and the readily exchangeable parts of these (Ch. III). The subsequent three chapters deal with the transport of alkali metal ions across body surfaces and with problems related to these phenomena: The handling in the kidney (Ch. IV), the handling in other exocrine glands (Ch. V), and the intestinal absorption (Ch. VI). The subjects of the last three chapters are: Intakes and general turnovers (Ch. VII), Effects of excesses and deficits (Ch. VIII), and Internal shifts and displacements (Ch. IX).

In the biology of multicellular organisms investigations at the cellular and the supracellular levels are complementary and equally important, since phenomena observed in systems of higher complexity are not adequately understood until they can be expressed in terms of underlying phenomena at the cellular or lower organizational levels, and since observations made at these levels only gain full significance when they can promote the understanding of phenomena observable in the intact organism. In the case of the alkali metal ions our understanding of phenomena observed in systems of high complexity has profited much from information supplied by more "basic" investigations. In several places in this part of the book references to sections in the first part will therefore be found. It must be admitted, however, that there are many more cases in which it has not yet been possible to account for the phenomena in the more complex systems in terms of their "basic components". While lack of imagination may be responsible for this shortcoming in some cases, the main reason is to be found in the fact that our knowledge at the different levels of organization is still too incomplete to permit integrations.

In the course of the preparation of the various sections of part II the authors have primarily had the human body in mind, and wherever available, preference has been given to observations made in man. The numerous gaps which for obvious reasons exist in our knowledge of this species, have been filled in with data and interpretations mostly derived from experiments on other mammals. — The fact that great interest has been paid to the alkali metals not only by physiologists but also by clinicians makes it desirable to pay due attention to the results of clinical studies. The line, generally followed, has been to include from clinical work such pieces of information which have greatly contributed to the elucidation of fundamental physiological processes. It is, however, considered outside the scope of this volume to deal with the pathogenesis and therapy of disorders of electrolyte metabolism. For such information the reader is referred to the many recent treatises, among others those by Danowski[1, 3], Gamble[2], Overman[4], Black[5], Selkurt[6], Hill[7], Welt[8], Elkinton and Danowski[9], Edelman and

NADELL[10], MOORE[11, 15], SCHWARTZ[12], BLAND[13], DARROW and HELLERSTEIN[14a] and the symposium on renal physiology in the Am. J. Med.[14b]*. For reviews of the recently defined clinical syndromes of primary hyperaldosteronism, hypoaldosteronism and adynamia episodica hereditaria reference should be made to the papers by CONN and LOUIS[16a], SKANSE and HÖKFELT[16b] HILLS,[16c] GAMSTORP et al.[17a] and SAGILD[17b].

The literature on the physiology of the alkali metals is so huge, that it is an unpracticable task to give a historical review and a complete set of references for every subject dealt with on the ensuing pages. The authors have, however, attempted such completeness wherever recent reviews of the subject are either lacking or incomplete. If modern and comprehensive review articles are available, main emphasis has been placed on covering the literature between the appearance of the review and the printing of this book, whereas extensive reference to older work has sometimes been omitted.

Since the alkali metals have often been termed as "bases", particularly in the older clinico-physiological literature, it should be emphasized that BRØNSTED's definition of acids and bases has been used throughout this text. According to this definition an acid is a proton donator, a base a proton acceptor. The alkali metals are termed cations. This terminology which has certain theoretical advantages is also advocated in recent American treatises[14a, 18].

[1] DANOWSKI, T. S.: Newer concepts of the role of potassium in disease. Amer. J. Med. 7, 525—31 (1949).

[2] GAMBLE, J. L.: Chemical anatomy, physiology, and pathology of extracellular fluid. Cambridge, Mass: Harward University Press 1950.

[3] DANOWSKI, T. S.: Newer concepts of the role of sodium in disease. Amer. J. Med. 10, 468—80 (1951).

[4] OVERMAN, R. R.: Sodium, potassium and chloride alteration in disease. Physiol. Rev. 31, 285—311 (1951).

[5] BLACK, D. A. K.: Sodium metabolism in health and disease. Oxford: Blackwell 1952

[6] SELKURT, E. E.: Sodium excretion by the mammalian kidney. Physiol. Rev. 34, 287 — 333 (1954).

[7] HILL, F. S.: Practical fluid therapy in pediatrics. Philadelphia: W. B. Saunders 1954

[8] WELT, L. G.: Clinical disorders of hydration and acid-base equilibrium. Boston: Little, Brown & Co 1955.

[9] ELKINTON, J. R., and T. S. DANOWSKI: The Body Fluids-Basic Physiology and Practical Therapeutics. Baltimore: Williams & Wilkins Comp. 1955.

[10] EDELMAN, I. S., and J. NADELL: Recent progress in the study of potassium metabolism. Stanford med. Bull. 13, 511—25 (1955).

[11] MOORE, F. D. (ed.): Symposium on water and electrolytes. Metabolism 5, 367—518 (1956).

[12] SCHWARTZ, W. B.: Potassium and the kidney. New Engl. J. Med. 253, 601—608 (1955).

[13] BLAND, J. H.: Clinical recognition and management of disturbances of body fluids. 2. ed. Philadelphia: W. B. Saunders: 1956.

[14a] DARROW, D. C., and S. HELLERSTEIN: Interpretation of certain changes in body water and electrolytes. Physiol. Rev. 38, 114—37 (1958).

[14b] MUDGE, G. H., and J. V. TAGGART (ed.): Symposium on renal physiology. Amer. J. Med. 24, 661—804 (1958).

[15] MOORE, F. D.: Common patterns of water and electrolyte change in injury, surgery and disease. New Engl. J. Med. 258, 277—285 (1958) and following issues.

[16a] CONN, J. W., and L. H. LOUIS: Primary aldosteronism, a new clinical entity. Ann. intern. Med. 44, 1—15 (1956).

[16b] SKANSE, B., and B. HÖKFELT: Hypoaldosteronism with otherwise intact adrenocortical function, resulting in a characteristic clinical entity. Acta endocr. (Kbh.) 28, 29—36 (1958).

[16c] HILLS, A. G.: Selective hypoaldosteronism. Amer. J. Med. 26, 503—507 (1959).

[17a] GAMSTORP, I., M. HAUGE, H. F. HELWEG-LARSEN, H. MJÖSNES, and U. SAGILD: Adynamia episodica hereditaria. Amer. J. Med. 23, 385—90 (1957).

[17b] SAGILD, U.: Hereditary transient paralysis. Copenhagen: Munksgaard 1959.

[18] WEST, E. S., and W. R. TODD: Textbook of Biochemistry 2. ed. New York: Macmillan Company 1956.

* The very recent book: SCHWAB, M., u. K. KÜHNS: Die Störungen des Wassers und Elektrolytstoffwechsels. Heidelberg: Springer 1959. Also gives a thorough discussion of these problems.

II. Distribution of alkali metals in body compartments and tissues

By

NIELS A. THORN

A. The sodium and potassium of the extracellular compartment (and some tissues built mainly of extracellular components)

a) Blood plasma

Since this fluid forms a rapid route of interconnection between the various parts of the extracellular compartment and tends to smooth out concentration differences that may exist among them, it is the natural starting point for a discussion of the distribution of sodium and potassium in the extracellular compartment.

Table 1a. *Concentrations of Na and K in the serum of normal persons belonging to different age-groups* (meq/l). Modified from ELKINTON and DANOWSKI[9]

Age group	Na		K	
	mean*	st. dev.	mean*	st. dev.
Newborn infants	143	3.3	5.9	1.4
Children	144	3.0	4.3	0.4
Young adults	146	2.6	4.4	0.3
Old-age group	144	3.2	4.6	0.4

* Number of determinations were not indicated.

In normal (human) subjects the sodium concentration of the plasma is most efficiently regulated. The average value is about 145 meq/l (Table 1a) with most observations falling within the range 140—150 meq/l. Concentrations below 132 or above 152 meq/l are exceedingly rare in normal subjects. Other mammalian species appear to have very similar concentrations; this applies at least to common lab. animals as dogs, cats, rabbits and rats (ALBRITTON[19]) (Table 1b).

In the case of potassium, the normal plasma concentrations are subject to considerably greater variations on a percentage basis. The average concentration is around 4.5 meq/l, with most observations falling within the range 3.7 to 5.3.

The greater variation for the potassium concentrations can be explained by the high ratio of intracellular to extracellular concentration of this ion. Small disturbances in the dynamic equilibrium between cells and extracellular fluid will profoundly influence the conc. in the latter.

Newborn infants seem to have a higher potassium concentration than individuals in other age groups (see Table 1a). To what extent this may be due to excitement and muscular activity during the blood sampling is not clear. Sex differences seem to be negligible for sodium and potassium. For an illustration of the day-to-day fluctuations in these concentrations the reader is referred to figure 4—11 in the book by ELKINTON and DANOWSKI[9]. Other reports on normal serum

---

[19] ALBRITTON, E. C. (ed.): Standard values in blood, p. 117. Philadelphia and London: W. B. Saunders 1952.

Table 1 b. *Concentrations of Na and K in the serum (S) or plasma (P) of various laboratory animals (meq/l). Modified from* ALBRITTON[19]

		Na			K	
		mean	range		mean	range
monkey	P	152	138—177	P	6.8	4.9—8.7
cat	S	151	147—156	S	4.3	4.0—4.5
dog	S	143	137—149	P	4.4	3.7—5.8
	P	150	135—160			
rabbit	S	141		P	5.1	
	P	136				
guinea pig				S	6.5	
rat	S	134	133—135	S	5.1	4.8—5.4
				P	5.9	5.4—6.4
chicken	P	154	140—175	P	6.4	4. 6—6.5

concentrations are those of FARBER et al.[20], TARAIL et al.[21a], RYSSING[21b] and WOOTOM and KING[22a]. In this latter paper it is stated that the distribution of normal serum sodium values is normal, that of potassium concentrations lognormal. A comparison of results obtained using different methods of analysis is found in the book by TELOH[22b].

It is sometimes preferred to present these concentrations per liter of plasma *water*. This way of presentation has the advantage of expressing directly the contribution of the particular cation to the osmolarity ("tonicity") of the fluid. Obviously, in the case of plasma, this is mainly of interest for sodium, which is the only component on the cation-side materially contributing to the osmolarity. In normal cases the concentrations per liter of *plasma water* can be calculated with sufficient accuracy by adding some 5% to the concentration per liter of *plasma*, since 100 ml (equal to approx. 104 g) of normal plasma contains very nearly 95 ml of water. In cases of pronounced lipaemia the application of such a fixed correction factor is not permissible, since in such cases there may be considerably less than 95 ml of water per 100 ml of plasma. Correspondingly, the sodium concentration per liter of plasma may well be low normal or subnormal, although the concentration per liter of plasma water is quite normal. This point has recently been discussed by ALBRINK, HALD and MAN[23] and ALBRINK, HALD, MAN and PETERS[24a].

[20] FARBER, S. J., E. D. PELLEGRINO, N. J. CONAN, and D. P. EARLE: Observations on the plasma potassium level of man. Amer. J. med. Sci. **221**, 678—87 (1951).

[21a] TARAIL, R., E. S. HACKER, and R. TAYMOR: The ultrafiltrability of potassium and sodium in human serum. J. clin. Invest. **31**, 23—26 (1952).

[21b] RYSSING, E.: Studier over den flammefotometriske metodes fejlkilder og anvendelighed til bestemmelse af kalium og natrium i blod og urin. København: Dansk Videnskabs Forlag 1952.

[22a] WOTTOM, I. D. P., and E. J. KING: Normal values for blood constituents. Hospital differences. Lancet **1**, 470—71 (1953).

[22b] TELOH, H. A.: Clinical flame photometry. Springfield, Ill.: C. C. Thomas 1959.

The high solid content of plasma should be kept in mind when comparisons are made between the conc. of the alkali metals in the plasma and in an ultra-filtrate of plasma. The decrease in the conc. caused by the high protein content approximately cancels the increase caused by the Donnan effect so that the conc. of the alkali metals in an ultrafiltrate are nearly the same as in the plasma when concentration is expressed as mass *per volume solution*[21a].

When the sodium concentration or the sum of cation equivalents per liter is used as an indicator of the tonicity of the plasma it may be wise to recall that in cases of extreme hyperglycaemia (800 mg of glucose per 100 ml of blood) glucose may contribute to the total osmolarity with more than 40 mosm/l or the equivalent of 20 meq of sodium plus matching monovalent anions per liter. Non-protein-nitrogen compounds also contribute to the total osmolarity. It seems, however, that there is a good correlation between serum sodium concentration (expressed as meq/l of serum water) and serum osmolarity when corrections have been made for the osmotic contributions of glucose and non-protein-nitrogen compounds[24b] (see also[14a]).

There are some additional points, which should be kept in mind in evaluating data on plasma concentrations of sodium and potassium.

The possibility of a redistribution of the ions should be kept in mind. The occurrence of an exchange of sodium and potassium between erythrocytes and plasma during the storage of blood is well known; on a percentage basis, such an exchange has the greatest effect on the potassium concentration of plasma. To prevent erroneously high potassium concentrations the plasma should therefore be separated from the corpuscles immediately following the withdrawal of the blood sample. For the same reason heparinization of the blood sample and centrifugation is to be preferred to setting aside a blood sample to await the separation of the clot and the serum. Hemolysis increases the concentration of potassium in the plasma considerably (BERNSTEIN[25]) see chapter on K in erythrocytes) — Disruption of platelets, especially when their number is increased, may have the same effect (see p. 222). — Leucocytes lose K on agitation of a blood sample (p. 103).

It should also be recalled that in the case of plasma potassium determinations, the subject must be kept under fairly standardized conditions for some time before the blood is sampled. Thus, the potassium concentration is lowered following an intake of carbohydrates while muscular exercise (either general or in muscles supplying blood to the vein from which the blood is sampled) may cause considerable rises, especially in untrained individuals (FARBER et al.[20], BLOCK[26], SRÉTER and FRIEDMAN[27a,b], GROB et al.[28] [see also (p. 95) part I of this book].

[23] ALBRINK, M. J., P. M. HALD, and E. B. MAN: Water content of hyperlipemic serum. J. clin. Invest. **33**, 914 (1954).

[24a] ALBRINK, M. J., P. M. HALD, E. B. MAN, and J. P. PETERS: The displacement of serum water by the lipids of hyperlipemic serum. A new method for the rapid determination of serum water. J. clin. Invest. **34**, 1483—1488 (1955).

[24b] EDELMAN, I. S., J. LEIBMAN, M. P. O'MEARA, and L. W. BIRKENFELD: Interrelations between serum sodium concentration, serum osmolarity and total exchangeable sodium, total exchangeable potassium and total body water. J. clin. Invest. **37**, 1236—56 (1958).

[25] BERNSTEIN, R.: Serum and plasma preparation for potassium analysis, effects of anticoagulants, storage time and temperature before separation, and haemolysis. Sth Afr. J. med. Sci. **18**, 99—104 (1953).

[26] BLOCK, J. D.: Effects of handling and eating on plasma electrolytes. Science **127**, 1056—57 (1958).

[27a] SRÉTER, F. A., and S. M. FRIEDMAN: The effect of muscular exercise on plasma sodium and potassium in the rat. Canad. J. Biochem. **36**, 333—38 (1958).

[27b] SRÉTER, F. A., and S. M. FRIEDMAN: Sodium, potassium and lactic acid after muscular exercise in the rat. Canad. J. Biochem. **36**, 1193—1201 (1958).

Reports in the literature on wider ranges of normal plasma concentrations than those mentioned above, may possibly be attributed to failure to consider some of these factors; this, in particular, applies to the higher potassium values reported.

As with other plasma electrolytes, the state of the sodium and potassium — whether "free" or somehow "bound" to plasma constituents, in particular the proteins — has been the object of some dispute. [For a general discussion of protein-binding of the alkali metals, the reader is referred to Part I chapter II (i).] (References to papers showing that Li is not protein-bound are found on p. 223.)

The experimental approach to this problem has been to determine whether the GIBBS-DONNAN ratios calculated from the distributions of these ions between plasma (serum) and an ultrafiltrate or equilibrium dialysate are equal to those of other ions and to the calculated theoretical ratio.

As is well known, DONNAN's law requires the following relationships between diffusable (filterable) monovalent ions

$$r = \frac{[A^-]_P \cdot f_P^{A^-}}{[A^-]_F \cdot f_F^{A^-}} = \frac{[C^+]_F \cdot f_F^{C^+}}{[C^+]_P \cdot f_P^{C^+}}$$

where the signs in brackets indicate concentrations *(per volume of water)* of any diffusible monovalent cation (C^+) or Anion (A^-) in plasma (subscript P) or ultra-filtrate (subscript F), and the f signs the activity coefficients of these ions in the two phases.

The calculation of the theoretical Donnan ratio (cf. VAN SLYKE et al.[29]) requires knowledge of the cation equivalency of the plasma proteins ("protein-bound base" in the old terminology, i. e. the number of equivalents of cations matching the excess of negative charges on the plasma proteins) and further involves the assumption of identical activity coefficients for the major diffusible ions in both phases.

The theoretical Donnan ratio, thus calculated for plasma and a protein-free filtrate is approximately 0.96 for monovalent ions, but subject, of course, to some variation with p_H, CO_2 tension and protein concentration.

When the Donnan ratios for various ions calculated from their observed total *concentrations* in the two phases are found to differ from each other and from the theoretical value it indicates the existence of differences between the activity coefficients in the two phases (which is just another way of saying that the motility of the ion in question is reduced to different degrees in the two phases by some kind of binding to other molecules).

Donnan ratios for sodium and potassium have been calculated in this way both for equilibrations across collodion membranes and natural membranes, especially those of the serous cavities (peritoneal, pleural and pericardiac). A considerable number of such data have recently been collected and recalculated by MANERY[30]. The reader is referred to that review for the detailed data; however, the average values and the ranges of the observed ratios are given in Table 2, together with the calculated theoretical ratios.

From these data it is apparent that in the case of sodium the ratios calculated from the observed concentrations correspond on the whole very closely to the

[28] GROB, D., A. LILJESTRAND, and R. J. JOHNS: Potassium movement in normal subjects. Amer. J. Med. **23**, 340—55 (1957).

[29] SLYKE, D. D. VAN, H. WU, and F. C. McLEAN: Studies of gas and electrolyte equilibria in the blood. V. Factors controlling the electrolyte and water distribution in the blood. J. biol. Chem. **56**, 765—849 (1923).

[30] MANERY, J. F.: Water and electrolyte metabolism. Physiol. Rev. **34**, 334—417 (1954).

theoretical values. This, together with the observation that the same also applies to the ratios for chloride (average 0.97) and bicarbonate (average 0.99), must be taken as an indication that *sodium — as well as chloride and bicarbonate — are almost exclusively present in plasma in the "free" ionic state* and that the activity coefficients of these ions in plasma do not differ very much from those applying to a protein-free filtrate. The tendency of the ratio for sodium to be a little too low may mean, however, that the activity coefficients of these ions are slightly lowered in the presence of proteins.

The Donnan ratios for potassium (average about 0.75) are seen to deviate considerably more from the theoretical value (0.96). The correct interpretation of these deviations is still a matter of dispute. It is already apparent from the ranges presented in Table 2 that the magnitude of the observed deviations differs

Table 2. *Donnan ratios for Na and K calculated from concentrations in plasma (serum = S) and ultrafiltrates (= F).* Modified from MANERY[30]

Conditions of equilibration	$\dfrac{Na_F}{Na_S}$	$\dfrac{K_F}{K_S}$	Calculated theoretical ratio (average)
A. Distribution across collodion membranes (filtrate practically protein-free)	0.91 (0.906—0.922)	0.76 (0.71—0.82)	0.96
B. Distribution between plasma and transudates			
a) transudates with less than 1% protein	0.95 (0.936—0.978)	0.74 (0.537—0.944)	0.956
b) transudates with more than 1% protein	0.95 (0.928—0.967)	0.80 (0.75—0.85)	0.97

considerably from one investigation to another. The same discrepancy appears from other data in the literature. Thus potassium ratios considerably below the theoretical have been reported from *in vitro* experiments by RICHTER-QUITTNER[31] and ROTSCHILD[32]. On the other hand, potassium ratios very close to the theoretical value have been observed by RONA et al.[33] and TARAIL et al.[21a] in *in vitro* experiments and by EICHELBERGER and RONA[34] and by FOLK et al.[35] in *in vivo* studies. The possibility that the observed deviations may be due to methodical short-comings must therefore be given serious consideration. At present the question must be held *sub judice*. If future *in vitro* studies confirm the earlier observed low potassium ratios, then we shall have to accept the occurrence of a binding of potassium in preference to sodium to the proteins (or differently stated: that the negative charges of the plasma proteins have K/Na ion selectivity coefficients above one). Quite apart from the general interest which attaches to ion selectivities exerted by charged macromolecules (see p. 5,9) this question also has significance for the problem of renal excretion of potassium by filtration versus tubular secretion.

[31] RICHTER-QUITTNER, M.: Zur Methodik der chemischen Blutanalyse III. Biochem. Z. **124**, 106—113 (1921).
[32] ROTSCHILD, G.: Die nicht-ultrafiltrierbare Fraktion des Kaliums im Blutserum normaler und adrenalectomierter Tiere. Thesis Basel 1939.
[33] RONA, P., F. HAUROWITZ u. H. PETOW: Beitrag zur Frage der Ionenverteilung im Blutserum. II. Biochem. Z. **149**, 393—398 (1924).
[34] EICHELBERGER, L., and M. RONA: An unusual case of generalized anasarca appearing in an impounded dog with cirrhosis of the liver. J. Lab. clin. med. **31**, 785—792 (1946).
[35] FOLK, B. P., K. L. ZIERLER, and J. L. LILIENTHAL jr: Distribution of potassium and sodium between serum and certain extracellular fluids in man. Amer. J. Physiol. **153**, 381—385 (1948).

Changes in the concentrations, besides being due to changes in water content of the extracellular fluid compartments, may be caused by loss or gain from the outside or to internal deposition or mobilization. Stores of a considerable capacity, at least for sodium (some 480 meq) exist in bone and seem possibly to function as a "buffer" with a large capacity in the regulation of the sodium concentration of the extracellular fluid (see p. 213).

There is no definite correlation between the plasma concentrations of sodium or potassium and the total body contents of these metals (see discussion or page 232). The question whether, then, the serum potassium concentration reflects the potassium need of patients, has recently been discussed by SCRIBNER and BURNELL[40a]. — There is a high degree of correlation, however, between serum sodium concentration (meq/l of serum water) and the ratio of total exchangeable sodium + total exchangeable potassium to total body water[24b]. For a discussion of the use of this relation as a basis for a classification of hypo- and hypernatremic states the reader is referred to[24b].

Plasma from rats acclimatized to cold (5° C) had a higher Na concentration (139.5 $\pm$ 1.6 meq/l) than control rats kept at 26° C (134.5 $\pm$ 1.5 meq/l). No change in K conc. was found[39b].

The plasma half-life of Na^{22} obviously differs with sodium intake (OPDYKE and CLARK[40c]). In humans on an intake of 13.7 gm NaCl/day it was 8 days, on 1.7 g NaCl 25 days. In small dogs on a intake of 3.88 gm of NaCl daily the half-life of Na^{22} was 6 days.

Acute respiratory acidosis and acute respiratory alkalosis produce a rise and a fall, respectively, in the concentration of potassium in the serum (SCRIBNER et al.[36], HICKAM et al.[37]).

In the rhesus monkey hypophysectomy is associated with a small, but significant reduction in the serum sodium concentration and a rise in the concentration of potassium[38].

Norepinephrine and epinephrine infusions produce an elevation of the serum potassium concentration and a decrease in the concentration of sodium. For a discussion of the mechanisms of this action, the reader should consult the paper by MUIRHEAD et al.[39a].

Effects of other hormones on plasma conc. are discussed on p. 537.

In a recent review some causes and effects of abnormalities in the concentration of sodium in the serum were discussed (DARROW and HELLERSTEIN[14a]).

b) Lymph

It is generally held that fluid leaves the blood capillaries by a process of ultrafiltration. Also, there is general agreement that it is not an ideal but an incomplete ultrafiltration since the capillary walls are somewhat permeable to the plasma proteins.

For a tissue which is in a metabolic steady state and which has no excretory or absorptive function the amount of water leaving it by way of the lymph vessels must equal the net amount entering from the blood capillaries plus the oxidation water.

---

[36] SCRIBNER, B. H., K. FREMONT-SMITH, and J. M. BURNELL: The effect of acute respiratory acidosis on the internal equilibrium of potassium. J. clin. Invest. **34**, 1276—1285 (1955).

[37] HICKAM, J. B., W. P. WILSON, and R. FRAYSER: Observations on the early elevation of serum potassium during respiratory alkalosis. J. clin. Invest. **35**, 601—606 (1956).

[38] KNOBIL, E., and R. O. GREEP: Serum electrolytes in the hypophysectomized rhesus monkey. Endocrinol. **62**, 61—63 (1958).

[39a] MUIRHEAD, E. E., A. GOTH, and J. JONES: Sodium and potassium exchanges associated with nor-epinephrine infusion. Amer. J. Physiol. **179**, 1—4 (1954).

[39b] HANNON, J. P., A. M. LARSON, and D. W. YOUNG: Effect of cold acclimatization on plasma electrolyte levels. J. appl. Physiol. **13**, 239—240 (1958).

The same also applies to the amounts of inorganic constituents, with the possible exception of bicarbonate, viz. if there is a steady production or breakdown of acids in the tissue. Consequently, as long as we are dealing with such a tissue the concentrations of sodium and potassium in the lymph will be equal to those in the net filtrate from the blood capillaries. A deviating composition is to be expected in lymph draining from excretory and absorptive tissues as well as tissues which are not in metabolic equilibrium. There are no data on the composition of lymph from a variety of organs and plasma, determined simultaneously. Some average figures, however, representing a considerable number of analyses on thoracic duct lymph, cervical lymph and blood serum from dogs, are given in Table 3a.

Table 3a. *Composition of lymph and blood serum (dogs)* (Na, K: meq/l, protein: gm/100 ml). Modified from MANERY[30]

Constituent	Serum	Thoracic duct lymph	Cervical lymph
Na	148	144	150
K	3.3	4.8	4.0
Protein	6.83	4.41	3.06

3b). *Composition of thoracic duct lymph and blood serum (patient with lung cancer)* (meq/l). Modified from LINDER and BLOMSTRAND[40b]

Constituent	Serum	Fasting lymph	Lymph collected during fat absorption
Na	142	138	140
K	4.7	3.3	4.2
Cl-	98	97	94

It appears that the sodium concentration of the lymph is quite close to that of an ideal ultrafiltrate, despite the fact that neither the thoracic duct lymph nor the cervical lymph originate exclusively from tissues without excretory or absorptive functions. The potassium concentrations of the lymph samples are, however, somewhat higher than might be expected for a plasma ultrafiltrate. Various explanations may be offered to account for this deviation. Most likely it is caused by a lack of a steady state which obviously is easily upset in the case of potassium, due to its high intra-extracellular concentration ratio (see section on plasma). Addition of lymphocytes from the lymph glands and secretion or absorption of fluids with potassium concentrations deviating from that of the blood plasma are other possibilities. Finally, blood and lymph samples were not always collected simultaneously. It is noteworthy that fasting human thoracic duct lymph collected by the method of LINDER and BLOMSTRAND had a conc. of potassium that was lower than that of fasting serum[40b] (Table 3b).

From the above argumentation and from the data cited as well as others it is reasonable to assume that, as regards its inorganic composition, lymph corresponds very closely to that of an ultrafiltrate of plasma.

c) Interstitial spaces

From the close similarity of the lymph to a plasma ultrafiltrate it follows that there must exist in the interstitial spaces a fluid phase which has an inorganic composition like an ultrafiltrate of plasma. This phase is subject to continuous replacement by inflow and outflow of fluids of similar composition.

Evidently, the existence of such a "movable" fluid phase in the interstices does not exclude, by any means, the co-existence of another fluid phase, which is

[40a] SCRIBNER, B. H., and J. M. BURNELL: Interpretation of the serum potassium concentration. Metabolism 5, 468—479 (1956).

[40b] LINDER, E., and R. BLOMSTRAND: Technique for collection of thoracic duct lymph of man. Proc. Soc. exp. Biol. (N. Y.) 97, 653—657 (1958).

[40c] OPDYKE, D. F., and I. CLARK: Plasma half life of Na^{22} in dogs. Proc. Soc. exp. Biol. (N. Y.) 88, 207—209 (1955).

more fixed and which does not ordinarily participate in the net movements of fluid into and out of the interstices. In fact the possibility exists that such a second phase may, in some cases, contain even a major part of the fluid present in the interstices.

At the present moment, it is unfortunately impossible to form a clear idea of how large amounts of such "fixed" fluid there exist in the interstitial spaces of various tissues, and what the composition of such fluid would be.

It is, however, unquestionable that the interstitial spaces of many tissues contain various charged macromolecules which — at least for the purpose of the present considerations — may be regarded as permanently present there. The fixed charges of such macromolecules (e.g. hyaluronic acid, chondroitin sulfate[41]) or structural components (e.g. collagenous fibrils) will have small ions of the opposite charges attached to them as counter-ions (see p. 6).

To the extent that these matching ions are osmotically active they will in turn attract water from the surrounding fluid until the activity of water in the fluid phase encircling the macromolecule (+ any possibly tension exerted by the macromolecule due to swelling caused by water entrance) is equal to the activity of water in the surrounding "free" fluid. Consequently we must count on the existence of a phase of "fixed" fluid adhering to such macromolecules. The amount of this fluid and its composition must depend upon the numbers and types of charges on the macromolecule, and the p_H and ionic composition of the surrounding fluid in the same way as has been borne out by numerous studies on synthetic and natural resins (cf. e.g. the symposium edited by MINER[42]). The possibility exists that a particular macromolecule may have both small cations and anions attached to it, viz. if it acts as a mixed cation-anion exchange resin by means of acidic and basic groups spaced sufficiently apart to exclude mutual interaction. If the isoelectric point of a macromolecular compound is observed to be, say, definitely below the p_H of the surrounding free fluid the only information thereby provided will be that an excess of cations are attached to it. There may be an additional attachment of both cations and anions.

With regard to the above mentioned terms "attached ions" and "fixed water" it should be understood that the linkages in question are fairly loose, and that these components are easily exchangeable with other ion and water molecules from the surrounding fluid. Consequently, they will be included in determinations of the "exchangeable" water and sodium (potassium) contents by means of isotope dilution methods if sufficient time is provided to allow equilibration to take place between the blood plasma and the "free" fluid surrounding the macromolecules.

It is obvious that determinations of plasma ultrafiltrate concentrations of alkali metals do not give any true picture of the conc. in such parts of the extracellular fluid where binding to polyelectrolytes occurs.

Relation of the "sodium space" to the extracellular space

This is not the place for a detailed discussion of the measurement of the volume of distribution of sodium (and potassium), and the relation of the sodium space to the extracellular space, measured by various substances (such as inulin or sucrose) considered to remain in the extracellular fluid. Generally it may be said, that the sodium space is somewhat larger than the inulin or sucrose space.

[41] FARBER, S., and M. SCHUBERT: The binding of cations by chondroitin sulfate. J. clin. Invest. **36**, 1715—1722 (1957).

[42] MINER, A. W. (ed.): Ion exchanges resins in medicine and biological research. Ann. N. Y. Acad. Sci. **57**, 61 (1953).

For discussions of these problems the reader is referred to the papers by Burch et al.[43], Berson and Yalow[44] and the review by Darrow and Hellerstein[14a].

The concept that the Cl space on the whole is an indicator of the extracellular space, originally put forward by Harrison et al.[45], has recently received new attention by the study of Cheek et al.[46]. It was found that 87.3% of the body chloride in rats was present in the extracellular fluid, the bulk of the rest being present in erythrocytes and the gut lumen. There was a very close similarity between the extracellular fluid volume calculated from corrected extracellular fluid chloride and corrected extracellular fluid sodium (see also p. 212, 509).

d) Tendon

Average values for analyses of rabbit and dog tendons are given in Table 4.

From these data it is apparent that the contents of sodium and chloride per liter of tendon water are very close to those of an ideal plasma ultrafiltrate — and parenthetically the same appears to hold for bicarbonate. The Cl. conc. is somewhat higher. The potassium concentration is a good deal higher, but not more than might be explained by the occurrence of a small cell phase with a high potassium concentration.

Table 4. *Analyses of tendons. Electrolyte concentrations are given per liter of tendon water; Donnan ratios are calculated from these concentrations and the concentrations per liter of serum water. Adapted from* Manery[30]

Tendons from	H_2O %	Na meq/l water	$\frac{Na_T}{Na_S}$	K meq/l water	Cl meq/l water	$\frac{Cl_S}{Cl_T}$
Rabbits	61.8	124.7	0.83		121	0.88
Dogs	66.8	139.8	0.91	9.1	102.8	0.99

The electrolyte composition of the extracellular fluid of tendons appears then to be very similar to that of an ideal plasma ultrafiltrate. This, of course, does not imply that electrolytes and water could not, in part, be "attached" to the structural elements of the interstitial space. It means, however, that if such attachment takes place to any appreciable extent, water and electrolytes must be attached in proportions very similar to those at which they occur in blood plasma.

At present, it is not known if and to what extent such attachment exists. The isoelectric point of collagen, which comprises some 90% of the organic constituents of tendons, has recently been reported to be at p_H 7—8 (Gustavson[47]). This implies that no appreciable *excess* of cations or anions should be associated with collagen, but obviously does not exclude some association of equimolar amounts of both types with free amino and carboxyl groups. Tendomucoid for which an isoelectric point of 4.5 has been reported (Day[48a]) must have an excess of cations

[43] Burch, G. E., C. T. Ray, and S. A. Threefoot: Some theoretic considerations of electrolyte space measured by the tracer method in intact man. J. Lab. clin. Med. **42**, 34—57 (1953).

[44] Berson, S., A. and R. S. Yalow: Critique of extracellular space measurements with small ions, Na24 and Br82 spaces. Science **121**, 34—36 (1955).

[45] Harrison, H. E., D. C. Darrow, and H. Yannet: Total electrolyte content of animals and its probable relation to the distribution of body water. J. biol. Chem. **113**, 515—529 (1936).

[46] Cheek, D. B., C. D. West, and C. C. Golden: The distribution of sodium and chloride and the extracellular fluid volume in the rat. J. clin. Invest. **36**, 340—351 (1957).

[47] Gustavson, K. H.: Advanc. Protein Chem. **5**, 353 (1949).

[48a] Day, T. D.: The mode of reaction of interstitial connective tissue with water. J. Physiol. **109**, 380—391 (1949).

associated with it, but this could hardly be expected to have appreciable effect on the overall composition, since tendomucoid accounts for only a few per cent of the total tendon weight.

AUDIA[48b] recently reported that the Na conc. in rat tail tendon water is somewhat lower than in an ultrafiltrate of plasma.

e) Corium

Determinations of the sodium and potassium content of corium present great difficulties, mainly due to the problem involved in separating the corium from the lowest layer of the epidermis and from the fat-rich tissue on which it is often layered. Hairs and skin glands are inevitably included also. It is obvious that admixture of cells from the Malphigian layer will cause the greatest disturbances in the determination of potassium, whereas admixture of fat tissue with its very low water content causes a more general reduction in the concentrations of the electrolytes when they are determined on a fresh tissue weight basis.

Some of the most reliable analyses of corium available seem to be those of EICHELBERGER and ROMA[49] in dogs in which heating to 50° C (the method of BAUMBERGER et al.[50]) was used for separation of the layers. Table 5a shows the average concentrations.

For a long time there has been a standing discussion whether skin functions as a depot for chloride, that is whether Cl^- ions are stored "dry" in the skin. MANERY in a recent review[30] discussed evidence which seemed to exclude this possibility. — Recently great losses in the sodium content of skin have been produced in the sodium depleting experiments of NICHOLS and NICHOLS[51] as well

Table 5a. *Concentrations of Na and K in whole skin, corium and epidermis of dogs* (meq/100 g of fat-free solids). Adapted from EICHELBERGER and ROMA[49]

	Na	K	Cl
Whole skin	34.2	8.5	30.2
Corium	34.6	8.1	30.7
Epidermis	31.0	12.2	26.8

Table 5b. *Concentrations of Na and K in the cornea and aqueous humour of the ox* (meq/kg of water). Modified from DAVSON[130]

	Na	K
Cornea . . .	147.2	29.4
Aqueous humour	149.5	7.1

as in those of WOODBURY[52]. In the first, some 25% of the sodium of skin was removed by acute sodium depletion produced by vivodialysis. There was a fairly similar loss of water from the skin. — These losses are apparently satisfactorily accounted for as losses of interstitial fluid and there appears, at the moment, not to be convincing evidence for the existence of depots of "fixed" ions or water.

f) Cornea

A comparison of the Na and K conc. of the ox cornea and aqueous humour is shown in Table 5b.

[48b] AUDIA, M.: Sodium and chloride spaces and water content of tendon in normal and depleted rats. Amer. J. Physiol. **195**, 702—704 (1958).

[49] EICHELBERGER, L., and M. ROMA: Electrolyte and nitrogen distribution in whole fat-free skin and heat-separated corium and epidermis. J. invest. Derm. **12**, 125—138, (1949).

[50] BAUMBERGER, J. P., V. SUNTZEFF, and E. V. COWDRY: Methods for the separation of epidermis from dermis and some physiologic and chemical properties of isolated epidermis. J. nat. Cancer Inst. **2**, 413—423 (1942).

[51] NICHOLS, G. jr., and N. NICHOLS: Changes in tissue composition during acute sodium depletion. Amer. J. Physiol. **186**, 383—392 (1956).

[52] WOODBURY, D. M.: Effect of acute hyponatremia on distribution of water and electrolytes in various tissues of the rat. Amer. J. Physiol. **185**, 281—286 (1956).

The high concentration of K is probably due to the fact that the epithelium constitutes some 15—20% of the weight of the ox cornea.

The question of the regulation of the state of hydration of the cornea has not been answered satisfactorily yet. However, the fact that various procedures which decrease the rate of metabolism of the cornea are accompanied by a swelling of the cornea would indicate the possibility of the existence of an active transport mechanism of some sort in the cornea epithelium. — This does not seem to involve Na since recent studies of the transport of Na[24] in both directions across the cornea of rabbits *in vivo* (MAURICE [53a, 53b]) were "consistent with the hypothesis that each of the epithelial and endothelial layers behave as an inert membrane".

B. The sodium and potassium of cartilage and bone

a) Cartilage

Probably the most comprehensive analyses of the composition of cartilage are those published by EICHELBERGER et al.[53c, 53d]. A selection of their average data is presented in Table 6. For a detailed discussion of the influence of age on these values the reader should consult[53c]. Other data — which agree well with them — may be found in the review by MANERY[30].

Table 6. *Composition of hyaline cartilage from diverse sources.* Electrolyte concentrations are given both as meq/kg of wet tissue and (in parenthesis) as meq/l of cartilage water. Sulfate is given in millimols and from this the chondroitin sulfate content (CS) has been calculated. F signifies "fiber solids" which is almost exclusively (about 90%) collagen. Modified from MANERY[30]

Source	H_2O gm/kg	Solids g/kg		Cl meq	Na meq	K meq	Ca meq	Mg meq	SO_4 mM
Trachea (adult beef)	710*	290*	F:147 CS:80	34.4 (48.5)	273 (385)	25 (35)	35 (49)	20 (29)	170 (240)
					total:(498)				
Costal (puppies 7—10 weeks)	745	255	F:133 CS:51	52.3 (70.2)	230 (309)	57.6 (77.3)	25.5 (34.2)	19.2 (25.8)	109 (146)
					total:(446)				
Articular (puppies 7—10 weeks)	764	236	F:109 CS:47.5	55.8 (73)	214 (280)	52.8 (69.2)	26 (34)	16.5 (22)	102 (133)
					total:(405)				

* Assumed values.

The most striking feature appearing from the data of Table 6 is the occurrence of very high concentrations of cations. As expressed in the parentheses of this table — per liter of cartilage water — the total cation concentrations amount to some 450 meq/l. This means that if they were all completely osmotically active, the cations *alone* would confer to the fluids of cartilage an osmolarity well above that of blood plasma (some 290 mosm/kg of water). Clearly, a considerable frac-

---

[53a] MAURICE, D. M.: The permeability to sodium ions of the living rabbit's cornea. J. Physiol. **112**, 367—391 (1951).

[53b] MAURICE, D. M.: The permeability of the cornea. Ophthal. Literature (Lond.) **7**, 3—25 (1953).

[53c] EICHELBERGER, L., T. B. BROWN, and M. ROMA: Histochemical characterization of inorganic constituents, connective tissue and the chondroitin sulphate of extracellular and intracellular compartments of hyaline cartilage. Amer. J. Physiol. **166**, 328—339 (1951).

[53d] EICHELBERGER, L., W. H. AKESON, and M. ROMA: Biochemical studies of articular cartilage I. Normal values. J. Bone Jt. Surg. **40**-A, 142—152 (1958).

tion of the cations must be bound in such a way that their osmotic activity is
appreciably reduced.

No doubt the chondroitin-sulfate containing chondromucoid, which is present
in cartilage in considerable quantities (cf. Table 6), is responsible for this binding.
Such binding is suggested by the parallellism of changes which occur in chondroitin-sulfate and sodium content with age. The chemical character of the
complex has been discussed in the papers by MATHEWS[54, 55] and by FARBER and
SCHUBERT[41] (see also p. 8).

BOYD and NEUMAN[56], who studied the cation-(Na, Ca and Ba) binding capacity
of veal costal cartilage* have provided evidence that the ester sulfate and glucuronate groups of chondroitin sulfate could account for virtually all of the cation
binding capacity of cartilage. If we consider e.g. the articular cartilage of Table 6,
102 mM of ester sulfate could bind 102 meq of cations and a similar amount could
be bound by the glucuronate groups, making a total of 204 meq per kg of wet
tissue. This accounts, as may be seen, for some $2/3$ of the total cations. It is not
too certain what proportions of the individual cations are bound in this way.
It is most likely, however, that most of the calcium and the major part of the
sodium is bound ("excess" sodium) (see bone p. 211) since the sulfate groups have a
great affinity to the calcium and since sodium is by far the predominant cation
in the free fluid equilibrating with the interstitial structures. Probably small
amounts of potassium and magnesium will also be bound. The amount of water
which is "attached" to the chondromucoid together with the cations is of course a
function of the degree to which the osmotic activity of the counter-cations is
lowered by the electrovalent forces, and of any possible tension developed in the
chondromucoid.

The remaining sodium (say some 60 meq/kg of articular cartilage) may be
visualized as occurring with most of the chloride in a fluid containing both in
similar concentrations as in plasma ultrafiltrate. Such fluid could be associated
in part with the collagen (cf. composition of tendon, above) and in part it could be
present as free fluid.

The major part of the potassium and magnesium could be attributed to the
intracellular phase, being matched there mostly with organic phosphate and
protein anions.

If the ions of the two latter phases are assumed to be completely osmotically
active, a total of nearly 700 gm of water would be required to ensure isotonicity. This,
as may be seen, would leave rather little water to be attached to the chondromucoid.

The association of sodium (and other cations) may therefore be characterized
as a dry storage ("rétention sèche"), i.e. a storage with less water than would be
required to produce isotonicity with the cations in question if they were completely
osmotically active. — A mobilization of such stores would therefore cause an
increase in the tonicity of the body fluids or increase in their volume if the tonicity
remains constant.

EICHELBERGER et al.[53c, 53d] have attempted a more refined subdivision of cartilage in various phases. The justification of such refinements may, however, be
questioned considering the number of assumptions involved in the calculations.

---

[54] MATHEWS, M. B.: Chondroitin sulphuric acid — a linear polyelectrolyte. Arch. Biochem.
a. Biophys. 43, 181—193 (1953).

[55] MATHEWS, M. B., and I. LOZAITYTE: Sodium chondroitin sulfate-protein complexes of
cartilage I. Molecular weight and shape. Arch. Biochem. 74, 158—174 (1958).

[56] BOYD, E. S., and W. F. NEUMAN: The surface chemistry of bone V. The ion-binding
properties of cartilage. J. biol. Chem. 193, 243—251 (1951).

* See also the paper by J. R. DUNSTONE: Some cation-binding properties of cartilage.
Biochem. J. 72, 465—473 (1959).

There is an essential difference between the availability of the "excess" sodium of cartilage and that of bone (see later). In contrast to the "excess" sodium of bone that of cartilage is more readily soluble in water, acids and alkalis and it can all be freely exchanged with radiosodium in the plasma (MANERY and BALE[57]).

The potassium concentration in cartilage decreases with age (IOB and SWAN-SON[58]. This seems to be in good agreement with the demonstration by ROSENTHAL et al.[59] that the number of cells in cartilage decreases with age.

b) Bone

During the last decade many reports have appeared on sodium and potassium in bone. Although some information has been obtained, much more is needed, especially about the function of the Na and K in bone, their availability for general metabolism in the body and the nature of the mechanisms which control the level of sodium and potassium in bone.

For recent detailed discussions of the general structure and function of bone the reader is referred to McLEAN et al.[60], GREEP et al.[61] and NEUMAN and NEU-MAN[62].

Amount of sodium in bone. A considerable part (approximately $1/3$) of total body sodium is contained in bone (HARRISON et al.[45], EDELMAN et al.[63], CHEEK et al.[46]). The content increases with age (BERGSTROM and WALLACE[64], MUNRO et al.[65a], FORBES et al.[66a]) but shows a slight decrease in senile rats[66b].

Table 7a shows some results obtained in recent analyses of bone, others are found in the review by MANERY[30]. It should be stressed that discrepancies in the results of analyses can be expected due to the difficulty of analysis (interference from Ca in flame photometric determination etc.), differences in the regions from which the samples have been taken and differences in the age of the animals. For a list of measurements of the Na content of rat bone from different regions and treated differently the reader is referred to MUNRO et al.[65a]. — Very recently AGNA et al.[65b] have performed a careful study of the mineral content of *normal*

[57] MANERY, J. F., and W. F. BALE: The penetration of radioactive sodium and phosphorus into the extra- and intracellular phases of tissues. Amer. J. Physiol. **132**, 215—132 (1941).

[58] IOB, V., and W. W. SWANSON: The extracellular and intracellular water in bone and cartilage. J. biol. Chem. **122**, 485—490 (1938).

[59] ROSENTHAL, O. J., M. A. BOWIE, and G. WAGONER: Studies in metabolism of articular cartilage, respiration and glycolysis of cartilage in relation to its age. J. cell. comp. Physiol. **17**, 221—233 (1941).

[60] McLEAN, F. C., and M. R. URIST: BONE: An Introduction to the Physiology of Skeletal Tissue. University of Chicago Press. Chicago 1955.

[61] GREEP, R. O. (ed) and others: Recent advances in the study of the structure, composition, and growth of mineralized tissues. Ann. N. Y. Acad. Sci. **60**, 541—805 (1955).

[62] NEUMAN, W. F., and M. W. Neuman: The nature of the mineral phase of bone. Chem. Rev. **53**, 145 (1953).

[63] EDELMAN, I. S., A. H. JAMES, H. BADEN, and F. D. MOORE: Electrolyte composition of bone and the penetration of radiosodium and deuterium oxide into dog and human bone. J. clin. Invest. **33**, 122—131 (1954).

[64] BERGSTROM, W. H., and W. M. WALLACE: Bone as a sodium and potassium reservoir. J. clin. Invest. **33**, 867—873 (1954).

[65a] MUNRO, D. S., R. S. SATOSKAR and G. M. WILSON: The exchange of bone sodium with isotopes in rats. J. Physiol. **139**, 474—488 (1957).

[65b] AGNA, J. W., H. C. KNOWLES, and G. ALVERSON: The mineral content of normal human bone J. clin. Invest. **37**, 1357—1361 (1958).

[66a] FORBES, G. B., G. L. MIZNER, and A. LEWIS: Effect of age on radiosodium exchange in bone (rat). Amer. J. Physiol. **190**, 152—156 (1957).

[66b] FORBES, G. B.: Effect of low sodium diet on sodium content and radiosodium exchange in rat bone. Proc. Soc. exp. Biol. (N. Y.) **98**, 153 —155 (1958).

human skull, rib and ilium. Some of their results are given in Table 7b. They are in agreement with earlier analyses (quoted by them) of bone in *pathological* conditions. It is especially noted that skull contains significantly greater amounts of Na and Ca and less K and N than ilium.

Nature of sodium in bone. Water makes up some 20—30% of bone (MANERY[30]), and since the cells of bone represent only a minute fraction of the volume, practically all the water must be located extracellularly. On the assumption

Table 7a. *Composition of bone.* The data from humans and dogs are from EDELMAN et al.[63]. The data for rats are from LEVITT et al.[84a]

Source	solids g/kg	meq per kg of tissue solids			
		Cl	Na	K	Ca
Human	478—866	29	234		12490
Dog	681—816	19	229		11650
Rat (bone cortex) . .	819	33	288	20	

that this water had the composition of a plasma ultra-filtrate it would contain only some 7% of the total bone sodium in adults (but some 33% in young animals (FORBES et al.[66a])]. Evidently far the greater part of bone sodium must be present extracellularly in an osmotically inactive state. — A comparison of the sodium and chloride concentrations leads to the same conclusion. The Na/Cl ratio is evidently much higher in bone than in a plasma ultra-filtrate. Therefore, even if all the chloride were present as free ions in a mobile extracellular phase with the composition of a plasma ultrafiltrate, this phase would only contain a small fraction of the total sodium. (Actually, all the chloride does not appear to be present in this form since it has been demonstrated (STOLL and NEUMANN[67]) that the hydrated shells of the crystals are freely permeable to Cl]. — It is beyond doubt that far the major part of this "excess" Na is present in crystalline deposits in the bone matrix, but there is little information on the nature of the binding of the "excess" sodium. There is some evidence that it is bound to the inorganic part of bone. Thus there is always a fairly constant ratio between Ca conc. and "excess" Na in bone ash in animals of the same age and on a constant Na intake, and bone Na is much less soluble in strong base than cartilage Na. The constant ratio between Na and Ca in bone (0.02) has been demonstrated by BERGSTROM[68] by CHEEK et al.[46] and by MUNRO et al.[65a]. (It was used by CHEEK et

[67] STOLL, W. R., and W. F. NEUMAN: The uptake of sodium and potassium ions by hydrated hydroxy-apatite. J. Amer. chem. Soc. **78**, 1585—1588 (1956).

[68] BERGSTROM, W. H.: The partipation of bone in total body sodium metabolism in the rat. J. clin. Invest. **34**, 997—1004 (1955).

Table 7b. *The composition of normal human skull, rib and ilium. Modified from AGNA et al.[65b].*

No. of samples	H₂O (wet bone) %	Fat (dry bone) %	Per Kilogram dry, fat-free bone								
			H₂O g	Ca eq	P g	CO₃ eq	N g	Cl meq	K meq	Na meq
Skull (10)	17.6±3.7	4.2±2.9	229± 63	12.5±0.27	111.1±3.7	1.70±0.06	48.1±4.5	28.3±6.1	16.4± 6.8	291±6.8
Rib (14)	21.6±6.4	6.4±5.3	319±143	11.6±0.47	104.5±4.7	1.63±0.10	53.4±3.1	35.3±9.0	34.0±11.6	268±8.3
Ilium (13)	25.8±4.0	14.1±7.3	448±139	11.4±0.64	100.5±5.1	1.61±0.08	56.0±3.9	41.1±8.6	38.9± 9.4	269±10.8

14*

al. as part of the correction employed to calculate extracellular sodium from total body Na in rats (see interstitial spaces p. 206). The hypothesis was advanced by NEUMAN et al.[69] (see also NEUMAN and NEUMAN[70]) that sodium and potassium is present at the crystal surface (ENGSTRÖM[71]) as a double salt of carbonate in a binding of the following type: $Ca-O-CO_2-Na$. This concept has been supported by BERGSTROM[72,73a] who reported equimolar losses of Na + K and carbonate from bone in acidosis. The hydrogen ions presumably act with the carbonate to form Na^+ and bicarbonate. The nature of bone carbonate has recently been discussed by BUCHANAN and NAKAO[73b].

"Availability", function of sodium in bone. Not all the Na of bone is readily exchangeable with radiosodium. Values given for the exchangeable sodium of adult bone are about 30—40% (for a list of references see BERGSTROM[68] and FORBES et al.[66a]). Acidosis produced by intraperitoneal injection of ammonium chloride or observed in patients can be associated with mobilization of maximally a similar part of the bone sodium (BERGSTROM[73a]). Since the extracellular fluid phase of sodium of bone only constitutes some 10% this must mean that part of the "excess" Na is exchangeable; on the other hand it also shows that a determination of the volume of distribution of Na without considerable corrections cannot give a true measure of the total amount of extracellular fluid (see p. 206).

In young animals a much larger fraction of skeletal sodium is exchangeable (FORBES et al.[66a]). This difference in the exchangeability of sodium in young and old animals can be explained as due to the difference in hydration and compactness of the bone crystals (NICHOLS and NICHOLS[74]) (see also p. 230).

From the foregoing it may thus be seen that Na seems to exist in bone in 3 phases: 1) the "fluid phase Na", 2) the "exchangeable" part of the "crystal phase Na" and 3) the "unexchangeable" part of the "crystal phase Na". There is a very great interest attached to the possible function of the "excess" (crystal phase) sodium. Because of the great amount represented in this fraction, mobilizations from it would cause considerable changes in the osmolar concentration of the extracellular fluid, or — if isotonicity is maintained — in the volume of this fluid (see cartilage 209).

In the papers by NICHOLS and NICHOLS[74, 75, 76a] a number of references can be found to studies demonstrating the effects of loading and restricting sodium on the Na content of bone. An approximate 6—13% of bone Na can be mobilized in adult animals by hyponatremic stimuli. (WINTHERS et al.[76b] have recently sug-

[69] NEUMAN, W. F., M. W. NEUMAN, E. R. MAIN, J. O'LEARY and F. A. SMITH: The surface chemistry of bone II. Fluriode deposition. J. biol. Chem. 187, 655—661 (1950).

[70] NEUMAN, W. F., and M. W. NEUMAN: Emerging concepts of the structure and metabolic functions of bone. Amer. J. Med. 22, 123—131 (1957).

[71] ENGSTRÖM, A.: Structure of bone from the anatomical to the molecular level in: Ciba Found. Symposium: Bone Structure and Metabolism. p. 3—13 London: Churchill.

[72] BERGSTROM, W. H.: The relationships of Na and K to carbonate in bone. J. biol. Chem. 206, 711—715 (1954).

[73a] BERGSTROM, W. H.: The skeleton as an electrolyte reservoir. Metabolism 5, 433—437 (1956).

[73b] BUCHANAN, D. L., and A. NAKAO: Studies on the nature of bone carbonate. Arch. Biochem. Biophys. 77, 168—180 (1958).

[74] NICHOLS, G., and N. NICHOLS: The role of bone in sodium metabolism. Metabolism 5, 438—446 (1956).

[75] NICHOLS, G. jr., and N. NICHOLS: Changes in tissue composition during acute sodium depletion. Amer. J. Physiol. 186, 383—392 (1956).

[76a] NICHOLS, N., and G. NICHOLS jr.: Effect of large loads of sodium on bone and soft tissue composition. Proc. Soc. exp. Biol. (N. Y.) 96, 835—839 (1957).

[76b] WINTHERS, R. W., R. T. WHITLOCK, J. L. DE WALT and L. G. WELT: Effect of alterations of the sodium concentration of the serum upon the content of sodium in bone. Amer. J. Physiol. 195, 691—701 (1958).

gested that the stimulus for mobilization in these cases was a simultaneous acidosis).
An approximate increase of 9% was observed after loading rats with Na [A
maximum change in the concentration of sodium in bone (20% of bone sodium)
would mean release of a total amount of some 480 meq].

The exchangeable part of bone sodium seems to function as a reservoir for
body Na. This depot can be mobilized after sodium loss due to vivodialysis
(NICHOLS and NICHOLS[76a]) after intraperitoneal glucose and ammonium chloride
(WOODBURY[77], MUNRO et al.[65a] and possibly under influence of adrenocortical
hormones (LUFT et al.[78], FLANAGAN et al.[79a], MUNRO et al.[79b]*, whereas it is
uninfluenced by thyroxine or (surprisingly) by parathormone[79c]. Despite severe losses
of sodium in the studies of MUNRO et al., the conc. of sodium in the extracellular
fluid (at least in the young animals) remained unchanged. — RENWICK et al.[80a] did
not observe any change in the serum sodium level even after 30 days of severe Na
restriction in man. This must indicate reservoir function or contraction of extracellular fluid volume. FORBES et al.[66a] stated that in diabetic acidosis, the net changes
in crystal Na content closely parallelled changes in the exchangeable fraction. This
was also the case in young rats reared on a low sodium diet[66b]. (These results were
in disagreement with those of MUNRO et al.[65a].)

It should be stressed that FORBES et al.[80b] in their recent studies on the response
of bone sodium to acute changes in extracellular fluid composition in cats found
only small declines in bone sodium after short term infusions of various acids,
alkalies and glucose solutions. The nature of the stimulus for the small release
of Na could not be identified since there was no correlation between the release
and changes in blood p_H, plasma Na conc. or total ECF Na content. — Sodium
loading caused no deposition of Na in bone.

As might be expected, the "unchangeable" fraction of sodium does not
seem to function as any very labile reservoir. If this were so, one would expect
large discrepancies between the results of metabolic balance studies and isotope
dilution methods. This was not found in the studies of WILSON et al.[81].

Also the "unexchangeable" part of bone sodium can, however, be "utilized",
but much more slowly than the exchangeable part. Uptake of Na[22] in the "unexchangeable" part has been demonstrated in man (MILLER et al.[82]) and in rats
(GREEN et al.[83]). Mobilization from this fraction was demonstrated by MUNRO et al.[65a].

[77] WOODBURY, D. M.: Effect of acute hyponatremia on distribution of water and electrolytes in various tissues of the rat. Amer. J. Physiol. 185, 281—286 (1956).
[78] LUFT, R., B. SJÖGREN, D. IKKOS, H. LJUNGGREN, and H. TARUKASKI: Clinical studies
on electrolyte and fluid metabolism. Rec. Progr. Horm. Res. 10, 425—470 (1954).
[79a] FLANAGAN, J. B., A. K. DAVIS, and R. R. OVERMAN: Mechanism of extracellular
sodium and chloride depletion in adrenalectomized dog. Amer. J. Physiol. 160, 89—102 (1950).
[79b] MUNRO, D. S., R. S. SATOSKAR, and G. M. WILSON: The effect of adrenalectomy on
bone sodium J. Physiol. 142, 438—446 (1958).
[79c] MUNRO, D. S., R. S. SATOSKAR, and G. M. WILSON: Bone calcium and sodium content
and the exchange of radiosodium in bones from rats treated with thyroxine and parathormone
J. Physiol 142, 447—452 (1958).
[80a] RENWICK, R., J. S. ROBSON, and C. P. STEWART: Observations upon the withdrawal
of sodium chloride from the diet in hypertensive and normotensive individuals. J. clin. Invest.
34, 1037—1043 (1955).
[80b] FORBES, G. B., R. B. TOBIAN and H. LEWIS: Response of bone sodium to acute changes
in extracellular fluid composition (cat). Amer. J. Physiol. 196, 69—73 (1959).
[81] WILSON, G. M., J. M. OLNEY, L. BROOKE, J. A. MYRDEN, M. R. BALL, and F. D. MOORE:
Body sodium and potassium II. A comparison of metabolic balance and isotope dilution
methods of study. Metabolism 3, 324—333 (1954).
[82] MILLER, H., D. S. MUNRO, and G. M. WILSON: The human use of Na[22]. Lancet 272, 734
(1957).
* See also p. 535 and the paper by F. O. DOSEKAN: The effect of alterations of plasma sodium
on the sodium and potassium contents of bone in the rat. J. Physiol. 147, 115—123 (1959).

The great capacities of the bones for storing sodium should be kept in mind in evaluations of states with abnormal serum concentrations of sodium as altogether in evaluations of the homeostasis of sodium. It should thus be recalled that a hyponatremia can be due to an external loss or internal sequestration in bone and that likewise the possibility exists that a hypernatremia may be due to an increased mobilization from bone provided that no secondary regulation has taken place to reestablish isotonicity (in which case an increase in fluid volume would ensue).

The concentration of potassium in bone seems to be higher than what could be present in the mobile extracellular phase and in the minute intracellular space. — Part of it is likely to be present in a similar state as the excess sodium of bone (BERGSTROM[73]).

For a list of chemical analyses of dentine and enamel the reader is referred to BOWES and MURRAY[84b] and LOGAN[85]. — The unexchangeable fraction of Na in incisor teeth of rats is approximately 60% (BAUER[86]). (ALEXANDER and associates[87] did not find any lithium in human bone.)

C. The sodium and potassium of fluids contained in special extracellular fluid cavities

a) Synovial fluid

For a detailed discussion of the physiology of synovial fluid the reader should consult BAUER et al.[88]. These authors favour the hypothesis that synovial fluid is a dialysate from the blood capillaries with added albumin and globulin due to the permeability of the vessel wall and with mucin added from the tissue lining the synovial cavity.

Table 8. *Concentrations of Na and K in synovial fluid of cattle* (meq/kg of water). Modified from BAUER et al.[88]

	joint fluid	plasma
Na	145	156
K	4.0	5.4

The concentration of sodium and potassium in normal joint fluid from cattle is seen in Table 8. The concentrations are very close to those of an ultrafiltrate of plasma. — The cation equivalent to the hyaluronic acid anions in the synovial fluid seems to be predominantly calcium. Probably no appreciable binding of sodium occurs.

The rate of exchange of sodium over the synovial membrane of the knee has been studied in normal humans by JACOX et al.[89]. It was slower than in muscle and subcutaneous tissue. — This is most likely due to the poorer vascularization. —

[83] GREEN, D. M., T. B. REYNOLDS, and R. J. GIRERD: Effects of diet, salt intake and salt loading on tissue sodium concentration and turnover. Amer. J. Physiol. 181, 97—104 (1955).

[84a] LEVITT, M. F., L. B. TURNER, A. Y. SWEET, and D. PANDIRI: The response of bone, connective tissue, and muscle to acute acidosis. J. clin. Invest. 35, 98—105 (1956).

[84b] BOWES, J. H., and M. M. MURRAY: The composition of human enamel and denture. Biochem. J. 29, 2721—2727 (1935).

[85] LOGAN, M. A.: Composition of cartilage, bone, dentin and enamel. J. biol. Chem. 110, 375—389 (1935).

[86] BAUER, G. C. H.: Metabolism of bone sodium in rats investigated with Na²². Acta physiol. scand. 31, 334—350 (1954).

[87] ALEXÁNDER, G. V., R. E. NUSBAUM, and N. S. MacDONALD: The boron and lithium content of human bones. J. biol. Chem. 192, 489—496 (1951).

[88] BAUER, W., M. W. ROPES, and H. WAINE: Physiology of articular structures. Physiol. Rev. 20, 272—312 (1940).

[89] JACOX, R. F., M. K. JOHNSON, and R. KOONTZ: Transport of radioactive sodium across synovial membrane of normal subjects. Proc. Soc. exp. Biol. (N. Y.) 80, 655—657 (1952).

There was a significantly more rapid clearance of Na^{24} from the knee joint of women than of men, and the clearance was more rapid in the early days of the menstrual cycle. This fact might suggest the existence of a hormonal control of synovial permeability to Na^{24}. — No data are available on the rate of exchange of potassium. Measurements of electric potentials in relation to electrolyte transport over the synovial membrane have not been done.

Synovial fluid from patients with rheumatoid arthritis has an elevated K concentration — correlated with the activity of the disease. This may be due to the increased cell content of the fluid in this condition. Cortisol decreased the K concentration in proportion to the clinical effect (MÄKINEN and KULONEN[90]).

b) Cerebrospinal fluid

There is no general agreement on whether the cerebrospinal fluid is formed as an ultrafiltrate of plasma or by a secretory process, but evidence in favour of the latter seems to be in overweight. — For a detailed discussion of the mechanism of formation the reader should consult MERRITT and FREMONT-SMITH[91], FLEXNER[92a], DAVSON[92b] and the symposium edited by WOLSTENHOLME and O'CONOR[92c]. Contributions from the latest years are also the papers by OLSEN and RUDOLPH[93, 94].

Recently the concentrations of sodium and potassium in cerebrospinal fluid and serum have been determined *simultaneously* in 20 normal persons (COOPER et al.[95]). The results are shown in Table 9. These values are in close agreement with earlier reports of the concentrations in cerebrospinal fluid alone (see SHAW and HOLLEY[96] and HELMSWORTH[97] for lists of references). The low potassium concentration is noticeable. The K concentration was unchanged in patients with cerebral hemorrhage and also in patients with hyper- or hypokalemia. Experimental elevation and lowering of the serum K concentration in dogs did not cause any change in the concentration of potassium in the spinal fluid in these animals whereas changes in the concentration of sodium in the serum were reflected in the spinal fluid. Results of a comparable nature were seen

Table 9. *Concentrations of Na and K in cerebrospinal fluid and serum determined simultaneously in 20 normal persons* (meq/l). Modified from COOPER et al.[95]

	K		Na	
	mean	st. dev.	mean	st. dev.
CSF	2.96	0.45	141.2	6.0
Serum . . .	4.46	0.45	140.6	7.4

[90] MÄKINEN, P., and E. KULONEN: Synovial fluid potassium. Scand. J. clin. Lab. Inv. 9, 388—390 (1957).

[91] MERRITT, H. H., and F. FREMONT-SMITH: The Cerebrospinal fluid. Philadelphia: W. B. Saunders 1937.

[92a] FLEXNER, L. B.: The chemistry and nature of the cerebrospinal fluid. Physiol. Rev. 14, 161—187 (1934).

[92b] DAVSON, H.: Physiology of the ocular and cerebrospinal fluids. London: Churchill 1956.

[92c] WOLSTENHOLME, G. E. W., and C. M. O'CONNOR (ed): The cerebrospinal fluid. Production, Circulation and Absorption. London: J. & A. Churchill 1958.

[93] OLSEN, N. S., and G. G. RUDOLPH: Transfer of sodium and bromide ions between blood, cerebrospinal fluid and brain tissue. Amer. J. Physiol. 183, 427—432 (1955).

[94] RUDOLPH, G. G., and N. S. OLSEN: Transfer of potassium between blood, cerebrospinal fluid and brain tissue. Amer. J. Physiol. 186, 157—160 (1956).

[95] COOPER, E. S., E. LECHNER, and S. BELLET: Relation between serum and cerebrospinal fluid electrolytes under normal and abnormal conditions. Amer. J. Med. 18, 613—621 (1955).

[96] SHAW, C. W., and H. L. HOLLEY: Sodium and potassium concentration in human cerebrospinal fluid. J. Lab. clin. Med. 38, 574—576 (1951).

[97] HELMSWORTH, J. A.: Potassium content of normal cerebrospinal fluid. J. Lab. clin. Med. 32, 1486—1490 (1947).

in the experiments of DUNKER[98] in dogs. Neither oxygen deficit, nor reduction of blood supply to the brain, produced any significant increase in the K conc. (although the serum K conc. was markedly elevated), and the introduction of fluids with high respectively low K conc. into the cerebral ventricles was soon followed by a reestablishment of the normal concentration. — These findings thus seem to indicate the existence of a very effective regulatory mechanism for the maintenance of the concentration of potassium in the cerebrospinal fluid. — The processes involved are, however, obscure. Interesting results may be expected from experiments (reported in progress by DUNKER) of the kinetics of exchange, involving measurements of electric potential differences over the membranes. — Changes induced in liquor concentration of potassium have striking effects on the vasomotor system (LEUSEN[99]). Injection of potassium chloride into the cerebral ventricles of unanaesthetized cats produce increased alertness and an acceleration of movements, in larger doses tonic seizures (FELDBERG and SHERWOOD[100]). — A somewhat similar picture was seen in man by STERN[101].

The slow exchange of Na^{24} between blood and cerebrospinal fluid was shown in the experiments of MILLER and WILSON[102] and OLSEN and RUDOLPH[93]. — For a discussion of the present state of our knowledge of the kinetics of exchange of K^{42} between blood, cerebrospinal fluid and brain tissue, the reader is referred to RUDOLPH and OLSEN[94].

c) Aqueous humour

The composition of the aqueous humour of the ant. and post. chambers of the eye of rabbits as compared to plasma is shown in Table 10.

Table 10. *Comparison of the composition of aqueous humour of the anterior and posterior chambers of the eye and the plasma in rabbits.* (meq/l of water [except K which is counts p. m.]). Modified from KINSEY[106,107]

	plasma	ant. chamb.	post. chamb.	ratio ant/post
Na . . .		146.5	144.5	1.01
K	1545	1154	1307	0.85
Cl	111.8	105.1	100.0	1.05
HCO$_3$ . .	24.0	27.7	34.1	0.81

The high conc. of bicarbonate in the post. chamber in Kinsey's opinion reflects secretion of bicarbonate into the posterior chamber.

In humans the total amount of aqueous humour is very small, yet the circulation seems to be very rapid (some 4 μl/min, KINSEY and GRANT[103]).

Since the problems involved in the formation of aqueous humour and the kinitics of exchange of sodium and potassium have very recently been thoroughly discussed in the review by LANGHAM, the reader is referred to that article for such information[104]. Aqueous humour is formed both by

[98] DUNKER, E.: Über Elektrolytverschiebungen in der extracellulären Hirnflüssigkeit. Pflügers Arch. ges. Physiol. **265**, 66—74 (1957).

[99] LEUSEN, I.: The influence of calcium, potassium and magnesium ions in cerebrospinal fluid on the vasomotor system. J. Physiol. **110**, 319—29 (1949).

[100] FELDBERG, W., and S. L. SHERWOOD: Effects of calcium and potassium injected into the cerebral ventricles of the cat. J. Physiol. **139**, 408—416 (1957).

[101] STERN, L.: Direct chemical action upon nerve centres in biology and medicine. Nature (Lond.) **156**, 7—9 (1945).

[102] MILLER, H., and G. M. WILSON: The measurement of exchangeable sodium in man using the isotope Na^{24}. Clin. Sci. **12**, 97—111 (1953).

[103] KINSEY, V. E., and W. M. GRANT: Mechanism of aqueous humour formation inferred from chemical studies on blood-aqueous humor dynamics. J. Gen. Physiol. **26**, 131·—149 (1942).

[104] LANGHAM, M. E.: Aqueous humour and control of intraocular pressure. Physiol. Rev. **38**, 215—242 (1958).

diffusion across the iris and the ciliary processes and by secretory activity, dependent on carbonic anhydrase and located to the ciliary processes.

Carbonic anhydrase inhibitor (Diamox) reduces the intraocular pressure of normal rabbits and dogs (and is used therapeutically in man to reduce intraocular pressure in patients with glaucoma). The percentage of animals responding can be influenced by regulation of dietary salt intake or administration of aldosterone and other corticoids (KINSEY et al.[105a]).

d) Vitreous humour

There are very few studies on the alkali metal metabolism of the vitreous humour which is mainly characterized by its high content of hyaluronic acid. The concentrations of Na and K in the vitreous humour of the horse as compared to aqueous humour and serum is shown in Tab. 11.

Table 11. *Concentrations of Na and K in the vitreous humour of the horse as compared to aqueous humour and serum.* (Solids: water: g. per 100 cm^3, Na, K : meq/l. (Modified from [105b])

	vitreous	aqueous	serum
water	99.6813	99.6921	93.3238
solids (dried at 100° C) . .	1.1087	1.0869	9.5362
Na . . . . , . .	118.8	121.2	145.7
K	4.9	4.8	5.1

Recently MAURICE[108] in a comprehensive paper reported studies on vitreous-blood and vitreous-humour-aqueous exchanges of Na^{24}. 90% of the Na^{24} injected into the vitreous body of rabbits was lost from the eye in 24 hours; of this 60% left by way of the anterior chamber. All exchange between aqueous humour and vitreous humour could be explained on the basis of free diffusion across the boundary between them. The membrane between vitreous humour and blood (the external limiting membrane of the retina) probably is a membrane of fairly low permeability.

e) Endolymph, perilymph

Endolymph is unique among extracellular fluids by having a high K and a low Na concentration. Table 12 shows the concentration of Na and K in the guinea pig endo- and perilymph.

Cerebrospinal fluid from the same animals had concentrations very similar to those of the perilymph. — The Cl concentration of endolymph was 90% of that of perilymph and cerebrospinal fluid.

For a discussion of the transport mechanism possibly involved the reader is referred

Table 12. *Concentrations of Na and K in the endo- and perilymph of guinea pigs.* (meq/l). Adapted from SMITH et al.[109]

	Na	K
Endolymph	15	140
Perilymph	150	6

[105a] KINSEY, V. E., E. CAMACHA, G. A. CAVANAUGH, M. CONSTANT and D. A. McGINTY: Dependance of IOP-lowering effect of acetazoleamide on salt. A. M. A. Arch. Ophthal. 53, 680—685 (1955).

[105b] ADLER, F. H.: Physiology of the eye. St. Louis: C. V. Mosby Comp. 1950.

[106] KINSEY, V. E.: Unified concept of aqueous humour dynamic and maintenance of intraocular pressure; elaboration of secretion-diffusion theory. Arch. Ophthal. 44, 215—235 (1950).

[107] KINSEY, V. E.: Comparative chemistry of aqueous humour in posterior and anterior chambers of rabbit eye; its physiologic significance A. M. A. Arch. Ophthal. 50, 401—417 (1953).

[108] MAURICE, D. M.: The exchange of sodium between the vitreous body and the blood and aqueous humour. J. Physiol. 137, 110—125 (1957).

[109] SMITH, C. A., M. L. WU, and O. H. LOWRY: The electrolytes of the endolymph and perilymph. Science 116, 529 (1952).

to part I, page 141. No suggestions have appeared for the possible significance of these electrolyte-concentrations for the function of the inner ear. — The relation of electrolyte disturbances to Menière's disease was discussed by PERLMAN et al.[110].

f) Amniotic fluid

For a detailed discussion of the processes involved in the formation of human amniotic fluid the reader is referred to HANON et al.[111] and to GARBY[112].

The amniotic fluid at term has a volume of approximately 1 l. There has been some dispute whether foetal urine contributes to the formation of this fluid at term. The possibility should be kept in mind in discussions of the composition of the amniotic fluid. The concentrations of sodium and potassium in amniotic fluid at term in man have been given as 127 and 4 meq/l, respectively (HANON et al.[111] and 125 and 3.9 meq/l, respectively, by HUTCHINSON et al.[113]). — The total osmolar concentration of amniotic fluid at term is less than that of plasma. (Values of 269 mosm/l (amniotic fluid) and 290 mosm/l (plasma) were found by HANON et al.[111]). This has been interpreted as due to admixture of foetal hypotonic urine. In agreement with this, in 1 case the amniotic fluid of a 6 week embryo examined by HANON et al. had concentrations of sodium and potassium of 138 and 5 meq/l respectively. (Foetal urine from different species have different osmolarity. It is hypotonic in man and sheep, but hypertonic in the guinea-pig (BOYLAN et al.[114], ALEXANDER et al.[115]).

Studies on the exchange of Na and K over the amnion membrane in humans have been done using 2 different techniques*. One represented by FLEXNER et al.[116] who withdrew a single sample of amniotic fluid after i.v. injection of the isotope. It was shown by this technique that there was a rapid transfer of labelled sodium, the sodium of the amniotic fluid being turned over once every 14.5 hr. COX and CHALMERS[117a] found results of the same order of magnitude. Na^{24} appeared in the amniotic fluid within 6 min after i.v. injection into the mother. In the guinea pig[117b] the rate at which water is delivered to the amniotic fluid is such that a volume of water equal to the volume of amniotic fluid is exchanged on the average about once an hour (during the last $2/3$ of the pregnancy). The rate of transfer of Na^{24} to the amniotic fluid on the average is some 50 times less rapid.

In the studies of PLENTL and associates[118, 119a] a catheter was inserted into the amniotic sac at term by a transabdominal amniotomy, thus permitting sampling

[110] PERLMAN, H. B., J. M. GOLDINGER, and J. O. CALES: Electrolyte studies in Menière's disease. Laryngoscope **63**, 640—651 (1953).

[111] HANON, F., M. COQUIN-CARNOT et P. PIGNARD: Le Liquide Amniotique. Paris: Masson et Cie 1955.

[112] GARBY, L.: Studies on transfer of matter across membranes with special reference to the isolated human amniotic membrane and the exchange of amniotic fluid. Acta physiol. scand. **40**, Suppl. 137 1—87(1957).

[113] HUTCHINSON, D. L., C. B. HUNTER, E. D. NESLEN, and A. PLENTL: The exchange of water and electrolytes in the mechanism of amniotic fluid formation and the relationship to hydramnios. Surg. Gynec. Obstet. **100**, 391—396 (1955).

[114] BOYLAN, J. W., E. P. COLBOURN, and R. A. McCANCE: Renal function in the foetal and new-born guinea pig. J. Physiol. **141**, 323—31 (1958).

[115] ALEXANDER, D. P., D. A. NIXON, W. F. WIDDAS, and F. X. WOHLZOGEN: Gestational variations in the composition of the foetal fluids and foetal urine in the sheep. J. Physiol. **140**, 1—13 (1958).

[116] FLEXNER, L. B., D. B. COWIE, and G. J. VOSBURGH: Studies on capillary permeability with tracer substances. Cold Spr. Harb. Symp. quant. Biol. **13**, 88—98 (1948).

[117a] COX, L. W., and T. A. CHALMERS: The transfer of sodium across the human placenta determined by Na^{24} tracer methods. J. Obstet. Gyn. Brit. Emp. **60**, 203—213 (1953).

[117b] FLEXNER, L. B., and A. GELLHORN: The transfer of water and sodium to the amniotic fluid of the guinea pig. Amer. J. Physiol. **136**, 757—761 (1942).

* See also the very recent paper by D. L. HUTCHINSON et al.: The role of the fetus in the water exchange of the amniotic fluid of normal and hydramniotic patients. J. clin. Invest. **38**, 971—980 (1959).

over a longer period. The use of the isotopes Na^{24} and Na^{22} made possible the estimation of transfer ratios in both directions simultaneously. An average of 26 moles of water, 13 meq of Na and 0.5 meq of K were exchanged per hour. — This exchange was independent of the volume of the amniotic fluid.

It was pointed out by GARBY[112], however, that the assumption of uniform mixing (an internally homogenous compartment) for the calculation of the exchange could not hold for the blood since venous samples were used. — The exchange rates were thus minimal values. Previous experiments on the transport of the alkali metals over the amnion membrane *in vivo* were on the whole criticized by GARBY for the undefined relations between self-diffusion flow and net-flow, this fact in his opinion allowing no conclusions as to the mechanism of the transfer.

No studies of relations between ion transport and electric potential differences seem to be available.

g) Transport over placenta

There are very few reports on the transport of the alkali metals across the placenta and no data at all allowing the formation of any concepts of the mechanisms of these transports.

FLEXNER et al.[116, 117b] demonstrated a correlation between the number of cell layers in the placenta of various animals and the transfer of Na^{24}. The rate of transfer per unit weight of the placenta of Na^{24} increased 70 times from the 9th to the 36th week of gestation. — GELLHORN et al.[117c] found increases in the transfer of Na per 100 g of placenta per hour from 3,3 meq at a gestation age of 10 weeks to 23,1 at a gestation age of 38 weeks. COX and CHALMERS[117a] injected Na^{24} to 20 pregnant women shortly before delivery. The quantity of sodium transferred per 100 g of placenta per hour was 5,7—24 meq, an amount much greater than that needed for the growth increase of the foetus. Increases in the rate of transfer of Na^{24} during pregnancy have also been shown in the goat[119b] and swine[119c].

In studies of the transfer of K^{42} in rats and guinea pigs DE SILVA and HARRISON[120] found evidence of a rapid exchange of K in the placenta combined with a slow blood flow.

The only study involving transport of other alkali metals than Na and K across the placenta seems to be that of HOOD and COMAR[121] in which it was demonstrated that foetal tissue accumulation of cesium did not take place since the ratio of cesium isotope conc. (Cs^{137}) in the foetus to conc. in the blood of the dam was 1.

D) The sodium and potassium of different tissues mainly composed of cells

a) Introduction

Since the physiological problems involved in the metabolism of the alkali metals in the various tissues have been so thoroughly dealt with in the first part of this book, this chapter will only contain some additional information as well as references to the above mentioned sections.

For tables with analyses for Na and K of all tissues from the few human bodies for which total analyses have been done, the reader is referred to FORBES and LEWIS[122] and DARROW and HELLERSTEIN[14a]. — Several factors must be taken into

[117c] GELLHORN, A., L. B. FLEXNER and L. M. HELLMAN: The transfer of sodium across the human placenta. Amer. J. Obstet. Gynec. 46, 668—672 (1943).

[118] NESLEN, E. D., C. B. HUNTER, and A. A. PLENTL: Rate of exchange of sodium and potassium between amniotic fluid and maternal system. Proc. Soc. 86, 432—435 (1954).

[119a] PLENTL, A. A.: Isotope tracer studies on the mechanism of amniotic fluid formation. Tendences actuelles en gynécologie et obstétrique. p. 518—522. Genève: Librairie de l'Université Georg & Cie, S.A. 1955.

consideration when analysing tissues. For some e.g. lung, spleen and highly vascularized endocrine glands, the blood content completely dominates the tissue, and true analyses of the blood-free tissue is extremely difficult. For others as e.g. skin and uterus, it is very difficult to separate the various anatomically and functionally different components of which they are built, e.g. analyses of uteri have often been made without separation of the gland-containing endometrium from the myometrium (and even without considering the phase of the menstrual cycle). The varying admixture of fat is another source of error. The question of expression of results (on a wet-weight basis; dry-weight basis; fat-free; fat-free, bone-solid free tissueweight basis etc.) and other similar problems have recently been discussed thoroughly in the reviews by Manery[30] and Darrow and Hellerstein[14a] *.

The disturbances in electrolyte composition of tissues caused by cell damage are discussed on p. 70.

The reader should consult page 229 for information on the rate of exchange of Na and K between plasma and the various tissues.

b) Epidermis, lens

Epidermis. Data for the concentration of sodium and potassium in the epidermis of dogs are listed in Table 5a in the section on corium (p. 207). The measurements have the same difficulties as were discussed for corium. In addition the varying thickness of the epidermis is a factor which should be remembered.

The difficulties of such studies are well illustrated by the discrepancies from the data of Eichelberger and Roma found by Carruthers and Suntzeff, in the distribution of the various cations contributing to the total cation content. For a discussion of these discrepancies the reader is referred to the review by Carruthers and Suntzeff[123].

Table 13. *Concentrations of Na and K in normal human lens.* Modified from [124]* and [125]**

	meq/100 g wet weight*	meq/100 g dry weight**
Na	4,0	16,7
K	4.4	16,3

Lens. The concentrations of Na, K and Cl in the normal human lens are shown in Table 13. There is a concentration gradient for sodium within the lens (of calves) in the way that the conc. of Na in the nucleus is approximately 1/5 of that in the cortex. This might indicate active Na transport from each successive layer of lens fibers toward the cortex (Amoore et al.[126]).

[119b] Pohl, H. A., L. B. Flexner, and A. Gellhorn: Transfer of radioactive sodium across placenta of goats. Amer. J. Physiol. **134**, 338—343 (1941).

[119c] Gellhorn, A., L. B. Flexner, and H. A. Pohl: Transfer of radioactive sodium across placenta of swine. J. cell. comp. Physiol. **18**, 393—400 (1941).

[120] Silva, J.L. de, and R. I. Harrison: The distribution of K in the uterus of pregnant rats and guinea pigs. J. Embryol. exp. Morph. **1**, 357—368 (1953).

[121] Hood, S. L., and C. L. Comar: Metabolism of Cesium-137 in rats and farm animals. Arch. Biochem. Biophys. **45**, 423—433 (1953).

[122] Forbes, G. B., and A. M. Lewis: Total sodium, potassium and chloride in adult man. J. clin. Invest. **35**, 596—600 (1956).

[123] Carruthers, C., and V. Suntzeff: Biochemistry and physiology of epidermis. Physiol. Rev. **33**, 229—243 (1953).

[124] Salit, P. W.: Mineral constituents of sclerosed human lenses. Arch. Ophthal. **30**, 255—258 (1943).

[125] Mackay, G., C. P. Stewart, and J. D. Robertson: Note on inorganic constituents of normal and cataractous human crystalline lenses. Brit. J. Ophthal. **16**, 193—201 (1932).

[126] Amoore, J. E., W. Bartley and R. van Heyningen: Distribution of sodium and potassium within cattle lens. Biochem. J. **72**, 126—133 (1959).

* For a discussion of the influence of hemorrhage on tissue Na and K see E. M. Widdowson and D. A. T. Southgate: Hemorrhage and tissue electrolytes. Biochem. **72**, 200—204 (1959).

The data on the composition of the human lens should be taken with some reservation because of the postmortem changes which take place. In the evaluation of these data it should also be remembered that the lens contains about 35% of solids. The concentrations of the ions per 100 g of lens water are consequently some 50% higher than those in the table.

One human lens weighs about 200—250 mg and yields 1—2 mg of total ash.

HARRIS and coworkers[127, 128, 129a, b] in a number of experiments on isolated rabbit lenses provided evidence for the existence of an active transport mechanism for Na or K or both over the lens surface. Interestingly enough, the uptake of K was increased by the presence of glutamate. This phenomenon is also seen for the retina (see part I, p. 104).

Further discussions of the alkali metals in ocular fluids are found in the books by DAVSON[130] by PIRIE and van HEYNINGEN[131] and by ADLER[105b].

c) Muscular tissues

Since this subject has been thoroughly discussed in the various chapters of part I of this book, this section will only contain some additional comments, especially applying to *in vivo* studies. The sodium and potassium concentrations of normal human skeletal muscle (rectus abdominis) can be seen in Table 14 modified from NICHOLS[132]. References to other similar studies may be found in that paper. — In magnesium deficiency produced experimentally in rats[133] the K-concentration of skeletal muscle fell to 80% of the initial

Table 14. *Concentrations of Na and K in human rectus abdominus muscle tissue removed at operations. Mean and st. dev. from 6 normal subjects (meq/kg fat free solids). Modified from* NICHOLS[132]

Na		K	
mean 185	stand. dev. 40	mean 421	stand.dev. 28

content after 64 days. The mean concentration of muscle Na increased in the deficient group by 51 meq/kg from the control value of 92 meq/kg.

The various factors which influence the function of skeletal muscle *in situ* in relation to potassium metabolism have recently been treated in the paper by GROB et al.[28] and that by GREEN et al.[83]. The existence of a homeostatic regulation of the intracellular conc. of Na in heart muscle as contrasted to skeletal muscle was suggested by DOSEKUN and MENDEL[134] on the basis of studies of rats.

The electrophysiology of the heart has been dealt with in a recent review[135].

[127] HARRIS, J. E., and L. B. GEHRSITZ: Aqueous plasma steady state ratios; their variations and significance. Amer. J. Ophthal. 34, 113—120 (1951).

[128] HARRIS, J. E., J. D. HAUSCHILDT, and L. T. NORDQUIST: Lens metabolism as studied with the reversible cation shift. I. The role of glucose. Amer. J. Ophthal. 38, 141—147 (1954).

[129a] HARRIS, J. E., J. D. HAUSCHILDT, and L. T. NORDQUIST: Lens metabolism as studied with the reversible cation shift. II. The effect of oxygen and glutamic acid. Amer. J. Ophthal. 38, 148—151 (1954).

[129b] HEINRICKS, D. J., and J. E. HARRIS: Lens metabolism as studied with the reversible cation shift III. The effect of lens (size). Arch. Ophthal. (Chicago) 57, 207—213 (1957).

[130] DAVSON, H.: Some considerations on salt content of fresh and old ox corneas. Brit. J. Ophthal. 33, 175—182 (1949).

[131] PIRIE, A., and R. van HEYNINGEN: Biochemistry of the eye. Oxford: Blackwell 1956.

[132] NICHOLS, N.: Intracellular glycogen and electrolyte concentrations in human skeletal muscle. Proc. Soc. exp. Biol. (N. Y.) 97, 363—366 (1958).

[133] MacINTYRE, J., and O. DAVIDSON: The production of secondary potassium depletion, sodium retention, nephrocalcinosis and hypercalcaemia by magnesium deficiency. Biochem. J. 70, 456—62 (1958).

[134] DOSEKUN, F-O., and D. MENDEL: The effect of alterations of plasma sodium on the sodium and potassium content of muscle in the rat. J. Physiol. 140, 190—200 (1958).

[135] HECHT, H. H. (ed.): The electrophysiology of the heart. Ann. N. Y. Sci. 65, 653—1146 (1957).

For a discussion of the relation between the metabolism of sodium and potassium and the electrocardiogram the reader should consult the review by BELLET[136a].

Smooth muscle has also been treated in part I (see also the paper by DANIEL[136b]).

As discussed on p. 195 there is some evidence that the K ione or K/Na ratio of the aorta is essential for the maintenance of the blood pressure[1591].

d) Blood cells

Erythrocytes, leucocytes. Since the physiology of the sodium and potassium of erythrocytes and leucocytes has been very thoroughly discussed in part I of this book (chapter VII, B), this subject will not be treated here.

Thrombocytes. Quite recently a report has appeared on the sodium and potassium content of human thrombocytes (HARTMANN et al.[137]). The results are shown in Table 15. They seem to indicate that the platelets in their composition are somewhat similar to red cells with a high potassium and a low sodium content. The mechanism of the maintenance of these concentrations and the possible involvement of active transport mechanisms have not been studied. — Coagulation and disruption of platelets by freezing releases potassium from the thrombocytes. This in cases of thrombocytoses may involve so large quantities that a "spurious" hyperkalemia ensues.

Table 15. *Concentrations of Na and K in human blood platelets* (meq/l of platelet water). Averages and ranges for 7 normal subjects. Modified from HARTMANN et al.[137]

Na		K	
mean	range	mean	range
33.7	31.6—35.0	86.4	81.1—88.8

e) Neural tissues

For discussions of the problems involved in this subject the reader should consult chapter VIII of part I in this book. — A discussion of the exchange of Na and K between plasma and brain and between brain and cerebrospinal fluid is found on p. 229 and 215, respectively.

f) Glandular tissues

The alkali metal content of the exocrine glands are discussed in chapter V.

g) Miscellaneous

Uterus. As stated in the introduction to this chapter, many analyses of the electrolyte content of uteri have been done without any due regard to the hormonal state of the organism and without separation of the glandular from the muscular layer.

The conc. of Na and K in the myometrium and its dependence on the influence of estrogens and progesterone has been discussed in chapter VIII in part I of this book. — For a discussion of the Na and K

Table 16. *Concentrations of sodium and potassium of testes* and ovaries. (meq/kg fresh tissue). Modified from MANERY and HASTINGS[138]

	Na	K
Testes (rats) . .	40.7	92.3
Ovaries (rabbits)	50.7	58.9

[136a] BELLET, S.: The electrocardiogram in electrolyte imbalance. Arch. intern. Med. **96**, 618—638 (1955).

[136b] DANIEL, E. E.: Smooth muscle electrolytes. Canad. J. Biochem. Physiol. **36**, 805 to 818 (1958).

[137] HARTMANN, R. C., J. V. AUDITORE, and D. P. JACKSON: Studies on thrombocytosis. I. Hyperkalemia due to release of potassium from platelets during coagulation. J. clin. Invest. **37**, 699—707 (1958).

[138] MANERY, J. F., and A. B. HASTINGS: The distribution of electrolytes in mammalian tissues. J. biol. Chem. **127**, 657—676 (1939).

of the glandular layer and the glandulars secretion the reader is referred to chapter V.

Testes, ovaries. Table 16 shows the concentrations of Na and K in the testes and ovaries of rats and rabbits, respectively. Both Na and K exchange very slowly between plasma and testes (see chapter III).

E) Distribution of lithium, rubidium and cesium

Distribution of naturally occurring lithium. On the whole the concentration of lithium in the various parts of the mammalian organism are small. — The concentration in human blood has been found to be 0.003—0.009 meq/l. TALSO and CLARKE[139] and FOULKS et al.[140] have shown that lithium is not bound to plasma protein.

KEILHOLZ[141] found the concentration in several human organs, including liver, to be 0.01—0.03 meq/kg wet weight. The values of 0.2—0.6 meq/kg wet weight found by LUNDEGÅRD and BERGSTRAND[142] for human liver are much higher than the values found by other authors. In muscle and kidneys of rabbits BERTRAND[143] found 0.016 and 0.12 meq/kg dry weight, respectively. SCHOU[144] in tissues of rats found a concentration of 0.05—0.10 meq/kg wet tissue. Minute amounts are present in other tissues (for further references see SCHOU[145]).

Distribution of lithium after administration. After injection of Li to rats, dogs and monkeys RADOMSKI et al.[146] found that its average volume of distribution was close to total body water. This was confirmed by TALSO and CLARKE[139] whereas FOULKS et al.[140] found an even greater value indicating intracellular accumulation of Li. DAVENPORT[147] found that lithium was rapidly taken up by liver, kidney and skin, but slowly by the brain (Table 17). Recently SCHOU[144] studied the distribution of lithium between serum and various tissues in rats (kept on a low sodium diet) at intervals from $^1/_4$—48 hr after i.v. injection of 5 meq/kg. Lithium passed rapidly into the kidney, more slowly into liver, bone and muscle, and very slowly into brain. After equilibrium had been established, the intra/extracellular conc. ratio in the liver and muscle was found to be 0.36 and 2.15

Table 17. *Distribution of lithium in rat plasma, brain and muscle* [meq/kg wet wt. (for muscle: fat free) *after i. p. injection of LiCl* (5 mmol/kg) to rats]. Modified from DAVENPORT[147].

hr after inj.	plasma	muscle	brain
1	7.6±0.6	3.3±0.2	0.7±0.1
24	2.0±0.1	2.6±0.2	2.0±2.0

[139] TALSO, P. J., and R. W. CLARKE: Excretion and distribution of lithium in the dog. Amer. J. Physiol. **166**, 202—208 (1951).

[140] FOULKS, J., G. H. MUDGE, and A. GILMAN: Renal excretion of cation in the dog during infusion of isotonic solutions of lithium chloride Amer. J. Physiol. **168**, 642—649, (1952).

[141] KEILHOLZ, A.: De opsporing van eenigen metalen en van arsenicum in plantardije en menschelijke organen. Pharm. Weekbl. **58**, 1482—1495 (1921).

[142] LUNDEGÅRDH, H., and H. BERGSTRAND: Spectral-analytical investigations into the content of mineral substances in the liver. Nova Acta Soc. Sci. Upsal. **12**, 5—43 (1940).

[143] BERTRAND, D.: Sur la diffusion du lithium chez les animaux. C. R. Acad. Sci. (Paris) **218**, 84—86 (1944).

[144] SCHOU, M.: Lithium studies. 3. Distribution between serum and tissues. Acta pharmacol. (Kbh.) **5**, 115—124 (1958).

[145] SCHOU, M.: Biology and pharmacology of the lithium ion. Pharmacol. Rev. **9**, 17—58 (1957).

[146] RADOMSKI, J. L., H. N. FUYAT, A. A. NELSON, and P. K. SMITH: The toxic effects, excretion and distribution of lithium chloride. J. Pharmacol. Z. exp. Ther. **100**, 429—444 (1950).

[147] DAVENPORT, V. D.: Distribution of parenterally administered lithium in plasma, brain and muscle of rats. Amer. J. Physiol. **163**, 633—641 (1950).

respectively. Also kidney, bone and brain had a conc. of Li significantly higher than that of serum. This shows that lithium is not distributed evenly across the cell wall in all tissues. — Schou et al.[148] in 6 maniac patients, treated for one or two weeks with lithium, found a concentration ratio between cerebrospinal fluid and serum of 0.47. Similar findings had been reported by others. — In 2 humans, died from lithium intoxication Treutner et al.[149] found concentrations of some 5 meq/kg of tissue in heart, lung, kidney, brain and skeletal muscle.

Distribution of naturally occurring rubidium. Analyses for naturally occurring rubidium in the body are very few. Bertrand and Bertrand[150] found human

Table 18. *Conc. of Rb in various organs of rabbit* (mg/kg dry weight). Modified from Bertrand and Bertrand[151]

organ	conc.
femoral muscle .	0.40
kidney	0.16
liver	0.48

Table 19. *The approximate concentrations of rubidium in various human organs* (% of dry weight). Modified from Sheldon and Ramage[152]

liver	0.0016—0.004
pancreas	0.0016—0.0024
spleen.	0.0016—0.005
kidney	0.0024—0.005
suprarenals . . .	0.0016—0.004
heart	0.0016—0.006
lung	0.0016—0.006
muscle	0.0024—0.006

plasma to contain 0.006—0.02 meq/l. The conc. in the erythrocytes was some 3 times higher. In various organs of rabbits Bertrand and Bertrand[151] found the conc. listed in Table 18. Sheldon and Ramage[152] who did spectrographic analyses of human tissues found Rb in all tissues except bone. The approximate concentration are listed in Table 19.

Distribution of rubidium after administration. This subject has been treated in a recent review by Relman[153]. Zipser et al.[154] studied the distribution and turnover in blood and urine of 3 humans after injection of 20 μC of Rb[86]. Within 2 days some 10% of the dose was concentrated in the total erythrocyte mass. The plasma retained appr. 0.5%. The red cell/plasma ratio was 20/1. The rate of urinary excretion was slow, only 14% of the dose being excreted by the urine during 12 days.

Relman et al.[155] for a period of 2 or 3 weeks gave rats a mixture of 20 meq/l of potassium and 20 meq/l of rubidium in the drinking water. After 2 weeks, the mean concentration in plasma and muscle were a shown in Table 20b. This

[148] Schou, M., N. Juel-Nielsen, E. Strömgren, and H. Voldby: The treatment of manic psychoses by the administration of lithium. J. Neurol. Neurosurg. Psychiat. 17, 250—260, 1954.

[149] Treutner, E. M., R. Morris, C. H. Noack, and S. Gershou: The excretion and retention of ingested lithium and its effect on the lithium balance of man. Med. J. Aust. 42, 280—291 (1955).

[150] Bertrand, G., and D. Bertrand: Sur la repartition du rubidium du sang entre le plasma et les globules. C. R. Acad. Sci. (Paris) 232, 131—133, 1951.

[151] Bertrand, G., and D. Bertrand: Sur la présence générale du rubidium chez les animaux. Ann. Inst. Pasteur 72, 805—809 (1946).

[152] Sheldon, J. H., and H. Ramage: A spectrographic analysis of human tissues. Biochem. J. 25, 1608—1627 (1931).

[153] Relman, A. S.: The physiological behaviour of rubidium and cesium in relation to that of potassium. Yale J. Biol. Med. 29, 248—262 (1956).

[154] Zipser, A., H. B. Pinto, and S. Freedberg: Distribution and turnover of administered rubidium (Rb[86]) carbonate in blood and urine of man. J. appl. Physiol. 5, 317—322 (1953).

[155] Relman, A. S., A. T. Lambie, A. M. Roy, and B. A. Burrows: The nature of the cation accumulation by muscle cells, the displacement of potassium by rubidium and cesium. Clin. Res. Proc. 4, 150 (1956).

was interpreted to show preference of Rb to K in an inward transport or to mean a selective intracellular binding of Rb. (see also p. 44) — The difference between the potassium dilution space and the rubidium dilution space is discussed on p. 230.

Distribution of naturally occurring cesium. Very limited information is available on this subject. The presence of cesium has been demonstrated spectrographically in the retina of oxen, sheep and pigs[156]. In the carcasses of vertebrates BERTRAND and BERTRAND[157] reported a concentration of 0.24 meq/kg dry substance.

Distribution of cesium after administration. The distribution and excretion of Cs[137] in rats and various farm animals has been studied by HOOD and COMAR[121] (see also p. 526).

Table 20a. *Concentrations of potassium, cesium and sodium in the plasma* (meq/l) *and muscle* (meq/l of water) *of rats given for 2 weeks 20 meq/l of K and Cs in the drinking water*

	K	Cs	Na
plasma	2.0± 0.6	0.5± 0.1	146.2±3.5
muscle	74.5±14.6	94.1±11.6	10.4±4.5

Table 20 b. *Same for potassium, rubidium and sodium in rats given 20 meq/l of K and Rb.* Modified from RELMAN[155]

	K	Rb	Na
plasma	1.95± 0.36	0.8± 0.5	141.4±5.2
muscle	75.4 ±11.7	90.7±11.8	4.2±2.6

A remarkably constant pattern of distribution was found in each species. The Cs[137] was accumulated in the tissues against a concentration gradient. The greatest accumulation and retention was found in the muscles (Table 21). This agrees well with the findings of HAMILTON[158] that an accumulation of 45% occurred in the muscles. The accumulation of the long-life isotopes in farm animals might render their tissues unfit for use as food. — RELMAN et al.[155] for a period of 2 or 3 weeks gave rats a mixture of 20 meq/l of potassium and 20 meq/l of cesium in the drinking water. After 2 weeks the mean concentration in plasma and muscle were as shown in Table 20a. This was interpreted to show preference of Cs to K in an active inward transport or to mean a selective intracellular binding of

Table 21. *Distribution of Cs[137] in rat tissues* (mean % dose/g) *1,7 and 28 days after injection.* Modified from HOOD and COMAR[121]

Tissues	days after injection		
	1	7	28
whole blood . .	0.068	0.041	0.00055
gastrocnemius muscle	0.37	0.44	0.020
liver	0.46	0.15	0.0043
spleen	0.39	0.16	0.0019
kidney	0.57	0.23	0.0069
lung	0.33	0.15	0.0017
brain.	0.083	0.13	0.0057
skin	0.15	0.089	0.0028
femur	0.20	0.13	0.0016
small intestine. .	0.51	0.29	0.0067
large intestine .	0.63	0.26	0.028
gonads	0.45	0.18	0.0074

Cs. The Cs accumulation was more pronounced than that of Rb so that the authors suggested that the skeletal muscle of the rat accumulates the 3 cations in the following order of preference: Cs > Rb > K (see above).

[156] SCOTT, G. H., and B. L. CANAGA: Cesium in mammalian retina. Proc. Soc. exp. Biol. (N. Y.) **40**, 275—276 (1939).

[157] BERTRAND, G., and D. BERTRAND: Existence normal du cesium chez les animaux. C. R. Acad. Sci. (Paris) **229**, 609—610 (19 49).

[158] HAMILTON, J. G.: The metabolism of the fission products and the heaviest elements. Radiology **49**, 325—343 (1947).

III. Total body contents of sodium and potassium
Total exchangeable sodium and potassium

By

Niels A. Thorn

A. Total body contents

There are altogether few data on the total body contents of the alkali metals in humans. — As regards sodium and potassium, a limited number of measurements have been reported. Although these can provide some idea about the problem, no reliable conclusions can be drawn concerning the range of normal variations, variations with sex and age etc.

One of the best studies of the total body contents of sodium and potassium in adult man is that of FORBES and LEWIS[122]. Analyses of the carcasses of 2 males in an apparently normal state of hydration showed the values listed in Table 22. It is noteworthy, that the closely corresponding potassium concentrations (66.5, 66.6 meq/kg on a fat-free basis) were similar to that recorded in a survey of earlier studies by SHOHL[159], and not very different from values given by WIDDOWSON, MCCANCE and SPRAY[160]. However, the sodium concentrations (78.2, 82.6 meq/kg on a fat-free basis) differ considerably from the results found in those 2 earlier reports, there being respectively 47.7 and 96.5 meq/kg on a fat-free basis. — For the older data this discrepancy might be due to deficiencies in analytical technique. — The value of 47.7 meq/kg (fat-free basis) or 39 meq/kg body weight quoted by SHOHL, seems unlikely since data from the isotope dilution technique (which underestimate the total sodium content (see later), show a total exchangeable sodium higher than or at least equal to the figures of SHOHL (see p. 231). — The possibility has been suggested that the one *normal* subject studied by WIDDOWSON et al. might have aspirated sea-water, this explaining the high figure of 96.5 meq/kg (the person, a female aged 42, committed suicide by drowning).

With few exceptions there was in 5 species — including man — a linear regression between body weight and total body Na or (for adults only) K, when these parameters were plotted on a double log scale grid[161].

No data exist for total body K in human infants and children, but in young adults a number of measurements have been done[161].

There is a considerable difference between the total body contents of Na in infants and adults (being 51 and 38 meq per 100 g fat-free, bone-salt free solids respectively). For a discussion of this question and the total body contents of Na and K in animals the reader is referred to a recent review by DARROW and HELLERSTEIN[14a].

Lithium has been found in minute amounts in numerous human tissues (see p. 223) — but there are no data on the total body contents.

[159] SHOHL, A. T.: Mineral metabolism, p. 19. New York: Reinhold Publ. Corp. 1939.
[160] WIDDOWSON, E. M., R. A. MCCANCE, and C. M. SPRAY: The chemical composition of the human body. Clin. Sci. 10, 113—125 (1951).
[161] FORBES, G. B.: Inorganic chemical heterogony in man and animals. Growth 19, 75—87 (1955).

For a detailed description of the occurrence of cesium and rubidium in animals the reader is referred to p. 224. For neither of these metals are there any data on the total body contents.

B. Total exchangeable sodium and potassium (Na$_e$, K$_e$)

The total body contents of sodium and potassium are of less interest for their biological function than the pools of these elements, the part "available" to the body in the homeostasis (total exchangeable sodium and potassium, Na$_e$, K$_e$), determined by the isotope dilution method. For a general discussion of this principle, the reader is referred to EDELMAN et al.[162] and MOORE et al.[163]. Some limitations and possible errors in the method were discussed by BURCH et al.[43], MARTIN and WALKER[164] and by FLEAR et al.[165, 166].

The physical properties of the various isotopes of Na and K are described in chapter II in part I of this book. — Besides the method applying the naturally occurring isotope K^{40} — and which assumes that no radioactivity from any other element is included in the measurement (e.g. BURCH and SPIERS[167], RUNDO and SAGILD[168], MILLER and MARINELLI[169]), the measurements have been done with K^{42} (e.g. ROBINSON et al.[170]), and Na^{24} (e.g. MILLER and WILSON[171]) and Na^{22} (e.g. MARTIN and WALKER[164]), respectively.

The latter long-life isotope (t $^1/_2$:2.6 years) permits the determinations of changes in Na$_e$ in the course of time if a continous measurement is made of the amount of tracer excreted. — The total body contents of isotope is measured by a whole-body counting technique. — The biological half-life of this isotope has been claimed by one group to be so short that no hazard is involved in its use in man (MARTIN et al.[172]). — MILLER et al.[82] however, pleaded for caution in the use of Na^{22} in clinical investigation in man.

Na$_e$ and K$_e$ have been determined either separately or simultaneously. The latter has been done by 1) a differential counting technique (Na^{24}, K^{42}, ROBINSON

---

[162] EDELMAN, I. S., J. M. OLNEY, A. H. JAMES, L. BROOKS, and F. D. MOORE: Body composition. Studies in the human being by the dilution principle. Science **115**, 447—454 (1952).

[163] MOORE, F. D., J. D. McMURREY, H. V. PARKER, and J. CARYL MAGNUS: Body composition. Total body water and electrolytes: Intravascular and extravascular phase volumes. Metabolism **5**, 447—467 (1956).

[164] MARTIN, M. M., and G. WALKER: Studies with Na^{22} — an assessment of sodium balance and distribution. Metabolism **6**, 466—478 (1957).

[165] FLEAR, C. T. G., R. CAWLEY, W. T. COOKE, and A. QUINTON: The relationships between change in renal activity and the ratio between radioactive and non-radioactive sodium and potassium in the urine. Clin. Sci. **17**, 105—112, 1958.

[166] FLEAR, C. T. G., R. CAWLEY, A. QUINTON, and W. T. COOKE: The simultaneous determination of total exchangeable sodium and potassium and its significance with particular reference to congestive cardiac failure and the steatorrhoea syndrome. Clin. Sci. **17**, 81—104 (1958).

[167] BURCH, P. R. J., and F. W. SPIERS: Radioactivity of the human being. Science **120**, 719—720 (1954).

[168] RUNDO, J., and U. SAGILD: Total and "exchangeable" potassium in humans. Nature (Lond.) **175**, 774 (1955).

[169] MILLER, C. E., and L. D. MARINELLI: Preliminary observations on the potassium content of the human body. Argonne National Laboratory Report on biological, medical and biophysics program, July 1955, p. 120.

[170] ROBINSON, C. V., W. L. ARONS, and A. K. SOLOMON: An improved method for simultaneous determination of exchangeable body sodium and potassium. J. clin. Invest. **34**, 134—140 (1955).

[171] MILLER, H., and G. M. WILSON: The measurement of exchangeable sodium in man using the isotope Na^{24}. Clin. Sci. **12**, 97—111 (1953).

[172] MARTIN, M. M., G. WALKER, and M. CHAPMAN: Sodium balance studied with Na^{22} and an external counter for measuring whole body radioactivity. Lancet **1957 I**, 653—656.

et al.[170], FLEAR et al[165]), by 2) using the differences in decay rates and radiation (Na^{22}, K^{42}, VEAL et al.[173]), 3) chemical separation (Na^{24}, K^{42}, JAMES et al.[174]) or 4) utilizing ion exchange chromatography (Na^{24}, K^{42}, ARONS et al.[175]).

The following approximate average values have been reported for K_e: Males 46.8 meq/kg (range of reported values: 41.7—51.1); females 41.2 meq/kg (range of reported values: 31.5—42.4) — (see the tables in LJUNGGREN et al.[176], ELKINTON and DANOWSKI[9], FLEAR et al.[166]).

The following approximate average values have been reported for Na_e: males 41.6 meq/kg (range of reported values: 36.7—43.7) females 40.2 meq/kg range of reported values: 37.7—42.3) (see the tables in ELKINTON and DANOWSKI[9], FLEAR et al.[166]. — The Na_e found in a group of young males in the very recent study of COOPER et al.[177] agrees well with the above figure. K_e decreases in both males and females with age (SAGILD[178]).

The considerable variations in the values reported for K_e and Na_e may be due to several reasons. — For sodium, only part of which is readily exchangeable, there might be a "reservoir" effect of the "unexchangeable" fraction. However, evidence against this possibility was found in the studies of WILSON et al.[81]. — Individual differences in body build are a significant cause of variation. MOORE et al. considered the expression meq per unit body mass the most suitable, but others (ARONS et al.[175]) have suggested the use of the ratio Na_e/K_e. CORSA et al.[179] found that K_e was better correlated with daily creatinine excretion than with any other parameter. IKKOS et al. have suggested the use of the expression milli-equivalents per liter of total body water (see COOPER et al.[177]). (Na_e and total body water (tritium space) were determined simultaneously by their method). Great difficulties are encountered in disease states because of changes in body composition. This made FLEAR et al.[166] suggest the use of the expression meq per unit height in these cases. As discussed on p. 509 variations in gastrointestinal contents may cause considerable errors in the determinaton of exchangeable Na.

The lower values for K_e in women and old age are most likely due to the fact that fat constitutes a higher proportion of the body in these cases. — Lack of standardization of the diet and cyclic hormonal changes in women are other causes of variation.

2 main problems in the method are the time which should be allowed for establishing equilibrium between the injected isotope and the Na and K of the body, and the problem of obtaining at equilibrium a "body sample" represent-

[173] VEAL, N., H. J. FISHER, J. C. M. BROWN, and J. E. S. BRADLEY: An improved method for clinical studies of total exchangeable sodium. Using ^{22}Na and a whole-body counting technique. Lancet. 1955 I, 419—422.

[174] JAMES, A. H., L. BROOKS, I. S. EDELMAN, J. M. OLNEY, and F. D. MOORE: Body sodium and potassium I. The simultaneous measurement of exchangeable sodium and potassium in man by isotope dilution. Metabolism. 3, 313—323 (1954).

[175] ARONS, W. L., R. J. VANDERLIND, and A. K. SOLOMON: The simultaneous measurement of exchangeable body sodium and potassium utilizing ion exchange chromatography. J. clin. Invest. 33, 1001—1007 (1954).

[176] LJUNGGREN, H., D. IKKOS, and R. LUFT: Studies on body composition I. Body fluid compartments and exchangeable potassium in normal males and females. Acta endocr. (Kbh.) 25, 187—198 (1957).

[177] COOPER, J. A. D., N. S. RADIN, and C. BORDEN: A new technique for simultaneous estimation of total body water and total exchangeable body sodium using radioactive tracers. J. Lab. clin. Med. 52, 129—137 (1958).

[178] SAGILD, U.: Total exchangeable potassium in normal subjects with special reference to changes with age. Scand. J. clin. Lab. Inv. 8, 44—50 (1956).

[179] CORSA, L. jr., D. GRIBETZ, C. D. COOK, and N. B. TALBOT: Total body exchangeable water, sodium and potassium in „hospital normal" infants and children. Pediatrics 17, 184—191 (1956).

ative of the ratio between radioactive and stable isotope (the specific activity) in the exchangeable pool as a whole.

12—24 hr have usually been considered sufficient for establishing equilibrium after the injection of the isotope (in hydropic individuals considerably longer time is required (O'MEARA et al.[180]). HLAD et al.[181] have recently claimed that reliable space measurements can be obtained after a continuous infusion of Na^{22} for 30 min, using an equation derived by them, in which sodium space equals the Na^{22} infusion rate divided by the slope of the curve resulting from a plot of Na^{22} versus time.

Both for sodium and for potassium, however, the total exchangeable content consists of fast and slow components.

The distribution kinetics of i.v. injected radiopotassium (K^{42}) in rats was studied carefully by GINSBURG and WILDE[182]. 4 major rate groups were distinguished: 1) kidney, lung and intestine equilibrated with plasma in 4—10 min 2) liver, skin and spleen in about 100 min 3) muscle and testes took 600 min, whereas 4) brain and erythrocytes did not reach equilibrium even after 24 hr.

The slow exchange in the brain has also been shown by KATZMAN and LEIDERMAN[183]. It has been suggested that the slowly exchangeable K of the brain tissue is located to the mitochondria[185]. This may seem less likely since the K of mitochondria under normal conditions exchanges rapidly (part I chapter IV). Lipid binding has been suggested by others[183].

For a discussion of the exchange of potassium in isolated systems and its dependance on metabolic activity and temperature the reader is referred to p. 42, for sodium to p. 44 and 133.

On the basis of experiments in dogs GELLHORN et al.[184] formed a hypothesis for the transcapillary exchange of Na^{24}. It stated that there are 2 rates at which Na is exchanged across the vascular membrane in the various areas of the animal organism.

There have been disagreements regarding the time taken for reaching equilibrium after injection of radiosodium. MANERY and BALE[57] studying the penetration of radiosodium into the extracellular and intracellular phases of the tissues of rats found rapid uptake in skin, kidney, liver and muscle, but delayed entrance into testes, femur and brain.

MILLER and WILSON[171] in studies of the distribution of Na^{24} in humans reported that exchange with the available Na^{23} was "practically completed after 12 hr". In cerebrospinal fluid drawn by lumbar puncture, however, equilibrium was not reached until at least 36 hr after injection. The slow equilibration with the cerebrospinal fluid has been confirmed in experiments in dogs with Na^{24} (OLSEN

[180] O'MEARA, M. P., L. W. BIRKENFELD, F. A. GOTCH and I. S. EDELMAN: The equilibration of radiosodium (Na^{24}), radiopotassium (K^{42}) and deuterium oxide (D$_2$O) in hydropic human subjects. J. clin. Invest. 36, 784—792 (1957).

[181] HLAD, C. J., jr., E. R. HUFFMAN, and H. ELRICK: Observations on a new method for measuring sodium space. Metabolism 7, 322—332 (1958).

[182] GINSBURG, J. M., and W. S. WILDE: Distribution kinetics of intravenous radiopotassium. Amer. J. Physiol. 179, 63—74 (1954).

[183] KATZMAN, R., and P. H. LEIDERMAN: Brain potassium exchange in normal adult and immature rats. Amer. J. Physiol. 175, 263—270 (1953).

[184] GELLHORN, A., M. MERRILL and R. M. RANKIN: Rate of transcapillary exchange of sodium in normal and shocked dogs. Amer. J. Physiol. 142, 407—427, 1944.

[185] HOLLAND, W. C., and G. V. AUDITORE: Distribution of potassium in liver, kidney and brain of the rat and guinea pig. Amer. J. Physiol. 183, 309—313 (1955).

and Rudolph[93]). — Edelman et al.[186, 187] however, from various facts concluded that equilibrium had actually been reached after 24 hr.

With doses within accepted tolerance limits observations with the isotope Na^{24} cannot satisfactorily be extended beyond 48 hr. The biological decay rate of Na^{22} after i.v. injection was studied by Threefoot et al.[188]. Recently it has been demonstrated in studies employing Na^{22} that Na_e increases with time during 72 hr. This suggests the existence of a slowly exchanging body sodium compartment (Martin and Walker[164]). — Veal et al.[173], also found that 10% of the total exchangeable sodium took several days for complete equilibration. It has been suggested (Martin and Walker[164]) that this slowly exchangeable sodium is located to the bones (see chapter IIB).

It seems that all the sodium of bone is eventually exchangeable however, when sufficient time is allowed for equilibration. This took approximately 14 weeks in rats[83] (see p. 213).

In contrast to what is the case for sodium, no suitable long half-life isotope of potassium is available (see part I chapter II a). However, Rb^{86} has a convenient half-life and radiation. Attempts have been made at calculating K_e from measurements of the K and the Rb^{86} of an intracellular compartment (erythrocytes) (Threefoot et al.[189]) or by applying small amounts of non-radioactive Rb^{85}. (Ansel and Zimmermann[190]). The distribution of mixtures of K^{42} and Rb^{86} injected i.v. to rats was studied by Kilpatrick et al.[191]. The Rb^{86} was not evenly distributed throughout the K in the body. It was concentrated more than K^{42} in liver, kidney, intestine, heart and spleen and less in brain and bone. In muscle and red cells the 2 isotopes were present in equal proportions. The Rb^{86} space was significantly larger than the K^{42} space. This is in accordance with the fact that cells establish higher conc. gradients for Rb than for K and it was concluded that although in some ways the 2 cations may behave similarly, Rb has its own characteristics and cannot be used as a reliable tracer for K in the whole organism.

Often a single sample of urine has been applied as the "body sample", in the determination of K_e or Na_e. For a discussion of the reliability of this procedure and suggestions for improvement the reader is referred to the paper by Flear et al.[165]. These authors essentially suggest the use of several urine samples and standardization of factors that may affect renal function.

In young rats a much larger fraction of skeletal sodium exchanges with radiosodium than in old ones, but since the skeleton of the old animal has a much higher concentration of Na, the total amount of Na per unit skeletal weight which is available for exchange does not vary appreciably with age[66a]. — It is in agree-

[186] Edelman, I. S., A. H. James, H. Baden, and F. D. Moore: Electrolyte composition of bone and the penetration of radiosodium and D_2O into dog and human bone. J. clin. Invest. 33, 122—131 (1954).
[187] Edelman, I. S., A. H. James, L. Brooks, and F. D. Moore: Body sodium and potassium IV. The normal total exchangeable sodium; its measurement and magnitude. Metabolism. 3, 530—538 (1954).
[188] Threefoot, S. A., G. E. Burch, and P. Reaser: The biological decay periods of sodium in normal men, patients with congestive heart failure and in patients with the nephrotic syndrome as determined by Na^{22} as the tracer. J. Lab. clin. Med. 34, 1—13 (1949).
[189] Threefoot, S. A., C. T. Ray, and G. E. Burch: Study of the use of Rb^{86} as a tracer for the measurement of Rb^{86} and K^{39} space and mass in intact man with and without congestive heart failure. J. Lab. clin. Med. 45, 395—407 (1955).
[190] Ansell, J. S., and B. Zimmermann: The use of stable rubidium for measurement of total exchangeable body potassium. Surg. Forum 5, 529—532 (1954).
[191] Kilpatrick, R., H. E. Renschler, D. S. Munro, and G. M. Wilson: A comparison of the distribution of ^{42}K and ^{86}Rb in rabbit and man. J. Physiol. 133, 194—201 (1956).

ment with this that FORBES and PERLEY[192] reported that Na_e in young infants was of a similar magnitude as the total body contents (see Table 22), but decreased rapidly in its ratio to the total body contents during the first 2 years of life, see also[179]. — In contrast, K_e for infants, children and young adults has a fairly constant value of 40 meq/kg of body weight (CORSA et al.[179]).

There is evidence for increase of exchangeable sodium in normal pregnancy (GRAY and PLENTL[193,194a]). — Prolonged corticotropin treatment in patients with rheumatic fever did not increase Na_e (AIKAWA and RHYNE[194b]). Myxoedema is associated with a high Na_e, this probably being due to excessive deposits of hyaluronic acid (AIKAWA[195a]) (see the chapter on Na and K in interstitial spaces p. 205).

The most common changes in Na_e and K_e in disease are an elevation of Na_e or a decrease of K_e. — For references to a number of papers dealing with Na_e and K_e in disease states and the interpretation of such data, the reader is referred to FLEAR et al.[166] and DEMARRET et al.[195b].

C. Relation between total body contents and total exchangeable contents

As discussed in the previous section the ratio between the exchangeable contents of sodium and potassium and the total body contents of these ions will

Table 22. *Comparison between total body contents of Na and K and total exchangeable Na and K.*
(Man)

Total body contents of Na and K								Total exchangeable Na and K (Na_e, K_e)		
*Adults**										
				fat-free basis		fresh wt. basis				
Age	sex	wt kg	% fat	Na	K	Na	K	Age	Na_e	K_e
				meq/kg		meq/kg			meq/kg	
46	male	53.8	18.1	82.6	66.5	67.6	54.4	young	41.9	46.3
60	—	73.5	27.0	78.2	66.6	57.1	48.6	adults	± 5.6	± 4.3
*Young infants***										
wt. range (g)					fresh wt. basis Na meq/kg			wt. range (g)	Na_e meq/kg	
2476—3360						av. 75.9		1795—3665	av. 76.4	

*Modified from FORBES and LEWIS[122].
**Modified from FORBES and PERLEY[192].

---

[192] FORBES, G. B., and A. PERLEY: Estimation of total body sodium by isotope dilution II Studies on infants and children. An example of a constant differential growth ratio. J. clin. Invest. **30**, 566—574 (1951).

[193] GRAY, M. J., and A. A. PLENTL: The variation of the sodium space and the total exchangeable sodium during pregnancy. J. clin. Invest. **33**, 347—353 (1954).

[194a] McGILLIVRAY, I., and T. J. BUCHANAN: Total exchangeable sodium and potassium in non pregnant women and in normal and pre-eclamptic pregnancy. Lancet **1958** II, 1090 to 1093.

[194b] AIKAWA, J. K., and M. B. RHYNE: The effect of prolonged corticotropin therapy for rheumatic fever on the exchangeable sodium content and body weight. Circulation **2**, 891 to 896 (1955).

[195a] AIKAWA, J. K.: The nature of myxoedema: Alterations in the serum electrolyte concentrations and radiosodium space and in the exchangeable sodium and potassium contents. Ann. intern. Med. **44**, 30—39 (1956).

[195b] DEMARRET, J. C., E. ENGEL and R. S. MACH: Etude du sodium et du potassium exchangeable par le Na[24] et le K[42] en clinique. Schweiz. med. Wschr. 88, 1180—1185 (1958).

depend on the time which has been allowed for equilibration, since complete equilibration will probably eventually occur for both. It has been a widespread practise, however, to determine the exchangeable Na or K (Na_e, K_e) 12 or 24 hr after the injection of the isotope. The commonly used expression "total exchangeable" sodium or potassium should thus be understood on this background as an expression of the fairly *rapidly* exchangeable part of these ions.

In Table 22 the data from dilution studies cited by FORBES and LEWIS[122] have been included for comparison with the data on the total body contents. The major part of K seems exchangeable. (MOORE et al.[163] give the figure from 90—98%, RUNDO and SAGILD[168] from 75—93%). Supporting this is the fact that it has been found[9] that the total exchangeable K and the K-balance varied parallelly.

It should be noted that only 68% of the total sodium seems readily exchangeable in adult man (this figure corresponds to values reported by DAVIES et al.[196] for rabbits. The unexchangeable part of the body sodium is located to the bones[212]. — As earlier discussed, the Na_e in young infants is very close to the total body contents (see Table 22 and FORBES and PERLEY[192]). This is due to the fact that all the Na of bone in young mammals is readily exchangeable with radiosodium[66a].

D. Relation between isotope dilution data and data from metabolic balance studies

WILSON et al.[81] found agreement between isotope dilution data with Na^{24} and K^{42} and metabolic study balance data. They stressed the advantage of the isotope dilution method in studies of body composition, especially for serial sequential observations over a long period of time or at the start of a study to give a picture of body composition. The dilution method does not lead to cumulative error and does not require hospitalization. There seems to be agreement between serial measurements of total exchangeable Na^{22} and data from metabolic balance studies in the same persons (MARTIN and WALKER[164]). Small discrepancies could be explained as due to losses in sweat (MARTIN et al.[172]).

E. Relation between Na_e and K_e and serum concentrations

MOORE et al.[197] studying Na_e and K_e in a series of patients with a variety of pathological conditions demonstrated that there was no definite correlation between serum levels and the corresponding measurements of Na_e and K_e. The two varied independently. It should be kept in mind that several factors (such as e.g. water and fat content of the body) independently affect these two values. — Very recently it has been shown by EDELMAN et al.[24b] that a close correlation exists between serum conc of Na (meq/l of serum water) and the ratio of $Na_e + K_e$ over total body water (see also p. 203).

---

[196] DAVIES, R. E., H. L. KORNBERG, and G. M. WILSON: Relation between total and exchangeable sodium in the body. Nature (Lond.). **170**, 979 (1952).

[197] MOORE, F. D., I. S. EDELMAN, J. M. OLNEY, A. H. JAMES, E. BROOKS and G. M. WILSON: Body sodium and potassium III. Inter-related trends in alimentary, renal and cardiovascular disease, lack of correlation between body stores and plasma concentration. Metabolism **3**, 334—350 (1954).

IV. Handling of alkali metal ions by the kidney

By

POUL KRUHØFFER*

A. Introduction

This section is intended to cover several aspects of renal function.

First of all, the predominant role played by the kidneys in the regulation of the total body contents of sodium and potassium must be dealt with. This involves consideration of the sequence of renal processes which determine the rates of excretion of these ions.

In some of these processes, transfer of sodium and potassium ions is, however, so intimately connected with the transfer of other ions (anions, hydrogen ions, ammonium ions) that it would be impossible to deal with the first without also considering the latter.

The renal processes determining the rate of excretion of water also deserve consideration, partly because tubular reabsorption of sodium ions (and associated anions) appears to be responsible for a major part of the tubular reabsorption of water, and partly because renal excretion of water and sodium in different proportions is one of the principal factors in the regulation of the sodium concentration in the extracellular fluid.

These few examples will suffice as a partial explanation of the fact that this chapter has become quite extensive, and perhaps disproportionally so as compared to others. There are, however, additional reasons.

In recent years a voluminous literature has appeared dealing with changes in the rates of excretion of sodium (and water) caused by a variety of factors. The discussions of the mechanisms by which such changes could be explained have most often centered on whether they should be attributed to changes in "the filtered load" (amount of sodium — or water — filtered in the glomeruli per minute) or to changes in the rate of tubular reabsorption. It now appears that such interpretations have been based on too loose grounds, and that quite often, they may have been misleading.

First of all, several authors have neglected the simple fact, that *a priori* it is impossible to attribute a change in the rate of excretion of a substance — say sodium — to any one of the above two factors, unless the change exceeds the error with which the rate of filtration of that substance (plasma concentration times filtration rate) can be determined. Since this error is hardly ever much below 5%, it is evident that the limitations of the clearance technique are such that the data from a considerable series of experiments would have to be considered, before changes in the rate of excretion of sodium within the "physiological range" could be ascribed to changes in the filtered load or in tubular reabsorption. This fact has recently been stressed by SELKURT[6] and in a thorough review by WESSON[198].

* This section, originally completed in October 1956, was brought up to date upon the writer's return to his home country in 1958. The writer wishes to express his grateful appreciation to Dr. NIELS A. THORN for valuable assistance during the revision.

[198] WESSON, L. G.: Glomerular and tubular factors in the renal excretion of sodium chloride. Medicine **36**, 281—296 (1957).

It appears, however, that even if data on the rates of filtration and excretion of such substances as sodium and water could be obtained without errors, we might still not be in a position to decide whether changes in the rates at which they are excreted are due to primary changes in the rates at which they are filtered or in those at which they are reabsorbed. This is so because it now seems that — in contrast to the apparent assumption even in recent publications (cf. e.g. review by SELKURT[6]) — the rate of filtration of sodium and water may not at all be independent of the rate of tubular reabsorption of these substances. On the contrary, tubular reabsorption of fluid (sodium salts + water) is probably a major factor determining the rate of filtration of water (and sodium). Hence, it appears that a thorough re-interpretation of data on renal excretions of sodium, the principal anions and water is required. As a background for the discussion of these problems, one of the following sections is reserved for a fairly detailed, although crude, consideration of the hydrodynamics of the nephron.

It will soon be apparent from this discussion that an undisputable explanation can hardly be offered for any change in urinary sodium or potassium excretion. There are just too many indeterminable variables.

From a pessimistic point of view it is quite justified, to say that we can explain nothing. On the other hand, our inability to obtain information on essential points leaves ample room for speculations, and by an *ad hoc* arrangement of a complex of assumptions, the less critical person may have an unfounded feeling of ability to explain almost everything.

This chapter has been written in an attempt to keep an intermediate course between complete negativism and over-optimism. More reserve might have been expressed on several points but this has been avoided for the sake of readability.

Rather much attention has been paid to the possible causes of the acute and marked changes in excretion rates which may be produced by various experimental procedures, since the understanding of the mechanism of such changes would seem to be a prerequisite for intelligible interpretations of slower and less pronounced changes. It should be borne in mind, however, that even very acute effects may be masked by quickly mobilized compensatory processes, and their demonstration furthermore be rendered difficult by distortions introduced by dead space errors, etc.

B. Processes involved in tubular transport of water and the predominant ions of plasma; their nature and localization

The terms proximal and distal tubules have been used rather ambiguously. In the present survey the term "proximal tubule" will be taken to mean the convoluted tubule of first order while the remainder of the tubular system i.e. from the thin segment of Henle's loop to the papilla will be considered under the collective term *"distal tubular system"*.

a) The proximal tubules

The most direct evidence of the nature of the transfer processes occurring in the proximal tubules in mammals is furnished by the fundamental studies of WALKER and OLIVER and their associates[199]. They resumed the ingenious work previously carried out by RICHARDS and his school on frogs and Necturi (cf.

[199] WALKER, A. M., P. A. BOTT, J. OLIVER, and M. C. MACDOWELL: The collection and analysis of fluid from single nephrons of the mammalian kidney. Amer. J. Physiol. **134**, 580—595 (1941).

RICHARDS[200] and WALKER et al.[201, 202]) and extended the micropuncture technique to various mammals. Tubular fluid was collected from various sites afterwards carefully located in the nephron and the composition was studied by ultramicrochemical procedures.

The concentration of creatinine was found to increase markedly along the proximal tubules and rather similarly in different tubules. Furthermore, the percentage rise in concentration above concurrent plasma (and ultrafiltrate) level was observed to be identical along the tubule for creatinine and glucose when phlorizin-poisoned animals were used.

Although it has not been universally accepted, the only intelligible interpretation of these findings would seem to be the one offered by the authors themselves: that water is reabsorbed along the proximal tubules, causing a rise in the concentration of non-reabsorbable substances such as creatinine. The progressive rise in creatinine concentration was consequently used by the authors to estimate the proportion of water reabsorbed in the proximal tubules. Since the distal part of the proximal tubule was inaccessible to puncture, due to its location deep in the kidney, such an estimate had to be based upon an extrapolation. By assuming that water reabsorption proceeded in the inaccessible parts in the same way as the rise in creatinine concentration ratio indicated it did in the first accessible half, the conclusion was arrived at that at least 80 % of the filtered water was reabsorbed in the proximal tubules.

When the osmotic pressure of the puncture fluid was measured, it was found that regardless of the site of puncture the fluid was isotonic with (or possibly slightly hypotonic to) the plasma. Consequently, it was concluded that the fluid reabsorbed had itself been isotonic with (or slightly hypertonic to) the plasma, since the capsular fluid had been demonstrated to be isotonic with plasma.

The sodium concentration in the puncture fluid was only determined on a few occasions; it was found to correspond — within the accuracy of the analytical method — to that of plasma. A fairly large number of chloride determinations were made; they indicated that the chloride concentration rose early in the proximal tubule to remain about 40 % above the level of the plasma concentration in the remainder of the accessible part.

However admirable the puncture experiments are, the results obtained should not be accepted without some reserve. It must be realized that to obtain tubular fluid unmodified, from a certain site, demands that the puncture itself causes no change in the hydrodynamic resistance to the escape of tubular fluid from the site of puncture. It seems most likely that the introduction of the puncture cannula — by providing an alternative route of escape — causes a reduction in the resistance. In this case, glomerular filtration would be favoured in proportion to reabsorption occurring in the tubular segment lying proximal to the puncture site. Consequently, it seems likely that the reabsorptions calculated to have taken place here are somewhat too low estimates.

These objections, however, hardly invalidate the main conclusion drawn from the micropuncture experiments: *That by far the major part of water, Na^+ and matching anions (Cl^- and HCO_3^-) of the glomerular filtrate is reabsorbed in the*

[200] RICHARDS, A. N.: Processes of urine formation. Proc. roy. Soc. London, Ser. B, **126**, 398—432 (1938).
[201] WALKER, A. M., C. L. HUDSON, T. FINDLEY, jr., and A. N. RICHARDS: The total molecular concentration and the chloride concentration of fluid from different segments of the renal tubule of amphibia: the site of chloride reabsorption. Amer. J. Physiol. **118**, 121 to 129 (1937).
[202] WALKER, A. M., and C. L. HUDSON: The reabsorption of glucose from the renal tubule in amphibia and the action of phlorizin upon it. Amer. J. Physiol. **118**, 130—143 (1937).

proximal tubules as a solution approximately isosmotic with plasma. Experimental support has thus been furnished to the suggestion previously made by REHBERG[203] and by SMITH[204]: that a major part (the "obligatory" reabsorption in Smith's terminology) of the filtered fluid is reabsorbed proximally.

It should be emphasized that WALKER et al. obtained their results under a set of rather fixed experimental conditions: moderate diuresis induced with saline or sucrose in anaesthetized animals. Caution must be displayed in applying the results to other experimental conditions. E.g. in extreme osmotic diuresis the above figures for percentage proximal water reabsorption are obviously no more applicable; on the other hand it may still be true that whatever reabsorption occurs remains of the "isosmotic type". Our further conceptions of the nature of the proximal reabsorption of water and electrolytes are mostly based upon indirect information obtained by "clearance studies".

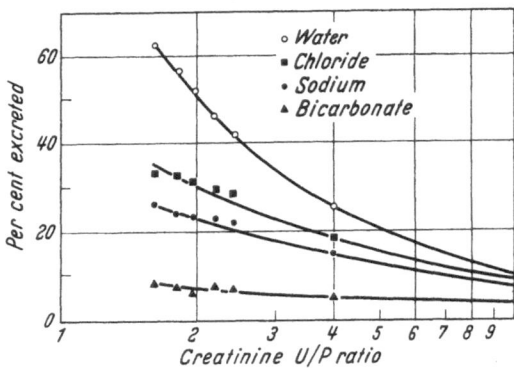

Fig. 1. *The relationship between the excretion percentages for water, sodium, chloride and bicarbonate and the creatinine urine/plasma ratio.* Plotted from data from an experiment in a dog in which increasing osmotic diuresis was induced by infusion of 25 per cent mannitol solution at a rate of 13.4 ml/min for 50 min. (From WESSON and ANSLOW[205])

Various investigators have carried out experiments in which heavy osmotic diuresis was evoked by such poorly reabsorbable non-electrolytes as mannitol and urea (WESSON and ANSLOW[205] in dogs; KRUHØFFER[206] in rabbits). By such means rates of urine flow as high as 60—70% of the simultaneous filtration rate (creatinine or inulin clearance) were obtained. The observation was made, however, that the excretion percentage for sodium was far below that of water, or stated otherwise: that the sodium concentrations in the urine fell to values far below those in the plasma (cf. Fig. 1). Since it was felt that the distal tubules (with assumedly small reabsorptive capacities) could hardly seriously modify the composition of a fluid passing through them at such high rates, these findings were taken as evidence that the predominant electrolytes (sodium and matching anions) had been reabsorbed against a concentration gradient in the proximal tubules. Granting the correctness of this interpretation the conclusion must be drawn that WALKER et al.'s finding, that the proximal tubular fluid remains isosmotic with plasma, cannot be accounted for by an active reabsorption of water and secondary reabsorption of the predominant electrolytes of the filtrate. On the contrary, reabsorption of the predominant electrolytes must be considered the primary active process which leads to a secondary reabsorption of water by osmosis through cells which are easily permeable to water.

In principle, the experimental results reported above can be explained either by an active reabsorption of sodium ions and concomitant reabsorption of anions

---

[203] REHBERG, P. B.: Studies on kidney function. I. The rate of filtration and reabsorption in the human kidney. Biochem. J. **20**, 447—482 (1926).

[204] SMITH, H. W.: Physiology of the kidney. London: Oxford Univ. Press 1937.

[205] WESSON, L. G., and W. P. ANSLOW: Excretion of sodium and water during osmotic diuresis in the dog. Amer. J. Physiol. **153**, 465—474 (1948).

[206] KRUHØFFER, P.: Studies on water-electrolyte excretion and glomerular activity in the mammalian kidney. Rosenkilde and Bagger, Copenhagen 1950.

or by an active reabsorption of the predominant anions of the glomerular filtrate and concomitant reabsorption of sodium ions. Various studies seem to indicate that the reabsorption of sodium ions should be considered as the active and primary process in the proximal tubules and the reabsorption of chloride and bicarbonate as secondary events. [This concept has very recently been supported by the studies of S. SOLOMON (summarized in part I, chapter VII (f)]. The finding of a potential gradient over the proximal tubular cells of rats of some 30 mV (lumen negative) would indicate active reabsorption of sodium.]

If the proximal reabsorption of sodium were a primary active process and the reabsorption of anions secondary and due to the electrical forces created by its transfer, then one should expect a competition betwen small, easily diffusible anions for accompanying the sodium ions. KRUHØFFER[206] therefore surveyed the literature on the effect of "foreign" anions on the excretion of chloride in the urine. Considerable experimental work had been carried out at the beginning of this century with administration of nitrates, thiocyanates, sulphates, phosphates, ferrocyanates etc. (see e.g. LOEWI[207] and SOLLMAN[208]). Although the conclusions which were drawn are not tenable in the light of present knowledge, yet the valuable information was obtained that as regards their ability to promote urinary excretion of chloride these anions fall into two groups: one represented by sulphate, phosphate, etc. and one represented by nitrate, thiocyanate etc. From the literature it was further apparent that when salts of anions of the latter group were administered over prolonged periods they would replace a very large part of the body chloride (HIATT[209], found that up to 70% could be replaced in dogs by infusion of sodium nitrate). In contrast, the infusion of, for instance, sodium sulphate (with a larger ion diameter) would only replace a smaller part (e.g. AMBERSON et al.[210] found that only some 25% of the chloride in dogs could be replaced by sulphate by this procedure, and similar observations were made by SCHOU[211] during his work on sulphate diuresis in rabbits).

KRUHØFFER therefore drew the conclusion that easily diffusible anions (such as chloride, bromide, thiocyanate, nitrate and iodide) are reabsorbed passively, and in mutual competition, by the electrostatic forces created by the reabsorption of sodium ions. The particular capacity of such anions to promote the excretion of chloride must therefore primarily be attributed to their ability to "take the place" of chloride in proximal electrolyte reabsorption. Sulphate for which the tubules are virtually passively impermeable is unable to do so, and the unmistakable chloruretic effect which it exerts must be ascribed to other mechanisms such as reduction in hydrodynamic resistance in the nephron, increase in glomerular propulsive pressure, etc. (see below in section on osmotic diuresis, p. 282). Further support for this hypothesis has been added by recent studies by SAUGMAN[212] in which it was shown (in dogs and rabbits) that the excretions of chloride, thiocyanate, nitrate and iodide followed a similar pattern (ratios between the excretion percentages) whenever an increase in the excretions was induced by loading with

[207] LOEWI, O.: Untersuchungen zur Physiologie und Pharmakologie der Nierenfunktion. Arch. exp. Path. Pharmak. 48, 410—438 (1902).

[208] SOLLMAN, T.: The effect of diuretics, nephritic poisons, and other agencies on the chlorides of the urine. Amer. J. Physiol. 9, 425—453 (1903).

[209] HIATT, E. P.: Extreme hypochloremia in dogs induced by nitrate administration. Amer. J. Physiol. 129, 597—609 (1940).

[210] AMBERSON, W. R., T. P. NASH, A. G. MULDER, and D. BINNS. The relations between tissue chloride and plasma chloride. Amer. J. Physiol. 122, 224—235 (1938).

[211] SCHOU, P. B.: Experimentelle Undersøgelser over Sulfatdiuresen. Danish Thesis. Copenhagen 1942.

[212] SAUGMAN, B.: Let diffusible anjoners udskillelse i pattedyrnyren. Danish thesis. Busck. Copenhagen 1957. (Summary in English.)

salts of any of these anions or with nonelectrolytes. An inverse relationship between the readiness with which these anions replaced chloride in the (proximal) reabsorbate ($SCN^- > NO_3^- > I^-$) and their ability to produce osmotic diuresis was also observed.

The above hypothesis raises the question whether bicarbonate should also be considered capable of replacing chloride ions in the process of proximal electrolyte reabsorption.

A number of studies from recent years have demonstrated a reciprocal relationship between the tubular reabsorptions of chloride and bicarbonate. Thus PITTS and LOTSPEICH[213] made the observation in dogs that bicarbonate infusion causing frank excretion of this anion in the urine led to increase in chloride excretion and a decrease in the amount of chloride reabsorbed per 100 ml of filtrate, whereas bicarbonate reabsorption on the same basis increased. Conversely, sodium chloride infusion led to a decrease in bicarbonate reabsorption (per 100 ml of filtrate) and an increased bicarbonate excretion. Similar observations were made by PITTS, AYER and SCHIESS[214] in human subjects (under conditions of rather constant filtration rates) and by KRUHØFFER[206] in rabbits.

Although theoretically explainable on the basis of a mutual competition between chloride and bicarbonate ions in a proximal reabsorption process, such a reciprocal relationship does not *per se* provide sufficient evidence to accept this explanation, since bicarbonate has the exceptional property that it may be removed as carbon dioxide. And, as discussed below, there are several reasons to believe that a removal as carbon dioxide actually accounts for at least an important part of the bicarbonate reabsorption in the proximal tubules.

From a consideration of the size of the bicarbonate and chloride ions one would *a priori* expect that *chloride* would be favoured in a proximal reabsorption involving a mutual competition among these ions. There is, however, a considerable body of evidence that the opposite is actually the case.

As mentioned above WALKER and OLIVER and their associates[199] made the observation that the chloride concentration in the proximal tubular fluid increased to values some 40% above the concurrent plasma concentration. Even when it is taken into consideration that the chloride concentration of the glomerular filtrate exceeds that of plasma due to Donnan forces and differences in water contents such a finding must imply that nearly all of the other principal anion of the filtrate, bicarbonate was reabsorbed in the proximal tubule. This means that bicarbonate was reabsorbed greatly in preference to chloride. It is possible that the experimental conditions, especially the use of deep anaesthesia, may have accentuated the difference since hypercapnia is now known to promote bicarbonate reabsorption (BRAZEAU and GILMAN[215]; RELMAN et al.[216]; DORMAN et al.[217]); this, however, does not invalidate the argument. Further evidence for a preferential proximal reabsorption of bicarbonate (and other anions) in proportion to chloride has come from stop-flow analyses. In fact, a proximal tubular secretion of chloride

[213] PITTS, R. F., and W. D. LOTSPEICH: Bicarbonate and the renal regulation of acid-base balance. Amer. J. Physiol. 147, 138—154 (1946).

[214] PITTS, R. F., J. L. AYER and W. A. SCHIESS: The renal regulation of acid-base balance in man. III. The reabsorption and excretion of bicarbonate. J. clin. Invest. 28, 35—44 (1949).

[215] BRAZEAU, P., and A. GILMAN: Effect of plasma CO_2 tension on renal tubular reabsorption of bicarbonate. Amer. J. Physiol. 175, 33—38 (1953).

[216] RELMAN, A. S., B. ETSTEN and W. B. SCHWARTZ: The regulation of renal bicarbonate reabsorption by plasma carbon dioxide tension. J. clin. Invest. 32, 972—978 (1953).

[217] DORMAN, P. J., W. J. SULLIVAN, and R. F. PITTS: The renal response to acute respiratory acidosis. J. clin. Invest. 33, 82—90 (1954).

was recently suggested by MALVIN et al.[218] to explain very high chloride concentrations in the effluent from proximal tubular sections, but the evidence for this is not conclusive. (It should be noted, on the other hand, that GIEBISCH[219] has suggested that the high tubular fluid/serum ratios observed for chloride may be artifacts caused by omission of deproteinizing the tubular fluid prior to the chloride determination.)

A similar conclusion can be drawn from some experiments by ELLINGER[220], who administered fluorescein to rats and made microscopical observations on exposed nephrons employing this substance as a p_H indicator during its passage along the tubules. The observation of a decrease in p_H in the proximal tubules namely to 7—6.2 in untreated and 6.5—6 in rats pre-treated with ammonium chloride, can only be interpreted to mean that bicarbonate was reabsorbed in preference to chloride. [It is noteworthy, however, that ELLINGER also observed considerable falls in p_H in the proximal tubules of frogs by the same technique, whereas such changes have not been observed by other investigators, using either *in situ* observations by means of other indicators (RICHARDS[221]) or direct p_H measurements (MONTGOMERY and PIERCE[222]).]

A more indirect support of the occurrence of a preferential proximal reabsorption of bicarbonate comes from the observations made by WESSON and ANSLOW[205] during mannitol diuresis in dogs. With increasing diuresis only slight increases were observed in the excretion percentage for bicarbonate, whereas that of chloride rose to considerable values (cf. Fig. 1). Assuming the bicarbonate reabsorptive capacity of the distal tubules to be of a rather limited and fixed capacity in such acute experiments, such findings indicate a preferential reabsorption of bicarbonate in the proximal tubules. Further support for this may be inferred from studies on the effect of potent carbonic anhydrase inhibitors such as acetazoleamide (Diamox) on renal function. Thus the fact that the excretion percentage for bicarbonate may rise to 40—60% (from initial values of virtually zero) following the administration of large doses of this drug (10—100 mg/kg/hr) to dogs (BERLINER et al.[223]; BERLINER[224]) can hardly be accounted for by blockade of a distal bicarbonate reabsorbing process, which normally must be assumed to account for the reabsorption of only a small fraction of the filtered bicarbonate (confer the figure of 15% of the filtrate assumed to be delivered to the distal tubules). The significant fall in the filtration rate, generally induced by such heavy dosage of acetazoleamide, also points to an inhibition of a proximal electrolyte reabsorption (cf. p. 263). Finally, it is pertinent to mention that a considerable increase in the rate of water excretion accompanies the increased rate of bicarbonate excretion induced by this drug, even when the subjects are in a state of

[218] MALVIN, R. L., W. S. WILDE and L. P. SULLIVAN: Bicarbonate reabsorption along renal tubules. Proc. Soc. exp. Biol. (N. Y.) 98, 448—450 (1958).

[219] GIEBISCH, G.: Measurements of p_H, chloride and inulin concentrations in proximal tubule fluid of Necturus. Amer. Y. Physiol. 185, 171—174 (1956).

[220] ELLINGER, P.: The site of acidification of urine in the frog's and rat's kidney. Quart. J. exp. Physiol. 30, 205—218 (1940).

[221] RICHARDS, A. N.: Methods and results of direct investigations of the function of the kidney. Beaumont lectures. p. 60. 1929.

[222] MONTGOMERY, H., and J. A. PIERCE: The site of acidification of the urine within the renal tubule in amphibia. Amer. J. Physiol. 118, 144—152 (1937).

[223] BERLINER, R. W., T. J. KENNEDY, jr., and J. ORLOFF: Relationship between acidification of the urine and potassium metabolism, effect of carbonic anhydrase inhibition on potassium excretion Amer. J. Med. 11, 274—284 (1951).

[224] BERLINER, R. W.: Tubular secretion of potassium and acid. Transact. of the 3rd Conf. New York: Josiah Macy Foundation 1952.

maximal water diuresis (WELT et al.[225]). This implies that bicarbonate reabsorption does not exclusively occur in a segment of the tubules, where salts may be reabsorbed without water, and together with the above evidence speaks for the existence of a preferential proximal reabsorption of bicarbonate, involving a similar $Na^+ - H^+$ exchange process as that assumed to underly acidification in the distal tubules. The apparent ability of carbonic anhydrase inhibitors to cause a partial blockade in proximal bicarbonate reabsorption demands the existence of carbonic anhydrase in the proximal tubules, but, to the knowledge of the author, no data have yet been published on the distribution of this enzyme in various segments of the tubular system. High concentrations have been demonstrated in whole renal cortex by DAVENPORT and WILHELMI[226].

Altogether, the above findings provide rather convincing evidence that a $Na^+ - H^+$ exchange process backed by carbonic anhydrase activity is responsible for a greater part, if not all, of the proximal reabsorption of bicarbonate. According to this view bicarbonate is removed from the tubular fluid by combining with the exchanged hydrogen ions, the carbon dioxide being formed leaving by diffusion. The reciprocal relationship between bicarbonate and chloride reabsorptions may very well be accounted for on the basis of such a mechanism since bicarbonate "reabsorption" would still be dependent upon active sodium reabsorption, and since a competition would be expected between chloride ions for joining the sodium ions and hydrogen ion for being exchanged with them. The preferential absorption of bicarbonate could then be attributed to the existence of a much smaller resistance to transfer of hydrogen ions than to the transfer of chloride ions through the proximal tubular cells.

Until recently we had no definite knowledge of the fate of potassium in the proximal tubules. Micropuncture studies in rats by WIRZ and BOTT[227] have, however, provided evidence that not only does potassium reabsorption occur in the proximal tubules, but that potassium may actually be reabsorbed against a concentration gradient. In eight of nine experiments the potassium concentration in fluid collected from the middle third of the proximal convolution was found to be lower than in plasma (fluid/plasma concentrations ranged from 0.26—0.86 in these cases and had the value of 1.14 in the ninth case). Proximal reabsorption of potassium is therefore dependent upon active cellular forces (if sodium reabsorption may be counted as being a primary active process). It is still unknown whether there is a specific transfer mechanism for potassium reabsorption or whether, e.g. potassium may be reabsorbed by the same mechanism which is responsible for sodium reabsorption. — That the reabsorption of potassium in the proximal tubules is essentially complete has recently been suggested by the experiments of DAVIDSON et al.[228]. The fact that the excretion of potassium was independent of the filtered load when the distal load of sodium for exchange (see later) was adequate, is in agreement with such a hypothesis. The above-mentioned views on proximal ion transfers are illustrated in Fig. 4a, p. 253.

[225] WELT, L. G., D. T. YOUNG, O. A. THORUP, jr., and C. H. BURNETT: Renal tubular phenomena under the influence of a carbonic anhydrase inhibitor. Amer. J. Med. **16**, 612 (1954)

[226] DAVENPORT, H. W., and A. E. WILHELMI: Renal carbonic anhydrase. Proc. Soc. exp. Biol. (N. Y.) **48**, 53—56 (1941).

[227] WIRZ, H., and P. A. BOTT: Potassium and reducing substances in proximal tubule fluid of the rat kidney. Proc. Soc. exp. Biol. (N. Y.) **87**, 405—407 (1954).

[228] DAVIDSON, D. G., N. G. LEVINSKY and R. W. BERLINER: Maintenance of potassium excretion despite reduction of glomerular filtration during sodium diuresis. J. clin. Invest. **37**, 548—555 (1958).

On the basis of stop-flow experiments MALVIN et al. [229] have recently suggested that a *passive mechanism*, not a cellular sodium pump, should be responsible for the proximal reabsorption of sodium and water. More specifically, they assumed, like LUDWIG, that the colloid osmotic pressure of the plasma in the peritubular capillaries should be the ultimate driving force for the reabsorption. However, their arguments are not acceptable.

In the first place they make the erroneous assumption that the sodium concentration in the proximal reabsorbate during stopped flow can be calculated on the basis of differences in the amounts of sodium (respectively water) reabsorbed in the formation of 1 ml of "proximal" stop flow urine and 1 ml of free flow urine. Differences between amounts of sodium (water) reabsorbed in the formation of urine samples containing identical amounts of creatinine would have provided a better basis.

Quite apart from this the result which they arrive at (viz. that the proximal reabsorbate during mannitol diuresis should have a sodium concentration equal to that of the plasma, and thus be hypotonic to the plasma) is inconsistent with the hypothesis of the colloid osmotic pressure as the ultimate driving force for the proximal reabsorption of (salt + water). This is so because the reabsorption of a hypotonic solution from an originally isotonic proximal fluid would soon make the latter sufficiently hypertonic (by elevation of the mannitol concentration) to arrest any further reabsorption by such weak driving forces as the colloid osmotic pressure (around 30 mm of Hg).

Since a major task of the proximal tubules must be to maintain a high rate of reabsorption of "salt" and water (thus serving the purpose of maintaining a high filtration rate, cf. p. 263) it would be reasonable if the proximal tubular walls had a *rather* high permeability to Na^+ and Cl^-, thus offering only a moderate restraint on their joint reabsorption. This, on the other hand, would mean that the sodium reabsorption pump, even if it had a high transfer capacity, would only be able to work up limited sodium (and chloride) concentration gradients between the plasma and the proximal tubular fluid when non-reabsorbable solutes, as mannitol, are present in the tubular fluid (because back-diffusion of Na^+ and Cl^- counteracts the creation of higher gradients). We must assume, however, that the ratio: ion permeability/capacity of the sodium pump, is still much smaller in the proximal tubules than in the jejunum, since, apparently, much higher ion gradients can be created by the proximal tubules than by the jejunum (cf. Part I, p. 133).

Summary. The above discussion of the events in the proximal tubules may now be briefly summarized. It is emphasized that much of the evidence upon which these statements are based is indirect and inconclusive. Proximal tubular reabsorption of the predominant ions of the glomerular filtrate is, in all probability, dependent on a primary active reabsorption of sodium ions. Concomitant reabsorption of chloride occurs by the electric forces thereby created, but the same forces also tend to carry hydrogen ions into the tubular fluid where they react with bicarbonate ions and form carbon dioxide, which diffuses away. Mutual competition between these secondary ion transfers accounts for an *apparent* competion between chloride and bicarbonate ions for accompanying the actively reabsorbed sodium ions. Actual competition on this basis occurs between chloride ions and other rather easily diffusible anions, which are normally only present in plasma in trace amounts (bromide, thiocyanate, nitrate, iodide).

Reabsorption of potassium ions is apparently active, but whether it occurs by a specific process or by the same transfer mechanism which is responsible for reabsorption of sodium ions is not known.

---

[229] MALVIN, R. L., W. S. WILDE, A. J. VANDER and L. P. SULLIVAN: Localization and characterization of sodium transport along the renal tubules. Amer. J. Physiol. **195**, 549—557 (1958).

Reabsorption of water is secondary to the reabsorption of the electrolytes (and other solutes); and the reabsorption of water by osmosis keeps pace very well with the solute reabsorption, so that an almost isosmotic fluid is left behind in the proximal tubules.

Under fairly normal conditions (and only then) the following percentages of the filtered amounts may roughly be assumed to be reabsorbed in the proximal tubules: water 85, sodium 85, chloride 75, bicarbonate 90—95 and potassium 90—95%.

b) The distal tubular system

Distal tubular processes concerned with water (and salt) reabsorption According to the above-mentioned analyses by WALKER and OLIVER and associates on proximal tubular fluid some 15% of the filtered water and sodium (and matching anions) should be delivered to the distal tubules as a fluid approximately isosmotic with plasma. If one accepts these findings to apply not only to the experimental conditions but also to "normal" conditions, it may be inferred that sodium and water should normally be reabsorbed in the distal tubular system at rates approaching 15% of the rate at which they are filtered. This follows from the fact that only up to a few per cent of the amounts filtered are normally excreted.

The exact localization, the intimate nature and the mutual interrelationship of these reabsorptions have been the subject of considerable debate for several decades. Recent studies have significantly increased our factual knowledge, but our present views are still, to a large extent, based upon inferential evidence from rather crude experimental observations.

A main fact which any hypothesis must be able to account for is that the mammalian kidney is able to produce both extremely hypotonic and markedly hypertonic urine. Since sodium and the matching anions constitute by far the greater part of the osmotically active solutes of the glomerular filtrate, the production of appreciable amounts of *hypotonic* urine obviously means that a significant part of the reabsorption of sodium and matching anions has occurred against a considerable concentration gradient. It also means that the cells responsible for this reabsorption, as well as any that might be located further distally, have resisted reabsorption of water by osmotic forces, i.e. have been highly impermeable to back-diffusion of water. (These statements obviously disregard the possibility of a net secretion of water in the tubules). The states of "water diuresis" and diabetes insipidus, in which about $1/_7$ of the filtered water may be excreted as a urine with exceedingly low sodium concentration are too wellknown to require any detailed discussion, but the findings of POTOR[230] may be quoted as an illustrative example. He found that the excretion of sodium in the urine became less than 40 mg per day in a patient with diabetes insipidus receiving a sodium-free diet, even if the rate of urine flow was as high as 9 l a day.

Although the hypothesis has recently been forwarded that some distal tubular secretion of urea takes place in certain mammals (SCHMIDT-NIELSEN[231]), it is generally agreed that the production of hypertonic urine signifies the existence of a tubular process by which water may be removed from the tubular fluid without removal of osmotically active solutes (or at least with less than osmotically equivalent amounts of these).

Another pertinent point is the fact that copious excretion of hypotonic urine, induced in normal subjects by water drinking or spontaneously occurring in patients with diabetes insipidus, may be converted to a low rate of excretion of a

[230] POTOR, A.: Renal regulation of sodium exchange. J. clin. Invest. **25**, 931 (1946).
[231] SCHMIDT-NIELSEN, B.: Urea excretion in mammals. Physiol. Rev. **38**, 139—168 (1958).

distinctly hypertonic urine by administration of small doses of the antidiuretic hormone of the neurohypophysis (a few tenths of a milliunit/hr/kg body weight). It is further noteworthy that such reductions in diuresis may occur without any *greater* changes in the rate of sodium excretion (cf. p. 345) and also without any measurable change in renal blood flow and filtration rate (MAXWELL and BREED[232]). The latter finding argues against a reduction in glomerular capillary pressure as being an essential element in the antidiuretic effect and the first suggests that the principal action of the antidiuretic hormone is to enhance tubular reabsorption of water without directly influencing sodium reabsorption.

It is now generally accepted that the tubular processes by which great deviations in the tonicity of the urine from that of plasma are produced are located in the distal tubular system and that the degree of action of the antidiuretic hormone on this part of the nephron is the major factor determining whether there will be produced little, but hypertonic or much, but hypotonic urine. It may well be that even these modest statements are incomplete, and that the action of the antidiuretic hormone is not entirely limited to the distal tubules, but that some action of a similar character may *also* be exerted on the proximal segments.

The mode of action of the antidiuretic hormone is evidently a problem of fundamental importance to our understanding of the subject under discussion. Various possibilities offer themselves to account for its ability to enhance water reabsorption. One would be that it commands an entirely independent process by which water should be selectively reabsorbed in the distal tubular system either with or, if the case may be, also against a concentration gradient. There are, however, certain reasons which render this possibility less likely. One derives from the fact that urine becomes extremely hypotonic in the absence of antidiuretic hormone action upon the kidney. As mentioned above this means that under such conditions the cells in the most distal parts of the tubular system must be remarkably little permeable to water. Since the antidiuretic hormone eliminates the hypotonicity of the urine, it seems logical to conclude that it has acted by increasing the permeability of these tubular cells to water. In other words, that it has permitted water to follow, by osmosis, the solutes being reabsorbed in the distal parts of the tubular system. These solutes are obviously mainly sodium and the matching anions. Some support for the view that the action of the antidiuretic hormone is to increase the permeability to water may be found in the fact that such an effect has been observed by KOEFOED-JOHNSEN and USSING[233a] in toad skin (cf. Part I,p. 128). Another factor which speaks somewhat in favour of the permeability hypothesis is that water reabsorption by osmosis demands no additional energy, whereas reabsorption by an independent process would do so. (For a recent hypothesis, that hyaluronidase, produced by the collecting duct cells in response to vasopressin, and acting on the intercellular cement and the basement membrane, should be responsible for the increased permeability, cf. GINETZINSKY[233b].)

Obviously, the permeability hypothesis per se can only account for reabsorption of water up to isotonicity of the remaining tubular fluid and one will have to assume

[232] MAXWELL, M. H., and E. S. BREED: The effect of the intravenous administration of Pitressin on renal function in man. J. Pharmacol. exp. Ther. **103**, 190—195 (1951).

[233a] KOEFOED-JOHNSEN, V., and H. H. USSING: The contributions of diffusion and flow to the passage of D_2O through living membranes. Effect of neurohypophyseal hormone on isolated anuran skin. Acta physiol. scand. **28**, 60—76 (1953).

[233b] GINETZINSKY, A. G.: Role of hyaluronidase in the reabsorption of water in the renal tubules: the mechanism of action of the antidiuretic hormone. Nature (Lond.) **182**, 1218—1219 (1958).

the existence of another type of distal tubular mechanism by which hypertonic urine may be formed. Logically, whatever the intimate nature of this concentrating mechanism is, it must confer hypertonicity to the urine in a tubular segment which is located distally to that in which a hormone-induced increase in water permeability allows water to be reabsorbed by osmosis until the remaining fluid becomes isotonic with normal plasma. It seems reasonable to identify these segments with the collecting tubules and the distal convoluted tubules, respectively.

A two-component system of this type has been proposed by SMITH, WESSON and ANSLOW (cf. WESSON and ANSLOW[234]). They introduced the designations T_{Na}^d for distal sodium reabsorption and $T_{H_2O}^d$ for the amount of water which may be reabsorbed by the osmotic forces created by the reabsorption of this amount of sodium (and matching anions) provided the tubules are under the influence of optimal antidiuretic hormone action. The other process was denoted $T_{H_2O}^c$ (c for concentration). This was visualized as "simply" a reabsorption of water against a concentration gradient occurring in very distal parts of the tubular system. As further discussed below the mechanism of formation of hypertonic urine does not appear to be as simple as this.

At present it is not quite clear whether the concentrating mechanism is operating autonomously or only under the influence of the antidiuretic hormone. The reader is referred to a review by THORN[235] for a thorough discussion of this problem, but it may be mentioned that various findings point towards autonomy. Thus, it has been found by several authors that cats and dogs, which were presumably completely deprived of antidiuretic hormone producing tissue, were capable of producing distinctly hypertonic urines at low rates when subjected to severe dehydration. More convincingly, it has recently been demonstrated by BERLINER and DAVIDSON[236] that constriction of one renal artery in unanaesthetized, water-loaded dogs causes slow production of a somewhat hypertonic urine from the same side, while the water diuresis persists on the other side*.

One way in which attempts have been made to measure the capacity of the process by which water may be passively reabsorbed with sodium salts in the distal tubules has been to determine the alterations in the rate of urine flow which results from changing from minimal to optimal stimulation of water reabsorption by antidiuretic hormone. A few such experiments were done by HARE et al.[237] who

---

[234] WESSON, L. G., jr., and W. P. ANSLOW: Effect of osmotic and mercurial diuresis on simultaneous water diuresis. Amer. J. Physiol. **170**, 255—269 (1952).

[235] THORN, N. A.: Mammalian antidiuretic hormone. Physiol. Rev. **38**, 169—195 (1958).

[236] BERLINER, R. W., and D. G. DAVIDSON: Production of hypertonic urine in the absence of pituitary antidiuretic hormone. J. clin. Invest. **36**, 1416—1427 (1957).

[237] HARE, R. S., K. HARE, and D. M. PHILLIPS: The renal excretion of chloride by the normal and by the diabetes insipidus dog. Amer. J. Physiol. **140**, 334—348 (1944).

* While these studies indicate the existence of some concentrating capacity in the absence of vasopressin, the fact remains that the overall concentrating capacity of the kidney is greatly diminished under such conditions. The very low permeability of the distal convoluted tubules and the collecting tubules under such conditions (see later) provide one obvious explanation for this, but apparently other factors must also be involved. If namely such permeability changes were the only immediate consequences of a lack of vasopressin, one would expect at least as great a hypertonicity of the medulla in water diuresis as in vasopressin antidiuresis, which is contrary to the findings of ULLRICH et al. reported in p. 248. It appears therefore that, if a slowing-down of the concentrating pump of the loops of HENLE does not take place on passing from vasopressin antidiuresis to water diuresis, then at least one of the following changes must occur: (1) A reduction in the water permeability of the proximal tubules, resulting in the delivery of a somewhat hypotonic fluid to the distal system, (2) An increase in medullary blood flow disturbing the production of medullary hypertonicity by the loops of HENLE.

administered Pitressin to diabetes insipidus dogs in which a pronounced solute diuresis had been induced by sodium chloride loading. A reduction in urine flow was obtained which according to their Table 3 and Fig. 8 amounted to some 10% of the concurrent filtration rate; since the latter was somewhat increased by the salt loading, the change in urine flow probably corresponds to nearly 15% of the normal filtration rate. Apart from the facts that the antidiuretic hormone may also have activated the concentration mechanisms, and that some water may have been reabsorbed distally together with the sodium salt already in the pre-administration period, such experiments may give erroneous values even for the amounts of water that may be reabsorbed under the influence of antidiuretic hormone. This is so, because, the estimates rest upon the assumption that the increased distal reabsorption of water induced by antidiuretic hormone does not affect the rate at which water is delivered to the distal tubules. As discussed in a later section (p. 345) this may be the case by a coincidence of opposing effects, but it cannot *a priori* be assumed to hold.

Another approach which is subject to fewer objections has been introduced by WESSON and ANSLOW[234]. They determined what is called the *positive free water clearance*, which simply means the amount of water one has to remove from a one minute sample of hypotonic urine to make the remaining fluid isotonic with plasma. Provided a specific concentrating mechanism has not been operating, this signifies the amount of water which was unable to follow (by osmosis) the solutes being reabsorbed. If it may be further assumed that under conditions of maximal water diuresis no water at all is reabsorbed in the distal tubules by osmosis whereas the proximal tubular fluid remains isosmotic, the maximum positive free water clearance obtained under such conditions would signify the amount of osmotically active solutes, mainly sodium salts (expressed as the number of ml of isotonic fluid containing it), which is reabsorbed in the distal tubules under such conditions. Assuming that optimal stimulation by antidiuretic hormone permits complete reabsorption of water by osmosis, this figure would also signify the amount of water that may be reabsorbed "isotonically" per min under the influence of antidiuretic hormone. Evidently a number of assumptions are required for the interpretation of such data, but it is at least noteworthy that the magnitude of the distal water reabsorption (inducible by antidiuretic hormone) as measured by this method corresponds very well to that obtained by the method of HARE et al.; this is also directly apparent from WESSON and ANSLOW's data, which also include information on the increase in urine flow obtained upon stopping the administration of antidiuretic hormone to dogs under conditions of a mixed maximal water diuresis and urea diuresis. The latter authors also made the observation that the size of the positive free water clearance was independent of the level of urea diuresis induced.

Although the interpretation of the above findings is perforce uncertain, the fact that a similar magnitude of distal sodium and water reabsorbing capacities is arrived at as by WALKER et al.'s approach must strengthen the view that the reabsorption capacity of the distal tubules for these substances normally constitutes only a small fraction of the total capacity of the tubular system. The sodium reabsorbing processes will be further discussed below, but it may be appropriate to point out here that sodium reabsorption which occurs in exchange with potassium and ammonium does not give rise to any positive free water clearance.

Attempts to measure the capacity of the concentrating mechanism ($T^c_{H_2O}$) have been made by determining what has been called the *negative free water clearance*, which means the number of ml of water which must be added to a one minute sample of a hypertonic urine to lower the osmotic pressure to that of plasma. If under certain conditions it may be assumed that a completely isotonic tubular fluid is delivered to the segment where the concentrating mechanism operates, and that no reabsorption of solutes takes place there or further distally, then this figure obviously measures the amount of water that has been removed per min from the tubular fluid by the concentrating mechanism.

In the belief that these conditions may be fulfilled when ample amounts of antidiuretic hormone are acting upon the kidney, ZAK et al.[238] determined the negative free water clearance in normal human subjects during exogenous or endogenous pituitary antidiuresis. They reported that the negative free water clearance remained constant (about 4—5 ml/min) when various degrees of mannitol diuresis were induced. This observation confirms KRUHØFFER's[206] finding that the rate of urine flow multiplied by the difference between the osmolar concentrations of the urine and the plasma remained approximately constant in rabbits subjected to various levels of sodium chloride diuresis and given a continuous infusion of antidiuretic hormone. Observations essentially suggesting a relationship of this sort had previously been reported by GALEOTTI[239], who found the difference between the osmotic pressures of urine and plasma to decrease gradually in dogs as the rate of urine flow was raised by intravenous infusion of hypertonic sodium chloride or glucose solutions. Similar observations were made by McCANCE et al.[240] in dehydrated human subjects during administration of sodium chloride, potassium chloride and urea.

If it can be assumed that the conditions mentioned above are fulfilled, we must conceive of the concentrating mechanism as a process or complex of processes in the distal tubular system which are capable of removing a maximum of some 4—5 ml of water per minute (in human subjects) from the tubular fluid against a concentration gradient, regardless of the rate at which fluid is delivered from the proximal segments. As mentioned above it is not quite clear to what extent this mechanism is also operating when hypotonic urine is being formed and especially when antidiuretic hormone is lacking. Less than the maximum amount of water will be removed when the osmolarity of the final urine reaches an upper value ("osmotic barrier") which varies from one species to another.

The concentrating mechanism has been suggested to be a "simple" active reabsorption of water by cells located far distally in the tubular system (possibly in the collecting ducts). There are, however, a number of arguments which support the idea of a more complex mechanism in which the loops of HENLE play an essential part.

Suggestive evidence for this view is provided by the fact that hypertonic urine is only formed by the kidneys of such animals, mammals and birds, which possess this structure (CRANE[241]). Furthermore, by the fact that the development of the loops in various mammals seems to be correlated with the concentrating power of their kidneys (PETER[242]; and later work which seems to indicate that the thickness of the renal medulla and the length of the loop is particularly large in desert mammals,

    [238] ZAK, G. A., C. BRUN, and H. W. SMITH: The mechanism of formation of osmotically concentrated urine during the antidiuretic state. J. clin. Invest. **33**, 1064—1074 (1954).

    [239] GALEOTTI, G.: Über die Arbeit, welche die Nieren leisten um den osmotischen Druck des Blutes auszugleichen. Arch. Anat. u. Physiol. Abtheil. f. Physiol. **1902**, 200.

    [240] McCANCE, R. A., W. F. YOUNG, and D. A. K. BLACK: The secretion of urine during dehydration and rehydration. J. Physiol. **102**, 415—428 (1944).

    [241] CRANE, M. M.: Observations on the function of the frog's kidney. Amer. J. Physiol. 81, 232—243 (1927).

    [242] PETER, K.: Untersuchungen über Bau und Entwicklung der Niere. Part I p. 334 to 336. Jena: Gustav Fischer 1927.

cf. SCHMIDT-NIELSEN and SCHMIDT-NIELSEN[243]). Finally, by the correlation between the development of the loops (cf. PETER[242]) and the increasing concentrating power in early life.

PETER, CRANE and also BURGESS et al.[244] suggested that a water reabsorption leading to the formation of hypertonic urine actually occurred in the thin segment of the loop. This view has, however, hardly many adherents to-day, and it is clearly inconsistent with WALKER et al.'s[199] finding in two cases of distinctly hypotonic fluid in the distal convoluted tubules under conditions where the bladder urine simultaneously formed was definitely hypertonic. The latter findings have recently been confirmed and extended by WIRZ[245]. During water diuresis the fluid was definitely hypotonic throughout the distal convoluted tubules. During dehydration-antidiuresis definite hypotonicity still existed in the first part of the distal convoluted tubules, whereas isotonicity was approached but never exceeded in the last part of this segment. Some authors have adopted the view, then, that the loops are not at all directly involved in the formation of hypertonic urine. Thus, SMITH[246] has attributed to the thin segment merely the role of permitting further osmotic equilibration of the proximal tubular fluid with the blood plasma.

It appears, however, that such a trivial function could hardly offer a satisfactory explanation for the existence of such unique structures as the loops. It is therefore of great interest that HARGITAY and KUHN[247] have advanced a hypothesis which assigns to the loops an essential part in the formation of hypertonic urine without assuming any net reabsorption of water in this portion of the nephron.

According to this hypothesis a movement of water is assumed to take place from the fluid in the descending limbs of the loops into that of the adjacent parts of the ascending limbs, the tubular walls and the interstitium forming a semipermeable membrane. By the additive effect of subsequent sections of the loop the fluid remaining in the loops would thus become increasingly hypertonic deeper in the medulla. During the passage of fluid in the collecting tubules through this region a small amount of water is then assumed to be removed by osmosis and returned to the loops of HENLE, making possible the formation of hypertonic final urine. Thus the fluid entering the distal convoluted tubules from the loops should equal that entering the loops from the proximal tubules *plus* the water returned from the collecting tubules and thus it should be somewhat hypotonic. In the distal convoluted tubules the major part of the solutes (salts) and water of this fluid is then assumed to be reabsorbed under ordinary conditions, leaving consequently only a small amount of fluid to be passed on to the collecting tubules.

HARGITAY and KUHN gave a mathematical treatment of a system working according to the "Multiplikationsprinzip", and in model experiments with a "Haarnadel-Gegenstrom" arrangement, imitating the loop, they demonstrated that successive concentration could actually be obtained on this principle.

As evidence for the occurrence of a similar mechanism in the kidney they referred to the findings of WIRZ, HARGITAY and KUHN[248] that the freezing-point

[243] SCHMIDT-NIELSEN, K., and B. SCHMIDT-NIELSEN: Water metabolism of desert mammals. Physiol. Rev. **32**, 135—166 (1952).

[244] BURGESS, W. W., A. M. HARVEY and E. K. MARSHALL, jr.: The site of the antidiuretic action of the pituitary extract. J. Pharmacol. exp. Ther. **49**, 237—249 (1933).

[245] WIRZ, H.: Der osmotische Druck in der corticalen Tubuli der Rattenniere. Helv. physiol. pharmacol. Acta **14**, 352—362 (1956).

[246] SMITH, H. W.: The kidney. Structure and Function in health and disease. p. 246. New York: Oxford Univ. Press 1951.

[247] HARGITAY, B., u. W. KUHN: Das Multiplikationsprinzip als Grundlage der Harnkonzentrierung in der Niere. Z. Elektrochem. **55**, 539—558 (1951).

[248] WIRZ, H., B. HARGITAY u. W. KUHN: Lokalisation des Konzentrierungsprozesses in der Niere durch direkte Kryoskopie. Helv. physiol. pharmacol. Acta **9**, 196—220 (1951).

depression of the tissue, as determined by cryoscopy on kidney slices, increases markedly through the medulla towards the papillae and to previous studies by LJUNGBERG[249]. The latter author determined the chloride concentration in serial sections of a cylinder punched out of the frozen kidneys of rabbits. An average chloride concentration of 449 mg per 100 ml of tissue was found in the inner zone of the medulla. From histological examinations of alternate sections which permitted an estimation of the tubular fluid present in the section, a correction could be applied for the latter (assuming it to have the tonicity of final urines). This led to the conclusion that the chloride concentration in the epithelial cell and/or the interstitial spaces in this region must have had a chloride concentration

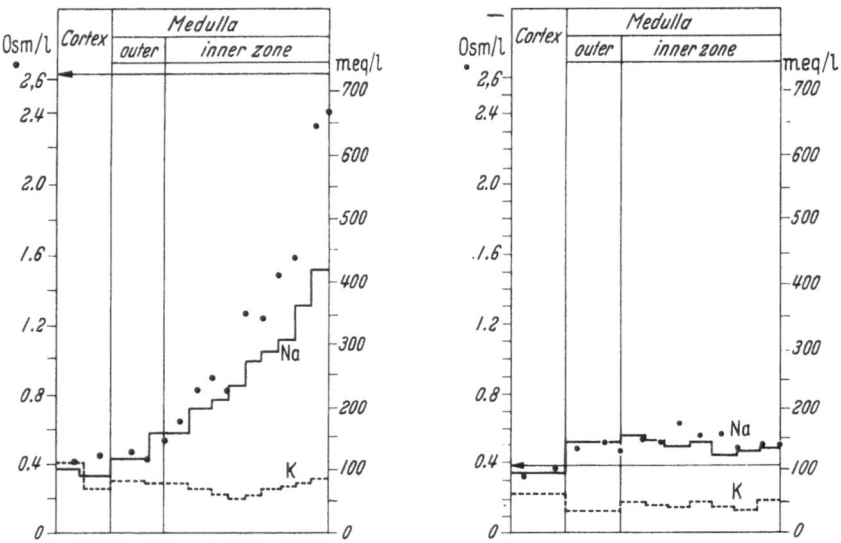

Fig. 2a and b. *"Osmotic Pressure"* (left ordinates, and given by dots) *and sodium and potassium concentrations* (right ordinates) *in slices from various regions of dogs' kidneys.* Fig. 2 a from animals deprived of water for four days; osmolarity of the urine formed immediately before killing: 2.66 osmol/l. Fig. 2 b from animals in a state of pronounced water diuresis; osmolarity of final urine: 0,37 osmol/l. (From ULLRICH et al.[250])

considerably above that in the blood plasma. To this evidence may be added the findings of ULLRICH et al.[250]. Slices were prepared from various regions of the kidneys of dogs which were acutely killed in different states of diuresis. By immersion in sodium chloride solutions of different concentrations that concentration was determined at which slices from a particular region neither gained nor lost weight. This was assumed to represent intracellular tonicity. According to this criterion kidney cortex was regularly slightly hypertonic (0.3—0.42 osmolar), whereas the osmolarity of the medullary cells rose gradually towards the papilla to values about 5 times higher, when slices from dehydrated dogs were studied. Under such conditions a parallel increase in the sodium concentration (up to 425 meq/l of tissue fluid) was also observed (cf. Fig. 2a). In slices from dogs in a state of pronounced water diuresis the tonicity of the medulla did not rise, but still it was found to be somewhat above that of the blood, and the sodium concentration too was somewhat higher than that of plasma (cf. Fig. 2b). Further

[249] LJUNGBERG, E.: On the reabsorption of chlorides in the kidney of the rabbit. Acta med. scand. Suppl. 186 (1947).
[250] ULLRICH, K. J., F. O. DRENCKHAHN u. K. H. JARAUSCH: Untersuchungen zum Problem der Harnkonzentrierung und -verdünnung. Arch. ges. Physiol. 261, 62—77 (1955).

evidence has recently been added by analyses of fluid collected by micropuncture from the bend of the loop of HENLE (GOTTSCHALK and MYLLE[251]). These authors found that, in the concentrating hamster kidney, this fluid had practically the same osmotic pressure as fluid from a collecting tubule at the same level (while fluid collected from the distal tubules was hypotonic or isotonic with plasma).

HARGITAY and KUHN's hypothesis has been criticized on the grounds that the blood supply to the medulla would interfere with the concentrating mechanism. The hypertonicity of the medulla — during formation of hypertonic urine — is however a well-established experimental fact, and the above criticism is also unwarranted. This is so because the passage of blood through the medulla is not a one-way traversal, but an into-and-back passage in vascular loops (vasa recta). Thus, while water would pass by osmosis from the blood of the descending limbs of the vascular loops into the interstices, it would also have the opportunity to go back by the same forces to the (now hypertonic) blood returning in the ascending vascular limbs. Such an osmotic equilibration between blood and interstitial fluid would be favoured by the probably slow linear flow in the sinusoidal vasa recta, and, if complete at each level of the medulla, the blood flow would not disturb an existing medullary hypertonicity. In this connection it is worth noticing that WIRZ[252] has found the blood from the deepest parts of the medulla to be markedly hypertonic.

HARGITAY and KUHN's hypothesis is attractive in so far as it is capable of accounting for the above-mentioned experimental facts (hypertonicity of the medulla, hypotonicity of the fluid in the distal convoluted tubules) at the same time as it places the actual formation of hypertonic urine in the most distal parts of the tubular system and offers an explanation to the correlation between the development of the loops and the concentrating power of the kidney.

In their formulation of the hypothesis the authors did not, however, make it clear which forces should be held responsible for the short-circuiting of water from the descending to the ascending limbs of the loops of HENLE and for the reabsorption of water from the fluid in the collecting tubules. It is, of course, theoretically possible that the tall cells of the ascending limb has a (limited) capacity for water secretion, by which they could work up at each medullary level a small osmotic gradient between their tubular fluid and the interstitial fluid. Concentration of the latter would then be the primary consequence and movement of water by osmosis from the descending limbs and the collecting tubules to the interstices would be secondary events. The limitation of the concentrating mechanism would be referable to a limited water secretory capacity of the cells of the ascending limbs.

This is, however, not the only mechanism which can account for all the above-mentioned facts. In the writer's opinion a more likely mechanism is a reabsorption of sodium and chloride by the loops without proportional reabsorption of water, leading to medullary interstitial hypertonicity and, in turn, reabsorption of water from the collecting tubules by osmosis. Fig. 3 illustrates how this mechanism could be assumed to operate; for a detailed explanation the reader is referred to the legend accompanying the figure. He is also invited to consult recent reviews by THORN[235] and BERLINER et al.[253] for discussions of the loop mechanism.

[251] GOTTSCHALK, C. W., and M. MYLLE: Evidence that the mammalian nephron functions as a countercurrent multiplier system. Science 128, 594 (1958).

[252] WIRZ, H.: Der osmotische Druck des Blutes in der Nierenpapille. Helv. physiol. pharmacol. Acta 11, 29—29 (1953).

[253] BERLINER, R. W., N. G. LEVINSKY, D. G. DAVIDSON and M. EDEN: Dilution and concentration of the urine and the action of antidiuretic hormone. Amer. J. Med. 24, 730 to 744 (1958).

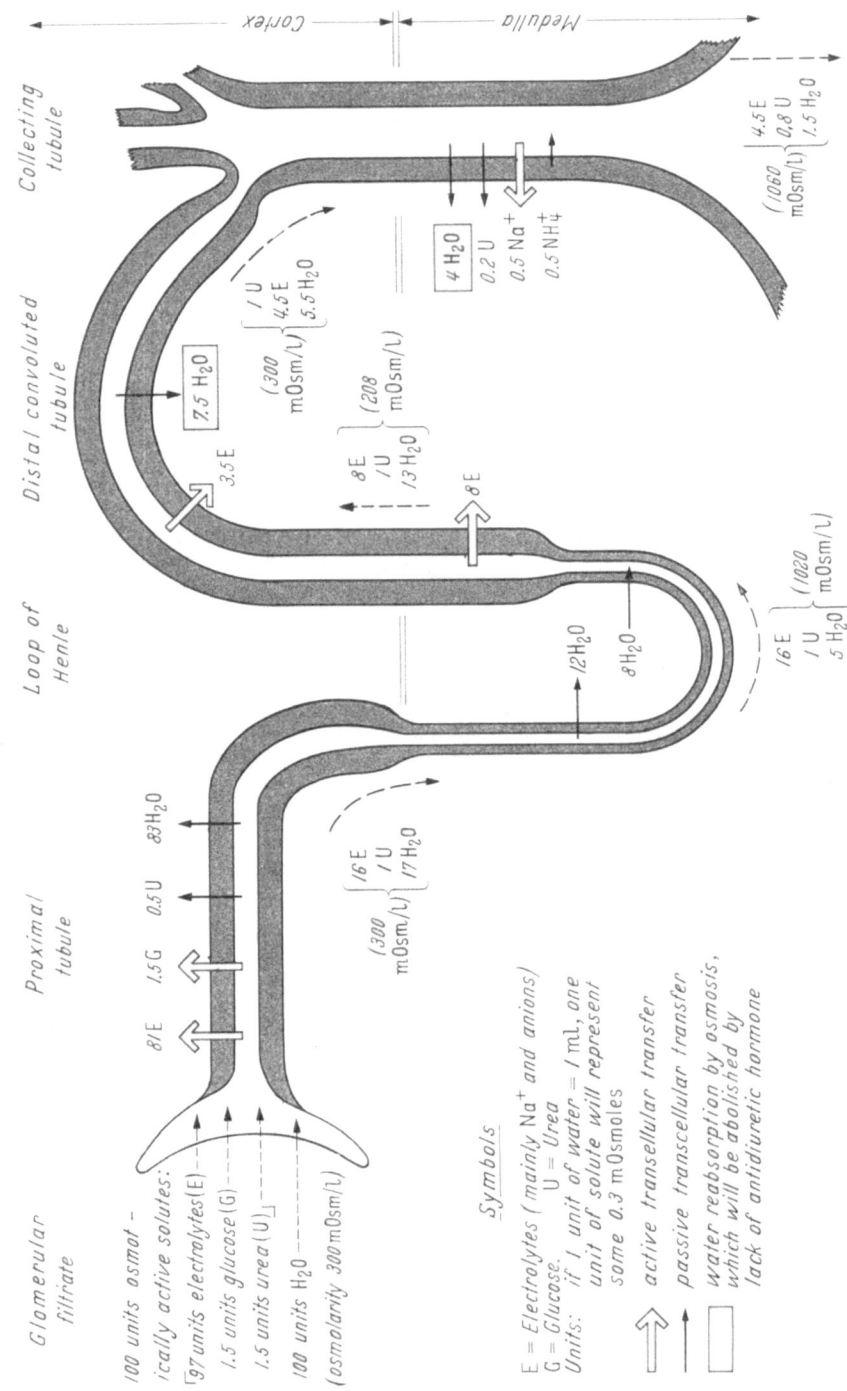

Fig. 3. Diagram illustrating processes possibly involved in the production of hypertonic (and hypotonic) urine

The figures shown for solute and water transfer in the nephron are for a case of maximal pituitary antidiuresis under conditions of moderate salt diuresis. For the sake of clarity only electrolytes = E (mainly sodium and matching anions), urea = U, glucose = G and water are considered, and the amounts transferred are given in arbitrary units rather than in absolute figures. If 1 unit of water = 1 ml (i.e. 100 ml filtered within the period considered) then 1 unit of osmotically active solute will be about 0.3 mOsmoles (i.e. the osmolarity of the glomerular filtrate = 300 mOsm/l). Active (primary) transcellular transfers are indicated by heavy arrows, passive transfer (osmosis, diffusion) by light arrows. Amounts of substances flowing from one tubular segment to another are shown by stippled arrows.

Isosmotic reabsorption of 83% of the glomerular filtrate is shown to take place in the proximal tubule, leaving 17% of isotonic fluid to enter the loop of HENLE. Here electrolytes (sodium and chloride) are reabsorbed in excess of water (the walls of the thick segment of the ascending limb of HENLE's loop being assumed to be almost impermeable to water), thus conferring hypertonicity to the medullary interstitial fluid and leaving a hypotonic fluid to enter the distal convoluted tubule. In the latter segment further electrolyte reabsorption occurs, and a reabsorption of water by osmosis until the remaining fluid becomes isotonic with the plasma (since antidiuretic hormone makes the tubular walls easily permeable to water). The greatly reduced amount of isotonic fluid then enters the collecting tubule and, in passing through the medulla, loses water by osmosis to the hypertonic interstitial fluid, leaving a small amount of hypertonic urine to enter the pelvis. The $Na^+ \rightleftharpoons NH^+_4$ exchange shown to take place in the collecting tubules represents a further addition of osmotic activity to the medullary interstitial fluid (cf. p. 260) which makes possible some additional reabsorption of water by osmosis from the collecting tubules. Also shown to occur in the collecting tubules is a slow back-diffusion of urea, which will maintain the urea concentration in the medulla almost as high as in the collecting tubule urine at the same level (since the urea is not easily lost from the medulla due to the countercurrent flow arrangement of the vascular and tubular loops)*.

As apparent from the figure the numbers of units of substances added to or removed from the medullary interstitial fluid in the period considered are as follows: 8 E, 0.5 Na^+, 0.2 U and (12 + 4) H_2O were added, and 8 H_2O were removed, representing together a net addition of hypertonic fluid (8 units of 326 mOsm/l). The addition of this fluid, which is removed by the blood passing through the vasa recta, ensures that high concentrations of Na, Cl and urea can be maintained in the interstices even if full equilibration between these and the blood is not achieved at each level.

It is readily seen that in the case illustrated the negative free water clearance will be (4.5 + 0.8) — 1.5 = 3.8 ml per 100 ml of filtrate.

If water-permeability of the distal convoluted tubules and the collecting tubules were entirely dependent upon the antidiuretic hormone, lack of this hormone should abolish the reabsorption of 7.5 and 4 ml of water (per 100 ml of fitrate). As explained elsewhere (p · 344) it cannot a priori be expected that this diminution in water reabsorption shall give rise to an exactly equal increment in urinary output and no other changes. If it did, the urinary output would become: 4.5 E, 0.8 U, (1.5 + 7.5 + 4) H_2O, or 13 ml of 100 mOsm/l urine (per 100 ml of filtrate), and the positive free water clearance would become 13 — 4.5 — 0.8 = 7.7 ml (per 100 ml of filtrate).

Distal reabsorption of sodium (and secretion of potassium). From the discussion above it appears that under fairly normal conditions some 15% of the filtered sodium and water is delivered to the distal tubules, which will reabsorb far the greater parts of these amounts leaving only minor fractions to be excreted. In other words, one must assume that some 2.5 meq of sodium is reabsorbed per minute in the distal tubular system in a normal human adult. If it can also be accepted that the proximal reabsorption of chloride is normally less complete on a

---

* This fact, that a high urea concentration can be obtained in the collecting tubule urine with practically no urea concentration gradient across the collecting tubule wall, simply by back-diffusion of a small fraction of the filtered urea, means that practically no concentrating power is spent on concentrating the urea in the collecting tubule urine. It explains therefore why higher urine osmolarities can be reached if urea is excreted in the urine at high rates than at low rates [cf. e. g. A. HENDRIKX and F. H. EPSTEIN: Effect of feeding protein and urea on renal concentrating ability in the rat. Amer. J. Physiol. **195**, 539—542 (1958)]. The osmolarity of the urea is so to speak superimposed upon that which one would obtain by mere action of the "sodium concentrating pump", if no urea entered into the glomerular filtrate.

percentage basis than that of sodium, it follows that somewhat more than 2 meq of sodium should be reabsorbed distally per minute *in combination with chloride*, and only a small fraction of a meq in another way. It is being widely held now that the latter reabsorption takes place as an *exchange process* by which sodium ions being reabsorbed are exchanged for other cations being secreted. As discussed above these two reabsorptions must be assumed to provide the forces by which water can be passively reabsorbed in the distal tubules, when these are acted upon by the antidiuretic hormone (the latter process could, however, only be effective in this respect to the extent that sodium ions were exchanged for hydrogen ions and only fully when the latter reacts with bicarbonate in the tubular fluid).

Current views of these processes are all based on inferential evidence, but since great importance must be attributed to them in the regulation of sodium and potassium excretions some of the basic features of these views will be made the subject of a brief discussion here, while consideration of the details is deferred to later sections.

The distal Na+ exchange process. The first indication of the occurrence of a reabsorption of sodium ions in exchange for other cations came from studies on the acidification of urine.

MONTGOMERY and PIERCE[222] had shown that when a $1/_3$ M sodium phosphate solution of p_H 7.5 was introduced into a distal tubule of a frog's kidney it underwent a change to p_H about 6.8 within only one minute. In a discussion of this finding SMITH[204] pointed out that it could hardly be accounted for by the classical theories of urinary acidification. One, that of selective reabsorption of bicarbonate, was excluded by the experimental conditions. The other, according to which the acidification is due to selective reabsorption of HPO_4^{--} (leaving $H_2PO_4^-$ behind), also seemed very unlikely as an explanation because it would demand the reabsorption of phosphate at a rate immensely exceeding that at which it is normally reabsorbed in a tubule during frank phosphaturia. Therefore, SMITH considered a secretion of hydrogen ions in exchange for sodium ions the only plausible explanation of the observed acidification.

Very convincing evidence for the existence of a similar process in the mammalian kidney was provided by PITTS and ALEXANDER[254]. In experiments in dogs, in which acidosis was produced by administration of hydrochloric acid and the buffer content of the urine greatly increased by intravenous infusions of phosphates (or creatinine), they were able to show that the excretion of titratable acidity in the urine might become 3 to 4 times greater than the sum of acid equivalents which might have originated from the CO_2 of the glomerular filtrate and from reabsorption of phosphate as HPO_4^{--} exclusively. The conclusion was therefore drawn that (at least) the large balance in acid equivalents had been added to the urine from the tubular cells by another process. The authors considered the most likely source of these large quantities of hydrogen ion equivalents (up to 0.4 meq per min) to be H_2CO_3, since it seemed unlikely to them that other acids would be available to the cells in such quantities. They found confirmation of this view in the fact that the administration of sulphanilamide (which had been shown by MANN and KEILIN to inhibit carbonic anhydrase *in vitro*) produced a very considerable decrease in the excretion of titratable acid. The possibility that hydrogen ions might be secreted in combination with an anion was considered most unlikely since no other anions than phosphate were excreted in significant amounts in these experiments. Among the remaining two possibilities: a reabsorption of metal

---

[254] PITTS, R. F., and R. S. ALEXANDER: The nature of the renal tubular mechanism for acidifying the urine. Amer. J. Physiol. **144**, 239—254 (1945).

cations plus hydroxyl ions and an exchange of metal cations for hydrogen ions, PITTS and ALEXANDER favoured the latter as being responsible for the acidification of the urine. This view has been almost universally accepted to-day. Considering the large hydrogen ion gradient that may exist across the luminal border of the distal cells the exchange at this place must be conceived of as dependent upon a cation exchange mechanism with marked selectivity for hydrogen ions.

For some time it was believed that the acidification process was confined to the distal tubules of mammals, mostly because acidification of urine (and ammonia secretion) had been shown to occur at this site in the amphibian kidney. As discussed above (p. 239) there is, however, increasing and rather convincing evidence that a sodium ion-hydrogen ion exchange does also take place in the proximal tubules. In fact, it appears that only a smaller part of the capacity for this exchange is located in the distal tubular system.

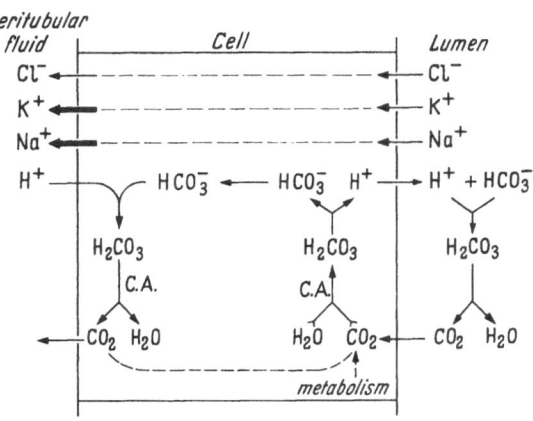

Fig. 4a. Diagram of processes presumably involved in proximal transfers of major ions

Although such thinking belongs completely to the realm of speculation it seems to make best sense in several respects if one assumes that the distal cells involved in the process of $Na^+ - H^+$ exchange differ in principle from the proximal by being virtually completely impermeable to chloride and similar anions. According to this view chloride ions could not compete with hydrogen ions for secondary transfer, so that the drag of the electric forces would be concentrated upon exchangeable cations. In this case distal reabsorption of chloride

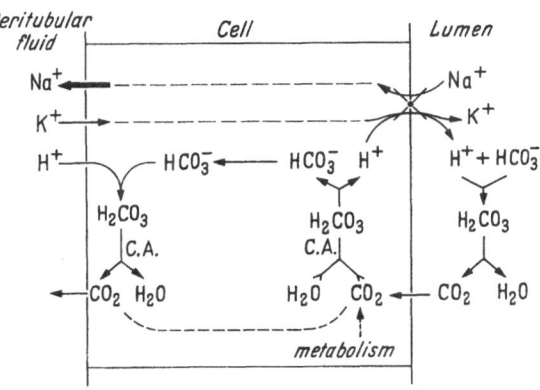

Fig. 4b. Diagram of processes involved in distal $Na^+ \rightleftarrows K^+$ or H^+ exchange processes

would have to occur by an independent process and probably in other cells (cf. the discussion below). If we assume that both the luminal and basal borders of the distal cells involved in $Na^+ - H^+$ exchange are virtually impermeable to anions (permselective), and take into consideration the depressive effect of carbonic anhydrase inhibitors on this exchange, we arrive at a concept of the events involved as portrayed in Fig. 4b (cf. PITTS[255]).

According to this diagrammatic representation sodium ions which are actively dragged through the cell (by an extrusion process operating at the basal end of the

[255] PITTS, R. F.: Modern concepts of acid-base regulation. Arch. intern. Med. 89, 864 to 876 (1952).

cell) exchanges with hydrogen ions at both borders. At the luminal border hydrogen ions are continuously provided for exchange by the action of carbonic anhydrase (C. A.). The bicarbonate ions simultaneously formed accompany the sodium ions on their passage through the interior of the cell but upon arrival at the basal end they combine again with hydrogen ions entering the cell from the peritubular space (in exchange for sodium ions). The carbonic acid thus formed is rapidly converted by carbonic anhydrase into carbon dioxide which may either diffuse into the blood or back to the luminal border. (If one assumed the basal border to be permeable to bicarbonate ions these would leave the cells together with the sodium ions and no exchange would have to occur at this site.)

According to this scheme the carbonic anhydrase may not only be of importance by speeding up the delivery of hydrogen ions for the exchange process in the luminal end. It is probably of equal importance that this enzyme also accelerates the delivery of an anion (bicarbonate) at this place which can accompany the sodium ion through the cell and *be disposed of* at the basal end. This double effect of the enzyme would seem to offer a satisfactory explanation of such phenomena as the very marked effect of carbonic anhydrase inhibitors and variations in the carbon dioxide tension in the blood (and the cells) upon the rate at which the $Na^+ - H^+$ exchange operates. Thus a rise in the carbon dioxide tension within the exchanging cells would accelerate this exchange partly by ensuring a more rapid delivery of hydrogen ions at the luminal end which would counteract a drop in hydrogen ion concentration at this site, and partly by making the fellow-travellers of the sodium ions, bicarbonate ions, more readily available. It must further be assumed that under conditions where the distal tubular fluid becomes distinctly acid, the hydrogen ion concentration gradient between this fluid and the cellular fluid will act as a factor limiting the exchange of sodium ions for hydrogen ions (and promoting the exchange for other cations). Other factors which will influence the rate of the $Na^+ - H^+$ exchange are the energy available for sodium ion transfer through the cells and the relative availability of other cations for exchange.

In the tubular fluid the fate of the hydrogen ions secreted may be one of the following: 1) a minute fraction may remain as free hydrogen ions, 2) some will react with bicarbonate ions to form carbonic acid and next (slowly) carbon dioxide, which diffuses back through the cells, 3) some will be bound (as titratable acidity) to the buffers of the urine and finally 4) some may combine with ammonia, if the latter gains access to the tubular fluid by diffusion (see below).

The formation of ammonia in the tubular cells — by deamination of glutamine and certain amino acids (VAN SLYKE et al.[256]; LOTSPEICH and PITTS[257]; KAMIN and HANDLER[258]) — and its subsequent secretion constitutes a very important supplement to the tubular secretion of hydrogen ions. Thanks to this process the body may rid itself of hydrogen ion equivalents by way of the urine at a rate several times that otherwise possible, and considerable amounts of sodium and potassium may be saved from excretion when a non-respiratory acidosis develops and induces an excretion of large amounts of anions of "strong" acids in the urine.

---

[256] SLYKE, D. D. VAN, R. A. PHILLIPS, P. B. HAMILTON, R. M. ARCHIBALD, P. H. FUTCHER, and A. HILLER: Glutamine as source material of urinary ammonia. J. biol. Chem. **150**, 481—482 (1943).

[257] LOTSPEICH, W. D., and R. F. PITTS: The role of amino acids in the renal tubular secretion of ammonia. J. biol. Chem. **168**, 611—622 (1947).

[258] KAMIN, H., and P. HANDLER: The metabolism of parenterally administered amino acids. III Ammonia formation. J. biol. Chem. **193**, 873—880 (1951).

The exact nature and localization of the ammonia secretion process in the mammalian kidney has not yet been definitely established. Experiments by RYBERG[259] — and similar ones more recently performed by others, cf. e. g. SCHWARTZ et al.[260] — have clearly indicated that the secretion of ammonia is dependent upon a reabsorption of sodium ions. RYBERG found that an appreciable increase in the excretion of ammonia (but reduction of urinary ammonia *concentration*) and a lowering of the p_H of the urine occurred when an increased urinary excretion of sodium was induced in an acidotic person, whose sodium excretion had been reduced to very low values by sodium depletion. A further important implication of these findings is that ammonia secretion must occur as far distally as the process for definite acidification, or possibly further distally if diffusion of ammonia gas is involved in the secretion. This would mean in the distal convoluted tubules, or rather — as discussed below — in the collecting tubules.

As regards the ways in which ammonia might enter into the urine, RYBERG's findings would also seem to reduce the possibilities to two: 1) an exchange of sodium ions for ammonium ions formed within the tubular cells from ammonia and hydrogen ions, or 2) a diffusion of ammonia gas from the cells into the tubular fluid in which the ammonia tension is kept low by a lowering of the p_H by hydrogen ion secretion. According to the latter possibility, suggested by SARTORIUS et al.[261] and by KRUHØFFER[206], ammonia might very well be formed in other cells than those engaged in exchange of hydrogen ions for sodium ions.

At present it seems impossible to make a well-founded choice between these two possibilities. A very conspicuous feature of the ammonia excretion is the inverse relationship between the ammonia excretion and the p_H of the urine which is well-established at least in experiments with acute changes in urinary p_H. Both mechanisms may account for this relationship. The diffusion hypothesis obviously by a greater diffusion gradient being created by a lowering of the ammonia tension in the tubular fluid at lower p_H values. The ammonium ion secretion hypothesis by pointing out that low tubular fluid p_H values would reduce hydrogen ion exchange by imposing an unsurmountable concentration difference; ammonium ions would then be favoured in the exchange process.

The p_H of the distal tubular fluid (and the rate at which it flows past the cells) is, of course, only one factor determining the rate of ammonia excretion. Obviously the NH_3 tension (or the NH_4^+ concentration) in the cells must also be a major factor. This is determined by 1) the absolute and relative activities of the enzymes which release ammonia from glutamine and amino acids and of those responsible for re-amination processes, 2) the amounts of substrates available for the enzymes. It is well-known that a gradual rise in ammonia excretion occurs over several days when acidifying salts are administered even though the urinary p_H reaches minimal values at a much earlier time. It seems established now that this continued rise is due to enzyme "adaptation", since DAVIES and YUDKIN[262] have shown that kidney slices from adapted animals show an increased capacity

[259] RYBERG, C.: The importance of sodium ions for the excretion of ammonium and hydrogen ions in the urine. Acta physiol. scand. 15, 161—172 (1948).

[260] SCHWARTZ, W. B., R. L. JENSEN, and A. S. RELMAN: Acidification of the urine and increased ammonium excretion without change in acid-base equilibrium: sodium reabsorption as a stimulus to the acidifying process. J. clin. Invest. 34, 673—680 (1955).

[261] SARTORIUS, O. W., J. C. ROEMMELT, and R. F. PITTS: The renal compensations of acid-base balance in man. IV. The nature of the renal compensations in ammonium chloride acidosis. J. clin. Invest. 28, 423—439 (1949).

[262] DAVIES, B. M. A., and J. YUDKIN: Studies in biochemical adaptation. The origin of urinary ammonia as indicated by the effect of chronic acidosis and alkalosis on some renal enzymes in the rat. Biochem. J. 52, 407—442 (1952).

for ammonia production, and several others have observed increased glutaminase activity in the renal tissue. The interpretation of such findings is, however, not quite unambiguous because of the complexity of the enzyme systems involved.

The capacity of the distal sodium exchange process and the availability of other cations (in particular potassium) for exchange are other factors which must determine the rate of ammonia excretion.

Several authors have questioned the importance of low urinary p_H as a major stimulus to ammonia secretion (DE OLIVEIRA[263]; SCHWARTZ and RELMAN[264]; LEONARD and ORLOFF[265]) mainly because they have failed to observe a definite fall in ammonia excretion at high urinary p_H values. This argument does not, however, definitely disprove the hypothesis since some of the other factors which enhance the ammonia secretion may have increased in importance at the same time. That the capacity of the enzyme system may increase in cases of body acidosis even though the urinary p_H is high has thus been observed by several investigators, e.g. by RECTOR et al.[266] in experiments with prolonged treatment of rats with acetazoleamide. It is still uncertain what constitutes the immediate stimulus to an adaptation of the ammonia producing enzymes, but a lowered intracellular p_H in the ammonia producing cells deserves serious consideration. This could account for the adaptation in primary non-respiratory acidosis, and the adaptation occurring in potassium deficiency (characterized by intracellular acidosis together with extracellular alkalosis and rather high urinary p_H) would also be consonant with this view. The occurrence of an adaptation during prolonged acetazoleamide treatment is not necessarily at variance with it, since the ammonia might be produced in other cells than those in which acetazoleamide would increase the p_H by inhibition of the carbonic anhydrase.

A further discussion of the subject of ammonia secretion would be beyond the scope of this treatise; a more comprehensive discussion and bibliography may be found in recent papers by ORLOFF and BERLINER[267] and MILNE et al.[268].

It is now well-established from studies in several mammalian species that *potassium may be excreted in the urine by tubular secretion.*

Remarkably high potassium clearances — 8 to 15 ml/min — were found as early as 1907 by BOCK[269] when rabbits were loaded with potassium salts, but since this was before measurements of the filtration rate were introduced, his conclusion that potassium (and other salts) are excreted by tubular secretion was not well-founded according to our present criteria.

Shortly after the introduction of the inulin clearance as a measure of the filtration rate, isolated reports of potassium clearances exceeding the simultaneously determined inulin clearances in diseased human subjects began to

[263] OLIVEIRA, H. L. DE: Excretion of ammonium in cases of acute tubular necrosis with acidosis and alkaline urine. Metabolism. **2**, 36—46 (1953).

[264] SCHWARTZ, W. B., and A. S. RELMAN: Metabolic and renal studies in chronic potassium depletion resulting from overuse of laxatives. J. clin. Invest. **32**, 258—271 (1953).

[265] LEONARD, E., and J. ORLOFF: Regulation of ammonia excretion in the rat. Amer. J. Physiol. **182**, 131—138 (1955).

[266] RECTOR, F. C., jr., D. W. SELDIN, A. D. ROBERTS, jr., and J. H. COPENHAVER: Relation of ammonia excretion to urine p_H. Amer. J. Physiol. **179**, 353—363 (1954).

[267] ORLOFF, J., and R. W. BERLINER: The mechanism of the excretion of ammonia in the dog. J. clin. Invest. **35**, 223—235 (1956).

[268] MILNE, M. D., B. H. SCHREINER, and M. A. CRAWFORD: Non-ionic diffusion and the excretion of weak acids and bases. Amer. J. Med. **24**, 709—729 (1958).

[269] BOCK, J.: Untersuchungen über die Nierenfunktion. I. Über die Ausscheidung der Alkalimetalle nach Injektion von Kaliumsalzen. Arch. exp. Path. Pharmak. **57**, 183—213 (1907).

appear. McCance and Widdowson[270] described a case of alkalosis resulting from treatment of a pyloric stenosis with "alkaline powder"; in this case the inulin clearance was reduced to about $1/6$ of the normal value, and the potassium clearance was 24% higher than the inulin clearance. Keith et al.[271] mention, without presenting any experimental data, that in normal subjects who were treated with fairly large doses of potassium salts to produce dehydration, the inulin clearance decreased while the potassium clearance increased, until finally the potassium clearance was the higher. They reported, moreover, that in several patients with chronic renal insufficiency, the potassium clearance was much higher than the urea clearance. Several later studies have established that in such diseases the potassium clearance also often exceeds the inulin clearance (Sirota and Kroop[272]; Nickel et al.[273]).

The occurrence of a tubular secretion of potassium has been demonstrated by systematic experiments in several mammalian species. Wirz[274] has reported potassium/inulin clearance ratios as high as 1.5 in adrenalectomized cats at a time when the inulin clearance was very low. Berliner and Kennedy[275] and Mudge et al.[276] have observed similar ratios well above unity in normal dogs during intravenous infusion of potassium chloride and during extreme urea diuresis. Similar evidence for potassium secretion was obtained by Kruhøffer[206] in normal rabbits during loading with potassium chloride, and more recently sheep have been added to the list of species in which potassium secretion may occur (Denton et al.[277]).

According to current views tubular secretion of potassium ions takes place in exchange for sodium ions and in the same distal cells which are involved in the exchange of hydrogen ions for sodium ions. [For a discussion of this exchange see also part I, chapter VII (i).] The view that potassium ions are secreted in exchange for sodium ions is mainly based on the observations that the excretion of potassium is markedly reduced when the excretion of sodium reaches low levels, and that, under such conditions, it may be appreciably raised when an increase in the excretion of sodium is induced by one of several different procedures (at least under conditions when sodium retaining mechanisms are activated). Detailed discussion of this evidence will, however, be deferred to the section on the interrelationship between urinary acidification and sodium and potassium excretion (p. 286). The rapidly growing evidence that potassium competes with hydrogen ions in the distal exchange of the latter for sodium will also be presented and discussed at the same place.

[270] McCance, R. A., and E. M. Widdowson: Alkalosis with disordered kidney functions. Lancet 233, 247—249 (1937).

[271] Keith, N. M., H. E. King, and A. E. Osterberg: Serum concentration and renal clearance of potassium in severe renal insufficiency in man. Arch. intern. Med. 71, 675—701 (1943).

[272] Sirota, J. H., and I. G. Kroop: Evidence suggesting renal tubular excretion of potassium in man during recovery from acute renal insufficiency. J. clin. Invest. 30, 1082 to 1088 (1951).

[273] Nickel, J. F., P. B. Lowrance, E. Leifer, and S. E. Bradley: Renal function, electrolyte excretion and body fluids in patients with chronic renal insufficiency before and after sodium deprivation. J. clin. Invest. 32, 68—79 (1953).

[274] Wirz, H.: Untersuchungen über die Nierenfunktion bei adrenalektomierten Katzen. Helv. physiol. pharmacol. Acta 3, 589—612 (1945).

[275] Berliner, R. W., and T. J. Kennedy, jr.: Renal tubular secretion of potassium in the normal dog. Proc. Soc. exp. Biol. (N. Y.) 67, 542—545 (1948).

[276] Mudge, G. H., J. Foulks, and A. Gilman: The renal excretion of potassium Proc. Soc. exp. Biol. (N. Y.) 67, 545—547 (1948).

[277] Denton, D. A., I. R. Donald, J. Munro, and W. Williams: Excess Na$^+$ substraction in the sheep. Aust. J. exp. Biol. med. Sci. 30, 213—250 (1952).

It is a common belief to-day that practically all of the filtered potassium is reabsorbed, so that nearly all that appears in the urine is derived from tubular secretion (BERLINER, KENNEDY, ORLOFF[223]). While no definite proof for the correctness of this view can be delivered at present it does not appear unreasonable, considering WIRZ and BOTT's[227] demonstration that the potassium concentration in the proximal tubular fluid is regularly below that of the blood plasma. MOREL[278] injected radioactive potassium into rabbits during mannitol diuresis and found the ratio between the specific activities of urine and plasma potassium to deviate markedly from unity during phases of rapidly rising or falling specific activities of the plasma potassium. He considered this finding as evidence that the major part of the potassium excreted in the urine was secreted by the tubules from a cellular potassium pool which only equilibrated with the plasma potassium with a certain time-lag. His argumentation is, however, not really convincing, partly because dead space errors were not definitely excluded and partly because the possibility was not considered that there might be a rapid exchange of potassium between the tubular fluid and the cell fluid. BLACK et al. (see BLACK and EMERY[279]) found that the specific activity of the potassium of the arterial blood for some time after a K^{42} injection differed from that of renal venous potassium, which, on the other hand, resembled the specific activity of the urinary potassium. While this indicates that renal tissue potassium was a major source of the potassium ions appearing in both urine and renal venous blood, it does not prove that a *net* tubular secretion is the major source of urinary potassium, since rapid exchanges of potassium, without a net secretion, could produce the same result. For further criticism see the recent review by BRADLEY and WHEELER[280].

Although it is true that all we actually know is that the amount of potassium excreted equals the amount filtered less the amount reabsorbed plus the amount secreted, it appears that BERLINER's view gives the most satisfactory explanation of the variations in potassium excretion observed under a variety of conditions. The possibility that the (proximal) reabsorption may become less complete under certain conditions should not, however, be completely lost sight of (cf. p. 288). BERLINER's view has recently been supported by the results found in experiments on the excretion of potassium at different glomerular filtration rates (DAVIDSON et al.[228]). — It would be expected that the potassium secretion in the distal tubules would be dependent on the availability of sodium ions for exchange. If the proximal reabsorption of filtered potassium is complete, the rate of excretion of potassium should be independent of the filtered load of potassium, provided an adequate distal load of sodium is maintained. This was actually found to be so in dogs in which the filtered load was changed by reduction of the filtration rate by means of an inflatable cuff placed around one renal artery.

Distal reabsorption of Na^+ and Cl^-. It remains to discuss the distal mechanism of joint reabsorption of chloride and sodium ions. Our present knowledge on this point is very meager, e.g. it is not even known which of these ions is transferred actively. Certain experimental findings have, however, aroused a good deal of speculation both as regards the location and the nature of this process.

OKKELS[281] demonstrated the existence of markedly argentophilic cells in the distal convoluted tubules and collecting tubules of the mammalian kidney.

[278] MOREL, F.: Les modalités d'excrétion du potassium par le rein, étude expérimentale à l'aide du radio-potassium chez le lapin. Helv. physiol. Acta **13**, 276—294 (1955).

[279] BLACK, D. A. K., and E. W. EMERY: Tubular secretion of potassium. Brit. med. Bull. **13**, 7—10 (1957).

[280] BRADLEY, S. E., and H. O. WHEELER: On the diversities of structure, perfusion and function of the nephron population. Amer. J. Med. **24**, 692—708 (1958).

These findings were confirmed by FEYEL and VIEILLEFOSSE[282] who also found, in experiments in rats, that both the number and distribution of these cells increased considerably when the plasma concentration of chloride was low; they took these findings as an indication that the cells were involved in active reabsorption of chloride. LJUNGBERG[249] thought it likely that such argentophilic cells were responsible for the very high chloride concentrations which he had observed in renal medullary tissue from rabbits (cf. p. 248), and he, too, attributed to these cells a role in active reabsorption of chloride.

Obviously a high concentration of a substance, in this case chloride, in an epithelial cell is no proof of an active transport of this substance through the cell, and all that one can say at present is that the argentophilic tubular cells may or may not be involved in an active transport of chloride (*plus* sodium and possibly also potassium).

In studies on the renal excretion of various anions in dogs, rabbits and human subjects SAUGMAN[212] has recently made certain observations which may suggest the existence of a selective reabsorption of chloride in the distal tubules. During osmotic diureses or pituitary antidiureses (i.e. under conditions where the distal reabsorption of water must be assumed to follow distal salt reabsorption) the excretion percentage of thiocyanate was consistently lower than that of chloride. During water diuresis which affected the chloride excretion very little, the excretion percentage for thiocyanate rose markedly (approximately as much as that of water). On the basis of the findings obtained during antidiuresis SAUGMAN assumes that thiocyanate ions are more completely reabsorbed in the proximal tubules than chloride. The fact that its excretion goes up markedly during water diuresis (in contrast to that of chloride) is suggested to mean that chloride is reabsorbed distally by a primary active process by which some chloride ions may be exchanged for thiocyanate ions until the rise in thiocyanate concentration in the tubular fluid arrests further exchange. That diffusion of thiocyanate as the free acid between tubular fluid and plasma should be responsible for the close parallelism between the reabsorptions of water and thiocyanate was rejected by SAUGMAN, since the pK of the acid is quite low.

These findings are, evidently, only suggestive of a selective and primary active distal reabsorption of chloride. If such a process actually exists, most of the chloride would, of course, be reabsorbed together with sodium, but there is no reason why potassium could not also be concomitantly reabsorbed. If so, one would probably have to assume that the distal reabsorption of chloride should occur at a more proximal site than that where potassium may be secreted by exchange. This is consonant with the view, discussed in p. 250, that an appreciable reabsorption of Na + Cl in the ascending limb of HENLE's loop should be the major driving power for the concentrating mechanism of the kidney. It should be emphasized, however, that our knowledge of the fate of the chloride ion in the distal part of the nephron remains little known. The findings of S. SOLOMON [cf. part I, chapter VII (f)] indicate the existence in the *superficial* distal tubules of rats of an electric potential gradient which would favour transport of chloride ions passively ("downhill") towards the blood in these tubular segments; they do not exclude, however, the existence of a reverse potential gradient in deeper parts, such as the ascending limbs of HENLE's loop.

---

[281] OKKELS, H.: Différences entre les diverses cellules du troisième segment du tube urinaire, chez les vertébrés. Bull. Histol. appl. Physiol. **6**, 12—33 (1929).

[282] FEYEL, P., et R. VIEILLEFOSSE: Les sécrétions rénales de l'urée et des chlorures. Arch. Anat. micr. **35**, 5—53 (1939).

Concluding remarks. It will be apparent from the foregoing discussion that a fairly well-defined picture of the various processes taking place in the nephron has emerged. It is equally clear that a number of problems concerning the location and in particular the intimate nature and interaction of the tubular transfer processes remain to be solved before a really comprehensive and thrustworthy conception can be formulated. Recent progress in the sampling of tubular fluid, such as the micro-catheterization of the collecting tubules (JARAUSCH and ULL-RICH[283]), and the "stop flow analysis" (MALVIN et al.[284]; PITTS et al.[285]) may prove to be important tools to the solution of, in particular, the localization problems. The results so far obtained with these methods have not revealed anything demanding modifications of the general views expressed above. In the hands of ULLRICH and coworkers (HILGER et al.[286]; KLÜMPER et al.[287]; ULLRICH et al.[288]) micro-catheterization experiments have given the following results as regards processes occurring in the collecting tubules:

1) Some active reabsorption of sodium.
2) Reabsorption of water, presumably by osmosis.
3) No evidence of potassium transfers.
4) A certain loss of urea, presumably by diffusion.
5) Ammonia secretion (in good agreement with reported high contents of glutaminase in the inner renal medulla).

The sodium reabsorption observed in the collecting tubules would, as pointed out by the authors, contribute to the hypertonicity of the medullary interstitial fluid, and it would thus serve the urinary concentrating mechanism in the same way as a sodium reabsorption in the loop of HENLE. It might *a priori* seem that nothing would actually be gained in this respect since the loss of sodium from the urine in the collecting tubules would cause a reduction in urine tonicity. It should be recalled, however, that this is not so if the sodium reabsorption was exclusively one of exchange with NH_4^+ ($H^+ + NH_3$); if so Na^+ in the urine would simply be replaced with another cation with no resulting change in the tonicity. As far as the osmotic activity of the medulla is concerned the production *plus* secretion of NH_4^+ ($NH_3 + H^+$) should by itself cause no change, since a glutamate ion would replace a glutamine ion, or an α-keto acid ion replace an α-amino acid ion. The sodium ions reabsorbed (in exchange) would therefore represent a net gain in medullary osmotic activity.

As to the nature of the tubular transfers of electrolytes it is apparent from the above discussion that the present trend is to consider a "sodium pump" in various modifications as underlying the major part of these transfers. It might be tempting at this place to relate sodium reabsorption to oxygen consumption (cf. Part I, p. 120). If

---

[283] JARAUSCH, K. H., u. K. J. ULLRICH: Zur Technik der Entnahme von Harnproben aus einzelnen Sammelröhren der Säugetierniere mittels Polyäthylen-Capillaren. Pflügers Arch. ges. Physiol. **264**, 88—94 (1957).

[284] MALVIN, R. L., W. S. WILDE and L. P. SULLIVAN: Location of nephron transport by stop flow analysis. Amer. J. Physiol. **194**, 135—142 (1958).

[285] PITTS, R. F., R. S. GARD, R. H. KESSLER, and K. HIERHOLZER: Localization of acidification of urine, potassium and ammonium secretion and phosphate reabsorption in the nephron of the dog. Amer. J. Physiol. **194**, 125—134 (1958).

[286] HILGER, H. H., J. D. KLÜMPER u. K. J. ULLRICH: Wasserrückresorption und Ionen-transport durch die Sammelrohrzellen der Säugetierniere. Pflügers Arch. ges. Physiol. **267**, 218—237 (1958).

[287] KLÜMPER, J. D., K. J. ULLRICH u. H. H. HILGER: Das Verhalten des Harnstoffs in den Sammelrohren der Säugetierniere. Pflügers Arch. ges. Physiol. **267**, 238—243 (1958).

[288] ULLRICH, K. J., H. H. HILGER u. J. D. KLÜMPER: Sekretion von Ammoniumionen in den Sammelrohren der Säugetierniere. Pflügers Arch. ges. Physiol. **267**, 244—250 (1958).

is assumed that some 99% of the sodium filtered is reabsorbed by active processes, this would mean that some 14 000 μeq/min or some 3700 μeq/100 g kidney/min are actively reabsorbed. If it is further assumed that the oxygen consumption of the anuric kidney [some 2 ml/100 g kidney/min (MUNCK[289])] represents the rate at which oxygen is normally expended on processes other than tubular transfers, and that practically all the additional oxygen consumed under normal conditions is being spent on tubular transport of sodium, some 4 ml of O_2 per 100 g of kidney/min must be used for this function (MUNCK[289]). 4 ml of oxygen or 180 μM are equivalent to 720 μeq valents. It is seen that a ratio of sodium transport to excess oxygen uptake of 5 or more is reached. This is in the upper end of the range found in other tissues (cf. Part I, p. 120 and Part II, p. 435).

It may also be pointed out at this place that if the major part of the oxygen consumption of the kidney is serving sodium (and thus water) reabsorption, then a close parallelism might be expected between the rate of oxygen consumption and the rate of fluid reabsorption. This again would mean that, under conditions where only a small fraction of the filtered electrolytes and water is excreted, a parallelism between the rate of oxygen consumption and the glomerular filtration rate could be expected. The writer feels that this concept deserves careful consideration in the evaluation of previous, and in the planning of future, studies on renal oxygen consumption.

C. Transport of fluid in the nephron as a whole (relationship between glomerular and tubular factors)

As previously mentioned this section has been included to discuss coherently, although only in broad terms, the relationship between those glomerular and tubular factors which determine the rates of excretion of sodium, principal anions and water.

Two fundamentally different types of forces are involved in fluid transportation in the nephron: 1) hydrostatic forces, generated by the heart and responsible for the formation of glomerular filtrate and for its further propulsion within the tubular lumina, and 2) active cellular forces responsible for absorption of fluid from the tubular lumina.

A (distal) tubular secretion of water has recently been postulated (WEST et al.[290] and other papers by the same group; BERGMANN et al.[291]), but since no convincing evidence has been provided, the possibility of a tubular secretion of water will be disregarded here.

The processes of tubular reabsorption of the predominant electrolytes (Na^+, Cl^-, HCO_3^-) and water were described in the preceding section. As mentioned there, under conditions not deviating too much from "normal" the major parts of these components of the filtrate (around 85%) are thought to be reabsorbed in the proximal tubules, while smaller or larger fractions of the remainder are reabsorbed in the distal tubules.

It is generally conceded that the fluid in BOWMAN's capsules (capsular fluid) is formed by ultrafiltration of plasma through the glomerular capillaries.

The quantitative aspects of the process of ultrafiltration through capillary walls and artificial membranes of similar pore diameters (40—100 Ångström) have

[289] MUNCK, O.: Renal circulation in acute renal failure. p. 25. Oxford: Blackwell 1958.
[290] WEST, C. D., S. A. KAPLAN, S. J. FOMON, and S. RAPOPORT. Urine flow and solute excretion during osmotic diuresis in hydrated dogs: Role of distal tubule in the production of hypotonic urine. Amer. J. Physiol. 170, 239—254 (1952).
[291] BERGMANN, F., S. DICKSTEIN, J. MENCZEL, and T. D. ULLMANN: Renal clearance of uncharged particles, as exemplified by thioureas. J. Physiol. 145, 22—36 (1959).

recently been thoroughly dealt with by PAPPENHEIMER[292]. In such artificial membranes the net flow of fluid across the membrane is proportional to the difference between the hydrostatic and colloid osmotic pressure gradients, and data from experiments on hind limbs, mesentery, etc., indicate that this relationship also holds for ultrafiltration through various capillaries. In the case of the glomerular capillaries direct testing has not yet been possible, but there is hardly any reason to question that the same relationship also applies to this case.

Consequently, the flow of fluid 1) through the glomerular membrane and 2) further along the tubular lumina for various distances must be considered to be maintained by a common pressure head, viz. the amount by which the difference (hydrostatic pressure in the glomerular capillaries — oncotic pressure of the plasma) exceeds the renal pelvic pressure. It is proposed to call this pressure head the *glomerular propulsive pressure*.

Some part of this pressure head, viz. (glomerular propulsive pressure — capsular pressure) = effective filtration pressure, is used for the formation of capsular fluid, and the remainder for the further propulsion within the tubular lumina.

It is a matter of great importance to our understanding of the interrelationship between the filtration, reabsorption and excretion of water and the principal electrolytes to know what the relative magnitudes of the hydrodynamic resistances in the glomerular membrane and in the various parts of the tubules are. Knowledge on this point has, however, only begun to be gained very recently, and the fact that it is still incomplete makes it reasonable to consider the problems from a theoretical point of view before the available evidence is discussed.

The problems involved are well illustrated by considering two extreme theoretical cases, viz. one in which the hydrodynamic resistance in the tubules is negligible in comparison with that in the glomerular membrane and another in which the resistance in the glomerular membrane is negligible as compared with the resistance in the tubules.

In the discussion of these cases reference is made to Fig. 5 which illustrates some basic features of the transport of fluid in a nephron. The horizontal tubing represents the nephron. It starts with a constriction which represents the hydrodynamic resistance in the glomerular membrane (R_{mb}). Then follows the tubules: proximal, Henle's loop and distal, ending in the renal pelvis. The resistances in the tubules are arranged in series with the glomerular resistance, and the resistance in the total length of the tubules is indicated by R_{tub}. Fluid is driven through these resistances by means of the glomerular propulsive pressure, which is indicated on the pressure reservoir as glomerular capillary pressure *minus* the oncotic pressure of plasma. Some fluid which becomes final urine is passed through all of the resistances, whereas some (and normally a much larger quantity), which is reabsorbed in the tubules, is driven through only some fraction of the total resistance in the nephron. The energy for the reabsorption process is assumed to be provided entirely by the tubular cells, and this process is therefore indicated by syringes, the plungers of which must be imagined to move downwards by extraneous forces.

In the first extreme case to be considered — that in which the tubular resistance is assumed to be negligible — it is immediately apparent that glomerular filtration and tubular fluid reabsorption would be independent variables. Assuming a constant resistance in the glomerular membrane the filtration rate would be solely determined by — and proportional to — the glomerular propulsive pressure, and uninfluenced by changes in tubular conditions such as changes in the rate of

[292] PAPPENHEIMER, J. R.: Passage of molecules through capillary walls. Physiol. Rev. **33**, 387—423 (1953).

fluid reabsorption or in tubular luminal diameters. Changes in the rate of excretion of water (and electrolytes) could therefore be effected by entirely independent variations in the rate of filtration and the rate of reabsorption.

In the second extreme case — with a negligible membrane resistance — it is readily seen that the following features would characterize the function of the nephron: 1) An increase in the rate of sodium and fluid reabsorption in the most proximal part of the tubular system (syringe no. 1) would lead to an almost identical increase in the rate at which fluid was filtered, since the pressure required to drive an additional amount of fluid down to this site of reabsorption would be very small compared with that needed to drive it throughout the nephron. For

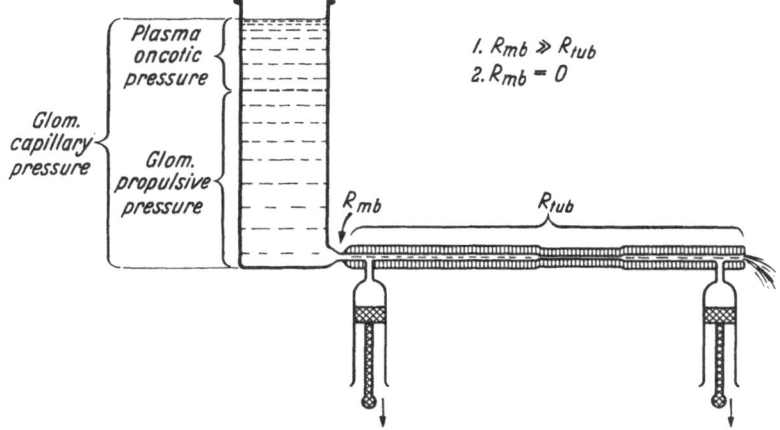

Fig. 5. Simplified diagram of the hydrodynamics of a nephron

the same reason the reduction in urine flow (and sodium excretion) would be much smaller than the increase in fluid reabsorption. 2) In contrast, an increase in the rate of fluid reabsorption in the most distal part of the tubular system (syringe no. 2) would greatly diminish the rate of urine flow, whereas it would have only very little effect upon the filtration rate, since the pressure requirements for driving fluid to an extremely distal site of reabsorption or all the way through to excretion would be nearly identical. 3) An increase in glomerular propulsive pressure — as an isolated alteration — would lead to an increase in the filtration rate and to an equally large increase in the rate of urine flow (and salt excretion). The increase in filtration rate would, however, not be nearly as large on a percentage basis as the increase in glomerular propulsive pressure since any additional fluid being filtered would have to pass the entire resistance in the nephron which greatly exceeds the average resistance passed by fluid being reabsorbed. 4) Finally it is evident that a reduction in the hydrodynamic resistance in the tubules corresponding to a widening of the tubular lumina could lead to a considerable increase in the filtration rate and a similar increase in urine flow (and salt excretion).

From these considerations the following conclusions may then be drawn as regards the second extreme case: The filtration rate would be greatly influenced by changes in tubular conditions such as changes in proximal reabsorption of sodium and fluid and changes in luminal diameters in tubular segments offering considerable resistance to flow. A suppression of the proximal reabsorption of sodium (and water) should therefore lead to a retention of such substances as urea the excretion of which is largely dependent upon glomerular filtration. The rates of excretion of sodium and water would be relatively little affected by changes in proximal reabsorption of sodium and water, but would be greatly influenced by changes in distal reabsorption of these components and by changes in tubular luminal diameters.

Although the problems have been dealt with here in a very simplified manner it is apparent that if the actual conditions in the nephrons approached the second extreme case considered, a considerable number of factors would have to be accounted for in order to provide satisfactory explanations of observed changes in the rates of filtration, reabsorption and excretion of water and electrolytes.

The actual conditions in the nephrons must obviously lie somewhere between the two extreme cases considered, but our present knowledge does not yet allow any definite conclusions as to whether they are closer to one or the other of the extreme cases.

The resistance in the glomerular membrane has never been measured directly, but attempts have been made to measure it by indirect methods. On the basis of observations on the glomerular sieving of myoglobin and ovalbumin in dog experiments PAPPENHEIMER[293] calculated the filtration coefficient of the glomerular membranes (i.e. the filtration rate per unit of effective pressure drop accross the glomerular membranes) to 1.9—4.5 ml/min per mm of Hg and 100 g of kidney, with an average value of 3.1. This latter value corresponds to an effective filtration pressure of 20 mm of Hg across the membrane at a normal filtration rate (62 ml/min per 100 g of kidney). From similar calculations based on the glomerular sieving of dextran fractions of various molecular sizes WALLENIUS and GARBY (personal communication) arrived at a value for the effective filtration pressure of only a few mm of Hg, suggesting that the glomerular resistance should be considerably smaller than indicated by PAPPENHEIMER's calculations. Both of these approaches are subject to objections, PAPPENHEIMER's because the possible effect of electric charges on the protein molecules was neglected and a spherical form of these molecules had to be assumed, and WALLENIUS and GARBY's because the dextran fractions did not contain molecules of only one particular size, but rather molecules within a certain size range. It would be of great interest to see the results of similar investigations carried out with more ideal indicator substances, and, in particular, it would be interesting to learn if any changes in the glomerular filtration coefficient could be demonstrated during osmotic diuresis or in other cases of profuse diuresis.

The hydrodynamic resistance in the different segments of the tubular system under normal conditions is not definitely known either, but recent micropuncture studies, so far only performed in rats, have provided some information on intra-tubular pressures which allows certain conclusions to be drawn as regards some of the tubular resistances at least in that species. WIRZ (cf. WIRZ[294] for a survey) has found an average pressure of 14.8 mm of Hg in the first two-thirds of the proximal tubules of moderately hydrated rats; this pressure was not significantly different from that observed in the peritubular capillaries and it was not significantly affected when a pitressin-antidiuresis was induced. A very similar value was observed by GOTTSCHALK and MYLLE[295] in normally hydrated rats, and no

[293] PAPPENHEIMER, J. R.: Über die Permeabilität der Glomerulummembranen in der Niere. Klin. Wschr. 33, 362—365 (1955).

[294] WIRZ, H.: Die Druckverhältnisse in der normalen Niere. Schweiz. med. Wschr. 86, 377—382 (1956).

[295] GOTTSCHALK, C. W., and M. MYLLE: Micropuncture study of pressures in proximal tubules and peritubular capillaries of the rat kidney and their relation to ureteral and renal venous pressures. Amer. J. Physiol. 185, 430—439 (1956).

definite correlation was observed by these investigators between the intratubular pressure and the distance from the glomerulus. Since a considerable part of the filtered fluid will be flowing through the first part of the proximal tubules, the latter finding indicates that the resistance in the proximal tubules must normally be small in comparison with the resistance in the glomerular membrane, if PAPPEN-HEIMER's conclusion is correct, that as much as some 20 mm of Hg is required to drive fluid through the glomerular membranes at a normal filtration rate.

The above-mentioned pressures indicate, however, also that there must be a considerably larger resistance in more distal segments of the tubular system, since there exists a pressure drop of some 15 mm of Hg across this part of the tubular system in spite of the fact that fluid is flowing through it at a rate amounting to only a small fraction of the filtration rate. WIRZ has measured the pressure within the distal tubules of a few rats. During moderate water diuresis there was a pressure fall from the proximal to the distal tubules of some 5 mm Hg. Injection of Pitressin caused no change in the proximal pressure, but it reduced the urine flow to $1/3$ of the previous value and reduced distal tubular pressure to near atmospheric pressure. — These findings are in essential agreement with later and more detailed studies by GOTTSCHALK and MYLLE[296]. In rats anaesthetized with pentobarbital and — most likely — in endogenous antidiuresis, the mean proximal tubular pressure was 12.5 ± 2.2 mm Hg, distal tubular pressure 6.7 ± 1.6 mm Hg. Pelvic pressure was around 1 mm Hg. Osmotic diuresis produced visible dilatation of the proximal and distal tubules, and the distal intratubular pressure rose to values close to the (now generally elevated) level of the proximal intratubular pressure. These results were interpreted by the authors to mean that the collecting tubule system is a limiting factor in the outflow of urine from the kidney and is an important determinant of intratubular pressure at high rates of urine flow. They suggested that the pressure fall over the thin limb of HENLE at low urine flows was due to a constriction of the nephron, that over the collecting tubules at high urine flows was due to a high degree of confluence of these structures.

The above studies do not permit any definite conclusions to be drawn as regards the relative size of the glomerular and tubular resistances. If, however, PAPPENHEIMER's figure of an effective pressure drop of some 20 mm of Hg across the glomerular membrane is assumed to apply to rats also, the tentative conclusion may be drawn that the tubular resistance is normally some 5 times higher than that in the glomerular membrane and that it is mainly located in the most distal parts of the nephron.

If this conclusion is correct it follows that the features which were concluded above to characterize the function of the nephron in the second extreme case (negligible membrane resistance) would also largely apply to the actual nephrons.

Until otherwise disproven it seems therefore reasonable to assume that the proximal reabsorption of sodium and water is normally of considerable importance as a factor determining the magnitude of the filtration rate. Likewise it seems justified to suppose that changes in proximal reabsorptions of sodium and water have considerably less effect on the rates of sodium and water excretions than similar changes in the rates of distal reabsorptions of sodium and water.

Alterations in tubular luminal diameters must also be considered a potential source of changes in filtration rate and urine flow (and salt excretion), but to be of importance in this respect, such alterations must lead to a perceptible change in the total resistance in the nephron. Alterations in luminal diameters would therefore

[296] GOTTSCHALK, C. W., and M. MYLLE: Micropuncture study of pressures in proximal and distal tubules and peritubular capillaries of the rat kidney during osmotic diuresis. Amer. J. Physiol. 189, 323—328 (1957).

have the greatest effect when they occur in tubular segments which normally have the highest resistance. According to the studies cited above this would seem to be the most distal parts of the distal convoluted tubules or segments further distally.

Although the nature of the resistance in this part of the nephron is not definitely established, it seems quite likely that it is mainly due to a partial collapse caused by pressure from the outside, as suggested by WINTON[297]. The existence of such a collapsed section in the tubular system is strongly suggested by WINTON's observation, that the filtration rate and the rate of urine flow is not significantly reduced during increasing ureter pressure before the latter reaches a value of some 15 mm Hg. This finding as well as GOTTSCHALK and MYLLE's observation that the proximal intratubular pressure does not start to rise before the ureter pressure has reached this value is most readily explained by assuming a gradual dilatation of a previously collapsed distal tubular segment in response to a rising ureter pressure. The presence of a considerable resistance in a collapsed tubular segment means that the resistance in the nephron contains an element which is readily altered by changes in intra- and extratubular pressures. This may well be a factor of importance to the control of water and electrolyte excretions, but it is hardly possible at present to state how and to what extent.

From the above discussion it is apparent that certain experimental findings may be predicted if it were correct that the resistance in the tubules is normally appreciably larger than that in the glomerular membrane. Some of the pertinent literature is briefly discussed below.

One would expect, for instance, that an abolition of the tubular reabsorption of sodium and fluid would cause a very appreciable diminution in the filtration rate. This is actually what has been found in perfusion experiments on dogs' kidneys when cyanide was added to the blood (BAYLISS and LUNDSGAARD[298]) or when the kidney was cooled (BICKFORD and WINTON[299]). Reductions in creatinine clearance to around 10—15 % of the normal values were observed, even though tubular reabsorption of fluid was not completely abolished. Very marked falls in creatinine and inulin clearances have also been observed in animals poisoned with drugs known to cause lesions in the (proximal) tubules but no perceptible changes in the glomeruli (e.g. dichromate nephritis in rabbits, SCHOU[211]; sublimate nephritis in rabbits, GUKELBERGER and TSCHUMI[300]). Furthermore very appreciable reductions in inulin clearance have been observed following transient clamping of the renal artery, a procedure causing anoxic damage to the tubular cells.

Another prediction would be a tendency to a parallelism between the (proximal) rate of fluid reabsorption and the filtration rate. Such a parallelism has been observed by several investigators in different species (e.g. by MOUSTGAARD[301], in dogs on diet of varying protein content; by WESSON et al.[302], in dogs following parenteral administration of saline, and by KRUHØFFER[206], in rabbits in various states of hydration). The fact that the glucose Tm does not change significantly

[297] WINTON, F. R.: Hydrostatic pressures affecting the flow of urine and blood in the kidney. Harvey Lect. 21—52 (1951—1952).

[298] BAYLISS, L. E., and E. LUNDSGAARD: The action of cyanide on the isolated mammalian kidney. J. Physiol. 74, 279—293 (1932).

[299] BICKFORD, R. G., and F. R. WINTON: The influence of temperature on the isolated kidney of the dog. J. Physiol. 89, 198—219 (1937).

[300] GUKELBERGER, M., u. H. TSCHUMI: Die Nierenfunktion bei der Sublimatdiurese. Schweiz. med. Wschr. 74, 33—34 (1944).

[301] MOUSTGAARD, J.: Om Proteinstoffernes Indflydelse på Nyrefunktionen hos Hund. (Danish Thesis) Copenhagen 1948.

[302] WESSON, L. G., jr., W. P. ANSLOW, jr., L. G. RAISZ, A. A. BOLOMEY, and M. LADD: Effect of sustained expansion of extracellular fluid volume upon filtration rate, renal plasma flow and electrolyte and water excretion in the dog. Amer. J. Physiol. 162, 677—886 (1950).

under similar conditions would seem to indicate that the covariation is a property of each particular nephron and that it does not simply reflect activation — inactivation of nephrons.

It may also be predicted that a certain change in the glomerular propulsive pressure should lead to a change in the filtration rate which is much smaller on a percentage basis than the change in propulsive pressure. It is in keeping with this prediction that BOJESEN[303] was unable to detect any significant change in inulin or creatinine clearance when the oncotic pressure of the plasma of dogs was reduced by as much as 8 mm of Hg by means of rapid intravenous injection of a Ringer-like solution. It is also noteworthy that the oncotic pressure had to be reduced by as much as some 4 mm of Hg to produce an increase in urine flow of 1 ml/min. Although with considerable reserve this finding may be interpreted to mean that the total resistance in the nephrons were about 4 mm of Hg/ml/min, a figure greatly exceeding that (about $^1/_3$ mm of Hg/ml/min) calculated by PAPPEN-HEIMER as the resistance in the glomerular membranes.

The fact that the above experimental findings are predictable on the assumption that the tubular resistance is normally considerably larger than that in the glomerular membrane can obviously not prove but only suggest, that the conditions in the nephrons actually are of this character. Alternative explanations are, indeed, possible.

In the above discussion reference has constantly been made to the events in a single nephron, and, as has often been done before, it has been tacitly implied that the overall function of the kidneys is simply the phenomena occurring in a single nephron multiplied by the number of nephrons in the kidney. This concept obviously represents an oversimplification, since completely identical function of the different nephrons is already precluded by their variable development (BRADLEY and WHEELER[280]). Still it might of course be that fairly parallel changes occurred in the nephrons.

According to the "cell-separation hypothesis" recently proposed by PAPPEN-HEIMER and KINTER[304] this may not even be the case. This hypothesis was formulated to account for certain peculiarities concerning the "dynamic haematocrit" of the blood in the kidney, viz. that it was normally only about half that of the haematocrit of the blood entering and leaving the kidney, and that it approached the value of the latter, when this was either abnormally high or abnormally low or when the renal arterial pressure was appreciably reduced (from 140 to 53 mm of Hg on an average). It was assumed that a "skimming" occurs in the interlobular arteries by which the afferent vessels at the base is supplied mainly with plasma, leaving the cell rich core-stream in the interlobular arteries to supply the terminal branches and thus the superficial glomeruli. Since an intrarenal haematocrit lower than that of the blood entering and leaving the organ would mean that the erythrocytes are passing the kidney faster than the plasma, it was further assumed that the cell-rich blood is passed directly to the interlobular veins by special short channels which do not communicate with the peritubular vascular bed. The authors feel that a scheme of the renal circulation of this type does not only account for the above observations on the intrarenal haematocrit, but also (due to variations in the degree of cell separation) for such phenomena as the relative constancy of the renal blood flow and the glomerular filtration rate when

---

[303] BOJESEN, E.: The renal mechanism of "dilution diuresis" and salt excretion in dogs. Acta physiol. scand. **32**, 129—147 (1954).

[304] PAPPENHEIMER, J. R., and W. B. KINTER: Hematocrit ratio of blood within mammalian kidney and its significance for renal hemodynamics. Amer. J. Physiol. **185**, 377—390 (1956).

the renal arterial pressure varies around its normal value (cf. also KINTER and PAPPENHEIMER[305]).

According to the cell-separation hypothesis the haematocrit of the blood supplied to the glomeruli becomes an important and variable factor determining the function of the nephron. Thus the glomeruli in the outer cortex, which are assumed to receive little plasma under normal conditions, are considered to contribute relatively little to the total filtration rate under such conditions, but their contribution is believed to increase when the skimming becomes less effective at falling renal arterial pressure or when the haematocrit of the systemic blood is reduced.

Although the occurrence of some skimming of the type proposed does not seem unlikely, the writer feels that the cell-separation hypothesis and its alleged implications should be looked at with considerable reserve, partly because the calculations of the "dynamic haematocrit" rest upon some very questionable extrapolations, and partly because the interpretation of these calculated values is based upon the assumption of renal vacular channels for which there is no anatomical evidence.

For recent discussions of the cell-separation hypothesis the reader should consult WINTON[306] and the chapter in Ann. Rev. Physiol. 1958.

In concluding this chapter it should be pointed out that the pressure relations in the various segments of the nephron in man are unknown. The only pressure measured in man is the wedged renal vein pressure. This pressure in normal subjects averaged 17.7. mm Hg (MUNCK[289]). It should also be stressed that safe conclusions may not be drawn from one species to another. This has been illustrated by the demonstration by GOTTSCHALK (see WINTON[306]) that "needle pressures" are higher and much more variable within a single kidney in the dog than in the rat.

D. Physical factors (pressures) affecting sodium (and water) excretion

Very prompt changes in the rate of urinary excretion of sodium and water can be induced by changing 1) the colloid osmotic pressure of plasma, 2) the renal arterial pressure, 3) the renal venous pressure or 4) the ureteral pressure. A change in glomerular propulsive pressure would seem to be a common denominator in all these cases.

It is a frequent experience in biological work, especially when whole animals are used, that the immediate effects of a change in one or another factor tend to be "blurred" with time by the interference of secondary reactions. Since this also holds for the complex systems determining urinary electrolyte excretions it follows that to get as undistorted a picture as possible of the effects of changes in any of the above pressures, studies must be carried out as soon as possible after the changes have been established.

Accurate determinations of rapidly changing rates of electrolyte excretions are, however, hampered by the occurrence of a continuous mixing of the urine in the renal pelves on its way to the bladder. This problem has recently been thoroughly discussed and procedures devised by which the errors originating in pelvic mixing can be appreciably reduced (BOJESEN[307]); when the rate of urine flow and plasma concentrations are rapidly changing, appreciable residual errors may, however, persist even when such corrections have been applied.

[305] KINTER, W. B., and J. R. PAPPENHEIMER: Role of red blood corpuscles in regulation of renal blood flow and glomerular filtration rate. Amer. J. Physiol. 185, 399—406 (1956).

[306] WINTON, F. R. (ed.): Modern views on the secretion of urine. London: Churchill 1956.

[307] BOJESEN, E.: The transport of urine in the upper urinary tract. Acta physiol. scand. 32, 39—62 (1954).

a) Effect of changes in the oncotic pressure of plasma

It is an old observation that a considerable increase in water and salt excretion may be induced within few minutes by intravascular infusion of large quantities of isotonic saline. (MAGNUS[308, 309], in dogs; KNOWLTON[310], in rabbits). The same phenomenon has been observed in isolated perfused kidneys by diluting the perfusion blood with saline (DREYER and VERNEY[311], EGGLETON et al.[312]), and the designation "dilution diuresis" applied to it, since it was attributed to the reduction produced in the protein concentration and thus in the oncotic pressure of the plasma.

As mentioned above (p. 267) this phenomenon has recently been very carefully studied by BOJESEN[303], in dogs, with special attention to the events occurring within the first 10 or 15 min following the "dilution". In order to evoke as little

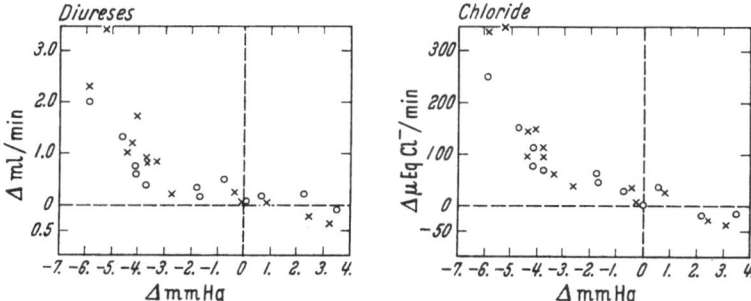

Fig. 6. *The relationship between changes in oncotic pressure of plasma and changes in the rate of water* (left) *and chloride* (right) *excretion*. Data from experiments in two dogs (× and ○). Dogs were given 200—300 ml intravenously of a Ringer-like solution with or without concentrated plasma proteins to raise or lower the oncotic pressure of plasma. The recorded changes in oncotic pressure (abscissae) and in excretion rates (ordinates) are all from observations made within 15 to 20 min after the injections. (From BOJESEN[303])

change as possible in the non-colloid composition of the plasma, a Ringer-like solution was used instead of isotonic saline as a diluting solution. In other experiments the antidiuretic effects of increasing the oncotic pressure was studied by infusion of RINGER's solution containing a high concentration of the dog's own plasma proteins, prepared from blood taken at an earlier occasion. Careful determinations (including the above-mentioned corrections for pelvic mixing) of the filtration rate and rates of excretion permitted the conclusion that no detectable changes occurred in the filtration rate or the rate of reabsorption of sodium in the early periods following the changes in plasma protein concentrations.

Furthermore, a direct proportionality between the changes in plasma oncotic pressure and the changes in rate of water (and sodium) excretion was observed over a wide range of the former (cf. Fig. 6). As mentioned above (p. 263) these findings are readily explainable from the alterations in the glomerular propulsive

[308] MAGNUS, R.: Über die Veränderung der Blutzusammensetzung nach Kochsalzinfusion und ihre Beziehung zur Diurese. Arch. exp. Path. Pharmak. 44, 68—126 (1900).

[309] MAGNUS, R.: Über Diurese. III. Über die Beziehungen der Plethora zur Diurese. Arch. exp. Path. Pharmak. 45, 210—222 (1901).

[310] KNOWLTON, F. P.: The influence of colloids on diuresis. J. Physiol. 43, 219—231 (1911).

[311] DREYER, N. B., and E. B. VERNEY: The relative importance of the factors concerned in the formation of the urine. J. Physiol. 57, 451—456 (1923).

[312] EGGLETON, M. G., J. R. PAPPENHEIMER, and F. R. WINTON: The mechanism of dilution diuresis in the isolated kidney and the anesthetized dog. J. Physiol. 98, 336—360 (1954).

pressure produced by the changes in the oncotic pressure, if one assumes that the hydrodynamic resistance of the glomerular membrane is small in comparison with the tubular resistance and that no changes occur in the active reabsorption of sodium (and associated reabsorption of water) in the tubules.

It is worth noticing that in subsequent periods of BOJESEN's experiments (extended over several hours) considerable increases occurred in the filtration rate and the rate of reabsorption of sodium (and water) as well as in renal blood flow. Such delayed changes have also been observed by other workers (BALDWIN et al.[313] and WESSON et al.[302] in dogs), who did not, however, take particular interest in recording the immediate response to saline infusion. These delayed changes are obviously not explainable from an increase in glomerular propulsive pressure caused by reduction of the oncotic pressure of plasma. It appears that they are elicited by some yet not clearly defined extrarenal changes related to expansion of the plasma volume, extracellular space etc. (cf. p. 368), but the nature of the renal mechanism by which they are brought about is uncertain. It is noticeable, as also observed by WESSON et al., that the increase in filtration rate is rather closely paralleled by a rise in renal blood flow. As a possible explanation of this relationship BOJESEN suggested that the rise in filtration rate is a consequence of an increased rate of (proximal) reabsorption of salt and fluid which in turn is caused by the increase in renal blood flow by way of an increased supply to the tubular cells of some hypothetic substances stimulating fluid reabsorption. Other explanations are obviously possible. Thus an alternative explanation could no doubt be formulated on the basis of the "cell separation hypothesis" briefly discussed above (p. 267). CRAWFORD and LUDEMANN[1506] claimed that the delayed increases in renal blood flow and filtration rate following saline infusions are much less pronounced and that the diuretic-saluretic response is smaller and more variable in man than in dogs. Recently, however, MARKLEY et al.[1505] produced evidence that man reacts in same way as dogs.

The antidiuretic and antinatriuretic effect of increasing the oncotic pressure of plasma by infusion of hyperoncotic, salt-poor serum albumin has been observed by several authors (GOODYER et al.[314]; WELT and ORLOFF[315]; PETERSDORF and WELT[316]). Considerable reductions in rates of excretion of water, total solutes and sodium and chloride were observed in healthy human subjects and diabetes insipidus patients following the infusion of 200—500 ml of 25% human serum albumin in saline, while the glomerular filtration rate seemed essentially unchanged as judged from determinations of the endogenous creatinine clearance. This response was particularly pronounced following rapid infusions, and it seems likely that with time the expansion of the plasma volume may bring other factors into action which may mask the immediate effects produced by the lowering in glomerular propulsive pressure. Thus it is noteworthy that considerable increases in renal plasma flow have been observed repeatedly following infusions of serum albumin; these may well have been accompanied by some rise in glomerular capillary pressure.

[313] BALDWIN, D., E. M. KAHANA, and R. W. CLARKE: Renal excretion of sodium and potassium in the dog. Amer. J. Physiol. 162, 655—664 (1950).
[314] GOODYER, A. V. N., E. R. PETERSON, and A. S. RELMAN: Some effects of albumin infusions of renal function and electrolyte excretion in man. J. appl. Physiol. 1, 671—682 (1949).
[315] WELT, L. G., and J. ORLOFF: The effects of an increase in plasma volume on the metabolism and excretion of water and electrolytes by normal subjects. J. clin. Invest. 30, 751—761 (1951).
[316] PETERSDORF, R. G., and L. G. WELT: The effect of an infusion of hyperoncotic albumin on the excretion of water and solutes. J. clin. Invest. 32, 283—291 (1953).

The mechanism of the paradox response (diuretic and more or less natriuretic effect) which has regularly been observed in nephrotic patients (LUETSCHER et al.[317]; ORLOFF et al.[318]; EDER et al.[319]) is not clearly understood. Our present knowledge of the renal pathology of this syndrome is still very scarce. It seems quite possible that the only primary renal defect is the increased permeability of the glomerular membrane to albumin, and that tubular changes are secondary effects of extensive protein reabsorption. Also, this disorder has a very fluctuating course and it appears that the said effect of albumin administration was generally obtained in phases of oedema formation. In such cases there is apparently a reduced plasma volume, reduced renal blood flow and increased excretion of sodium-retaining corticoid and antidiuretic substances. The possibility should be considered that restoration of the plasma volume might lead to elevation of glomerular capillary pressure and to a decreased production of these sodium and water retaining factors.

b) Effect of changes in renal arterial pressure

According to the views presented in the section on "Transport of fluid in the nephron as a whole", a local elevation in renal arterial pressure should be expected to cause an increase in the rates of excretion of sodium and water by raising glomerular capillary and thus glomerular propulsive pressure. Conversely, a reduction in renal arterial pressure should cause a decrease in sodium and water excretion. (It should be noted, however, that the so-called *autoregulation* of the renal circulation makes it unlikely that changes in the renal arterial pressure should result in changes of the same percentile magnitude in the glomerular capillary pressure. For instance, an increase in renal arterial pressure is accompanied by an increase in intrarenal vascular resistance, and, if this is mostly located in the pre-glomerular vessels, the increase in the glomerular capillary pressure will be smaller than that in the renal arterial pressure, even on a percentile basis.)

Such results were actually obtained by a number of investigators in experiments on dogs and human subjects. SELKURT[320] produced a progressive reduction in the right renal arterial pressure in dogs by a tourniquet around the abdominal aorta between the renal arteries; the left kidney thus served as a control. A reduction in femoral (and right renal) arterial pressure from 145 to 88 mm caused no demonstrable decrease in filtration rate (creatinine clearance) but a considerable lowering in the rate of sodium excretion ($0.097 \rightarrow 0.027$ meq/min). Further lowering of the arterial pressure caused additional decrements in sodium excretion but also in the filtration rate. The function of the left kidney remained practically unchanged. Similar results have been obtained by BLAKE et al.[321]; MUELLER et al.[322] and THOMPSON and PITTS[323].

[317] LUETSCHER, J. A., jr., A. D. HALL, and V. L. KREMER: Treatment of nephrosis with concentrated human serum albumin. II. Effects of renal function and on excretion of water and some electrolytes. J. clin. Invest. **29**, 896—904 (1950).

[318] ORLOFF, J., L. G. WELT, and L. STOWE: The effects of concentrated salt-poor albumin on the metabolism and excretion of water and electrolytes in nephrosis and toxemia of pregnancy. J. clin. Invest. **29**, 770—780 (1950).

[319] EDER, H. A., H. D. LAUSON, R. P. CHINARD, R. L. GREIF, G. C. COTZIAS, and D. D. VAN SLYKE. A study of the mechanism of edema formation in patients with the nephrotic syndrome. J. clin. Invest. **33**, 636—656 (1954).

[320] SELKURT, E. E.: Physical factors in relation to electrolyte and water excretion. Transact. 3rd. Conf. on Renal Function. New York: Josiah Macy jr. Foundation 1952.

[321] BLAKE, W. D., R. WEGRIA, H. P. WARD, and C. W. FRANK: Effect of renal arterial constriction on excretion of sodium and water. Amer. J. Physiol. **163**, 422—429 (1950).

[322] MUELLER, C. B., A. SURTSHIN, M. R. CARLIN, and H. L. WHITE: Glomerular and tubular influences on sodium and water excretion. Amer. J. Physiol. **165**, 411—422 (1951).

The effect of an acute increase in the arterial pressure to one kidney has been studied in the dog by SHIPLEY and STUDY[324] who supplied one renal artery with arterial blood from the dog itself by means of a pumping device. An increase in arterial pressure from approx. 80 to 180 mm Hg produced a very large increase in the rate of urine flow but no appreciable increase in inulin clearance or renal blood flow.

In man information on the effect of acute changes in arterial pressure has been obtained by EPSTEIN et al.[325] in experiments involving manual closure of arterio-venous fistulae. In 17 cases of post-traumatic fistulae in the neck and extremities occlusion led to an average rise of 11 mm Hg in mean arterial pressure but to no change in renal venous pressure (according to measurements in 6 cases). Within 10—15 min a significant increase in sodium excretion was detected (average from 0.185 to 0.267 meq/min), but this was unaccompanied by any consistent changes in inulin clearance, endogenous creatinine clearance or PAH-clearance.

It is of special interest to note in these studies that considerable changes in sodium and water excretion can be produced by changes in renal arterial pressure without any appreciable changes in filtration rate (or renal blood flow). The pattern is therefore identical with that observed by BOJESEN during the early phase of a dilution diuresis, and as in that case, changes in glomerular propulsive pressure seem to provide the simplest explanation.

The effects of more chronic reductions in renal arterial pressure on sodium and water excretions have also been studied experimentally in dogs. MUELLER et al.[322] found that with maintenance of a moderate partial occlusion of one renal artery over a period of several weeks, the rate of sodium excretion would remain permanently reduced even when there was no measurable change in filtration rate or renal blood flow. With more complete occlusion a reduction in filtration rate and renal blood flow occurred and the rate of sodium excretion was further reduced to only a few per cent of that of the unligated kidney. When the latter was removed, a gradual rise in the water and sodium output occurred from the ligated kidney, accompanied by appreciable rises (but certainly not a doubling) in renal plasma flow and glomerular filtration rate. The experiments of MUELLER et al. were confirmed by SURTSHIN and LATORRE[326].

c) Effect of increase in ureteral (pelvic) pressure

According to the views presented above an increase in ureteral (and thus in pelvic) pressure should reduce the rates of urine flow and sodium excretion by reducing the glomerular propulsive pressure (i.e. [glomerular capillary pressure — plasma oncotic pressure — pelvic pressure]).

This effect has been firmly established by experiments performed on intact animals as well as on isolated kidneys, and the causal relationship mentioned above was in fact already suggested by LUDWIG who considered increased ureter pressure to reduce urine flow by exerting back pressure on the glomerular membrane thus reducing the rate of filtrate formation.

[323] THOMPSON, D. D., and R. F. PITTS: Effects of alterations of renal arterial pressure on sodium and water excretion. Amer. J. Physiol. **168**, 490—499 (1952).

[324] SHIPLEY, R. E., and R. S. STUDY: Changes in renal blood flow, extraction of inulin, glomerular filtration rate, tissue pressure and urine flow with acute alterations of renal artery blood pressure. Amer. J. Physiol. **167**, 676—688 (1951).

[325] EPSTEIN, F. H., R. S. POST, and M. McDOWELL: The effect of an arteriovenous fistula on renal hemodynamics and electrolyte excretion. J. clin. Invest. **32**, 233—241 (1953).

[326] SURTSHIN, A., and G. LATORRE: Effects of contralateral nephrectomy on renal function depressed by previous unilateral renal arterial constriction Amer. J. Physiol. **182**, 524 to 530 (1955).

In more recent time this phenomenon has been studied on the isolated perfused dog kidney by WINTON and coworkers (cf. WINTON[297], for review). In some earlier experiments (WINTON[327]) it was observed that the urines produced by each of a pair of perfused kidneys remained practically indistinguishable as regards urea and chloride concentrations when equal reductions in urine flow were evoked on one side by raising ureter pressure and on the other by lowering arterial pressure. This observation suggests that the same fundamental mechanism is the basis of both types of antidiuresis, and in fact the ratio between such increases in ureter pressure and in arterial pressure which counterbalanced in regard to effect on urine flow was proposed for calculation of the ratio between glomerular capillary pressure and arterial pressure.

The above findings were essentially confirmed in later experiments (EGGLETON PAPPENHEIMER and WINTON[328]). The additional observation was made that simultaneous increases in arterial pressure and ureter pressure causing no change in the rate of urine flow and chloride excretion lead to some 5—15% reduction in creatinine clearance. At present it can hardly be decided whether this finding means that a decrease in salt and water reabsorption (and thus in filtration rate) occurred or that there was leakage of creatinine from the tubules. The former, however, seems the most likely explanation.

The results obtained in experiments in intact dogs agree closely with those from experiments on perfused kidneys. SHARE[329] found that elevation of the ureter pressure to 15 mm Hg was without any apparent effects on renal function. This agrees with WINTON's observation on perfused kidneys that no reduction in urine flow was produced before the ureter pressure reached some 10 mm Hg. As suggested by WINTON this lack of effect of a small rise in ureter pressure may be due to dilation of tubular lumina, previously more or less collapsed by the interstitial renal pressure acting on their outside. If this dilatation of *distal* tubules leads to a reduction in the hydrodynamic resistance in the tubules of similar magnitude as the reduction in glomerular propulsive pressure caused by the increase in ureter pressure, the latter would obviously be without effect on the rate of urine flow. With higher ureter pressures (20—30 mm Hg) SHARE observed considerable and rather parallel reductions in the rates of urine flow and sodium excretion, while there was a smaller percentile reduction in potassium excretion. Rather proportional and in some cases quite considerable decreases in creatinine and p-aminohippurate clearance were found, but considering the shortness of the urine collecting periods (2×10 min) such decreases may partly be due to errors caused by urine mixing in the pelvis.

SELKURT et al.[330] who also worked on pentobarbital anaesthetized dogs reported results which are in good keeping with those of SHARE. The effects of raising ureter pressure to 36 and 52 cm saline pressure (eq. to approx. 27 and 39 mm Hg) were studied. At the latter pressure the following average percentile reductions were observed: rates of water and sodium excretion 45%; potassium excretion 20%;

[327] WINTON, F. R.: The influence of increase of ureter pressure on the isolated mammalian kidney. J. Physiol. 71, 381—390 (1931).
[328] EGGLETON, M. G., J. R. PAPPENHEIMER, and F. R. WINTON: The relation between ureter, venous and arterial pressures in the isolated kidney of the dog. J. Physiol. 99, 135—152 (1940).
[329] SHARE, L.: Effect of increased ureteral pressure on renal function. Amer. J. Physiol. 168, 97—106 (1952).
[330] SELKURT, E. E., M. BRANDFONBRENER, and H. M. GELLER: Effects of ureteral pressure increase on renal hemodynamics and the handling of electrolytes and water. Amer. J. Physiol. 170, 61—71 (1952).

inulin or creatinine clearance 15%; p-aminohippurate clearance 5%. Some of their results are summarized in Fig. 7.

It is noteworthy that the rise in ureter pressure (even beyond 10—15 mm of Hg) needed to bring about a certain change in the rate of urine flow (or salt excretion) is very much higher than the change in oncotic pressure of plasma needed to cause a similar change according to experiments reported in p. 267.

Theoretically this difference might be due to the existence of different states in the kidneys in the two kinds of experiments, viz. that the static hydrodynamic resistance of a whole nephron were on an average much larger in the ureter pressure experiments than in the oncotic pressure experiments.

Since one would rather expect the reverse (because dilatation of otherwise collapsed distal tubular segments by the first 10—15 mm of Hg elevation of the ureteral pressure should reduce the resistance), it appears that the difference must have been caused by other factors. Probably several factors are involved: (1) The fact, that a decrease in tubular fluid reabsorption occurred as the ureteral pressure was being raised, would by itself counteract a fall in fluid excretion, since it means that less and less pressure would be spent on propulsion of fluid being reabsorbed, meaning again a saving of pressure for the excretion of fluid. (2) It is also likely that an elevation of the ureteral pressure causes a rise in glomerular capillary pressure (by increasing the pressure resting on the postglomerular capillaries) so that any increment in ureteral pressure results in a considerably smaller decrement in glomerular propulsive pressure. (3) Finally, a diminution of the tubular hydrodynamic resistance from a progressive distension of the tubules with rising ureteral pressure must be considered as another factor possibly counteracting a drop in fluid excretion with increasing ureteral pressure.

It should be noted that the occurrence of such changes in the nephrons in response to elevations of the ureter pressure would invalidate WINTON's calculations of the ratio between glomerular pressure and arterial pressure (see above). Since changes in intrarenal vascular resistances in response to changes in renal arterial pressure (cf. remarks on autoregulation on p. 271) also invalidate the procedure, little importance can be attached to figures derived from such calculations.

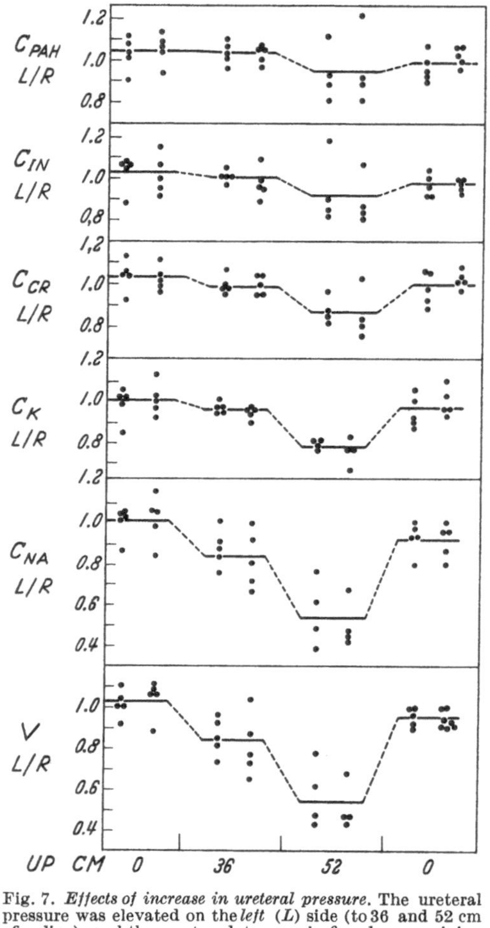

Fig. 7. *Effects of increase in ureteral pressure.* The ureteral pressure was elevated on the *left* (*L*) side (to 36 and 52 cm of saline) and then restored to zero in five dogs receiving isotonic Ringer's infusions. Data are given as ratios of experimental (*L*) to control (*R*). C_{PAH} para-aminohippurate clearance. C_{IN} inulin clearance. C_{CR} creatinine clearance. C_K Potassium clearance. C_{Na} sodium clearance. V rate of urine flow. (From SELKURT, BRANDFONBRENER and GELLER 1952[330])

d) Effect of elevation of renal venous pressure

LUDWIG suggested that an increase in renal venous pressure would exert an antidiuretic action by transmission of the elevated pressure to the fluid within the tubules; this would mean an increased backpressure opposing glomerular filtration. It seems preferable to express these thoughts in a slightly different way: that increased pressure in the peri-tubular vessels would cause compression of the

tubules with a narrowing of the tubular lumens and thus an increased hydrodynamic resistance to the formation of urine. Thus an effect basically similar to
that obtained by increasing ureter pressure should be expected.

Experimental support for this view has been provided by WINTON and coworkers
from studies on perfused kidneys, along similar lines as those mentioned above
in connection with the effect of increasing ureter pressure.

Several studies on the effects of a local unilateral increase in renal venous
pressure in whole animals have been performed in recent years (SELKURT, HALL
and SPENCER[331]; HALL and SELKURT[332]; BLAKE et al.[333]; JEANNERET[334]). All
investigators have agreed that even with small increases (of some 10 cm of saline)

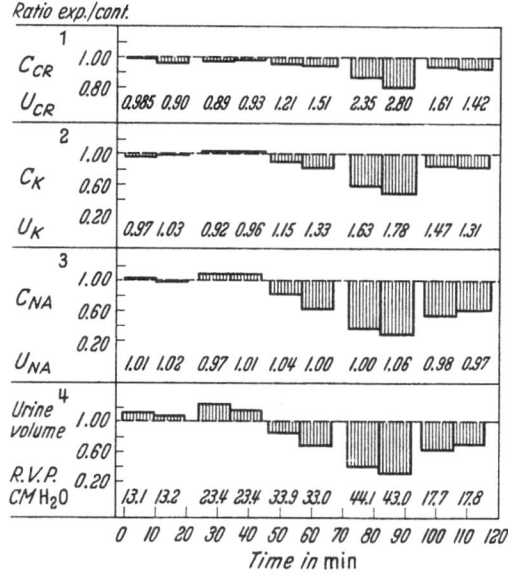

above the control pressures (i.e.
10—15 cm of saline) there is generally a significant reduction in the
rate of excretion of sodium and
water. With further increase in
renal venous pressure more ·mark-
ed effects are obtained. There
has been some disagreement as to
whether reductions in glomerular
filtration rate and renal plasma
flow invariably accompany the
reductions in rates of excretion
of water and sodium. While SEL-
KURT and his group appear to think
that they do (in contrast to BLAKE
et al.) it is nevertheless apparent
from several of their data that significant decreases in water and
sodium excretions occurred when
no measurable reductions in blood
flow or filtration rate were observed. With *large* increases in renal
venous pressure unquestionable
falls in blood flow and filtration
rate were observed by both groups
of investigators.

Fig. 8 from HALL and SEL-
KURT's article shows the results
from a typical experiment in which

Fig. 8. *Effects of acute unilateral increase in renal venous
pressure on kidney function.*(Data from a typical experiment.)
Graded increases in left renal venous pressure (figures given
at the bottom above the time abscissa) were produced by
gradual occlusion of the left renal vein in an anaesthetized
dog. Data are given as ratios between left experimental and
right control kidney. C_{CR}, C_K and C_{Na} are clearances of creatinine, potassium and sodium. U_{CR}, U_K and U_{Na} are
urinary concentrations of these substances. (From HALL
and SELKURT 1951[332])

the renal venous pressure on one side was raised by three consecutive increments (each of 10 cm saline) above the control level, and then returned to the
latter. It is apparent that the observed effects are quite similar to those obtained
by raising the ureter pressure.

The effects of a more sustained elevation of renal venous pressure has also been
studied experimentally. In dogs, JEANNERET[334] placed a ligature around the

[331] SELKURT, E. E., P. W. HALL, and M. P. SPENCER: Response of renal blood flow and
clearance to graded partial obstruction of the renal vein. Amer. J. Physiol. **157**, 40—46 (1949).

[332] HALL III., P. W., and E. E. SELKURT: Effects of partial graded venous obstruction
on electrolyte clearance by the dog's kidney. Amer. J. Physiol. **164**, 143—154 (1951).

[333] BLAKE, W. D., R. WEGRIA, R. P. KEATING, and H. P. WARD: Effect of increased renal
venous pressure on renal function. Amer. J. Physiol. **157**, 1—13 (1949).

inferior vena cava between the origins of the right and left renal veins. Sufficient constriction was used to cause the venous pressure distal to the constriction to rise to 200—300 mm of saline. Urine was collected separately from the two ureters by application of a special capsule to the explanted bladder. A diminution in sodium excretion of at least one months duration was observed on the side at which the kidney was exposed to the elevated venous pressure. The renal plasma flow also remained somewhat below that on the control side, whereas the filtration rate was almost unaffected. Changes therefore were similar to those observed in acute experiments. Similar findings have been reported by SIROTA and NABATOFF[335] in a case of Laennee's cirrhosis studied some 9 months after a splenorenal vein anastomosis had been made; adequate controls were, however, lacking in this case. Several studies have been performed in which both renal veins participated in an increased venous pressure; in these cases compensatory reactions soon brought electrolyte excretions up to normal levels (cf. the above papers for references).

e) Effects of pressures acting on the outside of the kidney

HERMAN and WINTON[336] have studied the effects of increasing or reducing the pressure acting on the outside of the isolated, kidney perfused at constant arterial pressure. The kidney was enclosed in a chamber into which were passing cannulae inserted into the artery, vein and ureter. The pressure in the chamber could be raised above or lowered below atmospheric pressure. Their results are exactly as one would expect from the above-mentioned concept of the mechanism of the antidiuretic and antinatriuretic effects of elevations of ureter and renal venous pressures. Exposure to subatmospheric pressures caused increased urine flow and chloride (and sodium?) excretion with increase in renal blood flow and possibly a small increase in creatinine clearance. Supraatmospheric pressure had the opposite effects. HERMAN and WINTON were apparently inclined to believe that the effects were due to mediation of the external pressure changes to the tubules through the renal parenchyme. Although this may be correct, it appears that a change in the pressure within the pelvis and the renal veins may also have contributed to the results, at least during periods of increased extrarenal pressure.

The effect of raising extrarenal pressure has also been studied in human subjects by compression of the abdominal wall by means of a pneumatic girdle. In this case external pressure will of course not be restricted to the kidney, the renal veins and the ureter. Other intraabdominal structures, such as the inferior vena cava, will also be exposed, thus complicating the picture by venous stasis in the lower extremities, etc.

Such experiments were made by BRADLEY and BRADLEY[337] who observed that application of an external compression pressure of 80 mm of Hg raised the pressure in the inferior vena cava to some 20 mm Hg (from a normal level of around 5 mm of Hg), clearly indicating that only a small part of the external pressure was transmitted to the abdominal cavity. As might be expected, the effects of this procedure

[334] JEANNERET, P.: A modified procedure for assessing separate kidney function in chronic dog preparations with observations on the effect of chronic unilateral venous congestion. J. Lab. clin. Med. 38, 604—412 (1951).

[335] SIROTA, J. H., and R. A. NABATOFF: Effects of unilateral renal vein hypertension secondary to splenorenal vein anastomosis on individual kidney function. Amer. J. Med. 13, 242—246 (1952).

[336] HERMAN, F. G., and F. R. WINTON: The interaction of intrarenal and extrarenal pressures. J. Physiol. 87, 77 (1936).

[337] BRADLEY, S. E., and G. P. BRADLEY: The effect of increased intraabdominal pressure on renal function in man. J. clin. Invest. 26, 1010 (1947).

were similar to those obtained by raising renal venous or ureter pressures. A rather parallel reduction (about 25%) in renal plasma flow and filtration rate was observed, accompanied by a considerable reduction in urine flow and an even greater fall in the rate of sodium excretion. In certain cases of ascites a similar mechanism may be a factor contributing to an impairment of the excretion of sodium.

In cases of elevated intraabdominal pressure impaired hepatic circulation with decreased inactivation of (mineralo-)corticoids may be a further complicating factor causing renal sodium retention. This is suggested by experiments by YATES[338], [339] demonstrating that rats in which the posterior vena cava was constricted above the hepatic veins showed an increased sodium-retaining effect of desoxycorticosterone and that the reductive inactivation of cortisone, cortisol and desoxycorticosterone (and possibly aldosterone too) was impaired in homogenates of livers from such animals.

E. Effects of changes in plasma sodium (and chloride) concentration on sodium excretion

It has long been known that intravenous administration of strongly hypertonic sodium chloride solutions induces a much more copious natriuresis and also diuresis than corresponding volumes of an isotonic solution. Rather extensive studies on this phenomenon have been carried out in recent years in various mammalian species and have included measurements of the glomerular filtration rate and sometimes also effective renal plasma flow. (SELKURT and POST[340] in dogs; KRUHØFFER[206] in rabbits, MOKOTOFF et al.[341] in human subjects).

The natriuresis (and diuresis) has often (cf. SELKURT[6]) been interpreted in terms of a shift in the proportion between the filtered load of sodium (generally increased) and the rate of tubular reabsorption of sodium (sometimes reduced). While, by definition, correct, such interpretations do not account for the intimate nature of the phenomenon, and, in particular, they neglect the facts, that the rate of sodium excretion is influenced by tubular factors other than the rate of sodium reabsorption, and that the filtration rate is determined by a multitude of factors, including tubular conditions (cf. p. 263). Furthermore, it has been a common mistake of base the interpretations on data, which were obtained at a time when the function of the kidneys had become greatly modified by various secondary reactions.

In fact, experiments as those cited above are poorly suited to provide information on what we actually want to know: how elevations of the plasma sodium (and chloride) concentration, *as the only variable*, affects the handling of electrolytes and water in the kidneys. This is so because a number of complicating factors, which by themselves affect the excretion of salt and water, are set into action in such experiments, and in particular when they are extended over periods of more than some 15 min. Thus, the addition of a hypertonic sodium chloride solution to the blood will reduce the oncotic pressure of the plasma, not only by simple dilution, but also by causing osmotic transfer of water from the extravascular space to the plasma. Secondly, changes in renal blood flow are likely to occur. Overfilling of the

[338] YATES, F. E.: Effects of central venous congestion on sodium, potassium and water metabolism in the rat, response to desoxycorticosterone. Amer. J. Physiol. **194**, 57—64 (1950).

[339] YATES, F. E., J. URQUHART, and A. L. HERBST: Impairment of the enzymatic inactivation of adrenal cortical hormones following passive venous congestion of the liver. Amer. J. Physiol. **194**, 65—71 (1958).

[340] SELKURT, E. E., and R. S. POST: Renal clearance of sodium in the dog: Effect of increasing sodium load on reabsorptive mechanism. Amer. J. Physiol. **162**, 639—648 (1950).

[341] MOKOTOFF, R., G. ROSS, and L. LEITER: Renal plasma flow and sodium reabsorption and excretion in congestive heart failure. J. clin. Invest. **27**, 1—9 (1948).

cardiovascular system which generally will occur in the first phase after infusion of a hypertonic solution of sodium chloride may, by some volume receptor mechanism, cause a reflex dilation of the renal vessels and an elevation in glomerular capillary pressure. In a later phase, dehydration is apt to occur if the initial administration of strongly hypertonic solution is not followed up by continuous administration of less concentrated solutions in sufficient quantities to compensate for the renal losses; renal vasoconstriction may then result. Such vascular reactions could act as complicating factors not only by their effect on glomerular propulsive pressure, but also because they may somehow lead to more or less parallel changes in the rate of sodium reabsorption in the proximal tubules (cf. p. 270) and thus affect the glomerular filtration rate. Finally, the possibility must be considered that marked elevations of the plasma sodium concentration and changes in blood volume may affect the production of hormones, such as those of the adrenal cortex, which affect tubular reabsorption of sodium.

Since the influence of these complicating factors may vary considerably according to the experimental conditions and the time at which the measurements are undertaken, it is not surprising to find that the rate of tubular reabsorption of sodium has been reported to remain essentially unchanged in some experiments, but to rise or fall through the individual periods in others. As far as one can judge from real acute experiments on well-hydrated animals an elevation of the plasma sodium concentration does not *per se* cause any significant change in the rate at which sodium is reabsorbed by the tubules. This also appears to be the result of experiments in which the direct effect of a elevation in the plasma sodium (and chloride) concentration on the kidney could be studied with less interference of secondary reactions. GOODYER and GLENN[342] have shown that direct infusion of a hypertonic sodium chloride solution into one renal artery of a dog causes a marked and prompt natriuresis and diuresis from the corresponding kidney, with very little rise in the excretions from the other. Similar experiments have been reported by SELKURT[6] who studied the effect of a stepwise increase in the sodium chloride concentration of the infusion fluid, and also measured the filtration rate on the two sides (cf. Fig. 9). A marked rise in sodium and urine excretion was obtained on the side of injection, but there was no measurable change in the rate of reabsorption of sodium.

Clearly then, an elevation of the plasma sodium (and chloride) concentration exerts a direct natriuretic and diuretic effect on the kidney, a fact which can also be demonstrated in the isolated perfused kidney (F. KIEL, personal communication).

How shall we explain this effect, and also the fact that with extreme loadings of animals with hypertonic sodium chloride solutions some 40—50% (and in personal experiments in rabbits even 60%) of the filtered sodium and water may appear in the urine even when the filtration rate is at a higher than normal level, i. e. that the amounts excreted may approach those normally filtered.

The fact that such profuse natriuresis and diuresis *may* be obtained when there is no or virtually no decrease in the rates of reabsorption of sodium and water clearly indicate that a *diminution in tubular reabsorption of salt and water cannot be the only or even the most important cause of these changes.* A rise in glomerular capillary pressure and a reduction in the oncotic pressure of plasma, both leading to a rise in glomerular propulsive pressure, may well be of considerable importance to the natriuretic and diuretic response. Considering the much more moderate

---

[342] GOODYER, A. V. N., and W. W. L. GLENN: Excretion of solutes injected into the renal artery. Amer. J. Physiol. **168**, 66—76 (1952).

magnitude of the responses obtained when the glomerular propulsive pressure is altered during dilution diuresis (cf. p. 267) it seems, however, rather unlikely that such changes are the only major factors involved.

If this view is accepted it follows by way of exclusion that a diminution in the hydrodynamic resistance in the nephron must play an important role among the factors underlying the profuse diuresis and natriuresis obtained upon administration of large amounts of hypertonic sodium chloride solutions. To account for the very marked responses the diminution in resistance would obviously have to occur in those sections of the nephron which contribute most to the total resistance in the nephron under normal conditions. As discussed in p. 265 there is some indication that the greatest part of the resistance is normally located in some very distal parts of the tubular system, due to the fact that they are in a state of partial collapse. It is also possible that the glomerular membrane may be responsible for a significant although smaller contribution to the total resistance. The distribution of the resistance in the nephron has, however, not yet been fully clarified.

Histological examinations of fixed preparations made from kidneys during saluresis-diuresis induced by hypertonic sodium chloride solutions reveal similar changes in the tubules as those encountered during diuresis induced by osmotic diuretics such as mannitol and sulphate, i.e. a flattening of the tubular cells, and a corresponding widening of the tubular lumina (cf. Fig. 10 and 11, p. 283). Apparently the tubular cells, proximal as well as distal, respond to exposures to hypertonic sodium chloride by a shrinkage.

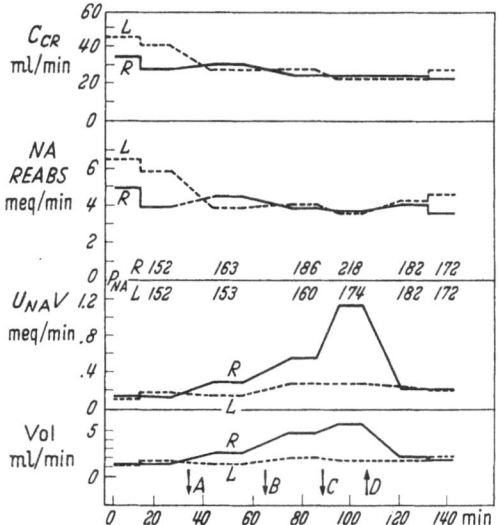

Fig. 9. *Effects of direct injection of hypertonic* NaCl *into one renal artery*. The experiment was performed by perfusing the right (R) kidney of an anaesthetized dog by way of an external circuit between a carotid and the right renal artery; on its way the blood passed through a mixing chamber into which hypertonic NaCl solutions were infused. Right renal arterial blood was sampled further downstream; femoral arterial blood was used for computing the clearances for the left kidney. Urine was collected separately from the two sides. At A, infusion of 5% NaCl began; B, changed to 8.7%; C, changed to 11,2%; at D, infusion stopped. Infusion rate: 2.17 ml/min. R right, experimental; L left, control. C_{CR}: creatinine clearance; P_{Na}: arterial plasma sodium concentrations (meq/l); $U_{Na}V$: rates of sodium excretion. Vol: rate of urine flow. (From SELKURT 1954[6])

ULLRICH et al.'s[250] observation (cf. p. 248) of changes in the weight of kidney slices upon immersion in sodium chloride solutions of different concentrations is evidence in the same direction.

It is easily realized that a widening of the lumina and a corresponding decrease in the resistance in appropriate segments of the tubules could lead to very marked diuresis and natriuresis if the hydrodynamic resistance in the tubules were normally considerably greater than that of the glomerular membrane. There are, however, certain difficulties in accepting cell shrinkage and consequent widening of the tubular lumina as a major factor in the production of the profuse diuresis-saluresis induced by loading with sodium chloride and osmotic diuretics. This is so in particular if the view is correct that the major part of the resistance in the nephron is located in partially collapsed distal tubules, since a diminution of this resistance could hardly be brought about by shrinkage of the cells in this segment. Still shrinkage of more proximally located cells could contribute to a diminution of the "collapse resistance", by facilitating the transmission of a higher pressure to the distal segments from the glomerulus.

Our present incomplete knowledge of the hydrodynamics of the nephron evidently prevents any definite conclusions to be drawn concerning the mechanism of the diuresis-saluresis induced by loading with hypertonic sodium chloride solutions. Probably the mechanism is quite complex even in experiments where the sodium and chloride concentration is elevated only in the plasma going to the kidney. It seems quite likely, however, that a reduction in the hydrodynamic resistance in the nephron plays an important role. Shrinkage of the tubular cells may account for such changes in the tubules. A reduction in the resistance of the glomerular membrane may also occur, and this too might be the result of a shrinkage of cellular elements (for results of electron microscopic studies on the membrane cf. BERGSTRAND [343]). The effect of the reduced hydrodynamic resistance is probably potentiated by an increase in glomerular propulsive pressure caused by dilatation of the renal vessels. A reduction in tubular reabsorption of salt and water may also potentiate the response, but it is not essential to its attainment.

It is an old experience that a smaller saluretic and diuretic response is obtained when hypertonic sodium chloride (or the salt itself) is given *by mouth*. An important factor in this case is undoubtedly that water will enter from the blood plasma into the intestinal tract; the resulting diminution in plasma volume and elevation in the oncotic pressure of plasma will tend to counteract the effect of the rise in plasma sodium (and chloride) concentration.

Just as an increase in the sodium concentration in the plasma is followed by several compensating processes, the interpretation of the effect of a decrease produced by water loading is quite complex. On the whole it may be stated, however, that moderate water loading has little effect on the rate of sodium excretion. [Very large loads of water may produce a rise in urinary sodium excretion (see section on diuretics and natriuretics).] Further discussion of this problem may be found in the survey by SELKURT [6].

F. "Osmotic diuresis" and sodium (and potassium) excretion

There is ample evidence, also from the older literature, that elevations of the plasma concentrations of filtrable non-electrolytes or anions which are poorly reabsorbed by the tubules lead to an increase in the rates of excretion of water and sodium. ("Osmotic diuresis" or "solute diuresis".)

Thus it was already recognized by MAGNUS[344] that in dogs and rabbits intravenous injection of a 7.85% sodium sulphate solution caused a considerably larger diuresis than a corresponding volume of a sodium chloride solution of similar osmolarity (4.90%). The marked diuretic effect of urea (and sucrose) was clearly demonstrated by LAMY and MAYER[345] in dogs.

A large number of subsequent studies have shown that a pronounced increase in sodium excretion generally accompanies the diuretic response. This is so when such anions as ferricyanate, sulphate or thiosulphate and to a lesser extent bicarbonate, nitrate or thiocyanate are administered and also when they are not

[343] BERGSTRAND, A.: Electron microscopic investigations of the renal glomeruli. Lab. Invest. **6**, 191—204 (1957).

[344] MAGNUS, R.: Über Diurese. II. Vergleich der diuretischen Wirksamkeit isotonischer Salzlösungen. Naunyn-Schmiedebergs Arch. exp. Path. Pharmak. **44**, 396—433 (1900).

[345] LAMY, H., et A. MAYER: Etudes sur la diurèse. III. Sur les conditions des variations du débit urinaires (sécrétion de l'eau par le rein). J. Physiol. Path. gén. **8**, 258—266 (1906).

given as sodium salts but as ammonium salts (West et al.[290]). Similarly, an increased rate of sodium excretion has been demonstrated to accompany the development of glycosuria in diabetic patients even before ketonuria was apparent (Atchley et al.[346]), and the glycosuria produced by infusion of large quantities of glucose in human subjects (Woodward[347]) and in rabbits (Kerpel-Fronius[348]). Further a natriuresis has been observed during urinary excretion of various sugars not normally present in the body and during mannitol diuresis (Holmes[349]).

To illustrate how marked the effects may be the data from a few representative experiments have been collected in Table 23.

Table 23. *Typical data from experiments with excessive osmotic diureses*

Osmotic Diuretic	Species	Filtration rate (ml/min)	Rate of urine flow ml/min	Excr. % for water	Excr. % for sodium	References
Mannitol	rabbit	17.5	10.2	58	35	Kruhøffer[206]
	dog	50.2	31.6	63	27	Wesson and Anslow[205].
Urea	dog	61	28.8	47.2	34.4	Mudge, Foulks and Gilman[350]
Sodium sulfate	rabbit	24.5	16.25	66	51*	Schou[211]

* Excretion-percentage for chloride (instead of sodium).

It is apparent that when there is a pronounced loading of the body with sulphate, urea or mannitol the rate of urine flow may rise to very high values, and in extreme cases may amount to considerably more than half the filtration rate. Since a considerable increase in filtration rate generally accompanies the rise in diuresis (if dehydration and other complications are prevented) this means that the rate of urine flow may approach the magnitude of the filtration rate in the normal well-hydrated state. Simultaneously the rates of sodium excretion are greatly increased, although (as previously mentioned, p. 236) in the case of non-electrolyte induced diuresis the percentage of filtered sodium excreted remains considerably below the percentage of filtered water excreted.

In attempting to explain the mechanism of the osmotic diuresis and natriuresis phenomenon several radically different views have been presented. In seeking an explanation for the natriuresis induced by mannitol and other non-electrolytes Wesson and Anslow[205] proposed that the "uphill" sodium concentration gradient which develops in the tubules under such conditions, might retard further reabsorption of sodium. Mudge et al.[350] arrived at a similar conclusion from their studies on the urea-induced diuresis in dogs, although in contrast to Wesson and Anslow they found no evidence for the existence of an upper limit of sodium concentration difference which could not be surpassed.

[346] Atchley, D. W., R. F. Loeb, D. W. Richards jr., E. M. Benedict, and M. E. Driscoll: On diabetic acidosis. A detailed study of electrolyte balances following the withdrawal and reestablishment of insulin therapy. J. clin. Invest. 12, 297—326 (1933).

[347] Woodward, K. F.: Diuresis produced by injections of dextrose. Its effect on nitrogen balance and on metabolism of fixed acids and bases in normal infants. Amer. J. Dis. Child. 47, 513—520 (1934).

[348] Kerpel-Fronius, E.: Zur Frage des diabetischen Salzmangelzustandes. Klin. Wschr. 16, 1466—1468 (1937).

[349] Holmes, H. J.: Studies of water exchange in dogs with reduced serum electrolyte concentration. Amer. J. Physiol. 129, 384—385 (1940).

[350] Mudge, G. H., J. Foulks, and A. Gilman: Effect of urea diuresis on renal excretion of electrolytes. Amer. J. Physiol. 158, 218—230 (1949).

In contrast, to these views which, in agreement with older opinions, assume a purely renal origin of the osmotic diuresis, an extrarenal mechanism has been proposed by SELDIN and TARAIL[351] on the basis of more moderate loading experiments in human subjects. These authors focused attention on the observation that injections of hypertonic solutions of urea into normal human subjects caused considerably less increase in the rate of sodium excretion than injections of glucose and mannitol solutions which apparently caused no larger excretions of non-electrolytes in the urine. Since glucose and mannitol, in contrast to urea, do not readily penetrate into the body cells, the opinion was expressed that the natriuretic effect of the former two is somehow brought about by cellular dehydration. While such a vaguely defined mechanism cannot be excluded as a contributory factor, it appears equally likely that the observed differences in natriuretic power might be caused by other mechanisms. It seems rather futile to speculate on this point at present, but, for instance, the greater expansion of the extracellular and the plasma volumes caused by mannitol and glucose might somehow be responsible e.g. by way of a "reflex" affecting sodium reabsorption in the distal tubules. Or the difference in natriuretic effect might be explainable on the level of direct effects on the tubular cells.

However that may be, there is no doubt that the diuretic and natriuretic response to a poorly reabsorbable non-electrolyte, be it urea or mannitol, is to a large extent dependent upon a direct action on the kidney since it may readily be produced in the isolated perfused kidney or by injection of the osmotic diuretic into one renal artery (GOODYER and GLEEN[352]).

The most important problem therefore seems to be to provide an explanation of how the osmotic diuretics are at all capable of producing profuse diuresis and natriuresis by direct action on the kidney. With regard to WESSON and ANSLOW's suggestion that a *diminution of the proximal reabsorption* of sodium (caused by an uphill concentration gradient) should be responsible for these effects, it appears that it is entirely inadequate as an explanation. This is apparent from the fact that profuse osmotic diuresis *may* be obtained without any significant reduction in the total rate of tubular reabsorption of sodium. Collateral evidence is provided by the fact that even nearly complete abolition of sodium and water reabsorption does not lead to urine flow rates of similar magnitudes (cf. p. 266).

As in the case of the profuse diuresis and natriuresis produced by marked elevations of the plasma sodium (and chloride) concentration, the conclusion seems unescapable that a marked reduction in the hydrodynamic resistance in the nephron must also play a major role in the production of osmotic diuresis. The possible location of this reduction in resistance in the nephron was discussed in connection with sodium chloride-induced diuresis and similar reflections are applicable in the case of osmotic diuresis.

As mentioned before, a flattening of the tubular cells and a corresponding widening of the tubular lumina is readily demonstrated in fixed sections of kidneys from animals in which osmotic diuresis has been induced by mannitol, sulphate, etc. (cf. Fig. 10 and 11). Such changes have previously been observed by others (BRODIE[353]; JESSEN[354]). The mechanism of the shrinkage of the tubular cells is not known,

[351] SELDIN, D. W., and R. TARAIL: Effect of hypertonic solutions on metabolism and excretion of electrolytes. Amer. J. Physiol. **159**, 160—174 (1949).

[352] GOODYER, A. V. N., and W. W. L. GLENN: Excretion of solutes injected into the renal artery of the dog. Amer. J. Physiol. **168**, 66—76 (1952).

[353] BRODIE, T. B.: Croonian Lecture. A new conception of the glomerular function. Proc. roy. Soc., Ser. B **87**, 571—592 (1914).

[354] JESSEN, J.: Histologiske studier over experimentelle nefriter (Danish Thesis) Copenhagen 1923.

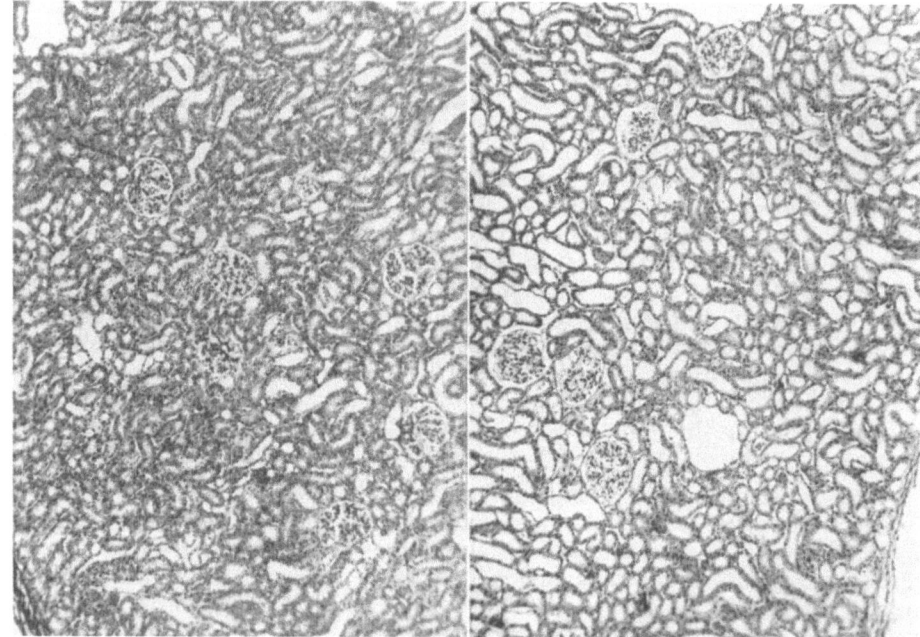

Fig. 10 and 11. *Histological changes in the kidney during osmotic diuresis*

Fig. 10. From an experiment in a dog. One kidney was removed from a normally hydrated, nembutal-anaesthetized dog; the kidney was rapidly cut into slices which were immediately fixed in formaline *(left side)*. Then 75 ml of a 20 per cent mannitol solution was injected intravenously, followed by a continous infusion of a slightly hypertonic solution of mannitol and NaCl and NaHCO₃ (8—10 ml/min). 10 min later when a diuresis of 4 ml/min had been obtained the other kidney was removed and treated in the same way as the first *(right)*

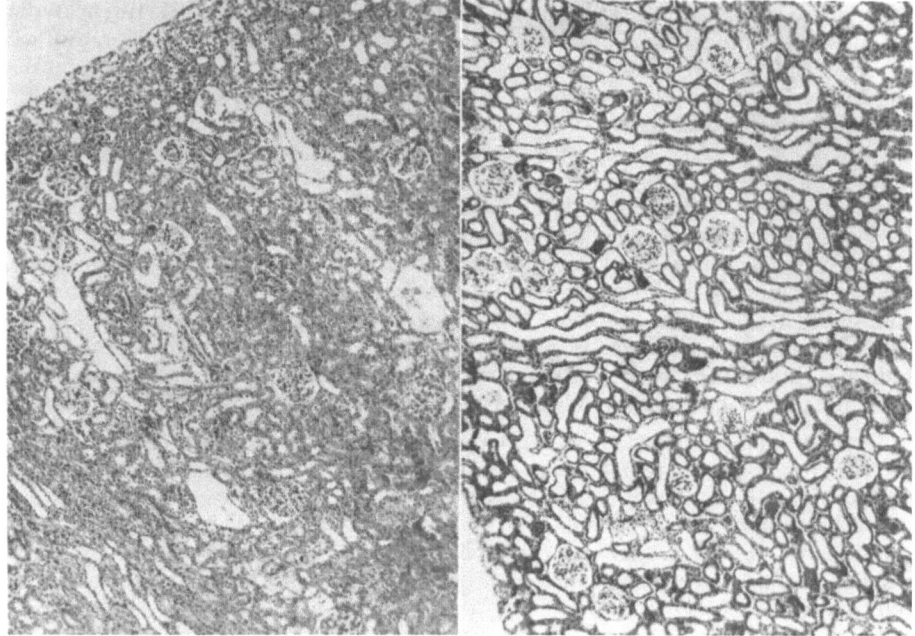

Fig. 11. From experiments in rats. *Left* is from a kidney removed from a nembutal-anaesthetized rat in a normal state and treated as mentioned above. *Right* is from a rat in which a sulphate diuresis of 0.5 ml/min was produced by intravenous injection of 3 ml of 15 per cent Na₂SO₄, 10 H₂O followed by continous infusion of a slightly hypertonic mixture of Na₂SO₄ and NaCl (0.6 ml/min) for 8 min. Marked flattening of both proximal and distal tubular cells is apparent in both types of experiments

nor how it is related to the shrinkage observed when the plasma sodium and chloride concentrations are raised. Although one can think of certain systems from which a cell shrinkage might be inferred, such speculations seem unwarranted considering our present lack of knowledge of the nature and location of the processes involved in electrolyte transfers through the tubular cell. The possibility should, however, be considered that the cell shrinkage (and the osmotic diuresis) might be related to a lowering of the concentration of sodium matched by easily reabsorbable anions (chloride and bicarbonate) in the tubular fluid. Such a lowering of the concentration of "movable" sodium in the tubular fluid will result from the administration of all those substances — nonelectrolytes and electrolytes — which are capable of producing a profuse diuresis even without an increase in the osmolarity of the plasma. In diuresis induced by sodium chloride a lowering in the concentration of "movable" sodium does obviously not occur, but it may be pertinent to note that in this case a profuse diuresis can only be obtained by increasing the osmolarity of the plasma far above its normal level.

As discussed in the preceding section there are certain difficulties in accepting cell shrinkage and consequent widening of the tubular lumina as the major factor in the production of profuse solute diureses. In this connection it should also be mentioned that GOTTSCHALK and MYLLE[295] observed *a rise* in the pressure in the proximal tubules when an osmotic diuresis was induced in rats by intravenous injection of hypertonic glucose. This observation lends no support to the view that a reduction in hydrodynamic resistance in the nephron distal to the site of puncture should be the major cause of the diuresis. Rather it points towards a rise in glomerular propulsive pressure or a reduction in the resistance in the glomerular membrane as the responsible factor. It should be noted, however, that the interpretation of these observations is difficult because no close correlation of intratubular pressure and rate of urine flow was observed; in fact the intratubular pressure had come almost back to the pre-injection level before maximum diuresis was reached. In recent micropuncture experiments in rats, however, GOTTSCHALK and MYLLE[296] demonstrated that in osmotic diuresis the clear-cut difference between proximal and distal intratubular pressure disappears, indicating the disappearance of a resistance in an intervening section, and the persistence of an appreciable resistance in the most distal parts of the tubular system. As apparent from the authors' diagrams on distal tubular pressure/urine flow relationships even the latter resistance did, however, drop considerably when an osmotic diuresis started, whereas it remained fairly constant at the lower value as the rate of urine flow increased further. Altogether it is apparent from the above discussion that we are still far from having any clear knowledge of the mechanism of the impressive phenomenon of osmotic diuresis. A reduction in the hydrodynamic resistance in the nephrons should, however, be taken into consideration as a possibly important factor until convincing evidence against it is produced.

Normal blood plasma does not contain any substances in concentrations sufficient to exert appreciable osmotic diuretic effect. Under pathological conditions urea may, however, reach concentrations which make it an effective osmotic diuretic, and in certain disease states, characterized by a diminished renal blood flow and probably a reduced glomerular capillary pressure, urea may well play a role in preserving some urine production in spite of otherwise unfavourable conditions.

Abnormal sodium (and potassium) losses induced by osmotic diuretics are most commonly encountered in cases of glycosuria and ketonuria, and, of course, especially when both of these phenomena are combined in severe diabetes.

Several studies (cf. also p. 246) have shown that during increasing osmotic diuresis the osmolarity of the urine approaches that of the plasma. A rather fixed relationship has been shown to exist (in the dehydrated state) between the rate of urine flow and the (effective) osmolarity of the urine independent of the nature of the substance used for induction of osmotic diuresis (cf. WEST and RAPOPORT[355]). From this finding it might be expected that relatively more sodium would be lost at a given rate of urine flow when an osmotic diuresis is induced by salts with di- and multivalent anions than when salts with monovalent anions are used; experimental observations confirmed this expectation (RAPOPORT and WEST[356]).

The mechanism of increased renal losses of *potassium* during osmotic diuresis is not definitely known. Some of the more moderate increases may well be due to an increase in the amounts being filtered without a corresponding rise (or even a decrease) in the amounts being reabsorbed. In cases where much larger increases in the excretion percentage ("tubular rejection fraction") for potassium are met with, tubular secretion is probably involved (cf. for instance MUDGE et al.[350]). In these cases the distal potassium-sodium exchange mechanism (cf. p. 252) must either be assumed to be activated prior to the induction of the osmotic diuresis or to become activated as a consequence of the loading with the osmotic diuretics (by dehydration etc.). In the first case it must further be assumed that before the induction of the osmotic diuresis the rate of potassium secretion has been limited by a scarce supply of sodium to the most distal parts of the tubules (cf. p. 286) whereas a more plentiful supply of sodium becomes available for exchange during the osmotic diuresis.

An increased renal excretion of *hydrogen ions* has recently been demonstrated during osmotic diuresis in persons in whom the distal $Na^+ - H^+$ exchange mechanism was presumably activated after the intake of ammonium chloride during a few days. This effect is presumably also due to an increased delivery of sodium to the distal tubules during the diuresis and thus increased availability of Na in the $Na^+ - H^+$ exchange (BECK[357]).

G. Interrelationship between urinary acidification and sodium and potassium excretion

The fundamental features of the tubular processes concerned with the acidification of the urine and with tubular transfer of potassium have been discussed in a previous section (p. 234). The processes involved were considered to be:

1) An active proximal reabsorption of potassium, by which the great majority of the filtered potassium is ordinarily assumed to be reabsorbed.

2) An active proximal reabsorption of sodium ions which may occur either with concomitant reabsorption of chloride or in exchange for hydrogen ions. In the latter case bicarbonate will be reabsorbed from the tubular fluid as carbon dioxide formed from the hydrogen and bicarbonate ions. Potassium ions are not supposed to compete with hydrogen ions in these transfers. Carbonic anhydrase must be assumed to be of importance to the hydrogen ion exchange (cf. Fig. 4a on p. 253).

3) A process localized far distally by which sodium ions are actively reabsorbed and exclusively in exchange for other cations, primarily hydrogen ions or potas-

[355] WEST, C. D., and S. RAPOPORT: Urine flow and solute excretion of hydropenic dog under "resting" conditions and during osmotic diuresis. Amer. J. Physiol. **163**, 159—174 (1950).

[356] RAPOPORT, S., and C. D. WEST: Excretion of sodium and potassium during osmotic diuresis in the hydropenic dog. Amer. J. Physiol. **163**, 175—180 (1950).

[357] BECK, R. N.: Osmotic diuresis and the base sparing function of the kidney. Clin. Sci. **17**, 37—42 (1958).

sium ions, which are mutually competing in this exchange. Here too carbonic anhydrase is assumed to be essential for a maximum rate of exchange of hydrogen ions by speeding up the rate at which hydrogen ions are made available in the luminal end of the cells for exchange with sodium ions across the cell membrane (and bicarbonate ions for concomitant transfer with the sodium ions through the cells). The possibility was mentioned that ammonium ions, formed intracellularly from hydrogen ions and ammonia, might also compete in the exchange for sodium ions, but that it is also possible that ammonia passes from tubular cells into the tubular fluid by diffusion (cf. Fig. 4 b on p. 253).

If it is correct that the major part of the potassium filtered is reabsorbed in the proximal tubules even when a net secretion of potassium takes place (K clearance > inulin clearance), then it may be inferred almost with certainty that the major potassium secretion takes place in the distal convoluted tubules. A secretion by the intramedullary parts of the distal tubular system would demand medullary plasma flow rates exceeding the inulin clearance, which seems most unlikely. As mentioned in p. 260 ULLRICH et al. found abundant secretion of ammonia in the collecting tubules, but no evidence for potassium secretion there; it is therefore quite likely that potassium and ammonium exchange secretions occur at different places, in which case there would be no competition between the two cations.

The present section is devoted to a more detailed discussion of various experimental studies which have contributed further to our understanding of the factors governing the acidification of the urine and the excretion of potassium (and sodium).

a) Potassium excretion as related to sodium excretion

A reasonable starting-point for this discussion is the now well-established facts that the excretion percentage of potassium is generally quite low under conditions where only *minute* quantities of sodium are excreted, and that it may rise to very high values when a moderate augmentation of the excretion of sodium is evoked in one or another way at the end of a period of sodium deprivation (or a period in which some other procedure has been applied to activate renal sodium retaining mechanisms).

Observations to this effect have been made by several authors, thus by RY-BERG[259] who observed an appreciable rise in potassium excretion when persons slightly depleted of sodium were given a hypertonic sodium chloride solution to drink, and by BOJESEN[303], who found that the increment in potassium excretion often exceeded the increment in sodium excretion when dilution diuresis was produced in dogs with a previously low sodium excretion. Probably the observation by TARAIL et al.[358] that an osmotic (glucose) diuresis induced a parallel rise and fall in the excretions of sodium and potassium has a similar origin.

Even more striking effects were obtained by SCHWARTZ et al.[260], who observed a very marked increment in potassium excretion (21,497 μeq over a period of $2^{1}/_{2}$ hr) when 1 l of slightly hypertonic, alkaline sodium sulphate solution was administered to healthy adults previously stimulated to retain sodium by sodium-free diets, administration of desoxycorticosterone or hydrocortisone, or both. Only a small increment in potassium excretion (2,618 μeq/$2^{1}/_{2}$ hr) resulted in control subjects maintained on a normal diet.

An increase in potassium excretion may also accompany a natriuresis induced by *therapeutic* doses of mercurial diuretics, and characteristically it is more

[358] TARAIL, R., D. W. SELDIN, and A. V. N. GOODYER: Effects of injection of hypertonic glucose on metabolism of water and electrolytes in patients with edema. J. clin. Invest. **30**, 1111—1119 (1951).

pronounced in patients, such as those with congestive heart failure, in whom the sodium retaining mechanisms are activated (cf. p. 382).

Another pertinent information is that desoxycorticosterone and cortisone have been found to be unable to produce any increase in the excretion of potassium in human subjects and rats when they were kept on sodium-free diets (SELDIN et al.[359]; WELT et al.[360]), whereas it is well-known that these substances induce an appreciable augmentation of the potassium excretion when given to subjects who are excreting sodium freely in the urine. It is also important to note that administration of potassium to sodium-depleted dogs have been found to cause profound and prolonged hyperkalaemia that may be dangerous (LARAGH and CAPECI[1518]) (see chapter on excesses and deficits, p. 522).

These experimental findings are most reasonably interpreted to mean that tubular secretion of potassium ions is dependent upon simultaneous reabsorption of sodium ions (as indicated above for process no. 3) and that it takes place at a locus far distally in the tubular system. Similar arguments were discussed above (p. 255) in the case of final acidification of the urine and secretion of ammonia, and points to a similar localization of the processes by which sodium ions are exchanged for hydrogen (and ammonium ?) ions and potassium ions. The possibility that hydrogen ions and potassium ions might compete in the same exchange process is therefore already suggested by these findings.

This view, which was first clearly expressed by BERLINER[361, 362], has been greatly strengthened as it has been found suitable to account for the changes in urinary acidification and potassium excretion observed under a variety of experimental conditions.

Before these findings are discussed it seems, however, appropriate to remind of the fact that it is by no means a new observation that an increased intake of sodium salts may cause an increased excretion of potassium in the urine, in fact it was demonstrated some 100 years ago. The literature pertaining to this phenomenon is, however, too extensive to be considered in detail here. (References may be found in the papers referred to below.)

In only a few of these investigations were the more acute effects of the administration of sodium salts studied. ELKINTON and WINKLER[363] found that the infusion of 2,000—3,000 ml of a 5% sodium chloride into dogs resulted in a considerable increase in the potassium excretion, whereas infusions of corresponding volumes of hypotonic or isotonic solutions were almost without such effect. Hypertonic urea solutions did, however, induce an increase in potassium excretion. Results in close agreement with these findings were obtained by WOLF[364] in experiments in human subjects. Infusions of hypertonic sodium chloride solutions (162—344 meq/l) caused a rise in the rate of potassium excretion up to twice the normal rate, infusions of hypotonic solutions had no such effect.

It does not seem unlikely, that in cases like these, where an osmotic diuresis has been produced, the rise in potassium excretion may have been due to another

[359] SELDIN, D. W., L. G. WELT, and J. H. CORT: The effect of pituitary and adrenal hormones on the metabolism and excretion of potassium. J. clin. Invest. 30, 673 (1951).

[360] WELT, L. G., D. W. SELDIN, and J. H. CORT: The effects of the pituitary and adrenal hormones on the metabolism and excretion of sodium and water. J. clin. Invest. 30, 682 (1951).

[361] BERLINER, R. W., T. J. KENNEDY, jr., and J. ORLOFF: Relationship between acidification of the urine and potassium metabolism. Amer. J. Med. 11, 274—282 (1951).

[362] BERLINER, R. W.: Tubular secretion of potassium and acid. Renal function. Transact. 3rd Conf. New York: Josiah Macy Found 1952.

[363] ELKINTON, J. R., and A. W. WINKLER: Transfers of intracellular potassium in experimental dehydration. J. clin. Invest. 23, 93—101 (1944).

[364] WOLF, A. V.: Renal regulation of water and some electrolytes in man, with special reference to their relative retention and excretion. Amer. J. Physiol. 148, 54—68 (1947).

mechanism than an increased Na⁺—K⁺ exchange. KRUHØFFER[206] suggested that a diminution of the percentage proximal reabsorption of potassium might account for these findings, since he observed that there was a rather parallel rise in the excretion percentages of potassium and water when osmotic diuresis of increasing magnitude was produced in rabbits by loading with hypertonic sodium chloride, sodium sulphate or mannitol. A similar mechanism may also have been contributing to the rise in potassium excretion observed by DARROW and YANNET[365] upon intraperitoneal injection of hypertonic sodium chloride solution into dogs which had previously been made salt-deficient. In this case potassium secretion is, however, more likely to have been the major factor since the preceding period of sodium deprivation must be assumed to have activated the distal sodium reabsorption process responsible for the secretion of potassium. It is also quite possible that the increased excretion of potassium observed in the other cases, where hypertonic solutions were administered, was due to an increased secretion of potassium, since a dehydration leading to activation of sodium retaining mechanisms was most likely induced by these procedures.

The older literature contains an abundance of reports on rather moderate increments in potassium excretion following rather small additions of sodium chloride to a standard diet; just a few may be referred to here (OEHME[366]; WILEY et al.[367]; GLATZEL and MECKE[368]).

After this digression we may turn to consider a number of alterations in the renal handling of electrolytes which are most readily accounted for on the basis of the three types of transfer processes listed above.

There are three groups of phenomena to be considered: 1) The effects of primary changes in the "acid-base status" of the body fluids. 2) The effects of potassium depletion and of potassium excess. 3) The effects of carbonic anhydrase inhibitors.

The assumptions that have been made to account for these effects are the following: 1) That a competition takes place in the proximal tubules between hydrogen ions and chloride ions, the former tending to exchange for sodium ions, the latter to join them. 2) That a distal competition — in a process of much smaller capacity — takes place between hydrogen and potassium ions, both tending to exchange for sodium ions. 3) That the rates of each of these secondary ion transfers is mainly determined by the relative "availability" (i.e. concentration) of the ion in question at the cell membranes, and, of course, by the rate of the sodium ion transfer.

b) The effects of primary changes in the acid-base status of the body fluids

Hyperventilation (respiratory alkalosis). It has been known since early in this century that hyperventilation induced by hypoxia causes a rise in the p_H of the urine and an increased excretion of bicarbonate in the urine. It was also soon realized that these reactions would serve the purpose of counteracting the rise in

---

[365] DARROW, D. C., and H· YANNET: Metabolic studies of the changes in body electrolyte and distribution of body water induced experimentally by deficit of extracellular electrolyte. J. clin. Invest. 15, 419—427 (1936).

[366] OEHME, C.: Der Wasser-Salzbestand des Menschen in Beziehung zum Säure-Basen-Haushalt. Naunyn-Schmiedebergs Arch. exp. Path. Pharmak. 104, 115—141 (1924).

[367] WILEY, F. H., L. L. WILEY, and D. S. WALLER: The effect of the ingestion of sodium, potassium, and ammonium chlorides and sodium bicarbonates on the metabolism of inorganic salts and water. J. biol. Chem. 101, 73—82 (1933).

[368] GLATZEL, H., u. W. MECKE: Untersuchungen über den Mineralstoffwechsel des Nierenkranken. IV. Die Mineralausscheidung des Gesunden bei länger dauernder Zufuhr äquivalenter Mengen von KCl und NaCl. Z. ges. exp. Med. 91, 504—522 (1933).

plasma p_H caused by the lowering of the carbon dioxide tension (pCO_2), cf. e.g. DAVIES et al.[369].

Since the plasma bicarbonate concentration is lowered by hyperventilation, the occurrence of an increased excretion of bicarbonate obviously signifies that a smaller percentage of the bicarbonate filtered is reabsorbed, and, if no appreciable change in the filtration rate has occurred, also that the absolute rate of bicarbonate reabsorption has decreased.

Several authors, who have used voluntary hyperventilation to produce a lowering of pCO_2 have established that the rate of bicarbonate reabsorption is greatly diminished whether measured in absolute terms (meq/min) or relative terms (meq/l of glomerular filtrate): OCHWADT[370] and STANBURY and THOMSON[371] in human subjects and BRAZEAU and GILMAN[215] in dogs.

According to current views the reduced rate of bicarbonate reabsorption is explained by a diminished rate of hydrogen ion secretion, and the latter is attributed to a diminished concentration of hydrogen ions in the tubular cells and probably also to a diminished rate of formation of these ions by the carbonic anhydrase. Considering the large magnitude of the changes in reabsorption rate the major effect must be attributed to the proximal tubules.

As a further consequence one would expect that the reabsorption of chloride ions would be favoured in the proximal tubules and the secretion of potassium ions in the distal tubules. Also, since the transfer of chloride and potassium ions is likely to meet with a greater resistance than hydrogen ions there should be a greater restraint on the reabsorption of sodium. Consequently, one would expect an increase in the excretion of potassium and sodium. Such changes have been reported by several groups of workers.

In experiments where voluntary hyperventilation was used to lower the pCO_2 an increased excretion of sodium and potassium was observed by McCANCE and WIDDOWSON[372] and by STANBURY and THOMSON[371]. Both groups of workers obtained a much smaller increase in sodium and potassium excretion (or even a decrease) in experiments on sodium-depleted subjects. In these latter cases the urine also failed to become alkaline and a considerable drop was observed in urine flow, urea clearance and creatinine excretion. To the present writer this would seem to indicate a diminished renal blood flow, possibly induced by the hypocapnia by way of a fall in the blood pressure.

An increase in sodium and potassium excretion (although smaller and less constant) has also been observed in experiments where hyperventilation was induced by hypoxia (LEWIS et al.[373], AXELROD and PITTS[374] and FERGUSON and SMITH[375] in dogs; BERGER et al.[376] in human subjects). The fact that the results

[369] DAVIES, H. W., J. B. S. HALDANE, and E. L. KENNAWAY: Experiments on the regulation of the blood's alkalinity. J. Physiol. 54, 32—45 (1920).

[370] OCHWADT, B.: Über Rückresorption und Ausscheidung von Bicarbonat durch die Niere während der Hyperventilationsalkalose. Pflügers Arch. ges. Physiol. 252, 529—536 (1950).

[371] STANBURY, S. W., and A. E. THOMSON: The renal response to respiratory alkalosis. Clin. Sci. 11, 357—374 (1952).

[372] McCANCE, R. A., and E. M. WIDDOWSON: The response of the kidney to alkalosis during salt deficiency. Proc. roy. Soc. London, Ser. B 120, 228—239 (1936).

[373] LEWIS, R. A., G. W. THORN, G. F. KOEPF, and S. S. DORRANCE: The role of the adrenal cortex in acute anoxia. J. clin. Invest. 21, 33—45 (1942).

[374] AXELROD, D. R., and R. F. PITTS: Effects of hypoxia on renal tubular function. J. appl. Physiol. 4, 593—601 (1952).

[375] FERGUSON, F. P., and D. C. SMITH: Effects of acute decompression stress upon plasma electrolytes and renal function in dogs. Amer. J. Physiol. 173, 503—510 (1953).

[376] BERGER, E. Y., M. GALDSTON, and S. A. HORWITZ: The effect of anoxic anoxia on the human kidney. J. clin. Invest. 28, 648—652 (1949).

are very similar to those obtained by voluntary hyperventilation might seem to indicate that the reduction in pCO_2 — and not the hypoxia as such — is the main factor determining the changes in urine composition resulting from exposure to (moderately) low oxygen tension in the atmosphere. Recent studies in dogs by SELKURT[377] indicate, however, that local effects of the hypoxia in the kidney may also be a contributory factor. By means of a pump, one kidney, in situ, was perfused alternately with arterial blood and with venous blood from the right ventricle. In periods of perfusion with venous blood there was usually an increase in the excretion of sodium and frequently also in the excretion of potassium. It is pertinent to mention that there was also regularly an increase in the para-aminohippurate clearance in the hypoxic periods (and usually some decrease in creatinine clearance). Since similar signs of renal hyperaemia have been observed in intact animals and human subjects exposed to moderately reduced oxygen pressures, it appears that vascular factors may also be of some importance to the increased rates of electrolyte excretions during hypoxia. Several authors believe that hormonal and nervous mechanisms are also involved. Evidently, the renal reactions to hypoxia are too complex to be soundly interpreted at the present time.

Increased pCO_2 (respiratory acidosis). As might be expected the effects of an elevation in the pCO_2 of the body fluids (including those in the tubular cells) are the reverse of those obtained with a reduction of the pCO_2.

Since the plasma bicarbonate concentration rises when the pCO_2 is elevated and since the urine produced under such conditions tends to be more acid and to contain less bicarbonate it would *a priori* be expected that the rate of tubular reabsorption of bicarbonate was increased.

That this is actually the case, and that it also applies to the maximal rate expressed in absolute terms has been ascertained by several groups of workers, who measured the filtration rate and raised the plasma bicarbonate concentration by infusion of sodium bicarbonate to ensure frank excretion of bicarbonate both under normal conditions and when the pCO_2 was elevated by inhalation of gas mixtures of high CO_2 content. Such results have been obtained in human subjects by SINGER et al.[378], in sheep by DENTON et al.[379] and in dogs by RELMAN et al.[380], DOWDS et al.[381], BRAZEAU and GILMAN[215] and DORMAN et al.[382]. It was clearly demonstrated that the rate of reabsorption of bicarbonate varied directly with the plasma pCO_2 over a wide range, and that the important factor determining the rate of bicarbonate reabsorption was the pCO_2, not the p_H of the plasma.

The changes in urinary excretion of sodium and potassium induced by hypercapnia, have not been studied as extensively as the changes in bicarbonate reabsorption, but moderate decreases in the excretions of both of these ions have been reported by DOWDS et al. and by SINGER et al. The interpretion of these

[377] SELKURT, E. E.: Influence of hypoxia on renal circulation and on excretion of electrolytes and water. Amer. J. Physiol. **172**, 700—708 (1953).

[378] SINGER, R. B., J. R. ELKINTON, E. S. BARKER, and J. K. CLARK: Transfers of cellular cations during acute respiratory alkalosis and acidosis experimentally produced in man. J. clin. Invest. **32**, 604 (1953).

[379] DENTON, D. A., M. MAXWELL, I. R. McDONALD, J. MUNRO, and W. WILLIAMS: Renal regulation of the extracellular fluid in acute respiratory acidaemia. Aust. J. exp. Biol. med. Sci. **30**, 489—510 (1952).

[380] RELMAN, A. S., B. ETSTEN, and W. B. SCHWARTZ: The regulation of renal bicarbonate reabsorption by plasma carbon dioxide tension. J. clin. Invest. **32**, 972—978 (1953).

[381] DOWDS, E. G., E. W. BRICKNER, and E. E. SELKURT: Renal response to hypercapnia. Proc. Soc. exp. Biol. (N. Y.) **84**, 15—20 (1953).

[382] DORMAN, P. J., W. J. SULLIVAN, and R. F. PITTS: The renal response to acute respiratory acidosis. J. clin. Invest. **33**, 82—90 (1954).

changes as well as those in bicarbonate reabsorptions is, of course, the reverse of that discussed above in the case of hyperventilation.

For further studies on the effects of acute respiratory alkolosis and acidosis (confirming those mentioned above) the reader should consult a recent paper by BARKER et al. [383]. That changes in bicarbonate reabsorption and potassium excretion, like those described above, may result from changes in pCO_2 confined to the renal tubules has been demonstrated by ORLOFF[384], by means of injections of acetic acid or sodium hydroxide containing solutions into the renal-portal circulation of one kidney in the chicken.

Effects of non-respiratory ("metabolic") alkalosis on potassium excretion.

In 1946 DARROW[385] reported that the potassium concentration was considerably reduced in muscles from rats in which an isolated chloride deficiency (and a non-respiratory alkalosis) had been produced by intraperitoneal injection of a sodium bicarbonate solution and subsequent re-aspiration. Similar findings were reported by MUDGE and VISLOCKY[386] in clinical cases of non-respiratory alkalosis. These findings indicated, although not conclusively, that large quantities of potassium had been lost from the body, and in DARROW's experimental studies, the kidneys were the only route by which such a loss could have occurred.

Later studies have amply confirmed that non-respiratory alkalosis greatly increases the renal excretion of potassium. McCANCE and WIDDOWSON[270] had described a single clinical case (cf. p. 257) in which the potassium clearance exceeded the inulin clearance, but severe dehydration was a complicating factor which made interpretations uncertain. The same applies to the high potassium-inulin clearances ratios (not, however, exceeding unity) observed by BURNETT et al.[387]. in patients who had suffered from loss of upper gastrointestinal contents.

Acute experimental studies in animals have clearly shown that very severe renal losses may be induced by a non-respiratory alkalosis. Potassium clearances almost identical with the inulin clearance were observed by KRUHØFFER[206] in rabbits during infusions of sodium bicarbonate solutions; simultaneously the plasma potassium concentration dropped to quite low values (2—2.5 meq/l). Activation of a tubular secretion of potassium was suggested to account for these findings. Very similar results were obtained by ROBERTS et al.[388] in dogs which received an infusion of 0.6—2.0 meq/min of sodium bicarbonate over a period of some hours. The final proof that tubular secretion of potassium may be activated by a metabolic alkalosis was delivered by FRANGLEN et al.[389], who observed potassium excretion rates well exceeding those at which potassium was calculated to be filtered. Dogs were used in these experiments and the alkalosis produced either by peritoneal dialysis with a solution high in bicarbonate and low in chloride concentration, or by infusion of bicarbonate solutions.

[383] BARKER, E. S., R. B. SINGER, J. R. ELKINTON, and J. K. CLARK: The renal response in man to acute experimental respiratory alkalosis and acidosis. J. clin. Invest. 36, 515—529 (1957).

[384] ORLOFF, J.: The rôle of the kidney in the regulation of acid-base balance. Yale J. Biol. Med. 29, 211—228 (1956).

[385] DARROW, D. C.: Changes in muscle composition in alkalosis. J. clin. Invest. 25, 324—330 (1946).

[386] MUDGE, G. H., and K. VISLOCKY: Electrolyte changes in striated muscle in acidosis and alkalosis. J. clin. Invest. 28, 482—486 (1949).

[387] BURNETT, C. H., B. A. BURROWS, R. R. COMMONS, and B. T. TOWERY. Studies of alkalosis. II. Electrolyte abnormalities in alkalosis resulting from pyloric obstruction. J. clin. Invest. 29, 175—186 (1950).

[388] ROBERTS, K. E., M. G. MAGIDA and R. F. PITTS: Relationship between potassium and bicarbonate in blood and urine. Amer. J. Physiol. 172, 47—54 (1953).

[389] FRANGLEN, G. T., E. McGARRY, and A. G. SPENCER: Renal function and the excretion of potassium during alkalosis. J. Physiol. 121, 35—45 (1953).

According to the views discussed above the activation of the potassium secretion must be attributed to an elevation of the p_H in the distal tubular cells involved in cation exchange. Potassium ions would be favoured in this exchange by the lower concentration of hydrogen ions (and possibly by an inhibition of the carbonic anhydrase).

The renal losses of potassium induced by "metabolic" alkalosis are of considerable clinical importance. The potassium deficiency often observed in pyloric stenosis is only partly explainable by a loss of potassium in the vomitus; the increased urinary excretion induced by the alkalosis is undoubtedly of no smaller importance. Another case where this factor should be kept in mind is the treatment of diabetic coma. As the ketone bodies are oxidized, and hydrogen ions thereby removed from the body fluids, a metabolic alkalosis tend to develop and, of course, in particular when infusions of sodium bicarbonate are also given. The latter treatment therefore involves the risk adding one more factor to several others which tend to produce a dangerous hypokalaemia.

Potassium excretion in non-respiratory acidosis. From what has been said above about potassium excretion in non-respiratory alkalosis it may seem paradoxical that rather high rates of potassium excretion are also sometimes encounted in cases of non-respiratory acidosis. And, indeed, there are several cases which cannot be adequately accounted for.

In endogenous acidosis with ketonuria a less efficient reabsorption imposed by the osmotic diuretic effect of the excess of ketone body anions defying reabsorption may possibly be involved. A tubular secretion of potassium, induced by activation of the distal cation exchange mechanism, may well have been responsible in several cases (including those with ketonuria) in which a sodium depletion (and dehydration) probably existed. It might also be expected that in cases with a strongly acid urine, and especially before the ammonia production has reached its peak level, the exchange of hydrogen ions would be hampered by the high concentration gradient against which they have to pass; an exchange for potassium ions might then take place even though the intracellular conditions would not *per se* favour such a "second choice". Further speculations are hardly warranted at this time.

c) The effects of potassium deficiency and potassium excess

It has already been discussed in some detail (p. 256) that the kidneys of normal subjects are capable of *excreting potassium* at a high rate *by tubular secretion when potassium salts are administered* in large quantities. It was also mentioned (p. 286), that a certain excretion of sodium in the urine is a prerequisite for any greater secretion of potassium to occur.

The potassium excretion in response to an additional potassium intake is also greatly diminished in potassium deficient subjects as has clearly been shown by MILNE et al.[390]. Apparently the tubular cells responsible do not take up the additional potassium offered before the general deficit has been paid, or they do not get an impulse for potassium secretion (from the adrenal cortex?) before this has happened.

The kidneys of normal mammals are also able to *conserve potassium* quite effectively *when a potassium deficiency develops*, although possibly not quite as well as in the case of sodium. Urinary potassium concentrations below the coincident plasma concentration have now been reported by so many authors that it is

---

[390] MILNE, M. D., N. C. H. JONES, and B. M. EVANS: Electrolyte excretion in states of potassium depletion in man. The kidney. Proc. Symp. Ciba Foundation and Renal Association 1953. Eds.: LEWIS, A. A. G., and G. E. W. WOLSTENHOLME. London: Churchill, Ltd. 1954.

beyond doubt that the kidney can reabsorb potassium against a concentration gradient. Virtually potassium-free urine was claimed by ORENT-KEILES and MCCOLLUM[391] to be produced by rats reared on a diet containing as little as 0.01% of potassium. In man urinary potassium concentrations, below the concurrent plasma level have been recorded by DANOWSKI[1], LOWE[392], FOURMAN[393] and several others.

The time-course and the efficiency of renal conservation of potassium have been studied by several authors. FOURMAN[393] used an acid loaded cation-exchange resin to produce a potassium deficiency while BLACK and MILNE[394] and BLAHD and BASSETT[395] used diets very low in potassium, viz. less than 10 meq and 14 meq per day respectively. In all studies a gradual decline in urinary excretion of potassium to quite low values was observed, so that all authors, agree that renal conservation is quite effective. It is noteworthy, however, that BLAHD and BASSETT observed that potassium balance was not attained during a 55 days period of dietary potassium restriction. Consequently, the renal conservation of potassium could not be considered quite successful at their level of potassium intake. From the studies of WESTON et al. it seems that the kidneys may restrict urinary potassium loss to as little as 1 meq per day. This problem is further discussed in p. 531.

An appreciable potassium deficiency is, however, most unlikely to develop merely from a too low content of potassium in the diet, since it is very difficult to compose a diet with a potassium content of less than 1 g (25 meq) per day (see p. 516).

Variations in the intake of *potassium affects the renal handling of electrolytes in other ways* than by changing the rates of potassium excretion. We shall consider separately the effects of a diminished and an increased intake of potassium salts.

Effects of potassium deficiency upon bicarbonate reabsorption. It is now well-established that potassium depletion may lead to, or at least promote, the development of an extracellular alkalosis, and as further discussed elsewhere (p. 538) there is evidence that under such conditions hydrogen ions move from the extracellular fluid into the cells with a consequent lowering of the p_H inside the cells and an elevation of the extracellular p_H. This may provide a satisfactory explanation of how the extracellular alkalosis originates in potassium deficiency, but it does not directly explain how the plasma bicarbonate is stabilized at an elevated level. Clearly, the kidney must be contributing by a more efficient excretion of hydrogen ion equivalents.

This has been confirmed in recent studies by ROBERTS et al.[396] who demonstrated that the maximal rate of tubular reabsorption of bicarbonate was appreciably increased (from about 28 to 33 meq/l of glomerular filtrate) in human subjects in whom a rather moderate potassium deficiency (180—280 meq) was produced by maintaining them on a low potassium diet for a period of 5—19 days. The increase in bicarbonate reabsorption was absolute (meq/min) and in this case also relative

[391] ORENT-KEILES, E., and E. V. MCCOLLUM: Potassium and animal nutrition. J. biol. Chem. **140**, 337—352 (1941).

[392] LOWE, K. G.: Metabolic studies with protein-free, electrolyte-free diet in man. Clin. Sci. **12**, 57—62 (1953).

[393] FOURMAN, P.: The ability of the normal kidney to conserve potassium. Lancet **262**, 1042—1044 (1952).

[394] BLACK, D. A. K., and M. D. MILNE: Experimental potassium depletion in man. Clin. Sci. **11**, 397—415 (1952).

[395] BLAHD, W. H., and S. H. BASSETT: Potassium deficiency in man. Metabolism **2**, 218—224 (1953).

[396] ROBERTS, K. E., H. T. RANDALL, H. L. SANDERS, and M. HOOD: Effects of potassium on renal tubular reabsorption of bicarbonate. J. clin. Invest. **34**, 666—672 (1955).

(i.e. increased reabsorption percentage), and it was shown that it could not be accounted for by elevations of plasma pCO_2.

According to current views an increased reabsorption of bicarbonate means an increased tubular secretion of hydrogen ions, and it appears that the above findings are most reasonably explained by assuming that a potassium deficiency causes a lowering of the p_H in the tubular cells from which hydrogen ions are secreted (proximal as well as distal). Thus hydrogen ions would be more readily available for exchange with sodium ions. It has been shown that the p_H in muscle cells is lowered during potassium deficiency (GARDNER et al. [397]), and it seems quite likely that the same may apply to the (proximal) tubular cells. Some support to this view has recently been delivered by ANDERSON and MUDGE[398]. These authors showed that slices of rabbit kidney cortex which had been incubated for 35 min in a potassium-free medium contained appreciably less bicarbonate than control slices incubated in a medium with a high potassium concentration (10 meq/l).

If potassium deficiency makes (easily movable) hydrogen ions more readily available for exchange with Na^+ the restraint on sodium reabsorption should be reduced and an enhanced reabsorption of sodium (reduced excretion) might be expected. Such results have been reported by several authors, e.g. ROBERTS et al.[396] and FITZGERALD and FOURMAN[399]. Other mechanisms may obviously also be involved.

As in other cases where a long-standing lowering of the p_H in the tubular cells must be assumed to exist the glutaminase activity in the kidney has been found to be increased in potassium deficiency. This probably explains why the ammonia excretion is typically increased even though the urinary p_H may be rather high. The existence of a high rate of ammonium excretion, representing a loss of H^+ from the body without reabsorption of bicarbonate, accounts in turn for the fact that an alkalaemia can exist in spite of increased urinary losses of bicarbonate (which are frequently observed). For further references cf. the review by RELMAN and SCHWARTZ[1578].

Effects of administration of potassium salts (potassium excess). It has been known since the work of LOEB et al.[400] that when potassium salts are administered, the urine becomes less acid and often definitely alkaline (see for instance WOLF[364], for a summary of the literature).

A closer study of this phenomenon was undertaken by ROBERTS et al.[388]. These authors observed that an infusion of 0.67—1.0 meq/min of potassium chloride into dogs produced an increased excretion of bicarbonate in the urine. Since a considerable fall in plasma bicarbonate concentration occurred simultaneously, the increased excretion was clearly the result of a reduced rate of bicarbonate reabsorption. Similar results were obtained by FULLER and MACLEOD[401] who also showed that the rate of bicarbonate reabsorption remained suppressed when the plasma bicarbonate concentration was brought up to normal levels by bicarbonate infusions.

[397] GARDNER, L. I., E. A. MACLACHLAN, and H. BERMAN: Effect of potassium deficiency on carbon dioxide, cation and phosphate content of muscle, with a note on (the) carbon dioxide content of human muscle. J. gen. Physiol. **36**, 153—159 (1952).

[398] ANDERSON, H. M., and G. H. MUDGE: The effects of potassium on intracellular bicarbonate in slices of kidney cortex. J. clin. Invest. **34**, 1691—1697 (1955).

[399] FITZGERALD, M. G., and P. FOURMAN: The renal factor in the alkalosis of potassium deficiency. Lancet II, 848—850 (1955).

[400] LOEB, R. F., D. W. ATCHLEY, D. W. RICHARDS, E. M. BENEDICT, and M. E. DRISCOLL: On the mechanism of nephrotic edema. J. clin. Invest. **11**, 621—639 (1932).

[401] FULLER, G. R., and M. B. MACLEOD: Effect of potassium infusion on renal tubular reabsorption of bicarbonate. Fed. Proc. **13**, 49—50 (1954).

The interpretation of these findings is the reverse of that discussed above in the case of potassium deficiency. The entrance of an excess of potassium ions into the body cells is assumed to be accompanied by a loss of hydrogen ions from the cells, and consequently an increase in the p_H of the intracellular fluid (cf. p. 538). The same is assumed to happen in the tubular cells involved in hydrogen ion secretion, with the result that this process is slowed down since hydrogen ions are "less available" for exchange.

These changes are probably also, at least in part, responsible for the well-known fact that an additional intake of potassium salt produces an *increased excretion of sodium* in the urine. As mentioned before concomitant reabsorption of chloride ions probably meet with a greater resistance than the exchange for hydrogen ions. Consequently, when hydrogen ions are less available the reabsorption of sodium ions must be assumed to meet with a greater restraint, and the reabsorption is apt to be less complete. Another factor which may be involved is a displacement of cellular sodium with potassium and a consequent small rise in plasma sodium concentration.

The natriuretic effect of potassium was demonstrated in self-experiments by BUNGE[402], who considered that it explained the craving for sodium chloride displayed by herbivorous animals. Considering the rather small and transient increase in sodium excretion produced by potassium salts and our present conceptions of the sequence of tubular processes involved in sodium and potassium excretion it seems rather unlikely that even large excretions of potassium could induce serious losses of sodium in the urine. Rather it appears that the importance of a reasonable sodium intake must be attributed to the fact, previously mentioned (p. 286), that the excretion of potassium by distal tubular secretion demands the presence of a certain amount of sodium (for exchange) in the distal tubular fluid.

The number of reports on increased excretion of sodium following administration of potassium salts is too large to be considered here in detail. In the case of potassium chloride the phenomenon has been reported in human subjects by MEYER and COHN[403], GLATZEL and MECKE[368], MacKEY and BUTLER[404] and by WOLF[364]. In rabbits it has been demonstrated by BOCK[405], in dogs by WHELAN[406] and in pigs and rats by MILLER[407, 408]. When other potassium salts have been used a possible natriuretic effect of the associated anion must be considered (cf. "osmotic" diuresis, p. 280).

The natriuretic effect has more recently been studied in human subjects by LIDDLE et al.[409], who also demonstrated that administration of potassium salts abolishes the sodium-retaining effect of ACTH.

[402] BUNGE, G.: Über die Bedeutung des Kochsalzes und das Verhalten der Kalisalze im menschlichen Organismus. Z. Biol. **9**, 104—143 (1873).

[403] MEYER, L. F., and S. COHN: Klinische Beobachtungen und Stoffwechselversuche über die Wirkung verschiedener Salze beim Säugling. Z. Kinderheilk. **2**, 360 (1911).

[404] MacKEY, F. M., and A. M. BUTLER: Studies of sodium and potassium metabolism. The effect of potassium on the sodium and water balances in normal subjects and patients with Bright's disease. J. clin. Invest. **14**, 923—939 (1935).

[405] BOCK, J.: Untersuchungen über die Nierenfunktion. I. Über die Ausscheidung der Alkalimetalle nach Injektion von Kaliumsalzen. Naunyn-Schmiedebergs Arch. exp. Path. Pharmak. **57**, 183—213 (1907).

[406] WHELAN, M.: The effect of intravenous injection of inorganic chlorides on the composition of blood and urine. J. biol. Chem. **63**, 585—620 (1925).

[407] MILLER, H. G.: Potassium in animal nutrition. I. Influence of potassium on urinary sodium and chlorine excretion. J. biol. Chem. **55**, 45—59 (1923).

[408] III.: Influence of potassium on total excretion of sodium, chlorine, calcium and phosphorus. J. biol. Chem. **67**, 71—77 (1926).

[409] LIDDLE, G. W., L. L. BENNETT, and P. H. FORSHAM: The prevention of ACTH induced sodium retention by the use of potassium salts, a quantitative study. J. clin. Invest. **32**, 1197—1207 (1953).

Table 24. *Relationship between presumed intracellular* p_H *in the renal tubules and measured bicarbonate reabsorption (and potassium excretion).* Modified from ROBERTS et al.[396] Up-turned arrow indicates increase, down-turned decrease; $\pm$ signifies: no consistent change

Conditions	Renal alterations				
	Intracellular			Rate of bicarbonate reabsorption (H+ secretion)	Rate of potassium excretion
	pCO_2	potassium	p_H		
Respiratory acidosis	↑	±	↓	↑	(↓)
Potassium deficiency with extra-cellular alkalosis	±	↓	↓	↑	↓
Respiratory alkalosis (hyperventila-tion)	↓	±	↑	↓	↑
Potassium "excess"	±	↑	↑	↓	↑
Carbonic anhydrase inhibition . . .	↓*	±	↑	↓	↑
Non-respiratory (metabolic) alkalosis			↑		↑
Non-respiratory (metabolic) acidosis			↓		± or ↑

    * by secondary respiratory regulation.

The changes in the renal handling of electrolytes so far considered in this section may now be summarized. This is adequately done by referring to Table 24 (adopted from ROBERTS et al.[396]). This table must be read with the view in mind that *the common denominator underlying the changes in reabsorptions and excretions is a change in* p_H *in the tubular cells ("availability of hydrogen ions for exchange").* Whether the changes in intracellular p_H may also be of importance to the hydrogen ion exchange by influencing the activity of the carbonic anhydrase is not yet clear, since, apparently the effect of p_H on the activity of renal carbonic anhydrase has not yet been determined. According to ROUGHTON and BOOTH[410] the activity of carbonic anhydrase from red blood cells has a rather flat minimum about p_H 6.4, but the authors were not quite certain that the rise in activity observed below this value was entirely due to a p_H effect.

d) The effects of carbonic anhydrase inhibitors

It remains to discuss the effects on the renal handling of electrolytes of carbonic anhydrase inhibitors, the detection of which has contributed greatly to current conceptions of the nature of the processes involved in tubular transfer of hydrogen and alkali metal ions.

It has been known since the work of MANN and KEILIN[411] that various sulfon-amides with an unsubstituted sulfonamide group exert a marked inhibitory effect on carbonic anhydrase. The observation that such substances also affect the excretion of bicarbonate, sodium and potassium by the kidney was first made with sulfanilamide. Upon the administration of this substance to human subjects SOUTHWORTH observed a drop in the CO_2-combining capacity of plasma, and in a subsequent paper (STRAUSS and SOUTHWORTH[412]) he reported in addition a definite

[410] ROUGHTON, F. J. W., and V. H. BOOTH: The effect of substrate concentrations, p_H and other factors upon the activity of carbonic anhydrase. Biochem. J. **40**, 319—330 (1946).

[411] MANN, T., and D. KEILIN: Sulphanilamide as a specific inhibitor of carbonic anhydrase Nature (Lond.) **146**, 164—165 (1940).

[412] STRAUSS, M. B., and H. SOUTHWORTH: Urinary changes due to sulfanilamide-adminis-tration. Bull. Johns Hopkins Hosp. **63**, 41—45 (1938).

increase in urine flow and in the renal excretion of sodium and potassium. The latter findings were confirmed by BECKMAN et al. [413]. A decrease in the carbon dioxide content of plasma and a fall in plasma p_H was observed in dogs by MARSHALL et al. [414], who also made the important observation that a rise in the p_H of the urine occurred. These authors therefore suggested that sulfanilamide depressed the tubular reabsorption of bicarbonate and that this might be the main cause of the plasma acidosis.

The significance of these findings was, however, not fully understood at that time, and due to its rather low activity as a carbonic anhydrase inhibitor, and the side effects of large doses, sulfanilamide never became of practical value as a saluretic.

It has already been mentioned (p. 252) that the ability of sulfanilamide to increase urinary excretion of bicarbonate and reduce the excretion of titratable acidity, was used by PITTS and ALEXANDER as an argument for considering carbonic acid as the major source of the hydrogen ions which they had shown to be secreted in the tubules. At that time, as also mentioned, tubular secretion of hydrogen ions was, however, generally believed to be a process of rather small capacity which was only responsible for the reabsorption of a rather small fraction of the bicarbonate present in the glomerular filtrate.

The usefulness of sulfonamides as a physiological tool gained further when other members of much greater potency were synthesized (MILLER et al.[415]) which could be used in doses sufficient to obtain almost complete inhibition of carbonic anhydrase in vivo, without detrimental side-effects. These properties also account for the fact that some of these substances are now being used (in smaller doses) as saluretics. The best known is 2-acetylamino-1,3,4-thiadiazole-5-sulfonamide = acetazoleamide = Diamox (first called 6063) which has been extensively studied.

The effect of a single therapeutical dose of acetazoleamide on the renal excretion of electrolytes is illustrated in Table 25 showing data from one of BERLINER et al.'s[223] experiments in dogs.

Table 25. *Effect of acetazoleamide (6063) on urine acidification and electrolyte excretions in dog.* From BERLINER et al.[223]

Time min	Urine flow ml/min	Urine p_H	Excreted Titr. Acid μeq/min	Excreted HCO_3 μeq/min	Excreted Na μeq/min	Excreted K μeq/min
—112	Infusion: Creatinine 20 mg/min; PAH 25 mg/min; H_2O 2.2 ml/min. Prime: 2 g creatinine, 0.9 g PAH					
0— 20	0.64	5.25	60	0.1	8	34
20— 41	1.03	5.25	71	0.1	7	36
41— 63	1.51	5.25	69	0.3	9	38
68	6063 I. V. 10 mg/kg					
77— 96	5.25	7.70	0	326	240	181
96—113	5.62	7.72	0	340	319	155
113—130	3.83	7.76	0	278	320	125

[413] BECKMAN, W. W., E. C. ROSSMEISL, R. B. PETTENGILL, and W. BAUER: A study of the effects of sulfanilamide on acid-base metabolism. J. clin. Invest. **19**, 635—644 (1940).
[414] MARSHALL, E. K., W. C. CUTTING and K. EMERSON: The toxicity of sulfanilamide. Amer. med. Ass. **110**, 252—257 (1938).
[415] MILLER, W. H., A. M. DESSERT, and R. O. ROBLIN: Heterocyclic sulfonamides as carbonic anhydrase inhibitors. J. Amer. chem. Soc. **72**, 4893—4896 (1950).

It is apparent that qualitatively the effects are similar to those obtained by sulfanilamide: an increase in urine p_H and in the excretion of bicarbonate, sodium and potassium accompanied by a decrease in the excretion of titratable acidity. The excretion of chloride was not significantly changed.

This response is typical and, together with a decrease in the excretion of ammonia, has also been observed in other species including man (cf. e.g. COUNIHAN et al.[416]; LEAF et al.[417] and MAREN et al.[418]). It is generally agreed that within the therapeutic dosage range (3—15 mg/kg) there is a gradual increase in the response to increasing doses (cf. e.g. COUNIHAN et al.).

Opinions seem to differ, on the other hand, as to how much the response (in particular the excretion of bicarbonate) may be increased by further increases in dose. According to MAREN[419] it seems difficult to produce an increase in the excretion percentage for bicarbonate beyond 25%. BERLINER[362] has, however, reported that as much as 50% of the bicarbonate of the glomerular filtrate may be excreted when large doses of acetazoleamide are given to dogs, and more recently SCHWARTZ and RELMAN[420] have claimed to have observed excretion percentages as high as 80 in acute experiments in dogs given very large doses (500 mg/kg). In this latter case a very marked increase in the excretion percentage for chloride was, however, also observed.

It may also be mentioned that very high excretion percentages for bicarbonate have been observed by BECKER-CHRISTENSEN[421] under special conditions in rabbits. This author used rabbits subjected to a marked sulphate diuresis and the excretion percentage for bicarbonate was therefore already elevated (about 15%) prior to the administration of sulfanilamide. When 1—1.5 g of this drug was injected intravenously the excretion percentage for bicarbonate rose to 80% on an average, and simultaneously the excretion percentage for chloride went up from about 40 to 60%. It appears that the pre-existing state of the kidney is an important factor determining how great a fraction of the filtered bicarbonate may become excreted upon the administration of a carbonic anhydrase inhibitor. A pre-existing state of osmotic diuresis seems to be particularly favourable for obtaining a large excretion percentage.

As previously discussed (p. 239) the production of *very high* excretion percentages for bicarbonate by means of carbonic anhydrase inhibitors has been one of the main arguments for considering not only the distal acidification process but also the larger proximal reabsorption of bicarbonate as due to a secretion of hydrogen ions to a large extent derived from carbonic anhydrase action. This view will also be held here although it must be admitted that the support afforded by the results cited above is not quite incontestable.

It may be argued that when sulfonamide administration leads not only to an increase in bicarbonate but also in chloride excretion, one may have to do with effects on the tubular

[416] COUNIHAN, T. B., B. M. EVANS and M. D. MILNE: Observations on the pharmacology of the carbonic anhydrase inhibitor "Diamox". Clin. Sci. **13**, 583—598 (1954).

[417] LEAF, A., W. B. SCHWARTZ, and A. S. RELMAN: Oral administration of potent carbonic anhydrase inhibitor ("Diamox"). I. Changes in electrolyte and acid-base balance. New Engl. J. Med. **250**, 759—764 (1954).

[418] MAREN, T. H., B. C. WADSWORTH, E. K. YALE, and L. G. ALONSO: Carbonic anhydrase inhibition. III. Effects of Diamox R on electrolyte metabolism. Bull. Johns Hopkins Hosp. **95**, 277—321 (1954).

[419] MAREN, T. H.: Carbonic anhydrase inhibition. IV. The effects of metabolic acidosis on the response to diamox. Bull. Johns Hopkins Hosp. **98**, 159—183 (1956).

[420] SCHWARTZ, W. B., and A. S. RELMAN: The dependence of renal sodium reabsorption on hydrogen exchange. J. clin. Invest. **33**, 965 (1954).

[421] BECKER-CHRISTENSEN, P.: Undersøgelser over Sulfonamidernes Indvirkning paa Organismens Syre-Baseligevaegt. pp. 123. Thesis: Copenhagen 1948.

cells not entirely referable to carbonic anhydrase inhibition. On the other hand, it cannot *a priori* be excluded that an increased excretion of chloride obtained by large doses might not also be a secondary effect of carbonic anhydrase inhibition; the possibility should be considered, for instance, that a blockade of the exchange with the easily movable hydrogen ions may cause a reduction in tubular cell volumes, and thus a diuresis and chloruresis of a type similar to that observed in "osmotic" diuresis.

In principle, the explanation that may be offered to account for the changes in electrolyte excretions produced by unsubstituted sulfonamides is similar to that discussed in connection with the effects of hypocapnia. The inhibition of the carbonic anhydrase makes hydrogen ions less available in both proximal and distal cells where a hydrogen ion exchange takes place. The secretion of hydrogen ions is therefore reduced and consequently also the reabsorption of bicarbonate. In the proximal tubules the reabsorption of sodium is impeded together with that of bicarbonate, and a further factor tending to augment the excretion of sodium (and chloride) may possibly be a reduction in tubular hydrodynamic resistance. In the distal tubules the reduced availability of hydrogen ions for exchange tends to favour an exchange of potassium ions for sodium ions, but probably with a greater restraint on the transfer of sodium ions; the excretion of both sodium and potassium is therefore increased.

No doubt, these interpretations as well as those previously discussed in this section, represent at best oversimplifications of the actual mechanisms involved. Although crude, it seems, however, likely that they contain a fundamental element of truth, and as a working hypothesis, they have at least the advantage of correlating a great number of experimental observations which are otherwise not easily accounted for.

The view that the increase in potassium excretion produced by sulfonamides is due to an increased (distal) secretion of potassium and not to a reduced (proximal) reabsorption has received some support from experiments performed by BERLINER et al.[223]. Some of their data are presented in Table 26 from which it appears that when salyrgan was given first it caused a large increase in the excretion of sodium and chloride and fairly small changes in bicarbonate or potassium excretion. When acetazoleamide (6063) was subsequently given,

Table 26. *Effect of Salyrgan and acetazoleamide (6063) alone or together on electrolyte excretion in dog. From* BERLINER *et al.*[223]

Time min	Creatinine clearance ml/min	Excretion of			
		Cl^- μeq/min	HCO_3^- μeq/min	Na^- μeq/min	K^- μeq/min
— 58	Start infusion: Creatinine 15 mg/min, sodium phosphate (p_H 7.4) 200 μM/min, NaCl 450 μM/min in water at 5.1 ml/min				
0— 40	73	4	1	13	56
41	Salyrgan 200 mg I. V.				
64— 94	69	864	102	1060	68
99	6063 10 mg/kg and 20 mg/kg/hr I. V.				
108—139	55	832	481	1527	92
141	BAL 100 mg I. M.				
155—190	58	74	446	745	208

sodium and bicarbonate excretions rose strikingly while chloride and potassium excretions were only little affected. When finally BAL was given, which abolishes the effects of the mercurial and leaves the effects of the sulfonamide, the chloride excretion dropped towards normal values and a fall in sodium excretion of similar magnitude occurred; the bicarbonate excretion remained almost unchanged and finally, and of particular interest here, there was a great increase in potassium excretion. In other words, if we read the table from below and upwards: acetazoleamide caused a considerable increase in potassium excretion and salyrgan was capable of bringing it back towards normal again. If one assumed that acetazoleamide caused an increase in potassium excretion by inhibiting the reabsorption of potassium, one would have to postulate that salyrgan was capable of speeding up the reabsorption again. This seems most unreasonable, and consequently BERLINER et al.'s conclusion, that acetazoleamide promotes the *secretion* of potassium, must be accepted.

The magnitude of the increase in potassium excretion induced by sulfonamide may vary considerably. From what has previously been said (p. 286) one would expect a particularly large increase when the distal sodium exchange process is activated. This may possibly explain why METCOFF et al.[422] found nephrotic children to respond mainly by an increased excretion of potassium, whereas normal subjects generally react with preponderant excretion of sodium. The authors themselves appear, however, to favour other explanations. Conversely, the kaliuretic response might be expected to be only small when the distal sodium exchange process is proceeding slowly. This may possibly explain in part why administration of acetazoleamide (and other stimuli, such as hyperventilation and administration of bicarbonate, which normally produce a marked increase in potassium excretion) has been found to induce very little rise in potassium excretion in potassium depleted subjects, although a greater than normal increase in sodium and bicarbonate excretions was obtained (EVANS et al.[1571]). Other factors such as low availability of potassium and high availability of hydrogen ions in the tubular cells may of course also be of importance.

It is well-established that with continued administration of sulfonamides one obtains less and less increase in sodium and bicarbonate excretion with each new dose, and that a similar "resistance" may be produced acutely by administration of sufficient amounts of ammonium chloride (cf. MAREN[419], for a review of the literature). In both cases the degree of resistance (diminution in response) correlates well with the plasma bicarbonate concentration, but it was suggested by MAREN, that this correlation might be fortuitous, and the important factor be changes in the p_H of the tubular cells. This view was also expressed by KAYE[423] who stated that with a reduction in intracellular p_H "proportionally less of the secreted hydrogen ions would originate through the action of carbonic anhydrase". A similar interpretation was also proposed by this author to account for very small responses to acetazoleamide obtained in patients with nephrogenic acidosis.

A lowered intracellular p_H is not, however, acceptable *per se* as an explanation of the resistance, because it only signifies the presence of an additional cellular store of hydrogen ion equivalents (of limited capacity) at a certain moment. A continuous reabsorption of bicarbonate at an appreciable rate by exchange secretion of hydrogen ions not provided by enzymatic hydration of CO_2 demands a *continuous supply* of hydrogen ions to the cell from other sources.

---

[422] METCOFF, M. S., M. B. JAMES, G. GORDILLO, and I. ANTONOWICZ: Renal electrolyte transport in normal and nephrotic children. Effects of simultaneous infusion of carbonic anhydrase inhibitor and nonreabsorbable anion. J. Lab. clin. Med. **46**, 333—341 (1955).
[423] KAYE, M.: The effect of a single oral dose of the carbonic anhydrase inhibitor, acetazoleamide, in renal disease. J. clin. Invest. **34**, 277—284 (1955).

Apart from other intracellular metabolic sources, the possibility of hydrogen ions entering from the blood must be considered. A low plasma p_H would, of course, mean that hydrogen ions would be more readily available from this source.

H. Hormonal factors affecting the renal handling of sodium, potassium (and water)

a) Hormones of the adrenal cortex and other steroids

Effects of adrenocortical insufficiency. The study of clinical and experimental adrenocortical insufficiency has clearly shown that the hormones of the adrenal cortex exert a vitally important influence on the metabolism of sodium and potassium. There is increasing evidence that these hormones are, in fact, involved in shifts of ions between cells and extracellular fluid, mobilization of sodium from stores in bone as well as in the regulation of the secretion of alkali metals by various glands. — Without denying the significance of these effects it still appears that as regards vital importance they are overshadowed by the effects on the renal excretion of electrolytes.

The first to call attention to electrolyte abnormalities in adrenocortical insufficiency (in adrenalectomized cats and rabbits) were BAUMANN and KURLAND[424] who detected a reduction in the plasma sodium concentration and to a lesser extent in the plasma chloride, together with an increase in the plasma concentrations of potassium and magnesium. Shortly after, the observation was made that injections of sodium-containing fluids prolonged the survival time of adrenalectomized dogs (ROGOFF and STEWART[425]) and cats (MARINE and BAUMANN[426]), and the latter authors expressed the opinion that the beneficial effect was due to the sodium content.

The prolongation of life obtained in these studies was, however, quite moderate, a fact which may have been due to administration of inadequate amounts of sodium in combination with large intakes of potassium, since meat was offered the animals as food. Subsequent studies disclosed the important fact that life could be maintained "indefinitely" in adrenalectomized animals merely by proper adjustment of the salt content of the diet. Considerable amounts of sodium salts, preferably as a mixture of sodium chloride and an "alkaline" sodium salt such as the bicarbonate or the citrate (to control the acidosis), were found to be an essential element of such maintenance diets (HARROP et al.[427]; ALLERS and KENDALL[428]). The beneficial effect of sodium salts was also demonstrated in clinical cases of adrenocortical insufficiency (LOEB[429]; STAHL et al.[430]). In addition, the

---

[424] BAUMANN, E. J., and S. KURLAND: Changes in the inorganic constituents of blood in supraadrenalectomized cats and rabbits. J. biol. Chem. 71, 281—302 (1926—1927).

[425] ROGOFF, J. M., and G. N. STEWART: Studies on adrenal insufficiency IV. The influence of intravenous injection of Ringer's solution upon the survival period in adrenalectomized dogs. Amer. J. Physiol. 84, 649—659 (1928).

[426] MARINE, D., and E. J. BAUMANN: Duration of life after suprarenalectomy in cats and attempts to prolong it by injections of solutions containing sodium salts, glucose and glycerol. Amer. J. Physiol. 81, 86—100 (1927).

[427] HARROP, G. A., L. J. SOFFER, W. M. NICHOLSON, and M. STRAUSS: Studies on the suprarenal cortex. IV. The effects of sodium salts in sustaining the suprarenalectomized dog. J. exp. Med. 61, 839—860 (1935).

[428] ALLERS, W. D., and E. C. KENDALL: Maintenance of adrenalectomized dogs without cortin, through control of the mineral constituents of the diet. Amer. J. Physiol. 118, 87—94 (1937).

[429] LOEB, R. F.: Effect of sodium chloride in treatment of a patient with Addison's disease. Proc. Soc. exp. Biol. (N. Y.) 30, 808—812 (1932—1933).

[430] STAHL, J., D. W. ATCHLEY, and R. F. LOEB: Observations on adrenal insufficiency. J. clin. Invest. 15, 41—46 (1936).

observation was made (WILDER[431]) that a further improvement could be achieved by restricting the potassium content of the diet, and that, when this was done, the sodium content of the maintenance diet could be reduced. The occurrence of lowered plasma concentrations of sodium and chloride and the elevation of the plasma potassium concentration following adrenalectomy was soon confirmed in other mammals and a similar tendency reported in clinical cases of Addisons's disease. A decrease in the plasma bicarbonate concentration, implicit in the earlier finding of a greater fall in sodium than in chloride concentration, was demonstrated by HASTINGS and COMPÈRE[432].

A clear demonstration that these changes in the plasma concentrations of sodium and potassium were related to an impaired regulation of the renal excretions of these ions was furnished by LOEB et al.'s[433] balance studies in dogs, which showed that adrenalectomy leads both to a negative sodium balance due to an increased renal excretion of sodium and to a potassium retention due to a diminished renal excretion of potassium. Similar observations were made by HARROP et al.[434] when substitution therapy in adrenalectomized dogs was stopped, and they were amply confirmed by later investigators (cf. also LOEB et al.[435]; HARROP et al.[436]; LOEB[437]).

The fact that death could be prevented and a tolerable state of health maintained in cases of adrenocortical insufficiency when the sodium and potassium intakes were properly adjusted constituted clear evidence that the disturbances in the electrolyte metabolism are important factors in the pathogenesis of this condition. Accordingly, the view was held by many that the symptoms and the fatal outcome could be adequately accounted for as secondary manifestations of the renal loss of sodium and renal retention of potassium. The sequence of events was considered to be as follows: renal loss of sodium with accompanying loss of water → dehydration, with haemoconcentration and diminution of the interstitial fluid volume and the plasma volume → circulatory failure with hypotension → impairment of the function of vital organs as the kidneys, liver etc.

Although these factors are still considered to play an important role it has become increasingly clear that they are by no means the only ones involved. An important argument for this is the fact that normal animals are little affected by a sodium loss which proves fatal to adrenalectomized animals. Furthermore, adrenalectomized animals (or Addisonian patients) which are maintained merely on a diet of well-balanced electrolyte contents are far from being in an optimal state of health; their resistance towards different types of "stress", such as exposure to cold, trauma and haemorrhage, is greatly reduced (cf. SWINGLE and

[431] WILDER, R. M., A. M. SNELL, E. J. KEPLER, E. H. RYNEARSON, M. ADAMS, and E. C. KENDALL: Control of Addison's disease with a diet restricted in potassium: A clinical study. Proc. Staff. Meet. Mayo Clin. 11, 273—283 (1936).

[432] HASTINGS, A. B., and E. L. COMPÈRE: Effect of bilateral suprarenalectomy on certain constituents of the blood of dogs. Proc. Soc. exp. Biol. ((N. Y.) 28, 376—378 (1931).

[433] LOEB, R. F., D. W. ATCHLEY, E. M. BENEDICT, and J. LELAND: Electrolyte balance studies in adrenalectomized dogs with particular reference to the excretion of sodium. J. exp. Med. 57, 775—792 (1933).

[434] HARROP, G. A., A. WEINSTEIN, L. J. SOFFER, and J. H. TRESCHER: Studies on the suprarenal cortex. II. Metabolism, circulation and blood concentration during suprarenal insufficiency in the dog. J. exp. Med. 58, 1—16 (1933).

[435] LOEB, R. F., D. W. ATCHLEY, and J. STAHL: The role of sodium in adrenal insufficiency. J. Amer. med. Ass. 104, 2149 (1935).

[436] HARROP, G. A., W. M. NICHOLSON, and M. STRAUSS. Studies on the suprarenal cortex. V. The influence of the cortical hormone upon the excretion of water and electrolytes in the suprarenalectomized dog. J. exp. Med. 64, 233—251 (1936).

[437] LOEB, R. F.: Adrenal cortex and electrolyte behavior. Harvey Lect. 37, 100—128 (1941—1942).

REMINGTON[438]). It is also well-established that their working capacity, although it may be somewhat improved by sodium chloride treatment, remains only a small fraction of that of normal animals (INGLE[439]). The cause of this reduced ability of the salt-maintained adrenalectomized animal to meet "stress" is not yet fully understood. An important factor seems, however, to be a failure of the cardiovascular system to respond adequately to the additional demands imposed by the stress situation, even when the blood volume and the plasma sodium and potassium concentrations are normalized. Evidence for this view has been provided by LEVINE and his associates. These investigators (GOLDSTEIN et al.[440]) found that the failing work performance of the gastrocnemius muscle of adrenalectomized (desoxycorticosterone-treated) dogs during electric stimulation *in situ* was preceded by a fall in the blood pressure. This finding together with the previous observation that the *in vitro* work performance of muscles from adrenalectomized animals did not differ from that of muscles from normal controls, led to the conclusion that a circulatory maladjustment was involved. The further observation that the blood pressure raising response to single doses, and especially to repeated injections or continuous administration, of norepinephrine was greatly reduced in adrenalectomized dogs (RAMEY et al.[441]) directed attention to an unresponsiveness of certain parts of the peripheral vascular bed to norepinephrine as a possible explanation of the circulatory failure during stress. That such factors might be involved received some support by the observation (FRITZ and LEVINE[442]) that the blood vessels of the mesoappendix of adrenalectomized rats became unresponsive to the vasoconstrictor action of norepinephrine after a few topical applications of this drug, and that the responsiveness could be restored by local application or intramuscular injection of adrenal cortical extract (but not by desoxycorticosterone). For further work indicating influence of corticoids on vascular tone cf. ZWEIFACH et al.[443], BARCLAY and EBERT[444] and WYMAN et al.[445].

However important these observations may be, it would probably not be correct to attribute the latent circulatory failure of adrenocortical insufficiency to peripheral factors exclusively, since, as already pointed out by THOMAS ADDISON, there is also much evidence of a "remarkable feebleness of the heart's action". It is reasonable to relate the above discussion to the well-established facts that in the treatment of a cardiovascular crisis in an Addisonian patient electrolyte therapy and administration of desoxycorticosterone has only limited effect whereas treatment with adrenal cortex extract and "glucocorticoids" may have a dramatic

[438] SWINGLE, W. W., and J. W. REMINGTON: The role of the adrenal cortex in physiological processes. Physiol. Rev. **24**, 89—127 (1944).

[439] INGLE, D. J.: The work preformance of adrenalectomized rats maintained on a high sodium chloride, low potassium diet. Amer. J. Physiol. **129**, 278—282 (1940).

[440] GOLDSTEIN, M. S., E. R. RAMEY, and R. LEVINE: Relation of muscular fatigue in the adrenalectomized dog to inadequate circulatory adjustment. Amer. J. Physiol. **163**, 561—565 (1950).

[441] RAMEY, E. R., M. S. GOLDSTEIN, and R. LEVINE: Action of nor-epinephrine and adrenal cortical steroids on blood pressure and work performance of adrenalectomized dogs. Amer. J. Physiol. **165**, 450—455 (1951).

[442] FRITZ, I., and R. LEVINE: Action of adrenal cortical steroids and nor-epinephrine on vascular responses of stress in adrenalectomized rats. Amer. J. Physiol. **165**, 456—665 (1951).

[443] ZWEIFACH, B. W., E. SHORR, and M. M. BLACK: The influence of adrenal cortex on behavior of terminal vascular bed. Ann. N. Y. Acad. Sci. **56**, 626—633 (1953).

[444] BARCLAY, W. R., and R. H. EBERT: The effect of cortisone on the vascular reactions to serum sickness and tuberculosis. Ann. N. Y. Acad. Sci. **56**, 634—636 (1953).

[445] WYMAN, L. C., G. P. FULTON, and M. H. SHULMAN: Direct observations on the circulation in the hamster cheek pouch in adrenal insufficiency and experimental hypercorticalism. Ann. N. Y. Acad. Sci. **56**, 643—658 (1953).

effect. In this connection, it also deserves to be emphasized that SWINGLE et al.[446] have demonstrated that adrenalectomized dogs on a diet moderately low in sodium can remain active and vigorous when they are treated with a typical glucocorticoid (prednisolone, 5 mg per day) in spite of the fact that they develop a marked hyponatraemia.

Before leaving the subject of circulatory failure in adrenocortical insufficiency it seems appropriate to point out that it can by no means be excluded that the impairment of the circulatory system, and the beneficial effect of such substances as cortisone is related to shifts of electrolytes between the cells of the cardiovascular system and the extracellular fluid. It may be pertinent in this connection to remind of the fact that patients with Addison's disease often present an electrocardiogram showing the signs otherwise considered typical of potassium deficiency and that these changes may often be rapidly reverted by treatment with cortisone alone (SOMERVILLE et al. [447]). Another interesting point is that in normotensive or experimentally hypertensive rats, in which a lowering in the blood pressure has been induced by potassium depletion, cortisone treatment has been found to cause a rapid return of the pressure to the initial level (FREED et al.[448]; ROSENMAN et al.[449]).

Whatever the mechanism of the impairment of the circulatory system in adrenocortical insufficiency may be — and it is apparently quite complex — it must be expected that with increasing circulatory failure the same compensatory mechanisms will be activated as in other cases of circulatory dysfunction (cf. p. 369), with the obvious exception of an increased production of sodium-retaining steroids. These compensatory adjustments include a constriction of the renal vessels leading to a reduced glomerular capillary pressure (and a reduced renal blood flow). Since such changes counteract the sodium-losing defect produced in the kidney by the lack of corticoids the possibility exists that a new steady state with sodium balance may again be achieved if the sodium intake is not too small.

The extensive studies on the actions of adrenocortical steroids which have been carried out in the last few years have disclosed a number of other effects which can certainly not be accounted for as secondary events to renal losses of sodium or other defects in renal function, e.g. the effects on the lympoid tissue, the leucocytes, the mesenchymal tissue, etc. Although electrolyte shifts may be associated with such actions, there is no clear evidence that they are, and present knowledge of the mechanisms involved are in general very meager. (For a comprehensive review, see THORN et al.[450].)

Natural corticosteroids. *Chemical nature.* The history of the isolation and characterization of the steroids from the adrenal cortex is too extensive to be covered here in more than a very sketchy way. Several reviews are available[451-458].

[446] SWINGLE, W. W., J. P. DA VANZO, D. GLENISTER, H. C. CROSSFIELD, and G. WAGLE: Role of gluco- and mineralocorticoids in salt and water metabolism of adrenalectomized dogs. Amer. J. Physiol. **196**, 283—286 (1959).

[447] SOMERVILLE, W., H. C. LEVINE, and G. W. THORN: The electrocardiogram in Addison's disease. Medicine **30**, 43 (1951).

[448] FREED, S. C., R. H. ROSENMAN, S. ST. GEORGE and M. K. SMITH: Effect of cortisone and ACTH on blood pressure of hypotensive potassium-deficient rats. Circulat. Res. **2**, 41—44 (1954).

[449] ROSENMAN, R. H., S. C. FREED, and M. K. SMITH: Effect of cortisone on blood pressure of hypertensive rats deprived of dietary potassium. Amer. J. Physiol. **177**, 325—329 (1954).

[450] THORN, G. W., D. JENKINS, J. C. LAIDLAW, F. C. GOETZ, J. F. DINGMAN, W. L. ARONS, D. H. P. STREETEN, and B. H. McCRACKEN. Pharmacological aspects of adrenocortical steroids and ACTH in man. New Engl. J. Med. **248**, 232, 284, 323, 369, 414, 588 and 632 (1953).

[451] REICHSTEIN, T., and C. W. SHOPPEE: The hormones of the cortex. Vitamines and hormones. Vol. I p. 345. Ed. by HARRIS, R. S., and K. V. THIMANN. N. Y. 1943.

Following the demonstration that adrenal cortical extracts are capable of maintaining adrenalectomized animals alive on normal salt intakes (cf. SWINGLE[455] and HARTMAN[456]) an enormous piece of work has been done by chemists in this field, and has culminated in the isolation and chemical characterization of some 46 steroids. This prolific activity of the chemists presented the biologists with the difficult task of accounting for the biological importance of all these substances, and especially to answer the question which of them are normal secretory products of the gland.

As assayed by one or more of the methods currently in use most of these compounds have been found to be biologically inactive and it seems most likely that they are intermediates or degradation and "side-track" products in the biosynthesis of the actual hormones. There are also a small number of substances which are biologically active, but are unable to maintain adrenalectomized animals alive (with the possible exception of progesterone in large doses in certain species); these substances include progesterone, various androgenic compounds and oestrone. Among these progesterone is now considered to be a precursor of the cortical hormones proper (cf. HECHTER and PINCUS, 1954[457], HÜBENER[459], WETTSTEIN[458], for reviews on the biosynthesis of the cortical steroids). A secretion of various androgens is assumed to be a normal function of the cortex, since this would account for the fall in the urinary excretion of 17-ketosteroids following the removal of the adrenals, and for the persistence of some excretion of these steroids in castrated subjects. Whether oestrone is a normal secretory product is not clear.

In addition to these compounds, seven others have now been isolated which possess the ability to maintain the life of adrenalectomized animals. Their chemical formulae and trivial names are given in Fig. 12, which contains, in addition, the formula of the assumed mother compound, progesterone. Chemically these substances have the following features in common: 1) the attachment of a carbonyl oxygen atom at the C-3, 2) the presence of a double bond between the C-4 and C-5 of the A ring, and 3) the attachment of an α-ketol group at the C-17.

As one after another of these compounds were isolated (and synthesized) it was soon realized that there were marked differences between their biological activities, which could not be characterized simply as quantitative differences in potency. This was evidenced by the fact that the ratio between the scores in different bioassays on adrenalectomized animals (life maintenance test, liver glycogen test, work performance test, and others) varied considerably from one compound to another. Desoxycorticosterone which had been found in only small quantities in beef adrenal glands, but had early been made available in large quantities by synthesis, proved to be highly active in the life maintenance test relative to its

[452] SHOPPEE, C. W.: Symposium on the adrenal cortex. J. clin. Endocr. 5. Proc. XXXVII, 1947.
[453] HARTMAN, F. A., and K. A. BROWNELL: The adrenal gland. Philadelphia. Lea & Febiger 1949.
[454] WETTSTEIN, A., and G. ANNER: Advances in the field of adrenal cortical hormones. Experientia (Basel) 10, 397 (1954).
[455] SWINGLE, W. W.: The cortical hormone of the adrenal gland. Harvey Lect. 27, 33—56 (1931—32).
[456] HARTMAN, F. A., K. A. BROWNELL, and W. E. HARTMAN: A further study of the hormone of the adrenal cortex. Amer. J. Physiol. 95, 670—686 (1930).
[457] HECHTER, O., and G. PINCUS: Genesis of the adrenocortical secretion. Physiol. Rev. 34, 459 (1954).
[458] WETTSTEIN, A.: Biochemie der Corticoide. Mitteilung auf IV. Internat. Kongress für Biochemie, Wien 1958.
[459] HÜBENER, H. J.: Über den Stoffwechsel der Nebennierenrindenhormone. Experientia (Basel) 13, 210—216 (1957).

activity in the other tests. In the case of cortisone and cortisol the ratios between these activities were the reverse, and corticosterone held an intermediate position (cf. SWINGLE et al.[460] and DORFMAN[461]).*

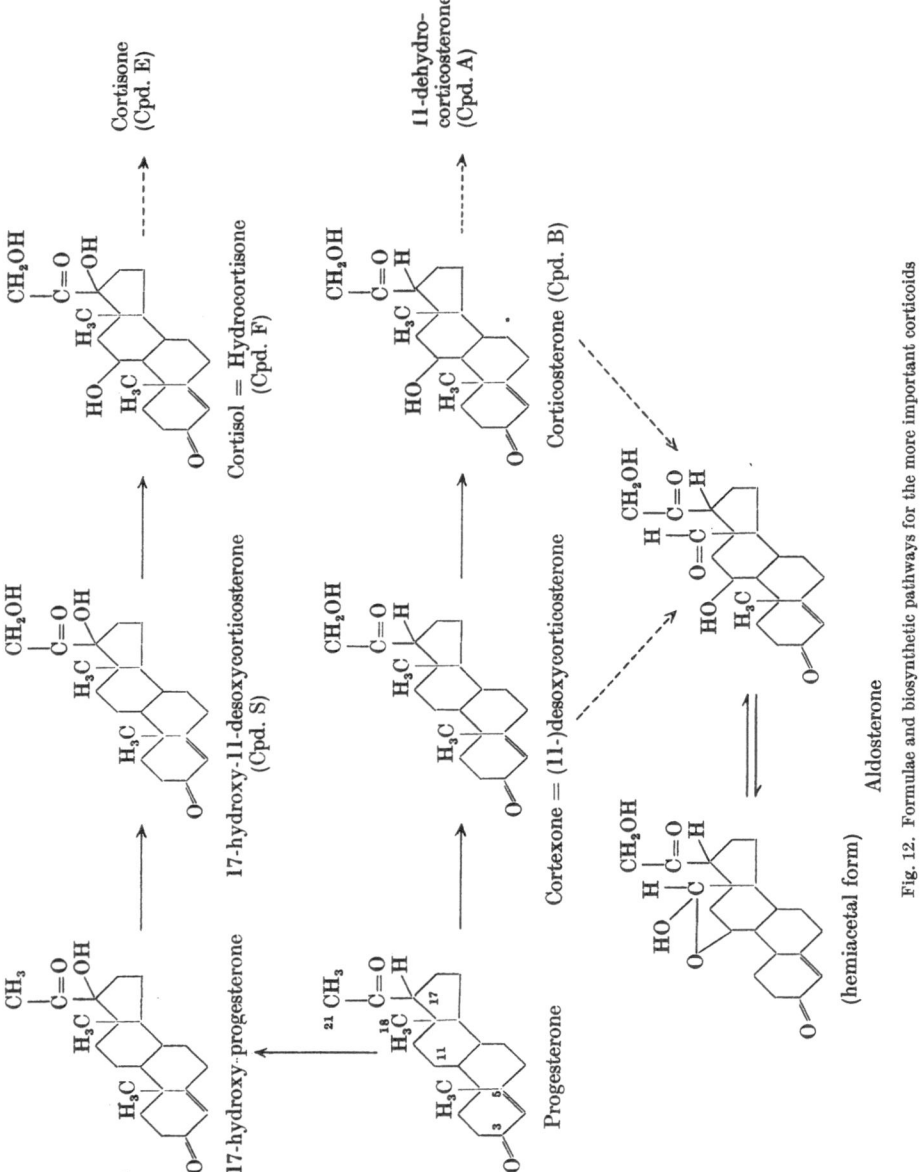

Fig. 12. Formulae and biosynthetic pathways for the more important corticoids

---

* The outcome of life maintainance tests is obviously greatly influenced by the salt intake; consequently the latter should be controlled and stated, but this precaution has sometimes been neglected.

[460] SWINGLE, W. W., E. COLLINS, G. BARLOW, and E. J. FEDOR: Bioassay and physiological effects of cortisone on adrenalectomized dogs. Amer. J. Physiol. **169**, 270—277 (1952).

[461] DORFMAN, R. I.: Bioassay of steroid hormones. Physiol. Rev. **34**, 138 (1954).

Shortly after the synthesis of desoxycorticosterone it became apparent that the life maintaining effect of this compound could be largely accounted for by its ability to correct the abnormalities in the renal handling of electrolytes, in particular the loss of sodium, induced by adrenocortical insufficiency. Desoxycorticosterone was therefore characterized as a *"mineralocorticoid"*, and other cortical steroids (with cortisol as a prototype), showing predominant effects on the organic metabolism(and work performance, mesenchymal tissues, etc.) as *"glucocorticoids"*.

Desoxycorticosterone was synthesized before it was isolated from the adrenal glands, and the demonstration of its remarkable sodium-retaining effect naturally prompted the belief that the actual salt-retaining factor of the adrenal cortex had been found. The correctness of this belief was, however, soon questioned partly because rather little of this substance was detected by REICHSTEIN and VON EUW[462] in the course of systematic fractionations of the steroids in adrenal cortex, and especially because various investigators found that the "amorphous fraction" remaining after crystallisation of various steroids had a stronger activity in life maintenance tests than desoxycorticosterone (for references cf. SWINGLE et al.[463]). Up to the present time it has been questioned whether desoxycorticosterone can at all be considered a normal secretory product of the adrenal cortex. HECHTER et al.[464] quoted some unpublished data of ZAFFARONI and AXELRAD, according to which beef blood should contain as much as 120 μg per 2 l (as compared to 360 and 400 μg of cortisol and corticosterone, respectively). The odd finding that the desoxycorticosterone concentration was found to fall to 35 μg/2 l upon a single passage through a beef adrenal gland, however, makes one wonder whether the compound so designated was actually (in its entirety) desoxycorticosterone. More recently FARRELL et al.[465] have reported smaller but certainly not insignificant concentrations (18.6 μg/l) in adrenal venous blood from acutely hypophysectomized dogs of a corticoid which they felt was "in all probability" desoxycorticosterone; a similar substance was not present in arterial blood in detectable concentrations. These authors therefore felt that desoxycorticosterone was a normal secretory product of some significance.

While the question of the importance of desoxycorticosterone as a secretory product must await the results of further studies, it is now generally agreed that the adrenal secretes a much more potent sodium-retaining steroid (aldosterone), and that much greater importance must generally be attributed to this secretion. This is clearly seen from Fig. 13 modified from FARRELL et al.[466]. Several early attempts at the purification of such a factor had failed. The success of recent studies must be ascribed to the introduction of chromatographic methods of separation and to the fact that bioassay methods were used in which the effects on renal excretion of sodium and potassium were directly tested. In 1952 SIMPSON

[462] REICHSTEIN, T., und J. VON EUW: Über Bestandteile der Nebennierenrinde. 20. Isolierung der Substanzen Q (Desoxy-corticosteron) und R sowie weiterer Stoffe. Helv. chim. Acta **21**, 1197—1210 (1938).

[463] SWINGLE, W. W., M. BEN, R. MAXWELL, C. BAKER, E. FEDOR, and G. BARLOW: Effect of the sodium-retaining factor of the adrenal cortex upon the serum electrolytes of adrenalectomized dogs. Endocrinology **54**, 698—705 (1954).

[464] HECHTER, O., A. ZAFFARONI, R. P. JACOBSEN, H. LEVY, R. W. JEANLOZ, V. SCHENKER, and G. PINCUS: The nature and biogenesis of the adrenal secretory product. Recent Progr. Hormone Res. **6**, 215 (1951).

[465] FARRELL, G. L., E. W. RAUSCHKOLB, P. C. ROYCE, and H. HIRSCHMANN: Isolation of desoxycorticosterone from adrenal venous blood of the dog. Effect of hypophysectomy and ACTH. Proc. Soc. exp. Biol. (N. Y.) **87**, 587—590 (1954).

[466] FARRELL, G. L., E. W. RAUCHKOLB, and P. C. ROYCE: Secretion of aldosterone by the adrenal of the dog. Effects of hypophysectomy and ACTH. Amer. J. Physiol. **182**, 269—272 (1955).

and TAIT[467] had devised a new method for testing corticosteroids according to this principle. In adrenalectomized rats given Na[24] and K[42] the ratio Na[24]/K[42] in the urine was found to be linearly related to the logarithm of the dose of desoxy-corticosterone for a range of 4—13 μg of this substance. With this method as a screening test a principle was chromatographically isolated from beef and hog adrenal extracts, which showed an activity some 60—80 times greater than that of desoxycorticosterone (TAIT et al.[468]; GRUNDY et al.[469, 470]). Shortly after, the occurrence of a substance of similar properties in adrenal venous blood from monkeys and dogs was announced (SIMPSON et al.[471]; FARRELL and RICHARDS[472]), constituting good evidence that the substance was a normal secretory product of the adrenal gland. There followed then in rapid succession: the isolation in pure chemical form (almost simultaneously by an Anglo-Swiss and an American group of workers, SIMPSON et al.[473]; MATTOX et al.[474]), the identification of the chemical structure (SIMPSON et al.[475]) and the synthesis by WETTSTEIN

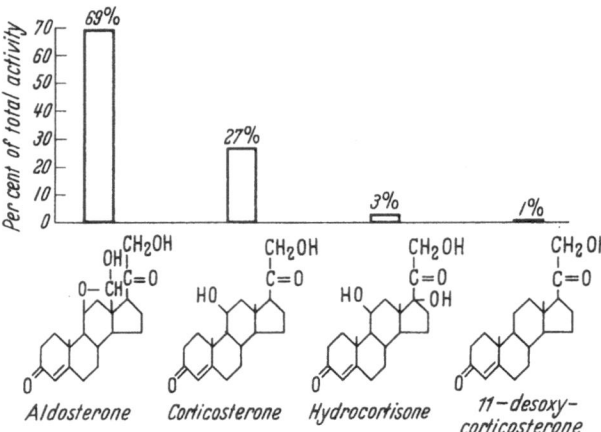

Fig. 13. Sodium retaining activity of steroids in adrenal venous blood of dogs

et al. (see [458]). When it became known that the substance contained an aldehyde group at the C-18 the name aldosterone was proposed to replace the name electrocortin, which had been in use for a short time.

Nature of corticosteroids secreted and normal rates of secretion. Recent research has provided valuable information concerning which corticoids are secreted by the adrenal glands, and what the normal rates of secretion are.

Two methods are available for such studies: a) Sampling and analysing the venous blood leaving the adrenal glands. 2) The in-vivo isotope dilution method

[467] SIMPSON, S. A., and J. F. TAIT: A quantitative method for bioassay of effect of adrenal cortical steroids on mineral metabolism. Endocrinology 50, 150—161 (1952).

[468] TAIT, J. F., S. A. SIMPSON, and H. M. GRUNDY: The effect of adrenal extract on mineral metabolism. Lancet 1, 122—129 (1952).

[469] GRUNDY, H. M., S. A. SIMPSON, and J. F. TAIT: Isolation of a highly active mineralocorticoid from beef adrenal extract. Nature (Lond.) 169, 795—796 (1952).

[470] GRUNDY, H. M., S. A. SIMPSON, J. F. TAIT, and M. WOODFORD: Further studies on the properties of highly active mineralocorticoid. Acta endocr. (Kbh.) 11, 119—220 (1952).

[471] SIMPSON, S. A., J. F. TAIT, and I. E. BUSH: Secretion of a salt-retaining hormone by the mammalian adrenal cortex. Lancet 2, 226—227 (1952).

[472] FARRELL, G. L., and J. B. RICHARDS: Isolation of a potent sodium-retaining substance from adrenal venous blood of the dog. Proc. Soc. exp. Biol. (N. Y.) 83, 628—631 (1953).

[473] SIMPSON, S. A., J. F. TAIT, A. WETTSTEIN, R. NEHER, J. VON EUW und T. REICHSTEIN: Isolierung eines neuen kristallisierten Hormons aus Nebennieren mit besonders hoher Wirksamkeit auf den Mineralstoffwechsel. Experientia (Basel) 9, 333—335 (1953).

[474] MATTOX, V. R., H. L. MASON, and A. ALBERT: Isolation of a sodium-retaining substance from beef adrenal extract. Proc. Staff Meet. Mayo Clin. 28, 596—576 (1953).

[475] SIMPSON, S. A., J. F. TAIT, A. WETTSTEIN, R. NEHER, J. VON EUW, O. SCHINDLER u. T. REICHSTEIN. Konstitution des Aldosterons, des neuen Mineralcorticoid. Experientia (Basel) 10, 132—133 (1954).

by which a labelled steroid of a known specific activity is infused at a known rate and the specific activity of the circulating or excreted steroid determined after an equilibration period.

As usually performed the first method is subject to the criticism that preceding operative procedures, etc. may have activated the secretion of corticotropin and possibly other mechanisms influencing the secretion of corticoids. As regards rates of secretion such studies may therefore, at least in certain cases, only provide information on maximal or near-maximal outputs. The isotope dilution method should be free of such objections, but systematic errors may be introduced by "recirculation" of activity, i.e. incorporation of radioactivity in the steroid produced by the adrenal cortex, or if the injected, labelled steroid is not handled in the body exactly in the same way as the endogenous.

The subject has recently been comprehensively reviewed by HECHTER and PINCUS[457]), REICHSTEIN[476] and BUSH[477] so that only a brief outline will be given here.

As far as the glucocorticoids are concerned it is generally agreed that cortisol and corticosterone make up by far the greater part of the steroids secreted by the adrenal cortex. The relative proportions of these two corticoids are reported to differ considerably in various species. Man and monkeys are reported to have very high cortisol/corticosterone ratios, dogs and cats somewhat lower ratios, cows ratios about one, and rabbits and rats ratios markedly below one. Data from dogs indicate considerable individual variations in the ratios. Remarkable rises in the ratio have been observed in rabbits during prolonged treatment with adrenocorticotropin (KASS et al.[478]).

In dogs the adrenal venous effluent method has given figures for total corticosteroid outputs in the order of 2 μg/min/kg body weight. These outputs are undoubtedly greatly elevated by an increased production of corticotropin; BUSH[479] and FARRELL et al.[465] have estimated that the corticosteroid output in hypophysectomized dogs is only one-fifth to one-tenth that of normal dogs (cf. also SWEAT and FARRELL[480]. The aldosterone concentrations (about 40 μg/l) observed by FARRELL et al.[481] in adrenal venous blood of dogs are in the order of $1/_{20}$ of those reported for total corticosteroids in adrenal venous blood of newly hypophysectomized dogs, and this figure may serve as a preliminary indication of the order of magnitude of the aldosterone production relative to that of the total corticoid output.

Isotope dilution methods have been used in human subjects to determine the 24 hr secretions of cortisol and corticosterone (PETERSON and WYNGAARDEN[482];

[476] REICHSTEIN, T.: Die wichtigsten Hormone der Nebennierenrinde. Acta endocr. (Kbh.) 17, 375—384 (1954).
[477] BUSH, I. E.: Recent work on the secretion of the adrenal cortex. Schweiz. med. Wschr. 85, 645—647 (1955).
[478] KASS, E. H., O. HECHTER, I. A. MACCHI, and T. W. MOU: Changes in patterns of secretion of corticosteroids in rabbits after prolonged treatment with ACTH. Proc. Soc. exp. Biol. (N. Y.) 85, 583—587 (1954).
[479] BUSH, I. E.: Species differences and other factors influencing adrenocortical secretion. Ciba Foundation Colloquia on Endocrinology 7, 21, London: Churchill 1953.
[480] SWEAT, M. L., and G. L. FARRELL: Decline of corticoid secretion following hypophysectomy. Proc. Soc. exp. Biol. (N. Y.) 87, 615—618 (1954).
[481] FARRELL, G. L., P. C. ROYCE, E. W. RAUSCHKOLB, and H. HIRSCHMANN: Isolation and identification of aldosterone from adrenal venous blood. Proc. Soc. exp. Biol. (N. Y.) 87, 141—143 (1954).
[482] PETERSON, R. E., and J. B. WYNGAARDEN: The miscible pool and turnover rate of hydrocortisone in man. J. clin. Invest. 35, 552—561 (1956).

PETERSON[483]; COPE and BLACK[484]) and aldosterone (AYRES et al.[485]). See also WETTSTEIN[458] for further references. Some of these recent results are shown in Table 27 together with recent determinations of the concentrations in peripheral blood. From the same studies the turnover times (time for complete renewal) of the circulating endogenous corticoids have been calculated. In the case of cortisol a period of some 25 min has been found, whereas the turnover of aldosterone appears to take place some three times faster.

Only small fractions of the corticoids secreted are excreted in the urine. In the case of aldosterone DAVIS et al.[486] estimated that only 1% or less was excreted in the urine in *unmodified* form. The smallness of this figure means that factors such as changes in the metabolic elimination of aldosterone (in the liver) and in its handling by the kidneys must be expected greatly to influence the magnitude of the fraction excreted. Great caution

Table 27. *Concentrations in peripheral blood (plasma) and rates of productions of various steroids in normal human subjects (compiled data; cf. ref. in the text)*

	Peripheral blood conc. µg/100 ml	Rate of production mg/24 h
Cortisol	(2.5)—8—14—(21)	14; 21
Corticosterone . .	0.4—1.6 (—8)	0.8 —2
Aldosterone . . .	0.03—0.16 (—0.47)	0.2

must therefore be exerted in using the rate of urinary excretion of aldosterone (and other corticoids) as a criterion for the rate of production.

The corticoids dealt with above are in all probability the most important ones secreted by the adrenal cortex, but there are several other active products being secreted. The possible secretion of desoxycorticosterone has been referred to above, and it should be mentioned that several other steroids, such as cortisone and 11-dehydrocorticosterone, have been isolated from adrenal venous blood. The continued appearance of reports on isolation of new biologically active steroids (and other substances) from adrenal cortex (cf. WETTSTEIN[458]) should serve to remind of the possibility that important aspects of the secretory activity of the adrenal glands may still await unveiling.

Control of the rates of secretion. Several findings provide evidence that the secretion of the "mineralocorticoids" and "glucocorticoids" are mutually remarkably independent, and that corticotropin has rather little effect on the former, whereas it is the major determining factor in the secretion of the latter.

It is well-known that hypophysectomy does not lead to such profound disturbances in the salt metabolism as does adrenalectomy, and this fact has been further emphasized by a number of recent studies. LANE and DE BODO[487] have shown that hypophysectomized dogs displayed an unimpaired ability to conserve sodium and that the renal mechanisms for excretion of intravenously administered potassium salts were essentially normal. Hypophysectomized rats have been shown to tolerate higher doses of potassium chloride than adrenalectomized,

[483] PETERSON, R. E.: The identification of corticosterone in human plasma and its assay by isotope dilution. J. biol. Chem. **225**, 25—37 (1957).

[484] COPE, C. L., and E. BLACK: The production of cortisol in man. Brit. med. J. **1958** I, 1020—1024.

[485] AYRES, P. J., J. BARLOW, O. GARROD, A. E. KELLIN, S. A. S. TAIT, J. F. TAIT, and G. WALKER: In MULLER and O'CONNOR (ED.): Int. Symp. Aldosterone. London: Churchill 1958.

[486] DAVIS, J. O., M. M. PECHET, W. C. BALL jr. and M. J. GOODKIND: Increased aldosterone secretion in dogs with right-sided congestive heart failure and in dogs with thoracic inf vena cava constriction. J. clin. Invest. **36**, 689—694 (1957).

[487] LANE, N., and R. C. DE BODO: Generalized adrenocortical atrophy in hypophysectomized dogs and correlated functional studies. Amer. J. Physiol. **168**, 1—19 (1952).

although not quite as high as normal animals (Collins[488]). In man extensive balance studies have demonstrated that the recently hypophysectomized patient is able to conserve sodium efficiently (Maclean et al.[489]).

Our present interpretation of these findings is that corticotropin is not necessary for the production of aldosterone by the adrenal cortex. This view has been strongly supported by a number of studies designed to test its validity. Thus it was found by Farrell et al.[481] that the aldosterone concentration in adrenal venous blood of dogs was little affected by hypophysectomy or corticotropin administration. By contrast, the cortisol concentration was greatly reduced some 6 hr after hypophysectomy, and it was greatly elevated after corticotropin administration. It is further noteworthy that Luetscher and Axelrad[490] and more recently Thorn et al.[494] found normal levels of urinary aldosterone output in patients with hypopituitarism (in contrast with greatly reduced urinary excretions of 17-hydroxycorticoids). In further agreement with these findings it has been observed by the latter investigators as well as by others (Liddle et al.[491]; Farrell et al.[492]) that whereas the suppression of corticotropin secretion leads to a marked drop in the secretion (or urinary excretion) of 17-hydroxycorticoids, the secretion (excretion) of aldosterone was not depressed. Furthermore such suppression treatment did not prevent an increase in aldosterone excretion in response to sodium deprivation.

Altogether the above findings permit the conclusion that endogenous corticotropin is not of any appreciable significance for the maintenance of a normal baseline production of aldosterone, nor is it necessary for increases in the production in response to certain physiological stimuli. [The observation of some authors (Hernando et al.[493]; Thorn et al.[494]) that some patients with panhypopituitarism may not respond to sodium deprivation with as large an increase in aldosterone excretion as do normal subjects is not incompatible with this conclusion. It is possible that these patients also had lesions in adjoining regions of the diencephalon which may regulate aldosterone secretion in response to such stimuli — see below.]

That (exogenous) corticotropin may not be entirely without effect on the secretion of aldosterone appears from Liddle et al.[491] and Venning et al.[495] demonstration of moderate, transient increases in the secretion following corticotropin administration and from the findings of Axerrad et al.[496] and Venning

[488] Collins, E. J.: Steroid-induced adrenal-pituitary hypofunction. Proc. Soc. exp. Biol. (N. Y.) 89, 443—445 (1955).

[489] Maclean, J. P., M. B. Lipsett, M. C. Li, C. D. West and O. H. Pearson: Regulation of salt metabolism after hypophysectomy in man. J. Clin. Endocr. 17, 346—355 (1957).

[490] Luetscher, J. A. jr., and B. J. Axelrad: Sodium-retaining corticoid in urine of normal children and adults and of patients with hypoadrenalism or hypopituitarism. J. clin. Endocr. 14, 1086—1089 (1954).

[491] Liddle, G. W., L. E. Duncan, and F. C. Bartter: Dual mechanism regulating adrenocortical function in man. Amer. J. Med. 21, 380—386 (1956).

[492] Farrell, G. L., R. C. Banks, and S. Koletshy: The effect of corticosteroid injection on aldosterone secretion. Endocrinology 58, 104—108 (1956).

[493] Hernando, L., J. Crabbé, E. J. Ross, W. J. Reddy, A. E. Renold, D. H. Nelson, and G. W. Thorn: Clinical experience with a physicochemical method for estimation of aldosterone in urine. Metabolism 6, 518—543 (1957).

[494] Dingman, J. F., K. Benirschke, and G. W. Thorn: Studies of neurohypophyseal function in man. Amer. J. Med. 23, 226—238 (1957).

[495] Venning, E. H., J. Dysenfurth, and J. C. Beek: Effect of corticotropin and prednisone on the excretion of aldosterone in man. J. clin. Endocr. 76, 1541—1553 (1956).

[496] Axelrad, B. J., B. B. Johnson, and J. A. Luetscher: Factors regulating the output of sodium-retaining corticoid of human urine. J. clin. Endocr. 14, 783 (1954).

et al.[497] of some increase in urinary aldosterone excretion under similar conditions. These responses were, however, quite small in comparison with the major increases in 17-hydroxycorticoid secretion (excretion) simultaneously observed.

If corticotropin (and the hypophysis in general) is not of (major) importance to the regulation of aldosterone secretion, the question presents itself: what non-pituitary factors are involved in the regulation ? At present no clear answer can be given, but various studies have suggested the direction in which it may be found.

Several recent studies on urinary corticoid excretions in human subjects or animals have shown that sodium deprivation leads to increased excretion of sodium-retaining steroids (aldosterone) without any evidence of increased production of other types of adrenal steroids (AXELRAD et al.[496]; LUETSCHER and AXELRAD[498]; STREETEN et al.[499]). Collateral evidence of an increased production of "salt-active" corticoids has been furnished by CONN and coworkers (cf. CONN and LOUIS[500]) who demonstrated a decrease in sodium and chloride concentrations in thermal sweat under such conditions.

Exactly how sodium-depletion becomes a stimulus for the secretion of aldosterone is not known. That a reduction in plasma sodium concentration should be involved appears to be excluded for the following reasons: 1) In simple sodium deprivation the changes in plasma sodium conc. are generally small and inconsistent. 2) Aldosterone excretion has been found actually to decrease when the plasma sodium conc. is lowered by water intake + pitressin administration. 3) Aldosterone excretion has been found to increase during simple dehydration in spite of the fact that the plasma sodium conc. increases to levels above normal (cf. BARTTER et al.[501]; DINGMAN et al.[494]).

Not only do these findings suggest that a lowering in plasma sodium concentration is not involved as a stimulus; they also make it unlikely that sodium depletion exerts its stimulating effect directly on the adrenal gland, since it is difficult to see how it could affect the adrenals directly except by way of a change in plasma sodium concentration.

From the above studies (cf. especially that of BARTTER et al.) it appears that the stimulus originates in the reduction of some part of the extracellular volume, or rather some part of the cardiovascular volume. It is in agreement with this view that FARRELL et al.[502], WOLFF et al.[503] and FINE et al.[504] have found that hypo-

[497] VENNING, E. H., A. CARBALLEIRA, and I. DYRENFURTH: Excretion of sodium-retaining substances. J. clin. Endocr. 14, 784 (1954).

[498] LUETSCHER, J. A. jr., and B. J. AXELRAD: Increased aldosterone output during sodium deprivation in normal men. Proc. Soc. exp. Biol. (N. Y.) 87, 650—653 (1954).

[499] STREETEN, D. H. P., J. W. CONN, L. H. LOUIS, S. S. FAJANS, H. S. SEITZER, R. D. JOHNSON, R. D. GITTHS, and A. H. DUBE: Secondary aldosteronism: I. The metabolic and adrenocortical responses of normal men to high environmental temperature. J. Lab. clin. Med. 46, 957—958 (1955).

[500] CONN, J. W., and L. H. LOUIS: Production of endogenous salt-active corticoids as reflected in the concentrations of sodium and chloride of thermal sweat. J. clin. Endocr. 10, 12—23 (1950).

[501] BARTTER, F. C., G. W. LIDDLE, L. E. DUNCAN jr., J. K. BARBER, and C. DELEA: The regulation of aldosterone secretion in man. The role of fluid volume. J. clin. Invest. 35, 1306—1315 (1956).

[502] FARRELL, G. L., R. S. ROSNAGLE, and E. W. RAUSCHKOLB: Increased aldosterone secretion in response to blood loss. Circulat. Res. 4, 606—611 (1956).

[503] WOLFF, H. P., KH. R. KOCZOREK u. E. BUCHBORN: Pathophysiologische und klinische Untersuchungen über sekundären Hyperaldosteronismus. Schweiz med. Wschr. 87, 163—167 (1957).

[504] FINE, D., L. E. MEISELAS, and T. AUERBACH: The effect of acute hypovolemia on the release of "aldosterone" and on renal excretion of sodium. J. clin. Invest. 37, 232—243 (1958).

volaemia produced by bleeding causes an increase in urinary excretion of aldosterone. It is at the moment not known in what part of the cardiovascular system
the volume receptors controlling aldosterone production may be located, nor is it
known whether they are the same which may cause sodium-saving by renal
vasoconstriction in various types of latent circulatory failure (cf. p. 369).

Granting the existence of cardiovascular volume receptors controlling aldosterone production, a next question becomes by which pathways their regulating
effect is mediated. Also to this question definite answers are missing. RAUSCHKOLB
and FARRELL[505] have suggested the existence of diencephalic centers controlling
aldosterone secretion on the grounds that the output of aldosterone was markedly
reduced in dogs following decapitation or midcollicular decerebration (with removal
of the brain rostral to the section), whereas it was not affected by decortication
or section of the neural connections between the head and the trunk. LOTSPEICH in
his review in Ann. Rev. Physiol., 1958 has questioned the validity of the authors'
conclusion, mainly by reference to the fact that the secretion of cortisol was also
diminished in exactly those case where a reduction in aldosterone secretion was
observed. However, this objection is not crucial, and the hypothesis of an independent central nervous control of the secretion of aldosterone has recently gained
further support by the findings of NEWMAN et al. [506], that disproportional changes
in the rates of secretions of cortisol and aldosterone could be produced by circumscribed lesions in the caudal diencephalon, the midbrain or in the rostral half of the
pons. With the last-named lesion, which did not affect the secretion of cortisol,
an *increase* in aldosterone production was actually observed. Furthermore,
the recent finding by FARRELL et al. (cited from WETTSTEIN[458]) that diencephalic
extracts are capable of producing an increase in the output of aldosterone in the
renal venous blood of decerebrate dogs suggests that FARRELL's view may be correct. ORTI et al.[507] have demonstrated the presence (in rat urine) of a thermolabile,
non-dialyzable substance stimulating aldosterone secretion. Whether this is
related to the diencephalic factor in not known*.

It is possible that some aspect of potassium metabolism can influence the
secretion of aldosterone, but the nature of the signal has not yet been established.
Several authors have reported that potassium administration may lead to some
increase in urinary aldosterone excretion (FALBRIARD et al.[508]; DINGMAN et al.[494]),
whereas others (JOHNSON et al.[509]) have reported that low potassium intake
decreases aldosterone excretion. It was found by LARAGH and STOERK[510] that
potassium intake did not lead to any marked rise in aldosterone excretion unless it
resulted in a significant rise in plasma potassium concentration (in their case

---

* Quite recent studies by G. FARRELL and associates [Federation Proc. 18, 44 and 113,
(1959)] on the effects of small diencephalic-mesencephalic lesions strongly suggest that a center
governing aldosterone secretion may be located in the pineal gland or its immediate vicinity.

[505] RAUSCHKOLB, E. W., and G. L. FARRELL: Evidence for diencephalic regulation of
aldosterone secretion. Endocrinology 59, 528—531 (1956).
[506] NEWMAN, A. E., E. S. REDGATE, and G. L. FARRELL: The effects of diencephalic-
mesencephalic lesions on aldosterone and hydrocortisone secretion. Endocrinology 63, 723—742
(1958).
[507] ORTI, E., E. P. RALLI, B. LAKEN, and M. E. DUMM: Presence of an aldosterone
stimulating substance in the urine of rats deprived of salt. Amer. J. Physiol. 191, 323—328
(1957).
[508] FALBRIARD, A., A. F. MULLER, R. NEHER and R. S. MACH: Etude des variations de
l'aldosteronurie sous l'effet de surcharges en potassium et de déperdations rénales et extra-
rénales de sel et d'eau. Schweiz. med. Wschr. 85, 1218—1220 (1955).
[509] JOHNSON, B. B., A. H. LIEBERMAN, and P. J. MULROW: Aldosterone excretion in
normal subjects depleted of sodium and potassium. J. clin. Invest. 36, 757—766 (1957).
[510] LARAGH, J. H., and H. C. STOERK: A study of the mechanism of secretion of the
sodium-retaining hormone (aldosterone). J. clin. Invest. 36, 383—392 (1957).

obtained by preliminary sodium restriction). These authors suggested therefore that the stimulating effect of potassium was mediated by the plasma potassium concentration, and as evidence for a direct effect on adrenal cortex they referred to the finding of ROSENFELD et al.[511] that perfusion of calf adrenals with solutions of a high K/Na ratio caused an increase in aldosterone output. This finding is, however, in contrast to the observation of ROSNAGLE and FARRELL[512] that potassium administration to dogs did not lead to any increase in the aldosterone output in the adrenal vein, and these authors have suggested that potassium administration may produce an increase in urinary aldosterone excretion by affecting the renal handling of the hormone rather than by influencing its production.

The importance of potassium in the regulation of aldosterone secretion remains therefore to be firmly established. There is, however, no reason why such a stimulus could not exist in addition to the "volume stimulus".

At one time it was suggested by Venning's group that growth hormone might increase the rate of secretion of aldosterone; this was not confirmed in studies by LUFT et al.[513].

Recently PITCOCK and HARTROFT[514a] have suggested that a trophic hormone stimulating the zona glomerulosa of the adrenal cortex to an increased production of aldosterone might be produced in the juxtaglomerular apparatus of the preglomerular arterioles. This idea was based upon the observation that, in animals on different salt intakes and in patients dying from various disorders the degree of granulation of these elements was found to be inversely related to the plasma sodium concentration. This suggestion is, of course, purely speculative, and other interpretations might seem equally justified. Nevertheless, these observations should serve to attract serious attention to the possibility that the juxtaglomerular apparatus *plus* the macula densa might somehow, directly or indirectly, be involved in reducing renal losses of salt and water. The complexity of the problem is illustrated by recent studies by TOBIAN et al.[514b] which suggest that changes in intrarenal arterial pressure may (also ?) affect the granulation of the juxtaglomerular cells.

For discussions of the regulation of aldosterone secretion the reader in referred to recent reviews by BARTTER[515], FARRELL[516b], GROSS[516c] LUETSCHER[516a] and the Internat. Symposium edited by MULLER and O'CONNOR[517].

Sites of production. There are a number of experimental observations which indicate that steroids with predominant effects on the electrolyte excretions are

[511] ROSENFELD, G., E. ROSEMBERG, F. UNGAR, and R. I. DORFMAN: Regulation of the secretion of aldosterone-like material. Endocrinology 58, 255—261 (1956).

[512] ROSNAGLE, R. S., and G. L. FARRELL: Alterations in electrolyte intake and adrenal secretion. Amer. J. Physiol. 187, 7—10 (1956).

[513] LUFT, R., D. IKKOS, and C. A. GEMZELL: Metabolic studies with human growth hormone. Abstr. IV, Acta endocr. Congress. Leiden 1958.

[514a] PITCOCK, J. A., and P. M. HARTROFT: The juxtaglomerular cells in man and their relationship to the level of plasma sodium and to the zona glomerulosa of the adrenal cortex. Amer. J. Pathol. 34, 863—883 (1958).

[514b] TOBIAN, L., J. THOMPSON, R. TWEDT, and J. JANECEK: The granulation of juxtaglomerular cells in renal hypertension, desoxycorticosterone and post-desoxycorticosterone hypertension, adrenal regeneration hypertension, and adrenal insufficiency. J. clin. Invest. 37, 660—671 (1958).

[515] BARTTER, F. C.: The role of aldosterone in normal homeostasis and in certain disease states. Metabolism 5, 369—383 (1956).

[516a] LUETSCHER, J. A.: Aldosterone. In Advanc. intern. Med. 8, 155—203 (1956).

[516b] FARRELL, G.: Regulation of aldosterone secretion. Physiol. Rev. 38, 709—728 (1958).

[516c] GROSS, F.: Die Steuerung der Aldosteronsekretion. Schweiz. med. Wschr. 89, 1—7 (1959).

[517] MULLER, A. F., and C. M. O'CONNOR (ed.): Aldosterone, an international symposium. Boston: Little, Brown and Co 1958.

mainly produced in the outermost layer or *zona glomerulosa* of the cortex, whereas the production of steroids which predominantly influence "the organic metabolism" takes place chiefly in the inner layers. These observations also indicate a considerable independence in the secretion of these two types of hormones. Whether there is also a difference between the steroids produced in each of the inner layers is not known.

It is well-known that hypophysectomy causes marked atrophy of the two inner layers, whereas the zona glomerulosa is affected later and much less (cf. e.g. LANE and DE BODO[487]); similarly administration of adrenocorticotropin is known to produce hypertrophy of the inner layers, but only moderate changes in the zona glomerulosa (cf. YOFFEY[518]). Further evidence of this has come from studies on animals treated with 1,1-dichloro-2,2-bis (p-chlorophenyl)-ethane (DDD). Prolonged treatment with this substance has been shown to cause atrophy and disappearance of the inner zones of the cortex, while the zona glomerulosa is left unaffected (NELSON and WOODARD[519]). Dogs (and rats) subjected to such treatment showed obvious signs of a reduced (or abolished) production of "glucocorticoids": increased insulin sensitivity, lack of development of hyperglycaemia when they were made alloxan diabetic (cf. NICHOLS and SHEEHAN[520]), as well as lack of signs of increased production of "glucocorticoids" in response to corticotropin (NICHOLS and GREEN[521]). They remained, however, in electrolyte balance, and administration of 10 g of potassium chloride, or twice as much as will cause a fatal crisis in adrenalectomized dogs, caused no recognizable effects. DEANE et al.[522] observed a broadening and a decrease of the cellular lipid content of the zona glomerulosa in rats subjected to a dietary deficiency of sodium. A similar picture, which was assumed to represent increased secretory activity, was obtained in animals given potassium chloride parenterally. Signs of a diminished activity (diminution of the zona with decrease in cell size, increase in the size on intracellular lipid droplets) were observed, on the other hand, in animals subjected to dietary potassium deficiency. The authors drew the conclusion that the ratio between the sodium and potassium intakes was an important factor controlling the secretory activity of the zona glomerulosa. DEANE et al. findings have been confirmed by PESCHEL and RACE[523], who also reported the occurrence of an increased zone width in human subjects (hypertensive patients) on a low sodium diet, and further confirmation was announced by HARTROFT and EISENSTEIN[524]. DEANE et al. made the additional observation that prolonged administration of desoxycorticosterone in large doses (2 mg daily) caused similar changes as

[518] YOFFEY, J. M.: The suprarenal cortex: The structural background in the suprarenal cortex. Proceed. 5th Symposium of the Golstan Research Society. Ed.: J. M. Yoffey. Butterworths Sci. Publ. London 1953.

[519] NELSON, A. A., and G. WOODARD: Severe adrenal cortical atrophy (cytotoxic) and hepatic damage produced in dogs by feeding 2.2.-bis (parachlorophenyl)-1.1-dichloroethane (DDD or TDE). Arch. Path. (Chicago) 48, 387—394 (1949).

[520] NICHOLS, J., and H. L. SHEEHAN: Effect of partial adrenal cortical atrophy on the course of alloxan diabetes. Endocrinology 51, 362—377 (1952).

[521] NICHOLS, J., and H. D. GREEN: Effect of DDD. Treatment on metabolic response of dogs to ACTH injection. Amer. J. Physiol. 176, 374—376 (1954).

[522] DEANE, H. W., J. H. SHAW, and R. O. GREEP: Effect of altered sodium and potassium intake on width and cytochemistry of zona glomerulosa of rat's adrenal cortex. Endocrinology 43, 133—153 (1948).

[523] PESCHEL, E., and G. J. RACE: Studies on the adrenal zona glomerulosa of hypertensive patients and rats. With special reference to the effect of dietary salt restriction. Amer. J. Med. 17, 355—364 (1954).

[524] HARTROFT, P. M., and A. B. EISENSTEIN: Alterations in the adrenal cortex of the rat induced by sodium deficiency: Correlation of histological changes with steroid hormone secretion. Endocrinology 60, 641—651 (1957).

dietary potassium deficiency i.e. signs of inactivity. ODENTHAL[525] was, however, unable to confirm the occurrence of a *selective* atrophy of the zona glomerulosa during desoxycorticosterone treatment; it is not clear to what extent this discrepancy may be explained by the fact that this author used considerably larger doses of desoxycorticosterone (10—15 mg daily), which may have caused a depression of the production of corticotropin, not encountered with smaller doses. If desoxycorticosterone in appropriate doses actually causes a selective depression of the activity of the zona glomerulosa it remains to be shown whether this is due to a direct action of this substance, to a sodium retention induced by its administration, or to an inhibition of a center controlling the activity of the zona glomerulosa.

The above hypothesis on the site of formation of aldosterone has recently received confirmation from in-vitro metabolic studies with separated "zones" of adrenal cortex from various animals. The capsule with the zona glomerulosa attached forms preferably aldosterone whereas the zona fasciculata forms 17-hydroxycorticoids (cortisol), and corticosterone is produced in both (cf. WETTSTEIN[458] for references).

In man only indirect evidence on the site of synthesis is available, and it is conflicting. There is some support of the zona fasciculata being the site of production in man. Thus the patients with primary hyperaldosteronism described by CHALMERS et al.[526] as well as by SKANSE et al.[527] showed an atrophy of the zona fasciculata of the uninvolved adrenal. This could be interpreted as a response to the sodium retention and potassium excretion caused by the aldosterone over-production in the diseased gland. In agreement with this concept VAN BUCHEM et al.[528] in their patient found an increase in the zona fasciculata of the gland which by hyperplasia caused the syndrome.

In contrast to the above findings PESCHEL and RACE[523] in hypertensive patients on a low sodium intake found a hypertrophy of the zona glomerulosa.

Evidently the question of the site of production of aldosterone in man remains to be solved.

Effects of corticoids on renal sodium and potassium excretions (and renal function in general). The conventional designations "mineralocorticoids" and "glucocorticoids" have been used in the above discussion to characterize corticoids which exert a predominant action on renal electrolyte excretions and organic metabolism, respectively. It should be emphasized that no strict distinction can be made in this respect between known steroids. It has been abundantly demonstrated that typical "glucocorticoids" such as cortisol and cortisone, are capable of inducing some renal retention of sodium under suitable experimental conditions. Conversely, several experiments have demonstrated that aldosterone, besides its remarkable sodium-retaining potency, also has considerable "glucocorticoid" activity, although the demonstration of such activity requires considerably higher doses than those necessary to produce marked sodium retention. Thus SCHULER

[525] ODENTHAL, I.: Zur Frage einer selektiven Atrophie der Zona glomerulosa der Nebennierenrinde nach Desoxycorticosteronzufuhr. Endokrinologie **29**, 305—311 (1952).

[526] CHALMERS, T. M., M. G. FITZGERALD, A. H. JAMES and H. SCARBOROUGH: Conn's syndrome with severe hypertension. Lancet **1956 I** 127—132.

[527] SKANSE, B., F. MÖLLER, K. GYDELL, S. JOHANSSON and H. B. WULFF: Observations on primary aldosteronism. Acta med. scand. **158**, 181—192 (1957).

[528] BUCHEM, F. S. P. VAN, H. DOORENBOS, and H. S. ELINGS: Conn's syndrome caused by adrenocortical hyperplasia. Pathogenesis of the signs and symptoms. Acta endocr. (Kbh.) **23**, 313—330 (1956).

et al.[529] have reported aldosterone to be one-third as active as cortisone in glycogen deposition tests, and a similar ratio between the activities of these corticoids was observed by eosinophil depletion tests by GAUNT et al.[530] and by SPEIRS et al.[531]. Indications of "glucocorticoid" activity were also reported by MACH et al.[532], who observed a reduction in glucose tolerance (and improved working capacity) in two Addisonian patents during treatment with aldosterone (150—300 μg/24 hr). Even desoxycorticosterone, which has long been considered the "mineralocorticoid" *par excellence* is not entirely devoid of "glucocorticoid" activity, as shown by VERZÁR and coworkers[533, 534].

Even if the various corticoids may not show any absolute differences in their actions, their relative potencies in various respects ("activity spectra") still differ sufficiently to justify a continued use of the terms "mineralocorticoids" and "glucocorticoids", if only it is kept in mind that even the prototypes of these classes show overlapping in activities (see table 28).

Difficulties encountered in evaluating the effects of corticoids on renal function. Corticoids in general are often described as causing a reduction in the renal excretion of sodium. Although this statement may be correct under some experimental conditions it nevertheless represents a great oversimplification.

There is considerable evidence that the corticoids influence the renal excretion of sodium in antagonistic ways. Exactly how these effects are established is not yet clear. It seems, however, most likely that the corticoids, and in particular the mineralocorticoids, stimulate distal tubular reabsorption of sodium and thus cause sodium retention. There is also evidence that corticoids, and apparently in particular the "glucocorticoids", stimulate proximal reabsorption of sodium and water, (i.e. increase the filtration rate) either by direct action on the tubular cells or indirectly through an augmentation of the renal blood flow. Whatever the mechanism for this latter effect may be it appears that, at least under suitable conditions, it may cause proximal tubular fluid to be delivered at a higher pressure to the distal tubular segments (or in the conventional mode of expression: increase the fluid load to the distal tubules). Whether this effect shall be ascribed to an increase in glomerular capillary pressure or to a decrease in the hydrodynamic resistance in the proximal parts of the nephron, or both, is not clear, but, whatever the mechanism may be, it might account for a tendency to cause an increased loss of sodium and to raise the ability to excrete water and sodium in response to water or sodium loading.

The existence of two different "sites of action" of corticoids in the kidney, one ("the proximal") to which the glucocorticoids are most readily attached and where they are particularly suited to "do the work", and another (distal) to which mineralocorticoids are readily bound and operating more efficiently, would seem to provide a satisfactory explanation to the fact that, under suitable conditions, these

[529] SCHULER, W., P. DESAULLES u. R. MEIER: Elektrocortin-Wirkung im Glykogentest. Experientia (Basel) **10**, 142 (1954).

[530] GAUNT, R., A. S. GORDON, A. A. RENZI, J. PADAWER, G. J. FRUHMAN, and M. GILMAN: Biological studies with electrocortin (aldosterone). Endocrinology **55**, 236—241 (1954).

[531] SPEIRS, R. S., S. A. SIMPSON, and J. F. TAIT: Certain biological activities of crystalline electrocortin. Endocrinology **55**, 233—235 (1954).

[532] MACH, R. S., J. FABRE, A. DUCKERT, R. BORTH, et P. DUCOMMUN: Action clinique et metabolique de l'aldostérone (electrocortine). Schweiz. med. Wschr. **84**, 407—418 (1954).

[533] SASS-KORTSÁK, A., F. C. WANG, and F. VERZÁR: Influence of desoxycorticosterone acetate on liver and muscle glycogen of adrenalectomized animals. Amer. J. Physiol. **159**, 256—262 (1949).

[534] WANG, F. C., and F. VERZÁR: Comparison between glycogenetic property of desoxycorticosterone, 11-dehydro-17-hydroxy-corticosterone (compound E) and adrenal cortical extract. Amer. J. Physiol. **159**, 263—268 (1949).

two groups of corticoids may have opposite effects on the renal excretion of sodium. It appears that several cases of so-called antagonism, which have been reported between cortisone (or corticotropin) and desoxycorticosterone (THORN et al.[543], WOODBURY et al.[535], DAVIS et al.[536]) or between cortisone and aldosterone (DESAULLES et al.[537], CONN[538], SKANSE et al.[527]) may be adequately explained by assuming that augmentation of the distal tubular load is the *principal* effect of glucocorticoids, whereas stimulation of distal tubular reabsorption of sodium is the *principal* effect of mineralocorticoids.

Table 28. *Mineralocorticoid* and glucocorticoid activity of natural and synthetic corticosteroids* (figures refer to activity in percentage of those of desoxycorticosterone and cortisol, respectively)

	Mineralocorticoid activity	Glucocorticoid activity
Cortisol	2— 4	100
Corticosterone	5—15	25— 50
Cortisone	2— 4	80— 90
Desoxycorticosterone	100	0
Aldosterone	1,000—4,000	25— 50
Δ^1-cortisol	0.1—1	300—500
9-α-fluorocortisol	2,000—4,000	200
9-α-fluoro-Δ^1-cortisol . . .	2,000—4,000	400—500
2-methyl-9-α-fluorocortisol . .	5,000	200

* Effect on renal, sodium retaining mechanisms.

"Antagonistic effects" might, however, also be accounted for on the basis of competition for sites of action. In the case of the two-site hypothesis competition would complicate matters if the two sites were not completely selective in their affinity for the "appropriate" corticoids. It might then be excepted that, for instance, an endogenous steroid might be displaced from its proper site by a less efficient administered corticoid, which, of course, should result in an "effect" of the administered corticoid exactly opposite to that of the displaced endogenous hormone. In some of the papers just referred to competition has been suggested as the basis for the antagonisms observed, but convincing evidence was not provided. There are however some indication that progesterone (cf. p. 339) and some newly synthesized steroids (cf. p. 418) may compete with aldosterone for its site of action. KLEIN et al.[539] have found that a non-identified, chloroform-extractable substance (believed to be a steroid from the adrenal cortex) from urines of premature infants and patients with congenital adrenal hyperplasia exerts a natriuretic effect when injected into rats. Whether competition is involved in this effect is not known.

The evaluation of the direct effects of the various corticoids is further complicated by a number of secondary events to which their administration may give rise. Thus the possibility exists that they may be converted to other active substances with a different activity spectrum. It is well established (although not

[535] WOODBURY, D. M., C. P. CHENG, G. SAYERS, and L. S. GOODMAN: Antagonism of adrenocorticotrophic hormone and adrenal cortical extract to desoxycorticosterone; electrolytes and electroshock treshold. Amer. J. Physiol. 160, 217—227 (1950).

[536] DAVIS, A. K., A. C. BASS, and R. R. OVERMAN: Comparative effects of cortisone and DCA on ionic balance and fluid volumes of normal and adrenalectomized dogs. Amer. J. Physiol. 166, 493—503 (1951).

[537] DESAULLES, P., W. SCHULER, and R. MEIER: Vergleich der Wirkung des Aldosterons auf das Fremdkörpergranulom der Ratte mit derjenigen von Cortexon, Cortison und Hydrocortison. Experientia (Basel) 11, 68—70 (1955).

[538] CONN, J. W.: Primary aldosteronism. A new clinical syndrome. J. Lab. clin. Med. 45, 6—17 (1955).

[539] KLEIN, R., P. TAYLOR, C. PAPADATOS, Z. LARON, D. KEELE, J. FORTUNATO, C. BYERS, and C. BILLINGS: Sodium losing material in human urine. Proc. Soc. exp. Biol. (N. Y.) 98, 863—866 (1958).

yet fully explored) that some transformations of this type may take place in the adrenal cortex; thus corticosterone is formed from desoxycorticosterone in the perfused bovine adrenal gland (cf. HECHTER and PINCUS[457]) and aldosterone may be formed from various other corticoids (cf. WETTSTEIN[458]). It is also possible that such transformations may occur in extra-adrenal tissues as suggested by KAHNT and WETTSTEIN's[540] and HÜBENER and AMELUNG's[541] observations with liver tissue and from observations on steroid excretions in adrenalectomized subjects treated with other steroids.

Another factor which must be taken into consideration is an inhibition of the normal secretion of the adrenal cortex by the administered compounds. One way in which this is known to occur is by a depression of the secretion of adrenocortico-tropin. The complications from this feed-back mechanism may not be so important, because the glucocorticoids are by far the most effective depressants of cortico-tropin production, and because this hormone in turn mainly controls the secretion of glucocorticoids. The administration of *very large* doses of desoxycorticosterone may, however, result in a perceptible glucocorticoid deficiency, probably by corti-cotropin depression.

A further complicating factor is the unquestionable ability of corticoids to cause "internal shifts" of electrolytes, and among these also sodium. Thus one of the effects of corticoids appears to be a mobilization of "fixed" sodium (and cal-cium) from the bones (cf. p. 213). An expansion of the extracellular fluid by such mobilized sodium would (as discussed elsewhere, p. 371) tend to increase the renal excretion of sodium, and this might in part explain the *negative* sodium balances which have been observed in some subjects during prolonged treatment with large doses of desoxycorticosterone (LUFT et al.[542]); it seems, however, quite likely that other factors are also involved.

In view of these complicating factors it is not too surprising that the effects of corticoids on renal electrolyte excretions vary not only from one corticoid to another, but also for a particular corticoid according to the experimental conditions. Thus animal species, the state of the adrenal cortex, the state of water and salt loading, the dosage and duration of the administration and a possible simultaneous treatment with other corticoids may greatly influence the response.

Effects of glucocorticoids and mineralocorticoids on renal excretion of Na *and* K. If one wants to generalize it appears that the most one can say is, that the mineralocorticoids (desoxycorticosterone, aldosterone) nearly always reduce sodium excretion and augment potassium excretion at least in shorter periods of treatment, whereas the effects of the *glucocorticoids* on sodium and potassium excretions are quite variable.

The latter part of this statement is abundantly documented in the literature, and only a few references will be made. Cortisol and cortisone was first reported by THORN et al.[543] to cause an increased excretion of sodium and chloride in short

[540] KAHNT, F. W., u. A. WETTSTEIN: Die 11-oxydation von Desoxy-corticosteron und Reichstein's Substanz *S* mit Hilfe tierischer Organhomogenate. Bildung von Corticosteron und 17-oxy-corticosteron. Helv. chim. Acta **34**, 1790—1805 (1951).

[541] HÜBENER, H. J., u. D. AMELUNG: Enzymatische Umwandlungen von Steroiden. I. Vergleich der Steroidumwandlung in Leber und Nebenniere. Z. physiol. Chem. **293**, 126—137 (1953).

[542] LUFT, R., B. SJÖGREN, D. IKKOS, H. LJUNGGREN, and H. TARUKOSKI: Clinical studies on electrolyte and fluid metabolism. Effect of ACTH, desoxycorticosterone acetate and cortisone; electrolyte and fluid changes in acromegali. Recent Progr. Hormone Res. **10**, 425 (1954).

[543] THORN, G. W., L. L. ENGEL, and R. A. LEWIS: The effects of 17-hydroxy-corticosterone and related adrenal corticoid steroids on sodium and chloride excretion. Science **94**, 348—349 (1941).

term experiments in normal or adrenalectomized animals. Prolonged administration of larger doses of cortisone was later reported (cf. INGLE et al.[544]) to cause some sodium retention and increased potassium excretion. The effect of a single dose of cortisol (intramuscularly as the free alcohol) on sodium excretion in adrenalectomized rats has recently been reported to vary with the dosage level. 1—10 μg per rat produced some retention of sodium, intermediate doses (50 to 500 μg) caused an increased excretion, and very large doses (1—25 mg) resulted again in retention (STREETEN et al.[545]). The authors feel that these findings may explain many earlier contradictory results. According to a recent preliminary report there may even be a reversal of the response with time following a single dose (0.5—1 mg) of cortisone or cortisol in adrenalectomized rats, viz. an initial retention followed by a considerable rise in sodium excretion (KAGAWA and ARMAN[546]). INGLE et al.[544] have reported that even corticosterone, which is generally considered to hold a position between the mineralocorticoids and the glucocorticoids, may cause a transient increase in sodium excretion when it is given in high doses (5 mg per day) to normal rats force-fed a high carbohydrate diet. It so happened, however, that this dosage also caused glycosuria, and the question may be raised whether the natriuresis was due to an osmotic diuresis.

Variations in the response to cortisone and cortisol have also been recorded in human subjects, and here too it appears that the response is greatly dependent on the dosage and the state of the subjects. An initial retention of sodium, later passing into a negative sodium balance during prolonged treatment with cortisone has been reported by SPRAGUE et al.[547]; LUFT et al.[542] and several others. In acute experiments, in which cortisol was administered intravenously to Addisonian patients at rates of 1 or 10 mg/hr LAIDLAW et al.[548] observed an increased excretion of sodium, which was especially marked at the 1 mg/hr level. ROBERTS and RANDALL[549], on the other hand, reported that intravenous administration of 1 mg of cortisone acutely (i.e. within an hour or so) reduced renal excretions of sodium and chloride in adrenalectomized dogs. Cf. also LIPSETT et al.[550].

As might be expected the effects of corticotropin are very similar to those of cortisone-cortisol. LUFT et al.[542] observed retention of sodium during the first week of treatment, but in the third week a net loss occurred. Both corticotropin and glucocorticoids generally cause a net loss of potassium which may continue even during prolonged treatment. It appears, however, that this loss can essentially be accounted for by a simultaneous negativity of the nitrogen balance, i.e. by a loss of protoplasma (cf. LUFT et al.). The potassium losses may therefore be

[544] INGLE, D. J., R. SHEPPARD, E. A. OBERLE, and M. H. KUIZENGA: A comparison of the acute effects of corticosterone and 17-hydroxycorticosterone on body weight and the urinary excretion of sodium, chloride, potassium, nitrogen and glucose in the normal rat. Endocrinology 39, 52—57 (1946).

[545] STREETEN, D. H. P., M. E. PONT, and J. W. CONN: Effects of hydrocortisone on urinary excretion of sodium in adrenalectomized rats. J. Lab. clin. Med. 46, 729—732 (1955).

[546] KAGAWA, C. M., and C. G. VAN ARMAN: Biphasic response in sodium excretion following 11,17-oxysteroid administration in adrenalectomized rat. Fed. Proc. 15, 443 (1956).

[547] SPRAGUE, R. G., M. H. POWER, H. L. MASON, A. ALBERT, D. R. MATHIESEN, P. S. HENCH, E. C. KENDALL, C. H. SLOCUMB, and H. F. POLLEY: Observations on physiologic effect of cortisone and ACTH in man. Arch. intern. Med. 85, 199—258 (1950).

[548] LAIDLAW, J. C., J. F. DINGMAN, W. L. ARONS, J. T. FINKENSTAEDT, and G. W. THORN: Comparison of the metabolic effect of cortisone and hydrocortisone in man. Ann. N. Y. Acad. Sci. 61, 315—323 (1955).

[549] ROBERTS, K. E., and H. T. RANDALL: The effect of adrenal steroids on renal mechanisms of electrolyte excretion. Ann. N. Y. Acad. Sci. 61, 306—314 (1955).

[550] LIPSETT, M. B., C. D. WEST, J. P. MACLEAN, and O. H. PEARSON: Adrenal function after hypophysectomy in man. J. clin. Endocr. 17, 356—363 (1957).

due to extrarenal effects alone, but on the other hand, it cannot be excluded that direct actions on the kidneys are also involved.

In contrast to the variable responses to the glucocorticoids, the effects of the typical *mineralocorticoids*, desoxycorticosterone and aldosterone, are much more consistent: a reduction of the renal excretion of sodium and an increase in potassium excretion, without a change in nitrogen balance which could account for the latter.

It is often mentioned that even desoxycorticosterone may exhibit antithetical effects (i.e. promote sodium excretion) under certain conditions. Some of the observations (McGavack et al.[551]; Zierler and Lilienthal[552]) which are quoted in support of this are similar to those of Luft et al. referred to on p. 319, i.e. experiments in which *prolonged* administration of desoxycorticosterone has been shown to cause a negative sodium balance after an initial period of sodium retention. The studies of Luft et al. have provided strong evidence for a mobilization of fixed sodium from bones, etc. in such cases, and it seems likely that desoxycorticosterone continues to exert a sodium-retaining effect at its site of action in the kidney, but, that this effect is overshadowed by a reverse effect, activated by the expansion of the extracellular fluid volume. A more acute paradoxical effect of desoxycorticosterone has been described by Soffer et al.[553, 554] in patients with Cushing's syndrome. These authors studied the natriuretic effect of an intravenous infusion of 200 ml of a 5% sodium chloride solution. Whereas an injection of 10 mg of desoxycorticosterone the day before the test caused a considerable reduction in the natriuresis in normal subjects, an increase in natriuresis was observed in 10 of 15 cases of Cushing's syndrome. The mechanism of this paradoxical response is obscure; transformation of the desoxycorticosterone into a natriuretic steroid is one of the possibilities to be considered. Another puzzling case of antithetical effect is that reported by Forsyth[555] who observed that smaller doses of desoxycorticosterone (below 5—10 μg) caused an increase in sodium excretion in sodium chloride-loaded, adrenalectomized mice, whereas higher doses reduced the excretion.

Aldosterone has now been shown in several species to be greatly superior to desoxycorticosterone as regards ability to induce renal retention of sodium. The ratio between the activities of these two steroids in this respect have tended, however, in more recent studies to be a little lower than that (60—80) reported by Simpson and Tait and their associates (cf. p. 308). Values around 25 were observed by Farrell and Richards[472] and by Desaulles et al.[556] on the basis of urinary excretion tests in adrenalectomized rats. A rather similar ratio was observed by

[551] McGavack, T. H., A. Saccone, M. Vogel, and R. Harris: Craniopharyngioma with panhypopituitarism: case report with clinical and pathological study. J. clin. Endocr. 6, 776—796 (1946).

[552] Zierler, K. L., and J. L. Lilienthal: Sodium loss in man induced by desoxycorticosterone acetate. Amer. J. Med. 4, 186—192 (1948).

[553] Soffer, L. J., G. Lesnick, S. Z. Sorkin, H. H. Sobotka, and M. Jacobs: The utilization of intravenously injected salt in normals and in patients with Cushing's syndrome before and after administration of desoxycorticosterone acetate. J. clin. Invest. 23, 51—54 (1944).

[554] Soffer, L. J., J. L. Gabrilove, and M. D. Jacobs: Further studies with the salt tolerance test in normal individuals and in patients with adrenal cortical hyperfunction. J. clin. Invest. 28, 1091—1093 (1949).

[555] Forsyth, B. T.: Sodium-excreting effect of desoxycorticosterone in adrenalectomized mice. Endocrinology 52, 65—72 (1953).

[556] Desaulles, P., J. Tripod, u. W. Schuler: Wirkung von Electrocortin auf die Elektrolyt- und Wasserausscheidung im Vergleich zu Desoxycortisosteron. Schweiz. med. Wschr. 83, 1088—1089 (1953).

SWINGLE et al.[557] between the minimum daily doses required to maintain normal serum sodium concentration, blood pressure and blood urea concentration in adrenalectomized dogs (about 10 μg of aldosterone as compared to 125—250 μg of desoxycorticosterone). A thorough study of the sodium retaining activities in dogs have been published by LIDDLE et al.[558]. These authors used adrenalectomized dogs maintained on a sodium rich diet and 5 mg of cortisone per day. The changes in the rates of excretions of sodium and potassium measured over a 5 hr period following hormone injections, were found to be linearly related to the log. dose of both desoxycorticosterone and aldosterone, but the ratio between the slopes of the curves indicated that aldosterone was 30 times more potent than desoxycorticosterone. According to the latter study aldosterone would then seem to be equally superior to desoxycorticosterone in producing sodium retention and potassium excretion. This contrasts with DESAULLES et al. finding that the activity of aldosterone in inducing potassium excretion is only 5 times greater than that of desoxycorticosterone, and also with SWINGLE et al. observation that, in the lower dosage range, aldosterone was less efficient in preventing hyperkalaemia than in preventing a drop in plasma sodium concentration. It is not clear to what extent this discrepancy may be due to the fact that LIDDLE et al. used animals on a sodium rich diet.

Although some qualitative differences are suggested by some of these studies, it seems reasonable for the present to assume that the direct actions of the two steroids on the kidneys are basically similar. Definite knowledge of these actions is lacking, but there is rather convincing evidence that *the principal action* of these *mineralocorticoids is to enhance distal tubular transfer* processes and in particular those responsible for an exchange of sodium ions with other cations.

A hint at such a distal site of action is already provided by the opposite effects on the excretions of sodium and potassium, which obviously could be readily accounted for by an increased exchange of sodium ions for potassium ions. According to current views the active element in this exchange is a reabsorption of sodium ions and a competition is believed to take place between potassium ions and hydrogen ions (and possibly ammonium ions) in the exchange (cf. p. 286).

It was therefore to be expected that a stimulation of the underlying sodium ion transfer should cause an increase of the secretion of not only potassium ions but also of hydrogen (and ammonium) ions. That such exchanges are accelerated by the corticoids is supported by various experimental and clinical observations. A decrease in the excretion of titratable acidity and ammonia has been observed in dogs during the development of adrenocortical insufficiency (ROBERTS and PITTS[559]), whereas SELDIN et al.[560] (see also [561]) have reported an increased excretion of titratable acids and ammonium when rats, subsisting on a potassium-deficient diet, were treated with desoxycorticosterone. During prolonged treatment with desoxycorticosterone the increased tubular secretion of hydrogen and

[557] SWINGLE, W. W., R. MAXWELL, M. BEN, C. BAKER, S. J. LeBRIE, and M. EISLER: Effect of aldosterone and desoxycorticosterone on adrenalectomized dogs. Proc. Soc. exp. Biol. (N. Y.) 86, 147—150 (1954).

[558] LIDDLE, G. W., J. CORNFIELD, A. G. T. CASPER, and F. C. BARTTER: The physiological basis for a method of assaying aldosterone in extracts of humane urine. J. clin. Invest. 34, 1410—1416 (1955).

[559] ROBERTS, K. E., and R. F. PITTS: Influence of cortisone on renal function and renal function and electrolyte excretion in adrenalectomized dogs. Endocrinology 50, 51—60 (1952).

[560] SELDIN, D. W., F. C. RECTOR jr., N. CARTER, and J. COPENHAVER: The relation of hypokaliemic alkalosis induced by adrenal steroids to renal acid secretion. J. clin. Invest. 33, 965—966 (1954).

[561] WILSON, J. D., and D. W. SELDIN: Effect of adrenalectomy on production of ammonia by the kidney. Amer. J. Physiol. 188, 524—528 (1957).

potassium ions result in a decrease in the plasma potassium concentration (KUHL-MAN et al.[562]; PERERA[563]; LUFT et al.[542], and others) and an increase in the plasma bicarbonate concentration (PERERA[563]; LUFT et al.[542], and others). To the author's knowledge similar changes induced experimentally by aldosterone administration, have not yet been reported. That such changes must occur is, however, clearly indicated by nature's own experiment, the newly discovered syndrome, *primary aldosteronism* (cf. CONN[564]), of which several cases have now been reported. Most cases of this syndrome in its pure form is caused by an adrenal cortex adenoma, which contains aldosterone in concentrations many times greater than normal cortex tissue; urinary aldosterone output is markedly increased. Characteristically, in this disorder one finds a pronounced alkalosis with elevated plasma p_H and bicarbonate concentration, a persistent hypokalaemia, and a tendency to hypernatremia. Similar, although generally less pronounced changes, have been described in several cases of CUSHING's syndrome (cf. e.g. CLUXTON et al.[565]; FORSHAM et al.[566]; TEABEAUT et al.[567]; PLOTZ et al.[568]). However, in most cases of CUSHING's syndrome such changes are not encountered and it appears that these are cases in which aldosterone is not produced in great excess whereas those accompanied by a significant hypokalaemic alkalosis are cases of mixed hyper-adrenocorticism, with excessive production of not only glucocorticoids but also of sodium-retaining corticoids.

It is important to emphasize that the development of an alkalosis (elevated plasma bicarbonate concentration) in cases of aldosteronism and during *prolonged* treatment with desoxycorticosterone should not be conceived of as exclusively a *direct* consequence of increased exchange secretion caused by hormonal stimulation of the coupled sodium reabsorption process. As mentioned elsewhere (p. 293) similar changes — alkalosis, often existing together with a high urinary p_H and urinary bicarbonate loss — are also encountered in potassium deficiencies other than those caused by mineralocorticoids. It is therefore most likely that when such changes occur in cases of prolonged impact of mineralocorticoids on the kidneys they will largely be secondary to a potassium deficiency (which also develops as a consequence of the hormonal stimulation of the sodium exchange-reabsorption process). The details of this mechanism are discussed in p. 294.

That the opposite changes (viz. hyperkalaemia and a reduction in plasma bicarbonate concentration) occur in adrenocortical insufficiency is well-known and has already been mentioned. The hyperkalaemia in this case is not however, necessarily entirely due to a reduced capacity for tubular secretion of potassium; it may also, in part at least, be explained by a more complete reabsorption of filtered potassium correlated to a greater percentage reabsorption of fluid in the

[562] KUHLMAN, D., C. RAGAN, J. W. FERREBEE, D. W. ATCHLEY, and R. F. LOEB: Toxic effects of desoxycorticosterone esters in dogs. Science 90, 496—497 (1939).

[563] PERERA, G. A.: Effect of continued desoxycorticosterone administration in hypertensive subjects. Proc. Soc. exp. Biol. (N. Y.) 68, 48—50 (1948).

[564] CONN, J. W.: Aldosterone in clinical medicine; past, present and future. Arch. intern. Med. 97, 135—144 (1956).

[565] CLUXTON, H. E., W. A. BENNETT, M. H. POWER, and E. J. KEPLER: Cushing syndrome without adenomatous or hyperplastic changes in the pituitary body or adrenal cortices and complicated by alkalosis. J. clin. Endocr. 5, 61—69 (1945).

[566] FORSHAM, P. H., E. FLINK, K. EMERSON jr., and G. W. THORN: Metabolic studies on Cushing's syndrome. J. clin. Invest. 28, 781 (1949).

[567] TEABEAUT, R., F. L. ENGEL, and H. TAYLOR: Hypokalemic, hypochloremic alkalosis in Cushing's syndrome. Observations on effects of treatment with potassium chloride and testosterone. J. clin. Invest. 10, 399—409 (1950).

[568] PLOTZ, C. M., A. I. KNOWLTON, and C. RAGAN: Natural history of Cushing's syndrome. Amer. J. Med. 13, 597—614 (1952).

proximal tubules which probably exists in this state. A marked hyperkalaemia could, however, not persist if there were not also an impairment of the tubular secretion of potassium. Another finding which is explainable by a diminished tubular cation exchange is the fact that adrenocortical insufficiency is associated with a diminished ability to respond to an acid load by an increased excretion of titratable acidity and ammonia (JIMINEZ-DIAZ[569]; SARTORIUS et al.[570, 571]). The cause of the lowered excretion of ammonia was further explored by WHITE and ROLF[572]. Since no changes in renal glutaminase activity were detected in adrenal-ectomized (or hypophysectomized) rats, and since the plasma glutamine levels were not affected either by adrenalectomy, it was felt that the lowered ammonia excretion was not due to a defect in the ammonia forming mechanism, but secondary to a failing ability to secrete "acid". A reduced capacity for ammonia excretion was also observed by WILSON and SELDIN[561] without evidence of defects in the glutaminase system or its ability to adaptation.

It has previously been mentioned (p. 287) that whereas administration of desoxycorticosterone causes kaliuresis and hypokalaemia in animals on a normal or high sodium intake, it fails to do so in animals on a low sodium intake. These findings have been confirmed in human subjects by LUFT et al.[542]. As may be recalled this phenomenon has been used as evidence for the occurrence of a $Na^+ - K^+$ exchange at a very distal site in the tubular system, the argument being that potassium cannot be secreted if sodium is not provided in ample amounts for exchange reabsorption. HOWELL and DAVIS[573] have made a further study of the phenomenon. They confirmed the earlier findings by showing that no kaliuresis was produced in dogs on a very low sodium intake (9 meq/day). In addition they made the interesting observation that a kaliuresis was not induced either by desoxycorticosterone in an *adrenalectomized* dog (with thoracic inferior vena cava constriction and ascites) even though the daily intake of sodium (and the rate of urinary sodium excretion before the desoxycorticosterone administration) was as high as 30 meq/day. Since the excretion of sodium as well as chloride fell to very low values in response to the desoxycorticosterone they explained the lack of kaliuresis by postulating that desoxycorticosterone had enhanced the reabsorption of sodium plus chloride and that this process was localized proximal to the sodium exchange process.

This view may well serve as an explanation for a lack of coincidence in time between the antinatriuresis and kaliuresis response to desoxycorticosterone, which has been reported by some workers and has been advanced as evidence that these phenomena should be due to separate actions of the hormone (cf. e.g. ROBERTS and RANDALL[549]). Another possible explanation is that the more easily movable hydrogen ions are the "first choice" in the exchange process, so that only when the reabsorption of sodium ions has reached a certain rate will potassium ions begin to participate in the exchange to an appreciable degree. The fact that renal retention of

[569] JIMINEZ-DIAZ, C.: Death in Addison's disease (functional renal failure). Lancet **1936** II, 1135—1139.

[570] SARTORIUS, O. W., D. CALHOON, and R. F. PITTS: The capacity of the adrenalectomized rat to secrete hydrogen and ammonium ions. Endocrinology 51, 444—450 (1952).

[571] SARTORIUS, O. W., D. CALHOON, and R. F. PITTS: Studies on the interrelationships of the adrenal cortex and renal ammonia excretion by the rat. Endocrinology **52**, 256—265 (1953).

[572] WHITE, H. L., and D. ROLF: Renal glutaminase in adrenalectomized and hypophysec-tomized rats, and plasma glutamine levels in normal and adrenalectomized rats. Amer. J. Physiol. **174**, 27—28 (1953).

[573] HOWELL, D. S., and J. O. DAVIS: Relationship of sodium retention to potassium excretion by the kidney during administration of desoxycorticosterone acetate to dogs. Amer. J. Physiol. **179**, 359—363 (1954).

potassium does not start as early as the increased excretion of sodium during a developing adrenocortial insufficiency (ROEMMELT et al.[574]) is not incompatible with an effect of the mineralocorticoids upon a $Na^+ \rightleftarrows H^+$ (or K^+) exchange process if it can be assumed that the urinary loss of potassium occurring under "normal" conditions is not caused by such an exchange to any appreciable extent, but by an incomplete reabsorption. The potassium retention would then be entirely dependent on an increase in the efficacy of the potassium reabsorption, which obviously need not coincide with a failing distal reabsorption of sodium. Rather it might be related to a reduction in renal blood flow and in glomerular propulsive pressure. The subject of potassium secretion should not be left without mentioning WIRZ'[575] observation that the potassium clearance may well exceed the (very low) inulin clearance of adrenalectomized cats. This observation indicates that corticoids are not a *sine qua non* for a potassium secretion ($Na^+ - K^+$ exchange).

The above discussion has centered on the assumed stimulating effect of the mineralocorticoids on the distal $Na^+ \rightleftarrows H^+$ (or K^+) exchange process. Although this effect generally dominates in a relative way so that bicarbonate saving is furthered proportionally more than that of chloride (and the HCO_3^-/Cl^- ratio of the blood plasma consequently raised) it is nonetheless clear that these hormones also exert a chloride-retaining effect. The mechanism of the latter is not definitely known, but it seems most reasonable to assume that it is due to a stimulation of a distal reabsorption of sodium plus chloride. The principal reason for assuming a distal site of action is that in acute experiments efficient sodium and chloride retention can be produced without any perceptible change in filtration rate. It would, however, be unrealistic not to admit that the problem is unsolvable on the basis of information gained by the "clearance technique", since the absolute changes in the rates of excretion of chloride (and sodium) caused by desoxycorticosterone amount to only a few per cent of the total rates at which it is filtered and reabsorbed. As a matter of fact a distal site of action has not been generally accepted. WOMERSLEY et al.[576] have argued for a proximal site of action, mainly on the grounds that intravenous administration of desoxycorticosterone glucoside under conditions of water diuresis reduces not only the rate of excretion of salt, but also the rate of excretion of water. JEANNERET et al.[577] have published results showing that in healthy human subjects, maintained on a salt-free diet and given 8—12 g of sodium bicarbonate, desoxycorticosterone (100 mg per day) can still induce a diminution in the urinary excretion of sodium (some 180 meq/day) as well as a smaller rise in potassium excretion (some 50 meq/day). Chloride excretion which was already very low (some 10 meq/day) was not appreciably diminished. These findings are certainly not adequate basis for the author's conclusion that desoxycorticosterone primarily affects sodium reabsorption and only secondarily chloride reabsorption. They only indicate that desoxycorticosterone can still stimulate a sodium $\rightleftarrows$ cation exchange if only sodium is available, even if the intratubular chloride concentration may be too low for a further promotion of the reabsorption of ($Na^+ + Cl^-$).

---

[574] ROEMMELT, J. C., O. W. SARTORIUS, and R. F. PITTS: Excretion and reabsorption of sodium and water in the adrenalectomized dog. Amer. J. Physiol. **159**, 124—136 (1949).

[575] WIRZ, H.: Untersuchungen über die Nierenfunktion bei adrenalektomierten Katzen. Helv. physiol. pharmacol. Acta **3**, 589—612 (1945).

[576] WOMERSLEY, R., O. A. THORUP jr., and L. G. WELT: The influence of enhanced sodium reabsorption by DOCA and compounds E and F on the rates of excretion of water, potassium, and ammonia. J. clin. Invest. **32**, 613 (1953).

[577] JEANNERET, P., A. F. ESSELIER u. H. J. HOLTMEIER: Über den Einfluß des Natriumions auf den Kalium-, Chlorid-, und Wasserhaushalt unter Mineralocorticoidwirkung. Helv. med. Acta **23**, 60—74 (1956).

At this point attention should also be called to recent studies (SIMMONS et al.[578, 579]) in which the course of the urinary sodium excretion during increasing mannitol diuresis has been followed in dogs under various conditions. *Briefly* stated these authors found that a higher degree of mannitol diuresis had to be induced in sodium-depleted dogs than in normally fed dogs in order to produce frank natriuresis. This might well be interpreted as due to a greater corticoid-activated reabsorption of sodium in the distal tubules. The fact that the authors were unable to demonstrate a similar difference between desoxycorticosterone-treated dogs and normal control dogs may well be due to the fact that a prolonged period of desoxycorticosterone was used. Thus it is likely that a new steady state with respect to sodium balance had been reached, in which the distal sodium reabsorption processes were again "saturated" already before mannitol diuresis was induced. Consequently their findings do not invalidate the view that desoxycorticosterone enhances distal sodium reabsorption. Similar experiments should be made in animals acutely treated with desoxycorticosterone.

As a last point strongly supporting the concept that aldosterone stimulates distal sodium reabsorption reference may be made to results from recent stop-flow experiments. It was shown that the sodium concentration in the effluent from distal tubular sections did not fall to nearly as low levels in adrenalectomized dogs as in normal animals, but aldosterone administration corrected this defect (VANDER et al.[580]). No data were given for chloride.

If the (Na + Cl) reabsorption process of the ascending limb of HENLE's loop, which apparently forms the basis of the urinary concentration process (cf. p. 250), were stimulated by aldosterone, then one would expect to find a reduced urinary concentrating capacity in cortical insufficiency. Apparently this question has not been studied by suitable technique (i. e. in terms of maximal negative free water clearance, cf. p. 245), but a few authors have stated that the urine from adrenalectomized animals could become "as concentrated" as that from normal controls.

The question, *how* aldosterone and other mineralocorticoids are able to stimulate distal sodium reabsorption, still remains unanswered. Several studies have indicated that there is an appreciable lag in the appearance of this effect. E. g. GANONG and MULROW[581] found a delay of some 5—30 min in the fall in sodium excretion and the rise in potassium excretion even when 5—10 μg of aldosterone was injected directly in the aorta or in a renal artery. This, and the fact that in the latter case no difference in the magnitudes of the effects on the two sides was detectable, suggest that either aldosterone is "taken up" rather slowly by the tubular cells or it has to undergo some change to become active. As regards the latter possibility one may remind of GLYNN's hypothesis, that corticoids should be converted to substances related to the cardiac glycoside aglucones before they become active (cf. Part I, p. 64). The structure of synthetic steroids blocking the renal action of aldosterone may also provide a hint in this direction (cf. p. 418).

Significance of corticoids for renal excretion of water and sodium loads. The defects in the renal handling of electrolytes and water in adrenocortical

[578] SIMMONS, D. H., R. B. HARVEY, and T. HOSHIKO: Effect of sodium intake on sodium loss due to mannitol diuresis. An empirical test for renal sodium-retaining activity. Amer. J. Physiol. **178**, 182—188 (1954).

[579] SIMMONS, D. H., R. B. HARVEY, and T. HOSHIKO: Role of adrenal and hypophysis in regulation of sodium excretion. Amer. J. Physiol. **181**, 379—389 (1955).

[580] VANDER, A. J., R. L. MALVIN, W. S. WILDE, J. LAPIDES, L. P. SULLIVAN, and V. M. McMURRAY: Effects of adrenalectomy on proximal and distal tubular sodium reabsorption. Proc. Soc. exp. Biol. (N. Y.) **99**, 323—325 (1958).

[581] GANONG, W. F., and P. J. MULROW: Rate of change of sodium and potassium excretion after injection of aldosterone into the aorta and renal artery of the dog. Amer. J. Physiol. **195**, 337—346 (1958).

insufficiency are not limited to impairments in the ability to retain sodium and chloride and in the ability to secrete potassium and hydrogen (ammonium)ions. It is well established that there is also a *reduced ability to excrete an additional load of sodium chloride* and a *reduced diuretic response to water* ingestion. The question of the possible cause of these defects and related phenomena has been the subject of considerable debate, and very different views have been expressed.

It is well-established that the ability to excrete a large load of sodium chloride is markedly reduced in adrenocortical insufficiency. Already suggested by early studies in adrenalectomized rodents, this phenomenon has more recently been thoroughly studied in adrenalectomized dogs by ROEMMELT et al.[574], and in patients with Addison's disease by BURNETT[582] and BURNETT et al.[583]. Sodium chloride administrered orally as well as by intravenous infusion of hypertonic solutions was found to be excreted much more slowly than by the normal controls. ROEMMELT et al. also showed, and emphasized, that at each particular elevated level of plasma sodium concentration, not only were the absolute rates of excretion of sodium and chloride smaller after adrenalectomy than before, but the same applied to the fractions of filtered sodium and chloride that were excreted. (This has often erroneously been cited as evidence that the absolute rates of reabsorption were greater after adrenalectomy than in the normal state. At comparable plasma sodium concentrations the glomerular filtration rate was, however, somewhat lower after than before adrenalectomy). In relation to these findings it is interesting to note that daily sodium chloride intake has to be within a narrow range to support optimal growth in adrenalectomized rats. Not only intakes below 350 mg, but also such above 1200 mg were found incapable of supporting growth and survival (ANDERSON[584]).

Since it was first demonstrated in adrenalectomized cats by SILVETTE and BRITTON[585], the existence of a *reduced diuretic response* to water administration in cases of adrenocortical insufficiency has been abundantly confirmed in many mammalian species including man (for a comprehensive list of references, see GAUNT et al.[586]). As is well-known this defect has been made use of as a differential-diagnostic test — the Robinson-Power-Kepler water test[587]; a normal water excretion in this test generally rules out Addison's disease (cf. also SIMPSON[588]; GARROD and BURSTON[589]).

It has been recognized for many years that the glomerular filtration rate is subnormal in untreated or inadequately treated cases of adrenocortical insufficiency, experimental as well as clinical. Some indication of this was already to be

[582] BURNETT, C. H.: Actions of ACTH and cortisone on renal function in man. In transaction of the 2nd conf. on renal function. Josiah Macy jr. Foundation. New York. 1951.

[583] BURNETT, C. H., D. W. SELDIN, and M. WALSER: Observations on the electrolyte and water metabolism in Addison's disease during oral salt loading. Transact. Ass. Amer. Physicians 66, 65—71 (1953).

[584] ANDERSON, E.: The physiology of the salt-treated adrenalectomized animal. Essays in Biology in Honor of HERBERT M. EVANS. Berkely: Univ. Calif. Press 1943.

[585] SILVETTE, H., and S. W. BRITTON: Effects of adrenalectomy and cortico-adrenal extract on renal excretion and tissue fluids. Amer. J. Physiol. 104, 399—411 (1933).

[586] GAUNT, R., J. H. BIRNIE, and W. J. EVERSOLE: Adrenal cortex and water metabolism. Physiol. Rev. 29, 281—310 (1949).

[587] ROBINSON, F. J., M. H. POWER, and E. F. KEPLER: Two new procedures to assist in recognition and exclusion of Addison's disease: a preliminary report. Proc. Staff Meet. Mayo Clin. 16, 577—583 (1941).

[588] SIMPSON, S. L.: Addison's disease and diabetes mellitus in three patients. J. clin. Endocr. 9, 403—425 (1949).

[589] GARROD, O., and R. A. BURSTON: The diuretic response to ingested water in Addison's disease and panhypopituitarism and the effect of cortisone thereon. Clin. Sci. 11, 113—128 (1952).

found in early observations of considerably increased blood urea concentrations in clinical (GAILLARD[590]) and experimental (MARSHALL and DAVIS[591]) cases, and in BEVIER and SHEVSHY's[592] observation of subnormal urea clearances in adrenal-ectomized rabbits. A fall in creatinine clearance to about one-third was observed by HARRISON and DARROW[593] in dogs passing into cortical insufficiency. Similar observations were made by WIRZ[575] in cats, and more recent studies by GAUDINO and LEVITT[594] have demonstrated a fall not only in inulin clearance but also in paraaminohippurate clearance in adrenalectomized dogs. Similar indications of reductions of glomerular filtration rate and renal plasma flow — sometimes to values below 50% of normal — have been observed in cases of Addison's disease by several groups of authors (TALBOTT et al.[595]; McGAVACK et al.[596]; SANDER-SON[597]; WATERHOUSE and KEUTMANN[598]; SLESSOR[599]; BURSTON and GAR-ROD[600]).

The apparent paradox that the capacity for excretion of salt and water loads is reduced in cortical insufficiency at the same time as there is a definite tendency to lose salt and water by way of the kidney has aroused much speculation. So far entirely satisfactory explanations of these and related problems have, however, not been provided, a fact which is not too surprising, in view of our incomplete picture of the function of the nephron and our limited possibilities to study its details.

The question may first be raised whether the reduced ability to excrete large water and salt loads is a consequence of a loss of sodium due to lack of secretion of sodium-retaining hormones. A failing water diuresis is known to accompany sodium depletion as evidenced by studies of McCANCE and WIDDOWSON[601] in human subjects, WILKINSON and McCANCE[602] in rabbits and HOLMES[603] in dogs. (cf. also CIZEK and HUANG[604], for a comparison between the effects of acute and chronic

[590] GAILLARD, L. M.: Insuffisance surrénale et azotémie. Bull. et mém. Soc. méd. Hôp. Paris **37**, 272—276 (1914).

[591] MARSHALL, E. K., and D. M. DAVIS: The influence of the adrenal on the kidneys. J. Pharmacol. exp. Ther. 8, 525—550 (1916).

[592] BEVIER, G., and A. E. SHEVSHY: Urea excretion after suprarenalectomy. Amer. J. Physiol. **50**, 191—203 (1919).

[593] HARRISON, H. E., and D. C. DARROW: Renal function in experimental adrenal in-sufficiency. Amer. J. Physiol. **125**, 631—643 (1939).

[594] GAUDINO, M., and M. F. LEVITT: Influence of the adrenal cortex on body water distribution and renal function. J. clin. Invest. **28**, 1487—1497 (1949).

[595] TALBOTT, J. H., L. H. PECORA, R. S. MELVILLE, and W. V. CONSOLAZIO: Renal func-tion in patients with Addison's disease and in patients with adrenal insufficiency secondary to pituitary pan-hypofunction. J. clin. Invest. **21**, 107—119 (1942).

[596] McGAVACK, T. H., A. SACCONE, M. VOGEL, and R. HARRIS: Craniopharyngioma with panhypopituitarism: case report with clinical and pathological study. J. clin. Endocr. **6**, 776—796 (1946).

[597] SANDERSON, P. H.: Renal function in Addison's disease. Clin. Sci. **6**, 197—206 (1948).

[598] WATERHOUSE, C., and E. H. KEUTMANN: Kidney function in adrenal insufficiency. J. clin. Invest. **27**, 372—379 (1948).

[599] SLESSOR, A.: Studies concerning the mechanism of water retention in Addison's disease and in hypopituitarism. J. clin. Endocr. **11**, 700—723 (1951).

[600] BURSTON, R. A., and O. GARROD: The variability of the lowered glomerular filtration rate in Addison's disease and panhypopituitarism and the effect of cortisone thereon. Clin. Sci. **11**, 129—139 (1952).

[601] McCANCE, R. A., and E. M. WIDDOWSON: The secretion of urine in man during experimental salt deficiency. J. Physiol. **91**, 222—231 (1937).

[602] WILKINSON, B. M., and R. A. McCANCE: The secretion of urine in rabbits during experimental salt deficiency. Quart. J. exp. Physiol. **30**, 249—261 (1940).

[603] HOLMES, H. J.: Studies of water exchange in dogs with reduced serum electrolyte concentration. Amer. J. Physiol. **129**, 384—385 (1940).

[604] CIZEK, L. J., and K. C. HUANG: Water diuresis in the salt-depleted dog. Amer. J. Physiol. **167**, 473—484 (1951).

salt-depletion). The increased susceptibility to water intoxication in such cases ("miner's cramp") is also well-known. In such cases there will also be a tendency to a fall in renal blood flow (and filtration rate) and it is natural to ask whether a reduced glomerular capillary pressure could account for the reduced water diuresis in both these cases and in cortical insufficiency. The objection may be raised that in simple sodium-depletion the secretion of sodium-retaining steroids is increased, whereas it is diminished or lacking in cortical insufficiency, and furthermore that the production of antidiuretic hormone may be increased when there is a diminution in blood volume even though the osmotic pressure of the extracellular fluids is lowered (cf. p. 351).

The similarity between the abnormalities in renal function in the above-mentioned cases and in cortical insufficiency may, of course, be fortuitous, and reference has only been made to these cases to emphasize that a reduced glomerular propulsion pressure or another renal defect with basically similar effects might, at least in part, be responsible for the reduced capacity for water and salt excretion in adrenocortical insufficiency (cf. ROSENBAUM et al.[605] for a comprehensive discussion of related problems).

If such defects were due entirely to a loss of sodium from the extracellular fluid (by way of the kidney and possibly also by internal shifts) it might be expected that the defects in renal function could be corrected by administration of sodium salts in appropriate amounts. The results which have been obtained in such studies are not quite uniform. HARRISON and DARROW[593] observed some rise in the filtration rate in adrenalectomized dogs during sodium chloride treatment, but normal values were never reached. ROEMMELT et al.[574], on the other hand succeeded in maintaining essentially unchanged renal blood flows and filtration rates in adrenalectomized dogs, which were maintained on desoxycorticosterone (and occasionally cortical extract) and saline, and deprived of all supportive measures except access to saline 3—5 days before the measurements; these dogs were amply hydrated since they were given $1/_2$ liter of saline per os prior to the measurements. As mentioned above they still showed a subnormal ability to excrete an additional load of salt. LOTSPEICH[606] have reported almost identical creatinine clearances in adrenalectomized rats maintained on a high salt diet and controls fed either the same diet or a normal diet, but the water diuresis response was not normalized. The latter finding was confirmed by KELLOGG and BURACK[607] who, however, found that the diuretic response to Ringer solution became normal. In Addisonian patients (cf. ref. above) the general impression has been that salt therapy is capable of preventing great falls in filtration rate and renal blood flow, whereas complete normalization of these functions is usually not achieved. Similarly, although some improvement may be obtained, the diuretic response to water ingestion remains definitely subnormal.

It appears that the above studies warrant the conclusion that salt therapy is inadequate to restore normal diuretic responses (at least to water) in adrenocortical insufficiency even though it may wholly or partially correct the deficiencies of the filtration rate and renal blood flow. Apparently the adrenals exert some influence on the renal handling of water and electrolytes besides its sodium-retaining effect.

[605] ROSENBAUM, J. D., W. P. NELSON III., M. B. STRAUSS, R. K. DAVIS, and E. ROSS-MEISSL: Variation in the diuretic response to ingested water related to the renal excretion of solutes. J. clin. Invest. **32**, 394—404 (1953).

[606] LOTSPEICH, W. D.: The effect of adrenalectomy on the renal tubular reabsorption of water in the rat. Endocrinology **44**, 314—316 (1949).

[607] KELLOGG, R. H., and W. R. BURACK: Comparison of Ringer diuresis and water diuresis in normal and adrenlectomized rats. Amer. J. Physiol. **163**, 724—725 (1951).

Considerable insight in the factors involved, although not in the mechanisms by which they work, has been gained from studies on substitution therapy with various corticoids.

Desoxycorticosterone has on the whole been found to be unable to restore water diuresis (GARROD et al.[608]), or at least its action in this respect has been found to be very weak (MOREL[609]; CHART et al.[610]). Results have been conflicting as regards its ability to restore a normal filtration rate and renal blood flow. From GARROD et al. studies in adrenalectomized dogs it appears that this steroid has no acute effects on the renal blood flow and the filtration rate, and these authors considered it likely that in those cases in which a rise in these functions had previously been recorded a net retention of sodium might have preceded the rises. *Aldosterone in doses sufficient to cause marked sodium retention* has also been reported not to normalize water excretion (cf. RENZI et al.[611]). From these and other results it appears that mineralocorticoids are unable to correct the deficiency in water excretion, at least in doses which are adequate to produce optimal sodium retention, and the conclusion must be drawn that the failing water diuresis is not fundamentally related to a lack of secretion of sodium-retaining corticoids.

It is apparent that the arguments already considered clearly point to the *glucocorticoids* as being of particular importance to the ability of the kidneys to rid the body of extraordinary loads of water and possibly also salt. Confirmation of this view has come from long series of studies on the effect of these corticoids in adrenocortical insufficiency. Thus cortisone treatment has been shown to be quite effective in restoring the water diuresis response in Addisonian patients (THORN et al.[612]; CHALMERS and LEWIS[613]; GARROD and BURSTON[589]). In adrenalectomized rats a similar effect of cortisone has been observed by MOREL[609], who, however, stated that desoxycorticosterone was also required for complete normalization of the diuretic response. Cortisol was also shown to be very effective in rats (RENZI et al.[611]), and CHART et al.[610] found that this also applied to prednisone and prednisolone, which are known to have a high "glucocorticoid" activity, but to be very weak "sodium-retainers". Acute restoration of water diuresis by cortisone in adrenalectomized dogs was observed by GARROD et al.[608].

In some of these studies the glucocorticoids were also found to cause elevation in the filtration rate and the renal blood flow (cf. also BURSTON and GARROD[600]). It should also be noted that aldosterone *in similar weight doses* has been found to be equally effective as cortisol in elevating the clearances of creatinine and para-aminohippurate in adrenalectomized rats and in raising the resistance of these animals to water intoxication (RENZI et al.). Such effects were actually to be expected, since, as mentioned above, aldosterone has definite glucocorticoid actions besides its dominating sodium-retaining activity. The doses of aldosterone required

[608] GARROD, O., S. A. DAVIES, and G. CAHILL jr.: The action of cortisone and desoxy-corticosterone acetate on glomerular filtration rate and sodium and water exchange in the adrenalectomized dog. J. clin. Invest. **34**, 761—776 (1955).

[609] MOREL, F.: Action synergique de la cortixone et de la désoxycorticostérone sur la diurèse provoqué du rat surrénalectomisé. C. R. Soc. Biol. (Paris) **146**, 202—207 (1952).

[610] CHART, J. J., N. HETZEL, and R. GAUNT: Effect of new adrenal steroids on electrolyte and water excretion. Proc. Soc. exp. Biol. (N. Y.) **91**, 73—75 (1956).

[611] RENZI, A. A., M. RENZI, J. J. CHART, and R. GAUNT: The effects of aldosterone and other steroids on water intoxication and renal function. Acta endocr. **21**, 47—56 (1956).

[612] THORN, G. W., P. H. FORSHAM, L. L. BENNETT, M. ROCHE, R. S. REISS, A. SLESSOR, E. B. FLINK, and W. SOMERVILLE: Clinical and metabolic changes in Addison's disease following the administration of compound E acetate. Trans. Ass. Amer. Physicians, **62**, 233—244 (1949).

[613] CHALMERS, T. M., and A. A. G. LEWIS: The effect of adrenocorticotropic hormone on the diuretic response to water in panhypopituitarism. Lancet **261**, 1158—1160 (1951).

to produce these effects are, however, much larger than those necessary to cause marked reduction in urinary excretion of sodium.

The above findings naturally bring up the question whether there exists a causal relationship between the ability of glucocorticoids to enhance diuretic responses and to elevate renal blood flow and glomerular filtration rate (the latter also signifying an increase in the rate of tubular reabsorption of sodium and fluid). Several of the above-mentioned investigators felt that there may well be a causal relationship between the latter phenomena and the known tendency of glucocorticoids to cause an increase in renal excretion of sodium. They did, however, consider it less likely that the enhanced diuretic responses should also be related to the ability of the glucocorticoids to increase the renal blood flow and the filtration rate, mainly because they failed to observe a close parallelism between the changes in these functions and the improvement in the diuretic response (CHALMERS and LEWIS; GARROD et al.).

It is, however, questionable whether the lack of complete parallelism is sufficient evidence to exclude a causal relationship. It is not actually necessary to visualize the latter as one in which a rise in renal blood flow or filtration rate constitutes the immediate cause of the improved diuretic response. It is equally — or possibly more — likely that the changes in all these functions may be referred to a common cause which may affect the individual functions to a variable degree. Obviously, a change in renal blood flow could not *per se* be the cause of an increased diuretic response. As discussed above (p. 263) the glomerular filtration rate cannot be considered as independently variable, and certainly a rise in filtration rate is not necessarily associated with the delivery of an increased fluid load to the more distal parts of the nephron which are generally believed to responsible for the production of hypotonic urine ("water diuresis"). The interpretation of the above findings is hampered, by the incompleteness of our general knowledge of the function of the nephrons, and more specifically by the fact that we quite ignorant of the mechanism by which the glucocorticoids produce an increase in renal blood flow and filtration rate. Any increase in filtration rate which is not accompanied by a similar increase in the urinary output of sodium and water obviously indicates an increased rate of tubular reabsorption of sodium and water. One way in which this could be brought about would be by a direct stimulation of the (proximal) reabsorption of sodium (+ water) by the glucocorticoids. The increased renal blood flow might then be a secondary event produced, for instance, by a vasodilatory effect of metabolic products from the tubular cells. On the other hand, the increased blood flow might be primary, and caused either by a direct effect of the glucocorticoids on the renal vessels (as suggested by DAVIS and HOWELL[614]) or by some sort of reflex activated by a general improvement of the state of the circulatory system. That the rise in glomerular filtration rate could be secondary to an improved renal circulation is apparent from the fact (cf. p. 271) that changes in renal blood flow produced by simple mechanical means may be accompanied by changes in the filtration rate in the same direction. — DINGMAN[615] has recently suggested, that the ability of glucocorticoids to increase the glomerular filtration rate should be a function of "keeping" water and solutes in the extracellular space. The present writer finds it difficult to see how this function is performed, and in his opinion the counterpart, i. e. the effect of the glucocorticoids on the elctrolyte composition of

---

[614] DAVIS, J. O., and D. S. HOWELL: Comparative effect of ACTH, cortisone and DCA on renal function, electrolyte excretion and water exchange in normal dogs. Endocrinology **52**, 245—255 (1953).

[615] DINGMAN, J. F.: Hypothalamus and the endocrine control of sodium and water metabolism in man. Amer. J. med. Sci. **235**, 79—99 (1958).

the intracellular phase, in particular that of the cardiovascular tissues, is more likely to be of importance. — Evidently it remains for the future to answer the questions how glucocorticoids cause a rise in the filtration rate and in the renal blood flow, and to what extent the same mechanism is also responsible for their ability to improve the diuretic response in cortial insufficiency. It may very well be that — as discussed below — other factors are involved in the latter phenomenon, but the possibility should still be considered that a delivery of fluid at a higher pressure to the distal tubules, either by an increase in glomerular capillary pressure (related to the augmentation in renal blood flow) or by a reduc-tion in hydrodynamic resistance in the proximal tubules (by diminution in cell volume) may also play an important role. Such changes would, of course, tend to increase the excretion of water as well as salt. Consequently, if a mechanism of this sort were to be held responsible for the increased capacity to excrete salt and water, one would obviously also have to assume that glucocorticoids enhance the rate of reabsorption of sodium in some part of the tubular system — presumably in the distal segments — although less intensely than the mineralocorticoids. Two effects like these, the first of which *may* be primarily extrarenal, would make it possible to account for the ability of glucocorticoids to increase the capacity for sodium excretion and to induce a rise in sodium excretion under some conditions as well as for their ability to induce sodium retention under other conditions.

Whether the net result of glucocorticoid administration would be an increase or a decrease in sodium excretion would then depend on the balance between the two effects. It seems reasonable to assume that each of these effects would vary with the preceding state of the underlying processes, which might account for the fact that the net response may vary considerably according to the experimental conditions, dosage level etc. (cf. p. 319). In such cases where the distal sodium reabsorption is already fully activated and the "proximal conditions" for sodium and water excretion are rather unfavourable, as for instance in congestive heart failure, it might be expected that the natriuretic effect of glucocorticoids would dominate. It is interesting to note in this connection that corticotropin (CAMARA and SCHEMM[616]) and possibly even more so prednisone (RIEMER[617]) have recently be found to be effective diuretics (natriuretics) in cases of refractory cardiac oedema. Cf. also VESIN and CATTAN[618].

Corticoids have also been shown to be capable of increasing renal blood flow and glomerular filtration rate in subjects with intact adrenals. In general these changes have only been observed after a certain period of treatment. Moderate increases in filtration rate (and less so in renal plasma flow) were observed by LEVITT and BADER[619] in human subjects during the first week of treatment with cortisone and corticotropin, and similar increases in filtration rate after some days treatment with corticotropin or cortisone were reported by INGBAR et al.[620]. 42 and 52% increases in filtration rate and renal plasma flow, respectively, were

---

[616] CAMARA, A., and F. SCHEMM: Corticotropin in heart disease. Its paradoxical effect on sodium excretion in resistent congestive failure. Circulation 11, 702 (1955).

[617] RIEMER, A. D.: The effect of prednisone in the treatment of refractory cardiac edema. Bull. Johns Hopkins Hosp. 98, 445—453 (1956).

[618] VESIN, P., et R. CATTAN: Mécanisme complexe de la diurese sodique dans les oedèmes traités par les corticoïdes. Bull. Soc. méd. Hôp. Paris 74, 605—610 (1958).

[619] LEVITT, M. F., and M. E. BADER: Effect of cortisone and ACTH on fluid and electrolyte distribution in man. Amer. J. Med. 11, 715—723 (1951).

[620] INGBAR, S. H., E. H. KASS, C. H. BURNETT, A. S. RELMAN, B. A. BURROWS, and J. H. SISSON: The effects of ACTH and cortisone on the renal tubular transport of uric acid, phosphorus and electrolytes in patients with normal renal and adrenal function. J. Lab. clin. Med. 38, 533—541 (1951).

observed by LITTLE et al.[621] during a period of administration of corticotropin to dogs. Considerable increases in these functions were also reported by DAVIS and HOWELL[614] during prolonged treatment of dogs with cortisone and corticotropin. These authors also observed smaller increases during treatment with desoxycortico-sterone, a finding which agrees with WINTER and INGRAM's[622] observation of a 20% increase in creatinine clearance during such treatment.

Prolonged intensive treatment with both glucocorticoids and mineralocorticoids may then cause an increase in intrarenal salt and water turnover (filtration-reabsorption). It is now also well-established that such treatment is often also followed by an increased water turnover in the body (water intake — urine flow (cf. discussion below on polyuria.)

Several authors have reported an increased content of antidiuretic substances in plasma and urine after adrenalectomy and BIRNIE et al.[623] thought they had provided evidence that the antidiuretic activity measured by their bioassay technique was actually due to vasopressin. These and other results obtained by similar techniques (intraperitoneal or subcutaneous injections in hydrated rats) however, have recently been severely criticized by VAN DYKE et al.[624]), who rightly pointed out that assay methods which give titers in blood from normal animals vastly above those which may be calculated to result from the distribution of a strongly antidiuretic dose of vasopressin in the blood volume "are so grossly inaccurate as to make valueless any conclusions that may have been reached".

Although an increased titer of vasopressin in cortical insufficiency may not have been validly demonstrated it is not excluded that it may exist. As discussed elsewhere (p. 349) there is considerable evidence that the production of vasopressin is also governed by reflexes from the cardiovascular system and it is possible that such reflexes (and VDM) may stimulate the production even though the subnormal tonicity of the plasma which generally exists in cortical insufficiency would tend to suppress it. There have also been claims that the rate of inactivation of vasopressin is diminished in cortical insufficiency, which of course would cause a prolongation of the effect of any vasopressin secreted. These claims have been based upon studies on the in vitro inactivation by liver extracts (cf. BIRNIE[625]), on the time course of the antidiuretic effect of pitressin in normal and adrenalectomized animals (LOCKETT[626]) and on a slower fall in the titer of the blood in adrenalectomized than in normal animals following the injection of very large doses — 100 mU/100 g of body weight — of vasopressin (cf. HELLER[627]) — Recently GAUNT et al.[628]

[621] LITTLE, J. M., W. M. KELSEY, and E. H. YOUNT jr.: Influence of the adrenal cortex on renal hemodynamics in the dog. Amer. J. Physiol. 185, 159—166 (1956).

[622] WINTER, C. A., and W. R. INGRAM: Observations on the polyuria produced by desoxy-corticosterone acetate. Amer. J. Physiol. 139, 710—718 (1943).

[623] BIRNIE, J. H., W. J. EVERSOLE, W. R. BOSS, C. M. OSBORN, and R. GAUNT: An antidiuretic substance in the blood of normal and adrenalectomized rats. Endocrinology 47, 1—12 (1950).

[624] DYKE, H. B. VAN, K. ADAMSON jr., and S. L. ENGEL: Aspects of the biochemistry and physiology of the neurohypophyseal hormones. Rec. Progr. Hormone Res. 11, 1 (1955).

[625] BIRNIE, J. H.: The role of the liver in water metabolism. Ciba Found. Colloquia on Endocrinology 4, 542—552 (1952).

[626] LOCKETT, M. F.: Preliminary studies on the sensitivity of adrenalectomized dogs to the antidiuretic hormone of the posterior pituitary gland. Ciba Found. Colloquia on Endo-crinology 4, 517—525 (1952).

[627] HELLER, H.: The influence of the suprarenal cortex on mineral and water metabolism. In the suprarenal cortex. Proc. 5th Symposium of the Colston Research Society. Butterworths Scientific Publ. London. 1953.

[628] GAUNT, R. C. W. LLOYD, and J. J. CHART: The adrenal-neurohypophyseal interrela-tionship. In H. HELLER (ed.): The Neurohypophysis, p. 233—251. London: Butterworths. 1957.

have reviewed studies on the relation between the neurohypophysis and the adrenal cortex. In experiments with simultaneous injections of cortisol and Pitressin to hydrated rats, cortisol seemed to inhibit the effect of Pitressin. However, they summed up their opinion on the neurohypophyseal — adrenocortical relation by stating that this relation is a complicated one. Cortisol seems to inhibit the release of vasopressin and also to increase its inactivation. — On the other hand, SOFFER et al.[629] in man could produce no increase in the rate of urine flow in water diuresis in patients with Addison's disease by giving ethanol which should inhibit the secretion of vasopressin. Even more convincing evidence against a vasopressin effect as responsible for the decreased capacity for water excretion in adrenocortical insufficiency has been produced by JONES et al.[630] who found that the decreased capacity also existed after adrenalectomy in rats with pre-existing diabetes insipidus.

Altogether it seems difficult at present definitely to exclude the possibility that an increased impact of vasopressin on the tubules or an increase in their sensitivity to this hormone may be of some importance to the phenomenon of diminished water diuresis in cortical insufficiency. Those supporting the view that such changes are of preeminent importance can, however, hardly expect to meet with general approval until they have accounted for the findings of SOFFER et al. and JONES et al., as well as the fact that water diuresis is also defective after hypophysectomy (GAUNT et al.[631]) or clinical loss of both adeno- and neurohypophyseal function (BURSTON and GARROD[600]). That the defective water diuresis response in panhypopituitarism is — at least in part due to secondary adrenocortical insufficiency is indicated by the fact that it has been possible to produce — or rather unmask — a diabetes insipidus by cortisone therapie in such cases (IKKOS et al.[632]; HOEL[633]). An increased distal salt-water load *plus* increased distal salt reabsorption would seem to provide a satisfactory explanation for this phenomenon. Cf. also the section on the adenohypophysis for a further discussion of related subjects.

Corticoid induced polyuria. The development of polydipsia-polyuria ("diabetes insipidus") during *prolonged* treatment with desoxycorticosterone was reported a few years after this corticoid was made available for therapy. The first observations were made on dogs (RAGAN et al.[634]; FERREBEE et al.[635], MULINOS et al.[636]) in which the rate of urine flow was found to increase gradually from the usual 400 ml per day up to 4—6 l. It was also clearly shown that the polyuria increased markedly

[629] SOFFER, L. J., A. GUTMAN, J. GELLER, and J. L. GABRILOVE: The role of adrenal steroids on renal function and electrolyte metabolism. Bull. N. Y. Acad. Med. **33**, 665—680 (1957).

[630] JONES, I. C., and A. WRIGHT: Some aspects of zonation and function of the adrenal cortex. IV. The histology of the adrenal in rats with diabetes insipidus. J. clin. Endocr. **10**, 266—272 (1954).

[631] GAUNT, R., J. W. REMINGTON, and M. SCHWEIZER: Some effects of intraperitoneal glucose injections and excess water in normal, adrenalectomized, and hypophysectomized rats. Amer. J. Physiol. **120**, 532—543 (1937).

[632] IKKOS, D., R. LUFT, and H. OLIVECRONA: Hypophysectomy in man: effect on water excretion during the first two postoperative months. J. clin. Endocr. **15**, 553—567 (1955).

[633] HOEL, J.: Cortisone induced recurrence in diabetes insipidus by total destruction of the hypophysis. Acta endocr. (Kbh.) **21**, 15—18 (1956).

[634] RAGAN, C., J. W. FERREBEE, P. PFYFE, D. W. ATCHLEY, and R. F. LOEB: A syndrome of polydipsia and polyuria induced in normal animals by desoxycorticosterone acetate. Amer. J. Physiol. **131**, 73—78 (1940).

[635] FERREBEE, J. W., D. PARKER, W. H. CARNES, M. K. GERITY, D. W. ATCHLEY, and R. F. LOEB: Certain effects of desoxycorticosterone. Amer. J. Physiol. **135**, 230—237 (1941).

[636] MULINOS, M. G., C. L. SPINGARN, and M. E. LOJKIN: A diabetes insipidus-like condition produced by small doses of desoxycorticosterone acetate in dogs. Amer. J. Physiol. **135**. 102—112 (1941).

when the salt intake was raised, and that no polyuria developed on a low sodium intake. Similar observations have been made in rats (for references see GAUNT et al.[586]); WINTER and INGRAM[622] confirmed the findings in dogs, but were unable to produce the syndrome in cats even with very large doses. In human subjects the development of a similar syndrome has at least been reported once (MOEHLIG and JAFFE[637]).

A typical finding in the syndrome of primary hyperaldosteronism has been a polyuria, resistent to vasopressin.

An apparently similar condition has more recently been shown to result from *prolonged* administration of glucocorticoids. The gradual development of polyuria in intact dogs during intensive cortisone treatment has been observed by SIREK and BEST[638], and DAVIS and HOWELL[614], and a similar state of polyuria and polydipsia has also been induced in adrenalectomized dogs by cortisone overdosage (SWINGLE et al.[639]). WINTER[640] has reported the development of a moderate polyuria in cortisone-treated rats; no absolute polydipsia was observed in these studies.

The mechanism of corticoid-induced polyuria appears to be quite complex, and only in part related to the ability of (gluco)corticoids to improve the capacity for salt and water excretion in cortical insufficiency. There are certain indications that the mechanisms of the polyurias induced by glucocorticoids and those induced by mineralocorticoids may be somewhat different. LEAF et al.[641] have suggested that some polyurias induced by corticotropin and cortisone (and thyroxin) may simply be osmotic diureses caused by an increased production of nitrogenous end products. It is quite likely that this mechanism may explain some of the moderate polyurias, but is cannot account for the more marked cases (apparently especially observed in dogs) in which the urine, as judged from specific gravity determinations, becomes less concentrated than it would be at comparable urine flow rates during exogenous osmotic diuresis. Nor could it account for the often more pronounced desoxy-corticosterone-induced polyuria since this corticoid has no appreciable catabolic effect.

In order to account for these latter cases it appears that one has to assume that one or both of the following mechanisms are operating: 1) A proximal mechanism (similar to that loosely outlined above) causing fluids to be delivered to the distal tubules at a higher pressure; the lack of an equivalent natriuresis must then be attributed to an increased distal rate of sodium reabsorption. 2) A reduced exposure of the (distal?) tubules to vasopressin or a decreased sensitivity to its water reabsorption promoting action.

The latter mechanism has received consideration in several publications, in which the reverse — exposure to higher concentrations of vasopressin or increased sensitivity — has generally also been suggested as an explanation of the reduced water diuresis response in cortical insufficiency. (Cf. GAUNT et al.[586], GAUNT[642]), cf. discussion above.

---

[637] MOEHLIG, R. C., and L. JAFFE: Syndrome simulating diabetes insipidus in dogs induced by desoxycorticosterone acetate. J. Lab. clin. Med. 27, 1009—1012 (1942).

[638] SIREK, O. V., and C. H. BEST: Intramuscular cortisone administration to dogs. Proc. Soc. exp. Biol. (N. Y.) 80, 594—598 (1952).

[639] SWINGLE, W. W., E. J. FEDOR, M. BEN, R. MAXWELL, C. BAKER, and G. BARLOW: Induction of diabetes insipidus in adrenalectomized dogs with cortisone. Proc. Soc. exp. Biol. (N. Y.) 82, 571—573 (1953).

[640] WINTER, C. A.: Comparison of the effect of cortisone acetate and of deoxycorticosterone acetate upon water balance. In Ciba Found. Colloquia of Endocrinology 4, 499—516 (1952).

[641] LEAF, A., A. R. MAMBY, H. RASMUSSEN, and J. P. MARASCO: Some hormonal aspects of water excretion in man. J. clin. Invest. 31, 914—922 (1952).

[642] GAUNT, R.: The interrelationship between the adrenal cortex posterior pituitary and anterior pituitary in water metabolism. Ciba Found. Colloquia on Endocrinology 4, 455—462 (1952).

With regard to the possibility that corticoid might change the sensitivity of the tubular cells to vasopressin it appears that such an effect is exerted by desoxy-corticosterone since it is generally agreed that polyuria induced by this corticoid is very resistent to vasopressin. On the other hand, opinions seem to differ considerably as regards the sensitivity of the cortisone-induced polyurias to vasopressin. SIREK and BEST[638] found that subcutaneous injection of 10 I.U. in oil was sufficient in polyuric dogs to reduce the daily urine volume from about 5 l to almost normal levels, whereas SWINGLE et al.[639] concluded that much larger doses were required (3 times 40 I.U.). Much smaller doses (2 times 10 milliunits per 100 g of body weight) was found by WINTER[640] to be effective in polyuric rats.

Recent studies on potassium deficiency has thrown new light on the phenomenon of corticoid induced resistance to vasopressin. It has been shown (cf. MILNE et al.[1579] and RELMAN and SCHWARTZ[605] for recent reviews) that potassium deficiency (of various origin) causes an increase in kidney weight and striking histological changes in the tubular system, in particular the distal parts (dilatation, vacuolization, granulation, degeneration). Simultaneously (or rather before) the ability to produce dilute and concentrated urine is reduced, and a resistance to vasopressin develops. It seems likely that such changes may play an important part in the development of polyuria from administration of corticoids (in particular the mineralocorticoids), since it is to be expected that potassium depletion has resulted from *prolonged* therapy with these substances. To the extent that this mechanism is involved the polyuria should be caused by a delayed, secondary effect of the corticoids rather than by immediate, direct effects. It remains to be studied to what extent corticoids are able to induce polyuria when the development of potassium deficiency is prevented.

Corticoid derivatives. In recent years steroid chemists have synthetized a number of analogues of naturally occurring corticoids. — Experimental and clinical work has shown that the activity spectra of some of these compounds may differ considerably from those of the parent substances. This highly interesting development might provide possibilities of learning more about the relation between molecular configuration and the mode of action. Likewise it may make possible the application of the principle of competitive inhibition to this branch of physiology. The following modifications of the corticoid molecules have resulted in compounds with interesting biological effects:

1) Introduction of a double-bond between carbon atom no 1 and 2.

2) Halogenation in the 9-α position.

3) Methylation at carbon atoms no 2 or 6. Combinations of these have also been made.

The sodium retaining effect on the kidney has been the mineralocorticoid effect mostly studied in these compounds. This effect seems to have been somewhat variable with the dosage employed. However, the following general statements can be made:

The Δ^1-analogues of cortisone and cortisol (prednisone and prednisolone) developed by HERZOG et al.[643] have a higher glucocorticoid potency than the parent molecule. Their outstanding characteristic is that the Na retaining effect is unchanged or reduced (STAFFORD et al.[644]). — The 9-α-halogen-steroids (esp. 9-α-

[643] HERZOG, H. L., A. NABILE, S. TOLKSDORF, W. CHARNEY, E. B. HERSHBERG, P. L. PERLMAN, and M. M. PESHET: New antiarthritic steroids. Science 121, 176 (1955).

[644] STAFFORD, R. O., L. E. BARNES, B. J. BOWMAN, and M. M. MEINZINGER: Glucocorticoid and mineralocorticoid activities of Δ^1-9-fluorohydrocortisone. Proc. Soc. exp. Biol. (N. Y.) 89, 371—374 (1955).

fluorocortisol) synthetized by FRIED and SABO[645] have increased glucocorticoid activity, but proportionally the mineralocorticoid activity is increased more. 9-α-fluorocortisol is about as strong as desoxycorticosterone in sodium retaining action in rats (BORMAN et al.[646]). It is about as potent as aldosterone in causing sodium retention in humans (GOLDFIEN et al. [647]). — STAFFORD et al.[644] have tested the activities of a compound with a combination of these modifications. There was no essential difference in sodium-retaining activity between this substance and 9-α-fluorocortisol but it had considerably larger glucocorticoid potency. — 2-methylanalogues of cortisol were developed by HOGG et al.[648]. They have been shown by BYRNES et al.[649] to be more potent than cortisol both in glycogen deposition and Na retaining effect in rats. LIDDLE, RICHARD and TOMKINS[650] have demonstrated increased Na-retaining effect in dogs and humans, possibly by increased tubular reabsorption of Na. — 2-methyl 9-α-fluorocortisone is more potent (about 3 times) than aldosterone in this respect and is thus the most potent sodium retaining steroid known so far. — A very characteristic property of the 2-methylated compounds seems to be the prolonged effect, persisting for appr. 48 hr in studies in humans as compared to a duration of the effect of a single oral dose of cortisol of less than 24 hr. This may be due to a difference in the metabolic breakdown of the compounds. LYSTER et al.[651] have reported on the metabolic effects of *6-methyl-Δ¹-cortisol* in rats. Whereas its glucocorticoid properties were 2—3 times stronger than those of prednisolone, this steroid produced Na excretion in the test animals.

Of these analogues especially prednisone and prednisolone have been used widely clinically, replacing cortisone and cortisol. However, the final place of the compounds in clinical therapy both for depression and substitution purposes remains to be established. For a recent comprehensive review cf. FRIED and BORMAN[652].

The elucidation of the basic mechanism of action of the corticoids has so far not been furthered by our knowledge of these synthetic analogues. They do undoubtedly compete with the natural corticoids for "attachment to the sites of action" of the latter, and their different activity spectra must be considered as resulting from differences in their affinities for these "sites" and from different abilities to perform the operations involved. Cf. also section on "antialdosterones", p. 417.

[645] FRIED, J., and E. F. SABO: 9-α-fluoro derivatives of cortisone and hydrocortisone. J. Amer. chem. Soc. **76**, 1455 (1954).

[646] BORMAN, A., F. M. SINGER, and P. NUMEROF: Growth-survival and sodium retaining activity of 9-halo derivatives of hydrocortisone. Proc. Soc. exp. Biol. (N. Y.) **86**, 570—573 (1954).

[647] GOLDFIEN, A., J. C. LAIDLAW, N. A. HAYDAR, A. E. RENOLD, and G. W. THORN: Fluorohydrocortisone and chlorohydrocortisone, highly potent derivatives of compound F. New Engl. J. Med. **252**, 415—421 (1955).

[648] HOGG, J. A., F. H. LINCOLN, R. W. JACKSON, and W. P. SCHNEIDER: The adrenal hormones and related compounds. III. Synthesis of 2-alkyl analogs. J. Amer. chem. Soc. **77**, 6401 (1955).

[649] BYRNES, W. W., L. E. BARNES, B. J. BOWMAN, W. E. DUBIN, E. H. MORLEY, and R. O. STAFFORD: Adrenal corticoid activities of 2-methylhydrocortisone acetate and 2-methyl-9 α-fluorohydrocortisone acetate. Proc. Soc. exp. Biol. (N. Y.) **91**, 67—70 (1956).

[650] LIDDLE, G. W., J. E. RICHARD, and G. M. TOMKINS: Studies of structure function relationships of steroids; the 2-methyl-corticosteroids. Metabolism **5**, 384—394 (1956).

[651] LYSTER, S. L., L. E. BARNES, G. H. LUND, M. M. MEINZINGER, and W. W. BYRNES: Adrenal corticoid activities of 6-methyl-Δ¹-hydrocortisone. Proc. Soc. exp. Biol. (N. Y.) **94**, 159—162 (1957).

[652] FRIED, J., and A. BORMAN: Synthetic derivatives of cortical hormones. In: HARRIS, R.S., and K. V. THIMANN (Eds): Vitamins and hormones. Vol. 16. Acad. Press. N. Y. 1958.

Licorice extract. Licorice extract has been shown to exert a mineralocorticoid-like action. It was found by Borst et al. (Borst et al.[653]; Molhuysen et al.[654]) to cause sodium and chloride retention and increased excretion of potassium in normal individuals.

Pelser et al.[655] reported that glycyrrhizinic acid as well as the corresponding aglucone, glycyrrhetinic acid (a triterpene) reduced the excretion of sodium and chloride and increased the excretion of potassium in Addisonian patients. More recently it has been reported by Kraus[656] that ammoniated glycyrrhizine induced sodium and water retention in rats, and in unilaterally nephrectomized rats treated with this substance or licorice and given 0.87% NaCl to drink Girerd et al.[657] have observed the development of hypertension, polyuria and similar cardiovascular and renal lesions as recorded following high doses of desoxy-corticosterone.

Whereas Pelser et al. claimed that glycyrrhizinic acid and glycyrrhetinic acid in doses of about 3—5 g daily (or some 20 g of licorice extract) maintained Addisonian patients in "electrolyte equilibrium" and working condition, Hudson et al.[658] found that glycyrrhizine alone was inadequate for maintenance of 3 (cancer) patients on whom bilateral adrenalectomy had been performed; cortisone administration could, however, be reduced to "dosages heretofore considered sub-normal". A similar conclusion was arrived at by Elmadjian et al.[659] who found that a daily dosage of 4 g of ammonium glycyrrhizinate was unable to maintain two adrenalectomized patients in a satisfactory state; the addition of as little as 10 mg of cortisol per day sufficed, however, to maintain them in excellent condition. Subsequent reduction of the glycyrrhizinate dosage to 2 g daily resulted in a deterioration of the clinical state.

The question of the mechanism of action of glycyrrhizine has not yet been solved. It is not converted to identifiable steroids in vivo. It is interesting that Atherden in recent experiments[660] have found that glycyrrhetic acid inhibits the destruction of progesterone and 11-desoxycorticosterone in rat liver homogenate. If this "protective" effect also extends to the glucocorticoids it would seem to provide a satisfactory explanation to the observations that glycyrrhizine alone seems to be ineffective in the treatment of *absolute* adrenal insufficiency, but to lower the glucocorticoid maintenance dosages. If glycyrrhizine does depress the breakdown of glucocorticoids the indications of a suppressive effect on the output

---

[653] Borst, J. G., G. G. Blomhert, J. A. Molhuysen, J. Gerbrandy, K. P. Turner, and L. A. de Vries: De uitscheiding van water en electrolyten gedurende het etmaal en onder invloed van succus liquiritice. Acta clin. belg. **5**, 405—409 (1950).

[654] Molhuysen, J. A., J. Gerbrandy, L. A. de Vries, J. C. de Jong, J. B. Lenstra, K. P. Turner, and J. G. G. Borst: A liquorice extract with deoxycortone-like action. Lancet **2**, 381—386 (1950).

[655] Pelser, H. E., A. F. Willebrands, M. Frenkel, R. M. van der Heide, and J. Groen. Comparative study of the use of glycyrrhizinic and glycyrrhetinic acids in Addison's disease. Metabolism **2**, 322—334 (1953).

[656] Kraus, S. D.: Desoxycorticosterone — mimetic action of ammoniated glycyrrhizin in rats. J. exp. Med. **106**, 415—422 (1957).

[657] Girerd, R. J., C. L. Rassaert, G. di Pasquale, and R. L. Krog: Production of experimental hypertension and cardiovascular-renal lesions with licorice and ammoniated glycyrrhizine. Amer. J. Physiol **194**, 241—245 (1958).

[658] Hudson, P. B., A. Mittelman, and M. Podberezec: Use of glycyrrhizine after bilateral adrenalectomy. New Engl. J. Med. **251**, 641—646 (1954).

[659] Elmadjian, F., J. M. Hope, and G. Pencus: The action of mono-ammonium glycyrrhizinate on adrenalectomized subjects and its synergism with hydrocortisone. J. clin. Invest. **16**, 338—349 (1956).

[660] Atherden, L. M.: Studies with glycyrrhetic acid: Inhibition of metabolism of steroids in vitro. Biochem. J. **69**, 75—78 (1958).

of corticotropin (cf. KRAUS) could be accounted for as secondary to an elevated level of glucocorticoids in the blood.

Progesterone. The effects of progesterone on urinary excretions of sodium, chloride and potassium have recently been studied in human subjects by LANDAU et al.[661]. 50—100 mg of progesterone daily (intramuscularly, approximately physiological amounts) was found to induce sharp rises in urinary sodium and chloride excretions in human subjects with normal adrenal function and even greater rises in Addisonians under treatment with cortisone and desoxycorticosterone. In an Addisonian patient not treated with corticoids but only with salt a similar dosage of progesterone caused no change in urinary sodium and chloride excretion.

To explain these findings, progesterone is suggested to inhibit the action of salt-retaining corticoids in the kidney. The salt-retention which followed immediately after the administration of progesterone was discontinued (but only in subjects with intact adrenals) was ascribed to a compensatory increase in adrenocortical secretory activity. No consistent changes in the urinary excretion of potassium were observed. The finding of a consistent natriuretic effect of progesterone was rather surprising since salt-retaining effects had previously been reported in intact dogs (and in adrenalectomized dogs, ferrets and calts). In the discussion of this discrepancy the authors were unable to suggest any other explanations than possible species differences and differences in dosages (relatively larger doses had been used in the animal experiments). For results of a recent extension of this work, cf. LANDAU et al.[662].

These findings stress the fact that other effects than such related to sexual functions should be kept in mind when dealing with this hormone.

The possible effect of progesterone as a competitive agent may have significance for the high secretion of aldosterone in pregnancy as well as the mechanism of congenital adrenal hyperplasia.

Oestrogens. The ovarial hormones would seem to be of only minor importance to the overall metabolism of electrolytes and water, since only minor disturbances follow ovariectomy (and menopause).

The association of premenstrual oedema with an increased urinary excretion of oestrogenic material (THORN et al.[663]) and the oedema of late pregnancy with a high oestrogen production has, however, suggested that oestrogen hormones may have sodium-retaining actions.

In careful water and electrolyte balance studies PREEDY and AITKEN[664] have recently demonstrated a small and transient (lasting some 4 days), but significant, decrease in the renal excretion of sodium and chloride in 11 normal subjects who received 10 mg of oestradiol monobenzoate in oil intramuscularly per day. Similar effects have previously been recorded in dogs (THORN and ENGEL[665]) and in

[661] LANDAU, R. L., D. M. BERGENSTAL, K. LUGIBIHL, and M. E. KASCHT: The metabolic effects of progesterone in man. J. clin. Endocr. **15**, 1194—1215 (1955).

[662] LANDAU, R. L., K. LUGIBIHL, and D. F. DIMIEK: Metabolic effects in man of steroids with progestational activity. Ann. N. Y. Acad. Sci. **71**, 588—598 (1958).

[663] THORN, G. W., K. R. NELSON, and D. W. THORN: A Study of the mechanism of edema associated with menstruation. Endocrinology **22**, 155—163 (1938).

[664] PREEDY, J. R. K., and E. H. AITKEN: The effect of estrogen on water and electrolyte metabolism. J. clin. Invest. **35**, 423—429 (1956).

[665] THORN, G. W., and L. L. ENGEL: The effect of sex hormones on the renal excretion of electrolytes. J. exp. Med. **68**, 299—312 (1938).

human subjects given half the above doses (KNOWLTON et al.[666]). DIGNAM etal.[667a] reported findings essentially similar to those of PREEDY and AITKEN[664]. — It remains to be shown whether the moderate sodium-retaining effect of oestrogens is due to renal or extrarenal actions or both. The fact that no change was found in K excretion might indicate that the adrenals are not involved. An extrarenal action is indicated by the fact that oestradiol treatment of mice causes an increase in the glucosamine content of the skin, and thus probably a deposition of hyaluronic acid (SCHMIDT[667b]). An extravascular "fixation" of Na^+ as counterions would accompany the deposition of the polyanions.

Androgens. It is well-known from several studies that androgens produce retention of nitrogen and calcium, and that this effect is generally accentuated in patients lacking an endogenous production of these hormones. Several balance studies with constant diets have shown that androgens also induce moderate retentions of sodium and generally also of potassium (THORN and ENGEL[665]; KNOWLTON et al.[666]; FOURMAN[668]). Like the oestrogens they differ therefore from the corticoids (and progesterone) by producing potassium retention rather than potassium loss. The potassium-retaining effect is probably caused by an extrarenal action associated with the anabolic effect. The nature of the sodium-retaining effect is still obscure. It seems certain, however, that it is not mediated through the adrenal cortex, since sodium retention has also been induced by androgens in patients with adrenal insufficiency (cf. FOURMAN for references).

Recently several analogues of androgens have been synthetized; among them 17-α-ethyl-17-hydroxy-19-nor-4-androsten-3-one is characterized by a very high anabolic/androgenic ratio (16/1) (SAUNDERS and DRILL[669]). Substances with a high anabolic/androgen ratio have been utilized to counteract the catabolic affects of corticoids used in long-time therapy.

b) Hormones of the adrenal medulla

The role of epinephrine and norepinephrine in the metabolism of sodium and potassium has been thoroughly discussed in p. 359 to which the reader is referred. In evaluating the effects of these substances in this field it should be recalled that (nor)epinephrine stimulates the production of corticotropin.

c) Hormones of the adenohypophysis

It is well established that the adenohypophysis exerts profound actions on the kidneys. This is apparent *inter alia* from a loss in kidney weight following hypophysectomy (McQUENN-WILLIAMS and THOMPSON[670]), and from the fact that hypo-

[666] KNOWLTON, K., A. T. KENYON, I. SANDIFORD, G. LOTWIN, and R. FRICKER: Comparative study of metabolic effects of estradiol benzoate and testosterone proprinate in man. J. clin. Endocr. 2, 671—684 (1942).

[667a] DIGNAM, W. S., J. VOSKIAN, and N. S. ASSALI: Effects of estrogens on renal hemodynamics and excretion of electrolytes in human subjects. J. clin. Endocr. 16, 1032—1042 (1956).

[667b] SCHMIDT, A.: The influence of cortisone and oestradiol on the amounts of hexosamine and water in skin. Acta. pharmacol. et toxicol. 14, 350—358 (1958).

[668] FOURMAN, P.: Effects of methyl testosterone and deoxycortone on electrolytes. Clin. Sci. 11, 387—396 (1952).

[669] SAUNDERS, F. J., and V. A. DRILL: Comparative androgenic and anabolic effects of several steroids. Proc. Soc. exp. Biol. (N. Y.) 94, 646—649 (1957).

[670] McQUEEN-WILLIAMS, M., and K. W. THOMPSON: The effect of ablation of the hypophysis upon the weight of the kidney of the rat. Yale J. Biol. Med. 12, 531—541 (1940).

physectomy prevents compensatory renal hypertrophy following unilateral nephrectomy (WINTERNITZ and WATERS[671]). It is also known that hypophysectomy — which causes no signs of permanent neurohypohyseal insufficiency — results in marked decreases in glomerular filtration rate, effective renal plasma flow and diodrast-Tm (WHITE et al.[672]; EARLE et al.[673]; EARLE et al.[674]).

The question what hormonal deficiencies are responsible for these functional impairments has been the subject of considerable debate. Administration of adrenocorticotropin (and cortisone and hydrocortisone) has been shown to be capable of restoring the filtration rate and the renal plasma flow partially towards normal (EARLE et al.[674]; LITTLE et al.[675]). Considerable increases in these quantities have also been observed in hypophysectomized dogs and normal dogs following the administration of growth hormone preparations (WHITE et al.[676]; DE BODO et al.[677]), but opinions differ as regards how completely the functions may be restored in hypophysectomized animals. Other adenohypophyseal hormones are also likely to play a role, but it is at present not clear how important each of them are. WHITE who has worked in this field for a long time has recently[678] summarized the available evidence as follows: "It is fair to say that the falls in kidney function observed after hypophysectomy can be explained only in part by a loss of thyreotropin; that loss of gonadotropin plays little or no part, that loss of growth hormone or some substance not yet separated from it plays an important part, and that loss of ACTH may play some part less important than of loss of growth hormone."

Considering the marked influence which the adenohypophysis exerts on the kidney it may seem astonishing that abnormalities in sodium and potassium metabolism are barely detectable after hypophysectomy. The ability of the kidneys to retain sodium (during sodium restriction) and to secrete potassium (following potassium administration) is nearly as good in hypophysectomized animals as in normals (EARLE et al.[673]). It should be recalled that — as previously discussed (p. 311) — hypophysectomy does not greatly influence the production of aldosterone, which must be considered of great importance to the most distal tubular transfers of electrolytes. The hormones of the adenohypophysis are apparently such which mainly enhance proximal electrolyte (and water) transfers by direct (probably growth hormone) or indirect (adrenocorticotropin) actions. The reduction in glomerular filtration rate following hypophysectomy is probably largely due to a fall in the rate of fluid reabsorption in the proximal tubules (cf. p. 263).

[671] WINTERNITZ, M. C., and L. L. WATERS: The effect of hypophysectomy on compensatory renal hypertrophy in dogs. Yale J. Biol. Med. 12, 705—709 (1940).

[672] WHITE, H. L., P. HEINBECKER, and D. ROLF: Effects of the removal of the anterior lobe of the hypophysis on some renal functions. Amer. J. Physiol. 136, 584—591 (1942).

[673] EARLE, D. P. jr., R. C. DE BODO, I. L. SCHWARTZ, S. J. FARBER, M. KURTZ, and J. GREENBERG. Effect of hypophysectomy on electrolyte and water metabolism in the dog. Proc. Soc. exp. Biol. (N. Y.) 76, 608—612 (1951).

[674] EARLE, D. P., S. J. FARBER, R. C. DE BODO, M. KURTZ, and M. W. SINKOFF: Effects of ACTH, cortisone and hydrocortisone on renal functions of hypophysectomized dogs. Amer. J. Physiol. 173, 189—198 (1953).

[675] LITTLE, J. M., W. M. KELSEY, and E. H. YOUNT, jr.: Influence of the adrenal cortex on renal hemodynamics in the dog. Amer. J. Physiol. 185, 159—166 (1956).

[676] WHITE, H. L., P. HEINBECKER, and D. ROLF: Enhancing effects of growth hormone on renal function. Amer. J. Physiol. 157, 47—51 (1949).

[677] DE BODO, R. C., I. L. SCHWARTZ, J. GREENBERG, M. KURTZ, D. P. EARLE, and S. J. FARBER: Effect of growth hormone on water metabolism in hypophysectomized dogs. Proc. Soc. exp. Biol. (N. Y.) 76, 612—618 (1951).

[678] WHITE, H. L.: Growth hormones and renal function. In: The Hypophyseal growth hormone, nature and actions. Eds.: R. W. SMITH, O. H. GAEBLER, and C. N. H. LONG. New York: The Blakiston Division. McGraw-Hill. 1955.

And it is well-known from other experimental conditions that considerable changes in the rate of (proximal) tubular reabsorption of fluid and in the filtration rate may occur without any marked influence on electrolyte excretions (for instance, when increases in tubular fluid reabsorption and (thus in) the filtration rate are produced by protein feeding in dogs).

Still it cannot be questioned that the adenohypophyseal hormones do exert some influence on the overall water and electrolyte status of the body. In the case of adrenocorticotropin such effects are clearly caused by changes in the production of corticoids, predominantly glucocorticoids, and they are at least to a large extent due to an action of these hormones on the kidneys (cf. section on corticoids).

Growth hormone has also been shown to affect renal excretion of sodium and potassium. WHITNEY et al.[679] found that the urinary excretions of sodium and potassium were reduced some 20% during a 5 to 7 days period in which a growth hormone preparation was administered to normal female rats maintained on a constant diet. The possibility that this effect might be mediated via the adrenal cortex (e.g. by contamination of the growth hormone preparation with corticotropin) was excluded by similar studies performed in adrenalectomized rats (STEIN et al.[680]). Similar sodium and potassium retentions were obtained whether the adrenalectomized rats were maintained with adrenal cortical extract or not.

Further evidence that growth hormone induces a retention of sodium and potassium was produced by a group of Swedish investigators in studies in acromegalic patients. (IKKOS et al.[681, 682]). Significant increases in total body water (antipyrine space), extracellular water (inulin, thiosulphate or bromide space) and total exchangeable sodium per kg body weight were observed, and also statistically significant increases in glomerular filtration rate (and probably in renal plasma flow). Similar effects were seen by these investigators after administration of a preparation of human growth hormone, isolated by starch-block electrophoresis. There was no increase in the rate of secretion of aldosterone in these studies (LUFT et al.[513]).

To what extent the sodium and potassium-retaining effect of growth hormone is due to a direct action on the kidney is not known. Considering the positive nitrogen balance produced by this hormone it seems likely that the retention of potassium is due to an extrarenal action by which potassium is deposited together with cellular protein. The retention of sodium may, however, well depend on a direct renal action.

d) Neurohypophyseal hormones

It is now being widely held that the neurohypophyseal hormones or some precursors of them are produced by neurosecretory cells in the hypothalamus and transported in the axons of the hypothalamo-pituitary tracts to other parts of the neurohypophyseal system where they are either secreted into the blood or stored. (For references see [235] and [683].) The pituicytes formerly believed to produce and

[679] WHITNEY, J. E., L. L. BENNETT, and C. H. LI: Reduction in urinary sodium and potassium produced by hypophyseal growth hormone in normal female rats. Proc. Soc. exp. Biol. (N. Y.) **79**, 584—587 (1952).

[680] STEIN, J. D., jr., L. LESLIE BENNETT, A. A. BATTS, and C. H. LI: Sodium, potassium and chloride retention produced by growth hormone in the absence of the adrenals. Amer. J. Physiol. **171**, 587—591 (1952).

[681] IKKOS, D., R. LUFT, and B. SJÖGREN: Body water and sodium in patients with acromegaly. J. clin. Invest. **33**, 989—994 (1954).

[682] IKKOS, D., H. LJUNGGREN, and R. LUFT: Glomerular filtration rate and renal plasma flow in acromegaly. Acta endocr. (Kbh.) **21**, 226—236 (1956).

[683] Zweites Internationales Symposium über Neurosekretion. Ed. W. BARGMAN, B. HANSTRÖM u. E. SCHARRER. Berlin: Springer 1958.

secrete the hormones, are now regarded as glia cells not even participating in the storage of the hormones.

Neurohypophyseal extracts have been shown to exert a variety of biological actions (oxytocic, avian depressor, milk-ejecting, mammalian pressor, mammalian antidiuretic) and there has been considerable debate on how many substances should be held responsible for these actions. Since the recent isolation, chemical identification and synthesis of vasopressin and oxytocin by DU VIGNEAUD and his group (cf. DU VIGNEAUD[684], VAN DYKE et al.[685]) it appears that all the named actions can be accounted for by these two substances. Up to recently it has, however, been questioned whether they can be independently secreted, since the content of both of them in the neurohypophyseal tissues have generally been found to change more or less in parallel in response to various stimuli which cause a release. As pointed out by VAN DYKE et al. this phenomenon need not indicate a parallel release of both hormones, but may very well be explained on the basis that the release and increased production of one of them depletes the neurohypophyseal system of a common precursor, which in term leads to decreased production of the other (or even a reversal of its process of formation ?). There are, however, also other experiments which indicate that vasopressin and oxytocin may not be released quite independently. For instance it has been observed by ABRAHAMS and PICKFORD[686] that uterine activity occurs in conscious dogs upon intracarotic (or intravenous) injection of hypertonic sodium chloride solutions, a stimulus generally considered specific for vasopressin release.

As late as 1953, HILD and ZETLER[687] have suggested that the vasopressor and the antidiuretic actions are caused by two different substances, since they found somewhat different ratios between these activities in extracts from different parts of the neurohypophyseal system. VAN DYKE et al. were, however, unable to confirm these findings, and attributed them to the use of inadequate bioassay procedures.

Vasopressin (antidiuretic hormone, ADH, β-hypophamine). *Renal action.* It is generally accepted that the variations in the release of this substance is a factor of the greatest importance to the regulation of the sodium concentration of plasma. As already discussed in a previous section (p. 243) this effect of the hormone must be attributed to an ability to increase the permeability to water in some part of the tubular system, which at least includes the distal segments. In the absence of an impact of the hormone on the kidney, these tubular cells become more or less impermeable to water, thus allowing the tubular fluid to become markedly hypotonic during the reabsorption of solutes ("water diuresis"). It seems reasonable to assume that the tubular cells do not become completely impermeable to water even if vasopressin is completely lacking; if so, the time factor becomes important, and it might be expected that when the rate of urine flow is reduced by other means, as for instance a reduction in the glomerular propulsive pressure, there would be less tendency to formation of hypotonic urine even in cases of complete diabetes insipidus. If the urinary concentrating process (cf. p. 244) is not dependent upon neurohypophyseal activity even hypertonic

[684] VIGNEAUD, V. DU: Hormones of the posterior pituitary gland: oxytocin and vasopressin. Harvey Lect. **50**, 1—26 (1954—1955).

[685] DYKE, H. B. VAN, K. ADAMSON, jr., and S. L. ENGEL: Aspects of the biochemistry and physiology of the neurohypophyseal hormones. Recent Progr. Hormone Res. **11**, 1 (1955).

[686] ABRAHAMS, V. C., and M. PICKFORD: Simultaneous observations on the rate of urine flow and spontaneous uterine movements in the dog, and their relationship to posterior lobe activity. J. Physiol. **126**, 329—346 (1954).

[687] HILD, W., u. G. ZETLER: Experimenteller Beweis für die Entstehung der sog. Hypophysenhinterlappenwirkstoffe im Hypothalamus. Pflügers Arch. ges. Physiol. **257**, 169 (1953).

urines might be formed in these cases; this might possibly account for the fact that SHANNON[688] has observed the formation of hypertonic urine during dehydration in dogs which apparently had been deprived of all vasopressin-forming tissue.

It is not known in how large a part of the tubular system vasopressin exerts an effect on the water permeability. According to the view most commonly held the action is limited to the distal section. There is, however, no convincing evidence for this view. Actually it is based entirely on the fact that maximal water diuresis amounts to some 15% of the simultaneous filtration rate and that WALKER et al. in their micropuncture experiments found evidence that some 80—85% of the filtered fluid is reabsorbed in the proximal tubules. The complementarity of these figures may well be fortuitous, and at present it is only possible to say that vasopressin exerts this effect on the distal segments and that it may or may not do it in the proximal segments.

It has previously been pointed out that a change in water reabsorption which occurs in the distal parts of the tubules will cause less change in other renal functions than a similar change occurring at a more proximal site. This follows from the fact the glomerular propulsive pressure required to drive 1 ml/min of fluid through the entire nephron does not differ so much from that required to drive it to a distal site of reabsorption as from that required to take it down to a proximal site. Nevertheless, if other tubular conditions remained unchanged the cessation of a distal reabsorption of water (as it occurs in water diuresis when the titer of vasopressin falls in the blood) would mean that a somewhat higher propulsive pressure would be needed for each ml of fluid that is filtered. If the glomerular propulsive pressure also remained unchanged a certain drop in filtration rate would occur, and since less sodium would thereby be presented to the tubules, it might also be expected that there should be a reduction in sodium excretion (assuming the rate of sodium reabsorption to remain unchanged).

How large changes in filtration rate could be expected on going from vasopressin antidiuresis to water diuresis (or *visa versa*) depends on what fractions of the total hydrodynamic resistance of the nephron are located proximal and distal to the site of action of vasopressin. If one assumes that the propulsion of 1 ml of fluid/min from the site of action of vasopressin to the renal pelvis requires only one-fourth of the pressure required for propulsion of 1 ml/min through the entire nephron it follows that a rise in urine flow from 1 to 17 ml/min (in a human subject) could only be expected to be associated with a fall in filtration rate of some 4 ml/min. Such small changes in filtration rate can obviously not be demonstrated with certainty. The corresponding changes in the rate of sodium excretion, amounting to a few per cent of the rate at which sodium is normally filtered would, however, be easily detectable. If vasopressin increases the cell permeability to water not only in the distal tubular segments, but also in the proximal tubules a greater change in filtration rate and thus in sodium excretion might be expected. Whether vasopressin acts in the proximal tubules too is not known, but the fact that ROSENBAUM[689] found water diureses above 30 ml/min in subjects treated with cortisone would seem to demand either such an action of vasopressin, or that the rate of distal reabsorption of sodium becomes as high as one-fourth of the normal rate of sodium filtration under the influence of cortisone therapy.

[688] SHANNON, J. A.: The control of the renal excretion of water. I. The effect of variations in the state of hydration on water excretion in dogs with diabetes insipidus. J. exp. Med. **76**, 371—386 (1942).

[689] ROSENBAUM, J. D., R. K. DAVIS, and B. C. FERGUSON: The influence of cortisone on water diuresis in man. J. clin. Invest. **30**, 668 (1952).

The question if and how vasopressin influences the rate of sodium (and chloride) excretion has been the subject of a very extensive literature. It seems reasonable to defer the discussion of the chaos of older reports a little, and to refer first to a few informative studies. SHANNON[690] and ANSLOW et al.[691] have found that administration of pitressin at a rate just sufficient to cause maximal antidiuresis in *hydrated* dogs (10—20 mU/hr) generally causes a significant increase in sodium and chloride excretion without detectable changes in the filtration rate. It appears that these *acute* changes in the rates of excretion of sodium and chloride, which only amounted to at most 2% of the rates at which they were filtered are most reasonably explained as suggested above. It is not unlikely, however, that the response is somewhat reduced by other effects of the vasopressin such as vascular actions causing changes in glomerular capillary pressure and changes in tubular cell volumes secondary to the changes in water permeability. Another factor possibly counteracting a natriuresis could be an increased distal reabsorption of sodium which might result from an increased epithelial permeability to ions accompanying the increased water permeability induced by vasopressin. (Compare Part I, p. 128 for such effects of vasopressin observed in the amphibian skin.) If vasopressin has also a proximal action, the assumption of such counter-balancing actions would be particularly required to account for the fact that this hormone has only a very moderate natriuretic effect. It was emphasized by ANSLOW et al. that doses of pitressin as those mentioned above were without effect on sodium and chloride excretion in non-hydrated normal dogs, a finding for which they suggested the plausible explanation that the tubules were already exposed to endogenous vasopressin in concentrations causing near-maximal antidiuresis.

The effect of prolonged administration of antidiuretic doses of vasopressin on sodium and chloride excretion has rather recently been carefully studied by LEAF et al.[692]. 10 subjects, including besides normal adults also cases of panhypopituitarism and diabetes insipidus, received a constant diet and fluid at various levels. Pitressin tannate in oil, 1 unit every 12 hr, was given over a period of 2 to 4 days to ensure continuous antidiuretic effect. If the fluid intake was made so high that a marked water retention occurred, a pronounced and progressive increase in sodium and chloride excretion occurred (although the serum concentrations were falling) whereas no significant change in these excretions were observed when the fluid intake was restricted. The authors therefore drew the reasonable conclusion that the increased loss of sodium and chloride in the first case was not caused by a direct effect of vasopressin, but by some homeostatic mechanism responding to the expansion of the body fluids. (Renal vasodilatation and reduced aldosterone secretion must be thought of, cf. p. 369 and p. 312). Similar findings were reported by WESTON et al. [693], by WRONG[694] and by LEVINSKY et al.[753]).

[690] SHANNON, J. A.: The control of the renal excretion of water. II. Rate of liberation of posterior pituitary antidiuretic hormone in the dog. J. exp. Med. **76**, 387—399 (1942).

[691] ANSLOW, W. P., jr., L. G. WESSON, jr., A. A. BOLOMEY, and J. G. TAYLOR: Chloruretic action of pressor-antidiuretic fraction of posterior pituitary extract. Fed. Proc. **7**, 3—4 (1948).

[692] LEAF, A., F. C. BARTTER, R. F. SANTOS, and O. WRONG: Evidence in man that urinary electrolyte loss induced by pitressin is a function of water retention. J. clin. Invest. **32**, 868—878 (1953).

[693] WESTON, R. E., I. B. HANENSON, J. GROSSMAN, G. A. BERDASCO, and M. WOLFMAN: Natriuresis and chloruresis following pitressin-induced water retention in non-edematous patients: Evidence of a homeostatic mechanism regulating body fluid volume. J. clin. Invest. **32**, 611 (1953).

[694] WRONG, O.: The relationship between water retention and electrolyte excretion following administration of anti-diuretic hormone. Clin. Sci. **15**, 401—408 (1956).

The literature on the effect of posterior pituitary preparations on the renal excretion of sodium and chloride is very contradictory. Although reports on a natriuretic or chloruretic effect are probably in the majority, several authors have reported either no effects or even reductions in chloride (or sodium) excretion. Several factors — including those already mentioned above — must be taken into consideration in the evaluation of these apparent discrepancies:

1) Different preparations were used, whole extracts as well as fractions thereof. Thus other pituitary substances may have interfered to a variable extent. It should be recalled in this connection that oxytocin has been found — at least when administered subcutaneously to rats — to cause diuresis and natriuresis (cf. p. 353).

2) Different dosages were used. It is well-known that vasopressin in larger doses has profound effects on the circulatory system, causing not only constriction in the peripheral capillaries and arterioles, but also a coronary vasoconstriction. Thus increases or decreases in arterial blood pressure may be obtained, depending on the dosage used and the preceeding state of the experimental subjects. I should be recalled that an increase in blood pressure is most likely to occur in anaesthetized subjects. An effect on glomerular capillary pressure through a direct vasoconstrictor action on the renal vessels must also be considered.

3) In some cases hydrated subjects were used, in others non-hydrated (cf. the discussion above). 4) Urine was collected over widely different periods. With short periods the dead space of the urinary tract may have lead to false results, while transient changes in the excretion must have escaped detection when very long collection periods were used. 5) In several long lasting experiments precautions were not taken to ensure a constant intake of salt (large variations in the amount of water drunk may represent considerable differences in salt intake).

It has been suggested that an antagonism between sodium-retaining corticosteroids and a natriuretic factor (probably vasopressin) from the neurohypophysis should be of great importance to the regulation of the body contents of sodium and chloride (cf. GAUNT et al.[628] and discussion on p. 334). It has even been suggested (ROEMMELT et al.[574]; SARTORIUS and ROBERTS[695]) that the renal loss of sodium in adrenocortical insufficiency should be due to unopposed and increased action of the neurohypophyseal factor. In the writer's opinion the natriuretic action, which can be exerted by vasopressin under certain conditions, is solely secondary to its water-retaining effect (or to vascular effects when larger doses are given). It is utterly unlikely that such an accidental action could serve as an important link in a vital regulation. The fact that animals and human subjects with diabetes insipidus do not reveal any notable signs of disturbances in the electrolyte metabolism if an adequate water intake is provided clearly indicates that vasopressin (and the neurohypophysis as a whole) can be of only minor importance for the regulation of sodium and chloride excretion. On the whole it appears that the question of whether vasopressin can act as a natriuretic has received much greater attention than it deserves. Consequently, the voluminous literature will only be very briefly reviewed here.

A definite reduction in chloride (and sodium) excretions has mostly been observed in patients with diabetes insipidus during prolonged treatment with posterior pituitary preparations (WEIR et al.[696]; SMITH and MACKAY[697]; THORN and STEIN[698]). The criticism 5) mentioned above applies to these studies.

---

[695] SARTORIUS, O. W., and K. ROBERTS: The effects of pitressin and desoxycorticosterone in low dosage on the excretion of sodium potassium and water by normal dog. Endocrinology 45, 273—283 (1949).

[696] WEIR, J. F., E. E. LARSEN, and L. G. ROWNTREE: Studies in diabetes insipidus, water balance and water intoxication. Arch. int. Med. 29, 306—330 (1922).

Several authors have failed to observe any significant change in sodium and chloride excretions following the administration of posterior pituitary preparations, even when an unmistakable antidiuresis was obtained.

In normal human subjects, doses of pituitrin which caused marked reduction in the diuresis in a 6 hr period produced no significant changes in the excretion of sodium, chloride, potassium and nitrogen (DANIEL and HÖGLER[699]). Similar results, as regards sodium and chloride, were obtained by ROBERT[700] who used both pituitrin and a vasopressin fraction and 8 hr urine collecting periods. LAVIETIES et al.[701] found no consistent changes in the 24 hr balance or in the 24 hr excretion of sodium and chloride in two patients with diabetes insipidus receiving doses of pituitrin with marked antidiuretic effect. A lack of effect on sodium and chloride excretions has also been observed in acute experiments. Thus, CHALMERS et al.[702] found virtually no change in chloride excretion when 1 mU of pitressin was administered intravenously to normal, hydrated human subjects, and doses of 20—100 mU intravenously generally caused a decrease in sodium and chloride excretion, and never an increase. 1 mU of pitressin per kg of body weight administered intravenously markedly reduced water diuresis in normal subjects, but had no consistent effect on sodium and chloride excretions (MURPHY[703]); similar results were obtained by 0.57 mU/kg by WHITE et al.[704], whereas NELSON and WELT[705] found that the usual response to total intravenous doses of 2.5 to 100 mU was a small reduction in sodium and chloride excretion. HARE et al.[706] found that pitressin was without effect on chloride excretion in diabetes insipidus dogs both under normal conditions and when 2.5% sodium chloride was constantly infused at a high rate.

Besides the studies referred to above, small increases in sodium or chloride excretions immediately following the administration of small doses of pitressin or pituitrin has been reported by BARCLAY et al.[707] and LADD[708] in human subjects and by SARTORIUS and ROBERTS[695] in dogs.

[697] SMITH, F. M., and E. M. MACKAY: Influence of posterior pituitary extracts on sodium balance in normal subject and patient with diabetes insipidus. Proc. Soc. exp. Biol. (N. Y.) 34, 116—118 (1936).

[698] THORN, G. W., and K. E. STEIN: Pitressin tannate therapy in diabetes insipidus. J. clin. Endocr. 1, 680—687 (1941).

[699] DANIEL, J., u. F. HÖGLER: Über die Diuresehemmung durch pituitrinum infundibulare (Infundibulin). Wien. Arch. inn. Med. 13, 481—508 (1927).

[700] ROBERT, F.: Über die Einwirkung von Hypophysin und seinen Fraktionen auf den Wasser-Salzstoffwechsel. Naunyn-Schmiedebergs Arch. exp. Path. Pharmak. 164, 367—382 (1932).

[701] LAVIETIES, P. H., L. M. D'ESOPO, and H. E. HARRISON: The water and base balance of the body. J. clin. Invest. 14, 251—265 (1935).

[702] CHALMERS, T. M., A. A. G. LEWIS, and G. L. S. PAWAN: The effect of posterior pituitary extracts on the renal excretion of sodium and chloride in man. J. Physiol. 112, 238—242 (1951).

[703] MURPHY, R. J. F.: Studies on the mechanisms of saline diuresis. J. clin. Invest. 29, 836 (1950).

[704] WHITE, A. G., G. RUBIN, and L. LEITER: Studies in edema. III. The effect of pitressin on the renal excretion of water and electrolytes in patients with and without liver disease. J. clin. Invest. 30, 1287—1297 (1951).

[705] NELSON, W. P., and L. G. WELT: The effect of pitressin on the metabolism and excretion of water and electrolytes in normal subject and patients with cirrhosis. J. clin. Invest. 31, 392—400 (1952).

[706] HARE, R. S., K. HARE, and D. M. PHILLIPS: The renal excretion of chloride by the normal and by the diabetes insipidus dog. Amer. J. Physiol. 140, 334—348 (1943—1944).

[707] BARCLAY, J. A., R. A. KENNEY, and M. E. NUTT: Effects of pituitrin and exercise on a water diuresis. J. appl. Physiol. 1. 609—613 (1949).

[708] LADD, M.: Renal excretion of sodium and water in man as affected by prehydration, saline infusion, pitressin and thiomerin. J. appl. Physiol. 4, 602—619 (1952).

The more pronounced increases in sodium and chloride excretions observed in dogs following the administration of larger doses of pituitrin (STEHLE[709]; UNNA and WALTERSKIRCHEN[710]) which were associated with a *diuretic* effect in animals not previously hydrated are probably due to an increase in arterial blood pressure or to oxytocin present in the pituitrin.

The increased excretions of sodium and chloride following *repeated* injections of pitressin to human subjects (MANCHESTER[711]; SMITH and MACKAY[712]) are probably of similar nature as those observed by LEAF et al. and WESTON et al. (vide supra).

The rate of secretion of vasopressin and its regulation. The rate of secretion of vasopressin has been evaluated by determining the rate at which the hormone must be administered by continuous intravenous infusion to cause graded antidiuresis. SHANNON[690] found that 1 to 5 mU/hr were required in diabetes insipidus dogs weighing 10 to 15 kg. In man an estimate of 7.5 to less than 50 mU/hr was reached by LAUSON[713]. 1 mU corresponds to about 1.7 mμg of pure hormone.

It is now generally agreed that some factor closely related to the total osmotic pressure of plasma serves as a major stimulus to the production of vasopressin by the neurohypophysis. Knowledge of the nature of this stimulus and the localization of the receptors has primarily been gained by a series of experiments performed by VERNEY and associates in dogs (for a review cf. VERNEY[714], THORN[235]). Injection of hypertonic solutions of sodium chloride, sodium sulphate or sucrose into the carotid artery was shown to inhibit water diuresis in doses which when given intravenously had no noticeable effect. Similarly no or very little antidiuretic effect was observed when the internal carotid artery had previously been ligated or the posterior pituitary lobe removed. From these observations the conclusion was drawn that the receptors are localized within the region supplied by the internal carotid artery. Hypertonic solutions of glucose were found to be less effective, and hypertonic solutions of urea had virtually no antidiuretic effect. This is assumed to be due to a greater permeability of the receptors to these substances than to those mentioned above. Thus the stimulus is considered to be an increase in the plasma concentrations of such substances and ions to which the receptors are virtually impermeable, and it is customary to speak of an effective osmotic pressure as the adequate stimulus. Under normal conditions this will mainly be made up of sodium and associated anions. The receptors are usually referred to as osmoreceptors, and although the exact localization has no yet been definitely proved they are generally believed to be the supraoptic and paraventricular neurones themselves which are characterized by a vesiculated structure (JEWELL[715]) and a rich blood

[709] STEHLE, R. L.: The diuretic-antidiuretic action of pituitary extract. Amer. J. Physiol. **79**, 289—296 (1927).

[710] UNNA, K., u. L. WALTERSKIRCHEN: Über den Zusammenhang zwischen Chlorid und Wasserausscheidung nach Pituitrin. Naunyn-Schmiedebergs Arch. exp. Path. Pharmak. **181**, 681—688 (1936).

[711] MANCHESTER, R. C.: Influence of posterior pituitary extracts on mineral and water exchange in children. Proc. Soc. exp. Biol. (N. Y.) **29**, 717—719 (1932).

[712] SMITH, F. M., and E. M. MACKAY: Influence of posterior pituitary extracts on sodium balance in normal subject and patient with diabetes insipidus. Proc. Soc. exp. Biol. (N. Y.) **34**, 116—118 (1936).

[713] LAUSON, H. O.: The problem of estimating the rate of secretion of antidiuretic hormone in man. Amer. J. Med. **11**, 135—156 (1951).

[714] VERNEY, E. B.: The antidiuretic hormone and the factors which determine its release. Proc. roy. Soc., London. Ser. B **135**, 25 (1947).

[715] JEWELL, P. A.: The occurrence of vesiculated neurones in the hypothalamus of the dog. J. Physiol. **121**, 167—181 (1953).

supply. DINGMAN[615], on the other hand, has suggested the posterior pituitary lobe to be the site of the osmoreceptors.

The ability of an increase in effective osmotic pressure to cause a release of vasopressin has been used by HICKEY and HARE[716] to test the functional capacity of the neurohypophysis. In patients with true diabetes insipidus injection of hypertonic saline causes no decrease in an existing water diuresis. Normal subjects and patients with polyuria due to primary polydipsia respond, however, with a considerable decrease in diuresis. Various modifications of the Hickey-Hare test have been proposed, cf. for instance WELT[717]).

It has become increasingly clear in recent years that the tonicity of the body fluids is by no means the only factor regulating the secretion of vasopressin.

BIRCHARD et al.[718] infused 1 l of 2% sodium chloride over a period of one hour in normal adults, and one hour after the completion of the infusion one litre of water was given to drink. Approximately one hour after the drinking of water the urine flow increased 2 to 4-fold, accompanied by a fall in urinary sodium concentration to 91 meq/l or lower. Since this "water diuresis" was obtained at a time when the plasma sodium concentrations were still above or equal to those observed in the initial oliguric periods it clearly indicated that factors other than the level of extracellular fluid tonicity are important determinants of water excretion. In the discussion reference is made to earlier related observations by BALDES and SMIRK, BAIRD and HALDANE, and H. W. SMITH. The first-mentioned authors suggested that *changes* in osmotic pressure rather than its absolute magnitude determined the onset of the diuresis. While this may play a certain role it seems more likely that an increase in the plasma volume has been the main factor responsible for the reduced secretion of vasopressin, as was also suggested by H. W. SMITH.

Further evidence that the plasma volume or rather the degree of filling of the cardiovascular system influences the secretion of vasopressin has come from other types of experiments. Several authors have reported that infusion (or ingestion) of a large volume of *isotonic* saline (or Locke's solution) may induce an increased flow of dilute urine (WESSON et al.[719]; BLOMHERT[720]; BLOMHERT et al.[721]; LADD[722]; STRAUSS et al.[723]). BLOMHERT reported that there are two phases of the diuretic response: a large flow of dilute urine in the first 1½ hr followed by a mild saline diuresis (cf. also WESSON et al.). STRAUSS et al. found that "water diuresis" could only be produced in recumbent, not in quitely seated subjects, by 1 to 2 l of

[716] HICKEY, R., and K. HARE: The renal excretion of chloride and water in diabetes insipidus. J. clin. Invest. 23, 768—775 (1944).

[717] WELT, L. G.: Clinical disorders of hydration and acid-base equilibrium. London: J. & A. Churchill. 1955.

[718] BIRCHARD, W. H., J. D. ROSENBAUM, and M. B. STRAUSS: Renal excretion of salt and water consequent to hypertonic saline infusion followed by water ingestion. J. appl. Physiol. 6, 22—26 (1953).

[719] WESSON, L. G., jr., W. P. ANSLOW, jr., L. G. RAISZ, A. A. BOLOMEY, and M. LADD: Effect of sustained expansion of extracellular fluid volume upon filtration rate, renal plasma flow and electrolyte and water excretion in the dog. Amer. J. Physiol. 162, 677—686 (1950).

[720] BLOMHERT, G.: Over de zogenaamde Waterdiurese. Thesis. Amsterdam: Scheltema & Holkema. 1951.

[721] BLOMHERT, G. J., GERBRANDY, J. A. MOLHUYSEN, L. A. DE VRIES, and J. G. G. BORST: Diuretic effect of isotonic saline solution compared with that of water. Influence of diurnal rhythm. Lancet 1951 II, 1011—1015.

[722] LADD, M.: The effect of prehydration on the response to saline infusion in man. J. appl. Physiol. 3, 379—387 (1950).

[723] STRAUSS, M. B., R. K. DAVIS, J. D. ROSENBAUM, and E. C. ROSSMEISL: „Water diuresis" produced during recumbency by the intravenous infusion of isotonic saline solution. J. clin. Invest. 30, 862—868 (1951).

isotonic saline. In a later publication (BIRCHARD and STRAUSS[724]) this finding was confirmed in normally hydrated subjects, but a prompt water diuresis was obtained in seated subjects who had ingested an excess of salt on the preceeding day (and whose extracellular fluid volume was presumably already expanded). "Water diuresis" has also been produced by expansion of the plasma volume by iso-oncotic solutions in saline (WELT and ORLOFF[725]).

It appears then that expansion of the plasma volume can suppress the secretion of vasopressin when there is no decrease (or even an increase) in effective osmotic pressure. As a counterpart various cases are known in which a decrease in blood volume or a redistribution of the blood is accompanied by an antidiuresis at normal body fluid tonicity or even in the face of a subnormal tonicity. Thus an accumulation of blood in the legs, produced by the assumption of the passive erect posture (BRUN et al.[726]) or by tourniquets on the thighs (WILKINS et al.[727]) in subjects undergoing water diuresis, has been found to cause a decrease in diuresis out of proportion to the reduction in salt excretion. The fact that the response is slight in patients with diabetes insipidus indicates that a release of vasopressin is mainly responsible for the antidiuresis in normal subjects (cf. also NOBLE and TAYLOR[728]). It is quite likely that a similar mechanism of vasopressin release is operating in a number of other conditions in which a diminution of the plasma volume (and the extracellular fluid volume) is a feature: haemorrhage, sodium depletion and dehydration with hyponatronaemia (LEAF and MAMBY[729]). How the antidiuretic substance(s) which has been observed in serum and urine in these cases (and several others with impaired circulation) is related to vasopressin is not yet clear. It should be recalled that the antidiuresis observed under these conditions is certainly not caused exclusively by the action of vasopressin and other substances with a selective action on water reabsorption. As discussed elsewhere (p. 369 and 312) the same conditions may also cause a marked reduction in the renal excretion of sodium, in part at least related to a reduction in renal blood flow, and this mechanism will obviously also produce a fall in urine flow.

It may be concluded that there exists a number of conditions, characterized by a change in blood volume or its distribution, in which factors other than the tonicity of the body fluids prove to be of importance in the regulation of the production of vasopressin. Since the new stimulus is apparently somehow related to the filling of some part of the cardiovascular system the phenomenon is often described by saying that a compromise is reached in which osmoregulation is sacrificed for volume regulation. It is probably more correct to say that there is a change in the relative importance of the two stimuli. Under conditions of sodium depletion the volume factor must be assumed to gain increasing importance and

[724] BIRCHARD, W. H., and M. B. STRAUSS: Factors influencing the diuretic response of seated subjects to the ingestion of isotonic saline solution. J. clin. Invest. **32**, 807—812 (1953).

[725] WELT, L. G., and J. ORLOFF: The effects of an increase in plasma volume on the metabolism and excretion of water and electrolytes by normal subjects. J. clin. Invest. **30**, 751—761 (1951).

[726] BRUN, C., E. O. E. KNUDSEN, and F. RAASCHOU: The influence of posture on the kidney function. I. The fall in diuresis in the erect posture. Acta med. scand. **122**, 315—331 (1945).

[727] WILKINS, R. W., C. M. TINSLEY, J. W. CULBERTSON, B. A. BURROWS, W. E. JUDSON, and C. H. BURNETT: The effects of venous congestion of the limbs upon renal clearances and the excretion of water and salt. I. Studies in normal subjects and in hypertensive patients before and after splanchnicectomy. J. clin. Invest. **32**, 1101—1116 (1953).

[723] NOBLE, R. L., and N. B. G. TAYLOR: Antidiuretic substances in human urine after haemorrhage, fainting, dehydration and acceleration. J. Physiol. **122**, 220—237 (1953).

[729] LEAF, A., and A. R. MAMBY: An antiuretic mechanism not regulated by extracellular fluid tonicity. J. clin. Invest. **31**, 60—71 (1952).

a new steady state will not be reached before some hyponatronaemia has developed. A mechanism of this sort would seem to be involved in the hyponatraemia observed both in cases of absolute sodium deficiency (Addison's disease, the "asymptomatic hyponatraemia" observed in some cases of pulmonary or debilitating disease (cf. Sims et al.[730]; Harrison et al.[731]) and other more common sodium-losing conditions) and in cases where there exists only a relative sodium deficiency (patients with congestive heart failure treated with a low sodium diet and/or natriuretics, but still oedematous; cf. Rubin and Braveman[732]).

Knowledge of the location and characteristics of the volume-sensitive receptors has only been gained very recently. Breathing against a positive pressure was found by Drury et al.[733] to cause antidiuresis, and negative pressure breathing has been demonstrated to evoke an increase in urine flow with little effect on the electrolyte excretions (Gauer et al.[734]; Gauer et al.[735]; Sieker et al.[736]). Since positive pressure breathing is associated with a decrease in intrathoracic blood volume and negative pressure breathing with an increase, the conclusion was tentatively drawn that the receptors are located somewhere in the walls of the pulmonary vessels or the heart. Further studies (Henry et al.[737]) have led to the conclusion that stretch receptors in the left atrium and/or terminal pulmonary veins are responsible for the "water diuresis" observed during negative pressure breathing. This conclusion was based on the fact that a diuresis could be produced by expanding the left atrium with a balloon, but not by distension of the pulmonary arterial tree (injection of plastic beads) or the entire pulmonary circulation (snares on the pulmonary veins). Other recent studies have characterized the discharge of the receptors in the left vago-sympathetic trunk of dogs, and it has been shown that manoeuvres which cause diuresis (distension of the left atrium with a balloon, negative pressure breathing and expansion of the blood volume with isotonic solutions) each cause a discharge in these fibres, whereas small haemorrhages decrease the activity (Henry and Pearce[738]).

Whether the atrial receptors are the only volume receptors involved in the control of the production of vasopressin is obviously not known. It appears, however, that they suffice to explain most of the changes in diuresis mentioned above. It is quite possible that an activation or inactivation of these receptors also plays a role in the diureses and antidiureses produced by a number of other factors which affect the circulatory system and thus may cause changes in the filling of the

---

[730] Sims, E. A. H., L. G. Welt, J. Orloff, and J. W. Needham: Asymptomatic hyponatremia in pulmonary tuberculosis. J. clin. Invest. 29, 1545—1557 (1950).

[731] Harrison, H. E., L. Finberg, and E. Fleischman: Disturbances of ionic equilibrium of intracellular and extracellular electrolytes in patients with tuberculous meningitis. J. clin. Invest. 31, 300—308 (1952).

[732] Rubin, A. L., and W. S. Braveman: Treatment of the low-salt syndrome in congestive heart failure by the controlled use of mercurial diuretics. Circulation 13, 655—663 (1956).

[733] Drury, D. R., J. P. Henry, and J. Goodman: The effects of continuous pressure breathing on kidney function. J. clin. Invest. 26, 945—951 (1947).

[734] Gauer, O. H., J. P. Henry, H. O. Sieker, and W. E. Wendt: Heart and lungs as a receptor region controlling blood volume. Amer. J. Physiol. 167, 786—787 (1951).

[735] Gauer, O. H., J. P. Henry, H. O. Sieker, and W. E. Wendt: The effect of negative pressure breathing on urine flow. J. clin. Invest. 33, 287—296 (1954).

[736] Sieker, H. O., O. H. Gauer, and J. P. Henry: The effect of continuous negative pressure breathing on water and electrolyte excretion by the human kidney. J. clin. Invest. 33, 572—577 (1954).

[737] Henry, J. P., O. H. Gauer, and J. L. Reeves: Evidence of the atrial location of receptors influencing urine flow. Circulation Res. 4, 85—90 (1956).

[738] Henry, J. P., and J. W. Pearce: The possible role of cardiac atrial stretch receptors in the induction of changes in urine flow. J. Physiol. 131, 572—585 (1956).

left atrium. A mechanism of this type must for instance be considered in relation to the diuresis produced by exposure to cold (cf. BADER et al.[739]; BASS[740]), and by administration of small doses of epinephrine.

The release of vasopressin is unquestionably influenced in other ways than by the tonicity of the body fluids and the atrial receptors. Emotional stress may influence it in different ways (O'CONNOR[741], HINKLE et al.[742]), and coitus (FRIBERG[743]) and pain exert an antidiuretic action. Various drugs cause antidiuresis via the neurohypophysis: morphine (DE BODO[744]), barbiturates (DE BODO and PRESCOTT[745]) and nicotine (BURN et al.[746]); and acetylcholin has been shown to produce this effect directly in the supraoptic nuclei. Alcohol, on the other hand, inhibits the release of vasopressin from the neurohypophysis and thus causes "water diuresis". (EGGLETON[747], LAMDIN et al.[748]). Breathing 5 to 7% CO_2 has also been found to cause a "water diuresis" in recumbent but not in sitting subjects. (BARFOUR et al.[749]). For a further discussion of factors influencing vasopressin release cf. THORN[235].

Reference may be made at the end to the fact that *tubular unresponsiveness to vasopressin* is known not only as a manifestation of renal disease (cf. WHITE et al.[750]) but also as a congenital anomaly (DANCIS et al.[751]). The fact that desoxycortisosterone may reduce the sensitivity of the tubules to vasopressin is discussed elsewhere (p. 336). According to recent reports (cf. RELMAN and SCHWARTZ[1578]) chronic potassium depletion is characterized by hydropic and degenerative changes in the tubular system, confined chiefly to the convoluted tubules, and by a vasopressin-resistant hyposthenuria (and other signs of renal tubular impairment). Recently it has been reported that patients with severe hyperthyroidism may fail to respond with antidiuresis and increase in urine osmolarity to 2 to 15 units of vasopressin (WESTON et al.[752]).

[739] BADER, R. A., J. W. ELIOT, and D. E. BASS: Hormonal and renal mechanisms of cold diuresis. J. appl. Physiol. 4, 649—665 (1952).

[740] BASS, D. E.: Electrolyte excretion during cold diuresis. Fed. Proc. 13, 8 (1954).

[741] O'CONNOR, W. J.: The effect of section of the supraoptico-hypophyseal tracts on the inhibition of water-diuresis by emotional stress. Quart. J. exp. Physiol. 33, 149—161 (1946).

[742] HINKLE, L. E. jr., C. J. EDWARDS, and S. WOLF: The occurrence of diuresis in humans in stressful situations and its possible relation to the diuresis of early starvation. J. clin. Invest. 30, 809—817 (1951).

[743] FRIBERG, O.: Antidiuretic effect of coitus in human subjects. Acta endocr. (Kbh.) 12, 193—196 (1953).

[744] BODO, R. C. DE: The antidiuretic action of morphine and its mechanism. J. Pharmacol. exp. Ther. 82, 74—85 (1944).

[745] BODO, R. C. DE, and K. F. PRESCOTT: The antidiuretic action of barbiturates (phenobarbital, amytal, pentobarbital) and the mechanism involved in this action. J. Pharmacol. exp. Ther. 85, 222—233 (1945).

[746] BURN, J. H., L. H. TRUELOVE, and I. BURN: The antidiuretic action of nicotine and of smoking. Brit. med. J. 1945I, 403—406

[747] EGGLETON, M. G.: The diuretic action of alcohol in man. J. Physiol. 101, 172—191 (1942).

[748] LAMDIN, E., C. R. KLEEMAN, M. RUBINI, and F. H. EPSTEIN: Studies on alcohol diuresis. III. The response to ethyl alcohol in certain disease states characterized by impaired water tolerance. J. clin. Invest. 35, 386—393 (1956).

[749] BARFOUR, A., G. M. BULL, B. M. EVANS, N. C. HUGHES JONES, and J. LOGOTHETOPOULOS: The effect of breathing 5 to 7% carbon dioxide on urine flow and mineral excretion. Clin. Sci. 12, 1—13 (1953).

[750] WHITE, A. G., M. KURTZ, and G. RUBIN: Comparative renal response to water and antidiuretic hormone in diabetes insipidus and in chronic renal disease. Amer. J. Med. 16, 220—230 (1954).

[751] DANCIS, J., J. R. BIRMINGHAM, and S. H. LESLIE: Congenital diabetes insipidus resistant to treatment with pitressin. Amer. J. Dis. Child. 75, 316—328 (1948).

[752] WESTON, R. E., H. B. HOROWITZ, J. GROSSMAN, I. B. HANENSON, and L. LEITER: Decreased antidiuretic response to β-hypophamine in hyperthyreoidism. J. clin. Endocr. 16, 322—337 (1956).

LEVINSKY et al.[753] have recently reported that the urine osmolarity achieved after vasopressin administration is reduced after a long period of vasopressin and water administration to dogs. It is not, however, quite clear from their data whether this indicates that the concentrating capacity of the kidneys is reduced under such experimental conditions, since the negative free water clearances were not given and the rate of urine flow did rise considerably as a consequence of the treatment. While further details are needed, this report, and others, seem to indicate that, under conditions of hyperhydration, the concentrating machinery of the kidneys may somehow be interfered with. How, and at what level in the machinery (sodium pump of Henle's loop, water permeability of the tubules, equilibrium in the medullary countercurrent system) this occurs is not known.

Oxytocin. Following the observation that crude posterior lobe extracts sometimes evoked a diuretic-chloruretic response, the question obviously presented itself whether such effects were caused by vasopressin or some other substance(s) present in the extracts.

In 1937 the observation was made by FRASER[754] that subcutaneous injection of pituitary preparations with a high oxytocin/low vasopressin activity into rats caused a diuretic-chloruretic response not obtained by vasopressin in the amounts contained in the injected extract. It was further noted that this response was more pronounced in non-hydrated than in hydrated rats. These results were confirmed and extended in a later study (FRASER)[755]. From this it appears that in non-hydrated rats a parallel increase in 4-hr diuresis and chloride excretion occurred following the administration of 0.0001 to 1.0 units of oxytocin activity per 100 g rat. The response increased with the doses in this interval and with the higher doses some seven times as much water and chloride was excreted by the oxytocin-treated rats as by the controls in which a similar volume of saline had been injected.

FRASER's findings have been confirmed by several other authors who also used rats, thus by KUSCHINSKY and BUNDSCHUH[756] and recently by BRUNNER et al.[757]. A diuretic-chloruretic effect was also obtained with synthetic oxytocin by JACOBSON and KELLOGG[758] in rats in which a steady state diuresis was produced by intravenous infusion of 0.12 ml of saline per minute; vasopressin under similar conditions gave a smaller chloruretic — but antidiuretic — response. The two hormones were also tested following infusions of hypo- or hypertonic sodium chloride solutions, and in the former case oxytocin had no consistent chloruretic effect. SAWYER[759] observed a natriuretic (and kaliuretic) response when pitocin was administered subcutaneously to rats which were hydrated by 0.05 N sodium

[753] LEVINSKY, N. G., D. D. DAVIDSON, and R. W. BERLINER: Changes in urine concentration during prolonged administration of vasopressin and water. Amer. J. Physiol. **196**, 451—456 (1959).

[754] FRASER, A. M.: The diuretic action of the oxytocin hormone of the pituitary and its effect on the assay of pituitary extracts. J. Pharmacol. exp. Ther. **60**, 89—95 (1937).

[755] FRASER, A. M.: The action of the oxytocic hormone of the pituitary gland on urine secretion. J. Physiol. **101**, 236—251 (1942).

[756] KUSCHINSKY, G., u. H. E. BUNDSCHUH: Über eine diuretische und Kochsalz ausschwemmende Substanz in Hypophysenhinterlappen-Präparaten. Naunyn-Schmiedebergs Arch. exp. Path. Pharmak. **192**, 683—700 (1939).

[757] BRUNNER, H., G. KUSCHINSKY, O. MÜNCHOW, and G. PETERS: Der Einfluß von Oxytocin auf Diurese und Salzausscheidung bei Ratte und Mensch. Klin. Wschr. **34**, 451—452 (1956).

[758] JACOBSON, H. N., and R. H. KELLOGG: Isotonic NaCl diuresis in rats. Antidiuresis and chloruresis produced by posterior pituitary extracts. Amer. J. Physiol. **184**, 376—389 (1956).

[759] SAWYER, W. H.: Posterior pituitary extracts and excretion of electrolytes by the rat. Amer. J. Physiol. **169**, 583—587 (1952).

chloride, but he obtained almost identical responses with similar doses of pitressin (0.001 to 1 units per 100 g rat). Cf. also DICKER[760] for a recent report showing that pitocin increases the rate of urinary excretion of osmotically active substances in rats.

From the available literature it may safely be stated that oxytocin has a rather strong chloruretic (natriuretic ?) action when it is administered to non-hydrated rats, and that this effect is not duplicated by vasopressin. In rats under other experimental conditions the difference between oxytocin and vasopressin in regard to chloride (sodium) excretion is apparently less striking.

The nature of the chloruretic action of oxytocin is not yet clear. DICKER and HELLER[761] found that 0.003 mU of pitocin per 100 g rat, which caused an appreciable increase in urinary chloride excretion in hydrated rats also produced a significant increase in inulin and diodrast clearances (on an average about 100%), whereas pitressin in similar doses caused no consistent changes in any of these parameters. It is uncertain to what extent the increases in the two clearances following oxytocin administration may be explained as dead space errors. If, however, they are partly real, this finding would seem to indicate that oxytocin reduces renal vascular resistance, and the possibility must be considered that the oxytocin saluresis-diuresis is caused by an increase in glomerular propulsive pressure. In this connection it may also be relevant to refer to recent studies by DEMUNBRUN et al.[762]. They observed striking (30—40%) reductions in glomerular filtration rate and renal plasma flow in dogs following complete destruction of the neurohypophysis (and the adjoining ventral tuberal and ventral anterior hypothalamus). In these dogs which had diabetes insipidus (but no obvious signs of adenohypophyseal dysfunction) oxytocin (pitocin) was found to restore the depressed renal functions to normal, whereas vasopressin had no such effect.

With regard to a possible physiological role the possibility has been considered that oxytocin — by virtue of its saluretic action-might act as an antagonist to the sodium-retaining corticoids. As mentioned above the relationship between the secretion of vasopressin and oxytocin in response to various stimuli has not yet been clarified. It may be noted that a reciprocal relationship would tend to stabilize the rate of excretion of sodium under conditions of varying osmotic stimulation (cf. discussion p. 344).

e) Hormones of the pancreas

Insulin. There are no indications that insulin exerts any direct effect on the renal excretions of alkali metal ions. The great losses of sodium and potassium which accompany the development of diabetic coma are adequately explained as caused by (glucose, and ketone body) osmotic diuresis and activation of $Na^+ — K^+$ exchange mechanism by shrinkage of the extracellular and plasma volume.

Changes in the excretions of these ions which accompany administration of insulin are well accounted for as secondary to the internal shifts produced by insulin.

Glucagon. Recent developments have strengthened the concept that glucagon has a status as a hormone of significance in carbohydrate metabolism. — BROMER et al.[763] have found that this substance — a polypeptide chain of 29

[760] DICKER, S. E.: Urine concentration in the rat during acute and prolonged dehydration. J. Physiol. **139**, 108—122 (1957).

[761] DICKER, S. E., and H. HELLER: The renal action of posterior pituitary extract and its fractions as analysed by clearance experiments on rats. J. Physiol. **104**, 353—360 (1946).

[762] DEMUNBRUN, T. W., A. D. KELLER, A. H. LEVKOFF, and R. M. PURSER, jr.: Pitocin restoration of renal hemodynamics to pre-neurohypophysectomy levels. Amer. J. Physiol. **179**, 429—438 (1954).

[763] BROMER, W. W., L. G. SINN, A. STAUB, and O. K. BEHRENS: Amino acid sequence of glucagon. J. Amer. chem. Soc. **78**, 3858—3860 (1956).

amino acids — has a marked enhancing effect on the renal excretion of Na and K both in the anaesthetized and the conscious dog. The action appears to be independent of its hyperglycemic effect and seems to be due to a direct action on the kidney (STAUB et al.[764]). Studies in man have indicated the same effect (ELRICK et al.[765]).

f) Miscellaneous

Renin and hypertensin. PICKERING and PRINZMETAL[766] found that injections of renin cause a conspicuous and parallel rise in urine flow and sodium and chloride excretion in rabbits on a low as well as a high intake of sodium chloride. As judged from the data the increment in urine must have been nearly isotonic with plasma. No constant effects on filtration rate were observed. In a later study similar results were obtained with hypertensin (HUGHES-JONES et al.[767]) and here the additional observation was made that the diodrast clearance was always reduced (whereas no consistent changes in inulin clearance were observed). Very similar observations have been made in rats (cf. SELLERS et al.[768]). The investigators were apparently inclined to attribute the natriuresis and diuresis to a depression in the tubular reabsorption of sodium, chloride and water. It appears, however, that the results may equally well be explained on the basis of a primary vascular effect, as for instance by a preferential constriction of the vasa efferentia, leading to a reduction in renal blood flow, but an increase in glomerular propulsive pressure. CROXATTO et al.[769] have found that the diuretic effect of renin in rats is abolished by adrenalectomy or hypophysectomy and restored by cortisone and desoxycorticosterone. How these findings shall be interpreted is not clear. It appears that there is a species difference in the response to hypertensin since this substance has been found to cause a *decrease* in sodium excretion and diuresis in man (NICKEL et al.[770]); in this case there was also a reduction not only in renal plasma flow, but also in filtration rate.

Serotonin. The effects of serotonin on the kidney have recently been reviewed by PAGE[771]. Experiments on unanaesthetized dogs have shown that serotonin can reduce renal sodium excretion[772]. In man studies by SCHNECKLOTH et al.[773] and by HULET and PERERA[774] have indicated that serotonin reduces sodium output but increases the excretion of potassium. The mechanism of action is unknown.

---

[764] STAUB, A., V. SPRINGS, F. STOLL, and H. ELRICH: A renal action of glucagon. Proc. Soc. exp. Biol. (N. Y.) **94**, 57—60 (1957).

[765] ELRICK, H., E. R. HOFFMAN, C. J. HLAD, jr., N. WHIPPLE, and A. STAUB: Effects of glucagon on renal function in man. J. clin. Endocr. 18, 813—824 (1958).

[766] PICKERING, G. W., and M. PRINZMETAL: The effect of renin on urine formation. J. Physiol. 98, 314—335 (1940).

[767] HUGHES-JONES, N. C., G. W. PICKERING, P. H. SANDERSON, H. SCARBOROUGH, and J. VANDENBROUCKE: The nature of the action of renin and hypertensin on renal function in the rabbit. J. Physiol. 109, 288—307 (1949).

[768] SELLERS, A. L., S. SMITH, III, H. C. GOODMAN, and J. MARMORSTON: Effect of renin on excretion of sodium, chloride and water in the rat. Amer. J. Physiol. **166**, 619—624 (1951).

[769] CROXATTO, H., L. BARNAFI, L. CAMAZON, and V. PARRA: Some endocrine factors in the polyuric action of renin. Endocrinology 54, 239—248 (1954).

[770] NICKEL, J. F., C. McC. SMYTHE, E. M. PAPPER, and S. E. BRADLEY: A study of the mode of action of the adrenal medullary hormones on sodium, potassium and water excretion in man. J. clin. Invest. **33**, 1687—1699 (1954).

[771] PAGE, I. H.: Serotonin (5-hydroxytryptamine); the last four years. Physiol. Rev. **38**, 277—335 (1958).

[772] BLACKMORE, W. P.: Effect of serotonin on water and electrolyte excretion. Fed. Proc. **16**, 282—283 (1957).

[773] SCHNECKLOTH, R., I. H. PAGE, F. DEL GRECO, and A. C. CORCORAN: Effects of serotonin antagonists in normal subjects and patients with carcinoid tumors. Circulation 16, 523—532 (1957).

[774] HULET, W. H., and G. A. PERERA: Effect of serotonin on renal excretion of sodium; possible relation to rauwolfia action. Proc. Soc. exp. Biol. (N. Y.) **91**, 512—514 (1956).

I. Effect of the renal nerves and sympathicomimetic amines on sodium and potassium excretion

a) The renal nerves

The kidneys receive a very rich supply of vasoconstrictor fibers from the sympathetic nervous system. In contrast, there is no convincing evidence of renal vasodilator fibers from either the sympathetic system or the vagi. An innervation of the tubular cells is claimed by some to be present (cf. DE MUYLDER[775]).

For many years much discussion has centered around the questions whether the renal nerves exert any influence on the excretory functions of the kidney under "normal conditions", and whether the renal nerves have any direct effect upon the function of the tubular cells, in particular on their electrolyte transfer processes. It appears that the last question should be answered in the negative since the alterations in water and electrolyte excretions accompanying changes in renal innervation would seem to be well accounted for in terms of changes in the constriction of the renal vessel. Hypothetical influences directly on the tubular cells should only be resorted to if experimental observations are made which cannot be explained by other means. The question whether the renal nerves exert any influence on the excretion of water and electrolytes under normal resting conditions or only under conditions of anaesthesia, emotional stress, etc. can still not be answered unequivocally; different results have been obtained even in recent research.

The classical experimental design for evaluation of the influence of the renal nerves on the excretory functions has been to denervate one kidney and use the other as a control. This approach was introduced in 1859 by CLAUDE BERNARD who observed that section of the splanchnic nerves on one side caused an increased urine flow on the operated side. This phenomenon of "denervation diuresis" was confirmed by several authors in similar acute experiments (for references to the older literature, cf. MARSHALL and KOLLS[776], who confirmed the enhanced urine flow and, in addition, observed an increase in the rate of chloride excretion from denervated kidneys).

Experiments comprising surgical procedures and anaesthesia immediately before and during the observation period can, of course, only provide information on the effects of the renal nerves under such particular conditions, deviating from the normal state. This also applies to those experiments of MARSHALL and KOLLS (and later studies by KRISS et al.[777], also in dogs) where denervation had been performed some time before the observation period, but in which surgical exposure of the ureters for cannulation under anaesthesia immediately preceded the observation period. In such experiments a greater urine flow and chloride excretion from the denervated kidney was also observed by KRISS et al., who, in addition, reported the finding of a significantly greater paraaminohippurate (and mannitol) clearance. Very similar observations were made by KAPLAN and RAPOPORT[778]

[775] DE MUYLDER: The "neurility" of the kidney. Springfield, Ill.: Charles C. Thomas. 1952.

[776] MARSHALL, E. K., jr., and A. C. KOLLS: Studies on the nervous control of the kidney in relation to diuresis and urinary secretion. I. The effect of unilateral excision of the adrenal, section of the splanchnic nerve and section of the renal nerves on the secretion of the kidney. Amer. J. Physiol. 49, 302—316 (1919).

[777] KRISS, J. P., P. H. FUTCHER, and M. L. GOLDMAN: Unilateral adrenalectomy, unilateral splanchnic nerve resection and homolateral renal function. Amer. J. Physiol. 154, 229—240 (1948).

[778] KAPLAN, S. A., and S. RAPOPORT: Urinary excretion of sodium and chloride after splanchnicotomy; effect on the proximal tubule. Amer. J. Physiol. 164, 175—181 (1951).

and Kaplan et al.[779] in acute denervation experiments in dogs under anaesthesia; these authors also demonstrated that the urine flow as well as the rate of excretion of chloride, sodium and potassium (and the mannitol clearance) remained greater from the denervated kidney during diuresis induced by hypertonic solutions of sodium chloride or mannitol. In later studies Kaplan et al.[780] also demonstrated that the increased excretions of these electrolytes could be made to fall to or below the level on the intact side by electric stimulation of the cut end of the greater splanchnic nerve. Less consistent rises in urine flow and sodium excretion upon unilateral splanchnicectomy under pentobarbital anaesthesia has more recently been reported by Page et al.[781]; in only 12 of 17 acute experiments in dogs receiving hypertonic saline infusions were such changes observed.

If surgery and anaesthesia is to be avoided immediately prior to and during the urine collection periods one kidney must be denervated and the ureters exteriorized some time ahead of the observation period. Dogs have been prepared in this way by several authors in the last few years and observations have been made on them in the unanaesthetized state as well as during anaesthesia.

Different results were obtained as regards the existence of any differences in the rate of excretion of sodium and water on the two sides in unanaesthetized dogs under normal resting conditions. Kaplan et al.[780] observed significantly higher excretions of water, sodium and potassium on the denervated side under conditions of a moderate sodium chloride or mannitol diuresis, whereas Surtshin et al.[782], Berne[783] and Surtshin and Hoeltzenbein[784] failed to find any consistent differences in the rates at which sodium was excreted from the two sides under varying conditions (mild dehydration, "normal" state, water diuresis, and diuresis induced by sodium chloride loading). A few results reported by Page et al.[781]. are less clear-cut; these authors did not use exteriorization of the ureters, but only ureter catheters brought to the outside through incisions in the flanks. In three of five cases in which observations were made a day or more after denervation the sodium excretion was found to be greater on the denervated side in the unanaesthetized state (and under pentobarbital anaesthesia).

In contrast to the diverging views as regards the normal, resting state, it is generally agreed that various types of "stress" may cause the sodium and water excretions from the innervated kidney to decline considerably below the level of those from the denervated kidney. This phenomenon was recorded by Surtshin et al. when ether anaesthesia or deep (but not light) pentobarbital anaesthesia was induced in dogs with chronic, unilateral denervation. Berne observed a similar effect of pentobarbital anaesthesia, and also reported that during the anaesthesia the renal plasma flow (and the filtration rate) was statistically smaller in the

[779] Kaplan, S. A., S. J. Fomon, and S. Rapoport: Effect of splanchnic nerve division on urinary excretion of electrolytes during mannitol loading in the hydropenic dog. Amer. J. Physiol. 166, 641—648 (1951).
[780] Kaplan, S. A., C. D. West, and S. J. Fomon: Effects of unilateral division of splanchnic nerve on the renal excretion of electrolytes in unanesthetized and anesthetized dogs: The mechanism of "crossed stimulation". Amer. J. Physiol. 175, 363—374 (1953).
[781] Page, L. B., C. F. Baxter, G. H. Reem, J. C. Scott-Baker, and H. W. Smith: Effect of unilateral splanchnic nerve resection on the renal excretion of sodium. Amer. J. Physiol. 177, 194—200 (1954).
[782] Surtshin, A., B. Mueller, and H. L. White: Effects of acute changes in glomerular filtration rate on water and electrolyte excretion: Mechanisms of denervation diuresis. Amer. J. Physiol. 169, 159—173 (1952).
[783] Berne, R. M.: Hemodynamics and sodium excretion of denervated kidney in anesthetized and unanesthetized dog. Amer. J. Physiol. 171, 148—158 (1952).
[784] Surtshin, A., and J. Hoeltzenbein: Excretion of sodium and water by the denervated canine kidney. Amer. J. Physiol. 177, 44—48 (1954).

innervated kidney. He also made the observation that emotional stress caused some diminution not only in urine flow (as was known from experiments of VERNEY and associates, cf. O'CONNOR[785]) but also in sodium excretion, filtration rate and renal plasma flow on the innervated side. Painful stimuli were found by SURTSHIN et al. to reduce the sodium excretion, renal plasma flow and filtration rate of the innervated kidney.

From this survey of the literature it is apparent that it cannot yet be definitely stated whether the renal nerves exert any depressing effect on the renal excretion of sodium in the normal state, but it may be considered as well-established that they may do so under various states of "stress". It is further apparent that in those cases where such measurements were undertaken, the renal plasma flow (and the filtration rate) tended to fall in the innervated kidney upon exposure to the "stress" situation. Such observations offer some support of the view that differences in renal vascular tone are responsible for the differences in sodium (and water) excretion which have been observed between denervated and innervated kidneys. This interpretation, which conforms with CLAUDE BERNARD's original proposal, has also been accepted by most of the authors who have recently worked in this field with the exception of KAPLAN and his group. According to the views previously discussed (p. 262) such changes in renal vascular tone must be assumed to cause alterations in the rate of sodium excretion by way of changes in the glomerular propulsive pressure, e.g. an enhanced constriction in the pre-glomerular vessels would reduce the glomerular capillary pressure and thus the propulsive pressure leading to a decrease in the renal output of sodium (and water). As previously discussed, the glomerular filtration rate *need not* vary in the same direction as the glomerular capillary pressure, since (normally) its magnitude is greatly dependent upon the rate of tubular reabsorption of fluid, which may be influenced independently by other factors. Changes in renal blood flow are more valuable as indicators of possible changes in glomerular capillary pressure, although, as has long been recognized, a parallelism cannot be expected if the underlying vasoconstriction occurs predominantly in the postglomerular vessels. A renal vasoconstriction with a sodium (and water) retaining effect is undoubtedly evoked by several other stimuli than those mentioned above, and in particular it must be assumed to be an important part of the sodium-retaining mechanisms which are activated in circulatory failure of various types. In these cases, which are discussed elsewhere (p. 368 and p. 378) inadequate filling of some part(s) of the cardiovascular system appears to activate reflexes in which the renal vasoconstrictors are (at least one of) the effectors. It should be emphasized, however, that the renal vasoconstrictors may be activated by these or other stimuli not only by way of the vasomotor nerves, but also by the humoral route, in particular by the sympathomimetic amines of the adrenal medulla.

The above discussion has been held in rather vague terms for the obvious reason that any more concise statements would reflect nothing but pure speculation. There are evidently several other aspects of renal circulation which should be considered in relation to electrolyte handling, and in which the renal nerves may play an important part. The "medullary shunt" phenomenon first reported by TRUETA and coworkers[786] is one such case. At present there still remains some doubt as to the reality of this phenomenon; not of course as regards the occurrence

[785] O'CONNOR, W. J.: The effect of section of the supraoptico-hypophyseal tracts on the inhibition of water-diuresis by emotional stress. Quart. J. exp. Physiol. **33**, 149—161 (1946).
[786] TRUETA, J., A. E. BARCLAY, P. M. DANIEL, K. J. FRANKLIN, and M. M. L. PRICHARD: Studies of the renal circulation. Oxford 1947.

of cases of extreme reductions of cortical blood flow, but as regards the existence of a simultaneous increase in the medullary blood flow of a similar order of magnitude. It is quite conceivable that an "opening up" of the medullary circulation could influence the function of the nephrons (by altering intrarenal pressures, by interfering with the HARGITAY-KUHN concentrating mechanism, etc.), although the simultaneous diminution in cortical flow and pressures would seem to be of greater importance. Another factor to be considered is the possible existence of intrarenal axon reflexes. At this time, there is, however, no clear evidence that such reflexes exist. Nor do we known what functions are carried out by such special structures as the juxta-glomerular· apparatus or intravenous nerve endings (cf. DE MUYLDER[775]). The problem whether the "autonomy" of the renal circulatory regulation depends on intrarenal nerve connections or is due to an inherent constriction response of the preglomerular vessels to dilatation also awaits its final answer.

b) Effects of sympathomimetic amines

Since norepinephrine is, in all probability, the mediator of the renal vasoconstrictor nerves, it might a priori be expected that administration of this substance (and epinephrine) would have similar effects as a stimulation of the renal nerves, i.e. a reduction in the rate of sodium (and water) excretion. This was also the response generally obtained in acute experiments in human subjects and dogs when proper doses of norepinephrine and epinephrine were given, but under certain conditions the opposite effects may be observed. It is in fact not too surprising that such "paradoxical" responses may be obtained even in acute experiments. One factor that may be responsible is a rise in systemic arterial pressure resulting from the profound effects of these substances on other parts of the vascular system. Such a rise would obviously counteract the decline in glomerular capillary pressure produced by a predominant constriction of the preglomerular vessels. Whether one or the other of these effects becomes decisive is, of course, greatly dependent upon the dosage used, and also on the pre-existing state of the circulation; conditions characterized by a low blood pressure and a pre-existing high renal vasomotor tone would presumably be most favourable for the observation of paradoxical responses. It is also possible that paradoxical responses may sometimes be accounted for merely from local effects in the kidney. According to an old view, which still has many adherents, (nor)epinephrine causes constriction of both the pre- and postglomerular vessels, and with smaller doses a predominant effect may be obtained on the latter leading to an actual increase in glomerular capillary pressure. In more prolonged experiments still other factors may be involved; the production of various hormones affecting renal handling of electrolytes and water may be influenced either by reflexes from the cardiovascular system or by more direct actions on the nervous centers controlling these productions.

The "typical" response, a decrease in sodium (or chloride) excretion, has been observed in many acute experiments on human subjects and dogs. A few of the more recent and thorough studies will be mentioned. JACOBSON et al.[787] observed a decrease in the rate of sodium excretion from an average of 145 to 74 μeq/min in 12 well-hydrated human subjects who received an intravenous infusion of 10 to 18 μg of epinephrine per minute. There was a well-marked fall in urinary potassium excretion, which was appreciably larger, on a percentage basis, than the fall in plasma potassium concentration simultaneously observed. A reduction in renal plasma flow was consistently observed, and in 9 of 12 experiments moderate falls in

---

[787] JACOBSON, W. E., J. E. HAMMARSTEN, and B. I. HELLER: The effects of adrenaline upon renal function and electrolyte excretions. J. clin. Invest. 30, 1503—1506 (1951).

filtration rate were recorded. Very similar changes in electrolyte excretions were observed by SMYTHE et al.[788] during intravenous infusion of either epinephrine, l-epinephrine or l-norepinephrine at similar rates as those used by JACOBSEN et al. (i.e. doses causing 25—30 mm of Hg increase in systolic pressure). A decrease in renal plasma flow was observed in all but one case, but no consistent changes in filtration rate were observed. It was further noted that the drop in sodium and potassium excretion was not paralleled by similar changes in the rate of urine flow, in fact the latter was usually increased somewhat during the infusion periods. These findings were confirmed in a later paper (NICKEL et al.[789]) in which it was emphasized in support of a vascular origin of the changes in sodium excretion, that no fall in the latter was observed in two cases where norepinephrine was administered, but in which no fall occurred in renal plasma flow. Typical responses were obtained in three cases of adrenocortical insufficiency and in four persons subjected to high spinal anaesthesia, indicating that the changes in electrolyte excretion are not mediated through the adrenal cortex nor through neural pathways. The authors made the further interesting observation that l-norepinephrine depressed both electrolyte *and water* excretions in a patient with diabetes insipidus. From this and other evidence the authors suggested that the increase in water excretion which often occurred after a certain lag period in normal subjects was due to a diminution of the production of antidiuretic neurohypophyseal hormone. Considering recent evidence for an effect of vascular "volume receptors" on the production of this hormone (cf. p. 351) such a secondary effect of (nor)epinephrine does not at all seem unlikely. There has also been claims in recent literature that (nor)epinephrine may inhibit the release of the antidiuretic hormone by a more direct action. [As an example of results differing from those just mentioned one might refer to the study of BRICKER et al.[790] who injected norepinephrine i.v. to each of twin young men in whom a transplantation had been done of a kidney from one (donor) to the other (recipient). In the denervated kidney of the recipient there was no change in the renal excretion of sodium whereas it tended to rise in the donor].

Results in essential agreement with those reported above for human subjects were obtained by BERNE et al.[791] in saline loaded *dogs* which were given l-epinephrine or l-norepinephrine intravenously at rates ranging from 0.2 to 2 $\mu g/kg/min$. The decrease in sodium excretion was generally somewhat larger in pentobarbital or chloralose anaestetized than in unanaesthetized animals and it was more pronounced in denervated kidneys, a fact which is explainable by sensitization of the vasoconstrictors to epinephrine. In keeping with this interpretation a greater fall in renal plasma flow was observed in denervated than innervated kidneys, and a fall in filtration rate was also a more regular finding in the denervated kidneys. The fact that cases were observed in which the sodium excretion dropped without any change or even with an increase in the filtration rate is not—as mentioned

[788] SMYTHE, C. McC., J. F. NICKEL, and S. E. BRADLEY: The effect of epinephrine (USP), l-epinephrine and l-norepinephrine on glomerular filtration rate, renal plasma flow, and the urinary excretion of sodium, potassium, and water in normal man. J. clin. Invest. **31**, 499—506 (1952).

[789] NICKEL, J. F., C. McC. SMYTHE, E. M. PAPPER, and S. E. BRADLEY: A study of the mode of action of the adrenal medullary hormones on sodium, potassium and water excretion in man. J. clin. Invest. **33**, 1687—1699 (1954).

[790] BRICKER, N. S., W. R. GUILD, J. P. REARDEN, and J. P. MERRILL: Studies on the functional capacity of a denervated homotransplanted kidney in an identical twin with parallel observations in the donor. J. clin. Invest. **35**, 1364—1380 (1956).

[791] BERNE, R. M., W. K. HOFFMAN, jr., A. KAGAN, and M. N. LEVY: Response of the normal and denervated kidney to l-epinephrine and l-norepinephrine. Amer. J. Physiol. **171**, 564—571 (1952).

above — incompatible with the view that the fall in sodium excretion can be accounted for by a reduction in glomerular capillary pressure. BERNE et al's findings are not in complete agreement with those of TOTH[792] and other earlier workers in this field, who found that doses about 5 μg/kg/min had to be administered to dogs to cause a decrease in chloride (and water) excretion, whereas an increase was observed with doses in the range employed by BERNE et al. A reversal of the response with varying doses was also observed by HANDLEY and MOYER[793] in pentobarbital anaesthetized dogs. When norepinephrine was infused at a rate that produced only moderate elevation in blood pressure the excretion of sodium, potassium and water was increased, whereas higher doses which increased the mean blood pressure to about 170 mm Hg resulted in decreased rates of excretion. Changes in renal plasma flow (and filtration rate) were generally parallel to those in sodium excretion. The actual doses employed were not stated.

The complexity of the renal response to epinephrine administration was recently emphasized by BLAKE[794] on the basis of a thorough study in dogs. At least three mechanisms were assumed to be involved: a direct (probably vasomotor) action on the kidneys — tending to depress sodium excretion, a fast indirect mechanism involving a carotid sinus reflex and tending to augment the sodium excretion and a delayed neurally mediated effect unrelated to the directional changes in the blood pressure.

A moderate increase in the rate of excretion of sodium (and chloride) has been a common finding in experiments in which epinephrine or norepinephrine were given subcutaneously or intramuscularly, and in which smaller but prolonged rises in blood concentrations must have occurred. This response was observed by DUNCAN et al.[795] in human subjects who were given 6 mg of epinephrine in oil intramuscularly per day for three days, and very similar results were obtained by BLISS et al.[796]. Both of these groups of investigators also made the observation that the potassium excretion was simultaneously moderately reduced. The significance of this finding, which together with the increase in sodium excretion represents a reversal of an aldosterone action, is not clear. The experiments were performed to study epinephrine as an adrenal cortex activator, and some indications of increased "glucocorticoid" and androgen production were obtained; this, of course, does not exclude a decrease in "mineralo-corticoid" production, since, apparently, the latter is not influenced by the adrenocorticotropic hormone.

An increase in urinary sodium (or chloride) excretion (and an augmented diuretic response to water intake) has also been observed in lower animals in response to subcutaneous or intramuscular injection of epinephrine or norepinephrine (GAUNT et al.[797] and EVERSOLE et al.[798], in rats; KRONENBERG and

[792] TOTH, L. A.: The effects of epinephrine on urine excretion in dogs. Amer. J. Physiol· 119, 140—148 (1937).

[793] HANDLEY, C. A., and J. H. MOYER: Changes in sodium and water excretion produced by vaso-active and by ganglionic and adrenergic blocking agents. Amer. J. Physiol. 178, 309—314 (1954).

[794] BLAKE, W. D.: Pathways of adrenaline action on renal function with observations on a blood pressure reflex regulating water and electrolyte excretion. Amer. J. Physiol. 181, 399—422 (1955).

[795] DUNCAN, L. E., jr., D. H. SOLOMON, M. P. NICHOLS, and E. ROSENBERG: The effect of the chronic administration of adrenal medullary hormones to man on adrenocortical function and the renal excretion of electrolytes. J. clin. Invest. 30, 908—915 (1951).

[796] BLISS, E. L., S. RUBIN, and T. GILBERT: The effect of adrenalin on adrenal cortical function. J. clin. Endocr. 11, 46—60 (1951).

[797] GAUNT, R., M. LILING, and M. CORDSEN: Adrenal medulla in water diuresis and water intoxication. Endocrinology 37, 136—146 (1945).

[798] EVERSOLE, W. J., F. A. GIERE, and M. H. ROCK: Effects of adrenal medullary hormones on renal excretion of water and electrolytes. Amer. J. Physiol. 170, 24—30 (1952).

OCKLITZ[799], in guinea pigs). We shall abstain from a further discussion of these studies, but it should be mentioned that EVERSOLE et al., finding no natriuretic effect of pure epinephrin, attributed the effect of commercial epinephrine from natural sources (adrenalin) to its content of norepinephrine.

The effects of other sympathomimetic drugs on urinary electrolyte excretions have received little experimental study. *Ephedrine* in doses sufficient to cause a perceptible rise in blood pressure, was found by NICKEL et al.[789] to augment the rate of excretion of sodium (and to reduce that of potassium!) in human subjects. In keeping with earlier studies (cf. MAXWELL et al.[800]) no significant changes in renal plasma flow were observed. If GADDUM's view, that ephedrine is not itself a vasoconstrictor, but acts only by inhibiting the enzymatic breakdown of epinephrine, is correct, the lack of depression in renal sodium excretion becomes understandable if one accepts the view that the renal vasoconstrictor nerves are almost or completely inactive in the normal resting state. There is as yet no well-founded explanation of the observed drop in potassium excretion.

J. Influence of the central nervous system on body contents and renal excretion of sodium (and water)

The eminent importance of the central nervous system in the regulation of the body content of *water* is well documented. The existence of a hypothalamic center for water conservation (in the region of the supraoptic nuclei) has been referred to elsewhere (p. 348). It has also been mentioned that this center, which exerts its effect on the renal tubules by way of vasopressin, is stimulated by hypertonicity of the blood, and that its activity is also modified by impulses reaching it through the vagi nerves (from left atrial volume receptors) and by impulses from other parts of the central nervous system. The existence of "drinking" or "thirst" centers more caudally in the hypothalamus has been firmly established in recent studies, notably those of ANDERSSON and associates (cf. [801, 802]), which further indicated that hypertonicity of the body fluids might also be of importance as a stimulus to this kind of water regulation centers.

The role played by the central nervous system in the regulation of the body content of *sodium* is much more uncertain, but there is some indication that it may be an important one. As discussed elsewhere (p. 368, p. 383 and p. 312) it appears, (1) that the cardiovascular system contains as yet undefined "volume receptors" which may respond when there is a general inadequate filling of that system or certain types of redistribution of the blood within it, and (2) that these receptors somehow elicit changes in the tone of the renal vessels, in the rate of production of aldosterone, and/or in other factors influencing the rate of excretion of sodium by the kidneys. How the gab between receptors and the "effectors" is being bridged is still obscure, but recent evidence seems to indicate that the diencephalon may also be involved in this case (at least as far as the regulation of the aldosterone secretion is concerned).

[799] KRONENBERG, G., and H. OCKLITZ: Adrenalindiurese und Kochsalzausscheidung. Naunyn-Schmiedebergs Arch. exp. Path. Pharmak. **207**, 491—499 (1949).

[800] MAXWELL, M. H., P. MORALES, and C. H. CROWDER, jr.: Effect of therapeutic doses of ephedrine on renal clearances in normal man. Proc. Soc. exp. Biol. (N. Y.) **77**, 539—542 (1951).

[801] ANDERSSON, B., and S. M. McCANN: A further study of polydipsia evoked by hypothalamic stimulation in the goat. Acta physiol. scand. **33**, 333—346 (1955).

[802] ANDERSSON, B., and S. M. McCANN: Drinking, antidiuresis and milk ejection from electric stimulation within the hypothalamus of the goat. Acta physiol. scand. **35**, 191—201 (1955).

If not only the intake and loss of water, but also the loss (and intake?) of sodium were subject to specific regulation by circumscribed regions of the central nervous system, then it might be anticipated that circumscribed lesions or stimulations of appropriate regions or their connections could give rise to selective and primary disturbances in the sodium status of the body (as well as in the water status).

Primarily we are, of course, concerned with the possible existence of salt-regulating centers and with disturbances resulting from their dysfunction. It is however appropriate, at this place, also to make some reference to the water regulating centers and the consequences of disturbances in their function. The main reasons for this is that such disturbances may lead to very marked changes in the plasma sodium concentration, and that changes of this origin have sometimes been misinterpreted as consequences of disturbances primarily affecting the sodium metabolism.

If the central nervous system contains centers selectively controlling the sodium content of the body as well as some controlling its water content, the we might expect to find the following types of changes in the salt-water status as a result of lesions or stimulations affecting the appropriate regions:

(1) *Primary neurogenic water deficit*, resulting from failure of the water conservation center (diabetes insipidus), or from inactivation of the thirst mechanism (neurogenic oligodipsia), or from a combination of both. In both cases dehydration and hypertonicity (hypernatraemia) would tend to develop, but whereas they will be rather mild in a conscious subject with uncomplicated diabetes insipidus (because of the effective compensatory action of the thirst mechanism), rather severe degrees might be expected in neurogenic oligodipsia. A combined defect could easily develop because of the proximity of the two centers.

(2) *Primary neurogenic water excess* would result from excessive thirst or from unbriddled secretion of antidiuretic hormone. The first case would be neurogenic polydipsia; no special name is available for the latter case. Both would be characterized by a tendency towards overhydration and hypotonicity (hyponatraemia). Only mild degrees could be expected in the former case (if uncomplicated), because an efficient compensation is exerted by the water conservation system. Since uncontrolled secretion of antidiuretic hormone could hardly be expected to be efficiently compensated by a reduction in thirst much more marked degrees of water retention and hypotonicity might be expected in the latter case (and the hypotonicity might be further aggravated by a renal loss of sodium induced via the volume receptors belonging to the sodium regulating system).

(3) *Primary neurogenic sodium deficit* ("neurogenic salt wasting") produced via an impaired renal retention of sodium (e. g. due to a change in renal haemodynamics and/or a reduced secretion of aldosterone). In this case there would be an initial period of negative sodium balance followed by a period in which the rate of urinary sodium loss exceeds that usually encountered in comparable sodium deficits of other origin. Hypotonicity of the body fluids would tend to develop, but it would be partly counteracted by secondary water depletion resulting from the reduced osmotic stimulus to the thirst and water conservation centers.

(4) *Primary neurogenic sodium excess* resulting from induced renal retention of sodium. Hypertonicity of the body fluids would tend to develop, causing secondary water retention by osmotic stimulation of the water conservation and thirst centers. Such water retention could not be expected completely to parallel the sodium retention *inter alia* because the resulting expansion of the blood volume might be anticipated to inhibit the production of antidiuretic hormone via the left atrial volume receptors.

Comments on neurogenic disturbances selectively affecting water metabolism. The fact that lesions of the hypothalamo-neurohypophyseal system may lead to a specific defect in water conservation (diabetes insipidus) is too common knowledge to require commentation.

From the fact, that excessive drinking may be induced by stimulation of a limited hypothalamic area, it might be excepted that *neurogenic oligodipsia* could develop as a rather isolated phenomenon from lesions in this area. Results from animal experiments have clearly substantiated this expectation. Thus it was found by STEVENSON et al.[803] that rats maintained on a dry diet and dependent on drinking for water intake developed chronic oligodipsia and hypernatraemia following bilateral lesions in the ventromedian nuclei of the hypothalamus. Similar observations were made by ANDERSSON and McCANN[804] in dogs following electrocoagulations in the hypothalamic drinking area, and satisfactory evidence was produced that, a least in several cases, diabetes insipidus was not a complicating factor. The authors found that such lesions might result in fatal dehydration unless supplementary water was forced upon the animals. When, on the other hand, such supplements were given no associated disturbances in sodium and chloride metabolism could be detected; this clearly indicated that the hypernatraemia otherwise observed was secondary to the dehydration resulting from inadequate water intake.

It seems also most likely that a primary neurogenic oligodipsia has been — at least partly — responsible for the dehydration-hypernatraemia-hyperchloraemia (sometimes associated with azotaemia, acidosis and hypokalaemia) which has been observed in clinical disorders of the hypothalamus (and the frontal lobes), and which was found to be alleviated merely by water (sometimes + Pitressin) administration (ENGSTRÖM and LIEBMAN[805], ANTHONISEN et al.[806], GORDON and GOLDNER[807]). Many of these cases appear, however, to have been complicated by some degree of diabetes insipidus, further promoting the development of water depletion.

Primary neurogenic polydipsia is a striking effect of artificial stimulation of the drinking area, but well-documented clinical cases of this phenomenon have apparently not been published. The genesis of habitual (psychogenic) excessive drinking (polyposia) is obscure. According to FOURMAN and LEESON[808] thirst during potassium deficiency or calcium excess is not always secondary to a polyuria of renal origin. Other problems concerning thirst and polyuria are reviewed in this recent paper.

Unbridled secretion of antidiuretic hormone was suggested by SCHWARTZ et al.[809] as an explanation to the hyponatraemia associated with persistent hypertonicity of the urine observed in two cases of bronchial carcinoma. Their interpretation is most likely correct, since a primary sodium depletion was seemingly excluded as the

[803] STEVENSON, J. A. F., L. G. WELT, and J. ORLOFF: Abnormalities of water and electrolyte metabolism in rats with hypothalamic lesions. Amer. J. Physiol. **161**, 35—39 (1950).

[804] ANDERSSON, B., and S. M. McCANN: The effect of hypothalamic lesions on the water intake in the dog. Acta physiol. scand. **35**, 312—320 (1955).

[805] ENGSTRÖM, W. W., and A. Liebman: Chronic hyperosmolarity of the body fluids with a cerebral lesion causing diabetes insipidus and anterior pituitary insufficiency. Amer. J. Med. **15**, 180—186 (1953).

[806] ANTHONISEN, P., T. HILDEN, and AA. C. THOMSEN: Electrolyte disturbances in cerebral lesions. Acta med. scand. **150**, 355—367 (1954).

[807] GORDON, G. L., and F. GOLDNER: Hypernatronemia, azotemia and acidosis after cerebral injury. Amer. J. Med. **23**, 543—553 (1957).

[808] FOURMAN, P., and P. LEESON: Thirst and polyuria. Lancet **1959 I**, 268—271.

[809] SCHWARTZ, W. B., W. BENNETT, S. CURELOP, and F. C. BARTTER: A syndrome of renal sodium loss and hyponatronemia probably resulting from inappropriate secretion of antidiuretic hormone. Amer. J. Med. **23**, 529—542 (1957).

cause of the hyponatraemia by the absence of any evidence of dehydration and by the failure to demonstrate any significant sodium deficit. The fact that the body stores of sodium may have been low normal is consistent with their conclusion, since it is well-known that moderate renal salt losses occur as secondary effects of a water retention induced by prolonged administration of vasopressin without restriction of the water intake (cf. the discussion p. 345). The authors were uncertain as to whether the hypersecretion should be attributed to a reflex elicited by the mediastinal tumors or to brain disorders, which also occurred in both cases.

Excessive release of antidiuretic hormone (from inflammatory stimulation of the supraoptic nuclei) was also proposed by NYHAN and COOKE[810] to explain the development of hyponatraemia and symptoms of water intoxication (dramatically relieved by administration of hypertonic saline) in five cases of acute bacterial or viral meningitis. Reduced capacity for water excretion, not attributable to dehydration, was characteristic to these patients. Similar findings reported by others (cf. McCRORY and MACAULAY[811] and CHEEK[812]) in cerebral disorders, in particular tuberculous meningitis, may well have a similar genesis, but final proof — by reliable determinations of the plasma vasopressin concentration — is still missing.

Comments on neurogenic disturbances primarily affecting sodium (salt) metabolism. It is still not definitely settled whether lesions and disorders of the central nervous system are capable of causing primary and specific disturbances in the body content of sodium.

Since the days of Bunge the phrase: "craving for salt" has been used to indicate the existence of some regulation of the salt intake. There is, however, no experimental evidence of the existence of "salt hunger" or "salt satiety" centers, and disturbances in "salt appetite" as consequences of experimental or pathological lesions of the central nervous system have not been reported.

There are, on the other hand, some experimental and clinical observations, which indicate that the renal loss of sodium is subject to control by the central nervous system, and that disturbances in the latter may lead to abnormal salt losses by way of the kidneys.

The central nervous system is obviously capable of influencing the rate of renal salt loss by affecting the tone of the renal vessels via the renal nerves (cf. p. 356). It remains, however, to be clarified whether the central nervous system contains a system of this ability, which is operating rather independently, and is doing so in a way serving the maintenance of a normal sodium status in the body. Control by the humoral route is another possibility, which must be reconsidered if recent work on diencephalic factors controlling the rate of aldosterone secretion (cf. p. 313) is confirmed.

Work on neurogenic salt wasting is rather sparse, and, in most cases, it suffers from the imperfection that data have been obtained on too few parameters to allow any definite conclusions to be drawn. Some of the evidence is briefly reviewed below.

JUNGMAN and MEYER[813] found that a transient chloruresis and polyuria developed in anaesthetized rabbits following a puncture lesion in the floor of the 4th

[810] NYHAN, W. L., and R. E. COOKE: Symptomatic hyponatremia in acute infections of the central nervous system. Pediatrics 18, 604—613 (1956).

[811] McCRORY, W. W., and D. MACAULAY: Ideopathic hyponatremia in an infant with diffuse cerebral damage. Amer. J. Dis. Child. 93, 51—57 (1956).

[812] CHEEK, D. B.: Hyponatronemia and central nervous system disease. Med. J. Aust. 44, 649—651 (1957).

[813] JUNGMANN, P., and E. MEYER: Experimentelle Untersuchungen über die Abhängigkeit der Nierenfunktion vom Nervensystem. Naunyn-Schmiedebergs Arch. exp. Path. Pharmak. 73, 49—80 (1913).

ventricle in front of the eminentia teres ("Salzstich"). The same response was obtained from both kidneys following a unilateral lesion. Since the response was not abolished by restricting salt and water intakes the saluresis is not the result of excessive intakes of salt or water. The saluresis, more or less paralleled by diuresis, could be due to either a change in renal vascular tone ("propulsion diuresis") or to a reduced sodium reabsorption with reduced water reabsorption as a secondary event. That it might be a vascular effect is suggested by the authors' finding, that, whereas cutting the sphlanchnic nerves by itself caused a similar saluresis and polyuria, no further response of this kind was obtained when the puncture was performed after the nerves had been cut. It is therefore possible that the saluretic response was due to severance of nerve tracts responsible for the maintenance of a (constrictory ?) tone in the (preglomerular ?) vessels of the kidney. In a later paper JUNGMAN[814] reported that the more caudally placed "Zuckerstich" (Claude Bernard's piqûre, in the median line between the acustic and vagal nuclei) caused a chloruresis of similar magnitude, and that this too failed to appear after sphlanchnicotomy.

The effects of transsection of the spinal cord may possibly be taken as further evidence that descending tracts are normally exerting a depressive action on renal losses of sodium. This question was recently studied by BALINT and FEKETE[815], who observed a moderate hyponatraemia in dogs some 5—30 days after transsection of the cord at the upper thoracic level. An impaired renal retaining capacity for sodium was suggested as the cause, since these dogs, in comparison with normal animals, responded to water deprivation with a smaller drop in urinary sodium and water output, and to water and saline loading with a greater increase in sodium and water output.

An increased excretion of sodium has recently been described by KOVACH et al. [816] as a response to elevation of the sodium concentration in the blood supplying the brain. The head of a dog was perfused by crossed circulation from another dog; the head was humorally isolated from the dog's own trunk, but the nervous connections by the spinal cord, the vagi (and the sympathetic nerves!) were left intact. When hypertonic sodium chloride (or phosphate) solutions were injected into the carotid blood going to the head an appreciable rise in the excretion of sodium by way of the kidneys was observed. Since the response was retained after denervation of the carotid sinuses and one kidney, but missing after adrenalectomy, the authors drew the conclusion that elevation of the sodium concentration somewhere in the brain elicits a reflex, which by action via the adrenals causes an increase in urinary sodium excretion. The effect of adrenal denervation was not studied. Blood pressure data were not given. Hypertonic solutions of mannitol gave no significant response. The writer is not convinced about the correctness of the conclusion, and he feels that the assessment must await the appearance of further experiments.

A syndrome of salt wasting (of variable duration) has been described as associated with various cases of cerebral disorders (encephalitis, bulbar polio, tumors, injury, cerebrovascular disease)[817, 818, 819]. These patients were apparently all suf-

---

[814] JUNGMANN, P.: Über die Beziehungen des Zuckerstiches zum sogenannten Salzstich. Naunyn-Schmiedebergs Arch. exp. Path. Pharmak. **77**, 122—148 (1914).
[815] BALINT, P., and A. FEKETE: Die Nierenfunktion des chronisch-spinalen Hundes. Pflügers Arch. ges. Physiol. **268**, 168—176 (1958).
[816] KOVÁCH, A. G. B., M. FÖLDI, N. PAPP, P. S. ROHEIM, and E. KOLTAY: Cerebral regulation of sodium excretion. Lancet **1959 I**, 338—340.
[817] PETERS, J. P., L. G. WELT, E. A. H. SIMS, J. ORLOFF, and J. NEEDHAM: A salt-wasting syndrome associated with cerebral disease. Transact. Ass. Amer. Phycns. **63**, 57—64 (1950).

fering from marked dehydration (and sodium deficit), and in spite of this and the low serum sodium levels they continued to loose sodium rapidly in the urine. Additional sodium chloride administered was quickly lost in the urine, and large quantities had to be given to correct the hyponatraemia. Impaired renal retention of sodium therefore seemed to be the immediate cause of an existing sodium deficit. As the ultimate cause the first group of authors suggested either interference with a central nervous mechanism controlling the secretion of (salt-active) adrenocorticoids or interference with a direct nervous influence on the renal vessels. In the later publications desoxycorticosterone was found incapable of arresting the renal loss of sodium, suggesting that the former explanation does not apply to the cases there studied. CORT therefore suggested that, in the case studied by him (a right posterior thalamic tumor), the condition might be due to "an interruption of hypothalamo-renal pathways affecting electrolyte reabsorption". Acceptable evidence for a direct effect of the renal nerves on the tubular reabsorption of salt and water has, however, never been presented, and, in fact, can hardly be gained with the methods now available (with the possible exception of the stop flow method). An interruption of pathways affecting renal haemodynamics therefore seems more likely.

Neurogenic impairment of renal salt retention was also held responsible for the hyponatraemia observed by RAPOPORT et al.[820] in three children with tuberculous meningitis. The persistence of natriuria and chloruria at the low plasma levels was used as an argument for the conclusion, but its validity may be questioned, since the existence of a sodium deficit and dehydration was apparently not proven. Uncontrolled secretion of antidiuretic hormone must therefore be regarded as an alternative explanation of the hyponatraemia. The authors also reported that the renal responses to various fluid loading procedures differed from those observed in normal subjects, but, at the present stage of our knowledge, it is difficult to see how these observations can be used for distinction between the existing possibilities.

Disturbances in the electrolyte metabolism associated with experimental or pathological lesions or with stimulation in the central nervous system have been reported in many papers not cited above. While some of these apparently fall within one or another of the categories described above, others are difficult to classify. Belonging to the latter are LEWY and GASSMANN's[821] findings that unilateral destruction of the paroptic ganglion in cats leads to hyperchloraemia and a decrease in urinary chloride concentration and output. The hyperchloraemia, which reached a summit value within a few hours, can hardly be explained by a disproportionate loss of water relative to chloride in the urine, since the occurence of an initial polyuria was not reported by the authors. Apparently the hyperchloraemia has resulted from an internal shift of water or/and electrolytes within the body, but the character of these movements is not borne out by the studies. The fall in urinary chloride output, which apparently sometimes outlasted the hyperchloraemia, may have had a different cause; the possibility exists that it was a "non-specific" effect of the anaesthesia and operation.

In LEWY and GASSMANN's paper the reader will find references to electrolyte disturbances following some other lesions. These findings are equally difficult to

[818] WELT, L. G., D. W. SELDIN, W. P. NELSON, W. J. GERMAN, and J. P. PETERS: Role of the central nervous system in metabolism of electrolytes and water. Arch. intern. Med. 90, 355—378 (1952).

[819] CORT, J. H.: Cerebral salt wasting. Lancet 1954 I, 752—754.

[820] RAPOPORT, S., C. D. WEST, and W. A. BRODSKY: Salt losing conditions, the renal defect in tuberculous meningitis. J. Lab. clin. Med. 37, 550—561 (1951).

[821] LEWY, F. H., and F. K. GASSMANN: Experiments on the hypothalamic nuclei in the regulation of chloride and sugar metabolism. Amer. J. Physiol. 112, 504—510 (1935).

interpret, and this also applies to WISE's[822] observation, that stimulation of the caudal part of the floor of the 4th ventricle by bipolar electrodes (0.5 volt, 5 sec) sometimes resulted in an increased urinary excretion of sodium, chloride and water, whereas a moderately stronger stimulus (1 volt) caused a decrease in the electrolyte excretion. The fact, that clonic cramps, presumably from stimulation of the pyramid tracts, were obtained with the stronger stimulus, indicates that a rather wide area was being stimulated. The observed changes in electrolyte excretions may therefore not have been direct and specific effects, but merely trivial consequences of e. g. changes in the arterial blood pressure (which was not recorded).

In his perusal of the literature the writer has met no indication that the counterpart of the neurogenic salt wasting, i. e. a neurogenic (renal) salt retention, has ever been demonstrated. Altogether, consultation of the literature shows that our knowledge of the role of the nervous system in electrolyte metabolism is scattered and uncertain. In the majority of the reports too few parameters have been recorded to allow sound interpretations and it appears that correction of this short coming is a pre-requisite to future advances.

K. Effects of changes in the state of the cardiovascular system on sodium excretion

The volume of the extracellular fluid is mainly determined by the body content of sodium (apart from that bound in the bones, etc.). This follows from the facts that sodium is the predominant cation in the extracellular fluid, and that the sodium concentration in this fluid is generally kept within fairly narrow limits by the efficient osmotic regulation of the hypothalamo-neurohypophyseal system.

Since the regulation of salt intake is a crude mechanism and since the extrarenal loss of sodium in the sweat is only incidental to other homeostatic functions than those concerned with the maintenance of body fluid composition and volume it is immediately apparent that the rate at which sodium is lost via the kidney is of pre-eminent importance to the regulation of the volume of the extracellular fluid.

There is growing evidence of the *existence of feedback mechanisms* by which the extracellular volume, or rather some parts of it, influence the renal excretion of sodium. Our present knowledge of these autoregulatory mechanisms is, however, still very fragmentary. This applies to the site of the receptors and the exact nature of the stimuli to which they respond as well as to the "reflex arches" involved, and, to some extent, even to the effector mechanisms in the kidney.

From a variety of experimental observations (to be discussed below) it appears reasonably safe to state that at least some of the important feedback mechanism are activated by changes in the degree of filling of some parts of the cardiovascular system. In its essentials this is not an entirely new concept; in rather vague terms it was already expressed by PETERS[823] who suggested that changes in the "fullness of the blood stream" might produce alterations in urine flow.

It is still uncertain in what part of the cardiovascular system such "volume receptors", as they are now most commonly called, are localized, and it may well be that they are situated in different places. Considering the particular importance of the cerebral circulation it is understandable that the possibility of an intracranial localization has been looked into. As we shall see there is some evidence, although not conclusive, that receptors may be present in the head. It appears, however, that there must be more important ones localized elsewhere, and the present trend

[822] WISE, B. L.: Relation of brain stem to renal electrolyte excretion. Proc. Soc. exp. Biol. (N. Y.) **91**, 557—560 (1956).

[823] PETERS, J. P.: Body water. Springfield and Baltimore: Charles C. Thomas 1935.

is to think of the heart itself and the large central vessels as the more likely site, although most investigators seem to agree that other sites are by no means excluded.

As already stated the exact nature of the renal effector mechanisms cannot be completely accounted for either. It appears, however, that both nervous and humoral factors are involved as efferent pathways. Sodium conservation may be effectuated rather promptly by a purely nervous reflex in which the renal vasoconstrictor nerves serve as the last part of the efferent pathway. Another way by which renal vasoconstriction and sodium conservation may be mediated is by an increased secretion of epinephrine from the adrenal medulla. In addition to these fast-reacting "vasomotor" mechanisms it also appears that alterations in tubular transfer activities are involved. As mentioned in the section on adrenal corticoids, there is growing evidence of an increased secretion of aldosterone under conditions of inadequate filling of the cardiovascular system and circulatory insufficiency. The mechanisms underlying the activation of this type of sodium conservation are still very much in the dark, but it seems reasonable to assume that this regulation is appreciably slower than the vasomotor mechanisms (cf. the delay in effect of injected aldosterone, mentioned in p. 326).

Only quite recently has there been produced some direct evidence as to the exact localisation of a "volume receptor" influencing the production of aldosterone. In pentobarbital anaesthetized dogs ANDERSON et al. [824] demonstrated that when the right atrium was exposed to a prolonged stretch the rate of aldosterone secretion was only about half the rate observed in intact dogs, sham-operated controls or dogs with the left atrium exposed to stretch. Right atrial stretch (distension) therefore apparently inhibits the secretion of aldosterone (probably by way of vagal fibres, although not tested). Increased or decreased activity of such inhibitory receptors could provide satisfactory explanations to the "slow" increases, respectively decreases, in urinary sodium excretion which are mentioned below in sections a—c as accompanying certain changes in the state of the circulatory system.

Other volume receptors influencing the secretion of aldosterone may very well exist, and it appears that they are definitely needed to explain the high (or at least normal) rates of secretion in congestive heart failure, a condition which typically is accompanied by a distension of the right atrium (see section d below). It also remains to be shown whether the right atrial receptors are capable of influencing the renal excretion of sodium by modifying the constriction of the renal vessels.

a) Effects of changes in total blood volume

It is well-known that acute severe *haemorrhage* leading to a fall in arterial pressure produces a fall in urine flow and sodium excretion. Even smaller or more gradual losses which may not cause any significant changes in blood pressure may, however, induce renal sodium retention. NETRAVISESH and WHITE[825] produced hypovolaemia in dogs by repeated bleedings on 3 to 4 successive days, during which 5.7 to 5.9% of the body weight was removed. A marked decrease in renal excretion of sodium was observed during the period of bleeding, but the rate of excretion returned to normal one or a few days after the last bleeding. Rather detailed studies on the acute effects of bleeding have been made by LOMBARDO et

---

[824] ANDERSON, C. H., M. McCALLY, and G. L. FARRELL: The effects of atrial stretch on aldosterone secretion. Endocrinology **64**, 202—207 (1959).

[825] NETRAVISESH, V., and H. L. WHITE: Effects of hemorrhage and transfusion on renal circulation and sodium excretion in dogs. Amer. J. Physiol. **161**, 442—447 (1950).

al.[826] in human subjects. Removal of small amounts of blood (2.5 ml/kg of body weight) from sitting subjects caused a moderate decline in sodium (and chloride) excretion, which could be prevented by neck compression (see below). Removal of larger amounts of blood (9 ml/kg) from recumbent subjects caused a very striking decline in the excretion of sodium, which could not be prevented by neck compression. There was no consistent relation between the changes in sodium excretion and in glomerular filtration rate; the maximum decline in sodium excretion occurred after the filtration rate had returned to the normal level.

Blood pressure determinations were not made in these studies, but it is unlikely that the declines in sodium excretion were simply reflections of a fall in arterial pressure; the continued decline in sodium excretion observed by LOMBARDO et al. after bleeding had been discontinued can undoubtedly not be accounted for in this way. Later studies by GOODYER et al. [827] have also clearly shown that even when the renal arterial pressure is maintained constant haemorrhage may produce a marked reduction in sodium excretion from innervated as well as denervated kidneys (and with little change in renal blood flow and filtration rate). Changes in the haemodynamics of the kidneys (vasoconstriction) or in tubular transfer mechanisms must evidently be important as mediators of the sodium conservation, and present evidende indicates that both are involved. Their relative importance is, however, not easy to evaluate at the moment.

As evidence that tubular mechanisms are involved it may be mentioned that FARRELL et al.[502] reported an increase in the concentration of aldosterone in the adrenal vein blood of dogs after blood withdrawal and that several authors (see WOLFF et al.[503]) have described an increase in the excretion of urinary aldosterone after bleeding in man.

That neurally induced vasoconstriction is also of considerable importance is suggested from experiments with unilateral renal denervation, in which it has been found that bleeding leads to a much less striking reduction in water and sodium excretion from the denervated than from the innervated kidney (BALINT et al.[828]).

Expansion of the blood volume might be expected to produce the opposite effects of those seen after bleeding, i.e. an increase in the rate of sodium excretion. The magnitude of the response which could be produced by way of a dilatation of the renal vessels would, however, depend upon the degree of pre-existing vasoconstrictor tonus in the renal vessels.

Apparently the effect of plasma or blood transfusions on the renal excretion of electrolytes has only been the subject of very limited experimental investigation. METCALF[829a] observed a very marked increase in urine flow when serum was infused in anaesthetized dogs, but unfortunately the urinary electrolyte excretions were not determined. Thus the greater part of the increase in urine flow may well have been of the "water diuresis" type (cf. p. 349), although the promptness of the response would rather seem to indicate a "propulsion" diuresis caused by an increased glomerular capillary pressure. NETRAVISESH and WHITE[825] reported very little if any rise in sodium excretion after transfusion of blood amounting to about

[826] LOMBARDO, T. A., S. EISENBERG, B. B. OLIVER, W. N. VIAR, E. E. EDDLEMAN, and T. R. HARRISON: Effects of bleeding on electrolyte excretion and on glomerular filtration. Circulation 3, 260—270 (1951).

[827] GOODYER, A. V., L. R. MATTIE, and A. CHETRICK: Renal response to non-shocking haemorrhage. Sodium retention at constant perfusion pressure. Proc. Soc. exp. Biol. (N. Y.) 97, 422—425 (1958).

[828] BALINT, P., A. FEKETE, and S. SZALAY: Tubular factors in the renal response to arterial hypertension. Experientia (Basel) 12, 228—229 (1956).

[829a] METCALF, W.: The fate and effects of transfused serum or plasma in normal dogs. J. clin. Invest. 23, 403—414 (1944).

2.5% of the body weight, but since they measured 24 hr outputs, they may have failed to observe a transitory rise. More detailed studies were made by BOJESEN[303] in unanaesthetized dogs. A moderate increase in sodium (chloride) excretion and urine flow was generally observed some 10—20 min after the intravenous injection of 200—300 ml of reconstituted serum; usually a delayed rise in renal plasma flow and filtration rate was detectable. ATKINS and PEARCE[829b] have recently reported similar findings in chloralosed dogs following infusions of plasma or isoncotic bovine albumin in Ringer-Locke solution in amounts of some 20% of the estimated blood volume. The natriuresis generally reached its maximum some 10—20 min before the diuresis, indicating the operation of two effector mechanisms. These responses were not consistently accompanied by elevations in arterial blood pressure; the authors felt that haemodilution could account for the increase in PAH clearance which usually occurred. Since bilateral vagotomy greatly reduced, but did not abolish, the natriuretic and diuretic responses, it was concluded that the vagi contribute to the renal response to blood volume expansion, but that receptors other than those of the cardiac atria must also be involved. The effects of a blood volume expansion caused by concentrated albumin has been discussed elsewhere (p. 270); it was emphasized that the delayed effects are variable, depending apparently upon the pre-existing state of hydration, etc. (cf. also ORLOFF and BLAKE[830]).

In addition to these rather clear-cut experiments we know of several other experimental conditions (and disease states) in which changes in blood volume may well be responsible for observed alterations in the renal excretion of sodium. These cases are, however, complicated by other changes (in interstitial fluid volume, oncotic pressure of the plasma, etc.), and thus the interpretation of the mechanisms involved is more difficult.

To this group belongs experiments in which ingestion or infusion of large volumes of isotonic or hypotonic saline (or RINGER's fluid) has been found to cause an increase in sodium excretion (WOLF[831]; LADD[832, 833]; STRAUSS et al.[834]; STRAUSS et al.[835]). It has previously been discussed that a dilution of the plasma proteins and a consequent fall in the oncotic pressure of plasma may be responsible for some increase in sodium excretion in such cases (cf. p. 269); in the same place it was also mentioned that other factors must be involved in the delayed rises in renal sodium excretion. It is noteworthy that even a *hypotonic* expansion of the extracellular volume may cause a rise in sodium excretion. Apparently the stimulus from a volume expansion is strong enough to produce increased sodium excretion in spite of the tendency towards a decrease caused by a lowering of the plasma sodium concentration. In this connection it is also pertinent to remind of LEAF et

[829b] ATKINS, E. L., and J. W. PEARCE: Mechanisms of the renal response to plasma volume expansion. Canad. J. Biochem. Physiol. **37**, 91—102 (1959).

[830] ORLOFF, J., and W. D. BLAKE: Effects of concentrated salt-poor human albumin on metabolism and excretion of water and electrolytes in dogs. Amer. J. Physiol. **164**, 167—174 (1951).

[831] WOLF, A. V.: The urinary function of the kidney. New York: Grune & Stratton 1950.

[832] LADD, M.: Effect of prehydration on the response to saline infusion in man. J. appl. Physiol. **3**, 379—387 (1951).

[833] LADD, M.: Effects of prehydration upon renal excretion of sodium in man. J. appl. Physiol. **3**, 603—609 (1951).

[834] STRAUSS, M. B., R. K. DAVIS, J. D. ROSENBAUM, and E. C. ROSSMEISL: "Water diuresis" produced during recumbency the the intravenous infusion of isotonic saline solution. J. clin. Invest. **30**, 862—868 (1951).

[835] STRAUSS, M. B., R. K. DAVIS, J. D. ROSENBAUM, and E. C. ROSSMEISL: Production of increased renal sodium excretion by the hypotonic expansion of extracellular fluid volume in recumbent subjects. J. clin. Invest. **31**, 80—86 (1952).

al.'s[692] observation that continual administration of pitressin over several days without restriction of the water intake was found to cause a marked increase in sodium and chloride excretion on the second or third day. It is not known whether the only important stimulus to natriuresis in these cases originates in an expansion of the blood volume, or whether the expansion of some part of the interstitial space is also of importance. The co-existence of renal sodium conservation and oedema in cases of nephrosis, and the natriuretic effect of hyperoncotic albumin solutions (causing plasma volume expansion and reduction of the interstitial fluid) in these cases would seem to indicate, however, that the intravascular fluid volume is of predominant importance.

Concordantly, a diminution of the blood volume is probably an important factor in the very effective renal conservation of sodium which is well-known to occur in cases of sodium deficiency or in severe cases of simple dehydration. The studies on the effect of sodium depletion on renal sodium excretion are too numerous to be considered here. Among the more recent experimental studies reference may be made to the work of BLACK et al.[836] in human subjects, and to those of CORT[837] and FRIEDEN et al.[838] on sodium depletion by peritoneal "dialysis" in dogs. As discussed elsewhere (p. 312) an increased secretion of aldosterone, causing enhanced distal tubular reabsorption of sodium, is undoubtedly an important factor in renal sodium conservation under conditions of sodium depletion. We are still without factual knowledge of the mechanisms by which sodium depletion stimulates the secretion of aldosterone, but it is reasonable to assume that volume receptors somewhere in the circulatory system are involved. Thus it is pertinent to note that BARTTER et al. [517] have found that an elevated urinary excretion, induced in healthy subjects by sodium deprivation, may be reduced by expansion of the plasma volume by infusion of salt-poor albumin. It remains to be shown whether changes in the activity of right atrial receptors suffice to explain such changes in aldosterone excretion.

b) Procedures causing redistribution of the blood volume

Congestive *accumulation of blood* in large parts of the *peripheral venous system* has been shown by several procedures to cause a decrease in sodium excretion and urine flow. In human subjects the usual procedure has been to inflate cuffs on both thighs to pressures just below the diastolic blood pressure. A marked and prompt fall in diuresis and sodium excretion following the inflation has been demonstrated by several groups of investigators (LEVITT et al.[839]; CHALMERS et al.[840]; WILKINS et al.[841]). The latter investigators found very similar responses in normal subjects and hypertensive patients. When the latter had been operated (bilateral lumbo-

---

[836] BLACK, D. A. K., R. PLATT, and S. W. STANBURY: Regulation of sodium excretion in normal salt and depleted subjects. Clin. Sci. 9, 205—221 (1950).

[837] CORT, J. H.: The renal response to extrarenal depletion of the blood volume. J. Physiol. 116, 307—319 (1952).

[838] FRIEDEN, J., L. RICE, and E. I. ELISBERG: Renal tubular sodium metabolism in sodium deficiency states. Amer. J. Physiol. 168, 93—96 (1952).

[839] LEVITT, M. F., L. B. TURNER, and A. Y. SWEET. The effect of experimental venous obstruction on salt and water distribution and excretion in man. J. clin. Invest. 31, 885—894 (1952).

[840] CHALMERS, T. M., A. A. G. LEWIS, and G. L. S. PAWAN: The effect of acute reduction of the glomerular filtration rate on sodium excretion in man. J. Physiol. 117, 218—221 (1952).

[841] WILKINS, R. W., C. M. TINSLEY, J. W. CULBERTSON, B. A. BURROWS, W. E. JUDSON, and C. H. BURNETT: The effects of venous congestion of the limbs upon renal clearances and the excretion of water and salt. I. Studies in normal subjects and hypertensive patients before and after splanchnicectomy. J. clin. Invest. 32, 1101—1116 (1953).

dorsal splanchnicectomy) there was still a very similar fall in water excretion, but there was generally a smaller fall in the excretion of the electrolytes (Na, K, Cl). (For similar observations during moderate mannitol diuresis cf. EPSTEIN[842].) The latter finding would seem to indicate that a neurogenic vasoconstriction of the renal vessels constitutes one part of the sodium conserving mechanism which is activated by a shift of blood from the central to the peripheral parts of the vascular system. These findings also suggest that the fall in renal excretion of water may partly be caused by other mechanisms than those responsible for the decrease in sodium excretion. Some further support for this view may be found in another observation made by the same group of investigators (not yet published in full): that patients with diabetes insipidus responded with a typical decrease in sodium excretion, but only with a very moderate fall in urine flow. Another finding (also unpublished in detail) of considerable interest is the fact that the fall in sodium and water excretion could be prevented by giving large blood transfusions. This shows clearly that the distension of the leg veins is not, *per se*, the cause of antisaluresis and antidiuresis; the stimulus for sodium and water conservation must somehow be related to the loss of blood from some other part of the circulation. Recently, results from the application of the same procedure in patients with congestive failure have been published (JUDSON et al.[843]). The observation was made that some patients showed the same response as normal subjects, while no changes or even appreciable increases in water and salt excretion occurred in others. The same variability in response was observed when about $1/_2$ l of blood was removed by venesection, and in both cases the patients responding atypically were also characterized by responding with a paradoxical increase in cardiac output or in arterial pressure.

Partial obstruction of the inferior or superior vena cava has been produced in human subjects by means of a special catheter with an inflatable balloon (FARBER et al.[844]). Partial obstruction which raised the vena cava pressure peripherally to the obstruction to 100—250 mm of saline, was found to cause a marked decrease in sodium and water excretion and less consistently in potassium excretion. No striking difference was observed between the responses to obstruction of the inferior vena cava above and below the renal veins. The renal plasma flow and the glomerular filtration rate usually decreased immediately after production of an obstruction, but returned towards control values while water and electrolyte excretions remained at their low levels or even decreased further. A similar lack of parallelism between the changes in sodium excretion and at least the glomerular filtration rate was reported in some of the above-mentioned studies. Thus CHALMERS et al.[840] noted that the sodium excretion continued to fall while the filtration rate increased when the venous obstruction was released. These findings would seem to indicate that the antisaluresis produced by *prolonged* venous obstruction is not mainly mediated by renal vasomotor changes.

Antisaluresis and antidiuresis have also been observed in dogs following the production of peripheral venous congestion in major veins. FRIEDEN et al.[845]

[842] EPSTEIN, F. H.: Renal excretion of sodium and the concept of a volume receptor. Yale J. Biol. Med. **29**, 282—298 (1956).

[843] JUDSON, W. E., J. D. HATCHER, W. HOLLANDER, M. H. HALPERIN, and R. W. WILKINS: The effects of venous congestion of the limbs and phlebotomy upon renal clearances and the excretion of water and salt. II. Studies in patients with congestive failure. J. clin. Invest. **34**, 1591—1599 (1955).

[844] FARBER, S. J., W. H. BECKER, and L. W. EICHNA: Electrolyte and water excretions and renal hemodynamics during induced congestion of the superior and inferior vena cava of man. J. clin. Invest. **32**, 1145—1162 (1953).

[845] FRIEDEN, J·, L. RICE, E. I. ELISBERG, B. EISENSTEIN, and L. N. KATZ: Effects of chronic peripheral venous congestion on renal sodium excretion. Amer. J. Physiol. **168**, 650—651 (1952).

produced *prolonged* venous pressure elevations by partial or complete ligation of various major veins (superior and inferior venae cavae; superior vena cava and vena azygos; inferior vena cava and femoral veins). When tested under conditions of continuous infusion of 1.5% NaCl at a rate of 6 ml/min these procedures invariably led to a fall in sodium excretory rate as long as the venous pressure in the obstructed segments remained elevated, whereas it returned to normal levels when collateral circulation was established. Since no consistent correlation was observed between the diminished ability to excrete sodium and renal plasma flow and filtration rate the authors concluded that the renal sodium conservation was effected by alterations in tubular reabsorption capacity. They also proposed that peripheral venous congestion, per se, should be the factor activating the sodium retaining mechanism. In the opinion of the present writer these conclusions, although they may be correct, are not adequately supported by the experimental findings, since the plasma sodium concentration may not have risen to as high levels in the animals with venous congestion and oedema as in normal controls following standard loading with hypertonic sodium chloride.

A reduced urinary sodium excretion rate was also observed by FRIEDMAN et al.[846] 24 hr after partial ligation of the inferior vena cava (or the left renal vein) at various levels in rats from which the right kidney and adrenal gland had previously been removed. Reduced excretory rates were also observed in totally adrenalectomized animals, and this also applied to the cases in which the inferior vena cava was ligated below the renal veins. This would seem to indicate that other factors than the secretion of adrenal hormones are involved in the sodium retention effected by venous congestion. As the authors pointed out themselves, the possibility exists, however, that the operative manipulations may have exerted a sodium retaining effect which was not entirely duplicated by sham operations.

The reduction in renal excretion of sodium following isolated elevation of the renal venous pressure has been discussed elsewhere (p. 274). When the inferior vena cava is obstructed cephalad to the renal veins this effect is added to that of peripheral venous congestion. This provides an adequate explanation of FRIEDMAN et al's finding that the reduction in sodium excretory rate was appreciably greater when ligation was made at this level than when it was made caudal to the renal vein. The fact that FARBER et al. were unable to demonstrate any striking difference would seem to be explainable by the moderate elevations in venous pressures which they produced; as also mentioned before an isolated elevation of renal venous pressure exerts no significant antisaluretic effect until a value around 200 mm of saline is reached.

When the inferior vena cava is partially ligated cephalad to the hepatic veins venous congestion also comprises the hepatic and splanchnic circulation and ascites is formed in addition to oedema. In dogs prepared in this way STAMLER et al.[847] found that a hypertonic sodium chloride load was excreted slower than in dogs in which comparable chronic elevations in renal venous and inferior vena cava pressure had been produced by partial ligation of the inferior vena cava just cephalad to the renal veins (cf. HWANG et al.[848]). The authors' conclusion, that the

[846] FRIEDMAN, S. M., M. NAKASHIMA, and C. L. FRIEDMAN: The role of the adrenal gland in sodium retention following acute venous obstruction. Canad. J. med. Sci. **30**, 585—509 (1952).

[847] STAMLER, J., H. GOLDBERG, A. GORDON, M. WEINSEL, and L. N. KATZ: Relationship of elevated renal venous pressure to sodium clearances and edema formation in unanesthetized dogs. Amer. J. Physiol. **166**, 400—407 (1951).

[848] HWANG, W., L. C. AKMAN, A. J. MILLER, E. N. SILBER, J. STAMLER, and L. N. KATZ: Effects of sustained elevation of renal venous pressure on sodium excretion in unanesthetized dog. Amer. J. Physiol. **162**, 649—654 (1950).

different ability of the animals in these two groups to excrete an extra load of sodium is due entirely to differences in tubular sodium reabsorption, is subject to the same criticism as mentioned above, that a standard loading with hypertonic sodium chloride may not have raised the plasma sodium concentration equally much in the two groups of animals. The presence of ascites would tend to diminish the elevation obtained. That a procedure as the one used by STAMLER may, however, cause a decreased inactivation in the liver of mineralocorticoids is supported by the recent experiments of YATES et al. discussed in p. 277. The very recent finding by DAVIS et al.[849], that an appreciable increase in aldosterone *secretion* was demonstrable after partial, acute constriction of the thoracic vena cava (and sometimes also following constriction above the level of the adrenals) indicates, however, that an impaired *inactivation* of aldesterone is not the only cause of an enhanced tubular reabsorption of sodium under these conditions. It is also interesting to note that the increased secretion of aldosterone was also observed when the "central" loss of blood was compensated by dextran infusions.

LEVY and BERNE[850] have shown that acute, graded occlusion of the pulmonary artery in dogs produces a reduction in renal sodium excretion. The mechanism of sodium retention produced by this procedure is undoubtedly closely related to that operating in congestive heart failure and since the latter is discussed in a separate section (p. 378) the discussion of these findings and others on experimental heart failure is deferred to this section.

c) Influence of posture

It has been known for a long time that in normal human subjects the rate of urine flow is greater in the recumbent than in the standing posture. References to the older literature on this subject may be found in the paper by WHITE et al.[851] who observed that the increase in water excretion on changing from the standing to the recumbent posture was accompanied by appreciable rises in chloride and bicarbonate (and therefore undoubtedly also sodium) excretions. These findings have been confirmed and extended in several recent studies. A decrease in the rate of water and sodium excretion on changing from the recumbent to the quiet standing posture has been reported by the following investigators: KATTUS et al.[852], EPSTEIN et al.[853], NETRAVISESH[854], PEARCE et al.[855]. Whereas KATTUS et al. found no evidence of a smaller urinary excretory rate in the sitting than in the recumbent posture, later worker all seem to agree that such differences exist at least when the subjects have been seated for some time (LEWIS et al.[856]; VIAR et

[849] DAVIS, J. O., B. KLIMAN, N. A. YANKOPOULOS, and R. E. PETERSON: Increased aldosterone secretion following acute constriction of the inferior vena cava. J. clin. Invest. **37**, 1783—1790 (1958).

[850] LEVY, M. N., and R. M. BERNE: Effects of acute reduction of cardiac output upon the mechanisms of sodium excretion in the dog. Amer. J. Physiol. **166**, 262—268 (1951).

[851] WHITE, H. L., I. T. ROSEN, S. FISCHER, and G. H. WOOD: The influence of posture on renal activity. Amer. J. Physiol. **78**, 185—200 (1926).

[852] KATTUS, A. A., B. SINCLAIR-SMITH, J. GENEST, and E. V. NEWMAN: The effect of exercise on the renal mechanism of electrolyte excretion in normal subjects. Bull. Johns Hopk. Hosp. **84**, 344—368 (1949).

[853] EPSTEIN, F. H., A. V. N. GOODYER, F. D. LAWRASON, and A. S. RELMAN: Studies on the antidiuresis of quiet standing: The importance of changes in plasma volume and glomerular filtration rate. J. clin. Invest. **30**, 63—72 (1951).

[854] NETRAVISESH, V.: Effects of posture and of neck compression on outputs of water, sodium and creatinine. J. appl. Physiol. **5**, 544—548 (1953).

[855] PEARCE, M. L., E. V. NEWMAN, and M. R. BIRMINGHAM: Some postural adjustments of salt and water excretion. J. clin. Invest. **33**, 1089—1094 (1954).

[856] LEWIS, J. M., jr., R. M. BUIE, S. M. SEVIER, and T. R. HARRISON: The effect of posture and of congestion of the head on sodium excretion in normal subjects. Circulation **2**, 822—827 (1950).

al.[857]; ROSENBAUM et al.[858]; NETRAVISESH[854]). Tilting motionless subjects to a 45 degrees head up position has also been reported to cause a pronounced fall in sodium excretion (HOLLAND and STEAD[859]).

The mechanisms of the antisaluresis and antidiuresis which follow the assumption of a more or less upright posture after reclining are undoubtedly the same as those activated by partial occlusion of larger parts of the venous system. In the erect position blood is shifted away from the central parts of the cardiovascular system and accumulated in the legs. Again the problems present themselves whether the accumulation of blood in peripheral veins and the increase in interstitial fluid in the congested areas or the diminished filling of some central or upper part of the vascular system constitute the stimuli to sodium and water retention. The crucial experiment — whether the ortostatic antisaluresis can be prevented by blood transfusions — has apparently not been performed in this case. PEARCE et al.[855] have shown that when the legs are wrapped with bandages before the standing posture is assumed the antisaluresis is inhibited, whereas the effect on the antidiuresis is variable. In similar vein, LUSK et al.[860] have shown that compression of the legs of sitting subjects, by means of elastic bandages, caused a significant rise in sodium excretion, reaching its maximum of some 60 % in the second hour of compression. Urine flow was not significantly altered. Alcohol, on the other hand, was found by PEARCE et al., to inhibit the antidiuresis but it enhanced the antisaluresis. Since alcohol is known to inhibit the release of the antidiuretic hormone the latter finding indicates that the orthostatic antidiuresis is, at least in part, effected by another mechanism than that effecting the antisaluresis. It seems reasonable to assume that that part of the orthostatic antidiuresis which can be prevented by alcohol intake may be due to diminished inhibition of the release of antidiuretic hormone by those neural pathways from the left atrium, which have now been found to cause "water diuresis" when stimulated by distension of the atrium (cf. p. 351).

As in the case of the antisaluresis caused by venous obstruction, it has not yet been settled by what mechanisms the orthostatic antisaluresis is effected. Some of the above-mentioned investigators have determined the glomerular filtration rate, but the opinions differ as to whether a reduction occurs when the standing or sitting position is assumed. It appears that there is at least no consistent relationship between the changes in sodium excretory rate and the filtration rate. Renal plasma flow which might be a somewhat better indicator of the glomerular capillary pressure was not determined in the above studies. Even a renal vasoconstriction resulting from increased concentrations of *circulating* epinephrine and norepinephrine may have to be considered (cf. SUNDIN[861]). An increased production of aldosterone may well be responsible for the slower and more persistent components of the antisaluresis, since MULLER, MANNING and RIONDEL[517]

[857] VIAR, W. N., B. B. OLIVER, S. EISENBERG, T. A. LOMBARDO, K. WILLIS, and T. R. HARRISON: The effect of posture and of compression of the neck on excretion of electrolytes and glomerular filtration; further studies. Circulation **3**, 105—115 (1951).

[858] ROSENBAUM, J. D., W. P. NELSON, III, M. B. STRAUSS, R. K. DAVIS, and E. C. ROSSMEISL: Variation in the diuretic response to ingested water related to the renal excretion of solutes. J. clin. Invest. **32**, 394—404 (1953).

[859] HOLLAND, B. C., and E. A. STEAD, jr.: Electrolyte excretion after single doses of ACTH, cortisone, desoxycorticosterone glucoside and motionless standing. J. clin. Invest. **33**, 132—135 (1954).

[860] LUSK, J. A., M. N. VIAR, and T. R. HARRISON: Further studies on the effects of changes in the distribution of extracellular fluid on sodium excretion. Observations following compression of the legs. Circulation **6**, 911—918 (1952).

[861] SUNDIN, T.: The effect of posture on the urinary excretion of adrenaline and noradrenaline. Acta med. scand. **161** (Suppl. 336) (1958).

observed an increased urinary excretion of aldosterone when normal subjects changed from the recumbent to the erect position. It remains to be shown to what extent a reduced inhibition of the secretion by right atrial receptors can account for this finding.

The effects of postural changes on urinary sodium excretion have been studied in patients with orthostatic hypotension by BACHMAN and YOUMANS[862]. These patients showed a much more marked decrease in urinary sodium excretion than normal subjects when the upright position was assumed following a period of recumbency. The authors felt that this difference could not merely be due to differences in vascular factors ("decreased filtered load"), but that changes in tubular reabsorption was also involved. This conclusion which may well be correct, was, however, only based upon the observation that the antisaluresis persisted for some time after the subjects had again assumed the recumbent posture, whereas the endogenous creatinine clearance returned to the original values much faster. Similar observations were in fact made by EPSTEIN et al.[853] in normal subjects.

One group of investigators (cf. VIAR et al.[857]) have reported that *compression of the neck* (by inflation of a cervical cuff to a pressure of some 20 mm of Hg) caused some increase (25—75%) in sodium and chloride excretion in sitting subjects, whereas it had little effect in recumbent subjects. No consistent changes were observed in potassium and water excretion or in creatinine clearance. As mentioned above the same group (LOMBARDO et al.[826]) also found that the moderate decline in sodium excretion produced by small blood losses could be prevented by compression of the neck. The authors suggested (cf. LUSK et al.[860]) that these findings as well as others might be explained by a single hypothesis: "that there exists an intracranial center which responds to a decrease in the intracranial extracellular volume by inducing sodium retention".

NETRAVISESH[854] was, however, unable to confirm the experimental finding that neck compression caused an increase in sodium excretion in sitting subjects. Furthermore, FISHMAN[863] failed to find any evidence of an intracranial, pressure-sensitive receptor influencing renal sodium excretion. This author found no significant alterations in sodium or water excretion (or creatinine and paraaminohippurate clearances) in anaesthetized dogs following neck compression (60 mm Hg) either singly or combined with cerebrospinal drainage to maintain unchanged cerebrospinal fluid pressure. Nor did an elevation in this pressure to 500 mm of water pressure by intracisternal injection of saline cause any significant changes in these parameters. These findings would seem to indicate that if there exists an intracranial receptor responding to changes in intracranial fluid volume or to dilation of the intracranial vessels, it could only be of subordinate importance in comparison with other factors in the regulation of sodium losses. In this connection it may also be mentioned that LOMBARDO[864] failed to obtain the usual response to neck compression — an increase in sodium excretion rate — in patients with congestive heart failure. It is well-known that such patients often also respond in a paradoxical way to venesections and on changing from the recumbent to the upright posture.

Before leaving the subjects of the effects of redistribution of the blood volume, attention may be called to the recent work of HILTON et al.[865]. These authors

[862] BACHMAN, D. M., and W. B. YOUMANS: Effects of posture on renal excretion of sodium and chloride in orthostatic hypotension. Circulation 7, 413—421 (1953).

[863] FISHMAN, R. A.: The failure of intracranial pressure-volume change to influence renal function. J. clin. Invest. 32, 847—850 (1953).

[864] LOMBARDO, T. A.: Effect of posture on excretion of water and sodium by patients with congestive heart failure. Circulation 7, 91—95 (1953).

studied the effect of opening a large artificial arteriovenous fistula in pentobarbital anaesthetized dogs. Shortly after the opening of the fistula the shunt was adjusted so as to cause no significant lasting lowering in mean aortic blood pressure. Nevertheless, the rate of sodium excretion dropped markedly and remained low, and a persistent drop in renal plasma flow was also observed. These findings are compatible with the view that a reduction in glomerular capillary pressure played an important role in the fall in sodium excretion, but obviously the experimental findings provides no clue to the mechanism by which renal vasoconstriction was effected, nor do they militate against humoral factors as being involved.

In experiments like these some blood has been displaced from the arterial into the venous system. Whereas, on a percentage basis, the gain of the venous system is small (and thus accompanied by little distension and pressure increase), the loss of the arterial system is appreciable. Since no drop occurred in (mean) arterial pressure the stiffness of the arterial walls must have increased by the contraction of intramural muscle fibres (probably as part of a response to blood pressure maintaining reflexes). While the arterial pressure per se was excluded as a stimulus to the renal retention of sodium, such a change in the state of the arterial walls could well mean a change in a stimulus acting upon intramural arterial receptors, and the possibility has to be considered, that such changes could play a role in eliciting renal sodium retention in these and other cases characterized by a tendency towards a reduced filling of the arterial system.

The question of the existence and nature of salt and water volume receptors has recently been discussed by HOMER SMITH[866] and by EPSTEIN[842].

d) Sodium retention in circulatory failure (formation of cardiac oedema)

One of the most frequent disturbances in sodium (and water) metabolism is the accumulation of abnormal quantities of sodium and rather proportional amounts of water in the extracellular space. Now that methods are available for the detection, it seems logical to include any abnormal increase in the volume of the interstitial fluid in the concept of oedema. It is, however, still customary to restrict the use of the designation oedema to only those cases which give rise to a visible deformation of the skin and in which "pitting" can be observed. Attempts to maintain a sharp distinction between clinical oedema in this sense and milder (and less localized) cases ("subclinical" or "latent" oedema) have brought many unrealistic arguments into the discussion of the mechanism of oedema formation. This is true in particular in the case of the most common type of generalized oedema, the oedema of cardiac failure.

Half a century has passed since STARLING gave a clear account for the factors determining the movement of fluid between the interstitial spaces and the plasma in the blood capillaries. Although the potential, immediate causes of formation and maintenance of oedema were thus delineated the pathogenesis of sodium and water retention in congestive heart failure is still the subject of much dispute and far from being fully understood. Different views have been expressed; these and extensive references to the pertinent literature may be found in a large number of reviews which have appeared in the last few years[867-880].

[865] HILTON, J. G., D. M. KANTER, D. R. HAYS, E. H. BOWEN, J. R. GOLUP, J. H. KEATING, and R. WEGRIA: The effect of acute arteriovenous fistula on renal functions. J. clin. Invest. **34**, 732—736 (1955).

[866] SMITH, H. W.: Salt and volume receptors. An exercise in physiologic apologetics. Amer. J. Med. **23**, 623—652 (1957).

[867] MERRILL, A. J.: Mechanisms of salt and water retention in heart failure. Amer. J. Med. **6**, 357—367 (1949).

Although there has been some dissent it seems almost universally accepted to-day that the positive sodium and water balance which characterizes the formation of cardiac oedema is due to an impaired renal excretion of sodium and water, and that among these two components sodium is the one primarily involved. PETERS[874] has suggested that impaired regulations on the intake side might be involved. To cite: "Volumes have been written about the failure of the kidneys to eliminate edema in various conditions, but continuation of thirst has aroused little curiosity". In support of the view that maladjustment of the intakes might be held responsible for the positive balances PETERS emphasized that anuric animals restrict their fluid intakes so that they do not become edematous. The value of this argument may be questioned since the uraemic state may have interfered with the mechanisms controlling the intake of water and salt. It is true, of course, that patients with congestive heart failure do not spontaneously reduce their salt intake to the very low levels often required to prevent the formation and maintenance of oedema, but this fact can hardly be used as an argument that dysregulation of the intake is the cause of the positive balance; no more than a permissive role can be attributed to the lack of spontaneous reduction of the intakes. The important fact is that in patients with congestive heart failure the kidneys fail to excrete sodium at a rate corresponding to normal or even greatly subnormal intakes until a considerable accumulation in the body has taken place; in healthy subjects, on the other hand, sodium intakes greatly exceeding normal are effectively counterbalanced by adjustment of the renal loss before any major accumulation occurs.

Thus it cannot be questioned that the cardiac patient accumulates sodium and water due to a defective renal excretion of sodium, and the real problem is what the precise nature of this defect is and how it is evoked.

Extensive studies have been carried out to answer these questions, but we are still far from having definite answers to them. It has, however, become increasingly clear that the mechanisms involved are closely related to those operating in threatening or manifest circulatory failure arising from other causes (cf. the first part of this section).

[868] STEAD, E. J., jr.: Circulatory factors in congestive heart failure. In: Factors Regulating Blood Pressure. 3rd Conference. Josiah Macy, jr. Found. 1949.

[869] NEWMAN, E. V.: Function of the kidney and metabolic changes in cardiac failure. Amer. J. Med. 7, 490—496 (1949).

[870] BRADLEY, S. E., and W. D. BLAKE: Pathogenesis of renal dysfunction during congestive heart failure. Amer. J. Med. 6, 470—480 (1949).

[871] STEAD, E. A., jr.: Renal factor in congestive heart failure. Circulation 3, 294—299 (1951).

[872] MILLER, G. E.: Water and electrolyte metabolism in congestive heart failure. Circulation 4, 270—277 (1951).

[873] LARAGH, J. H.: Mechanisms of oedema formation and principles of management. Amer. J. Med. 21, 423—433 (1956).

[874] PETERS, J. P.: The problem of cardiac edema. Amer. J. Med. 12, 66 (1952).

[875] DANOWSKI, T. S.: Electrolytes and congestive failure. Ann. intern. Med. 37, 453—464 (1952).

[876] NEWMAN, E. V.: Metabolic adjustments to normal and disturbed circulation in man. New Engl. J. Med. 250, 347—352 (1954).

[877] YOUMANS, W. B.: Renal function in congestive heart failure. Ann. intern. Med. 41, 739—746 (1954).

[878] BORST, J. G. G.: The characteristic renal excretion pattern associated with excessive or excessive or inadequate circulation. In: The Kidney. Ciba Found. Symposium. London: J. & A. Churchill 1954.

[879] BARGER, A. C.: The pathogenesis of sodium retention in congestive heart failure. Metabolism 5, 480—489 (1956).

[880] LIEBERMAN, A. H.: Current status of aldosterone in the etiology of edema. Arch. internal Med. 102, 990—997 (1958).

Cardiac failure, as compared with circulatory failure caused by other factors, is distinguished by the frequent occurrence of an elevated central (and peripheral) venous pressure. This phenomenon is too well-known to require any documentation, but it may be mentioned as an example that MAXWELL et al.[881] found renal venous pressures ranging from 12.7 to 30 mm of Hg (average 22.4) in nine patients with congestive heart failure while values between 10 and 14.6 (average 11.7) were observed in 17 normal subjects. As another indication of the elevated venous pressure one may also remind of STARR's[882] finding that immediately after death the equalized pressure in the vascular system was up to three times higher in patients dying with congestive heart failure than in those dying without heart disease.

Among the factors which may be listed as possible *immediate* causes of oedema formation (increased capillary hydrostatic pressure, increased permeability of capillaries to plasma proteins, decreased oncotic pressure of the plasma, reduced rate of drainage of interstitial fluid by way of the lymphatics and consequently building up of an increased oncotic pressure in the interstitial fluid) it is now generally held that an increased capillary hydrostatic pressure is the main causative factor in the production and maintenance of cardiac oedema. The other factors may contribute to a variable extent. An elevation in central venous pressures must almost with certainty give rise to an increased capillary pressure; a normal central venous pressure on the other hand does not preclude the existence of an elevated capillary pressure since the resistance in the peripheral veins may be increased by an augmented venous tone.

The frequent existence of increased venous pressures together with renal sodium retention in cases of congestive heart failure raises the question what mutual relationship there may be between the two phenomena. This question has been the subject of much dispute in the literature. Theoretically, there are three possibilities: 1) that the renal retention of sodium might be the cause of the increased venous pressures, 2) that the elevated central (and renal) venous pressure might be the cause of the impairment in renal excretion of sodium and water, and 3) that the two phenomena were mutually independent consequences of the failing function of the heart. Arguments for and against these possibilities have played a prominent part in recent discussions on the pathogenesis of cardiac oedema, and each of them has had its advocates.

According to the first possibility the sequence of events leading to the formation of cardiac oedema should be as follows: cardiac failure → reduced renal loss of sodium and water → increase in plasma volume → increased hydrostatic pressure in the systemic veins and capillaries → formation of oedema. If these were the steps involved one would expect a very considerable rise in plasma volume before any appreciable rise in venous pressure would occur, since the venous vascular bed has a very large capacity and distensibility (compliance). Very large increases in the plasma volume during a period of oedema formation are not, however, regularly observed, at least not before gross retention has occurred. Another point which militates strongly against the above mechanism as the only or major one involved is the fact that intravenous administration of saline to *normal* dogs in amounts sufficient to produce a doubling of the extracellular volume caused no or only very

[881] MAXWELL, M. H., E. S. BREED, and I. L. SCHWARTZ: Renal venous pressure in chronic congestive heart failure. J. clin. Invest. **29**, 342—348 (1950).

[882] STARR, I.: Role of the "static blood pressure" in abnormal increments of venous pressure, especially in heart failure. II. Clinical and experimental studies. Amer. J. Med. Sci. **199**, 40—55 (1940).

small increases in venous pressures (WARREN et al.[883]). It appears that other factors than mere accumulation of extracellular fluid and distension of a "passive" venous system must contribute to the increase in venous pressure in congestive heart failure.

According to the second possibility the following sequence of events should be operating: cardiac failure → increased venous tone → increased venous pressure → renal retention of sodium and water. → formation of oedema.

There is considerable evidence that a rise in renal venous pressure does not provide an adequate explanation of the impaired renal function in congestive heart failure. Thus, in healthy animals, production of a chronic rise in renal venous pressure to the levels encountered in patients with congestive heart failure does not produce any major retention of sodium and water (cf. p. 275). It is also pertinent to note that a rise in venous pressures does not always precede the retention of sodium as might be expected if a rise in central venous pressures was the cause of the sodium retention; the reverse order has been observed in several cases of cardiac failure (e.g. by WATTEN and STEAD[884]; NEWMAN and FISHEL[885]; GOLDMAN and BASSETT[886]). It is also noteworthy that the observed elevations in (renal) venous pressure are much too small to account for the large reductions in renal blood flow which have been reported by several authors in cases of congestive heart failure (see below); this strongly suggests that factors other than an elevated venous pressure may influence renal salt excretion.

From the above discussion it appears that both of the two first possibilities considered are by themselves inadequate to explain all of the changes in salt excretion and venous pressure which have been observed during developing congestive failure. This has naturally led to the conclusion that there are independent mechanisms by which renal retention of sodium and an elevation in venous pressure may be produced in congestive failure. Drawing this conclusion obviously does not imply that a causal relationship never exists between salt retention and an increase in venous pressure. A rise in venous pressure may obviously be a factor *contributing* to renal retention of sodium, and a retention of sodium and water would obviously tend to *promote* a rise in venous pressure.

A rise in *systemic* venous pressure without expansion of the blood volume must be brought about by an increase in venous tone, as emphasized by STARR and RAWSON[887] on the basis of studies on a mechanical circulation model. A redistribution of the blood volume could not produce a significant rise due to the large capacity and compliance of the systemic venous system. The increase in venous tone must be considered a compensatory reaction serving the purpose of raising or maintaining the filling pressure of the heart (primarily the right half) under conditions of threatening or manifest circulatory failure. The details of the mechanism by which the increase in tone is activated are, however, only vaguely understood.

[883] WARREN, J. V.. J. A, MERRILL, and E. A. STEAD, jr.: The role of the extracellular fluid in the maintenance of normal plasma volume. J. clin. Invest. 22, 635—641 (1943).

[884] WARREN, J. V., and E. A. STEAD, jr.: Fluid dynamics in chronic congestive heart failure. (An interpretation of the mechanisms producing edema, incresed plasma volume, and elevated venous pressure in certain patients with prolonged congestive failure.) Arch. intern. Med. 73, 138—147 (1944).

[885] NEWMAN, W., and L. FISHEL: Daily changes in venous pressure and weight in chronic congestive heart failure. Circulation 1, 706—711 (1950).

[886] GOLDMAN, R., and S. H. BASSETT: The relationship of sodium retention and venous pressures to edema formation. Circulation 12, 630—634 (1955).

[887] STARR, I., and A. J. RAWSON: Role of the "static blood pressure" in abnormal increments of venous pressure, especially in heartfailure. I. Theoretical studies on improved circulation schema whose pumps obey Starling's law of the heart. Amer. J. med. Sci. 199, 27—39 (1940).

It should be emphasized that whereas an impairment of the renal excretion of salt and water is a *sine qua non* in the formation of cardiac oedema, an elevation of the venous tone is also of major importance as a conditioning factor, because, by increasing the systemic venous pressure and the capillary hydrostatic pressure, it sets the stage for an extravascular rather than an intravascular accumulation of any fluid retained by the kidneys.

Our knowledge of the *mechanism* by which a *reduction in the renal loss of sodium* is effected is also very incomplete. This applies to the renal mechanism proper as well as to the extrarenal stimulus by which it is activated and the pathways along which the stimulus is mediated.

As regards the renal mechanism no agreement has been reached on the relative importance of glomerular and tubular factors, but it appears that both may be involved although to a variable degree in different cases.

Attention was focused on glomerular factors by A. J. MERRILL's[888] observation that the filtration rate was reduced to about one-half of normal in bed-ridden cardiac patients and that there was an even greater reduction in the (effective) renal blood flow (to values as low as one-fifth of normal). Similar findings have been reported by several other authors (e.g. MOKOTOFF et al.[889]; AAS and BLE-GEN[890]). From MERRILL's work and later studies it appears that the extraction ratio for para-aminohippurate may be somewhat lower in patients with congestive failure than in normal subjects; the difference is not, however, large enough to invalidate the PAH clearance as an approximate measure of the renal plasma flow.

MERRILL attached most importance to the low values for the filtration rate (or the filtered load of sodium) and thought they might be taken as an indication that the renal retention of sodium and water was due to an impairment of the glomerular function rather than to alterations in tubular function. As discussed in a previous section (p. 261) there are, however, good reasons to believe that the measurement of these parameters constitutes an inadequate basis for a distinction between glomerular and tubular factors, since the former are, apparently, by themselves greatly influenced by tubular function. According to this view, primary changes in the rate of (proximal) salt and water reabsorption are presumably capable of "setting" the filtration rate at different levels, and different rates of sodium (and water) excretion may be produced at each of these without appreciable changes in the filtration rate by alterations in the glomerular propulsive pressure (or in distal sodium reabsorption). A fixed correlation between the filtration rate (filtered sodium load) and sodium excretion could therefore not be expected to exist.

It was also soon realized that a correlation of this type was lacking in several cases of congestive heart failure. Cases of sodium retention and oedema formation in cardiac patients were reported in which the filtration rates were normal or near-normal (cf. for instance DAVIS and SHOCK[891]; WERKÖ et al.[892]) and so were cases

---

[888] MERRILL, A. J.: Edema and decreased renal blood flow in patients with chronic congestive heart failure. Evidence of "forward failure" as primary cause of edema. J. clin. Invest. **25**, 389—400 (1946).

[889] MOKOTOFF, R., G. ROSS, and L. LEITER: Renal plasma flow and sodium reabsorption and excretion in congestive heart failure. J. clin. Invest. **27**, 1—9 (1948).

[890] AAS, K., and E. BLEGEN: The renal blood flow and the glomerular filtration rate in congestive heart failure and some other clinical conditions. Scand. J clin. Lab. Invest. **1**, 22—32 (1949).

[891] DAVIS, J. D., and N. W. SHOCK: The effect of theophylline ethyldne diamine on renal function in control subject and in patients with congestive heart failure. J. clin. Invest. **28**, 1459—1468 (1949).

[892] WERKÖ, L., E. VARNAUSKAS, H. ELIASCH, J. EK, H. BUCHT, B. THOMASSON, and J. BERGSTRÖM: Studies on the renal circulation and renal function in mitral valvular disease. I. Effect of exercise. Circulation **9**, 687—699 (1954).

in which increased salt excretion and loss of oedema occurred without any discernible increase in the filtration rate (BRIGGS et al.[893]; SINCLAIR-SMITH et al.[894]). Failure to detect any significant fall in the filtration rate has also been reported in dogs in which various grades of cardiac failure and oedema were produced by constriction of the pulmonary artery and/or lesions of the pulmonary and tricuspid valves (BARGER et al.[895]).

From cases of clinical and experimentally produced congestive heart failure in which both the filtration rate and the renal blood flow have been measured it appears that not only is there a greater percentage reduction in the blood flow than in the filtration rate when both are lowered, but a reduction in the renal blood flow is almost invariably found even in those cases in which there is no significant reduction in the filtration rate. The latter finding is in keeping with the observation that a fall in the filtration rate may be lacking when moderate reductions in renal blood flow are produced by constriction of the renal arteries (cf. p. 271).

The reductions in renal blood flow which have been observed in severe cases of congestive heart failure (down to one-fifth of normal) are of such a magnitude that it is obvious that they cannot be accounted for by the observed increases in renal venous pressure, since the latter amount to only small fractions of the normal difference between the pressures in the renal arteries and the renal veins. The observed reductions in renal blood flow must therefore be due to an increased vascular resistance in the kidneys (cf. MAXWELL et al.[881]).

Together the above findings suggest that the renal retention of sodium might have a closer causal relationship to a constriction of the renal vessels than to the glomerular filtration rate. A fall in renal blood flow which were predominantly due to a constriction of the preglomerular(afferent) vessels would be associated with a fall in the glomerular capillary pressure and thus in the glomerular propulsive pressure. This might be the immediate cause of the reduced excretion of sodium and water regardless of whether there was a simultaneous reduction in glomerular filtration rate or not (the latter being mainly dependent on whether a reduction in the rate of tubular fluid reabsorption occurred). It appears that such a mechanism might provide an intelligible interpretation of many findings which are otherwise not readily accounted for. Obviously no more than a gross parallelism between the renal blood flow and sodium excretion may be expected, *inter alia* because constriction of the pre- and postglomerular vessels would have opposite effects on the glomerular propulsive pressure.

We have no definite information about the stimulus which causes vasoconstriction in the kidneys in congestive heart failure, nor about the pathways along which the stimulus is brought to act on the renal vessels. It is reasonable to believe that the stimulus is closely related to that (those) causing renal vasoconstriction in other cases of threatening or manifest circulatory failure (following blood loss or accumulation of blood in the peripheral vascular bed). As previously discussed in this section it is likely that the stimulus may be dependent upon the filling of some part of the cardiovascular system ("volume receptors").

[893] BRIGGS, A. P., D. M. FOWELL, W. F. HAMILTON, J. W. REMINGTON, N. C. WHEELER, and J. H. WINSLOW: Renal and circulatory factors in the edema formation of congestive heart failure. J. clin. Invest. **27**, 810—817 (1948).

[894] SINCLAIR-SMITH, B., A. A. KATTUS, J. GENEST, and E. V. NEWMAN: Renal mechanism of electrolyte excretions and metabolic balances of electrolytes and nitrogen in congestive cardiac failure, effects of exercise, rest and aminophyllin. Bull. Johns Hopk. Hosp. **84**, 369—394 (1949).

[895] BARGER, A. C., A. M. RUDOLPH, and E. F. YATES: Sodium excretion and renal hemodynamics in normal dogs, dogs with mild valvular lesions of the heart and dogs in frank congestive heart failure. Amer. J. Physiol. **183**, 595 (1955).

It is natural to think of the renal vasoconstrictor nerves as part of the pathways involved in the mediation of the stimulus. In an attempt to decide whether this is the case BERNE and LEVY[896] studied the effects of an acute reduction in cardiac output produced by partial constriction of the pulmonary artery in dogs in which the left kidney had previously been denervated. Almost identical reductions in renal blood flow, filtration rate and sodium excretion were observed in the normal and denervated kidneys. These observations do not, however, exclude a neurogenic renal vasoconstriction in congestive heart failure since the observed reductions in renal blood flow were no greater on a percentage basis than the decrease in mean arterial pressure, indicating that no vasoconstriction had occurred in either of the kidneys. MOKOTOFF and ROSS[897] thought that a neurogenic origin could be excluded on the basis of their finding that high spinal anaesthesia did not produce any significant improvement in renal blood flow (or filtration rate) in heart patients in whom the blood pressure was maintained by ephedrine. Ephedrine was chosen because it was believed that it would not act on the renal vessels under these conditions. The weight of the argument depends on whether this assumption is correct.

MOKOTOFF and ROSS suggested that a release of humoral agents were responsible for the renal vasoconstriction. In this connection it is natural to think of epinephrine released from the adrenal glands, but it may also be mentioned that BORST[898] has postulated that "the renal excretion of salt and water may be under the control of a substance that is formed in excess or inadequately eliminated under conditions where the metabolic requirements are not met by the circulation".

BORST made no suggestions concerning the possible site of action in the kidneys of his hypothetical antisaluretic substance. It must be admitted that although it seems a reasonable assumption that renal vasoconstriction and a consequent fall in glomerular propulsive pressure is an important factor in renal retention of sodium in congestive failure, this by no means precludes that other (tubular) factors may participate and that they may be of major importance in some cases. Thus it is pertinent to note that oedema and ascites without any depression in renal blood flow (or filtration rate) have been observed in dogs with experimental constrictive pericarditis (DAVIS et al.[899]).

Several authors have considered the possibility that an increased secretion of sodium-retaining corticoids might play a role in the retention of sodium in congestive heart failure. An increased excretion of such corticoids in the urine in patients with congestive failure was reported in various earlier studies (cf. for instance DEMING and LUETSCHER[900]; LASCHE et al.[901]), and improved methods have shown that aldosterone is excreted in increased amounts (LUETSCHER and CURTIS[902]; WOLFF et al.[903]). On the whole greatly elevated excretions have been found during phases of actual accumulation of oedema, whereas lower or even normal outputs have been observed in patients in a steady state (cf. WOLFF, KOCZOREK and BUCHBORN[517]). The interpretation of these findings is complicated by

[896] BERNE, R. M., and M. N. LEVY: Effect of acute reduction in cardiac output on the denervated kidney. Amer. J. Physiol. 171, 558—563 (1952).

[897] MOKOTOFF, R., and G. ROSS: The effect of spinal anesthesia on renal ischemia in congestive heart failure. J. clin. Invest. 27, 335—339 (1948).

[898] BORST, J. G. G.: In: The Kidney. Ciba Found. Symposium. London: J. & A. Churchill 1954.

[899] DAVIS, J. O., A. E. LINDSAY, and J. L. SOUTHWORTH: Mechanisms of fluid and electrolyte retention in experimental preparations in dogs. I. Acute and chronic pericarditis. Bull. Johns Hopk. Hosp. 90, 64—89 (1952).

[900] DEMING, Q. B., and J. A. LUETSCHER: Bioassay of desoxycorticosterone-like material in urine. Proc. Soc. exp. Biol. (N. Y.) 73, 171—175 (1950).

[901] LASCHE, E. C., W. H. PERLOFF, and T. M. DURANT: Some aspects of adrenocortical function in cardiac decompensation. Amer. J. med. Sci. 222, 459—467 (1951).

the fact that increased excretion of aldosterone has also been found to occur in normal persons subjected to sodium depletion (cf. p. 312). Since a sodium-depleting regime is generally used in the treatment of decompensated patients it might be argued that the increased excretion (secretion) of aldosterone represented only a result of such treatment, and not a characteristic of cardiac failure. This objection seems, however, unwarranted, since these patients are not depleted of sodium; on the contrary they contain abnormally large amounts. Rather it might be argued that the increased secretion of aldosterone in normal, sodium-depleted subjects is due to the fact that the sodium depletion has brought them in a state of (threatening) circulatory failure, and that this, by similar mechanisms as circulatory failure of cardiac origin, represents a stimulus for the secretion of aldosterone.

It might also be argued that the increased urinary excretion of aldosterone observed in cases of cardiac failure might not at all reflect an increased rate of secretion, but merely a depressed hepatic inactivation (from hepatic stasis) or an enhanced urinary excretion of the hormone. It is consonant with this view that DRISCOL et al.[904] failed to find any increased *secretion* of aldosterone in dogs in which experimental congestive heart failure had been produced by partial constriction of the pulmonary artery. A definitely increased aldosterone secretion was, however, observed by DAVIS et al.[905] in dogs in which dropsy had been produced by the same procedure. The reason for this discrepancy is not at all apparent, but it may have been a matter of differences in the degree of dropsy or in the phases (active accumulation *versus* steady state) during which the measurements were undertaken.

On this basis of the fact that, in dogs with experimental congestive heart failure, adrenalectomy causes loss of the oedema and ascites, and that considerably more than maintenance doses of desoxycorticosterone must be given to re-establish the same degree of sodium retention, DAVIS et al.[906] have argued that more than normal secretion of aldosterone is required for the maintenance of cardiac oedema. Although a more perfect substitution therapy (cortisol + aldosterone) could have been used, the argument still seems to carry some weight in favour of an *increased secretion* of aldosterone as an essential factor in the pathogenesis of cardiac oedema. (It may be mentioned in passing that an increased secretion of aldosterone, which would stimulate the tubular secretion of potassium would provide a satisfactory explanation to the potassium deficits and the high plasma bicarbonate/chloride ratios which have been reported in severe cases of congestive heart failure).

In considering the possible mechanisms by which such an increased secretion of aldosterone might be maintained, it must be noted that, whereas a reduced inhibition of the secretion by right atrial receptors might explain the increased secretion following sodium depletion or loss of blood, other factors (arterial receptors?) must be held responsible in the case of cardiac failure. In fact, in these latter cases the atrial receptors would depress the aldosterone secretion (and act as "safety valves" preventing too excessive sodium retention).

[902] LUETSCHER, J. A., and R. H. CURTIS: Relationship of aldosterone in urine to sodium balance and to some other endocrine functions . J. clin. Invest. **34**, 951 (1955).

[903] WOLFF, H. P., K. R. KOCZOREK, and E. BUCHBORN: Hyperaldosteronism in heart disease. Lancet **1957 II**, 63—66.

[904] DRISCOL, T. E., M. M. MAULTSBY, G. L. FARRELL, and R. M. BERNE: Aldosterone secretion in experimental congestive heart failure. Amer. J. Physiol. **191**, 140—144 (1957).

[905] DAVIS, J. O., M. M. PECHET, W. C. BALL jr., and M. J. GOODKIND: Increased aldosterone secretion in dogs with right-sided congestive heart failure, and in dogs with thoracic inferior vena cava constriction. J. clin. Invest. **36**, 689—694 (1957).

[906] DAVIS, J. O., D. S. HOWELL, and R. E. HYATT: Sodium excretion in adrenalectomized dogs with chronic cardiac failure produced by pulmonary artery constriction. Amer. J. Physiol. **183**, 263—268 (1955).

It appears that the formation of oedema in cardiac failure may be the resultant of the activation of several "compensatory" reactions. The relative importance of these in regard to oedema formation is difficult to evaluate at present, but it is likely that it varies from one case to another. The mechanisms by which the sodium-retaining reactions are activated are still very much in the dark. A diagrammatic representation of our fragmentary knowledge of the mechanism of formation of cardiac oedema has been attempted in Fig. 14. It should be recalled that cardiac oedema may be present even when failure of the heart as a pump occurs only intermittently during periods of the day when particular demands are made to the heart, especially during muscular exercise.

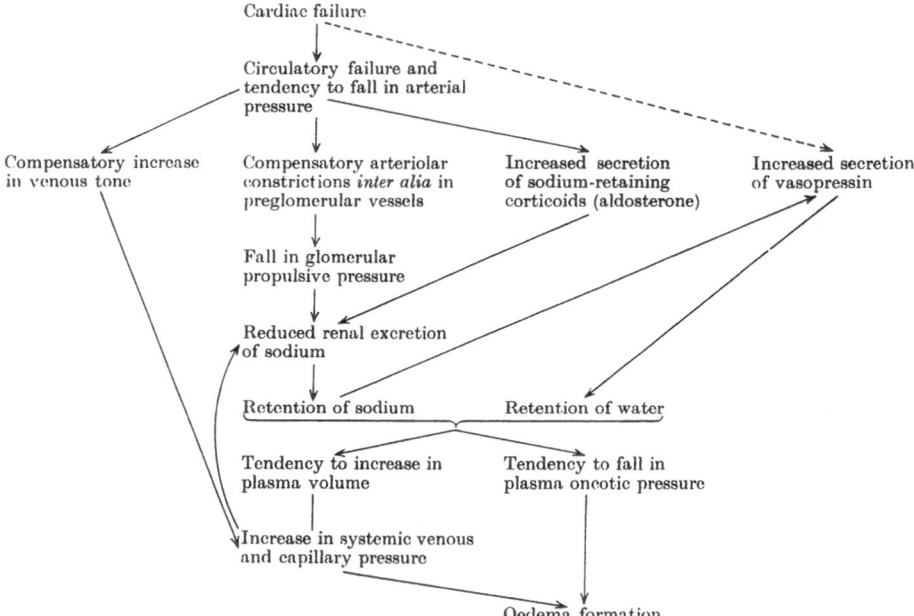

Fig. 14. Tentative diagrammatic representation of the mechanism of formation of cardiac oedema

The possibility that an increased production (or decreased inactivation) of antidiuretic substances such as vasopressin might be a primary and essential factor in the formation of cardiac oedema is declined by most authors. For a recent discussion reference should be made to the paper by THORN[235]. Sodium retention is generally held the essential event and water retention is considered to be superimposed upon it. In most cases of untreated congestive heart failure a proportionate retention of sodium and water is observed (plasma sodium concentration within the normal range), and in these cases water retention is readily explained as secondary to sodium retention, the latter providing a stimulus for the osmoreceptors. There are, however, several cases in which a hypotonicity of the body fluids exists. The existence of an excess retention of water relative to sodium in these cases does not necessarily imply that water retention plays a leading role in sodium retention. Rather it must be interpreted to mean that other stimuli than the tonicity of the body fluids have been brought to act on the centers controlling the secretion of vasopressin, or that a change has occurred in the sensitivity (threshold) of the osmoreceptors. In both cases osmoregulation may still be active, but at a new level. The mechanisms involved in this resetting have not been elucidated, but with regard to the first possibility atrial pressoreceptors and VDM should be considered (cf. section on vasopressin, p. 348). ELKINTON and DANOWSKI[9] have suggested that in protracted congestive failure a loss of osmotically active cellular constituents might occur and "that this is in turn reflected in generalized hypotonicity"; whether this is believed to happen by way of a change in the threshold of the osmoreceptors is not stated.

L. Effect of exercise on renal sodium excretion

Both moderate (KATTUS et al.[907]) and severe exercise (BARCLAY[908]) has been found to cause a decrease in the rate of urinary excretion of sodium in human subjects.

The mechanism of this phenomenon is not definitely known, but since marked reductions in renal blood flow have been observed during severe exercise it appears most reasonable to assume that a fall in glomerular propulsive pressure (due to renal vasoconstriction) is a major factor involved.

In dogs a similar phenomenon has not been observed, neither in moderate (BLAKE[909]) nor in severe exercise (CARLIN et al.[910]), and the latter authors also failed to observe any alterations in renal blood flow.

Experiments in human subjects (normal and patients with cardiac disease) have more recently been performed by FREEMAN et al.[911] but in such a way that the subject remained in the supine position during the exercise period. No consistent drop in sodium excretion or renal blood flow was observed in normal subjects or compensated cardiac patients. The authors suggested that the previously reported diminutions had been produced by assumption of the upright position rather than by the exercise itself. It would possibly be more correct to say that when the action of gravity is *added to* an arteriolar dilatation in a large part of the body a considerable sequestration of blood must take place in peripheral parts of the circulatory system, and that this results in similar renal effects as a passive venous congestion of the lower limbs.

M. Diurnal variations in the renal excretion of sodium and potassium

The existence of a diurnal rhythm in the renal excretion of sodium, potassium and water has been known for a long time (LAEHR[912]) and has been discussed recently in various reviews (ROSENBAUM et al.[913], SELKURT[6], STRAUSS[914] and

[907] KATTUS, A. A., B. SINCLAIR-SMITH, J. GENEST, and E. W. NEWMAN: Effect of exercise on renal mechanism of electrolyte excretion in normal subjects. Bull. Johns Hopk. Hosp. **84**, 344—368 (1949).

[908] BARCLAY, J. A., W. T. COOKE, R. A. KENNEDY, and M. E. NUTT: The effects of water diuresis and excercise on the volume and composition of the urine. Amer. J. Physiol. **148**, 327—337 (1947).

[909] BLAKE, W. D.: Effect of exercise and emotional stress on renal hemodynamics, water and sodium excretion in the dog. Amer. J. Physiol. **165**, 149—157 (1951).

[910] CARLIN, M. R., C. B. MUELLER, and H. L. WHITE: Effects of exercise on renal blood flow and sodium excretion in dogs. J. appl. Physiol. **3**, 291—294 (1950).

[911] FREEMAN, O. W., G. W. MITCHELL, J. S. WILSON, F. W. FITZHUGH, and A. J. FITZHUGH: Renal hemodynamics, sodium and water excretion in supine exercising normal and cardiac patients. J. clin. Invest. **34**, 1109—1113 (1955).

[912] LAEHR, H.: Versuche über den Einfluß des Schlafes auf den Stoffwechsel. Allg. Z. Psychiat. **46**, 286—317 (1890).

[913] ROSENBAUM, J. D., B. C. FERGUSON, R. K. DAVIS, and E. C. ROSSMEISL: The influence of cortisone upon the diurnal rhythm of renal excretory function. J. clin. Invest. **31**, 507—520 (1952).

[914] STRAUSS, M. B.: Body water in man. London: C. & A. Churchill 1957.

WESSON[198]), to which the reader is referred for detailed information. Normally, during the night, there is a retention of water and sodium and potassium, whereas the maximum rate of excretion is reached at daytime. This rhythm is very stable against changing the "day" to 22 hr or 14 hr. It is independent of posture and food intake. It does not seem to be due to a cyclic secretion of adrenocortical steroids. It may possibly be related to a cycle in the excretion of ammonia and hydrogen ions. There is disagreement on its relation to variations in glomerular filtration rate.

N. Diuretic and natriuretic agents
a) Introduction (definitions and types of diureses)

Strictly, a diuretic means a substance capable of evoking increased urine flow and a natriuretic means one enhancing the rate of sodium excretion by the urinary route. The phycician, however, uses these terms in a somewhat more restricted sense. His purpose for instituting "diuretic" therapy is to achieve a *net* reduction in the water content of the body, or, as is now clearly more important in cases of oedema, a *net* reduction in body sodium. Since the word "diuretics" is chiefly used in medical circles, we shall therefore choose to define diuretics and natriuretics as such substances which induce a *net* loss of water and sodium, respectively, by enhancing urinary excretions. In the discussion of these agents in the present section, the main emphasis will be placed upon those groups of substances which have proved to be of practical therapeutical value, and here again special attention will be paid to the possible mechanism of action of the different agents. Details about therapeutical use, toxicology, etc. will not be given. The reader interested in these aspects is referred to recent comprehensive reviews (PITTS and SARTORIUS[915]; MODELL[916]; PITTS[917] and a monography (VOGL[918])) which contain very extensive bibliographies.

As an introduction to the discussion it seems appropriate to summarize from previous sections those factors which may be responsible for a diuresis i.e. an increase in the rate of urine flow. From the composition of the urine two main types of diuresis may be distinguished: A) *Water diuresis*, characterized by a dilute, hypotonic urine and caused, in all probability, by diminished reabsorption of water in the distal tubules, without any (appreciable) change in tubular reabsorption of electrolytes (distal water rejection diuresis). B) *Solute diuresis*, characterized by a proportionate rise in the excretion of urinary solutes and water and accordingly, the excretion of a urine approaching isotonicity with increasing diuresis.

Several factors may lead to the production of this latter type of diuresis, which is generally accompanied by an increased excretion of sodium.

a) Such changes in the hydrodynamic conditions in the nephron which favour the propulsion of fluid through the nephron. This may be either an increase in the glomerular propulsive pressure (increased glomerular capillary pressure, fall in oncotic pressure) or a reduction in the hydrodynamic resistance (or differently expressed, increase in conductance) which the fluid meets during its passage through the glomerular membrane and the tubules (widening of the tubular lumens by tubular cell shinkage, etc.). For short, *"propulsion diuresis"* and *"conduction diuresis"*, respectively.

---

[915] PITTS, R. F., and O. W. SARTORIUS: Mechanism of action and therapeutic use of diuretics. Pharm. Rev. **2**, 161—226 (1950).

[916] MODELL, W.: Recent contributions to diuretic therapy. Amer. J. med. Sci. **231**, 564—596 (1956).

[917] PITTS, R. F.: Some reflections on mechanisms of action of diuretics. Amer. J. Med. **24**, 745—763 (1958).

[918] VOGL, A.: Diuretic therapy. Baltimore 1953.

b) A reduced tubular reabsorption of filtered solids, in particular sodium *plus* anions, with consequent reduction of water reabsorption, *("tubular rejection diuresis")*. As previously discussed a diminution in *distal* reabsorption of sodium plus anions and water must be assumed to result in a considerably greater increase in sodium and water excretion than a corresponding reduction in proximal reabsorption.

As we shall presently see, our knowledge of which of all these factors are responsible for the "diuretic" effect of the most commonly used diuretics, is still very meager.

According to the definitions given above for "diuretics" and "natriuretics", sodium salts would not be included among the natriuretics. When administered as sufficiently hypertonic solutions they would, however, still be diuretics, since the tonicity of the urine produced would be lower than that of the solutions administered. A considerable dehydration may be achieved by such means, but in general this procedure is without therapeutical applicability, since the diuretic effect is only achieved at the expense of an increase in sodium content of the body. In special cases in which marked hyponatronaemia has developed following rigorous sodium depletion therapy the administration of hypertonic salt solutions may, however, be useful even when oedema is present. In such cases correction of the hyponatronaemia sometimes leads to an improvement of conditions, including overall kidney function (cf. for instance WELT[8]).

b) Water

Under appropriate conditions *water* would still be a natriuretic and a diuretic. It has been shown that the administration of very *large quantities* of water may produce a significant rise in urinary salt excretion and a net loss of body water (MARSHALL[919]; STEWART and ROURKE[920]; WOLF[921]). This effect forms the basis of the regimen of high water intake recommended by SCHEMM[922, 923] in the management of oedema. This type of natriuretic and diuretic therapy is, however, of questionable practical value since: 1) the hyperhydration phase which must be passed through involves a risk of critical dilatation of the heart, in particular in cases of pre-existing weakening and dilatation, 2) only rather limited amounts of sodium can be removed from the body, and only when the sodium intake is rigorously restricted 3) the procedure is rather inconvenient to the patient.

There is, however, some evidence that the natriuretic response to the hydration procedure is especially large in some of those disorders in which oedema is apt to develop. Thus it is pertinent to note that EK[924] observed a threefold increase in the rate of urinary excretion of sodium in patients with (mostly essential) hypertension during intravenous infusion of 25 ml/min of a 3—5% glucose solution over a period of 100 min, while no significant rise in sodium excretion occurred in normal subjects under similar conditions, although they responded with a greater and more

[919] MARSHALL, E. K., jr.: The influence of diuresis on the elimination of urea, creatinine and chlorides. J. Pharmacol. exp. Ther. **16**, 141—154 (1920).

[920] STEWART, J. D., and G. M. ROURKE: Effects of large intravenous infusions on body fluid. J. clin. Invest. **21**, 197—205 (1942).

[921] WOLF, A. V.: Dehydrating effect of continuously administered water. Amer. J. Physiol. **143**, 567—571 (1945).

[922] SCHEMM, F. R.: High fluid intake in the management of edema, especially cardiac edema; the details and basis of the regime. Ann. intern. Med. **17**, 952—969 (1942).

[923] SCHEMM, F. R.: High fluid intake in the management of edema, especially cardiac edema; clinical observations and data. Ann. intern. Med. **21**, 937—976 (1944).

[924] EK, J.: The influence of heavy hydration on the renal function in normal and hypertensive man. Stockholm 1955.

prompt rise in urine flow. Simultaneously the hypertensive group showed a considerably greater rise (especially on a percentage basis) in renal plasma flow (PAH clearance) and filtration rate (inulin clearance) than did the normal subjects. This difference in responses is most readily explained by assuming that the (afferent) arterioles in the kidneys of hypertensive patients are subject to an abnormally high tonus, which is appreciably diminished by hyperhydration, leading to a considerable increase in renal blood flow and in glomerular propulsive pressure. Thus the response of these patients is one of a mixed propulsion and water diuresis. Normal subjects on the other hand would have a much smaller degree of pre-existing vascular tonus, and accordingly respond almost exclusively with a water diuresis. It is further noteworthy that WERKÖ et al.[925] observed a similar pronounced natriuresis when the above procedure of rapid intravenous infusion of glucose solutions was applied to cases of mitral stenosis. Here too (as discussed elsewhere, p. 378) there is much evidence for the existence of an increased tonus of the renal vessels.

The explanation suggested above for the hyperhydration natriuresis obviously raises the question whether it would be possible to cause natriuresis by abolishing an abnormal renal vascular tonus with some vasodilating drug. Unfortunately, the present armamentarium seems little promising, since we have not yet at our disposal a drug acting quite selectively on the renal vessels. Consequently, a dilatation of the renal vessels will generally be accompanied by a lowering in arterial blood pressure, which *per se* reduces glomerular propulsive pressure and thus counteracts a natriuresis (cf. however "xanthine diuretics" below, p. 411).

c) Osmotic diuretics

The assumed mechanism of osmotic diuresis and natriuresis has been discussed above (p. 280). It was emphasized that we are still without definite knowledge on this point, but that a reduction in the hydrodynamic resistance in the nephron deserves serious consideration as a possibly important factor. It remains for the present section, only to discuss briefly the therapeutical usefulness of such diuretics.

Several substances have been tried, mostly as remedies in the management of oedema, but for one or another reason they have only enjoyed limited use.

Among the non-electrolytes *sucrose* has been given as an intravenous infusion of 100—500 ml of a 50% solution. Such dosages cause a marked natriuresis (and diuresis) but reports (LINDBERG et al.[926]; ANDERSON and BETHEA[927]) on pathological changes (foamy swelling and even actual necrosis in the convoluted tubules) have apparently discouraged its further use, as judged from the lack of more recent reports.

Mole for mole *mannitol* (and sorbitol) has about the same efficacy as natriuretic and diuretic agents as sucrose, since upon injection they all remain almost completely confined to the extracellular space, and since none of them are reabsorbed in the tubules to any appreciable extent. They also have the property in common of being virtually non-absorbable from the intestinal tract which excludes their use by oral administration.

---

[925] WERKÖ, L., J. EK, H. BUCHT, and E. VARNAUSKAS: The influence of a rapid infusion of isotonic glucose on the pulmonary and renal circulation in normal individuals and cases with mitral stenosis. 2nd World Congress of Cardiology 1954. Abstracts of papers.

[926] LINDBERG, H. A., M. H. WALD, and M. H. BARKER: Renal changes following administration of hypertonic solutions. Arch. intern. Med. 63, 907—918 (1939).

[927] ANDERSON, W. A. D., and W. R. BETHEA: Renal lesions following administration of hypertonic solutions of sucrose J. Amer. med. Ass. 114, 1983—1987 (1940).

In the acute experiment a marked natriuresis may be produced by intravenous infusions of large quantities of mannitol (some 1 g/kg in the course of an hour) as evidenced by several studies previously referred to (p. 281). If strongly hypertonic solutions are used, a marked dehydration soon develops which somehow leads to a drop in renal plasma flow and a consequent marked reduction in salt and water excretion; simultaneously the plasma mannitol concentration rises and may reach intolerable levels.

Apparently mannitol has only found limited use as a natriuretic. Mannitol diuresis has been employed as an experimental tool in the study of various disorders. Thus BRODSKY and GRAUBARTH [928] reported that patients with arterial hypertension excreted much more sodium than normal subjects during mannitol diuresis. (Cf. EK's studies referred to in p. 389).

To the knowledge of the author, renal lesions similar to those seen with sucrose have not been reported following the use of mannitol.

Glucose (infusion) has also been suggested as a diuretic and natriuretic, but it has the disadvantage that it is only effective to the extent that the plasma concentrations are brought up above renal threshold values. Accordingly, comparable natriuretic effects are only achieved with a greater rise in the osmolarity of the body fluids than with say mannitol. Larger amounts are therefore needed, also because a rapid cellular uptake of glucose occurs at elevated plasma levels.

Among the non-electrolytes *urea* is no doubt the substance which has gained most common use as an osmotic diuretic, and in the beginning of this century it was used to quite some extent. The fact that some 30—50% of the filtered urea is ordinarily reabsorbed by back-diffusion tend to make urea a somewhat less efficacious diuretic and natriuretic agent than e. g. mannitol at similar osmolar concentrations in the blood plasma. This difference in efficacy tends, however, to disappear at very high plasma levels since only a very small percentage of the filtered urea will then be reabsorbed.

Urea has the distinct advantage over the above-mentioned non-electrolytes that it may be administered by the oral route since it is readily absorbed from the intestinal tract by diffusion. Furthermore, the great permeability of urea, which results in a distribution in the entire body water, accounts for another advantage: that no expansion of the extracellular compartment occurs at the expense of the intracellular fluids. On the other hand the greater permeability of urea, makes higher dosages necessary. The commonly accepted dosage for adult humans appears to be some 50—60 g per day, generally divided in 3—4 doses, and preferably given with the meals.

The main drawbacks of the urea therapy is the unpleasant taste which is difficult to mask and a tendency to cause gastrointestinal discomfort and nausea. Despite these difficulties, which could probably be somewhat reduced by giving smaller doses more frequently and as less concentrated solutions (40% has often been used), it appears that urea has so many virtues that it ought to regain wider use, at least as an adjunct to other sodium- and water depleting therapy.

d) Salts

The number of *salts* which may be used to produce natriuresis is rather limited, since sodium salts are excluded for obvious reasons and since the ions must be non-toxic in rather high doses. While magnesium sulfate has occasionally been proposed, most interest has been displayed in the *potassium salts*.

[928] BRODSKY, W. A., and H. N. GRAUBARTH: Excretion of water and electrolytes in patients with essential hyperthesion. J. Lab. clin. Med. 41, 43—55 (1953).

It is generally agreed that an increased intake of potassium induces an increased urinary excretion of sodium even when the potassium is administered with such anions as chloride or bicarbonate (or organic anions metabolically converted into the latter) which are readily reabsorbed in the tubules.

This effect was already observed in self-experiments by BUNGE[929] following the ingestion of 12 g of potassium as citrate (or phosphate). MEYER and COHN[930] observed a perceptible increase in the sodium excretion (and loss in body weight) following the administration of 8 g of potassium bicarbonate to infants over a period of two days. GLATZEL and MECKE[931] demonstrated an increased excretion of sodium in normal human subjects over a period of eight days, during which about 5 g of potassium chloride per day was added to a standard diet. MACKEY and BUTLER[932] made similar observations; but they emphasized that the negative sodium balance was less pronounced, occurred later and was more transient, if the diet was low in sodium. A natriuretic effect was also recorded by WOLF[933] in experiments of shorter duration on human subjects during the ingestion of large volumes of potassium chloride and bicarbonate solutions in different concentrations. Similar observations have been made in animal experiments.

All authors seem to agree that only a low grade natriuresis is achieved at least with the ordinary therapeutic doses of some 3—7 g of potassium per day. It also appears that the increase in sodium excretion is rather transient. Thus it was demonstrated by MILLER in pigs[934] and in rats[935] that an addition of potassium salts to the diet resulted in an appreciable increase in the renal excretion of sodium during the first 48 hr, after which, however, the excretion rapidly fell to the normal value. Similar transient effects are apparent from the charts illustrating KEITH and BINGER's[936] study on the effect of various potassium salts (chloride, nitrate, bicarbonate, acetate and citrate) in normal individuals and patients with various types of dropsy. From this study it also appears that a more lasting natriuretic effect may be obtained in certain types of dropsy.

The latter authors also maintained that the most satisfactory results were obtained with the nitrate. This in fact is what one would expect since the nitrate ion is not nearly as readily reabsorbed in the tubules as the chloride ion, and consequently is more apt to add the natriuretic effect of a common osmotic diuresis to that of any more specific effect of the potassium ion.

The mechanism by which potassium, even when administered as the chloride, exerts its natriuretic effect is by no means clear, a fact which is quite understandable considering our lack of definite knowledge of the processes by which the transfer of potassium takes place through the tubular walls, in particular in the

---

[929] BUNGE, G.: Über die Bedeutung des Kochsalzes und das Verhalten der Kalisalze im menschlichen Organismus. Z. Biol. **9**, 104—143 (1873).

[930] MEYER, L. F., u. S. COHN: Klinische Beobachtungen und Stoffwechselversuche über die Wirkung verschiedener Salze beim Säugling. Z. Kinderheilk. **2**, 360 (1911).

[931] GLATZEL, H., u. W. MECKE: Untersuchungen über den Mineralstoffwechsel des Nierenkranken. IV. Die Mineralausscheidung des Gesunden bei länger dauernder Zufuhr äquivalenter Mengen von KCl und NaCl. Z. ges. exp. Med. **91**, 504—522 (1933).

[932] MACKEY, E. M., and A. M. BUTLER: Studies of sodium and potassium metabolism. The effect of potassium on the sodium and water balances in normal subjects and patients with Bright's disease. J. clin. Invest. **14**, 923—939 (1935).

[933] WOLF, A. V.: The renal regulation of water and some electrolytes in man, with special reference to their relative retention and excretion. Amer. J. Physiol. **148**, 54—68 (1947).

[934] MILLER, H. G.: Potassium in animal nutrition. I. Influence of potassium on urinary sodium and chlorine excretion. J. biol. Chem. **55**, 45—59 (1923).

[935] MILLER, H. G.: III. Influence of potassium on total excretion of sodium, chlorine, calcium and phosphorus. J. biol. Chem. **67**, 71—77 (1926).

[936] KEITH, N. M., and M. W. BINGER: Diuretic action of potassium salts. J. Amer. med. Ass. **105**, 1584—1591 (1935).

proximal parts. If the active potassium reabsorption, which apparently occurs in the proximal tubules, was such that sodium and potassium were reabsorbed by a common transfer mechanism in mutual competition, one might of course speculate that an increased potassium concentration in the filtrate would diminish the reabsorption of sodium ions by displacing them from the common transfer mechanism. (For other possible mechanisms the reader is referred to the discussion p. 295).

From an assessment of the available literature it appears that potassium salts are of limited value as natriuretic agents, at least in such doses as have generally been used. This does not preclude that they may be of some value when used in combination other agents. In particular, they would appear to be a natural adjunct to natriuretic therapy with carbonic anhydrase inhibitors, such as Diamox, which may induce considerable urinary losses of potassium, and thus reduce the risk of toxic effects of potassium administration in cases of sodium deprivation.

Before leaving the subject of salts as natriuretics and diuretics, it may be mentioned in passing, although beyond the scope of this presentation, that sodium sulphate infusions have been proposed as a diuretic in the treatment of anuria developing following operations, burns or crush injuries. (MØLLER[937]; WENDT[938]; OLSON and NECHELES[939]; MAITLAND[940]). Although admittedly somewhat risky such therapy may have a certain rationale since it may prevent the formation of blocking precipitates and agglutinations in the tubules. It appears, however, that it should preferably be instituted before complete anuria has developed, and possibly it would be advantageous to carry out infusions over more prolonged periods with more dilute solutions. Urine analyses should be made with a view to checking potassium losses.

e) Acidifying diuretics

Ammonium chloride (and to a smaller extent ammonium nitrate and calcium chloride) has been used to a considerable extent during the last thirty years to produce acidosis with the aim of enhancing urinary losses of sodium. Such therapy has, however, generally been used in combination with other diuretics, especially mercurials, and the number of well controlled studies on the effects of the acidifying agents themselves are limited.

A very detailed study has, however, been made by SARTORIUS, ROEMMELT and PITTS[941], who tested the response of two healthy adult subjects to a total of 60 and 75 g of ammonium chloride administered over a five days period. The experimental subjects were maintained over 15 (16) days on a diet constant with respect to salt content and caloric value. The first five days served as a control period; during the next five the ammonium chloride was administered and during the last five (or six) days the recovery was observed. Detailed analysis of plasma electrolyte composition and 24 hr urinary excretions of all quantitatively important electrolytes were made. Some of the electrolyte excretions observed in one of these experiments are presented in Fig. 15.

[937] MØLLER, K. O.: Ein Fall von Urämie, behandelt mit intravenöser Infusion hypertonischer Natriumsulfatlösung. Klin. Wschr. 7, 165—168 (1928).

[938] WENDT, H.: Über die Behandlung der Azotämie beim extrarenalen Nierensyndrom mit intravenösen Natriumsulfatinfusionen. Klin. Wschr. 23, 107—108 (1944).

[939] OLSON, W. H., and H. NECHELES: Studies on anuria; effect of infusion fluid and diuretics on anuria resulting from severe burns. Surg., Gynec., Obstet. 84, 283—291 (1947).

[940] MAITLAND, A. I. L.: Crush injuries. Brit. med. J. 1941I, 570.

[941] SARTORIUS, O. W., J. C. ROEMMELT, and R. F. PITTS: The renal regulation of acid-base balance in man. IV. The nature of the renal compensations in ammonia chloride acidosis. J. clin. Invest. 28, 423—439 (1949).

It is apparent that a significant rise in sodium excretion occurred already on the first day of ammonium chloride administration, but in the course of the next two days sodium excretion again diminished to reach control levels already before ammonium chloride administration was stopped. A total of some 275 meq of sodium was lost in excess of the control excretion (125 meq/24 hr) within the first three days of acidosis. Potassium excretion, on the other hand, showed no significant rise on the first day of ammonium chloride administration, but then rose to reach a maximum on the third day (166 meq/24 hr as compared to 80 meq/24 hr in the control period). There was a rather parallel rise in the excretion of titratable acid and ammonia in the first days, but whereas the former reached a maximum value on the second or third day the ammonia excretion continued to rise throughout the period of ammonium chloride administration. At the end of this period the sum of the per day excretions of ammonia and titratable acid had almost risen to equality with the number of meq of ammonium chloride administered per day, meaning that rather little further net loss of metal cations was achieved. At this time there had occurred a total net loss of some 450 meq of sodium *plus* potassium, some two thirds of which was sodium.

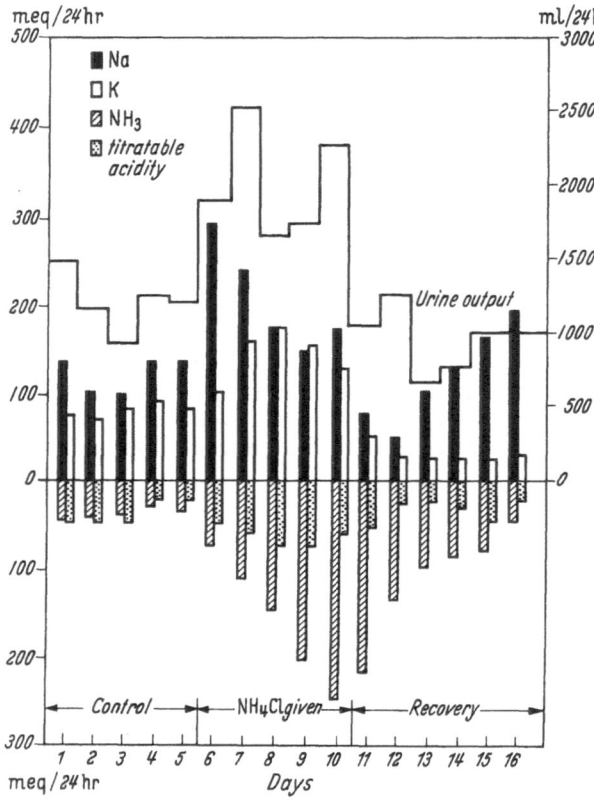

Fig. 15. *Urine output and urinary excretions of sodium, potassium ammonia and titratable acidity before, during and after administration of ammonium chloride. A healthy human subject received 15 g (ca. 280 meq) of ammonium chloride daily over a five-day period (6—10th day).*
(From SARTORIUS et al.[941])

From these data it may be learnt that a significant but moderate loss of sodium and potassium may be induced by administration of ammonium chloride in the usual therapeutical doses. This loss gradually diminishes as the capacity of the kidney for ammonia secretion builds up, and in fact, the lag of this process is a prerequisite for any urinary loss of metal cations.

The loss of sodium as well as potassium indicate that the cations derive from extracellular as well as intracellular sources. The fact that there is also an increased loss of calcium points to the bone minerals as a possible source of some of the sodium loss. In this connection it may also be pointed out that the loss in body weight was considerably below the 3 kg which one obtains from a 450 meq loss of sodium *plus* potassium by assuming 150 meq to represent one liter. This may be due to the fact that part of these cations has occurred in the body in an osmotically inactive state, from which they were released without any proportionate release of water (cf. p. 209 and 4—10).

The reciprocal changes in sodium and potassium excretions from the second day of ammonium chloride administration with no appreciable changes occurring in the plasma potassium concentration is strong evidence for a compensatory mechanism acting on the kidney. It seems reasonable to assume that it is activated by the sodium loss and that it may act by promoting distal tubular reabsorption of sodium in exchange with potassium (cf. p. 292).

During the "recovery" following the discontinuance of the acid load ammonia excretion remains high for several days thus enabling the body to re-accumulate sodium and potassium and at the same time to rid itself of the excess of hydrogen ion equivalents which it had accomodated.

The mechanism by which ammonium chloride induces a loss of sodium (and potassium) is not yet clear, and considering the small magnitude of these changes it also seems doubtful that any experimental approach to its clarification can be devised at present. The immediate effect of ammonium chloride administration is the substitution of some of the plasma bicarbonate (and some of the negative charges on the plasma proteins) with an equivalent amount of chloride. Possibly the most satisfactory speculation that one can offer at present is that chloride is not quite as readily reabsorbed in the proximal tubules as is bicarbonate, an exchange of hydrogen ions with the actively reabsorbed sodium ions meeting less resistance than a concomitant reabsorption of chloride ions. Thus, a substitution of plasma bicarbonate with chloride would tend to retard the reabsorption of sodium.

Furthermore, it should not be lost sight of that the urea formed from the ammonium chloride might be sufficient to produce a mild osmotic diuresis. That this mechanism can only account for part of the natriuresis induced by ammonium chloride, is borne out by the fact that a natriuresis may also be induced by administration of dilute *hydrochloric acid* (STEHLE[942]) as well as by *oral* intakes of *calcium chloride*.

It is well known that very considerable amounts of sodium and potassium may be lost in the urine during a state of *endogenous acidosis* viz. ketosis. Characteristically, in this case no greater losses appear until the renal thresholds of the ketone bodies are exceeded and ketonuria develops. As this happens, the excess of ketone bodies being filtered produces a typical osmotic diuresis by which not only sodium matched with ketone body anions but also an excess of sodium matched with chloride is delivered from the proximal to the distal tubules. The sodium and chloride reabsorptive capacities of this latter section is thus surpassed, and urinary losses of sodium and chloride increase. Part of the sodium reabsorbed in the distal tubules will be exchanged with ammonium and potassium ions which then appear in the urine. In diabetes mellitus the excretion of glucose further increases the osmotic diuresis, leading to additional urinary losses of cations. As cation depletion and dehydration develop compensatory reactions are, however, evoked which inter alia cut down renal blood flow and reduce glomerular propulsive pressure, thereby counteracting the natriuresis.

f) Mercurial diuretics

Although the diuretic effect of calomel was already known by PARACELSUS, and had been used in treatment of cardiac dropsy in the eighteenth century, it was not

---

[942] STEHLE, R. L.: A study of the effect of hydrochloric acid on the mineral excretion of dogs. J. biol. Chem. **31**, 461—470 (1917).

before the advent of the organic mercurial compounds, suitable for parenteral administration, that mercury came into common use as a diuretic.

When compared on the basis of the amounts of mercury excreted in the urine the organic mercurial compounds are much less toxic than inorganic compounds. Their diuretic efficacy, however, is also much smaller when assessed on the same basis, a fact which suggested to SOLLMAN et al.[943]) that the organic compounds may not be directly diuretic, but that their action is dependent upon a liberation of mercury ions. This apparently is a point on which there is not yet any general agreement. Some support to the view that organic mercurial compounds only obtain diuretic effect upon dissociation may possibly be found in the fact that such measures as alcalizing therapy and administration of 2,3-dimercaptopropanol (BAL) abolish the diuretic effect of inorganic as well as organic mercurial compounds. The observation of FARAH and MARESH[944], that monothiols such as cysteine and glutathione reduce the toxicity of organic mercurials to the heart without materially changing their diuretic effect or the doses required to cause death from renal lesions, is not necessarily inconsistent with this concept. It may only mean that these monothiols do not reach the renal site of action of mercury as well as does BAL, or that they are not so effective in preventing the binding of mercury at this particular site. It is, however, by no means excluded that the organic mercurials act as such. The discussion of the two possibilities has recently been resumed, but no conclusive evidence seems to have been produced (cf. PITTS[917], MUDGE and WEINER[945]).

A considerable number of organic mercurials has been used as diuretics; some of the most commonly used are (KING[946], TAGGART[947]):

> Mersalyl (Salyrgan, Diuregan).
> Novasurol (Merbaphen).
> Mercurin (Novurit).
> Mercuhydrin (Meralluride).
> Mercuzanthin (Mercurophyllin).
> Thiomerin (Mercaptomerin).
> Chlormerodrin.

All except the last are marketed for injection purposes with equimolar amounts of theophyllin to promote absorption and reduce local irritation upon intramuscular injection. These amounts of theophyllin are too small to exert any diuretic action by themselves. Thiomerin is mercuzanthin coupled with mercaptoacetate. The mercury content of these mercurials ranges from 25—35%, and their efficacies following intravenous administration are apparently very much alike. Therapeutic doses are $1/2$—$1^1/_2$ mg Hg/kg, while maximal natriuretic and diuretic responses has been reported in various animals with about 5 mg Hg/kg. With doses around 10—15 mg/kg lethal levels are reached.

The typical response to a fair, intravenous dose of a mercurial is characterized by a lag period of about $1/_2$ hr, with peak diuresis being reached in the second hour. The magnitude as well as the duration of the diuretic response increases with

[943] SOLLMAN, T., N. E. SCHREIBNER, H. N. COLE, J. A. GAMMEL, and J. E. RAUSCHKOLB: The diuretic effects of various mercurial treatments. J. Pharmacol. exp. Ther. **39**, 245 (1930).

[944] FARAH, A., and G. MARESH: Influence of sulfhydryl compounds on diuresis and renal and cardiac circulatory change caused by merssalyl. J. Pharmacol. exp. Ther. **92**, 73—82 (1948).

[945] MUDGE, G. H., and I. M. WEINER: The mechanism of action of mercurial and xanthine diuretics. Ann. N. Y. Acad. Sci. **71**, 344—354 (1958).

[946] KING, C. V. (ed.): Mercury and its compounds. Ann. N. Y. Acad. Sci. **65**, 357—652 (1957).

[947] TAGGART, J. V. (ed.): Chlorothiazide and other diuretic agents. Ann. N. Y. Acad. Sci. **71**, 321—478 (1958).

dosage and with the degree of hydration and the size of the body stores of sodium and chloride. (cf. PITTS and DUGGAN[948]). Characteristically, the extra fluid excreted above the pre-administration excretion is fairly close (cf. qualifying discussion below) to being isotonic with blood plasma and consequently the osmolarity of the urine approaches that of plasma with increasing diuresis, regardless of whether it was initially above or below the level of the latter. (BLUMGART et al. [949]; WESTON et al.[950]; DALE and SANDERSON[951]; GROSSMAN et al.[952] and further studies referred to below). It is a further characteristic of the mercurial diuresis that there are no consistent changes in ammonia excretion and only moderate changes in the excretion of titratable acidity (WESTON et al.[950]). Correspondingly, there is no change or only a very moderate increase in bicarbonate excretion (BERLINER et al.[953]). It follows that the increase in excretion of metal cations and chloride is very closely identical (equimolar). Except under rather special conditions, to be discussed below, sodium will make up by far the greater part of the additional cation loss, and thus be very nearly equal to the rise in chloride loss. (BLUMGART et al.[949]; MUDGE et al.[954]; DUGGAN and PITTS[955]; BRODSKY and GRAUBARTH[956]).

Mechanism of the renal response. The question how mercurials evoke a response as this has been the subject of considerable debate for many years. Although it is generally accepted that mercurials induce natriuresis and diuresis by a direct action on the kidney, the possibility still exists that they may also produce certain *extrarenal effects* of some importance to the diuretic response. Several authors (cf. CRAWFORD and McINTOSH[957]; SERBY[958]; MØLLER[959]; CALVIN et al.[960]) have reported that an increase in plasma volume may occur prior to the diuretic response and in particular when the latter is small or absent. There has been a good deal of discussion, mainly around 1930, about mobilization of tissue

[948] PITTS, R. F., and J. J. DUGGAN: Studies on diuretics. II. The relationship between glomerular filtration rate, proximal tubular reabsorption of sodium, and diuretic efficacy of mercurials. J. clin. Invest. **29**, 372—379 (1950).

[949] BLUMGART, H. L., D. R. GILLIGAN, R. V. LEVY, M. G. BROWN, and M. C. VOLK: Action of diuretic drugs. I. Action of diuretics in normal persons. Arch. intern. Med. **54**, 40—81 (1934).

[950] WESTON, R. E., J. GROSSMAN, and L. LEITER: The effect of mercurial diuretics on renal ammonia and titratable acidity production in acidotic human subjects with reference to site of diuretic action. J. clin. Invest. **30**, 1262—1271 (1951).

[951] DALE, R. A., and P. H. SANDERSON: The mode of action of a mercurial diuretic in man. J. clin. Invest. **33**, 1008—1014 (1954).

[952] GROSSMAN, J., R. E. WESTON, E. R. BORUN, and L. LEITER: Factors influencing the course of mercurial diuresis during pitressin infusion in normal subjects. J. clin. Invest. **34**, 1611—1624 (1955).

[953] BERLINER, R. W., T. J. KENNEDY, and J. ORLOFF: Relationship between acidification of the urine and potassium metabolism. Amer. J. Med. **11**, 274—282 (1951).

[954] MUDGE, G. H., J. FOULKS, and A. GILMAN: Effect of urea diuresis on renal excretion of electrolytes. Amer. J. Physiol. **158**, 218—230 (1949).

[955] DUGGAN, J. J., and R. F. PITTS: Studies on diuretics. I. The site of action of mercurial diuretics. J. clin. Invest. **29**, 365—371 (1950).

[956] BRODSKY, W. A., and H. N. GRAUBARTH: Mechanism of mercurial diuresis in hydropenic dogs. Amer. J. Physiol. **172**, 67—76 (1953).

[957] CRAWFORD, J. H., and J. F. McINTOSH: Use of novasurol in edema due to heart failure. J. clin. Invest. **1**, 333—358 (1925).

[958] SERBY, A. M.: The pharmacology and therapeutics of novasurol. Arch. intern. Med. **38**, 374—384 (1926).

[959] MØLLER, K. O.: Experimentelle Untersuchungen über die Pharmakologie des Salyrgans. I. Untersuchungen über die Salyrgandiurese bei Kaninchen. Naunyn-Schmiedebergs Arch. exp. Path. Pharmak. **148**, 56—66 (1930).

[960] CALVIN, D. B., G. DECHERD, and G. HERRMANN: Response of plasma volume to diuretics. Proc. Soc. exp. Biol. (N. X.) **44**, 529—531 (1940).

water and salts, supported by such evidence as accelerated flow of fluid from CURSCHMANN cannulae placed in oedematous tissus upon the administration of mercurials (TSCHERNING[961]; OFFENBACHER[962]). It has also been claimed that mersalyl exerts a similar "spreading effect" as hyaluronidase in subcutaneous tissues. (EDLUND and LINDERHOLM[963]).

The author finds it difficult to assess these findings (which have not been uniformly confirmed), and in particular what their significance may be in relation to the diuretic and natriuretic effect of mercurials.

The proof of a *direct action* upon the kidney was delivered by BARTRAM[964] who injected mercurials into one renal artery in anaestetized dogs which were kept hydrated by infusion of rather large volumes of saline. Upon the injection of some 0.5 mg/kg of novasural or 2 mg/kg of salyrgan a striking diuresis was obtained on the injected side, while no significant diuresis occurred from the other kidney. Somewhat larger doses caused diuresis on both sides, but earlier and more pronounced on the injected side. Still larger doses (i.e. some 15—20 mg of the two drugs) caused a depression in urine flow on the injected side; but a pronounced diuresis on the opposite side. Earlier failures to obtain similar results may have been due to mercurial overdosage. The observation of KUPFER et al.[965] that the injection of salyrgan (8 mg of Hg) on the arterial side of a pump-lung perfusion of a dog's kidney caused a prompt and very marked increase in vascular resistance in the kidney and marked diminution in diuresis, is probably pertinent to this and to the latter observations of BARTRAM. Upon addition of the mercurial to the outflow blood from the kidney KUPFER et al. generally observed a significant increase in natriuresis and diuresis and no significant change in renal vascular resistance or glomerular filtration rate. Aminophyllin abolished the vasoconstrictor effect of salyrgan. It is noteworthy that MØLLER[966] has reported the occurrence of an immediate reduction in kidney volume and a simultaneous diminution in urine flow following *intravenous* injection of salyrgan (3—9 mg Hg/kg) in dogs and rabbits. The much cited experiments by GOVAERTS[967], in which a kidney from a dog at the height of novasurol diuresis was anastomosed to the vessels in the neck of a normal dog and continued to show diuresis, is further evidence of a direct renal action. PITTS[917] has recently repeated BARTRAM's experiments and confirmed the faster and predominant saluretic-diuretic effect on the injected side; as regards the response from the other side he did, however, make certain observations which are not readily explained.

While a direct action of mercurials on the kidney is thus well-established, the exact site of action and the details about the mechanism of mercurial diuresis are still the subject of considerable debate, which has greatly intensified during the last few years. The concensus of opinion is that the action responsible for the

[961] TSCHERNING, R.: Über Salyrgan. Dtsch. med. Wschr. **53**, 1465—1466 (1927).

[962] OFFENBACHER, R.: Über die Behandlung anhydropischer Herzkranker mit Novosurol. Arch. Verdaukr. **42**, 487—489 (1928).

[963] EDLUND, T., and H. LINDERHOLM: The action of salyrgan on skin permeability — salyrgan as a spreading factor. Acta physiol. scand. **18**, 144—150 (1949).

[964] BARTRAM, E. A.: Experimental observations on the effect of various diuretics when injected directly into one renal artery of the dog. J. clin. Invest. **11**, 1197—1219 (1932).

[965] KUPFER, S., D. D. THOMPSON, and R. F. PITTS: The isolated kidney and its response to diuretic agents. Amer. J. Physiol. **167**, 703—713 (1951).

[966] MØLLER, K. O.: Experimentelle Untersuchungen über die Pharmakologie des Salyrgans. IV. Die Kreislaufwirkung des Salyrgans. Naunyn-Schmiedebergs Arch. exp. Path. Pharmak. **164**, 242—251 (1932).

[967] GOVAERTS, P.: Origine rénale ou tissulaire de la diurèse par un composé mercuriel organique. C. R. Soc. Biol. (Paris) **99**, 647—649 (1928).

diuretic effect is on the tubules, but whether proximal or distal or both still remains uncertain.

One way in which attempts have been made to localize the site of action in the tubules has been by histological and histochemical examinations of kidneys from animals exposed to diuretic or higher doses of mercurials. There is a considerable body of evidence that with minimal necrotizing doses of mercurials renal damage is confined to the proximal convoluted tubules, in particular the more distal portions ot these (cf. EDWARDS[968]; SIMONDS and HEPLER[969]; WACHSTEIN and MEISEL[970]). With larger doses necrosis also occurs in the distal convoluted tubules and the ascending limb of HENLE's loop. By histochemical methods using neotetrazolium for determination of succinic dehydrogenase, WACHSTEIN and MEISEL[971, 972] observed that the administration of high doses of mercuhydrin and novurit (10 mg of Hg/kg) to rats caused a reduction in this enzyme (and necrosis) in the terminal parts of the proximal tubules. From studies with a similar technique MUSTAKALLIO and TELKKÄ[973], however, reported that the earliest and most pronounced changes occurred in the ascending limb of HENLE's loop.

Another approach to the problem of the mechanism of mercurial diuresis has been to record alterations in renal function induced by mercurials. One group of these studies is concerned with such substances which are transferred by the renal tubules in such small quantities, that an interference with their transfer would be without any appreciable effect on the rate of urine flow, i. e. would be unable to account *per se* for more pronounced mercurial diureses.

Among the substances known to be transferred by the proximal tubular cells, glucose-Tm has been reported to be markedly depressed in man by therapeutic doses of organic mercurials (WESTON et al.[974]); McDONALD and MILLER[975] did not find any such depression, while they reported a marked depression in Tm for p-aminohippurate, a substance now also known to be secreted by the proximal tubules. This confirms the earlier findings of BRUN et al.[976], and BERLINER et al.[977] that therapeutic doses cause very appreciable reductions in Tm for p-amino-hippurate and diodrast in man.

Several authors have been unable to obtain similar effects with corresponding doses in the dog, although good diuretic responses were obtained. Thus BERLINER et al.[977], did not observe any depression in Tm for p-aminohippurate, and

[968] EDWARDS, J. G.: Renal tubule (nephron) as affected by mercury. Amer. J. Path. 18, 1011—1127 (1942).

[969] SIMONDS, J. P., and O. E. HEPLER: Experimental nephropathics. Quart. Bull. Northwest. Univ. Med. School. 19, 278—295 (1945).

[970] WACHSTEIN, M., and E. MEISEL: Protective action of certain amino acids on toxicity of mercurial diuretics in rats. Proc. Soc. exptl. Biol. (N. Y.) 76, 523—527 (1951).

[971] WACHSTEIN, M., and E. MEISEL: (a) Influence of experimental renal damage on histochemically demonstrable succinic dehydrogenase activity in the rat. Amer. J. Path. 30, 147—165 (1954).

[972] WACHSTEIN, M., and E. MEISEL: (b) Renal succinic dehydrogenase and mercurial diuretics. Experientia (Basel) 10, 495 (1954).

[973] MUSTAKALLIO, K. K., and A. TELKKÄ: Histochemical localization of the mercurial inhibition of succinic dehydrogenase in rat kidney. Science 118, 320—321 (1953).

[974] WESTON, R. E., J. GROSSMAN, I. S. EDELMAN, D. J. W. ESCHER, L. LEITER, and L. HELLMAN: Renal tubular action of diuretics; effects of mercurial diuresis on glucose reabsorption. Fed. Proc. 8, 164 (1949).

[975] McDONALD, R. K., and J. H. MILLER: Effect of mercury on renal tubular transfer of p-aminohippurate and glucose in man. Proc. Soc. exp. Biol. (N. Y.) 72, 408—410 (1949).

[976] BRUN, C., T. HILDEN, and F. RAASCHOU: On the effects of mersalyl on renal function. Acta pharmacol. (Kbh.) 3, 1—12 (1947).

[977] BERLINER, R. W., T. J. KENNEDY, and J. G. HILTON: Salyrgan and renal tubular secretion of para-aminohippurate in the dog and man. Amer. J. Physiol. 154, 537—541 (1948).

HANDLY et al.[978], did not observe it for this substance nor for glucose. The lack of uniformity in the relationship between diuretic effect and inhibition of tubular transfers of these substances obviously weaken the argument that observed inhibitions may be taken as evidence for a proximal site of action as responsible for the diuretic effect of mercurials.

The fact that the secretion of ammonia, which is known to occur in the most distal parts of the nephrons, is not influenced by diuretically effective doses of mercurials (WESTON et al.[950]) has been advanced as evidence against a distal site of action. Such a negative result does not, however, preclude that other distal processes may be affected. That this may actually be the case is suggested by the fact that mercurials apparently depress tubular secretion of potassium, a process which is also generally believed to be confined to the distal parts of the nephron. (BERLINER and KENNEDY[979]; MUDGE et al.[980]), see below.

It is evident that these results do not permit any conclusions as to whether the *diuretic* response to mercurials is due to an action in proximal or distal parts of the nephron. And, in fact, whatever relationship had been observed between diuretic response and inhibition of these transfers, such studies would only be capable of providing suggestive evidence since the tubular processes underlying these might have sensitivities to mercurials greatly different from those underlying the reabsorption of salt and water.

Other studies have dealt directly with the effect of mercurials on the handling by the kidney of water and the quantitatively most important electrolytes of the glomerular filtrate, i.e. sodium and the matching anions. During the last few years a great number of studies have been reported in which the experimental conditions prevailing at the time of administration of mercurials have been varied in several ways and to different degrees (hydration — dehydration, salt loading — salt deprivation, alkalosis — acidosis, etc.). Although these studies have not yet provided conclusive answers to the question of the mechanism of mercurial diuresis, it may safely be stated that they have carried us a good step forward, and that they have also provided results which must be given serious consideration in any hypothesis of renal handling of electrolytes in general.

From the description of the typical diuretic response to mercurials presented above it appears that we have to do with a solute diuresis, which is further characterized by very nearly equimolar increments in the excretions of sodium and chloride and (ordinarily) rather little change in the excretion of other solutes.

How could such a solute diuresis arise, in principle ?

Among the types mentioned in the introduction to this section (p. 388) a "propulsion diuresis" due to an increase in glomerular propulsive pressure seems rather unlikely, since there is no evidence that mercurials cause an increase in renal blood flow in the intact organism (PITTS and DUGGAN[948]) or in the perfused kidney (KUPFER et al.[965]). Also, an *uncomplicated* propulsion diuresis would be expected to cause some increase in the excretion of bicarbonate (as well as chloride) The latter argument also holds against an *uncomplicated* "conduction diuresis",(due to a reduction of the resistance to the flow of fluids through the nephron). Consequently, it seems most likely that a prominent factor in the diuretic response is an inhibition of tubular reabsorption of sodium and chloride, with little effect on the

[978] HANDLEY, C. A., J. TELFORD, and M. LaFORGE: Xanthine and mercurial diuretics and renal tubular transport of glucose and p-aminohippurate in the dog. Proc. Soc. exp. Biol. (N. Y.) **71**, 187—188 (1949).

[979] BERLINER, R. W., and T. J. KENNEDY: The renal tubular secretion of potassium. J. clin. Invest. **27**, 525 (1948).

[980] MUDGE, G. H., A. AMES, J. FOULKS, and A. GILMAN: Effect of drugs on renal secretion of potassium in the dog. Amer. J. Physiol. **161**, 151—158 (1950).

reabsorption of bicarbonate. It is well documented from a considerable number of experiments, in which glomerular filtration rate was measured, that a reduction in the rate of tubular reabsorption of sodium and chloride actually occurs during pronounced mercurial diuresis. (PITTS and DUGGAN[948]; and several other studies where a copious natriuresis was observed, without any significant changes in filtration rate). Data illustrating this effect are presented in Table 29 taken from the work of FARAH et al.

Now, according to current views, sodium and chloride are being reabsorbed in the proximal as well as the distal tubules, and in both places water reabsorption is dependent upon such reabsorptions. In principle, the natriuretic and diuretic response might therefore be due to an inhibition in the proximal as well as in the distal tubules. Several attempts have been made to argue for or against an action at each of these sites, on the basis of the magnitude of the reduction in tubular reabsorption of Na and water that may be obtained with maximally effective doses of mercury. DUGGAN and PITTS[955] found that in dogs pretreated with saline infusions (initial dose *plus* 10 ml/min) a reduction in tubular reabsorption of water and sodium amounting to some 17—21% of the normally filtered amounts could be obtained with mercurials at doses around 45 mg Hg. This suggested to them that the mercurial probably exerted its action on the distal tubular system, since the reabsorptive capacity of that part of the nephron was generally believed to be of this magnitude. That this identity in magnitudes was only fortuitous is clearly borne out by several more recent studies, in which considerably larger reductions in tubular reabsorption were observed. Thus, WESSON and ANSLOW[981] and FARAH et al., cf. Table 29, have reported excretion percentages (tubular rejection fractions) for sodium, chloride and water as high as 40% in dogs at normal filtration rates and pre-existing excretion percentages below 5%. If the — admittedly somewhat loosely founded — view, that distal capacities for sodium and water reabsorption amount to less than 20% of the rates at which sodium and water are normally filtered, is correct, such results must be taken to mean that at least part of the inhibition is exerted in the proximal tubules. Similar significance can not be attributed to excretion percentages of some 35% reported as obtained in cardiac patients by WESTON et al.[950]), since they were obtained at subnormal levels of filtration rates, for which reason they do not represent as large absolute reductions in tubular reabsorptions.

Further attempts to distinguish between proximal and distal sites of action have been made on the basis of determinations of the osmolarity of the extra amount of fluid excreted in response to mercurials, or, what actually amounts to the same, by determining "free water" clearances. As apparent from the discussion in a previous section (p. 242) the formation of hypotonic and hypertonic urines both depend on distal tubular functions. In both cases the reabsorption of sodium in the distal tubular system forms the backbone of the process, but a suitable state of permeability to water in the more distal parts of the system is a further essential requirement.

The formation of hypotonic urine signifies the reabsorption of "salt" in the ascending limbs of HENLE's loop, the distal convoluted tubules and the collecting tubules which is not accompanied by (proportional) reabsorption of water. The capacity of this process finds an expression in the "positive free water clearance", i. e. the number of ml of water which must be subtracted from a one minute sample of hypotonic urine to make the remaining solution isotonic which plasma. This would represent the amount of "salt" reabsorbed in these segments, if it might be assumed that: (1) they receive isotonic fluid from the proximal tubules, (2) no water

---

[981] WESSON, L. G., and W. P. ANSLOW: Effect of osmotic and mercurial diuretics on simultaneous diuresis. Amer. J. Physiol. **170**, 255—269 (1952).

Table 29. *Action of esidron acid on sodium excretion at high rates of saline infusion.*
Male dog, 39.8 kg, sodium pentobarbital anesthesis. Isotonic saline infused at a rate of 39.8 ml/min/m². All values are based on one m² of body surface. From A. FARAH, T. S. COBBEY jr., and W. MOOK[994]

Time min	Urine Flow ml/min	Plasma sodium mM/l	Sodium filtered mM/min	Sodium excreted mM/min	Sodium reabsorbed mM/min	Urine Sodium mM/l
0— 20	10.9	153.6	14.24	0.55	13.69	50.5
20— 40	9.8	155.2	13.01	0.44	12.57	44.4
40— 60	10.25	156.5	12.69	0.42	12.27	40.7
60— 80	9.9	157.1	12.31	0.41	11.90	41.0
80— 85	30 mg/kg esidron acid with cysteine (1 : 1 molar ratio)					
80—100	9.8	158.3	11.28	0.53	10.75	54.0
100—120	12.95	159	10.95	1.02	9.93	92.0
120—130	32.9	160.8	14.80	4.1	10.70	124.6
130—140	43.5	162	16.31	7.07	9.24	162.5
150—160	47.0	160	14.36	7.01	7.35	148.9
160—170	47.1	159	14.98	7.00	7.98	148.6
170—180	45.0	160	13.84	6.82	7.02	151.1
180—190	44.4	158	13.01	6.96	6.05	156.7
190—193						
BAL 4 mg/kg I.V.						
190—200	6.5	158	9.8	1.0	8.80	153.8
200—210	9.5	160	10.10	0.80	9.30	94.7
210—220	10.1	161	12.42	0.75	11.72	74.2
220—230	11.4	164	10.96	0.81	10.16	70.1

at all is reabsorbed along with the salt, (3) no other significant reabsorption of osmotically active solutes takes place in these segments.

Formation of hypertonic urine, on the other hand, is visualized to depend primarily upon active reabsorption of sodium without water by the ascending limbs of HENLE's loops which in turn makes possible a reabsorption of water by osmosis from the collecting tubules into hypertonic medullary interstices. This may give rise to a "negative free water clearance", i. e. the amount of water that must be added to a one minute sample of hypertonic urine to make it isotonic with plasma. Under conditions where both the distal convoluted tubules and the collecting tubules are highly permeable to water the magnitude of this clearance will grossly measure the rate at which salt has been reabsorbed unaccompanied by water by the loops of HENLE (as long as equilibrium is closely attained by the medullary vascular countercurrent system at each level of the medulla).

The effect of mercurials on the negative free water clearance has been determined by a few experimentators under conditions where it may reasonably be believed that the latter condition is fulfilled, viz. during the administration of optimal doses of antidiuretic hormone. In such experiments on saline loaded normal human subjects WELT et al.[982] and GROSSMAN et al.[952] found no appreciable changes in negative free water clearance during rises in diuresis from a few ml/min to 10—18 ml/min induced by therapeutic doses of thiomerin (80 mg Hg). Expressed in another way the *extra* excreted fluid was very nearly isotonic with plasma; in fact, from the latter work it was found to be slightly hypertonic at least for small rises in diuresis. From these observations it seems justified to conclude that the distal tubular process by which concentrated urines are produced is not affected by mercurials in doses, capable of producing sizable rises in diuresis.

[982] WELT, L. G., A. V. GOODYER, J. H. DARRAGH, W. A. ABELE, and W. H. MARONEY: Site of saluretic action of an organic mercurial compound. J. appl. Physiol. 6, 134—138 (1953).

Several investigators have determined the effect of mercurials on "positive free water clearances" under such conditions where these may be assumed to have their maximal value, viz. under conditions of water loading. WESSON and ANS-LOW[981] reported the results of four such determinations in dogs in a state of maintained water diuresis and two during a stabilized mixed water and urea diureses. In both cases mercurin was given in a dose corresponding to 10 mg Hg/kg. Although the authors conclude that the positive free water clearance was little affected by the mercurial, it rather appears from the data presented that in most cases there was an appreciable reduction. LADD[983] made similar studies in three patients prehydrated by some 2 l of water and subsequent infusion of saline at a fast rate. The administration of thiomerin (0.3—0.9 mg Hg/kg) was found to produce a decrease in positive free water clearance of 30—40%. Although free water clearances were not actually calculated the statements of CAPPS et al.[984] and of DALE and SANDERSON[951], that mersalyl in therapeutic doses did only cause a slight augmentation of a preexisting maximal water diuresis, while an appreciable rise in U/P ratios for sodium and chloride ensued implies that a decrease in positive free water clearance must have occurred. Altogether it appears that a decrease in positive free water clearance is a regular response to mercurials even in therapeutical doses. If the possibility could be excluded that the mercurials have caused a liberation of antidiuretic hormone the conclusion must be drawn that either mercurials increase the permeability of the (distal) tubular cells to water, or that they inhibit sodium and chloride reabsorptions in a portion of the tubules where the reabsorption of water is dependent upon these reabsorptions, but lagging behind them under conditions of water diuresis. Certainly, the latter alternative seems the most likely. Although not necessarily so, it also seems most likely that the tubular portion indicated above is identical with the distal tubular system.

From the experimental results so far discussed it appears that there is some indication that the diuretic-saluretic response to mercurials may be dependent upon an inhibitory action on sodium and chloride reabsorptions in the proximal as well as in the distal portions of the tubular system.

A similar conclusion has recently been drawn by SAUGMAN[212]. In dogs which had received and were excreting nitrate and iodide in amounts sufficient to cause a moderate osmotic diuresis he observed that the administration of salyrgan (3—4 mg Hg/kg) caused some increase in the excretion percentage (e.g. from 20 to 30, and from 27 to 40% for iodide and nitrate respectively) for these anions at fairly constant filtration rates. On the assumption that these anions are only reabsorbed in the proximal tubules — and in competition with chloride for concomitant reabsorption with the actively reabsorbed sodium — he concluded this increase was due to an inhibition of proximal sodium reabsorption. Since the rise in the excretion percentage for chloride simultaneously observed was somewhat greater than that observed to accompany a corresponding rise in the excretion percentages for nitrate and iodide during increasing osmotic diuresis he further felt that mersalyl had also exerted some inhibition upon a distal reabsorption process specific for chloride.

Very recently the stop-flow technique has been used in an attempt to clarify the tubular site of action of mercurials (KESSLER et al.[985], VANDER et al.[986]). Since

[983] LADD, M.: Renal excretion of sodium and water in man as affected by prehydration, saline infusions, pitressin and thiomerin. J. appl. Physiol. 4, 602—619 (1952).

[984] CAPPS, J. N., W. S. WIGGINS, D. R. AXELROD, and R. F. PITTS: The effect of mercurial diuretics on the excretion of water. Circulation 6, 82—89 (1952).

[985] KESSLER, R. H., K. HIERHOLZER, R. S. GURD, and R. F. PITTS: Localization of diuretic action of chlormerodrin in the nephron of the dog. Amer. J. Physiol. 194, 540—546 (1958).

[986] VANDER, A. J., R. L. MALVIN, W. S. WILDE, and L. P. SULLIVAN: Localization of the site of action of mercurial diuretics by stop flow analysis. Amer. J. Physiol. 195, 558—562 (1958).

the sodium concentration in the effluent from the distal tubular segments was found to be reduced to the same very low levels in the "mercurial periods" as in the control periods, the authors drew the conclusion that mercurials do not depress distal sodium reabsorption (but do exert an inhibitory action on the proximal reabsorption of sodium, chloride and water). These conclusions are not indisputable, in particular the objection may be raised that, whereas the said findings in the distal effluents show that the *concentration gradient* against which sodium can be reabsorbed in the distal segments is not reduced by diuretic doses of mercurials, they do not prove that the *reabsorption capacity* (meq/min) of these segments is uninfluenced.

How do these conclusions go with our present concepts of the tubular transfer processes and in particular with the picture of the hydrodynamics of the nephron sketched in a previous section (p. 261)?

If mercurials caused a sizable inhibition of proximal sodium reabsorption would we not expect an appreciable rise in not only chloride but also in bicarbonate excretion (the latter of which does not occur)? "Yes", would seem to be the answer if we visualize proximal reabsorption of sodium ions as a unitary process which may occur with either concomitant chloride ion transfer or hydrogen ion exchange (leading indirectly to a bicarbonate "reabsorption") in mutual competition. It must be recalled, however, that there is some evidence (cf. p. 238) that an exchange with hydrogen ions is "given some preference" or expressed in another way that the chloride transfer meets with a resistance greatly exceeding that encountered by an exchanging hydrogen ion. An inhibition of the primary transfer process (sodium reabsorption) might therefore well be accompanied by a preferential decrease in *that* secondary ion transfer (chloride reabsorption) which meets the greatest resistance. A preferential reduction in the transfer of chloride could also be visualized to arise from an increased resistance to secondary ion transfers induced by the mercurials.

Another question arises from the observation that very sizable reductions in the rate of tubular reabsorption of water and sodium has been reported to occur without any significant change or even with an increase in filtration rate, at least under conditions of an increased salt load (cf. Table 29; for further references see PITTS and SARTORIUS[915]; DUGGAN and PITTS[955]). Would we not expect a *reduction* in filtration rate to result from a decrease in proximal fluid reabsorption? Even if mercurials are mainly assumed to inhibit fluid reabsorption in the more distal portion of the proximal tubules, i.e. that portion in which changes in fluid reabsorption has the least effect on the filtration rate, we would still have to answer this question in the affirmative. However, only with the qualification that we were sure that there was no simultaneous change in propulsion pressure or nephron hydrodynamic resistance. But we are not sure, and it remains for the future to explore this field. In the meantime we may tentatively assume that mercurials in suitable doses may cause a reduction in the resistance to the flow of fluids through the nephron. Otherwise it may be difficult to account for the induction of urine flow rates as high as 40% of the filtration rate. One might speculate that such an assumed effect of mercurials could be bound up with the other effect suggested above, i.e. an augmentation of the resistance to cellular transfer of chloride. If namely the processes responsible for an active transcellular transfer of sodium are localized at the basal border of the tubular cells, i.e. a sodium extrusion, and if mercurials produce an increase in the resistance to the entrance of chloride across the luminal border, the general effect would be that the cells "pumped themselves out" for sodium and chloride. A reduction in cellular contents of these ions would in turn lead to a reduction in cell volume, if cellular isotonicity were maintained i.e.

to an increase in the diameter of the tubular lumens. The reduction in resistance to the flow of fluid through the tubules thereby created could counteract the drop in filtration rate which might be expected as the immediate result of a decrease in proximal reabsorptions of salt and water. Furthermore, it would promote diuresis. That mercurials might increase the conductance of the glomerular membrane is another possibility which deserves consideration.

Cellular site of action. The above speculations call on a few comments on the supposed site of action of mercurials in the cells. It may be stated at once that we have no definite knowledge on this point, and it is probably wise to keep in view that there may be more sites of action of importance to the diuretic response. It is a common view that the actions of mercurials responsible for their diuretic effect are exerted in the interior of the tubular cells. Sulfhydryl groups are known to have a high affinity to mercuric ions and mercurials with a free valence of mercury and the metabolic inhibitions observed in vitro in tissue preparations upon the addition of mercurials are generally attributed to a combination of mercury with sulfhydryl enzyme systems. A reduction in succinic dehydrogenase activity has been observed in kidney tissue from rats which had received sub-lethal doses of mercurials (for references see PITTS and SARTORIUS[915] and WACHSTEIN and MEISEL[971, 972]); inhibition of this and similar enzymes was suggested as an explanation of the diuretic effect. It has further been found by CAFRUNY and FARAH[987] that *diuretic* doses of mersalyl (10 mg/kg) lowered the concentration of protein-bound sulfhydryl in the terminal parts of the proximal tubules, the ascending limbs of Henle's loop and the collecting ducts, and that BAL restored these concentrations to control levels. COHEN[988] has observed a reduction in the incorporation of radioactive phosphate in kidney slices from rats which had received diuretic doses of salyrgan (about 5 mg Hg/kg); no reduction in oxygen uptake was demonstrable in the slices, but it did occur when lethal doses (15 mg Hg/kg) had been administered. COHEN suggested tentatively that mercurials impede the generation of high energy phosphate bonds and that a deficiency of such utilizable energy might be responsible for a reduction in tubular reabsorptions.

Although admittedly highly suggestive, such demonstrations of inhibitions of enzyme activities and supposedly secondary metabolic effects thereof, do not, of course, necessarily imply that such effects play a causative role in the mechanism of the diuretic response; they may be only parallel effects, or at least they may be only part of the explanation. The question of how mercurials are excreted by the kidneys is of some pertinence to this discussion. That the commonly used organic mercurials may be excreted by tubular secretion was postulated by BRUN et al.[976] on the grounds that they are known to be very rapidly excreted by the kidneys and that they are cyclic acids with similar pK values as various substances (phenol red, diodrast, penicillin etc.) known to be secreted by the (proximal) tubules. In a very thorough study it has later been shown by GROSSMAN et al.[989] that in patients to whom thiomerin or mercuhydrin had been administered the renal clearances of mercury amount to some $1/2 - 2/3$ of the glomerular filtration rate. Since major fractions of the organic mercurials are bound in plasma to proteins (i.e. are present in non-filterable form) these figures do not disprove — but rather

---

[987] CAFRUNY, E. J., and A. FARAH: Effects of the mercurial, mersalyl, on the concentration of protein-bound sulfhydryl in the cytoplasm of dog kidney cells. J. Pharmacol. exp. Ther. **117**, 101—105 (1956).

[988] COHEN, E. M.: On the mechanism of action of mercurial diuretics. Acta physiol. pharmacol. neerl. **3**, 45—58 and 59—70 (1953).

[989] GROSSMAN, J., R. E. WESTON, R. A. LEHMAN, J. P. HALPERIN, T. D. ULLMAN, and L. LEITER: Urinary and fecal excretion of mercury in man following administration of mercurial diuretics. J. clin. Invest. **30**, 1208—1220 (1951).

prove — tubular secretion of these substances. Such secretion has recently been conclusively demonstrated in chicken and dogs (WEINER et al.[990]; see PITTS[917]), and evidence for a proximal site of secretion has been provided. The existence of a tubular secretion of mercurials does obviously not necessarily imply that they exert their saluretic effect during the passage through the cells, and the fact that an organic mercurial without diuretic effects may be secreted by the tubules (KESSLER et al.[991]) urges to caution in drawing such conclusions. The preferential cell damage in the more distal parts of the proximal tubules (or further distally) following sublethal doses rather suggests that these substances may exert important actions (and possibly also saluretic actions) on the tubular cells from the luminal side. This finding seems to indicate that mercurials which enter the tubular fluid — be it by filtration or tubular secretion — must undergo some concentration before they exert cell damaging effects. Another point which lends some support to the view that the actual action of the organic mercurials is established upon their arrival in the tubular fluid is the fact that the existence of a proteinuria prior to the administration of mercurials exert a protective effect against the nephrotoxic action. This has been demonstrated by induced albuminuria in rats (LIPMANN[992]) and by induced haemoglobinuria in dogs (HAVILL et al.[993]). Inactivation of mercury by the presence of proteins in the tubular lumens suggests itself as an explanation; alternative explanations are, however, possible.

Factors influencing the diuretic response to mercurials. It has been known for a long time that the magnitude of the diuretic and saluretic response to mercurials is greatly dependent upon the state of hydration and in particular, on the *body stores of salt*, to which such terms as "availability of fluid for excretion" have been applied. Recent experimental studies have fully confirmed these views. Thus DUGGAN and PITTS[955] found that dogs only pre-treated with water responded with very small and shortlived diuresis following the administration of organic mercurials (generally in doses corresponding to some 45 mg of Hg) and that a fall in filtration rate occurred during the decline of the diuretic response. Dogs pre-treated with a preliminary dose and continued infusion of 10 ml/min of saline, however, showed a much larger and more lasting response and no fall in filtration rate. Analogous results were obtained by PITTS and DUGGAN[948] in normal human subjects. Without previous hydration or increased salt intakes the diuretic response was short and small and generally accompanied by some fall in glomerular filtration rate as well as in renal plasma flow. When saline was infused at a rate of 10 ml/min for $2^{1}/_{2}$ hr prior to the administration of the mercurin (80 mg of Hg) as well as during the remaining observation period very large diuretic responses ensued and actual increases in glomerular filtration rate and renal plasma flow were generally observed. These findings were confirmed by FARAH et al.[994] in their experiments in dogs.

More than one factor is probably involved in this apparently potentiating effect of salt administration on the diuretic-saluretic response to mercurials. If no salt has been administered prior to administration of the mercurial compensatory

---

[990] WEINER, I. M., A. F. BURNETT, and B. R. RENNICK: The renal tubular secretion of mersalyl (Salyrgan) in the chicken. J. Pharmacol. exp. Ther. **118**, 470—476 (1956).

[991] KESSLER, R. H., R. LOZANO, and R. F. PITTS: Studies of structure diuretic activity relationships of organic compounds of mercury. J. clin. Invest. **36**, 656—668 (1957).

[992] LIPMANN, R. W.: Effect of proteinuria on toxicity of mercurial diuretics in the rat. Proc. Soc. exp. Biol. (N. Y.) **72**, 682—687 (1949).

[993] HAVILL, W. H., J. A. LICHTY, and G. H. WHIPPLE: Tolerance for mercury poisoning increased by frequent hemoglobin injections. J. exp. Med. **55**, 627—635 (1932).

[994] FARAH, A., T. S. COBBEY, jr., and W. MOOK: Renal action of mercurial diuretics as affected by sodium load. J. Pharmacol. exp. Ther. **104**, 31—39 (1952).

reactions to the initial salt and water loss apparently develop, comprising *inter alia* a diminution in renal blood flow. In consequence, a reduction in glomerular propulsion pressure must be assumed to occur which tends to diminish the response. Apart from the fact that saline administration counteracts the development of a salt and water deficiency, it probably also enhances the diuretic-saluretic response in a more direct way. Probably as a response to an expansion of the plasma volume increased renal blood flow and an increased rate of proximal salt and water reabsorption (as evidenced by increase in filtration rate) has been induced by the saline infusions. As is further apparent from the experimental data some elevation in plasma sodium concentrations has been produced (cf. Table 29). Prior to the administration of mercurials the kidneys have therefore seemingly been in a state characterized by some increase in glomerular propulsion pressure (increased glomerular capillary pressure — lowered osmotic pressure of the plasma), some shrinkage in the (proximal) tubular cells (by hypertonicity of the body fluids), increased reabsorption activity in the proximal cells and saturation of the distal reabsorption processes. As a consequence of these factors rather high urine flow rates were present already in the control periods. Under such conditions the scene is so to speak set for great diuretic responses. Such would result from loading with even moderate amounts of osmotic diuretics and if mercurials act mainly by inhibiting proximal reabsorption of salts and water they too would be expected to produce greater diuretic responses. Conversely, it seems understandable that renal vasoconstriction with lowering of glomerular propulsive pressure and diminution of proximal fluid reabsorption, low tonicity of the body fluids and lack of saturation of distal reabsorption processes would create unfavourable conditions for responses to mercurial diuretics. WESTON et al.[995] have studied patients with unresponsiveness to mercurial diuretics and have — among other factors — emphasized the importance of "impaired renal haemodynamics" to failing responsiveness. They have further shown that a great increase in diuretic and natriuretic response may be obtained in such patients by intravenous administration of 0.48—0.72 g of aminophyllin some time after the administration of the mercurial. It is noteworthy that a considerable increase in renal plasma flow was induced by the aminophyllin. This finding confirms what has been known for many years, that theophyllin potentiates the diuretic effect of mercurials, but it may be appropriate to point out that since the effect of theophylline is short-lived it should be given shortly before the peak of the effect of the mercurial is expected i. e. some 1 to 2 hr after the latter has been administered.

Another factor which has long been known to influence the response to mercurial diuretics is what may loosely be called the *acid-base state of the body*. The administration of acidifying agents, such as ammonium chloride, prior to a mercurial has been used for many years to augment the action of the latter. That a true potentiation is obtained, not only an addition of effects, was shown by ETHRIDGE et al.[996], AXELROD and PITTS[997] and others. It is also known (cf. these studies and those by MUDGE and HARDIN[998]) that preliminary administration

[995] WESTON, R. E., D. J. W. ESCHER, J. GROSSMAN, and L. LEITER: Mechanisms contributing to unresponsiveness to mercurial diuretics in congestive failure. J. clin. Invest. **31**, 901—910 (1952).

[996] ETHRIDGE, C. B., D. W. MYERS, and M. N. FULTON: Modifying effect of various inorganic salts on the diuretic action of salyrgan. Arch. intern. Med. **57**, 714—728 (1936).

[997] AXELROD, D. R., and R. F. PITTS: The relationship of plasma pH and anion pattern to mercurial diuresis. J. clin. Invest. **31**, 171—179 (1952).

[998] MUDGE, G. H., and B. HARDIN: Response to mercurial diuretics during alkalosis: A comparison of acute metabolic and chronic hypokalemic alkalosis in the dog. J. clin. Invest. **35**, 155—163 (1956).

of sodium bicarbonate may greatly diminish or completely abolish the diuretic-saluretic response to mercurials.

It has been believed by many that the explanation to these observations should be sought in changes in the p_H of the extracellular fluids. It appears, however, that this conception must be abandoned, since it has been shown by HILTON[999], who administered ammonium chloride (6 g per day) to a human subject over a period of 30 days, that the diuretic and natriuretic response to mercuhydrin (80 mg Hg) remained unchanged even when the p_H and bicarbonate and chloride concentrations had returned to normal values at the end of this period by endogenous compensating reactions. The urine obviously remained acid throughout the period of ammonium chloride administration in HILTON's experiments and it might of course be, as others have suggested, that the factor responsible for the potentiating effect was a reduction in the p_H of the tubular fluid at some level. Thus an effect of the p_H of the urine upon the dissociation of the organic mercurial has been suggested. Recent reports by BENESCH and BENESCH[1000] that the reactions between organic mercurials and dithiols are markedly influenced by p_H may also be pertinent to this point.

The view that a lowering of the p_H of the tubular fluid is responsible for the potentiating action of ammonium chloride administration is not, however, easily reconciled with the fact that the diuretic-saluretic response to organic mercurials is not inhibited by preliminary administration of a carbonic anhydrase inhibitor, like Diamox, which renders the urin alkaline (BERLINER et al.[223]; AXELROD and PITTS[997]). MUDGE and HARDIN[998] made an interesting comparison between the diuretic-saluretic efficacy of a mercurial, mercuhydrin (39 mg of Hg), during extracellular alkalosis produced in one group of dogs by potassium depletion (low potassium diet combined with daily injections of 10 mg of DOCA) and in another by administration of sodium bicarbonate. Whereas almost complete refractoriness developed in the latter case, in the first group the chloruretic response was either similar to or somewhat higher than that observed in the normal state. Since the extracellular alkalosis of potassium depletion is known to be accompanied by an intracellular acidosis, which probably also comprises the tubular cells (cf. p. 538 and p. 394) the authors postulated that an increased acidity of the tubular cells facilitates the interaction between mercury and cellular components of the electrolyte transport mechanism. They realized, however, that since an acid urine (p_H about 6) was produced by the potassium deficient animals, their data did not exclude urinary p_H as a factor of importance.

Evidently, the potentiating action of ammonium chloride therapy upon mercurial diuresis cannot be fully accounted for at present, and it seems likely that not a single, but several of the changes induced by such therapy may be of importance. (For a further discussion cf. MUDGE and WEINER[945].)

Effects of mercurials on urinary potassium excretion. In the above presentation the effect of mercurial diuretics has been described as causing the excretion of nearly equivalent amounts of sodium and chloride and, unless a water diuresis was previously present, an excretion of water in nearly isotonic proportions. Mercurials are not, however, entirely devoid of effects on the excretion of other electrolytes, and under special conditions they may even induce major changes in the excretion of potassium.

[999] HILTON, J. G.: Potentiation of diuretic action of mercuhydrin by ammonium chloride. J. clin. Invest. **30**, 1105—1110 (1951).

[1000] BENESCH, R., and R. E. BENESCH: Reactions of thiols with organic mercury compounds. Arch. Biochem. **38**, 425—441 (1952).

That mercurials may affect urinary excretion of potassium one way or the other has been known for some time. It is, however, only with more recent studies that the conditions have been defined under which mercurials may induce increased and decreased urinary losses of potassium, respectively. MUDGE et al.[980] made the observation that in dogs under conditions of water diuresis, in which the urinary excretion of potassium was low (and the urine/plasma ratio for potassium regularly below 1) organic mercurial diuretics (some 40 + 40 mg of Hg) produced an increase in potassium excretion (rises in the excretion percentage from 5 to some 20—30% were observed). In dogs, which had been pretreated for several days with potassium chloride and which were given additional amounts of this salt during the experiments, similar dosages, however, caused a marked decrease in potassium excretion. In this latter group, potassium was subject to tubular secretion as evidenced by the fact that the potassium clearance regularly exceeded the exogenous creatinine clearance in the control periods. The abolition of at least this excess excretion by mercurials must have been due to an inhibition of tubular potassium secretion. Probably greater amounts of potassium than these were actually being secreted in the control periods and accordingly the observation, that the mercurials generally induced a fall in potassium clearance/inulin clearance ratios from 1.0—1.2 to 0.5—0.7, may reasonably be interpreted to mean that most of this fall was caused by an inhibition of potassium secretion. This is also the interpretation proposed by the authors, who furthermore suggest that the increased potassium excretions observed in the first group reflect a depression of tubular reabsorption of potassium exerted by the mercurials.

Whereas the correctness of the first interpretation is beyond doubt (similar depressions in potassium excretion have been observed by BERLINER and KENNEDY[979] and by BERLINER, KENNEDY and ORLOFF[223]) it seems more questionable whether an inhibition of the reabsorption should be held fully responsible for the increase in potassium excretion observed in the first group of experiments. As emphasized by GROSSMAN et al.[952], there is growing evidence that mercurials are particulary apt to cause an increased excretion of potassium in cases where sodium excretion is sparse and where sodium conserving mechanisms must be assumed to be activated (low sodium intake, cardiac and hepatic diseases, following adrenal cortical steroid administration, etc.). In such cases a greater part of the additional sodium delivered to the distal tubules in response to the proximal effects of mercurials, is assumed to be exchanged in the distal tubules for other cations: potassium, ammonium and hydrogen ions. It is noteworthy in this connection that SCHWARTZ and WALLACE[1001] have observed an increase in the excretion of potassium as well as some increase in ammonia excretion in response to mercurials in some cardiac patients belonging to this category.

It is also pertinent that these patients (8 out of 10) all became unresponsive to mercurials, probably because they were suffering from a circulatory insufficiency severe enough to induce marked constriction of the renal vessels. WESTON et al.[995] have reported that pretreatment of a patient with desoxycorticosterone over a period of four days changed the response to thiomerin (85 mg of Hg) in such a way that there was a smaller rise in sodium excretion than in chloride excretion; the difference was mainly accounted for by a more pronounced rise in potassium excretion.

Apparently, we must count on an exchange of sodium with potassium in the distal tubules as a factor responsible for an increased excretion of potassium during mercurial induced saluresis, and in particular in cases where distal sodium

[1001] SCHWARTZ, W. B., and W. M. WALLACE: Electrolyte equilibrium during mercurial diuresis. J. clin. Invest. **30**, 1089—1104 (1951).

conserving mechanisms are activated. Parenthetically, this is comparable to the phenomena observed when natriuresis is induced by other means, such as administration of sodium salts, osmotic diuretics etc. (cf. p. 286).

At first sight it may seem self-contradictory to assert that mercurials may promote potassium excretion by putting the distal potassium exchange mechanism to work and at the same time to claim that mercurials inhibit such exchange (potassium secretion). It appears, however, that these views are compatible and that the apparent paradox is satisfactorily explained by assuming that therapeutical doses of mercurials do not completely block distal cation exchange. It is apparent from MUDGE et al. studies, referred to above, that such doses did not depress potassium excretions to very low values; one may reasonably infer that potassium secretion was not entirely blocked. Thus, potassium exchange may — although possibly somewhat inhibited — increase somewhat in magnitude, when sufficient sodium is offered to saturate whatever exchange capacity remains uninhibited.

In summary, organic mercurials may or may not cause some inhibition of (proximal) potassium reabsorption. They definitely inhibit (distal) exchange of potassium for sodium, but under conditions where this exchange is activated (sodium deficiency, cardiovascular insufficiency, etc.) sufficient exchange of potassium for sodium may still occur during therapeutical mercurial saluresis to produce an appreciable increase in urinary excretion of potassium. This latter point is of considerable interest to the physician since it indicates that frequent use of mercurials in such cases may contribute to the development of a potassium deficiency. The alkalosis which also results from such therapy may further promote potassium losses (cf. p. 291).

g) Xanthine diuretics

In spite of the fact that the diuretic-saluretic action of methylated dioxypurines (caffeine, theobromine and in particular theophylline) have been known for a long time great uncertainty still prevails concerning the mechanism of this action. Research in this field was very active until the organic mercurials came into use; much less work has been done in recent years to elucidate the mode of action of the xanthines than that of the mercurials. The older work on xanthines was comprehensively reviewed by BOCK[1002] and certain aspects were critically discussed by CUSHNY[1003].

It is generally recognized that the maximum diuretic potency of the xanthine diuretics is definitely inferior to that of mercurials, and that theophylline is the most and caffeine the least effective of the group. Since the toxicity of the xanthines is negligible in comparison with that of the mercurials they are, however, still used rather extensively in the treatment of milder cases of cardiac oedema. Their use as adjuncts in mercurial therapy has been mentioned above. Theobromine and theophylline are mostly administered as conjugates with other substances which improve their solubility (e. g. theobromine sodium salicylate = diuretin, theophylline sodium acetate = theocin and theophylline ethylene diamine = aminophylline = theophyllamine). It is highly questionable whether any of the many theophylline derivates and conjugates which have been recommended offer any advantages over theophylline itself (apart from the greater solubility); the diuretic efficacy of conjugates appears to be identical with that of the parent substance (cf. MODELL[916]).

[1002] BOCK, J.: Die Purinderivate. *In*: Handbuch der experimentellen Pharmakologie Vol. II[1]. Berlin: Springer 1920.

[1003] CUSHNY, A. R.: The secretion of the urine. London: Longmans, Green and Co. 1926.

The magnitude of the diuretic-saluretic response to xanthines has been reported to vary greatly in different species; particularly large responses have been observed in rabbits, whereas failure to obtain diuretic responses have been reported in cats. Such differences in responsiveness may, in part at least, be due to differences in the experimental conditions, since it is well-known from studies in a single species that the magnitude of the diuretic response is greatly influenced by the state of hydration ("availability of extracellular fluid") and by anaesthesia, etc.

The typical response to a therapeutic dose of theophylline administered intravenously [(0.24)—0.48—(0.72) g in man] differs from that observed after therapeutic doses of mercurials by being more prompt, of shorter duration and generally of smaller magnitude. The urine flow generally reaches its maximum 10—20 min after the injection and returns to almost normal after 1 to 2 hr (DAVIS and SCHOCK[1004]). Considerably more protracted diuretic responses — up to 8 to 10 hr — have been reported by others (cf. e.g. BLUMGART et al.[1005]).

The increase in urine flow is rather closely paralleled by a rise in the urinary excretion of sodium and chloride and generally also in potassium (and calcium). It was emphasized by BLUMGART et al. and more recently also by EK[1006] that the *additional* fluid which is excreted during theophylline diuresis is rather similar to extracellular fluid as regards ionic composition. Xanthine diuresis is therefore, typically, a solute diuresis as is mercurial diuresis. It differs, however, from the latter by a definite tendency towards a smaller increment in chloride excretion than in sodium excretion (in mercurial diuresis the ratio: increment in chloride excretion (meq)/increment in sodium excretion (meq) is typically rather close to one). In other words the excretion of bicarbonate is frequently significantly increased in xanthine diuresis, whereas it is generally little affected in mercurial diuresis.

As regards **the mechanism of xanthine diuresis** it appears that we are almost as far from a clear understanding to-day as we were around 1930.

It is well-known that therapeutic doses of xanthines exert definite actions on several extrarenal tissues, *inter alia* on the cardiovascular system. Many studies have demonstrated that various xanthines, and in particular theophylline, increase cardiac output by direct stimulation of the myocardium (cf. for instance HOWARTH et al.[1007] and FOWELL et al. [1008]). Several authors have observed that theophylline may cause a considerable movement of salt and water from the tissues to the blood with a consequent increase in plasma volume (MØLLER[1009]; CURTIS[1010]; CALVIN et al.[1011]). Such movements were found by MØLLER to occur

[1004] DAVIS, J. O., and N. W. SCHOCK: The effect of theophylline ethylene diamine on renal function in control subjects and in patients with congestive heart failure. J. clin. Invest. **28**, 1459—1468 (1949).

[1005] BLUMGART, H. L., D.D. R. GILLIGAN, R. D. LEVY, M. G. BROWN, and M. C. VOLK: Action of diuretics in normal persons. Arch. intern. Med. **54**, 40—81 (1934).

[1006] EK, J.: The influence of heavy hydration on the renal function in normal and hypertensive man. Scand. J. clin. Lab. Invest. Suppl. 7 (1955).

[1007] HOWARTH, S., J. McMICHAEL, and E. P. SHARPEY-SCHAFER: The circulatory action of theophylline ethylene diamine. Clin. Sci. **6**, 125—135 (1947).

[1008] FOWELL, D. M., J. A. WINSLOW, V. P. SYDENSTRICKER, and N. C. WHEELER: Circulatory and diuretic effects of theophylline isopropanolamine. Arch. intern. Med. **83**, 150—151 (1949).

[1009] MØLLER, K. O.: Flüssigkeits- und Chloridaustausch zwischen Blut und Geweben nach Theophyllineingabe. Naunyn-Schmiedebergs Arch. exp. Path. Pharmak. **126**, 143—158 (1927).

[1010] CURTIS, G. M.: The action of the specific diuretics. J. Amer. med. Ass. **93**, 2016—2018 (1929).

[1011] CALVIN, D. B., G. DECHERD, and G. HERRMANN: Response of plasma volume to diuretics. Proc. Soc. exp. Biol. (N. Y.) **44**, 529—531 (1940).

very promptly and to be particulary pronounced (up to 25% increase in plasma volume) in nephrectomized animals (rabbits) or animals which failed to respond by diuresis, but sizable increases in plasma volume have also been found to precede the development of diuresis in animals and human subjects. Whether these fluid movements are caused by the vascular effects of the xanthine or they are due to a "mobilizing" action on the extravascular tissues is not clear.

The possibility must definitely be considered that these extrarenal actions may *contribute* to the diuretic-saluretic action of the xanthines. It is, however, beyond doubt that the xanthines also exert direct actions on the kidney and it is generally held that the diuretic-saluretic effect is mainly due to such actions.

That xanthines exert a diuretic action directly on the kidney is well-established by various experiments on perfused kidneys. A diuretic and chloruretic effect of caffeine was demonstrated by RICHARDS and PLANT[1012] in the perfused rabbit kidney (even when a constant rate of blood flow through the kidney was maintained). An indisputable diuretic-chloruretic effect of caffeine was also observed by VERNEY and WINTON[1013] when 50—200 mg of this substance was added to the circulating blood (approx. 700 ml) in heart-lung-kidney preparations of the dog. A diuresis and natriuresis was also observed by KUPFER et al.[1014] in several (but not all) experiments when some 50 mg of aminophylline was added to the blood of a pump-lung-kidney preparation of a dog. An attempt to demonstrate a direct action on the kidney was also made by CHRISTIAN and BARTRAM[1015] who studied the effect of injection of various xanthines into one renal artery on the urine flow from the two kidneys. With theobromine and caffeine no significant difference in diuretic response was observed between the two sides, and even theophylline did not give as clear-cut results as the mercurials. With smaller doses of this substance (3.3 mg/kg) the diuretic response did, however, tend to be greater on the injected side (whereas it was smaller with large doses of 19.6 mg/kg). This technique is obviously unsuited for demonstration of a direct renal action in the case of substances which are not avidly bound to the renal tissue, and failure to get a greater response on the injected side with proper doses does not exclude a direct action on the kidney.

The question, which renal actions are responsible for the diuretic-saluretic effect, has not yet been answered satisfactorily. There are two principal views. According to the first the diuretic effect is caused by an action on the renal vasculature or the glomerular membrane which enhances the glomerular filtration process. The second holds that it is due to a depressive action on the tubular reabsorption of salt and water.

Both of these views date back to the turn of the century. The concept of a dilatory action on the renal vessels as the causal factor was first clearly expressed by LOEWI[1016] on the basis of observations in oncometer experiments. The view that inhibition of tubular reabsorption processes is the cause of xanthine diuresis

[1012] RICHARDS, A. N., and O. H. PLANT: Urine formation by the perfused kidney: Preliminary experiments on the action of caffeine. J. Pharmacol. exp. Ther. 7, 485—509 (1915).

[1013] VERNEY, E. B., and F. R. WINTON: The action of caffeine on the isolated kidney of the dog. J. Physiol. 69, 153—170 (1930).

[1014] KUPFER, S., D. D. THOMPSON, and R. F. PITTS: The isolated kidney and its response to diuretic agents. Amer. J. Physiol. 167, 703—713 (1951).

[1015] CHRISTIAN, H. A., and E. A. BARTRAM: Experimental observations on the action of diuretics. Trans. Ass. Amer. Phycns 47, 292—303 (1932).

[1016] LOEWI, O., W. M. FLETCHER, u. V. E. HENDERSON: Untersuchungen zur Physiologie und Pharmakologie der Nierenfunktion. III. Über den Mechanismus der Coffeindiurese. Naunyn-Schmiedebergs Arch. exp. Path. Pharmak. 53, 15—32 (1905).

was first propounded by SOBIERANSKI[1017] following the demonstration of certain changes in the *in vivo* staining properties of the tubular cells during caffeine diuresis.

It is known that the xanthines reduce the renal vascular resistance by some action directly on the kidney. This is borne out by the above-mentioned experiments on perfused kidneys in which an appreciable reduction in the vascular resistance was observable whether a constant perfusion pressure or a constant perfusion flow was used. The occurrence of a renal vasodilation in the whole animal following the administration of xanthines was already indicated by the observation of an increase in the kidney volume in several old studies with the oncometer technique (for references see BOCK[1002] and CUSHNY[1003],) and LOEWI's demonstration of a similar effect in the denervated kidney pointed against a mediation via the renal nerves. The interpretation of the volume increase as evidence for a dilatation and reduced resistance in the renal vascular bed met with much criticism, but it was strongly supported by a considerable number of studies in which an increase in renal blood flow was observed without significant changes in arterial blood pressure. An increase in renal blood flow following caffeine administration was detected by a "venous outflow" method by CUSHNY and LAMBIE[1018] in dogs and by SCHMIDT[1019] in rabbits. An early rise in renal blood flow was also observed after intravenous injection of 12 mg of theophylline into rabbits by WALKER et al.[1020], using a thermostromuhr-method. Indications of an increased renal blood flow have also been obtained by various authors using the more indirect clearance methods which measure effective renal plasma flow; these findings are further discussed below.

The observation of a reduction in renal vascular resistance suggests that xanthine diuresis might be a "propulsion diuresis", caused by an increase in glomerular capillary pressure. Such a mechanism would be consistent with the finding that the additional fluid excreted during xanthine diuresis is similar in ion composition to extracellular fluid, and with the related finding of VERNEY and WINTON that the changes in the composition of the urine secreted under the influence of caffeine could be reproduced by inducing a similar increase in diuresis by a rise in perfusion pressure.

However, several authors have raised the objection against this view that a close correlation does not exist between renal blood flow and the magnitude of the xanthine diuresis. The increase in renal blood flow has frequently been found to be of only short duration, and to be greatly outlasted by the diuresis (CUSHNY and LAMBIE; SCHMIDT; WALKER et al.; DAVIS and SCHOCK, cf. references above). CHASIS et al.[1021] have even found renal plasma flow (diodrast clearance) to fall to subnormal values (after a transient increase) when a large dose of aminophylline or caffeine was given intravenously to normal human subjects.

[1017] SOBIERANSKI, W. v.: Über die Nierenfunktion und die Wirkungsweise der Diuretica. Naunyn-Schmiedebergs Arch. exp. Path. Pharmak. **35**, 144—180 (1895).

[1018] CUSHNY, A. R., and C. G. LAMBIE: The action of diuretics. J. Physiol. **55**, 276—286 (1921).

[1019] SCHMIDT, E.: Tierexperimentelle Untersuchungen über die Beeinflussung der Nierenfunktion durch intravenös einverleibtes Sublimat und Neosalvarsan unter besonderer Berücksichtigung des sogenannten Linserchen Gemisches (Neosalvarsan und Sublimat). Naunyn-Schmiedebergs Arch. exp. Path. Pharmak. **101**, 66—99 (1924).

[1020] WALKER, A. M., C. F. SCHMIDT, K. A. ELSOM, A. E. KENDALL, and C. G. JOHNSON: Renal blood flow of unanesthetized rabbits and dogs in diuresis and antidiuresis. Amer. J. Physiol. **118**, 95—110 (1937).

[1021] CHASIS, H., H. A. RANGES, W. GOLDRING, and H. W. SMITH: The control of renal blood flow and glomerular filtration in normal man. J. clin. Invest. **17**, 683—97 (1938).

Failure to observe a close parallelism between renal blood flow and urine flow does not, however, definitely exclude a rise in glomerular capillary pressure as a causal factor in xanthine diuresis. A return of the total renal vascular resistance to normal or supranormal levels (before the diuresis ceases) might still be associated with an increased glomerular capillary pressure if a constriction affecting predominantly the postglomerular vessels occurred as a secondary phenomenon. A rapid loss of fluid from the plasma through the kidneys might be a factor which could activate such a secondary vasoconstriction, and the preglomerular vessels might not participate in this constriction if the dilatory effect of the xanthines is confined to these vessels and still acting on them. In discussing possible vascular mechanisms of xanthine diuresis it may also be mentioned in passing that alternative explanations would seem to be possible within the frames of the cell-separation hypothesis of PAPPENHEIMER and KINTER (cf. p. 267).

Theoretically, a xanthine diuresis might also be caused by a reduction in the hydrodynamic resistance in the glomerular membrane. Such an effect of xanthines (plus a mobilizing action on the tissues) was once proposed (on very loose grounds) by ELLINGER[1022] to explain xanthine diuresis. It appears that no evidence for this view has later been added.

An increase in glomerular filtration rate (up to some 20%) following the administration of xanthine diuretics has been observed in animals and human subjects by several authors (Creatinine clearance in dogs by SCHMITZ[1023]; Creatinine clearance in humans by ROLLER and WIEDEMANN[1024]; inulin clearance in humans by CHASIS et al.[1021], DAVIS and SCHOCK[1004] and EK[1006]; inulin clearance in rabbits by KRUHØFFER). Several others have failed to observe any significant changes in filtration rate (WALKER et al.[1020]; BLUMGART et al.[1005]).

Changes in the filtration rate (or failure to observe any) have often been advanced as arguments in the discussion of glomerular *versus* tubular factors as the possible cause of xanthine diuresis. It appears, however, that determinations of the filtration rate do not allow such distinctions to be made, since tubular conditions seem to be of major importance as factors determining the filtration rate (cf. p. 263). A rise in filtration rate may therefore well be due to primary changes in tubular conditions (increased rate of fluid reabsorption, reduced tubular hydrodynamic resistance) and it cannot be taken as definite evidence that factors acting directly in the glomeruli have been altered in a direction favourable for the filtration. Similarly, a greater increment in urine flow (and sodium excretion) than in filtration rate does not necessarily imply that the reduction in tubular reabsorption of water (and sodium), which has occurred, has been the cause of the diuresis; in such cases a high glomerular propulsive pressure may have been mainly responsible for the increase in urine flow, and a concurrent fall in proximal fluid reabsorption may have tended to keep the filtration from rising without affecting the excretion of water and sodium to any greater extent.

It is apparent from the above discussion that we are not yet in a position to produce a well-founded explanation of the renal mechanism of xanthine diuresis. However, the different views are not mutually exclusive and it may be that both an increase in glomerular propulsive pressure and a reduced reabsorption of salt and water (and possibly also a reduced resistance in the nephron) may be involved.

[1022] ELLINGER, A.: Die Angriffspunkte der Diuretica. Klin. Wschr. 1, 249—253 (1922).
[1023] SCHMITZ, H. L.: Studies on the action of diuretics. I. The effect of euphyllin and salyrgan upon the glomerular filtration and tubular reabsorption. J. clin. Invest. 11, 1075—1097 (1932).
[1024] ROLLER, D., u. G. WIEDEMANN: Untersuchungen über das Verhalten der Nierenfunktion unter dem Einfluß von Theophyllinpräparaten. Z. klin. Med. 140, 566—592 (1942).

With reference to a depressed tubular reabsorption as a possible factor it is, however, pertinent to note that the literature contains various data according to which increases in filtration rate greatly exceeding concurrent increases in urine flow have been recorded (cf. CHASIS et al.[1021] and EK[1006].) In such cases, in which an *increase* in the total rates of reabsorption of salt and water occurred, the diuresis is at least not explainable by an overall depression of the tubular transfer of salt and water. A depression of distal reabsorptions (accompanied by an increase in proximal reabsorptions) might, however, still have been a factor of importance.

h) Diuretics chemically related to the xanthines

Several purine and pyrimidine derivatives have been tested in recent years for diuretic activity mainly in the hope of finding oral diuretics which cause larger and more protracted saluresis and less gastrointestinal distress than the xanthiness. Only a few of these have come into therapeutical use.

Among these one of a series of substituted 6-aminouracils, *1-allyl-3-ethyl-6-aminouracil* (aminometramide = aminometradine = Mictine) have received a fairly extensive study. Following a preliminary study in dogs, this substance (and the corresponding propyl-ethyl derivative) was shown by KATTUS et al.[1025] to possess a somewhat greater diuretic-saluretic potency in human subjects than a similar dose of theophylline by mouth. These findings were confirmed for the propyl-ethyl derivative by SPENCER and LLOYD-THOMAS[1026] and for the allyl-ethyl derivative by PLATTS and HANDLEY[1027]. In all of these studies a rather high incidence of gastrointestinal disturbances were observed, but it may be that the ratio between the diuretic and emetic potency is somewhat more favourable than in the case of theophylline.

Rather little has been done to clarify the mechanism of the diuretic action of these drugs, but it seems reasonable to assume that it is similar to that of the xanthines. KATTUS et al.[1025] found no consistent changes in glomerular filtration rate in dogs following the administration of aminouracil dervatives and a similar finding was reported by ARMAN and DETTELBACH[1028] who also failed to find any increase in renal blood flow. Further references to recent studies on aminometradine (and the related amisometradine = Rolicton) may be found in a recent review by BEYER[1029].

The chloruretic and diuretic activity of formoguanamine has been studied by LIPSCHITZ and STOKEY[1030] and that of isocytosines by VAN ARMAN[1031] and McKEEVER et al.[1032].

[1025] KATTUS, A., T. M. ARRINGTON, and E. V. NEWMAN: Clinical observations on a new oral diuretic 1-propyl-3-ethyl-6-aminouracil and preliminary studies on 1-allyl-3-ethyl-6-aminouracil. Amer. J. Med. **12**, 319—330 (1952).

[1026] SPENCER, A. G., and H. G. LLOYD-THOMAS: Clinical trial of a new diuretic. Brit. med. J. **1953 I**, 957—960.

[1027] PLATTS, M. M., and T. HANDLEY: Aminometradine in treatment of congestive heart failure. Brit. med. J. **1956 I**, 1078—1080.

[1028] ARMAN, C. G. VAN, and H. R. DETTELBACH: Diuretic effects of 1-ethyl-3-allyl-6-aminouracil. Fed. Proc. **14**, 392 (1955).

[1029] BEYER, K. H.: Nonmercurial organic diuretics. Arch. intern. Med. **102**, 1005—1015 (1958).

[1030] LIPSCHITZ, W. L., and E. STOKEY: Diuretic action of formoquanamine in normal persons. J. Pharmacol. exp. Ther. **92**, 131—139 (1948).

[1031] ARMAN, C. G. VAN: The diuretic activity of isocytosines. J. Pharmacol. exp. Ther. **111**, 285—292 (1954).

[1032] McKEEVER, W. P., C. R. HINES, and I. C. WINTER: Preliminary trial of new oral nonmercurial diuretic, SC-3858. J. Lab. clin. Med. **44**, 897—898 (1954).

i) Unsubstituted sulphonamides (carbonic anhydrase inhibitors)

The natriuretic and diuretic properties of these drugs have been discussed elsewhere (p. 296). Acetazoleamide (Diamox) which is some 100 times more potent as a carbonic anhydrase inhibitor than sulphanilamide is recognized as the most useful therapeutic agent in this group. p-sulphonamido-benzoic acid (Dirnate), once suggested, has been found to be too weak to be of practical value (LINDSAY and BROWN[1033]).

Acetazoleamide is only a moderately effective natriuretic but it seems to be a useful adjunct to other diuretic therapy. Since the efficacy of the mercurials is reduced by the alkalosis which they tend to produce, combination of these drugs with the acidosis-producing acetazoleamide seems rational. It should be recalled, however, that acetazoleamide, and under certain conditions also the mercurials, may cause considerable losses of potassium. Measures should therefore be taken against potassium depletion.

The fact that acetazoleamide produces large renal losses of potassium suggests its use in the treatment of hyperkalaemia (potassium intoxication). Actually its usefulness in this field is very limited since renal failure is by far the most frequent cause of hyperkalaemia. Whether the hyperkalaemia is caused by a complete renal shut-down or by renal lesions more specifically blocking tubular secretion of potassium, acetazoleamide — which owes its kaliuretic action to an acceleration of the potassium secretion — will obviously be ineffective as a remedy.

That acetazoleamide may have other renal actions than those immediately referable to its interference with the tubular formation and secretion of hydrogen ions is apparent from recent studies by HARRISON and HARRISON[1034]. These authors have found that treatment of rats with acetazoleamide causes a remarkable fall in urinary citrate excretion, and that prolonged administration (some 250 mg per 100 g food) leads to the formation of calcium phosphate precipitates in the kidneys.

j) Chlorothiazide (and derivatives)

Recently a new oral diuretic/saluretic, chlorothiazide, 6-chloro-7-sulfamyl--1,2,4-benzothiadiazine-1,1-dioxyde) has attracted considerable clinical interest. Still more recently a number of derivatives have appeared, which are about 10—20 times more potent as natriuretics than the mother compound: Hydrochlorothiazide (cf. RICHTERICH[1035]) and the 6-trifluoromethyl derivative (cf. KOBINGER[1036]).

The available literature has been comprehensively reviewed quite recently (TAGGART[947], BEYER[1029]), so that only some of the more important points need to be considered here.

In human subjects an oral dose of 1—2 g of chlorothiazide induces a natriuresis-diuresis of almost the same magnitude as the usual therapeutic doses of organic mercurials. The predominant effects of such doses are uniformly described as natriuresis and chloruresis (as in the case of mercurials). However, as one might

---

[1033] LINDSAY, A. E., and H. BROWN: Clinical experience with p-sulfonamido-benzoic acid, a carbonic anhydrase inhibitor, as a diuretic agent. J. Lab. clin. Med. **43**, 839—847 (1954).

[1034] HARRISON, H. E., and H. C. HARRISON: Inhibition of urine citrate excretion and the production of renal calcinosis in the rat by acetazoleamide (Diamox) administration. J. clin. Invest. **34**, 1662—1670 (1955).

[1035] RICHTERICH, R.: Natriuretic potency of hydrochlorothiazide in humans. Experientia (Basel) **14**, 458 (1958).

[1036] KOBINGER, W., and F. J. LUND: Investigations into a new oral diuretic, Rontyl ® (6-trifluoromethyl-7-sulfamyl-3,4-dihydro-1,2,4-benzothiadiazine-1,1-dioxide). Acta pharmacol. toxicol. **15**, 265—274 (1959).

expect from the free sulfonamide group of chlorothiazide, this agent has some inhibitory effect on carbonic anhydrase, a fact, which probably (cf. p. 299) accounts for a moderate kaliuresis even with therapeutic doses (prolonged therapy may, however, result in an appreciable potassium loss if a reasonably high potassium intake is not maintained).

These findings indicate that chlorothiazide owes its diuretic effect to something more than an inhibition of carbonic anhydrase in the tubules. This is further apparent from BEYER's studies in dogs in which it was demonstrated that in NH_4Cl induced acidosis chlorothiazide (contrary to acetazoleamide) still produces natriuresis and chloruresis, often together with a *decrease* in urinary p_H. (In the same studies it was also shown that chlorothiazide, contrary to the mercurials, is also natriuretic under conditions of an alkalosis produced by a high $NaHCO_3$ intake; under such conditions the urinary excretion of bicarbonate was, however, also greatly increased by chlorothiazide.)

The question, what other mechanisms than the very moderate carbonic anhydrase inhibitory action are responsible for the natriuretic effect of chlorothiazide and its derivatives, cannot be definitely answered at present. That chlorothiazide exerts a natriuretic effect directly upon the kidney is apparent from the fact that infusion of the drug into one renal artery (0.007—0.04 mg/min/kg body weight) causes a larger natriuresis from the same side (LAVENDER and PULLMAN[1037]).

VANDER et al.[1038] have interpreted their findings in stop flow experiments as evidence that chlorothiazide does not depress distal reabsorptions of sodium. These authors further believe that their data indicate an inhibitory effect on the proximal reabsorption of salt + water, but it appears that their findings might equally well be explained on the basis that chlorothiazide produces a "propulsion" or "conduction" diuresis.

PITTS[917] has interpreted the observation, that maximal saluretic doses of chlorothiazide and chlormerodrin, when given simultaneously, show additive effects, as an indication that these two drugs exert their saluretic effects by blocking different tubular processes engaged in the reabsorption of sodium. However, there is no reason why, theoretically at least, a similar finding could not be obtained if at least one of the two drugs owed its saluretic properties to a "propulsion or conduction effect". On the other hand, the few published determinations of renal blood flow during chlorothiazide diuresis provide no support for a propulsion type of diuresis.

Great effectiveness by the oral route and an assumed low toxicity have already made chlorothiazide very popular as a remedy in salt depletion therapy. Recent reports on thrombocytopenia during such treatment do, however, call for some caution.

k) Antialdosterones

The facts, that severe renal losses of sodium result from adrenalectomy, and that several types of clinical and experimental oedema disappear following adrenalectomy, suggest that it should be possible to bring about an effective sodium depletion therapy by preventing the action of corticoids, in particular aldosterone, on the kidneys. Recent investigations have indicated two ways in which this goal can be achieved by drugs.

Amphenone B (1,2-bis-[p-aminophenyl]-2-methyl-1-propane dihydrochloride) has been demonstrated to be an efficient inhibitor of the biosynthesis of corticoids,

[1037] LAVENDER, A. R., and T. N. PULLMAN: Effects of unilateral infusion of chlorothiazide. Fed. Proc. **17**, 93 (1958).
[1038] VANDER, A. J., R. L. MALVIN, W. S. WILDE, and L. P. SULLIVAN: Localization of the site of action of chlorothiazide by stop-flow. J. Pharmacol. exp. Ther. **125**, 19—22 (1959)

and among these aldosterone (HERTZ et al.[1039], RENOLD et al.[1040]). The high toxicity of this and related compounds has, however, prevented any extensive clinical use.

The second method, which aims at a competitive, specific inhibition of aldosterone at its tubular site of action, seems more promising. Recently chemists have developed two new synthetic *steroid-17-spirolactones:* [3-(3-oxo-17β-hydroxy-4-androsten-17α-yl) propionic acid γ-lactone] = SC-5233, and its more potent 19-nor-analogue, SC-8109, which exert a fairly powerful natriuretic effect in this way (KAGAWA et al.[1041], LIDDLE [1042]). Our present experience with these compounds, which is still quite limited, has very recently been reviewed by LIDDLE[1043].

As regards the mode of action of the "spirolactones" there is hardly any room for doubt that they are *true antagonists of aldosterone*. In the first place, their effects in intact animals "simulate the abrupt withdrawal of aldosterone", i. e. they cause an increase in urinary excretion of sodium, chloride and water, usually a slight decrease in potassium excretion, a very marked decrease in "H+" excretion, and a moderate decrease in ammonia excretion (LIDDLE[1043]).

Secondly, and more important as an argument, it has been shown that "the spirolactones" only exert their effects in the presence of mineralocorticoids. KAGAWA et al. [1041] showed that there is no effect in adrenalectomized rats, and LIDDLE[1042] made the same observation in adrenalectomized dogs. Consonant with these observations no saluretic effect was observed in Addisonian patients maintained merely on a high-sodium diet (without steroid therapy), but a typical response was obtained when they were given desoxycorticosterone in addition (LIDDLE[1043]). Other studies, by ROSS and BETHUNE[1044], have shown that intravenous infusions of SC-8109 is capable of suppressing the sodium retaining effects of exogenous aldosterone in normal human subjects [when given in doses some 1000 times as great as the amount of aldosterone infused (1 mg)].

Finally, it has been found by LIDDLE[1043] that short courses of treatment with "spirolactones" have no significant effect on the urinary output of aldosterone (and 17-keto and 17-hydroxycorticoids), a fact, which argues against a depressive action on aldosterone secretion as being partly responsible for the natriuretic effect in intact subjects.

It is interesting to note that the lactone bridge of the propionic acid provides the carbon 17 of the "spirolactones" with an attached ring structure, which make these steroids rather similar to the aglucones of the cardiac glycosides, substances which are known to interfere with alkali metal ion transports in other tissues (cf. Part I, p. 64).

The "spirolactones" do not produce massive saluresis-diuresis, a fact which is consonant with the concept, that aldosterone should be engaged in only a small part of the tubular reabsorption of sodium. On the other hand, it appears that continued administration of these substances (some 2 g orally per day) over several

[1039] HERTZ, R., W. W. TULLNER, J. A. SCHRICKER, F. G. DHYSE, and L. F. HALLMAN: Studies on amphenone and related compounds. Recent Progr. Hormone Res. 11, 119—147 (1955).
[1040] RENOLD, A. E., J. CRABBÉ, L. HERNANDO-AVENDANO, D. H. NELSON, E. J. ROSS, K. EMERSON, and G. W. THORN: Inhibition of aldosterone secretion by amphenone in man. New Engl. J. Med. 256, 16—21 (1957).
[1041] KAGAWA, C. M., J. A. CELLA, and C. G. VAN ARMAN: Action of new steroids in blocking effects of aldosterone and desoxycorticosterone on salt. Science 126, 1015 (1957).
[1042] LIDDLE, C. M.: Sodium diuresis induced by steroidal antagonists of aldosterone. Science 126, 1016—1018 (1957).
[1043] LIDDLE, G. W.: Aldosterone antagonists. Arch. intern. Med. 102, 998—1004 (1958).
[1044] ROSS, E. J., and J. E. BETHUNE: Antagonism between the effect of aldosterone and a synthetic steroid lactone on the renal excretion of sodium and potassium in man. Lancet 1959 I, 127—129.

days or more may produce completely satisfactory results in the treatment of oedema. The spirolactones have also been used successfully to correct the electrolyte disturbances in cases of primary hyperaldosteronism (SALASSA et al.[1045]).

Various 16α-hydroxylated steroids and in particular cyclic acetals or ketals of 16α, 17α-diol steroids have been found to possess natriuretic properties (Cf. FRIED and BORMAN[652]). Whether this is due to a true antialdosterone action or to their pronounced glucocorticoid activity remains to be shown.

o) The Renal Excretion of Lithium, Rubidium and Cesium

a) Lithium

Some years ago, when lithium chloride was rather popular as a taste substitute for sodium chloride in sodium-depletion therapy of patients with cardiac oedema, a number of cases of severe lithium intoxication, and even a few deaths, were reported in such patients (WALDRON[1046]; CORCORAN et al.[1047]; HANLON et al.[1048]; STERN[1049]).

These events and the discovery that lithium is useful in the treatment of manic phases of manio-depressive psychosis prompted new investigations on the toxicity of lithium. Although these also included studies on the renal elimination, the handling of lithium ions in the kidney and its relationship to other renal ion transports still remain incompletely understood.

The renal excretion of lithium has been studied in acute experiments in dogs by TALSO and CLARKE[1050], RADOMSKI et al. [1051], and FOULKS et al.[1052], and by SCHOU[1053, 1054] in rats.

The view that the urine is by far the most important route of excretion of lithium was clearly confirmed by TALSO and CLARKE, who found that, whereas some 60—80 per cent of an administered lithium dose was excreted in 48 hours in normal dogs, the serum lithium concentration of nephrectomized dogs remained essentially constant for more than 24 hours (after the lithium administered had reached distribution equilibrium in the course of 6—8 hours).

In the studies of FOULKS et al. the excretion fraction for lithium (i. e. the lithium/creatinine clearance ratio) was found to vary between 0.18 and 0.45 at serum lithium concentrations varying from 1 to 22 meq./l (with a slight tendency towards a fall in the excretion fraction at the higher concentrations). The authors therefore

[1045] SALASSA, R. M., V. R. MATTOX, and M. H. POWER: Effect of an aldosterone antagonist on sodium and potassium excretion in primary hyperaldosteronism. J. clin. Endocr. 18, 787—789 (1958).

[1046] WALDRON, A. M.: Lithium intoxication occuring with the use of a table salt substitute in the low dietary treatment of hypertension and congestive heart failure. Univ. Hosp. Bull., Ann. Arbor. 15, 9—10 (1949).

[1047] CORCORAN, A. C., R. D. TAYLOR, and I. PAGE: Lithium poisoning from the use of salt substitutes. J. Amer. med. Ass. 139, 685—688 (1949).

[1048] HANLON, L. W., M. ROMAINE, F. J. GILROY, and J. E. DEITRICK: Lithium chloride as a substitute for sodium chloride in the diet. J. Amer. med. Ass. 139, 688—692 (1949).

[1049] STERN, R. L.: Severe lithium chloride poisoning with complete recovery. J. Amer. med. Ass. 139, 710—711 (1949).

[1050] TALSO, R. J., and R. W. CLARKE: Excretion and distribution of lithium in the dog. Amer. J. Physiol. 166, 202—208 (1951).

[1051] RADOMSKI, J. L., H. N. FUYAT, A. A. NELSON, and P. K. SMITH: The toxic effects, excretion and distribution of lithium chloride. J. Pharmacol. exp. Ther. 100, 429—444 (1950).

[1052] FOULKS, J., G. H. MUDGE, and A. GILMAN: Renal excretion of cation in the dog during infusion of isotonic solutions of lithium chloride. Amer. J. Physiol. 168, 642—649 (1952).

[1053] SCHOU, M.: Lithium studies. 1. Toxicity. Acta pharmacol. toxicol. 15, 70—84 (1958).

[1054] SCHOU, M.: Lithium studies. 2. Renal Elimination. Acta pharmacol. toxicol. 15, 85—98 (1958).

concluded that the percentage reabsorption of filtered lithium is independent of its plasma concentration. Excretion fractions of similar magnitude, viz. 0.35 to 0.45, were observed by RADOMSKI et al. in three dogs at serum lithium concentrations ranging from 1.8 to 8.5 meq./l. The results obtained by TALSO and CLARKE were rather different; excretion fractions between 0.01 and 0.43 were observed at serum lithium concentrations ranging from 15 to below 1 meq./l, and the majority were below 0.2. It is further noteworthy that particularly low excretion fractions were observed at the lowest serum lithium concentrations (cf. the authors' fig. 1). In his recent studies in rats SCHOU observed just the reverse: at low plasma lithium concentrations (<1 meq./l) considerably higher excretion fractions (a few values above 0.8 were reported) were obtained than at higher plasma concentrations. At higher plasma levels the excretion fractions were in the same range as those observed by FOULKS et al., and here too the excretion fractions tended to fall with increasing plasma lithium concentrations (cf. fig. 16).

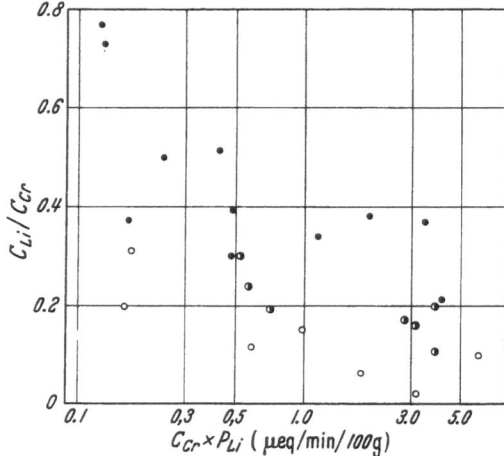

Fig. 16. *Lithium excretion in rats*. Relation between lithium/creatinine clearance ratio and filtered lithium load ($C_{Cr} \times P_{Li}$). *Open circles*: sodium excretion below 0.30 µeq./min/100 g; *semi-closed circles*: sodium excretion 0.30—1.00 µeq./min/100 g; *closed circles*: sodium excretion above 1.00 µeq./min/100 g. (From SCHOU[1054])

The reason for the discrepancy between the excretion fractions observed at low plasma lithium concentrations is not clear. Species differences and analytical shortcomings are, of course, among the possibilities to be considered.

The tendency towards falling excretion fractions with increasing plasma lithium concentrations, as observed by SCHOU (cf. fig. 16), can, however, hardly be attributed to analytical errors. It appears that these findings might result from graded changes in the function and permeability of the tubular cells, since marked morphological changes were observed by SCHOU in the proximal tubules of rats, during both the initial and final stages of lithium poisoning, while damage to the distal tubular system was reported by RADOMSKI et al. (One might e. g. imagine that the luminal boundery of the proximal tubular cells were normally rather impermeable to lithium ions, and that its permeability increases with advancing lithium poisoning. If the permeability of this boundary were a factor limiting the reabsorption of lithium, the latter would be enhanced by such changes and a fall in the excretion fraction could be expected.)

Whatever the reasons for the above deviations may be, the main conclusion must be, that the percentage of filtered lithium which is reabsorbed is largely independent of the plasma lithium concentration. This suggested to FOULKS et al. that the reabsorption of lithium might be accomplished by a passive back diffusion (as in the case of urea). This, however, is not the only mechanism by which the relative constancy of the excretion fraction could be accounted for. If lithium ions were actively reabsorbed by the same transfer mechanisms as sodium ions but less efficiently, the same outcome might be expected. This explanation was offered by SCHOU, who felt that competition between lithium and sodium ions for common transport systems in other cell membranes provided the most attractive explanation of the distribution of lithium ions between cell fluids and extracellular fluid.

The fact that the accidents referred to in the first paragraph occurred in patients on restricted sodium intakes, and with lithium doses considered non-toxic under normal conditions, already suggested that a low sodium intake might impede the renal excretion of lithium and thus increase its toxicity. This was confirmed by TALSO and CLARKE's studies, in which it was noted that dogs on a high sodium diet had generally higher lithium excretion fractions than those on a low sodium diet. Similar observations were made in rats by SCHOU (cf. fig. 16), who also found supporting evidence from other studies in which rats were given daily doses of lithium ranging from 0.5 to 10 meq./kg body weight while their sodium intakes were held at different levels. At certain intermediate doses of lithium a reversible, hypotonic polyuria developed, which apparently was due to insensitivity of the distal tubular system to antidiuretic hormone, since large doses of this hormone were incapable of preventing or counteracting it. When higher doses of lithium were given oliguria developed, and rapidly led to death in anuria, even if the lithium administration was stopped. A comparison of the series with different sodium intakes showed that larger doses of lithium were required to produce both the signs of reversible and irreversible renal impairment in animals on high sodium intakes than in those on low intakes, and it was furthermore apparent that high sodium intakes also exerted the effect of keeping the plasma lithium concentration at a lower level.

These results would hardly seem to leave any doubt that high sodium intakes reduce the toxicity of lithium by enhancing its renal excretion. SCHOU thought that this effect could be explained on the basis of a competition between sodium and lithium for tubular transfer, but it is hard to believe that increases of a few per cent in the plasma (and ultrafiltrate) concentration of sodium (from higher sodium intakes) could cause decreases in the lithium reabsorption of some 100 per cent simply by outplacing lithium from a common transport mechanism. It seems more likely that the lithiuretic effect of sodium depends upon its ability to increase the propulsion pressure and to reduce the hydrodynamic resistance of the nephron (cf. p. 278), thereby allowing less concentration of lithium to occur in the tubules and reducing the time available for reabsorption of any filtered lithium ion. This effect would be non-specific, i. e. it would be shared with other substances (e. g. mannitol) causing solute diuresis. In paranthesis it may be stated that the weak natriuretic effect of moderate lithium doses (cf. FOULKS et al. and SCHOU) probably has a similar mechanism.

A *kaliuretic effect of lithium* has been described by FOULKS et al. When isotonic lithium chloride was infused intravenously increases in the excretion fraction for potassium from 0.05—0.12 to 0.4—0.7 were observed. These rises in potassium excretion were unquestionably due to an increase in the tubular secretion of potassium, since they were almost abolished by the administration of a moderate dose of an organic mercurial. (If one would postulate that lithium had induced a less complete reabsorption of potassium, one would also have to postulate that mercurials cause an improvement of the reabsorption of potassium, which does not make sense.)

It is not quite clear how the lithium loading effected the augmentation in tubular secretion of potassium; it is possible that more than one mechanism was at work.

It is well-known that under conditions where the distal $Na^+ \rightleftharpoons K^+$ or H^+ exchange process is activated, the rate at which K^+ is secreted by this process may be limited by a sparse supply of sodium ions to the distal segments of the tubular system, and an increased supply of sodium ions may then call forth a rise in potassium secretion (cf. p. 286). It is quite possible that this mechanism was contributing to the kaliuresis observed by FOULKS et al., since in their experiments the rate of sodium excretion was *quite* low before lithium was administered, and it increased markedly during the administration.

As another mechanism by which lithium might cause kaliuresis BERLINER et al.[1055] suggested an inhibition of the urinary acidification process with an increased potassium secretion as a secondary event. In favour of this possibility the authors referred to the fact, that lithium administration had been found to cause a reduction in the excretion of titratable acidity in the urine and a rise in urine p_H, whereas one would expect exactly the reverse (together with increased potassium excretion) if the increase in potassium secretion was simply due to an increase in the supply of sodium to the distal tubules. It is easy to visualize, that if potassium and hydrogen ions in the distal tubular cells compete for exchange with sodium ions, an interference with the production of hydrogen ions in these cells would favour the exchange secretion of potassium ions (cf. the action of carbonic anhydrase inhibiting sulphonamides, p. 299). There is, however, no direct evidence that lithium inhibits carbonic anhydrase of renal origin, and in the case of carbonic anhydrase from erythrocytes FOULKS at al. found no inhibitory action with lithium concentrations as high as 0.2 M. It is not easy to see on what other points lithium could interfere with the "availability" of hydrogen ions for exchange. Evidently, further experiments are needed before BERLINER et al. hypothesis can be accepted.

b) Rubidium and Cesium

Since the distribution of rubidium and cesium between intra- and extracellular fluid has been found to imitate fairly closely that of potassium (cf. p. 224) it might be anticipated that they would also — at least qualitatively — share renal transport mechanisms with potassium.

The results of recent studies on the renal excretion of *rubidium*, mostly with Rb[86] as an indicator, seem to support this view. In such studies (RAY et al.[1056], TYOR and ELDRIDGE[1057], RELMAN[1058]) the rubidium clearances were on an average somewhat lower than those of potassium, but RELMAN reported variations in the rubidium/potassium clearance ratio from 0.3 to 1.8. RAY et al. found that the two clearances tended to vary concordantly under a variety of conditions, and further results to this effect were reported by RELMAN. Increases in the clearances of both rubidium and potassium could be evoked by both rubidium and potassium loading, as well as by the administration of acetazoleamide. During such procedures the rubidium clearance was frequently observed to exceed the inulin clearance, clearly indicating that rubidium can be subject to tubular secretion. It was stressed that in these cases the potassium clearance was still higher, and this was taken as evidence that rubidium is less efficiently secreted by the distal tubular cells than is potassium. RELMAN did not provide an explanation to the fact that the rubidium clearance *sometimes* greatly exceeded the potassium clearance, nor

[1055] BERLINER, R. W., T. J. KENNEDY, and J. ORLOFF: The relationship between potassium excretion and urine acidification. *In* Ciba Found. Sympos. on the Kidney. Eds.: LEWIS, A. A. G., and G. E. W. WOLSTENHOLME. London: J. & A. Churchill 1954.

[1056] RAY, C. T., S. A. THREEFOOT, and G. E. BURCH: The excretion of radiorubidium, Rb[86], radiopotassium, K[42], and potassium, sodium, and chloride by man with or without congestive heart failure. J. Lab. clin. Med. **45**, 408—430 (1955).

[1057] TYOR, M. P., and J. S. ELDRIDGE: A comparison of the metabolism of rubidium 86 and potassium 42 following simultaneous injection into man. Amer. J. med. Sci. **232**, 186—193 (1956).

[1058] RELMAN, A. S.: The physiological behavior of rubidium and cesium in relation to that of potassium. Yale J. Biol. Med. **29**, 248—262 (1956).

is it clear from his report whether this happened only in cases with low rates of excretion of the two cations. If so, the explanation might be that rubidium is also less readily reabsorbed (proximally) than potassium.

Cesium. According to THREEFOOT et al.[1059] the Cs^{134}/K^{39} clearance ratio was on an average between 0.43 and 0.52 in three dogs, but the ratio was subject to considerable variation. When alterations in the potassium clearance were produced by potassium loading and by desoxycorticosterone administration consistent covariation in the cesium clearance was not observed. This would seem to indicate that cesium is not subject to (distal) tubular secretion by a similar mechanism as potassium; this conclusion is, however, weakened by the facts that the clearances were averages for long periods and that *very* high potassium clearances were not obtained. The glomerular filtration rate was not measured in these experiments, but on assumption of reasonable values the excretion fraction of Cs^{134} must have been below 0.1. Provided the Cs^{134} of plasma is freely ultrafilterable this must mean that Cs^{134} is very effectively reabsorbed. (Cf. also p. 526 for other papers dealing with cesium excretion.)

c) Note on Thallous Ions

Although thallium does not belong to group I of the periodic table it may be appropriate to draw attention to the fact that recent studies on the renal excretion of thallous ions in rabbits suggest that these monovalent ions may be subject to tubular secretion by the same mechanism as potassium ions. The observation referred to was made by LUND[1060] who found that, whereas the clearance of thallous ions (Tl^{204}) varied from 30 to 70 per cent of the creatinine clearance when glucose or sodium sulphate was used to induce a mild diuresis, it exceeded the creatinine clearance when potassium sulphate was used as a diuretic.

P) Transport of sodium and potassium across the urinary bladder wall

Various investigators have been interested in the possibility of a passage of solutes from the lumen of the urinary bladder into the blood stream. — Recently HLAD et al.[1061] instilled solutions containing Na^{22} and K^{42} into the bladder of dogs. Some transfer, especially of Na^{22}, to the blood occurred. The rate of transfer was shown to be a function of the p_H of the bladder contents over a range of 5 through 8. Studies by VIVION et al.[1062a] have shown that Na^{24} is absorbed appreciably slower from the intact bladder in man. The mechanism is unknown. No measurementes of electric potential on the two sides were done. Two-directional isotope studies will be required before information on *net* transfers can be obtained by isotops. That significant net movements of Na, K, Cl and water (and urea and creatinine) may occur in the direction of the concentration gradients across the bladder and ureter walls has quite recently been demonstrated by controlled perfusions of these structures in dogs, using ordinary chemical methods for analysis (LEVINSKY and BERLINER[1062b]). The magnitude of the movements observed was large enough to introduce perceptible errors in renal excretion studies at low rates of urine flow.

[1059] THREEFOOT, S. A., G. E. BURCH, and C. T. RAY: The biological decay rates and excretion of radiocesium, Cs^{134}, with evaluation as a tracer of potassium in dogs. J. Lab. clin. Med. **45**, 313—322 (1955).

[1060] LUND, A.: Distribution of thallium in the organism and its elimination. Acta pharmacol. toxicol. **12**, 251—259 (1956).

[1061] HLAD, C. J., jr., R. NELSON, and J. H. HOLMES: Transfer of electrolytes across the urinary bladder in the dog. Amer. J. Physiol. **184**, 406—411 (1956).

[1062a] VIVION, C. G., C. J. HLAD, and B. EISEMAN: The absorption of sodium from the human urinary bladder. J. Urol. **79**, 471—473 (1958).

[1062b] LEVINSKY, N. G., and R. W. BERLINER: Changes in composition of the urine in ureter and bladder at low urine flow. Amer. J. Physiol. **196**, 549—553 (1959).

V. Handling of alkali metals by exocrine glands other than the kidney

By

Jørn Hess Thaysen

A wealth of factual information has accumulated within the last decades about the concentrations of the alkali metals in the secretions of the exocrine glands. In the present chapter special emphasis has been placed on comparing different glands with an attempt at elucidating as far as possible the reasons for the similarites and differences between the various secretory products. In a concluding section (section H, p. 503) the different data with a bearing on the mechanism of glandular electrolyte secretion are reviewed in the light of current knowledge of electrolyte transport in other systems.

A) The duct possessing glands

a) Introduction

The epithelia lining the ducts or tubules of the ductpossessing glands are highly differentiated and they differ morphologically from gland to gland (Fig. 17). It is therefore reasonable to assume that the ducts do not merely serve as pathways for the secretion formed in the acini, but that they contribute somehow to the elaboration of the final secretory product.

A "primary secretion" formed in the acini may well be modified by the secretory or reabsorptive functions of the glandular ducts in a similar fashion as the glomerular filtrate is modified during its passage down the renal tubules. Unlike the glomerular nephron, the glands do, however, not possess a membrane through which the primary secretion is formed as an ultrafiltrate of the plasma. Determination of the composition of the primary secretion and of the manner in which it is modified as it flows down the glandular duct system is therefore beset with considerable practical difficulties, and progress in our knowledge of the mechanism of glandular secretion has consequently been slower than progress in renal physiology.

Despite the complexity of the glandular duct systems there is a definite advantage in treating the secretory mechanism of all the duct-possessing glands under a common heading, since something may be learnt from relating structural and functional similarities and differences. This line of approach was first adopted by Merkel[1063] more than 70 years ago. Merkel compared various salivary glands and concluded that the different epithelia (cf. Fig. 17) had the following functions: 1) The *acini* form a viscous secretion with a high concentration of organic material. 2) The cuboidal epithelium of the *intercalary ducts* secretes primarily water, and 3) The rodded epithelium of the *striated intralobular ducts* (the „Speichelröhren" of Pflüger) secretes the salts of the saliva. The first two conclusions were based on examination of the viscosity and protein content of the secretory product and is in keeping with the fact that the sublingual gland, which has ample acinar epithelium but no intercalary ducts, secretes a viscous saliva, high in organic material, whereas the parotid gland, having relatively long intercalary ducts, produces a more watery type of salivary secretion. The submaxillary gland holds an

---

[1063] Merkel, F.: Die Speichelröhren. Rektoratsprogramm. Leipzig: Vogel 1883.

intermediate position with respect to the length of the intercalary ducts as well as to the viscosity of the secretory product. MERKEL's conclusion about the salt secreting functions of the striated epithelium of the ,,Speichelröhren" was not based on analysis of the saliva, but on morphological appearance and staining reactions only. MERKEL i. a. emphasized that the striated ducts of the glands resembled the convoluted tubules of the kidney and deduced that the two structures had similar functions. According to the then current concept of renal physiology the convoluted tubules were operative in the formation of a hypertonic urine by the secretion of various salts.

In 1886 WERTHER[1064] subjected MERKEL's hypothesis to experimental investigation. Contrary to expectation he found that those salivary glands, which had ample striated epithelium always produced a hypotonic secretory product, whereas glands, which were devoid of striated epithelium, produced a secretion which was isotonic with the plasma. These experiments thus disproved MERKEL's conclusion about the salt-secreting function of the striated ducts, and seemingly they also refuted his theory of a similarity in function between the histologically related structures in the glands and in the kidney.

During the following decades the function of the different epithelia of the glands was mainly studied by histological methods. BABKIN[1065] has reviewed this work, but definite conclusions as to the participation of the glandular ducts in the secretory process were not possible. BABKIN, therefore, emphasized the need for further physiological experimentation. Since then some progress has been made by a further extension of the old comparative studies of MERKEL and WERTHER, through the application of certain concepts from modern renal physiology and by the use of electrophysiological methods, relating changes in membrane potentials to ionic transfers. The following pages are devoted to a survey of this work and to the delineation of a hypothesis of the mechanism of sodium and potassium secretion by the duct-possessing glands.

Fig. 17 shows a comparison between the histological structure of the six main duct-possessing glands and their pattern of electrolyte secretion. Apparently the glands fall into two main groups with respect to sodium and potassium excretion:

Group 1, comprising the *sweat*, *submaxillary* and *parotid* glands. In the secretions of these glands the concentration of sodium varies with secretory rate and is always lower than the concentration of sodium in the plasma. The concentration of potassium is apparently independent of wide ranges of variation in secretory rate, but shows a definite rise at the very low rates of secretion.

Group 2, comprising the *pancreatic*, *lacrymal* and *sublingual* glands. In the secretions of these glands the concentration of sodium is independent of secretory rate and about equal to the concentration of sodium in plasma water. The concentration of potassium is, likewise, independent of secretory rate and shows no rise at the lowest rates as in the secretions of group 1.

The following hypothesis has been forwarded to account for the demonstrated differences in sodium and potassium secretion by the two groups of glands: All glands form "primary secretions" in which the concentrations of sodium and potassium are independent of secretory rate and in which the sums of sodium and potassium concentrations are about equal to the sums of the concentrations of the same two ions in plasma water (Table 30, p. 427). As these "primary secretions" flow down the glandular ducts, sodium is reabsorbed by a process of a limited

[1064] WERTHER, M.: Einige Beobachtungen über die Absonderung der Salze im Speichel. Pflügers Arch. ges. Physiol. **38**, 293—311 (1886).

[1065] BABKIN, B. P.: Secretory Mechanism of the Digestive Glands. 2nd Ed. New York: Hoeber 1950.

maximal capacity in the glands of group 1, but not in the glands of group 2 (NITTA[1066]; THAYSEN, THORN and SCHWARTZ[1067]; THAYSEN and THORN[1068]; THAYSEN[1069]; SCHWARTZ and THAYSEN[1070]; BULMER and FORWELL[1071]; BRO-RASMUSSEN, KILLMANN and THAYSEN[1072]; LUNDBERG[1073], THAYSEN[1074]). Like sodium, potassium is transferred into the secretions in a concentration which is independent of secretory rate, but differs from gland to gland. Unlike sodium, however, potassium is

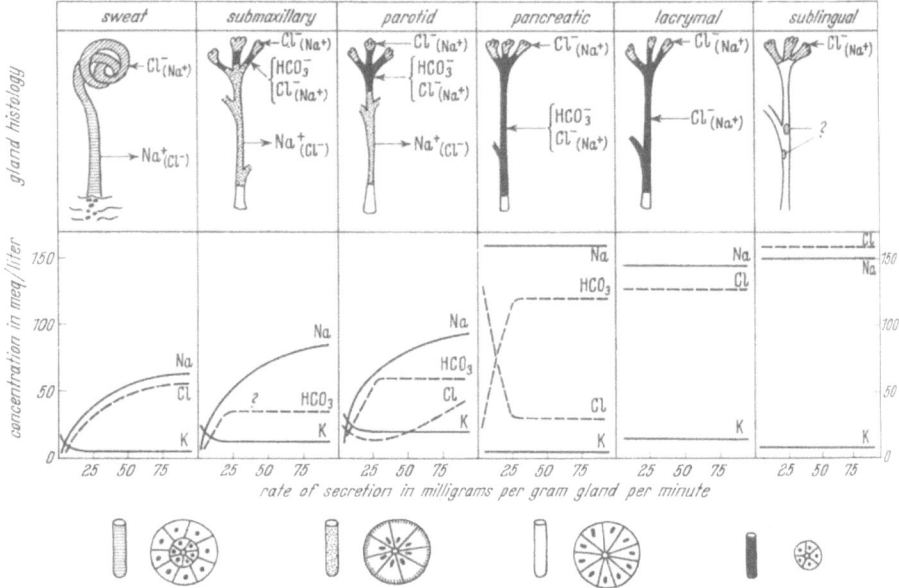

Fig. 17. *Comparison between the histological structure of the six main duct possessing glands and their excretion of electrolytes.* The cross-sections at the bottom of the figure are (from left to right): double layered epithelium of sweat duct; striated epithelium of intralobular ducts; high cylindrical epithelium of excretory ducts; low cuboidal epithelium of intercalary ducts

not reabsorbed in any of the glands. The gradual rise in potassium concentration at the low secretory rates in the glands of group 1 may be due to reabsorption of water in a region of the gland, which is relatively impermeable to potassium ions

[1066] NITTA, H.: On the possibility of a reabsorption in the excretory duct of the sweat gland. Nagoya Med. J. 1, 59—74 (1953).

[1067] THAYSEN, J. H., N. A. THORN, and I. L. SCHWARTZ: The excretion of sodium, potassium and carbon dioxide in human parotid saliva. Amer. J. Physiol. 178, 155—159 (1954).

[1068] THAYSEN, J. H., and N. A. THORN: The excretion of urea, sodium, potassium and chloride in human tears. Amer. J. Physiol. 178, 160—164 (1954).

[1069] THAYSEN, J. H.: Sekretionsstudier, Diss. J. Jørgensen and Co., Copenhagen 1955.

[1070] SCHWARTZ, I. L., and J. H. THAYSEN: Excretion of sodium and potassium in human sweat. J. clin. Invest. 35, 114—120 (1956).

[1071] BULMER, M. G., and G. D. FORWELL: The concentration of sodium in thermal sweat. J. Physiol. 132, 115—122 (1956).

[1072] BRO-RASMUSSEN, F., S.-Å. KILLMANN, and J. H. THAYSEN: The composition of pancreatic juice as compared to sweat, parotid saliva and tears. Acta physiol. scand. 37, 97—113 (1956).

[1073] LUNDBERG, A.: Electrophysiology of Salivary Glands. Physiol. Rev. 38, 21—40 (1958).

[1074] THAYSEN, J. H.: Glandular secretion of electrolytes. Ciba Foundation Colloquia on Ageing. Vol. 4. Water and Electrolyte Metabolism in Relation to Age and Sex. pp. 62—77. London: Churchill 1958.

(LANGSTROTH, McRAE and STAVRAKY[1075]; THAYSEN, THORN and SCHWARTZ[1067]) and/or to an exchange between sodium and potassium ions during the process of sodium reabsorption.

The outward transfer of electrolytes. Old work, showing that secretory pressure can exceed arterial blood pressure, and that the secretory process can continue for a certain period following complete occlusion of arterial blood supply (LUDWIG[1076]), clearly demonstrates that all theories of "pressure dialysis" or "ultrafiltration" have to be abandoned in considerations on the mechanism of the secretory process.

As demonstrated on the ensuing pages, there is, however, reasonably good evidence, that the secretions of the ductpossessing glands are elaborated by an active outward transport of electrolytes from plasma to glandular lumen, and that the outward transfer of water occurs in passive sequence of the osmotic gradient thus created. Such a mechanism must result in the formation of "primary secretions" which are either isotonic or hypertonic, depending upon the permeability of the secreting epithelia to water.

The osmolarity and the electrolyte composition on the primary secretions has never been measured by glandular micropuncture or other similar techniques. All statements about their physico-chemical properties are therefore still hypothetical. Table 30 shows the composition of the precursor secretionas according to the above mentioned hypothesis, which claims that the precursors are isotonic at all rates of formation and contain sodium as the chief cation.

Table 30. *The hypothetical precursor secretions.* (All values in meq/l)

gland	sweat	parotid	submax-illary	sublingual	lacrymal	pancreatic	extra-cellular fluid
Na conc. (meq/l)	155	140	148	152	145	155	155
K conc. (meq/l)	5	20	12	8	15	5	5
Na + K (meq/l)	160	160	160	160	160	160	160
Na/K	30	7	12	19	10	30	30

It is likely, that the sodium and potassium concentrations of all "primary secretions" are independent of the rate, at which the primary secretions are elaborated. There is, however, one exception to this generalization, i.e. "the potassium transient" described by BURGEN[1077]. BURGEN has shown that the submaxillary gland cells lose potassium and take up sodium in the initial phases of stimulation. In this phase potassium ions are lost towards the plasma perfusing the gland as well as towards the secretion, causing the potassium concentration of the first samples of saliva to exceed the concentration of potassium in the following samples. The phenomenon occurs independently of the rate at which the initial samples are secreted[1067,1068,1070,1077]. When the gland cells have lost a certain fraction of their potassium and taken up an almost equivalent amount of sodium (cf. Table 31, p. 434) glandular composition remains stable as long as stimulation is continued. In this steady state potassium appears in the secretion at a constant

[1075] LANGSTROTH, G. O., D. R. McRAE, and G. W. STAVRAKY: The secretion of protein material in the parasympathetic submaxillary saliva. Proc. roy. Soc. London, S. B. **125**, 335—347 (1938).

[1076] LUDWIG, C.: Neue Versuche über die Beihilfe der Nerven zur Speichelabsonderung. HENLE und PFEUFER: Z. rat. Med., N. F. 1, 255—277 (1851).

[1077] BURGEN, A. S. V.: The secretion of potassium in saliva. J. Physiol. **132**, 20—39 (1956).

concentration, which is independent of secretory rate, and all salivary potassium is now derived from the plasma perfusing the gland as indicated by an equivalent arteriovenous potassium deficit. When stimulation ceases, the gland cells extrude sodium in exchange for potassium and cellular concentrations revert to resting conditions within about 30—60 min.

Apparently a typical "potassium transient" is common to all duct-possessing glands, since an initial high concentration of potassium following stimulation has been found in the secretions of sodium-reabsorbing glands: Submaxillary (BURGEN[1077]) and parotid (THAYSEN et al.[1067]) as well as in the secretions of glands, which do not reabsorb sodium: Lacrymal (THAYSEN and THORN[1068]) and sublingual (LUNDBERG[1073]).

The rising potassium concentration at the low secretory rates is, however, specific to the secretions of the sodium-reabsorbing glands (Fig. 17, p. 426). This phenomenon cannot be explained on the basis of the potassium transient, but is most likely due to some mechanism, which the sodium-reabsorbing glands have in common as distinct from the glands that do not reabsorb sodium. The problem is discussed in further detail on page 433.

Electrophysiological studies by LUNDBERG[1078,1079,1080,1081] have thrown light on the mechanism of the outward transport of electrolytes in the glandular acini. LUNDBERG found resting membrane potentials over the inner (blood side) acinar cell membrane in cats' submaxillary and sublingual glands of 22 and 33 mV respectively (cell interior negative). On stimulation the inner acinar membrane hyperpolarizes by about 30 mV in both glands. The resting potential over the outer (luminal) gland cell membrane of the sublingual gland is a few mV larger than over the inner membrane (cell interior negative). On repetitive stimulation of the chorda there is initially little or no potential change over the outer membrane, but with continued stimulation the potential difference over the outer membrane usually, but not always increases by about 10—15 mV.

The origin of these potential changes is not clarified in detail. LUNDBERG[1073] has discussed the various possibilities and concluded that the hyperpolarization of the inner acinar membrane is due to an active transport of anion from the extracellular fluid into the cell. He was able to support this contention experimentally. When the isolated gland was perfused with sodium nitrate instead of with sodium chloride, secretory rate and secretory potentials decreased markedly. When sodium chloride was again added to the perfusate, secretory rate and secretory potentials reverted to normal. Bromide could be substituted for chloride without affecting the secretory activity of the gland, iodide could not.

Much work remains to be done before the mechanism of the outward transport of electrolytes and water in the glandular acini is clarified in detail. Further, it is important to realize that the acinar epithelia may not be the only cells participating in the formation of the "primary secretions". As discussed on p. 430 there is certain evidence that the cuboidal epithelia of the intercalary ducts are operative in the formation of isotonic fluids of low viscosity and protein-content. The cuboidal cells have, however, not been examined by electrophysio-

---

[1078] LUNDBERG, A.: Electrophysiology of the submaxillary gland of the cat. Acta physiol. scand. **35**, 1—25 (1955).
    [1079] LUNDBERG, A.: Secretory potentials in the sublingual gland of the cat. Acta physiol. scand. **40**, 21—34 (1957).
    [1080] LUNDBERG, A.: The mechanism of establishment of secretory potentials in sublingual gland cells. Acta physiol. scand. **40**, 35—58 (1957).
    [1081] LUNDBERG, A.: Anionic dependence of secretion and secretory potentials in the perfused sublingual gland. Acta physiol. scand. **40**, 101—112 (1957).

logical methods or other techniques, which could throw light on their role in the secretory process.

LUNDBERG's work demonstrates that the acinar cells of the sublingual gland are engaged in the active outward transport of chloride. It is apparent from Fig. 17 that chloride concentration of sublingual saliva equals the sum of sodium and potassium concentrations, indicating that chloride is the main, and perhaps the only, anion of that secretion. Several other secretions do, however, contain considerable quantities of bicarbonate in addition to chloride. In fact, the maximum bicarbonate concentration of submaxillary saliva, parotid saliva and pancreatic juice exceeds plasma bicarbonate concentration, indicating that the respective glands possess specific mechanisms for the excretion of this anionic species. The morphological site of bicarbonate secretion (cf. p. 430) and the nature of the secretory mechanism involved still remain obscure.

It is, known that the submaxillary, parotid (SAND [1082]) and pancreatic (VAN GOOR[1083,1084]) glands contain considerable quantities of carbonic anhydrase, which catalyzes the reaction: $CO_2 + H_2O \to H_2CO_3$. At the cellular p_H H_2CO_3 is almost completely dissociated into H^+ and HCO_3^-. In the presence of NaCl, which enters the cells during stimulation, $NaHCO_3$ is somehow secreted into the glandular lumen, leaving behind an equivalent amount of HCl. Possibly this hydrochloric acid causes the definite decrease in glandular p_H which was demonstrated by HAMMARSTEN and JORPES[1085] in the secretin stimulated pancreas. Eventually the HCl is transported (or diffuses ?) into the blood stream, causing venous p_H to be considerably lower than arterial, as observed by WILLS[1086] in the case of the canine submaxillary gland.

That the formation of HCO_3^- is catalyzed by carbonic anhydrase and of great importance for the production of a considerable fraction of the primary secretions of the pancreatic and of the two salivary glands is demonstrated by the finding, that the carbonic anhydrase inhibitor "diamox" does not only depress bicarbonate concentration in the respective secretions, but also the rate of secretion (p. 458 and 463).

According to STILL et al.[1087] and SAND[1082] the chief source of CO_2 for the formation of HCO_3^- is the metabolic CO_2 of the actively secreting gland. It is, however, likely that far more than 1 equivalent of sodium can be actively transported into the secretion for every mole of oxygen consumed (p. 435). In all probability the ratio between active sodium transport and oxygen consumption is so high, that the metabolic CO_2 cannot account for all the bicarbonate appearing in the secretions as sodium bicarbonate. It is of significance in this connection that STILL et al.[1087] have reported venous CO_2 tensions which are lower than arterial CO_2 tensions in the actively secreting pancreatic gland, indicating that CO_2 was withdrawn from the plasma perfusing the gland. Further the

[1082] SAND, H. F.: Source of the bicarbonate of saliva. J. appl. Physiol. **4**, 66—76 (1951).

[1083] GOOR, H. VAN: La répartition de l'anhydrase carbonique dans l'organisme des animaux. Arch. int. Physiol. **45**, 491 (1937).

[1084] GOOR, H. VAN: Die Verbreitung und Bedeutung der Carbonanhydrase. Enzymologia. **8**, 113—128 (1940).

[1085] HAMMARSTEN, E., and E. JORPES: Die Einwirkung der Pankreassekretion auf die Alkalireserve im Blute und auf die Wasserstoffionenkonzentration in der Drüse. Acta med. scand. **68**, 205—214 (1928).

[1086] WILLS, J. H.: Electrolyte changes in submaxillary glands during stimulation. Amer. J. Physiol. **135**, 164—174 (1941).

[1087] STILL, E. U., A. L. BENNETT, and V. B. SCOTT: A study of the metabolic activity of the pancreas. Amer. J. Physiol. **106**, 509—523 (1933).

experiments of BALL, TUCKER, SOLOMON and VENNESLAND[1088] show that at least some of the bicarbonate appearing in the pancreatic secretion may be derived directly from the plasma CO_2 or the plasma bicarbonate.

The mechanism of bicarbonate excretion is still imperfectly understood. It is of interest, however, and may prove fruitful, to relate the above theory to the current hypothesis of HCl secretion by the parietal cells of the gastric glands. Parietal secretion occurs in the "reverse direction" of bicarbonate secretion in the duct-possessing glands (i.e. HCl is transported into the lumen and bicarbonate into the blood), but it has first been pointed out by DAVIES[1089], that there are, nevertheless, several similarities between the two processes.

The morphological site of the outward transport of electrolytes. Very little is known about the morphological site (or sites) of the outward transport of electrolytes and water in the duct possessing glands. According to the old theory of MERKEL (p. 424) the glandular acini are operative in the secretion of enzymes or other protein material, whereas the cuboidal epithelia of the intercalary ducts secrete primarily water.

That *the acini* have a function in the formation of the secretory products has been confirmed by the work of LUNDBERG (p. 428), who was able to show that the acinar cells of the sublingual gland produce an isotonic secretion, and that the chief anion of this secretion in chloride.

If the hypothesis of MERKEL about a secretory function of *the intercalary ducts* is accepted, then it must be assumed that the intercalary secretion is isosmotic with the plasma and not plain water as originally suggested by MERKEL. It is apparent from Fig. 17 that the tonicity of a secretory product does not vary with the amount of intercalary epithelium in the gland producing it, but depends entirely upon the presence or absence of sodium-reabsorbing striated epithelium (p. 434). Our knowledge of the function of the cuboidal epithelium of the intercalary ducts has, however, not been extended much since the days of MERKEL, although certain experimental results on pancreatic secretion indicate, that the pancreatic acini form an isotonic secretion with chloride as the main anion and rich in enzyme, whereas the cuboidal cells of the pancreatic intercalary ducts form an isotonic secretion with bicarbonate as the chief anion and with little or no enzyme activity. With changes in overall glandular activity the two secretions mix in varying proportions, causing the characteristic rate dependent variations in the anionic composition of the final secretory product (cf. Fig. 17, and p. 462). This hypothesis of pancreatic secretion represents a parallel to a current view on gastric secretion, according to which the variations in acidity of the gastric juice are explained by the variable production of two components, a neutral and an acid, which are elaborated by different cells in the gastric mucosa (p. 478).

With the reservations that the paucity of experimental evidence requires, the best working hypothesis for the time being is to carry the above observations on sublingual and pancreatic secretion further, and state that the outward transport of electrolytes and water in *all* the duct-possessing glands is located to the acinar epithelium as well as to the cuboidal epithelium of the intercalary ducts. The *acinar cells* form an isotonic product with chloride as the chief anion, containing enzymes and other protein material elaborated in the acinar cells. The *cuboidal epithelium of the intercalary ducts* secretes a protein-poor isotonic product con-

[1088] BALL, E. G., HELEN F. TUCKER, A. K. SOLOMON, and BIRGIT VENNESLAND: The source of pancreatic juice bicarbonate. J. biol. Chem. **140**, 119—129 (1941).
[1089] DAVIES, R. E.: Doctoral Thesis. Univ. of Sheffield (1948); quoted from A. K. SOLOMON: Fed. Proc. **11**, 722—731 (1952).

taining chiefly bicarbonate or chiefly chloride, depending upon whether the tissue contains carbonic anhydrase.

This hypothesis agrees on several points with the relationship between glandular morphology and secretory composition, which is illustrated in Fig. 17. The sublingual gland contains acini, but no intercalary ducts. The secretion is protein-rich, viscous, and chloride concentration equals the sum of sodium and potassium concentrations. The submaxillary, parotid and pancreatic glands contain acini and intercalary ducts, and carbonic anhydrase activity has been demonstrated in all glands. In all three secretions the concentration of bicarbonate rises to a certain maximum with increasing secretory rate, whereas the concentration of chloride varies inversely with that of bicarbonate in such a manner that the sums of the concentrations of the two anions equal about 90 % of the sums of the concentrations of sodium and potassium at all rates[1072]. The maximum bicarbonate concentration increases (and the protein content of the secretions decreases[1065]) in the order: submaxillary saliva — parotid saliva — pancreatic juice, i.e. in the same order as there is an increasing length of the intercalary ducts of the glands in question.

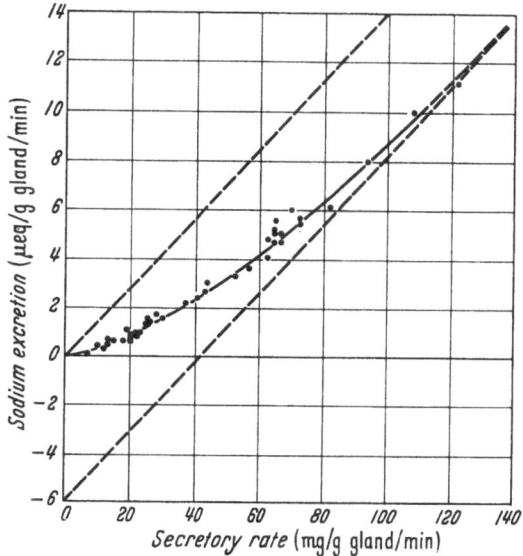

Fig. 18. *The rate of excretion of sodium in parotid saliva in relation to the rate of secretion.* (Redrawn from the data of THAYSEN, THORN and SCHWARTZ[1067])

The reabsorption of sodium. Although the composition of the secretory products has never been determined directly by micropuncture at various intervals along the glandular tubules, indirect evidence is accumulating, that sodium is being reabsorbed from the "primary secretions" in the ducts of the sweat, parotid and submaxillary glands. It must be assumed that sodium reabsorption occurs through epithelial membranes of low permeability to water, since the final secretory products are hypotonic.

Fig. 18 illustrates the rate of excretion of sodium in parotid saliva in relation to secretory rate as an example of the kinetics of sodium excretion in the glands of "Group 1". The fully drawn line, which represents the observed values from the experiments of THAYSEN, THORN and SCHWARTZ[1067] approaches, but does not quite reach, the dotted line, which represents the theoretical asymptote provided thatsodium concentration of the primary secretion is 140 meq/l (Table 30, p. 427), and provided that sodium reabsorption represents a constant quantity, independently of the rate at which the primary secretion is formed. The reason for this splay of the observed values from the theoretical relationship may be, that a certain quantity of water is moving back into the blood stream in sequence of active sodium reabsorption, and/or that the rate of sodium reabsorption decreases some with decreasing Na conc. of the fluid in the duct lumen (cf. p. 115).

When urea is used as a glandular "clearance substance" there is reasonable qualitative evidence to suggest that water is, in fact, being reabsorbed from the "primary secretions" of the sweat and parotid glands (submaxillary saliva has not yet been examined in a similar fashion).

It has been shown that the concentrations of urea in sweat, parotid saliva and tears remain proportional to the concentration of urea in the plasma within a wide range of variation in the latter. This finding indicates that urea is excreted in these secretions by a process of simple diffusion and not via a specific secretory mechanism, which might become saturated by increasing load. Potentially urea may therefore be used as a tracer for the movement of water within the secreting glands in a similar fashion as in the glomerular nephron (SCHWARTZ, THAYSEN and DOLE[1090], THAYSEN and THORN[1068] and ALBRECTSEN and THAYSEN[1091]).

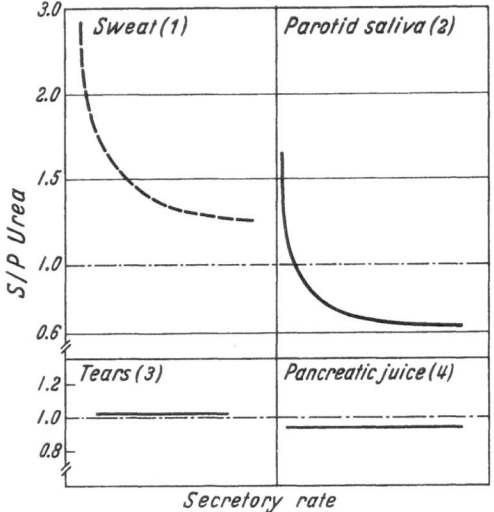

Fig. 19. *The relation between the S/P ratio for urea and secretory rate in sweat, parotid saliva, tears and pancreatic juice. From the data of:* (1) ARAKI and ANDO[1092]; (2) ALBRECTSEN and THAYSEN[1091]; (3) THAYSEN and THORN[1068] and (4) BRO-RASMUSSEN, KILLMANN and THAYSEN[1072]

Fig. 19 illustrates the relationship between the S/P (secretion/plasma) concentration ratio for urea and secretory rate in sweat, parotid saliva, pancreatic juice and tears.

In tears and in pancreatic juice S/P urea is close to 1.0 and independent of secretory rate. No internal circulation of water can thus be demonstrated with the use of "urea clearance" in these glands, which do not reabsorb sodium from their "primary secretions".

In sweat and in parotid saliva, however, S/P urea varies with the rate of secretion. In the sweat it decreases from 2—3 at low rates to about 1 when sweating becomes profuse (ARAKI and ANDO[1092]; BULMER[1093]). In parotid saliva S/P urea decreases from about 1.6 at low rates of secretion to about 0.6 when the flow of saliva is brisk (ALBRECTSEN and THAYSEN[1091]). Since no specific secretory mechanism for urea exists in either gland[1090, 1091], the hypothesis has been advanced that urea, which diffuses into the gland with some "primary secretion", is concentrated by reabsorption of water in a region of the gland which is relatively impermeable to urea[1090,1091,1092,1093]. The observed variations in S/P urea with secretory rate (Fig. 19) indicate that the quantity of water, which is being reabsorbed, must be relatively constant at all rates of secretory activity[1092, 1093], and it has been suggested that water diffuses from glandular lumen to plasma in passive sequence of the osmotic gradient created by the active reabsorption of solute, possibly of sodium[1090, 1091, 1093].

[1090] SCHWARTZ, I. L., J. H. THAYSEN, and V. P. DOLE: Urea Excretion in human sweat as a tracer for movement of water within the secreting gland. J. exp. Med. **97**, 429—437 (1953).

[1091] ALBRECTSEN, S. R., and J. H. THAYSEN: The excretion of urea by the human parotid gland. Scand. J. clin. Lab. Invest. **7**, 231—238 (1955).

[1092] ARAKI, Y., and S. ANDO: Urea, amino acid and ammonia in human sweat. Jap. J. Physiol. **3**, 211—218 (1952).

[1093] BULMER, M. G.: The concentration of urea in thermal sweat. J. Physiol. **137**, 261—266 (1957).

The variations in S/P urea have not been examined simultaneously with the variations in sodium concentration in any of the secretions. No attempt has therefore been made to determine, whether the splay of the observed values for sodium excretion from the asymptote of Fig. 18 is due exclusively to backdiffusion of water, or whether a certain decrease in the rate of sodium reabsorption does also occur with decreasing overall glandular activity. It is quite possible, however, that the question cannot be finally decided upon on the basis of the "glandular urea clearance", since the latter probably represents only a qualitative and not a quantitative measure of the movement of water within the secreting gland[1090].

Recently LUNDBERG[1073, 1078, 1079, 1080, 1081] has presented independent evidence in favour of the theory that cations are being reabsorbed from a primary secretion in some of the duct possessing glands of the cat. In the submaxillary gland, that produces a secretion in which sodium concentration varies in about the same manner as in the human glands of "group 1", LUNDBERG[1078] demonstrated that the lumen of the (striated?) ducts becomes negative as compared to the hilus, when the gland is activated by stimulation of the chorda. A similar internal duct negativity could not be demonstrated in the sublingual gland (LUNDBERG[1079]), which (like the other glands of "group 2") produces a secretion, that is isotonic with the plasma and has a total cation concentration of about 160 meq/l. Provided that the potential changes on stimulation can be regarded as the electrical signal of ionic transport, LUNDBERG concludes that there may well be a net transport of cation from the lumen to the blood side in the ducts of the submaxillary glands, but not in those of the sublingual gland.

Although the composition of the submaxillary secretion was not measured simultaneously with the potential difference between duct lumen and hilus, the potential appears large enough (about 40 mv) to accept, that reabsorption of anion may occur in merely passive sequence of active cation reabsorption. In all probability chloride is the chief anion reabsorbed in passive sequence of active sodium reabsorption. Evidently this must be the case in the sweat gland, which produces a "primary secretion" consisting chiefly of chloride salts. But also in the parotid and submaxillary glands, the primary secretions of which contain considerable quantities of bicarbonate, chloride ions are apparently reabsorbed in preference of bicarbonate ions — possibly due to the difference in the molecular size of the two anions (Fig. 17).

The rise in potassium concentration at the low secretory rates in submaxillary saliva (LANGSTROTH, McRAE and STAVRAKY[1075]), parotid saliva (THAYSEN, THORN and SCHWARTZ[1067], BURGEN[1077]), and sweat (KUNO[1094]) may be due to reabsorption of water from the primary secretion (LANGSTROTH, McRAE and STAVRAKY[1075]) and/or to an exchange between sodium and potassium ions during the process of sodium reabsorption. Glandular clearance techniques are not sufficiently refined to distinguish between these two possibilities.

Some recent experiments by ULLRICH[1095] are of considerable interest in relation to the present hypothesis of sodium reabsorption. ULLRICH demonstrated, that the oxygen consumption of isolated canine parotid gland slices increased, when the sodium concentration of the normal Ringer medium was augmented by 200 meq/l. The parotid tissue thus behaved in a fashion, which was qualitatively similar to tissue slices from the outer medullary zone of the glomerular kidney and from the colonic mucosa structures, which are both assumed to possess

[1094] KUNO, Y.: Human Perspiration. Springfield: C. G. Thomas 1956.
[1095] ULLRICH, K. J.: Aktiver Natriumtransport und Sauerstoffverbrauch in der äußeren Markzone der Niere. Pflügers Arch. ges. Physiol. **267**, 207—217 (1958).

mechanisms for active sodium reabsorption (cf. p. 241 and 509). In contrast, the respiration of pancreatic tissue slices was depressed by increases in the Na conc. of the medium — a type of reaction, which the pancreatic tissue had in common with e. g. uterine mucosa, liver, brain, muscle and adrenal gland.

The morphological site of sodium reabsorption. It is only possible to speculate on the morphological site of sodium reabsorption in the glands. It is, however, not unreasonable to assume that sodium reabsorption is located in the striated intralobular ducts (THAYSEN[1069]). Striated epithelium is present in the parotid and submaxillary glands, which apparently reabsorb sodium from their "primary secretions", but absent in the sublingual, lacrymal and pancreatic glands, which show no evidence of sodium reabsorption (Fig. 17). This hypothesis fits well with the old theory of MERKEL[1063] about a certain similarity in function between the striated ducts of the salivary glands and the convoluted tubules of the kidney. The main function of both structures is, however, not secretory as believed by MERKEL, but reabsorptive as was actually first indicated by the experiments of WERTHER (p. 425). With respect to the sweat gland evidence from data on the movement of water within the secreting gland (SCHWARTZ, THAYSEN and DOLE[1090]) suggests that sodium reabsorption takes place in the double layered epithelium of the duct.

The ionic transport in the striated ducts of the submaxillary and parotid glands and in the duct of the sweat gland is illustrated schematically in Fig. 17.

Glandular sodium and potassium balance during secretion. Determinations of glandular sodium and potassium content in the resting and stimulated state are few. It appears from Table 31 that the glands lose potassium in exchange for sodium when secretory activity is stimulated.

Table 31. *Alkali metals in resting and stimulated glandular tissue.*
(All data in meq/l of gland water)

Author	Gland	resting			stimulated		
		water (%)	K (meq/l of gland water)	Na (meq/l of gland water)	water (%)	K (meq/l of gland water)	Na (meq/l of gland water)
WILLS[1086]	cats submaxillary	76	113	54	78	100	74
WILLS[1086]	dogs submaxillary	76	139	22	77	131	64
BURGEN[1077]	dogs submaxillary	75	99	42	75	67	83
INGRAHAM and VISSCHER[1096]	dogs pancreatic	74	134	82	—	—	—
OLDFELDT[1097]	dogs pancreatic	—	147	89	unchanged		
SOLOMON[1098]	dogs pancreatic	—	105	45	—	—	—
LUNDBERG[1073]	cats sublingual	79	105	83	—	—	—

The most careful study of glandular sodium and potassium balance during stimulation has been performed by BURGEN[1077] on the dogs' submaxillary gland. His chief results are the following:

When a previously rested gland is stimulated to secrete, it goes through a transient phase during which it loses potassium ions in exchange for sodium ions. The potassium loss takes place over the outer (luminal) membrane as well as over the inner (blood side) membrane. Consequently the first samples of saliva collected have a higher potassium concentration than the following (the "potassium transient"). Further, potassium ions flow into the plasma, causing venous plasma

[1096] INGRAHAM, R. C., and M. B. VISSCHER: Analyses of gastric mucosa and pancreatic gland tissue of dog for Na, K, Cl and PO₄. Proc. Soc. exp. Biol. (N. Y.) **40**, 147—149 (1939).
[1097] OLDFELDT, C. O.: The alkali in the pancreatic secretion. J. Physiol. **102**, 362—366 (1943).
[1098] SOLOMON, A. K.: Electrolyte secretion in the pancreas. Fed. Proc. **11**, 722—731 (1952).

potassium concentration to exceed arterial plasma potassium concentration. When these initial exchanges have taken place a steady state is arrived at, during which glandular sodium and potassium content remains approximately constant. In the steady state all potassium appearing in the secretion must be derived from the plasma perfusing the gland, since a quantitative relationship was found between the salivary potassium excretion and the arterio-venous potassium deficit. The ratio between glandular plasma flow and rate of secretion was about 4—8 and the concentration of potassium in the saliva about three times that of the plasma. When stimulation ceases, the gland extrudes sodium ions in exchange for potassium ions and reaches its resting composition in the course of 30—60 min. When restimulated after the said interval, a typical "potassium transient" is obtained. When restimulated before the said interval the potassium transient is lacking or very small.

BURGEN only studied the sodium-reabsorbing submaxillary gland, but according to the discussion on p. 428 it is reasonable to assume, that a similar "potassium transient" is found also in glands, which do not reabsorb sodium.

Glandular oxygen consumption in relation to electrolyte transport. Table 32 shows determinations of the increase in oxygen uptake during maximal stimulation of three different glands. The values for oxygen consumption have been recalculated as microequivalents of oxygen per gram wet weight of gland per minute (1 μM of $O_2 = 4$ μeq). Since the volume and composition of the secretions was not measured simultaneously with oxygen uptake, the figures for electrolyte transport are based on the assumptions:

1. That maximal stimulation of the glands causes a secretory flow of 100 mg per gram wet weight of gland per minute (cf. Fig. 17).

2. That the formation of the "primary secretions" only involves active transport of anion (cations following passively) and that 16 μeq of anion are transported to form 100 mg of isotonic primary secretion (cf. p. 428 and Table 30).

3. That active sodium reabsorption in the parotid and submaxillary glands amounts to 6 μeq per gram wet weight of gland per minute (cf. Fig. 18).

The work of HEIDENHAIN[1101], ANREP[1102] and KOMAROV, LANGSTROTH and MCRAE[1103,1104] suggests that protein synthesis in the glands is a continuous process,

Table 32. *Relation between oxygen consumption and electrolyte transport*

Author	Gland	Oxygen uptake in microequivalents per gram wet weight of gland per min			Electrolyte transport in micro-equivalents per gram wet weight of gland per min	Ratio of electrolyte transport to increased oxygen uptake
		resting	stimulated	increase		
BARCROFT[1099]	dogs submaxillary	5.4	17.9	12.5	22 (16+6)	1.8
OHARA[1100]	dogs parotid	5.7	12.4	6.7	22 (16+6)	3.3
STILL etal.[1087]	dogs pancreatic	5.2	11.1	5.9	16	2.7

[1099] BARCROFT, J.: The Architecture of Physiological Function. Cambridge University Press 1938.

[1100] OHARA, K.: Studies on the oxygen consumption of human skin tissues with special reference to that of the sweat glands. Jap. J. Physiol. **2**, 11—18 (1951).

[1101] HEIDENHAIN, R.: Über sekretorische und trophische Drüsennerven. Pflügers Arch. ges. Physiol. **17**, 1—67 (1878).

[1102] ANREP, G. V.: The metabolism of the salivary glands. J. Physiol. **54**, 319—331 (1921).

[1103] KOMAROV, S. A., G. O. LANGSTROTH, and D. R. MCRAE: The secretion of crystalloids and protein material by the pancreas in response to secretin administration. Canad. J. Res. D **17**, 113—123 (1939).

[1104] LANGSTROTH, G. O., D. R. MCRAE, and S. A. KOMAROV: The synthesis and secretion of protein material by the pancreas. Canad. J. Res. D. **17**, 137—149 (1939).

which is apparently not accelerated, when the glands are stimulated to secrete. It is thus likely, that the synthesis of enzymes or other protein-material does not require excess oxygen consumption, when the gland is discharging. The ratios between active electrolyte transport and increased oxygen uptake in Table 32 are therefore calculated on the assumption, that the total superbasal oxygen consumption during the secretory process is available for active electrolyte transport.

The ratios of Table 32 indicate that 1.8, 3.3 and 2.7 μeq of electrolyte can be actively transported for every microequivalent of oxygen consumed in excess of basal requirements (i.e. 7.6, 13.2 and 10.8 μeq of electrolyte for every micromole of oxygen). It is of interest to compare these values with the findings of ZERAHN [1105,1106] on the frog skin (p. 120). ZERAHN showed that 4—5 μeq of sodium can be actively transported through the frog skin for every microequivalent of oxygen consumed in excess of basal requirements (i.e. 16—20 μeq of sodium for every micromole of O_2). The reader is also referred to the calculations of electrolyte transport in relation to oxygen consumption in the tubule of the glomerular nefron (p. 261).

These findings are of considerable interest because certain hypotheses advanced to explain active transport of ions claim that only one cation is transported for each electron being transferred to oxygen. It must be emphasized, however, that the present calculation of the conditions in the duct-possessing glands comprises several approximations, since oxygen uptake and secretory rate were not measured simultaneously.

Recently, TERROUX, SEKELJ and BURGEN [1107] determined blood flow and oxygen uptake in the canine submaxillary gland at secretory rest and at varying rates of salivary flow. They found a resting blood flow of 0.26 ml per gram gland per minute. During activity blood flow rose to about 8—10 times the corresponding salivary flow, but there appeared to be a poor correlation between blood flow on the one side and salivary flow and oxygen consumption on the other. Resting oxygen consumption was about 27 μl of O_2 (= 4.9 μeq of O) per gram gland per minute. During stimulation there appeared to be a linear correlation between superbasal oxygen consumption and the rate of saliva secretion within a range of variation in the latter from 40 to 380 μl per gram gland per minute. The superbasal oxygen consumption amounted to about 30 μl of O_2 per 100 μl of saliva formed (= 5.36 μeq of O per 100 μl of saliva, or a ratio between electrolyte transport and oxygen consumption of about 4 according to the present calculations). The linear correlation between oxygen consumption and rate of saliva secretion in the experiments by TERROUX et al. does not fit the present theory of a dual electrolyte transport mechanism in the submaxillary gland: One varying in simple proportion to secretory rate (outward transport) and another representing a relatively constant quantitiy at all rates of salivary flow (reabsorption). There was, however, a very considerable spreading of the individual observations.

Factors affecting sodium and potassium excretion by the duct-possessing glands. As in other systems, the cellular mechanism responsible for active transport of electrolytes in the glands remains unknown. Glandular sodium and potassium

[1105] ZERAHN, K.: Oxygen consumption and active sodium transport in the isolated and short-circuited frog skin. Acta physiol. scand. 36, 300—318 (1956).

[1106] ZERAHN, K.: Oxygen consumption and active transport of sodium in the isolated, short-circuited frog skin. Nature (Lond.) 177, 973—983 (1956).

[1107] TERROUX, K. G., P. SEKELJ and A. S. V. BURGEN: Oxygen consumption and blood flow in the submaxillary gland of the dog. Canad. J. Biochem. Physiol. 37, 5—15 (1958).

secretion is, however, known to be affected by a number of factors, which are discussed in detail in the following sections on the secretion of the individual glands. A short review comparing all glands is given here in so far as the findings can be discussed in the light of the above hypothesis of glandular electrolyte secretion.

The effect of ischemia. It was first demonstrated by LUDWIG[1076] that occlusion of the arterial blood supply to a gland causes an abrupt and marked decrease in the rate of secretion, but that secretory activity may continue at the lower rates for 30—60 min before it is completely arrested. Like the cells of the frog skin (p. 120) the gland cells are thus able to perform a limited amount of active electrolyte transport for a certain period following withdrawal of oxygen supply. Possibly the transport is energized by glycolysis in both systems as evidenced by an increased concentration of lactate in the medium in which the frog skin is suspended (p. 120) and in the secretory product of ischemic sweat glands (p. 443).

The effect of ischemia on electrolyte secretion has only been studied in the case of the sweat (p. 443) and submaxillary (p. 455) glands. It has been demonstrated that the concentration of sodium (chloride) in the secretions from these glands decreases less than should be expected from the decrease in secretory rate, when arterial blood supply is arrested. If arterial occlusion is of long duration, the concentration of sodium (chloride) in the secretion from the ischemic glands may even exceed that of control glands, despite a manifold difference in the rate of secretion.

These findings suggest that ischemia impairs the outward transport of electrolytes (i.e. the volume of secretion decreases) as well as sodium reabsorption (i.e. the sodium concentration of the final secretory product increases above the value to be expected from the normal flow-concentration relationship). The results may thus be regarded as yielding indirect evidence in favour of the hypothesis, that the formation of sweat and of submaxillary saliva involves active outward transport of electrolyte through epithelial membranes, which are readily permeable to water, as well as active reabsorption of sodium through epithelial membranes of low permeability to water.

The effect of ischemia on the volume and composition of secretions from glands, which do not reabsorb sodium, has not been studied. It is to be expected, however, that occlusion of the arterial blood supply to such glands would reduce the volume of secretion formed, without affecting its osmolarity.

The effect of variations in the plasma concentrations of sodium and potassium. It has been shown that the S/P (secretion/plasma) concentration ratio for potassium is independent of relatively wide ranges of variation in the concentration of potassium in the plasma. This applies to the sodium reabsorbing salivary glands (p. 455) and sweat glands (p. 443) as well as to the pancreatic gland (p. 462) which possesses no sodium-reabsorbing mechanism.

Variations in the plasma sodium concentration cause an immediate and almost parallel variation in the sodium concentration of pancreatic juice (p. 462), whereas the effect is less conspicuous in the secretions of the sodium-reabsorbing sweat (p. 443) and salivary glands (p. 455).

These results indicate that the Na and K concentrations in the "primary secretions" of all glands are affected by variations in the Na and K concentrations of the plasma. The reader is referred to similar studies on the effect of variations in plasma electrolyte concentrations and in plasma osmolarity on the gastric (p. 473) intestinal (p. 485) and hepatic (p. 489) secretions.

The effect of adrenal steroids. Adrenal steroids may well have a dual site of action in the glands, i.e. on the formation of the "primary secretions" as well as on the reabsorption of sodium in the ducts. A comparative study of the effect of aldosterone on sodium reabsorbing and non-sodium reabsorbing glands might shed some light on this problem, but has never been performed to the knowledge of the author. In fact, information on the effect of adrenal steroids on the concentrations of alkali metals in the pancreatic, lacrymal and lingual secretions is nil, whereas a copious body of literature has appeared on the effect of the steroids on the Na/K ratios of sweat and saliva. No decided standpoint can therefore be taken on the site of action of adrenal steroids within the glands. The fact that salivary (p. 457) and sweat (p. 444) potassium concentrations are significantly elevated in the steady state of secretion, when adrenal steroids are administered, however, suggests that the steroids do depress the Na/K ratio of the "primary secretions" besides having a possible accelerating effect on sodium reabsorption in the ducts.

Criticism of the present theory of sodium and potassium secretion has recently been forwarded by BURGEN and his collaborators[1108, 1109]. BURGEN and SEEMAN[1108] assume that the acini of the canine submaxillary gland form an isotonic primary secretion, consisting chiefly of potassium bicarbonate. As this primary secretion flows down the duct system, it is modified by reabsorption of potassium ions, which are — in part — replaced by sodium ions moving from the peritubular space to the duct lumen. The reabsorbed potassium ions are recycled to the acini via the peritubular capillaries, in which blood is assumed to flow in a direction counter to that of the saliva. The locus of sodium transfer from the peritubular capillaries to the duct lumen was investigated by BURGEN, TERROUX and GOUDER[1109] in the canine parotid gland. From measurements of secretory rate and of the appearance time for labelled sodium in the saliva and from an estimate of the glandular duct capacity (or "dead space") these authors arrived at the conclusion that sodium was transferred into the parotid saliva somewhere distally to the striated ducts, possibly in the large interlobular ducts. The validity of the statement rests on the correctness of the estimation of the glandular "dead space", which was 50—100 μl/g canine parotid gland according to BURGEN et al., but considerably smaller in the human parotid gland according to ALBRECTSEN and THAYSEN[1091].

b) The sweat glands

Due i.a. to the minute size of the sweat glands, methods for collection of sweat are less easily standardized than are methods for collection of the secretions of most other duct-possessing glands. For details regarding methodology the reader is referred to the review by ROBINSON and ROBINSON[1110], but it should be emphasized, once more, that experimental design must take into account all the different variables, which are discussed on the ensuing pages. Considerable confusion regarding interpretation of results can be avoided, when these variables are always carefully controlled. Of prime importance is exact determination of secretory rate, and it can hardly be stressed too much, that no way of stating the results (as the "Na/K-ratio" or otherwise) does permit the investigator to dispense with the necessity for measurement of sweating rate.

One further point is worthy of comment. The sweat harvested by most practicable methods represents the combined output of a great many sweat glands

[1108] BURGEN, A. S. V., and P. SEEMAN: The role of the salivary duct system in the formation of the saliva. Canad. J. Biochem. Physiol. **36**, 119—143 (1958).

[1109] BURGEN, A. S. V., K. G. TERROUX and E. GOUDER: The sites of transfer of sodium, potassium and iodide in the parotid duct system of the dog. Canad. J. Biochem. Physiol. **37**, 359—370 (1959).

[1110] ROBINSON, S., and A. H. ROBINSON: Measurement of sweating. In: Methods in Medical Research. Vol. 6, p. 100—120. Year Book Publ. Chicago 1954.

within a smaller or larger area of the skin. The density and secretory capacity of sweat glands varies between different skin regions in the same person and between identical skin regions in different persons (see i.a. Kuno[1111, 1094]). Comparable secretory rates per unit skin area do therefore not necessarily represent comparable mean secretory rates per gland, and no definite statement about the physiological significance of regional or individual variations in sweat composition is possible, unless the number of functioning glands is determined. Likewise, it is apparent that the relative contributions of individual sweat glands must be studied in relation to variations in overall secretory rate within any given skin area, if one wants to bridge the gap between results obtained on the skin as an organ of sweating and the physiology of its functioning units: The sweat glands. Examples of the significance of these considerations are presented on the following pages. A method for the collection of sweat, permitting simultaneous registration of the number of functioning glands, has been published by Dole and Thaysen[1112].

In the following sections alkali metal excretion by the sweat glands is considered in relation to the follwing variables:

1. Type of gland.
2. Rate of secretion.
3. Skin temperature.
4. Duration of secretion.
5. Type of stimulus.
6. Plasma concentration of the alkali metals.
7. Glandular blood flow.

8. Adaptation to salt depletion.
9. Adreno-cortical steroids.
10. Different drugs.
11. Individual differences.
12. The excretion of lithium, rubidium and cesium.
13. The effect of prolonged sweating on sodium and potassium metabolism.

Type of gland. The human sweat glands can be divided into:

1) *The apocrine glands* of the axillary and other regions, which respond chiefly to psychic stimuli and produce a somewhat milky, odorous secretion.

2) *The eccrine glands of the palms and soles* which respond mainly to psychic stimuli and secrete a watery non-odorous secretion. These glands are present also in animals otherwise devoid of a sweating mechanism and are possibly involved in the function of securing a firm stand or grasp.

3) *The eccrine glands of the general body surface*, responding chiefly to thermal stress and secreting a watery, non-odorous sweat.

Regarding structure, innervation and secretory pattern of these different gland types the reader is referred to the monographs by Kuno[1094, 1111] and to the recent reviews by Randall[1113] and Randall and Kimura[1114].

The composition of *palmar sweat* harvested in microcapillary tubes, has been examined by Lobitz[1115, 1116, 1117] and his collaborators. At high rates of secretion these investigators found a sodium chloride concentration of 385 mg-% (about 65 meq of sodium per liter), whereas the slow, intermittent secretion contained as much as 1091 mg-% (or about 190 meq of sodium per liter). The sodium concen-

[1111] Kuno, Y.: The Physiology of Human Perspiration. London: Churchill 1934.

[1112] Dole, V. P., and J. H. Thaysen: Variation in the functional power of human sweat glands. J. exp. Med. **98**, 129—144 (1953).

[1113] Randall, W. C.: The physiology of sweating. Amer. J. Phys. Med. **32**, 292—318 (1953).

[1114] Randall, W. C., and K. K. Kimura: The pharmacology of sweating. Pharmacol. Rev. **7**, 365—397 (1955).

[1115] Lobitz, W. C., and A. E. Osterberg: Chemistry of palmar sweat. Preliminary reports, apparatus and techniques. J. invest. Derm. **6**, 63—73 (1945).

[1116] Lobitz, W. C., and A. E. Osterberg: The chemistry of palmar sweat II: Chloride. Arch. Derm. Syph. **56**, 462—467 (1947).

[1117] Lobitz, W. C., and H. L. Mason: Chemistry of palmar sweat VII: Discussion of studies on chloride, urea, glucose, uric acid, ammonia nitrogen and creatinine. Arch. Derm. Syph. **57**. 907—915 (1948).

tration at high rates corresponds to that of the *eccrine glands on the general body surface* (see below). If evaporative loss from the minute quantities of sweat collected can be excluded with certainty, the palmar glands, however, differ from the other glands in secreting a hypertonic sweat at the lowest secretory rates. It is not clear why the palmar glands should show an inverse relationship between secretory rate and sodium concentration; and further investigation of the problem is needed.

Rate of secretion. The rate of secretion affects sodium and postassium concentrations differently.

Sodium. KITTSTEINER[1118, 1119] first demonstrated that the concentration of chloride in the sweat increases with secretory rate. This relation has been confirmed by several later investigators, and it has been shown that sodium follows the same general trend as does chloride (cf. the review by ROBINSON and ROBINSON[1120]).

From the data of many investigators ROBINSON and ROBINSON[1120] have computed the mean Na/Cl ratio to be 1.11. LOCKE, TALBOT, JONES and WORCESTER[1121] found the following relationship between sodium and chloride concentrations of the sweat: $Na = (1.12 \ Cl) + 3$ meq/l.

The range of variation in sodium concentration with secretory rate is from about 5 meq/l at low rates of secretion to about 60 (100) at high rates of secretion. Values higher than 100 meq/l reported in some papers are probably due to methodological factors or physiological variables other than secretory rate[1120].

The rate of change in sodium concentration with secretory rate was first examined by KITTSTEINER[1118], who states: ,,Es scheint mit wachsender Absonderungsgeschwindigkeit der Kochsalzgehalt sich einer bestimmten Grenze (etwa 0,5%) zu nähern, welche er nicht mehr überschreitet." Several later investigators claim that there is a linear relationship between sodium concentration and secretory rate, but HANCOCK, WHITEHOUSE and HALDANE[1122] and SCHWARTZ and THAYSEN[1070] found that the increase in sweat sodium concentration decreased with each successive equal increment in the rate of secretion, although no definite maximum was reached. A typical experiment from SCHWARTZ and THAYSEN's paper[1070] is shown in Fig. 17, p. 426.

These findings leave little doubt that the concentration of sodium in the sweat is strongly influenced by secretory rate. A statement of sodium concentration in the sweat without reference to the rate of secretion is therefore of little meaning, and considerable confusion may arise, especially in comparative work, if secretory rate remains undetermined.

In all the quoted experiments sweat was harvested from a smaller or larger area of the skin, comprising a great many individual sweat glands, which may apparently vary to a considerable extent in secretory capacity (DOLE and THAYSEN[1112]). The demonstrated variations in sodium concentration with secretory rate may therefore be due to either of two mechanisms:

1) All sweat glands produce a secretion of essentially similar nature with a sodium concentration that is dependent upon secretory rate.

[1118] KITTSTEINER, C.: Kochsalzgehalt und Reaktion des Schweißes. Arch. Hyg. **73**, 275—305 (1911).

[1119] KITTSTEINER, C.: Weitere Beiträge zur Physiologie der Schweißdrüsen und des Schweißes. Arch. Hyg. **78**, 275—326 (1913).

[1120] ROBINSON, S., and A. H. ROBINSON: Chemical composition of sweat. Physiol. Rev. **34**, 202—220 (1954).

[1121] LOCKE, W., N. B. TALBOT, H. S. JONES, and J. WORCESTER: Studies of the combined use of measurements of sweat electrolyte composition and the rate of sweating as an index of adrenal cortical activity. J. clin. Invest. **30**, 325—337 (1951).

[1122] HANCOCK, W., A. G. R. WHITEHOUSE, and J. S. HALDANE: The loss of water and salts through the skin. Proc. roy. Soc. London, S. B. **105**, 43—59 (1929).

2) Different sweat glands produce a secretion of different composition, and with an increase in overall secretory rate more and more glands are activated, which secrete a sweat of high sodium concentration.

Due to technical difficulties sweat from single glands has not been examined over a wide range of secretory rates. Comparative studies on the composition of sweat from glands of different secretory capacity are lacking. The only means to bridge the gap between the performance of the skin as an organ of sweating and the physiology of its individual glands is therefore to examine changes in sweat gland pattern in relation to changes in overall secretory rate. The work of KUNO and associates[1094, 1111], RANDALL[1123, 1124, 1125], and DOLE and THAYSEN[1112] indicates, that a change in overall secretory rate from a given skin area is mainly due to a change in mean flow per gland, and that the relative activities of different glands remain constant despite considerable variations in their combined output. These findings suggest, that the increase in sodium concentration with secretory rate is representative of individual sweat gland function.

Potassium. Reported values of potassium concentration in the sweat show considerable variations with a range from about 2 to about 15 meq/l (ROBINSON and ROBINSON[1120]). The results obtained regarding variations in potassium concentration with secretory rate are, likewise, conflicting. However, the general impression gained from a review of the recent literature is, that the concentration of potassium in sweat collected under standardized conditions is equal to or slightly larger than the concentration of potassium in the plasma, and that variations in potassium concentration with secretory rate are much less pronounced than in the case of sodium.

The first sample of sweat collected after stimulation of secretory activity usually has a higher concentration of potassium than the following ones (HANCOCK, WHITEHOUSE and HALDANE[1122]; KUNO[1111]; SCHWARTZ and THAYSEN[1070]). KUNO[1111] believes that the high potassium concentration at the onset of sweating may be due to washing out of potassium from the epidermis. This view is apparently supported by the findings of HANCOCK et al.[1122], who showed, that the phenomenon was most pronounced if the skin had not been carefully rinsed in advance of the experiment. It is, however, a question whether mixing of the newly formed sweat with sweat residues or other impurities on the skin surface is the only explanation for the phenomenon. THAYSEN and THORN[1068] also found a high potassium concentration of the first sample of tear fluid collected after stimulation of the lacrymal gland, and both THAYSEN, THORN and SCHWARTZ[1067] and BURGEN[1077] showed that the first saliva specimens collected after stimulation of the salivary glands had a higher concentration of potassium than the following ones (see p. 427). In the case of the salivary glands, BURGEN[1077] explains the phenomenon as being due to an initial cellular loss of potassium in exchange for sodium when the gland goes from the essentially resting to the stimulated state (p. 434).

Apart from the first sample(s) of sweat collected after stimulation, most authors agree that the concentration of potassium in the sweat is only slightly, if at all, affected by variations in the rate of secretion. At the very low secretory rates KUNO[1111] does, however, find a definite increase in potassium concentration in parallel to the findings on the secretions of other sodium reabsorbing glands (cf. Fig. 17, p. 426).

[1123] RANDALL, W. C.: Quantitation and regional distribution of sweat glands in man. J. clin. Invest. **25**, 761—767 (1946).

[1124] RANDALL, W. C.: Sweat gland activity and changing patterns of sweat secretion on the skin surface. Amer. J. Physiol. **147**, 391—398 (1946).

[1125] RANDALL, W. C., and W. McCLURE: Quantitation of the output of individual sweat glands and their response to stimulation. J. appl. Physiol. **2**, 72—80 (1949).

Skin temperature. KITTSTEINER[1118], [1119] first produced evidence that the concentration of chloride in the sweat is dependent not only upon sweating rate but also upon skin temperature. WEINER and VAN HEYNINGEN[1126] went even further and claimed that the chloride concentration of general body sweat (obtained by the "weight-change and wash-down" method) follows the skin temperature rather than the rate of sweating. Since there is a close connection between skin temperature and sweating rate (KITTSTEINER[1119]; LOCKE et al.[1121]), it is, however, difficult to draw definite conclusions from experiments in which these two parameters have not been varied independently. By a modification of KITTSTEINER's original technique, ROBINSON, GERKING, TURRELL and KINCAID[1127] produced local cooling or heating to one forearm (the other serving as a control) in persons sweating profusely in response to generalized heat. They collected and analyzed sweat from "arm bags" and found that, *independently of secretory rate* and independently of the stage of acclimatization of the men, the concentration of sodium and of chloride was significantly higher on the heated than on the cooled arm. They conclude that the effect of variations in skin temperature, which occurs within 30 min. of changing the temperature, is due to a direct effect on the sweat glands and not to a central or hormonal factor.

The demonstrated effect of skin temperature on sweat sodium and chloride concentrations may in part invalidate methods of sweat collection in which a rise of skin temperature is the consequence of deficient evaporation ("arm bag" and "collection chamber"). VAN HEYNINGEN and WEINER[1128] compared the composition of "arm bag" sweat to general body sweat and concluded that the higher concentration of chloride in arm bag sweat may be due to an abnormal rise in skin temperature on the enclosed arm. The relationship between skin temperature and potassium concentration of the sweat has not been examined.

The mechanism of the temperature effect on sweat sodium concentration remains unexplained. Temperature variations also affect electrolyte excretion by the salivary glands (p. 454) and have been shown to influence the "sodium pump" in isolated systems (p. 62).

Duration of secretion. Whereas KITTSTEINER[1119] found chloride concentration of the sweat to be independent of the duration of the secretion, later investigators have reported that sodium (chloride) concentration tends to increase in prolonged sweating[1139], [1129]. ROBINSON and ROBINSON[1120] state that this phenomenon may be due to a "fatigue of the sweat glands" with progressive incapacity of performing the osmotic work involved in the production of a hypotonic secretion. Glandular glycogen stores tend to become exhausted with prolonged stimulation, and the glandular reserve of anaerobic metabolism in response to excessive demands consequently decreases.

Whereas these explanations do not appear unlikely, it is still difficult to evaluate the reports in the literature, since a number of different factors may well have played a role for the observed increase in sweat sodium concentration during prolonged sweating. A *rise in secretory rate* on prolonged heat exposure is not unlikely, and the rate has not been controlled in all investigations. Similarly *a rise in skin temperature* may well occur in prolonged exposure to heat, a parameter which also remains uncontrolled in most studies. In this connection it is of some

---

[1126] WEINER, J. S., and R. E. VAN HEYNINGEN: Relation of skin temperature to salt concentration of general body sweat. J. appl. Physiol. 4, 725—733 (1952).

[1127] ROBINSON, S., S. G. GERKING, E. S. TURRELL, and R. K. KINCAID: The effect of skin temperature on salt concentration of the sweat. J. appl. Physiol. 2, 654—662 (1950).

[1128] HEYNINGEN, R. E., van and J. S. WEINER: Comparison of arm bag sweat and body sweat. J. Physiol. 116, 395—403 (1952).

[1129] LADELL, W. S. S.: Thermal sweating. Brit. med. Bull. 3, 175—179 (1945).

interest that LADELL[1129] found sweat chloride concentration to rise less with duration of sweating in acclimatized than in non-acclimatized persons. Acclimatized persons sweat more readily than non-acclimatized and may, *ceteris paribus*, keep skin temperature at a lower level. Finally, PEARCY et al.[1130] have shown that sweat chloride concentrations varies with *the manner in which sweat losses are replaced* (p. 449). If dehydration is induced in prolonged sweating, chloride concentration of the sweat tends to increase, whereas it decreases when the water loss is replaced.

It is apparent from this discussion that no definite information is yet available with respect to the relationship between duration of secretory activity *per se* and the excretion of sodium and chloride by the sweat glands.

Type of stimulus. The sweat glands may be stimulated reflexly as well as by parasympathomimetic and sympathomimetic substances (RANDALL[1113, 1114]). All kinds of stimulation have been used in work on man, but comparative investigations on the composition of the sweat with different stimuli are not available. SCHWARTZ and THAYSEN[1070] examined sweat produced after local intradermal injection of mecholyl on the forearm, and their results regarding sodium and potassium excretion are not significantly different from those of LOCKE et al.[1121], who collected sweat from the same region in response to thermal stress.

Plasma concentration of Na and K. AMATRUDA and WELT[1131] found a slight decrease in sweat sodium concentration despite increase in sweating rate following a water load (infusion of 3 l 5% glucose). Conversely sweat sodium concentration increased slightly despite definite decrease in the rate of sweating following injection of 430 meq of sodium chloride in 500 ml of water. Alkalosis caused slight decrease in potassium concentration of the sweat. Acidosis increased sweat potassium concentration. SCHWARTZ and THAYSEN[1070] found that the concentration of potassium in the sweat remains proportional to the concentration of potassium in the plasma within a range of variation in the latter from 3.7 to 5.6 meq/l.

Glandular blood flow. When the arterial blood supply of an arm is occluded during exposure to heat, sweating on the occluded arm continues, although at decreasing rates, for at least 30 min after arrest of blood supply. The ischemic sweat glands are even capable of a considerable increase in secretory rate, if radiant heat is applied directly to the skin (RANDALL et al.[1132, 1133]). VAN HEYNINGEN and WEINER[1134] have demonstrated that sweat chloride concentration on the occluded arm decreases less than should be expected from the decrease in secretory rate. If occlusion is of long duration, sweat chloride concentration may even rise over and above that of the control arm, despite a manifold difference in sweating rate. According to WEINER and VAN HEYNINGEN[1135], lactate concentration of the sweat shows a definite increase on the ischemic side, and cellular glycogen stores become reduced, indicating that the ischemic sweat glands depend upon glycolysis to perform the work of secretion (cf. the findings on the frog skin,

[1130] PEARCY, M., S. ROBINSON, D. I. MILLER, J. T. THOMAS JR., and L. DE BROTA: Effects of dehydration, salt depletion and pitressin on sweat. J. appl. Physiol. 8, 621—626 (1956).

[1131] AMATRUDA, T. T., and L. G. WELT: Secretion of electrolytes in thermal sweat. J. appl. Physiol. 5, 759—771 (1953).

[1132] RANDALL, W. C.: Local sweat gland activity due to direct effect of radiant heat. Amer. J. Physiol. 150, 365—371 (1946).

[1133] RANDALL, W. C., R. DEERING, and I. DOUGHERTY: Reflex sweating and the inhibition of sweating by prolonged arterial occlusion. J. appl. Physiol. 1, 53—59 (1948).

[1134] HEYNINGEN, R. E.VAN, and J. S. WEINER: The effect of arterial occlusion on sweat composition. J. Physiol. 116, 404—413 (1952).

[1135] WEINER, J. S., and R. E. VAN HEYNINGEN: Lactic acid and sweat gland function. Nature (Lond.) 164, 351 (1949).

p. 120). Since, besides chloride, there are considerable quantities of lactate in the sweat, it is quite possible that estimation of sodium concentration would have revealed even greater differences between the ischemic and the normal glands than did estimation of chloride.

VAN HEYNINGEN and WEINER[1134] showed that the effect of arterial occlusion is not due to alteration of skin temperature on the ischemic arm, since the phenomenon also occurred when the temperature of the skin on the ischemic arm was kept at the same level as that of the control. Apparently, the sweat glands need about one hour to recover normal function following prolonged ischemia. The mechanism of the effect of glandular ischemia on the volume and composition of the sweat is discussed on page 437.

Adaptation to salt depletion. A decrease in sweat sodium and an increase in sweat potassium concentration represents one of several physiological adjustments, which occur during adaptation to salt depletion (McCANCE[1136]). In practice, this adaptation of the sweat glands is frequently encountered during the process of acclimatization to work in hot environments, as shown by DILL et al.[1137] and many others[1138, 1139, 1140]. Adaptation of the sweat glands is, however, not an obligatory factor in acclimatization. It develops only when sweat sodium losses are inadequately replaced, and is also seen in non-acclimatized individuals, who have become sodium depleted for other reasons (ROBINSON et al.[1140]).

The adaptation of the sweat gland to salt depletion is both incomplete and delayed as compared to that of the kidney.

Under standard conditions with respect to sweating rate and other parameters, several of the above mentioned workers found that sodium (chloride) concentration may become halved or more than halved during adaptation. The concentration of potassium is doubled, and the "Na/K ratio" of the sweat decreases to one third or one fourth of the original value. Sodium excretion by the sweat glands is, however, not completely arrested even under conditions of severe sodium depletion, where urinary sodium concentration may drop to near zero.

The response of the sweat glands is not only incomplete as compared to the renal response, but also relatively slow. The kidneys react within hours, the sweat glands within days (McCANCE[1136]; ROBINSON et al.[1141]).

That the adaptation of the sweat glands during acclimatization is related to sodium depletion is clearly demonstrated by the experiments of ROBINSON et al.[1140]. These investigators showed that a typical reduction of sweat chloride concentration was evident from the first day of heat exposure, when the subjects had been on a low sodium diet in advance of the experiments. Further a low sweat chloride concentration was normalized in the course of 3 days, despite unchanged heat exposure, when fully adapted subjects were given a liberal addition of sodium chloride to their diet.

[1136] McCANCE R. A.: The effect of salt deficiency in man on the volume of the extracellular fluids and on the composition of sweat, saliva, gastric juice and cerebrospinal fluid. J. Physiol. **92**, 208—218 (1938).

[1137] DILL, D. B., F. G. HALL, and H. T. EDWARDS: Changes in composition of sweat during acclimatization to heat. Amer. J. Physiol. **123**, 412—419 (1938).

[1138] MICKELSEN, O., and A. KEYS: The composition of sweat with special reference to the vitamins. J. biol. Chem. **149**, 479—490 (1943).

[1139] JOHNSON, R. E., G. C. PITTS, and F. G. CONSOLAZIO: Factors influencing chloride concentration in human sweat. Amer. J. Physiol. **141**, 575—589 (1944).

[1140] ROBINSON, S., R. K. KINCAID, and R. K. RHAMY: Effects of salt deficiency on salt concentration of sweat. J. appl. Physiol. **3**, 55—62 (1950).

[1141] ROBINSON, S., J. R. NICOLAS, J. H. SMITH, W. J. DALY, and M. PEARCY: Time relation of renal and sweat gland adjustments to salt deficiency in man. J. appl. Physiol. **8**, 159—165 (1955).

LADELL[1142] and CONN et al.[1143, 1144, 1145, 1146] first demonstrated that the sweat glands react with a typical "adaptation response" to adrenocorticotropin and desoxycorticosterone, and they suggested that the effect of sodium depletion on the sweat gland is mediated via an increased adrenal secretion of salt conserving hormone. From the above discussion it appears that the sweat gland epithelium (like the epithelium of the salivary glands) responds less readily to aldosterone than do the cells of the renal tubule.

Adrenal cortical steroids. As mentioned above, CONN et al.[1143, 1144, 1145, 1146] first demonstrated that administration of adrenocorticotropin and desoxycorticosterone causes a decrease in sodium and an increase in potassium concentration of thermal sweat. These results have been confirmed by many later investigators, who also were able to verify CONN's original statement, that the Na/K ratio of the sweat is high in Addisons disease and low in Cushings disease. For a limited period of time, the "sweat test" acquired a certain clinical application in the diagnosis of conditions associated with increased or decreased adrenocortical function.

A review of the literature on the "sweat test" left the present writer with the impression that exact determination of secretory rate was far too often dispensed with. This certainly does invalidate the results, since it is quite obvious, that the "non-endocrine" variations in the "Na/K-ratio" with secretory rate are considerable and far larger than the "endocrine" variations. It cannot be stressed too much that standardization of experimental conditions with respect to secretory rate is a prerequisite for the use of the sweat test in any kind of comparative work. This is of equal importance whether the results are stated as absolute concentrations of sodium and potassium in the sweat or as the Na/K ratio (cf. Fig. 21, p. 457).

Drugs. For a recent review on the pharmacology of sweating, the reader is referred to the paper by RANDALL and KIMURA[1114]. Studies on variations in sodium and potassium excretion as related to drug action are not on record. DOLE, STALL and SCHWARTZ[1147] have designed a sweat collection method, which may permit a study of the reactivity of the sweat glands to local intradermal injection of drugs in doses that have little or no systemic effect.

Individual differences in sweat composition. *Regional variations* in the concentration of chloride in the sweat have i.a. been examined by MICKELSEN and KEYS[1138], who state the following values: Torso — 55 meq/l, face — 101 meq/l, thigh — 75 meq/l and arm — 55 meq/l. Methods of collection from the different regions were not similar and secretory rate is not stated, for which reason the results probably illustrate general trends only. It is well known that there is a considerable regional variation in the density[1111, 1094, 1112] and perhaps also in the mean secretory activity[1112] of the sweat glands. The whole question must be reexamined in relation to these parameters. It is, however, of great importance for practical work that the composition of sweat collected from any localized skin

[1142] LADELL, W. S. S.: The effect of desoxycorticosterone acetate on chloride content of sweat. J. Physiol. **104**, 13—14 P (1945).

[1143] CONN, J. W., M. W. JOHNSTON, and L. H. LOUIS: Acclimatization to humid heat. A function of adrenal cortical activity. J. clin. Invest. **25**, 912—913 (1946).

[1144] CONN, J. W., L. H. LOUIS, M. W. JOHNSTON, and B. J. JOHNSON: The electrolyte content of thermal sweat as an index of adrenal function. J. clin. Invest. **27**, 529—530 (1947).

[1145] CONN, J. W.: Electrolyte composition of sweat. Clinical implications as an index of adrenal cortical activity. Arch. intern. Med. **83**, 416—428 (1949).

[1146] CONN, J. W., and L. H. LOUIS: Production of endogenous "salt active" corticoids as reflected in the concentrations of sodium and chloride in thermal sweat. J. clin. Endocr. **10**, 12—23 (1950).

[1147] DOLE, V. P., B. G. STALL, and I. L. SCHWARTZ: Method for local induction and quantitative analysis of human sweat. Proc. Soc. exp. Biol. (N. Y.) **77**, 412—415 (1951).

area can hardly be regarded as representative of total body sweat and that the same regions (and collection methods) must be used in all comparative work.

Even under standardized conditions with respect to rate of secretion as well as to method and site of collection there are considerable *individual variations* in the concentration of sodium (or chloride) in the sweat (McCance[1136,1148]; Locke et al.[1121]; Schwartz et al.[1070]). Since the number of functioning glands remained undetermined in these studies, it is, however, not known, whether the demonstrated differences are merely due to the well-known variations in the density and distribution pattern of the sweat glands between persons (ref. Kuno[1111]), or whether there is also an individual difference in the physiological performance of single sweat glands.

McCance[1148] found a mean sodium concentration in the sweat of 9 men of 62 meq/l and of 7 women of 55 meq/l. The mean potassium concentrations were 6.1 and 5.5 meq/l, respectively. However, average secretory rate was greater in the men (1846 ml) than in the women (1219 ml) and may account for the apparent *sex difference* in sodium concentration. Similar results have been obtained by Darling[1149] and Davies and Clark[1150]. Tanaka[1151, 1152, 1153] has shown that the lower sweating rates in females than in males in response to the same thermal stress is due mainly to a smaller mean flow per gland in the females, and that this difference between the sexes is most pronounced in the reproductive years of the women, much less before puberty or after the menopause.

Reported *racial differences* in sodium and potassium excretion with the sweat are very hard to clarify in detail, since climatic conditions and dietary habits are subject to large variations. Apart from the fact that possible differences between races may thus be due merely to varying degrees of adaptation (see p. 444), there also appears to be a difference in the number of functioning sweat glands between individuals raised in the tropics and individuals raised in the temperate zones, independently of their origin (Kawakata and Sahamoto[1154]). Comparing West African Coal Miners to British soldiers in Iraq, Ladell[1155] was unable to demonstrate any significant difference in the chloride concentration of the sweat between the two races.

Salt losing sweat glands. The work of Kessler and Andersen[1156], Darling et al.[1157], di Sant'Agnese et al.[1158] and di Sant'Agnese[1159] has demonstrated,

[1148] McCance, R. A.: Individual variations in response to high temperature. Lancet **235**, 190—191 (1938).

[1149] Darling, R. C.: Some factors regulating composition and formation of human sweat. Arch. Phys. Med. **29**, 150—155 (1948).

[1150] Davies, D. F., and H. E. Clark: Hypertensive syndrome with relative adrenal cortical overactivity. Circulation **2**, 494—504 (1950).

[1151] Tanaka, M.: Studies on the functions of human sweat organs VI. Sexual differences in the ability to perspire. Mie med. J. **7**, 109—114 (1957).

[1152] Tanaka, M.: Studies on the functions of human sweat organs VII. Effect of sex hormones on the ability to perspire. Mie med. J. **7**, 115—122 (1957).

[1153] Tanaka, M., and A. Kawahata: Studies on the functions of human sweat organs V. Age as an important factor influencing the ability to perspire. Mie med. J. **7**, 101—107 (1957).

[1154] Kawahata, A., and H. Sakamoto: Sweating of the Aino. Jap. J. Physiol. **2**, 166—169 (1952).

[1155] Ladell, W. S. S.: Some physiological observations on West African Coal miners. Brit. J. Indust. Med. **5**, 16—20 (1948).

[1156] Kessler, W. R., and D. H. Andersen: Heat prostration in fibrocystic disease of the pancreas and other conditions. Pediatrics 8, 648 (1952).

[1157] Darling, R. C., P. A. di Sant'Agnese, G. A. Perera, and D. H. Andersen: Electrolyte abnormalities of the sweat in fibrocystic disease of the pancreas. Amer. J. med. Sci. **225**, 67—70 (1953).

[1158] Sant'Agnese, P. A. di, R. C. Darling, G. A. Perera, and E. Shea: Sweat electrolyte disturbances associated with childhood pancreatic disease. Amer. J. Med. **15**, 777—784 (1953).

[1159] Sant'Agnese, P. A. di: Fibrocystic disease of pancreas, a generalized disease of exocrine glands. J. Amer. med. Ass. **160**, 846—853 (1956).

that patients with fibrocystic disease of the pancreas are particularly liable to heat prostration due to an abnormally high sodium concentration in their sweat, whereas the renal salt-conserving mechanism appears to be intact. In a large series of patients DI SANT'AGNESE[1159] found the following composition of sweat from patients with fibrocystic disease (mucoviscoidosis) as compared to normal controls:

	Na (meq/l)		Cl (meq/l)	
	mean	(range)	mean	(range)
Patients	133	(80—190)	106	(60—160)
controls	59	(10—80)	32	(4—60)

Secretory rate was about equal in the two groups. The high Na conc. in the sweat of patients with fibrocystic disease was not depressed by salt-depletion nor by administration of desoxycorticosterone-acetate. The basic abnormality remains unknown, but further study of the condition may possibly shed some light on the mechanism of sodium conservation by the sweat glands.

The secretion of Li, Cs and Rb. The secretion of the alkali metals Li, Cs and Rb by the sweat glands has not been examined.

The effect of prolonged sweating on the homeostasis of water, sodium and potassium.

Water loss. The maximum secretory capacity of the sweat glands cannot be stated exactly. It varies with sex and age (TANAKA[1151, 1152, 1153]), with the climate in which the person gas been raised (KAWAKATA and SAHAMOTO[1154]), with the degree of acclimatization (DILL[1137]) and with little understood individual differences Sweating rates as high as 2—3 l per hour in response to severe thermal stress have been reported by LADELL[1129] and come close to the highest secretory rates obtained by SCHWARTZ and THAYSEN[1070] by maximal stimulation of the sweat glands with intradermal mecholyl. Apparently such maximal sweating rates may be followed by a decline in the secretory activity of the sweat glands, despite unaltered stimulus (KITTSTEINER[1119]; GERKING and ROBINSON[1160]; THAYSEN and SCHWARTZ[1161]) The maximum rate at which sweating can continue with unaltered intensity over longer periods is probably somewhere between 1 and 2 l per hour.

In practice, climatic conditions and the amount of physical activity vary considerably in the course of the day and the rate of sweat secretion fluctuates in parallel to the need for heat excretion. Average values for hourly sweating rates under different conditions are given in ADOLPH's monograph[1162]. Maximum 24 hr sweating rates in U.S. soldiers performing physical work in the desert were 11 l (ADOLPH), whereas KUNO[1111] reports maximum 24 hr sweating rates as high as 15 l Japanese soldiers in the tropics.

The rate of sweat secretion is chiefly geared to the need for heat dissipation and only slightly affected by the requirements of body water economy. Reports on the relationship between sweating rate and progressive dehydration are, however, somewhat conflicting. Thus, ADOLPH found sweating to continue with unaffected rate, despite progressive dehydration amounting to 8% of initial body weight in

[1160] GERKING, S. D., and S. ROBINSON: Decline in the rate of sweating of men working in severe heat. Amer. J. Physiol. **147**, 370—381 (1946).

[1161] THAYSEN, J. H., and I. L. SCHWARTZ: Fatigue of the sweat glands. J. clin. Invest. **34**, 1719—1725 (1955).

[1162] ADOLPH, E. F.: Physiology of Man in the Desert. New York. Interscience Publ. Inc. 1947.

the course of 8 hr. Similarly, LADELL[1163] found that dehydration by an amount of 2—3 kg did not affect the rate of sweating. Other workers (PITTS et al.[1164]; ROBINSON et al.[1165]), however, state that sweating rate declines measurably with moderate degrees of dehydration. ROBINSON et al.[1165] claim that there is a close relationship between the rise in serum chloride during progressive dehydration and the decline in sweating rate. The effect on the sweat glands is apparently not mediated via the increased secretion of antidiuretic hormone by the dehydrated men, since both AMATRUDA and WELT[1131] and PEARCY, ROBINSON, MILLER, THOMAS and DEBROTA[1130] have shown that pitressin is without the slightest effect on sweating rate in normally hydrated men.

Electrolyte loss. Sweat has a lower concentration of sodium and of chloride than the extracellular fluid. The sweat potassium concentration equals the concentration in the plasma or exceeds it slightly, especially in persons adapted to salt depletion.

The quantity of the different electrolytes lost with the sweat of course depends upon the volume of sweat secreted. Sweat electrolyte concentrations are, however, affected by such a variety of factors (p. 440 to 447) that no valid estimate of total electrolyte loss can be made by measurement of sweat volume only.

When sodium depletion is induced due to deficient replacement of salt to heavily sweating persons the concentration of sodium in the sweat is lowered. The response starts within 8—12 hr, but is not completed before several days. It develops more rapidly when water is replaced, than when dehydration is induced (ROBINSON et al.[1165]). The sweat glands thus respond to the needs of sodium economy of the body, but the response is incomplete, since sodium exretion is never completely arrested even during severe depletion, and the response is delayed as compared to the sodium conserving response of the kidney (p. 444).

Replacements. During maximal 24 hr sweating rates of 11—151 water turnover represents 25 % of total body water per day. Assuming an average sweat sodium concentration of 60 meq/l, the 24 hr sodium turnover represents 20—30 % of total exchangeable body sodium of an adult man. These turnover rates are so large that maintenance of normal homeostasis, even over short periods, rests almost entirely on a balanced replacement of water and sodium chloride losses by oral intake.

ADOLPH[1162] found that men living and working in the desert with liberal access to water and food adequately replaced water loss with the sweat as estimated from the relative constancy of urine volume between individuals and in the same individual from day to day. Actual "overdrinking" was rare, 24 hr urine volume on average slightly smaller (just below 1000 ml) than observed in the same men, when staying in a temperate climate.

Whereas the thirst mechanism is, thus, relatively well geared to the requirements of homeostasis, the same cannot be said about the craving for salt. The relatively frequent development of fatigue, muscular twitchings or actual "heat cramps" in profusely sweating men with free access to water and food has been shown to be due to a deficient replacement of sodium chloride losses with the sweat. The problem is of considerable practical importance in tropical and industrial medicine. For details the reader is referred to the monographs by DILL[1166],

---

[1163] LADELL, W. S. S.: The effects of water and salt intake upon performance of men working in hot and humid environments. J. Physiol. **127**, 11—46 (1955).

[1164] PITTS, G. C., R. E. JOHNSSON, and F. C. CONSOLAZIO: Work in heat as affected by intake of water, salt and glucose. Amer. J. Physiol. **142**, 253—259 (1944).

[1165] ROBINSON, S., R. T. MALETICH, W. S. ROBINSON, B. B. BOHRER, and A. L. KING: Output of NaCl by sweat glands and kidneys in relation to dehydration and salt depletion. J. appl. Physiol. **8**, 615—620 (1956).

[1166] DILL, D. B.: Life, Heat and Altitude. Cambridge. Mass.: Harvard University Press. 1938.

LEE[1167], ADOLPH[1162], NEWBURGH[1168] and KUNO[1111] as well as to the extensive clinical and physiological observations by LADELL[1129, 1142, 1155, 1163, 1169] and the recent work by ROBINSON and his colleagues[1127, 1130, 1140, 1141, 1165].

The effect of sweating without replacement of water and salt. *Sweating rate* decreases slightly as serum chloride goes up in response to progressive dehydration (ROBINSON et al.[1165]). The dehydrated person may, however, still react with increased sweat secretion to increments in the thermal stress (ADOLPH[1162]). Sweat sodium and chloride concentrations remain unchanged or increase slightly with progressive dehydration[1165].

Urine volumes decrease with progressive dehydration. ADOLPH[1162] found a decrease from 30 to 15 ml/hr with dehydration amounting to 6% of initial body weight. When dehydration reaches 15—20% anuria usually ensues. The concentration of chloride in the urine goes up and frequently exceeds plasma concentration (KUNO[1111]). Due to the decrease in urine volume the rate of urinary chloride excretion, however, drops (ADOLPH[1162]; ROBINSON et al.[1165]), and urinary sodium and chloride losses are usually quite insignificant in comparison to sweat losses. This appears clearly from the experiments of LADELL[1169], where urinary chloride losses only amounted to 1.3, 2.5, 3.5 and 9.0% of total chloride loss in 4 experiments with progressive dehydration and salt depletion.

Changes in volume and composition of the body fluids represent a combination of sodium depletion and simple dehydration. The first causes contraction of extracellular volume, the latter proportionate contraction of extra- and intracellular volume and rise in the osmolarity of the body fluids, as evidenced i.a. by rising serum concentrations of chloride and of sodium. Thus, under all conditions extracellular volume is contracted relatively more than intracellular volume. How much more depends on the sodium concentration of the sweat. LADELL's[1169] subjects who had high sweat chlorides (72—88 meq/l) showed calculated reductions of extracellular volume, which were not only relatively but also numerically larger than calculated reductions in intracellular volume. In ADOLPH's[1162] experiments the measured "volume of distribution of total water loss" averaged 40% of total body weight, indicating that intracellular water depletion was numerically larger, albeit still relatively smaller than was contraction of extracellular volume. This may have been due to a lower sweat sodium concentration in ADOLPH's subjects, but data on sweat electrolyte concentrations are not reported.

Serum chlorides remain stationary during moderate dehydration (ROBINSON et al.[1165]; KUNO[1111]), but rise in parallel to the degree to which simple dehydration is induced by progressive and unreplaced sweat loss (ADOLPH[1162]; LADELL[1169]).

The clinical picture of progressive dehydration and salt depletion is not to be described here. It should be emphasized, however, that "heat cramps" do not develop with this kind of depletion (LADELL[1169, 1163]). When sweat losses represent 10% of initial body weight symptoms of exhaustion and circulatory failure develop. When sweat loss approaches 20% death ensues in hyperthermia, circulatory collapse and complete anuria. In moderately severe cases the condition is rapidly improved by balanced replacement of sweat losses. In severe cases infusions have to be used, since the patient is unable to drink. If salt is not available it is safer to replace water loss only in part (theoretically by the amount that will

---

[1167] LEE, D. H. K.: A Basis for the Study of Man's Reaction to Tropical Climate. Univ. of Queensland Press 1940.

[1168] NEWBURGH, L. H.: Physiology of Heat Regulation and the Science of Clothing. Philadelphia: W. B. Saunders 1949.

[1169] LADELL, W. S. S.: The changes in water and chloride distribution during heavy sweating. J. Physiol. **108**, 440—450 (1949).

revert simple dehydration), since a drop in serum sodium and intracellular over-hydration will otherwise develop (see below).

The effect of sweating with replacement of water but not of salt. *Sweating rate* remains constant[1130, 1165]. Actual "overdrinking" does not increase sweating rate (KUNO[1111]). (The subjective feeling of accentuated sweating occasionally following water intake is only a very small quantity, when actually measured, and represents a reflex from the stomach wall rather than an effect of temporary hydremia. The increase occurs so promptly after drinking that no water can yet have been absorbed[1111]). Sweat sodium concentration decreases, but the adaptive response of the sweat gland epithelium is delayed and incomplete in comparison to that of the kidney (p. 444).

Urine volume may show a temporary and rather marked increase but decreases to control values within a few hours after onset of sweating. The initial diuresis may be accompanied by a small decrease in weight (ROBINSON et al.[1165]). Sodium and chloride concentrations of the urine drop within a few hours and the adaptive response of the kidneys is fully developed within 5—10 hr[1141].

Changes in the volume and composition of the body fluids are caused by the replacement of sodium chloride loss with pure water. The rapidity with which the abnormalities arise depends entirely on sweat sodium concentration. When sweat sodium concentration is low (as e.g.in acclimatized persons and at low sweating rates), substitution of sweat losses with pure water is of course considerably less deleterious than when sweat sodium concentration is high (as e.g. in non-acclimatized individuals and when sweat flows profusely). Substitution of sodium chloride loss with pure water causes contraction of the extracellular compartment, expansion of the intracellular compartment and drop in serum chloride and serum sodium (LADELL[1169]).

The clinical picture is characterized by progressive fatigue associated with muscular twitchings which may develop into actual "heat cramps". According to LADELL heat cramps only occur when a combination of hyponatremia and intra-cellular overhydration has been induced. This type of heat exhaustion is the one most commonly encountered in everyday life and was first described by EDSALL[1170]. The condition is cured by administration of sufficient sodium chloride to replace the deficit, and may be prevented if persons performing physical labour at high environmental temperature are encouraged to take a salt supplement.

The effect of sweating with replacement of salt but not of water loss. *Sweating rate* tends to decrease as in unreplaced sweat loss (ROBINSON et al.[1165]).

Urine volume decreases slightly as in unreplaced sweat loss. Urinary chloride concentration is high.

Changes in volume and composition of the body fluids are those of simple dehydration with proportionate contraction of extra- and intracellular volumes and rise in serum sodium and serum chloride concentrations.

The situation is artificial, but is approached if castaways at sea in the tropical zones attempt to relieve their thirst by drinking sea water.

c) The salivary glands

The mixed saliva of the oral cavity represents the combined secretions of the three large salivary gland pairs and of numerous smaller glands. The relative contributions of the different glands to the mixed saliva depend not only on their individual secretory capacity, but also to a certain extent on the intensity

---

[1170] EDSALL, D. L.: Two cases of violent true transitory myoclonia and myotonia apparently due to excessively hot weather. Amer. J. med. Sci. **128**, 1003—1016 (1904).

(SCHNEYER and LEVIN[1171, 1172]) and the kind (ZEBROWSKI[1173]) of stimulus applied. In the oral cavity the saliva is mixed with food debris and subjected to bacterial decomposition, resulting i.a. in a decrease in p_H (TULLAR[1174]). Caution should therefore be observed in drawing conclusions on salivary gland physiology from analysis of the mixed, contaminated and decomposed fluid in the mouth.

Collection of pure saliva, as it emerges from the opening of the glandular ducts, is beset with certain difficulties in work on man. Parotid saliva is rather easily obtained in "Lashley cups" (LASHLEY[1175]; CURBY[1176]), whereas the separation of submaxillary and sublingual saliva requires the use of "segregators", which have to be constructed separately for each individual (SCHNEYER[1177]). Most work on the secretion of individual salivary glands has therefore been performed on animals and is frequently referred to in the following, where data on humans are lacking or incomplete.

In the ensuing sections salivary excretion of sodium and potassium is considered in relation to the following variables:

1. Type of gland.
2. Rate of secretion.
3. Gland temperature.
4. Duration of secretion.
5. Type of stimulus.
6. Plasma concentration of the alkali metals.
7. Glandular blood flow.
8. Adaptation to salt depletion.
9. Adrenal cortical steroids.
10. Different drugs.
11. Individual variations.
12. The excretion of lithium, cesium and rubidium.

Type of gland. SCHNEYER and LEVIN[1171, 1172] have determined the relative secretory rates of the three large salivary gland pairs in man under different intensities of stimulation. At low secretory rates the three glands contributed the following percentages to the total amount of secretion formed: submaxillary 69, parotid 26 and sublingual 5%. When salivation was stimulated, the parotid increased its output relatively more than the two other glands. The percentages were: submaxillary 63, parotid 34 and sublingual 3%. SCHNEYER and LEVIN did not examine the different types of saliva chemically, and there are no data available in the literature on such comparative investigation in man.

1. *Parotid gland.* Pure parotid secretion of man was examined by THAYSEN, THORN and SCHWARTZ[1067] and by HILDES and FERGUSON[1178]. Their results are almost comparable. Sodium concentrations varied between 5 and 90 meq/l with secretory rate. Potassium concentrations were about 20 meq/l and independent of secretory rate at flows exceeding 0.5 ml/min. At lower rates of secretion, salivary potassium concentration showed a consistent and marked increase (cf. Fig. 17, p. 426). It is of interest, that the parotid saliva of sheep (DENTON[1191]) and rabbits

[1171] SCHNEYER, L. H., and L. K. LEVIN: Rate of secretion by individual salivary gland pairs of man under conditions of reduced exogenous stimulation. J. appl. Physiol. 7, 508—512 (1955).
[1172] SCHNEYER, L. H., and K. L. LEVIN: Rate of secretion by exogenously stimulated salivary gland pairs of man. J. appl. Physiol. 7, 609—613 (1955).
[1173] ZEBROWSKI, v.: Zur Frage der sekretorischen Funktion des Parotis beim Menschen. Arch. ges. Physiol. 110, 105—173 (1905).
[1174] TULLAR, P. E.: Acid formation in human saliva. J. Dent. Res. 32, 688 (1953).
[1175] LASHLEY, K. S.: Reflex secretion of the human parotid gland. J. exp. Psychol. 1, 461—493 (1916).
[1176] CURBY, W. A.: Device for collection of human parotid saliva. J. Lab. clin. Med. 41, 493—496 (1953).
[1177] SCHNEYER, L. H.: Collection of separate submaxillary and sublingual salivas in man. J. Dent. Res. 33, 683—684 (1954).
[1178] HILDES, J. A., and M. H. FERGUSON: The concentration of electrolytes in normal human saliva. Canad. J. Biochem. Physiol. 33, 217—225 (1955).

(WERTHER[1064]) differs in composition from the parotid saliva of man, dog and other species. The parotid secretion of sheep and rabbits is isotonic with the plasma and the concentration of sodium does not vary with secretory rate.

2. *Submaxillary gland.* Pure submaxillary saliva has not been examined in man. HILDES and FERGUSON[1178], however, compared the composition of pure parotid secretion with that of the mixed saliva from all other glands. As demonstrated above, about 95% of this saliva originates from the submaxillary glands. They found sodium concentration to be almost equal in parotid and "submaxillary" saliva and varying in a similar fashion with the rate of secretion. It is, however, difficult to compare secretory rates, since they were not calculated per unit weight of gland. Further, the "submaxillary" saliva was contaminated by small amounts of sublingual secretion, which has a high sodium concentration. Good comparative data from animal work are lacking. WERTHER[1064] and BAXTER[1179] compared the chloride concentrations of parotid and submaxillary saliva, but since the bicarbonate concentrations of these two secretions differ greatly (Fig. 17, p. 426) no conclusions can be drawn from such studies with respect to possible differences in sodium concentration. Since there is a definite difference in the length of the striated ducts in the parotid and submaxillary glands, exact comparative studies of the variations in sodium concentration with rate of secretion (per unit weight of gland) would be of considerable interest on the background of the hypothesis advanced on p. 431 to 434. HILDES and FERGUSON[1178] found that potassium concentration is considerably lower in human "submaxillary" saliva (10—15 meq/l) than in human parotid saliva (20—25 meq/l). In both secretions the concentration of potassium showed a significant increase at the low rates of secretion. BURGEN[1077] showed that canine parotid juice has, similarly, a higher concentration of potassium than canine submaxillary saliva.

3. *Sublingual gland.* Human data are lacking. WERTHER[1064] and LANGLEY and FLETCHER[1180] found sublingual saliva of the dog to be nearly isosmotic with the plasma. LUNDBERG[1080] states the following data on the cat: sodium: 159 meq/l, chloride: 161 meq/l and potassium: 9 meq/l.

4. *Mixed saliva* from man has been examined by a great many workers, mainly clinicians using salivary electrolyte composition as an index of adrenal cortical activity (p. 457). Sodium concentration of mixed saliva varies with secretory rate between 5 and 90 meq/l, whereas average potassium concentration is about 20 meq/l and independent of secretory rate, except at the very low flows, where a definite rise is usually observed. The best figures on mixed saliva are probably those of PRADER et al.[1181].

Rate of secretion. It was first shown by HEIDENHAIN[1101] that the concentration of inorganic material in dog's submaxillary and parotid saliva increases with increasing secretory rate. WERTHER[1064] showed that the main inorganic constituent of saliva was sodium chloride, the concentration of which varied almost in proportion to the variations in total ash. These relations have been confirmed by later investigators, working on animals (LANGLEY and FLETCHER[1180];

[1179] BAXTER, H.: Variations in the inorganic constituents of mixed and parotid gland saliva activated by reflex stimulation in the dog. J. biol. Chem. **102**, 203—217 (1933).

[1180] LANGLEY, J. N., and H. M. FLETCHER: On the secretion of saliva, chiefly on the secretion of salts in it. Phil. trans. roy. Soc. London **180 B**, 109—154 (1889).

[1181] PRADER, A., E. GANTIER, R. GANTIER, D. NÄJ, J. S. SEMER, and E. J. ROTSCHILD: The Na and K concentration in mixed saliva: influence of secretion rate, stimulation, method of collection, age, sex, time of day and adrenal cortical activity. Ciba Found. Colloquia on Endocrinol. **8**, 382—395 (1955).

GREGERSEN and INGALLS[1182]; BAXTER[1179]; LANGSTROTH, MCRAE and STAVRAKY[1075]) and on man (BROWN and KLOTZ[1183, 1184]; THAYSEN, THORN and SCHWARTZ[1067]; HILDES and FERGUSON[1178]). GREGERSEN and INGALLS[1182] first showed that the concentration of potassium in dogs submaxillary saliva was independent of salivary flow.

1) Sodium. The range of variation in sodium concentration with secretory rate in from about 5 meq/l at the lowest to about 90 meq/l at the highest rates of salivary flow. With possible small variations this applies to parotid as well as to submaxillary and to mixed human saliva. Sublingual saliva has not been examined in relation to rate of secretion. The constant finding of a sodium concentration of about 150—160 meq/l in different tests[1080], however, indicates that there is hardly any variation in sodium concentration with secretory rate.

The rate of variation in sodium concentration with secretory rate is subject to divergence of opinion. In his original description HEIDENHAIN[1101] states that the concentration of inorganic material increases to a certain maximum, following which further increase in secretory rate did not cause further increase in the concentration of ash. WERTHER[1064] found the same relationship for chloride. LANGLEY and FLETCHER[1180] emphasize that no maximum is reached, but "the increment in percentage of salts become less with each successive equal increment in the rate of secretion". GREGERSEN and INGALLS[1182], like HILDES and FERGUSON[1178], found an almost linear relationship between sodium concentration and secretory rate. The results of THAYSEN, THORN and SCHWARTZ[1067] on the variations in sodium concentration of human parotid saliva are in agreement with the findings of LANGLEY and FLETCHER[1180]. With increasing secretory rate the increase in sodium concentration of parotid saliva becomes progressively smaller, but no definite maximum is reached (cf. Fig. 17, p. 426).

The reason for this divergence of opinion regarding the rate-concentration relationship for sodium is not clear. Certain aspects of experimental design must, however, be taken into consideration:

1) The exact control of secretory rate. Most workers have used reflex stimulation, during which considerable fluctuations in secretory rate are unavoidable. Unless the individual collection periods have been of very brief duration, this fact may well have masked the exact rate-concentration relationship. THAYSEN et al.[1067] used a single subcutaneous injection of metacholine, which caused a pronounced increase in secretory rate followed by a rather steady decline. From each individual subject it was thus possible to collect many samples of saliva, obtained over a wide range of secretory rates, and it could be assumed that the secretory rate had varied but little within the individual collection period. Stimulation with metacholine is artificial, but differences in sodium excretion in "reflex saliva" and "metacholine saliva" have not been observed (p. 455).

2) The effect of the dead space of the glandular ducts and of the collection system. The former has been calculated[1091] and appears to be minimal in comparison to the volumes of secretion recovered by most workers, and THAYSEN et al. claim that the dead space of their collection system was very small.

[1182] GREGERSEN, M. I., and E. N. INGALLS: The influence of rate of secretion on the concentration of potassium and sodium in dog's submaxillary saliva. Amer. J. Physiol. 98, 441—446 (1931).

[1183] BROWN, J. B., and N. J. KLOTZ: Studies of the chemistry of mixed human saliva. Attempts to correlate chemical composition of mixed human saliva with rate of secretion. J. Dent. Res. 14, 435—438 (1934).

[1184] BROWN, J. P., and N. J. KLOTZ: Studies on the chemistry of mixed human saliva. III: Sodium, potassium and calcium in salivas secreted at widely varying secretory rates. J. Dent. Res. 16, 19—22 (1937).

No doubt, the experiments ought to be repeated under conditions where fluctuations in secretory rate and the effect of the dead space are both eliminated, e.g. with a modification of the technique recently advocated by ÖBRINK in the study of gastric secretion (p. 466).

2) Potassium. When the rate of salivation is brisk the concentration of potassium is independent of a wide range of variation in secretory rate. This has been found in work on animals (GREGERSEN and INGALLS[1182]; LANGSTROTH, McRAE and STAVRAKY[1075]; WILLS[1086]) and man (THAYSEN, THORN and SCHWARTZ[1067]; HILDES and FERGUSON[1178]). At low rates of secretion the concentration of potassium in parotid and submaxillary saliva rises considerably[1067, 1075, 1178]. The reader is referred to the discussion on p. 433 and to Fig. 17, p. 426

In animals as well as in man the concentration of potassium in the saliva from all types of glands is always greater than the concentration of potassium in the plasma.

At secretory rates exceeding 0.5 ml/min the following potassium concentrations have been observed:

Human parotid saliva: 20 meq/l[1067, 1178].

Human mixed submaxillary and sublingual saliva: 12 meq/l[1178].

Cats sublingual saliva: 9 meq/l[1080].

The flow-concentration relationship for potassium in the different types of salivary secretion is illutsrated in Fig. 17, p. 426.

The first sample of saliva obtained after stimulation of secretory activity in a previously "resting" gland always contains a higher concentration of potassium than average. This phenomenon is independent of the rate at which the first sample is secreted and has also been demonstrated in the sweat (p. 441) and in the tears (p. 464). BURGEN[1077] has examined the high initial salivary potassium concentration in relation to glandular potassium balance, and was able to demonstrate that it is due to a loss of potassium ions from the gland cells when secretory activity is stimulated. The "potassium transient" is discussed in further detail on p. 427 and 434.

Gland temperature. Variations in the composition of saliva with temperature have been studied by BURGEN[1077]. BURGEN found that the duration of the "potassium transient" was lengthened by a decrease in gland temperature and shortened by an increase in temperature. During steady state secretion a decrease in temperature caused a drop in secretory rate and a definite increase in potassium concentration of the saliva. An increase in temperature did not appreciably affect secretory rate, but potassium concentration of the saliva increased significantly. The secretion of sodium in relation to variations in gland temperature has not been studied. The reader is referred to the sections on the effect of temperature on other glandular secretions, notably the sweat (p. 442).

Duration of secretion. The concentration of protein-material in the saliva decreases on prolonged stimulation (HEIDENHAIN[1101]) and may eventually drop to zero, indicating that glandular stores of enzymes and other protein-material have become exhausted (ANREP[1102]). In contradistinction HEIDENHAIN found that the concentration of inorganic material remained practically constant on prolonged stimulation, showing no other variations than such a might be explained on the basis of fluctuations in secretory rate. Thus, apart from the initial "potassium transient", there is no indication that the duration of secretory activity has any influence on the secretion of electrolytes by the salivary glands. As in the case of the sweat glands (cf. p. 442) the problem does, however, require further experimental investigation with modern techniques before a definite statement can be made.

Type of stimulation. The significance of the double (parasympathetic and sympathetic) innervation of the salivary glands is not clearly understood. The reader is referred to the discussion in BABKIN's monograph[1065] and to the recent studies by EMMELIN[1185].

Conventional methods of stimulation in experimental work are:

Reflex stimulation: chewing of paraffin or application of dilute acids etc. to the tongue.

Electrical stimulation of the parasympathetic and sympathetic nerve supply (normally only possible in animals).

Chemical stimulation: injection of parasympathomimetic or sympathomimetic agents.

No systematic investigation has been carried out on the influence of different types of stimulation on alkali metal excretion. WILLS[1086] claims that canine submaxillary saliva, obtained in response to pilocarpine, has a higher concentration of sodium than saliva obtained in response to chorda stimulation, whereas potassium concentration is about equal with the two methods of stimulation. PRADER et al.[1181] have, however, shown that sodium concentration of human mixed saliva is similar after reflex and after pilocarpine stimulation, when differences in secretory rate are corrected for. Likewise, there is apparently no difference in sodium and potassium concentration of human parotid saliva obtained by reflex stimulation[1178] and by stimulation with mecholyl[1067]. As opposed to HEIDENHAIN[1101] both LANGLEY and FLETCHER[1180] and KESZTYUS and MARTIN[1186] claim that "sympathetic saliva" of animals contains more sodium and chloride than does "parasympathetic saliva" (corrected for differences in secretory rate).

Glandular blood flow. The arterial blood flow of the salivary glands in different animals has been estimatad by a number of investigators. A resting value of about $0.2-0.3$ ml/g gland/min is probably a fair average. When the glands are stimulated to secrete, blood flow may increase up to $2-4$ ml/g gland per min[1077], probably in part due to the release of vasodilator substance from the gladular tissue (see i. a. HILTON and LEWIS[1187]). Blood flow is, thus, always in considerable excess of the rate of salivary secretion. WILLS[1086] states a ratio of superbasal blood flow to salivary flow of about 12; TERROUX et al.[1107] found a ratio of $8-10$.

There is general agreement, that salivary flow drops, but does not cease altogether, when the arterial blood supply is cut off, a fact that was first demonsstrated by LUDWIG[1076]. When arterial occlusion is of long duration, secretion eventually is completely arrested. When glandular blood flow was completely or partially occluded LANGLEY and FLETCHER[1180] found an increase in the concentration of chloride in the saliva, despite the decrease in secretory rate. These findings are in agreement with the alterations in secretory rate and chloride concentration of sweat following arterial occlusion (p. 443) and are discussed in further detail on p. 437.

Plasma concentration of Na and K. LUDWIG[1076] first examined the composition of the saliva in relation to alterations of the salt concentration of the plasma. The results are, however, inconclusive. LANGLEY and FLETCHER[1180]

[1185] EMMELIN, N.: On the innervation of the submaxillary gland cells in cats. Acta physiol. scand. **34**, 11—21 (1955).

[1186] KESZTYUS, L., and J. MARTIN: Über den Einfluß von Chorda- und Sympaticus-Reizung auf die Zusammensetzung des Submaxillar-Speichels. Pflügers. Arch. ges. Physiol. **239**, 408. 418 (1938).

[1187] HILTON, S. M., and G. P. LEWIS: The mechanism of the functional hyperaemia in the submandibular salivary gland. J. Physiol. **129**, 253—271 (1955).

injected 0.2% NaCl intravenously in dogs (until hemoglobinuria occurred) and found a drop in the salt concentration of the saliva, despite increase in secretory rate. Conversely, injection of 20% NaCl was followed by an increase in salivary salt concentration, despite temporary decrease in the flow of saliva. DeBeer and Wilson[1188] state that injection of NaCl and KCl does not materially alter the concentration of the two elements in the saliva. There was, however, no good control of secretory rate, the total quantities of sodium and of potassium injected were smaller than those used by Langley and Fletcher and the resulting alterations in plasma concentrations were not stated. Recently Langley, Gunthorpe and Beall[1189] have clearly demonstrated that increases in plasma Na concentration (following injection of hypertonic NaCl) cause the sodium concentration of parotid saliva to increase at the same time as there is a marked decrease in the volume rate of salivary flow. Burgen[1077] found that both the initial potassium transient (p. 434) and the steady level potassium secretion are increased by a rise in plasma potassium concentration. The increase in the potassium transient is, however, smaller than that of the steady state secretion. In the steady state there is a linear correlation between saliva K and plasma K concentrations, although the slope varies between different animals and between different salivary glands in the same animal. The fact that the S/P ratio for K in the steady state secretion is independent of wide variations in plasma K concentration has been confirmed by Langley, Gunthorpe and Beall[1189], who also showed that the volume rate of parotid secretory flow increases with increasing plasma K concentration.

These findings on the relationship between saliva and plasma concentrations of Na and K are in agreement with the work of Amatruda and Welt [1131] on the sweat gland. The problem is discussed in further detail on page 437.

Salt depletion. McCance[1136] first demonstrated that salt depletion causes a drop in sodium and a rise in potassium concentration of unstimulated human

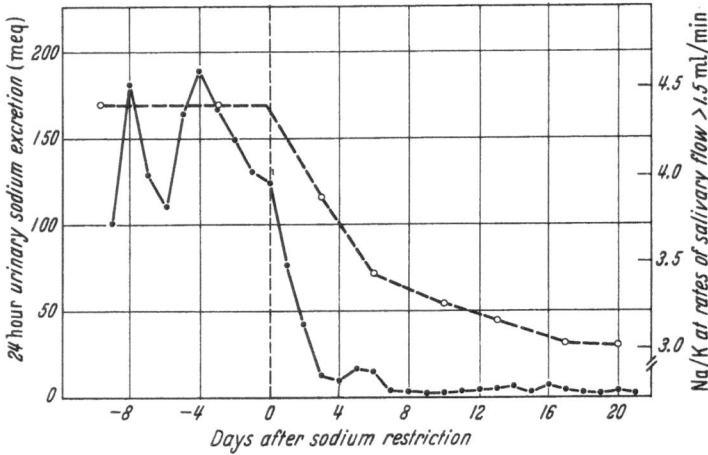

Fig. 20. *Salivary Na/K ratio and urinary Na excretion following sodium restriction* (redrawn from the data of Thorn, Schwartz and Thaysen[1190]). ●——● = Urinary Na excretion (meq/24 hrs). ○---○ = Na/K of saliva at rates of flow exceeding 1.5 ml/min

[1188] DeBeer, E. J., and D. W. Wilson: The inorganic composition of the parotid saliva of the dog and its relation to the composition of the serum. J. biol. Chem. **95**, 671—685 (1932).

[1189] Langley, L. L., C. H. Gunthorpe and W. A. Beall: Parotid clearance of sodium and potassium. Amer. J. Physiol. **195**, 693—696 (1958).

mixed saliva. The response of the salivary glands is, however, both delayed and incomplete as compared to that of the kidneys. In this respect there is a close similarity between the salivary glands and the sweat glands (p. 444). Fig. 20 redrawn from the data of THORN, SCHWARTZ and THAYSEN[1190], shows the adaptation of the human parotid gland and kidney to a low sodium intake.

The adaptation of the kidney was complete within 2 days, and urinary sodium concentration dropped to near zero. The adaptation of the parotid gland was first complete after 16 days, and the mean reduction of salivary sodium concentration (at secretory rates exceeding 50 mg/g gland/min) was from 82 ($\pm$6) to 60 ($\pm$8) meq/l only (cf. Fig. 21). Undoubtedly, the adaptation of both the parotid gland and the kidney might have proceeded more rapidly if the effect of the low sodium intake had been enhanced by increased sodium loss, but this does not deduce from the basic observation regarding the difference in response between the two organs.

It is well known that sodium depletion is followed by a decrease in serum sodium concentration, a contraction of plasma volume and total extracellular volume, a decreased mean arterial pressure and an increase in the adrenal secretion of salt conserving steroids, primarily aldosterone. In sodium depleted sheep DENTON[1191, 1192] examined the relative significance of these different factors in the adaptation process of the parotid gland. He showed that local changes in sodium concentration and volume of the blood perfusing the gland only played a minor role, whereas the adaptation process was completely obliterated in

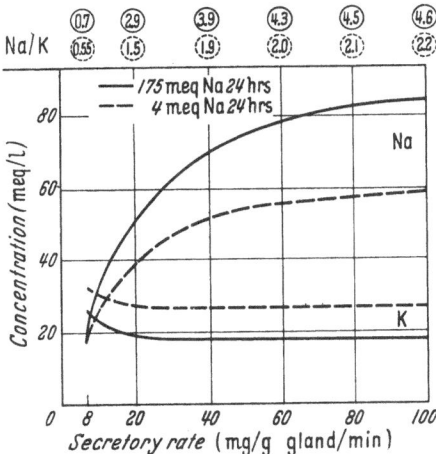

Fig. 21. *The effect of salt depletion on the sodium and potassiums concentrations of human parotid saliva.* (Redrawn from the data of THORN et al.[1190]). — — = high sodium intake, ——— = low sodium intake

adrenalectomized animals (GODING and DENTON[1193]). This conforms with the finding, that injection of aldosterone causes a significant depression of the Na/K ratio of human saliva and points to the adrenal gland as the main factor in the development of glandular adaptation to sodium depletion.

Adrenal cortical steroids. FRAWLEY and FORSHAM[1194], GRAD[1195], DREIZEN et al.[1196] and several others have shown that the administration of desoxycorti-

[1190] THORN, N. A., I. L. SCHWARTZ, and J. H. THAYSEN: Effect of sodium restriction on secretion of sodium and potassium in human parotid saliva. J. appl. Physiol. 9, 477—480 (1956).

[1191] DENTON, D. A.: The study of sheep with permanent unilateral parotid fistula. Quart. J. exp. Physiol. 42, 72—95 (1957).

[1192] DENTON, D. A.: The effect of variations in the blood supply on the secretion rate and composition of parotid saliva in Na depleted sheep. J. Physiol. 135, 227—244 (1957).

[1193] GODING, J. R., and D. A. DENTON: Adrenal cortex and the parotid secretion of sodium depleted sheep. Science 123, 986—987 (1956).

[1194] FRAWLEY, T. F., and P. H. FORSHAM: The salivary Na/K ratio and adrenal salt regulating factors: prolonged salt retention with desoxycorticosterone methylacetate. J. clin. Endocr. 11, 772—773 (1951).

[1195] GRAD, B.: The influence of ACTH on the sodium and potassium concentration of human mixed saliva. J. clin. Endocr. 12, 708—718 (1952).

[1196] DREIZEN, S., W. NIEDERMEIER, A. I. REED, and T. D. SPIES: The effect of ACTH and cortisone on sodium and potassium levels in human saliva. J. Dent. Res. 31, 271—280 (1952).

costerone, adrenocorticotropin or cortison is followed by a drop in sodium and an increase in potassium concentration of human mixed saliva. The effect is illustrated in Fig. 21, which shows the full adaptive response of the human parotid gland to a low sodium intake. This complete adaptive response was first attained 16 days following sodium restriction, but MACH et al.[1197] have shown that the salivary glands may react within 8 hr to an injection of aldosterone. The reader is referred to the results of similar studies on the sweat glands, cited on p. 445.

For a limited period of time the "saliva test" attained a certain clinical application in the diagnosis of conditions associated with adreno-cortical dysfunction[1198, 1199, 1200]. Most of the early work operated with the "Na/K-ratio" of "unstimulated" or "stimulated" mixed saliva. The range of variation in the Na/K-ratio of normals was, however, very large[1194] which set a definite limitation to the interpretation of the test. Among others, PRADER et al.[1181] have pointed out that this large variation in the normal Na/K-ratio is due to deficient standardization of experimental conditions with respect to secretory rate. It is quite obvious from a glance at Fig. 21, that the "non-endocrine" variation in Na/K with secretory rate is numerically larger than the "endocrine" variation, caused by complete adaptation to a low sodium intake.

Data with satisfactory standardization of secretory rate are scarce — probably because the practical importance of the saliva test has decreased in later years in parallel to the improvement of methods for determination of steroid hormones in plasma and urine.

The effect of various drugs. WHITE et al.[1199] found no effect of mercurial diuretics on the concentration of sodium and chloride in human mixed saliva. This result was to be expected since the mercurials are not concentrated in the glandular tubules. A dose sufficiently large to have an effect on glandular electrolyte secretion must therefore be sizeable and would in all probability cause severe and generalized toxic effects.

NIEDERMEIER et al.[1201] have shown that the administration of "diamox" (2-acetylamino-1,3,4-thiodiazole-5-sulfonamide) caused a decrease in sodium and bicarbonate concentration, but no change in potassium concentration of human mixed saliva.

Administration of bicarbonate and ammonium chloride has only a questionable effect on salivary bicarbonate concentration (SAND[1082]; YOSHIMURA et al.[1202]).

EMMELIN et al.[1203] injected various parasympathomimetic substances directly into the submaxillary duct of cats and dogs, and found the typical effects of these substances with minute doses that had no systemic action whatsoever. Possibly this route of application may prove useful in further studies of drug action on salivary secretion.

[1197] MACH, R. S., J. FABRE, A. DUCKERT, R. BARTH, and P. DU COMMUN: Action clinique et métabolique de l'Aldosterone. Schweiz. med. Wschr. 84, 407—415 (1954).
[1198] EISENMENGER, W. J., S. H. BLONDHEIM, A. M. BONGIOVANNI, and H. G. KUNKEL: Electrolyte studies on patients with cirrhosis of the liver. J. clin. Invest. 29, 1491—1499 (1950).
[1199] WHITE, A. G., P. S. ENTMACHER, G. RUBIN, and LOUIS LEITER: Physiological and pharmacological regulation of human salivary electrolyte concentrations. J. clin. Invest. 34, 246—255 (1955).
[1200] WHITE, H. G., H. GORDON, and L. LEITER: Studies in edema II: The effect of congestive heart failure on saliva electrolyte concentrations. J. clin. Invest. 29, 1445—1447 (1950).
[1201] NIEDERMEIER, W., R. E. STONE, S. DREIZEN, and T. D. SPIES: Effect of Diamox. Proc. Soc. exp. Biol. (N. Y.) 88, 273—275 (1955).
[1202] YOSHIMURA, J., W. TAKAOTIA, and T. MORI: Essential factors governing the acid-base balance of saliva. Jap. J. Physiol. 4, 154—168 (1954).
[1203] EMMELIN, N., A. MUREN, and R. STRÖMBLAD: Secretory and vascular effects of various drugs injected into the submaxillary duct. Acta physiol. scand. 32, 325—338 (1954).

Individual variations. In all comparative work on salivary electrolyte secretion it is of paramount importance that the experimental conditions are standarized with respect to secretory rate. It is apparent from the preceeding discussion that ideal requirements are not fulfilled by examination of "unstimulated saliva", nor by the use of the Na/K-ratio without reference to secretory rate. The results of studies, in which these parameters have been used as the basis for comparison, must therefore be taken with "a grain of salt". With respect to the developing organism, it appears likely that the standard for comparison should include some correction for the factor of growth (e.g. secretory rate per gram gland or per kilogram of body weight).

Time of day. Several investigators claim that there are diurnal variations in the Na/K-ratio, probably occurring in parallel to the well known fluctuations in adrenal cortical activity (GRAD[1204], MATHIS[1205]). With exacting control of secretory rate PRADER et al. found that salivary sodium concentration is always higher in the morning than during the rest of the day.

Age. MATHIS[1205] and GRAD[1204] found that the Na/K-ratio decreases until the age of 20—40 years, following which there is a gradual increase with the highest values reached during senescence. PRADER et al.[1181] found that the newborn baby has a very high sodium concentration in the saliva. From the age of about 3 months salivary sodium concentration (corrected for rate of secretion) is about equal to that of adults.

The age variations in salivary sodium and potassium secretion may be due to either of two mechanisms: 1) They may be caused by the well known variations in adrenal production of salt conserving hormone throughout the life span (cf. p. 301), and/or 2) they may be due to variations in the sodium reabsorbing capacity of the salivary ducts quite independently of adrenal activity. Until the reactivity of the glands to a standard dose of aldosterone has been tested at various ages, the decision as to which factor is the more important must be kept *sub judice*.

Sex. With good control of secretory rate, PRADER et al.[1181] found no consistent differences between the two sexes.

Individual differences. With good control of secretory rate both HILDES and FERGUSON[1178] and PRADER et al.[1181] demonstrated considerable variations in sodium concentration between individuals, whereas the variations in the same individual from day to day were only of borderline significance. Simultaneous collection of saliva from the two parotid glands in the same individual showed very uniform results[1178].

The secretion of Li, Cs and Rb. GOOD[1206] first showed that Li is excreted in the salivary secretion of cats. After administration of 1 gram of Lithium chloride he found 0.021 g in the total saliva produced from the time of administration and until the cat died from Li-intoxication. BERGER[1207] showed that Li makes its appearance in the urine 10—15 min and in the saliva 20—25 min following oral administration. BURGEN[1208] has made a careful study of salivary

[1204] GRAD, B.: Diurnal and age changes in the sodium and potassium concentration of human mixed saliva. J. Geront. 6 (suppl.3), 93 (1951).

[1205] MATHIS, H.: Beiträge zur Chemie des Speichels III: Über den Gehalt des gemischten Mundspeichels an den Kationen: Kalium, Kalzium und Natrium sowie an den Anionen: Chlor und Phosphor. Z. Stomat. 32, 1188—1209 (1934).

[1206] GOOD, C. A.: An experimental study of lithium. Amer. J. med. Sci. 125, 273—284 (1903).

[1207] BERGER, J.: Über die Ausscheidung des Lithiums im Harn und die Spaltung des Lithiumjodids im Organismus. Naunyn-Schmiedebergs Arch. exp. Path. Pharmak. 55, 1—15 (1906).

[1208] BURGEN, A. S. V.: The secretion of lithium in saliva. Canad. J. Biochem. Physiol. 36, 409—411 (1958).

Li excretion in the dog following constant intravenous infusion of LiCl. He found the S/P (secretion/plasma) concentration ratio for Li to vary between 2.5 at low rates of secretion and 1.0 at high secretory rates. The S/P ratio remained unaffected by variations in the concentration of Li in the plasma. Gland analyses showed that Li was not concentrated intracellularly (ratio Li in gland water to Li in plasma water was about 1), and there was no Li transient at the onset of secretion (compare intracellular K conc and K transient on page 434). The secretion of Cs and Rb by the salivary glands has apparently not been investigated.

d) The pancreatic gland

Due to the anatomical conditions pure pancreatic secretion of man can only be collected during duodenal surgery or in patients with pancreatic fistula[1209, 1210]. Duodenal contents consisting mainly of pancreatic juice, contaminated with minor quantities of bile and duodenal secretion, may however be obtained by the "secretin test", which was originally designed by ÅGREN and LAGERLÖF[1211] and LAGERLÖF[1212] and which has attained practical clinical application in the diagnosis of pancreatic dysfunction[1213, 1214, 1215, 1216].

On account of the technical difficulties involved in obtaining pure pancreatic secretion of man, most of our knowledge regarding the physiology of the pancreatic gland is derived from work on animals with acute or permanent pancreatic fistula. The first successful permanent pancreatic fistula, which was devised by PAVLOV, and its many later modifications are discussed in detail in the monograph by THOMAS[1217]. The permanent fistula have the advantage that pancreatic juice, uncontaminated by other secretions, may be obtained from unanesthetized animals, which have recovered completely from the stress of operation.

In the ensuing sections the excretion of sodium and of potassium with the pancreatic juice is considered in relation to:

1. Rate of secretion.
2. Duration of secretion.
3. Type of stimulus.
4. Plasma concentration of the alkali metals.
5. Activity of certain drugs.
6. Individual differences.

[1209] SCHUMM, O.: Über menschliches Pankreassekret. Z. physiol. Chem. 36, 292—332 (1902).

[1210] WATMAN, R. N.: Inhibition of human pancreatic secretion by carbonic anhydrase inhibitor. Surgery 39, 337—339 (1956).

[1211] ÅGREN, G., and H. LAGERLÖF: The pancreatic secretion in man after intravenous administration of secretin. Acta med. scand. 90, 1—29 (1936).

[1212] LAGERLÖF, H. O.: Pancreatic Function and Pancreatic Disease. Acta med. scand. suppl. 128 (1942).

[1213] DIAMOND, J. S., and S. A. SIEGEL: The secretin test in the diagnosis of pancreatic diseases with a report on 130 tests. Amer. J. Digest. Dis. Nutr. 7, 435—442 (1940).

[1214] DREILING, D. A., and F. HOLLANDER: Studies in pancreatic function I: Preliminary series of studies with the secretin test. Gastroenterology 11, 714—729 (1948).

[1215] DREILING, D. A., and F. HOLLANDER: Studies in pancreatic function II: A statistical study of pancreatic secretion following secretin in patients with and without pancreatic disease. Gastroenterology 15, 620—627 (1950).

[1216] DREILING, D. A.: The technique of the secretin test: Normal ranges. J. Mt. Sinai Hosp. 21, 363—372 (1955).

[1217] THOMAS, J. E.: The External Secretion of the Pancreas. Springfield, Ill.: Charles C. Thomas 1950.

Rate of secretion. The pancreatic juice is isosmotic with the plasma and remains so independently of the rate at which it is secreted[1218], [1219], [1220], [1221], [1222], [1212], [1103], [1072]

The concentration of *sodium* in secretion water is approximately equal to the concentration of sodium in plasma water[1221], [1072] and independent of secretory rate[1221], [1222], [1103], [1072]. The concentration of *potassium* is, likewise, about equal in secretion and plasma water and independent of secretory rate[1209], [1221], [1103], [1072]. The main anions of pancreatic juice are bicarbonate and chloride. At low secretory rates bicarbonate concentration is equal to (or slightly smaller than) plasma bicarbonate concentration. With increasing secretory rate bicarbonate concentration rises to a maximum, following which the concentration remains independent of further increases in the rate of secretion[1223], [1224], [1212], [1225], [1226], [1072]. The maximum bicarbonate concentration is subject to individual variation within an approximate range from 90 to 140 meq/l. The concentration of chloride varies inversely with that of bicarbonate (cf. Fig. 17). The sum of the concentrations of bicarbonate and chloride constitutes about 90—95% of the sum of the concentrations of sodium and potassium at all rates of secretion[1072].

Duration of secretion. Whereas the concentration of protein material in pancreatic juice decreases on prolonged secretory activity of the gland, it appears that the concentrations of sodium and potassium remain unaffected by the duration of the secretion (KOMAROW, LANGSTROTH and MCRAE[1103]).

Type of stimulation. The relative importance of the different humoral and nervous mechanisms involved in the stimulation of pancreatic secretion have hardly been clarified in detail. For a discussion the reader is referred to the monographs by BABKIN[1065] and THOMAS[1217].

In experimental work secretory activity is usually stimulated in one of the following manners:

1) Application of dilute acids, soap, meat extracts etc. to the duodenal mucosa.

2) Electrical stimulation of the parasympathetic and sympathetic nerves.

3) Injection of secretin (BAYLISS and STARLING[1227]), pancreozymin (HARPER and RAPER[1228]) and "mecholyl" (or other parasympathomimetic agents).

The concentration of sodium and of potassium in the pancreatic juice are apparently independent of the type of stimulus used and equal to the concen-

[1218] BABKIN, B. P., and W. W. SAWITSCH: Zur Frage über den Gehalt an festen Bestandteilen in dem auf verschiedene Sekretionserreger erhaltenen pankreatischen Saft. Z. physiol. Chem. **56**, 321—342 (1908).

[1219] WOHLGEMUTH, J.: Untersuchung über den Pankreassaft des Menschen. Biochem. Z. **39**, 302—323 (1912).

[1220] GAMBLE, J. L., and M. A. MCIVER: Acid-base composition of pancreatic juice and bile. J. exp. Med. **48**, 849—857 (1928).

[1221] BALL, E. G.: The composition of pancreatic juice and blood serum as influenced by the injection of inorganic salts. J. biol. Chem. **86**, 449—462 (1930).

[1222] BALL, E. G.: The composition of pancreatic juice and blood serum as influenced by the injection of acid and base. J. biol. Chem. **86**, 433—448 (1930).

[1223] SCHMIDT, C.: Über das Pankreassekret. Ann. Chem. u. Pharm. **92**, 33—41 (1854).

[1224] WOINAR, A. O.: Zur Frage nach der Rolle des Sekretins bei der Regulierung der Blutalkalireserven. Pflügers Arch. ges. Physiol. **221**, 144—149 (1928).

[1225] HART, W. M., and J. E. THOMAS: Bicarbonate and chloride of pancreatic juice secreted in response to various stimuli. Gastroenterology **4**: 409—420 (1945).

[1226] CONLY, S. S., J. O. CRIDER, and J. E. THOMAS: Relation of bicarbonate concentration of pancreatic juice to rate of secretion. Amer. J. Physiol. **182**, 97—99 (1955).

[1227] BAYLISS, W. M., and E. H. STARLING: The mechanism of pancreatic secretion. J. Physiol. **28**, 325—353 (1902).

[1228] HARPER, A. A., and H. S. RAPER: Pancreozymin, a stimulant of the secretion of pancreatic enzymes in extracts of the small intestine. J. Physiol. **102**, 115—125 (1943).

trations of the same two ions in plasma water. The volume of secretion formed and the concentrations of enzyme, chloride and bicarbonate in the pancreatic juice are, however, dependent upon the manner in which pancreatic secretion is stimulated.

Application of peptone to the duodenal mucosa (THOMAS and CRIDER[1229]), injection of mecholyl (COMFORT and OSTERBERG[1230], LAGERLÖF[1212] and others) and stimulation of the vagal nerve (MELLANBY[1231]) all produce a secretion of relatively small volume with a high concentration of enzyme and of chloride, but a low concentration of bicarbonate. Application of dilute acids to the duodenal mucosa (THOMAS and CRIDER[1229]) and injection of secretin (BAYLISS and STARLING[1227]; MELLANBY[1231]; LAGERLÖF[1212]; DREILING[1216] and others) produce a profuse watery secretion, low in enzyme and chloride, but high in bicarbonate. When the vagal nerve is stimulated during secretin administration it causes the concentration of enzyme in the juice to increase (MELLANBY[1231]).

Administration of atropine (MELLANBY[1231]; THOMAS and CRIDER[1232]) or section of the vagi (MELLANBY[1231]) diminishes enzyme secretion in response to any kind of stimulus, but does not affect the volume of juice produced, nor its bicarbonate concentration. Carbonic anhydrase inhibitors reduce the volume and the bicarbonate concentration of pancreatic juice obtained in response to secretin (p. 463).

These findings indicate, that two kinds of isotonic secretions, containing sodium and potassium in concentrations equal to those of plasma water, are formed within the pancreas:

1) A product secreted in comparatively low volume, containing chloride as the chief (or only) anion and with a high concentration of enzymes. The formation of this product is stimulated reflexly via the vagal nerve and by the injection of parasympathomimetic substances but not by secretin administration.

2) A product secreted in comparatively large volumes, containing bicarbonate as the chief anion, but with little or no enzyme activity. The formation of this product is stimulated reflexly via the vagal nerve, by the injection of parasympathomimetic substances and, preeminently, by secretin administration.

As is well known, the secretion of the gastric glands similarly consists of two components and there is a certain parallel between the response of the pancreatic gland to vagal versus secretin stimulation and the response of the gastric glands to vagal versus histamine stimulation (cf. p. 471). In the case of the gastric glands it is now generally accepted, that the neutral (enzyme rich) component is elaborated by the "non-parietal" cells, whereas the hydrochloric acid is elaborated by the parietal cells. Whether the two products of the pancreatic gland are also formed in different types of cells remains undetermined. Certain facts, especially the experiments with alloxan and ethionine referred below however, indicate that the enzyme-rich, chloride containing secretion is elaborated in the acini, whereas the enzyme-poor, bicarbonate containing secretion is elaborated in the cuboidal epithelium of the intercalary ducts.

Plasma concentration of the alkali metals. BALL[1221] and GILMAN and COWGILL[1233] first demonstrated that the concentration of sodium plus potassium in secretion

[1229] THOMAS, J. E., and J. O. CRIDER: Specific gravity and total nitrogen of pancreatic juice secreted in response to various stimuli. Amer. J. Physiol. 140, 574—577 (1944).

[1230] COMFORT, M. W., and A. E. OSTERBERG: Pancreatic secretion in man after stimulation with secretin and mecholyl. Arch. intern. Med. 66, 688—706 (1940).

[1231] MELLANBY, J.: The mechanism of pancreatic digestion. The function of secretin. J. Physiol. 60, 85—91 (1925).

[1232] THOMAS, J. E., and J. O. CRIDER: The secretion of pancreatic juice in the presence of atropine or hyoscyamine in chronic fistula dogs. J. Pharmacol. 87, 81—89 (1946).

[1233] GILMAN, A., and G. R. COWGILL: Osmotic relations between blood and body fluids IV: Pancreatic juice, bile and lymph. Amer. J. Physiol. 104, 476—479 (1933).

water of dog's pancreatic juice is equal to the concentration of sodium plus potassium in plasma water. Injections of hypertonic sodium chloride or potassium chloride solutions increased the concentrations of sodium or potassium in plasma water and secretion water to exactly the same degree. MONTGOMMERY, SHELINE and CHAIKOFF[1234] showed that labelled sodium made its appearance in dogs pancreatic juice as early as the first 3 min after the injection of the radioactive salt. Maximum concentration was found after 15 min. With the exception of the early periods the concentration of labelled sodium in the juice closely followed that of the serum.

The effect of certain drugs. The possible role of carbonic anhydrase in the secretion of bicarbonate by the pancreatic gland has been discussed on p. 429. The carbonic anhydrase inhibitor "diamox" (2-acetylamino- 1, 3, 4 thiodiazole-5-sulfonamide) causes a decrease in the bicarbonate concentration and a decrease in the volume of pancreatic juice produced by animals (BIRNBAUM and HOLLANDER[1235], [1236]) and by man (DREILING and JANOWITZ[1237], WATMAN[1210]).

It is of considerable theoretical interest that ethionine, which produces a lesion of the pancreatic acini, causes the enzyme concentration of pancreatic juice to decrease, but does not affect the volume of juice secreted, nor its bicarbonate concentration (KALSER and GROSSMAN[1238]). Conversely, alloxan gives rise to histological changes in the cuboidal epithelium and increases the treshold dose for secretin without affecting enzyme secretion (GROSSMAN and IVY[1239]).

Individual variations. Individual variations in sodium and potassium concentrations of the pancreatic juice are small. There are, however, individual differences in the total volume[1240] of juice produced and in its maximal bicarbonate concentration in response to a standard stimulus (for normal ranges in humans see ÅGREN and LAGERLÖF[1211], DIAMOND and SIEGEL[1213], LAGERLÖF[1212] and DREILING and HOLLANDER[1215]).

There are no data available on the effect of variations in blood flow, nor on the effect of adrenal steroids on pancreatic secretion of sodium and potassium. The secretion of Li, Cs and Rb has not been examined.

e) The lacrymal gland

The total osmolarity and the salt concentration of tears was disputed among early investigators, some claiming that the lacrymal fluid was hypotonic[1241], others

[1234] MONTGOMMERY, M. L., G. E. SHELINE, and I. L. CHAIKOFF: Elimination of sodium in pancreatic juice as measured by radioactive sodium. Amer. J. Physiol. 131, 578—583 (1941).

[1235] BIRNBAUM, D., and F. HOLLANDER: Inhibition of pancreatic secretion by the carbonic anhydrase inhibitor 2-acetyl-amino-1,3,4-thiodiazole-5-sulfonamide. Proc. Soc. exp. Biol. (N. Y.) 81, 23—25 (1952).

[1236] BIRNBAUM, D., and F. HOLLANDER: Inhibition of pancreatic secretion by the carbonic anhydrase inhibitor 2-acetyl-amino-1,3,4-thiodiazole-5-sulfonamide. Amer. J. Physiol. 174, 191—195 (1953).

[1237] DREILING, D. A., H. JANOWITZ, and M. HALPERN: The effect of diamox a carbonic anhydrase inhibitor on human pancreatic secretion, implications on the basic mechanism of pancreatic secretion. Gastroenterology 29, 262—279 (1955).

[1238] KALSER, M. H., and M. I. GROSSMAN: Pancreatic secretion in dogs with ethionine induced pancreatitis. Gastroenterology 26, 189—197 (1954).

[1239] GROSSMAN, M. I., and A. C. IVY: Effect of Alloxan upon external secretion of the pancreas. Proc. Soc. exp. Biol. (N. Y.) 63, 62—63 (1946).

[1240] HAMMARSTEN, E., G. ÅGREN, and H. LAGERLÖF: The relation between secretin dose and pancreatic effect in man. Acta med. scand. 92, 256—266 (1937).

[1241] MAGAARD, H.: Über das Sekret und die Sekretion der menschlichen Tränendrüse. Virchows Arch. path. Anat. 89, 258—271 (1882).

that it was hypertonic[1242, 1243, 1244] as compared to the plasma. KROGH et al.[1245] have explained the historical background for the erroneous, but, until recently, widespread statement in pharmacological textbooks, that tears are hypertonic, and that solutions for instillation in the conjunctival sack should be isosmotic with a 1.3 % solution of sodium chloride. In 1930 RIDLEY[1246] clearly demonstrated that tear fluid is isosmotic with the plasma, and that the concentrations of sodium and of chloride are about equal in the two biological fluids. This finding has been confirmed by several later workers[1245, 1247, 1248, 1068].

Rate of secretion. THAYSEN and THORN[1068] showed that the concentrations of sodium, chloride and potassium in the human tear fluid are independent of a 12-fold range of variation in the rate of lacrymation. They found the following concentrations: sodium 146 ($\pm$ 10) meq/l, chloride 128 ($\pm$ 5) meq/l, and potassium 15 ($\pm$ 3) meq/l. (cf, Fig, 17, p. 426).

Duration of secretion. GIARDINI and ROBERTS[1248] claim that the chloride concentration of tears tends to decrease with prolonged lacrymation from about 135 to about 110 meq/l. Other workers have not been able to confirm this finding[1068]. The first sample of tears collected after vigorous stimulation of secretory activity invariably has a higher potassium concentration than the following. This phenomenon occurs independently of the volume of the first sample. THAYSEN and THORN[1068] found the first samples to contain potassium in a concentration of 24 ($\pm$ 2) meq/l, the following samples had an average potassium concentration of 15 ($\pm$ 3.6) meq/l. A similar "potassium transient" has also been observed in the case of sweat (p. 441), parotid saliva and submaxillary saliva (p. 454) and is discussed in further detail on p. 427 and 434.

Plasma concentration. The following tear/plasma concentration ratios have been stated: sodium 1.0 ($\pm$ 0.07), chloride 1.2 ($\pm$ 0.05) and potassium 3.4 ($\pm$ 0.9)[1068] The composition of tears in relation to variations in the concentration of alkali metals in the plasma has not been examined.

The effect of gland temperature and of adreno-cortical steroids on the composition of the lacrymal secretion has not been examined. Individual variations are probably small, but have not been studied in detail.

The secretion of lithium, cesium and rubidium remains unknown.

B. The glands of the gastrointestinal tract.

a) The oesophageal glands

For details regarding structure and innervation of the oesophageal glands the reader is referred to the monograph by BABKIN[1065]. Uncontaminated oesophageal secretion of two dogs was examined by VINEBERG and KOMAROV[1249], who found

[1242] ARLT, F.: Über den Tränenschlauch. Arch. Ophthal. 1·2 135—160 (1855)

[1243] MASSART, J.: Sensibilité et adaptation des organismes à la concentration des solutions salines. Arch. Biol. (Liège) 9, 515—570 (1889).

[1244] WEISS, O.: Der intraokuläre Flüssigkeitswechsel. Z. Augenheilk. 25, 1—14 (1911).

[1245] KROGH, A., C. G. LUND, and K. PEDERSEN-BJERGAARD: The osmotic concentration of human lacrymal fluid. Acta physiol. scand. 10, 88—90 (1945).

[1246] RIDLEY, F.: The intraocular pressure and the drainage of the aqueous humour. Brit. J. exp. Path. 11, 217—240 (1930).

[1247] SMOLENS, J., J. H. LEOPOLD, and J. PARKER: Studies in human tears. Amer. J. Ophthal. 3 Ser. 32·1, 153—160 (1949).

[1248] GIARDINI, A., and J. R. E. ROBERTS: Concentration of glucose and total chloride in tears. Brit. J. Ophthal. 34, 737—743 (1950).

[1249] VINEBERG, A. M., and S. A. KOMAROV: The influence of the vagus nerve on oesophageal secretion. Amer. J. Physiol. 104, 73—80 (1933).

secretory rate from the entire viscus to vary between 1 and 8 ml/hr on vagal stimulation. From their detailed analysis and the composition of oesophageal mucus the following figures shall be quoted:

$$p_H: \quad 7.5 - \quad 8.3$$
$$Cl: 144 \quad -177 \text{ meq/l}$$
$$K: \quad 13 \quad - \quad 15 \text{ meq/l}$$
$$Ca: \quad 3.1 - \quad 3.5 \text{ meq/l.}$$

Apparently the electrolyte composition of oesophageal mucus is thus very similar to that of mucus secreted in other parts of the gastrointestinal tract (p. 471 and 485).

b) The gastric mucosa

During digestive work the stomach contains gastric juice, which is contaminated by swallowed saliva, oesophageal mucus, regurgitated duodenal contents and food debris, and this mixture is gradually being evacuated via the pylorus.

The quantitative recovery of pure gastric juice is therefore beset with considerable technical difficulties in work on the intact stomach of man and animals, and results obtained in most clinical studies should be taken with a "grain of salt".

The introduction of injectable stimulants of gastric secretion (histamine, metacholine, insulin etc.) represented a great advance, since the use of "test meals" could be avoided, and comparatively pure gastric juice obtained if swallowing of saliva was prevented and the stomach and the duodenum aspirated separately via indwelling catheters (LIM, MATHESON and SCHLAPP[1250], ÅGREEN and LAGERLÖF[1211], IHRE[1251]). These refined techniques have, however, not attained widespread application on humans, and consequently most data on the physiology of gastric secretion are derived from experiments on animals, in which the entire stomach or parts of it can be isolated surgically as "pouches" (for details see PAVLOV[1252] and BABKIN[1065]).

Clearly, the gastric juice obtained from such pouches is not contaminated by extragastric secretions, but certain technical details in the surgical procedure and in the handling of the pouches should be considered in order to avoid exsudation from the pouch stoma (see BABKIN[1065]) and inflammatory reactions of the mucosa. Since the electrolyte composition of gastric juice varies with the rate of secretion and with the method of stimulation it is of considerable importance that the pouch contents are drained in such a manner, that the samples obtained become truly representative of the applied stimulus and of the rate at which they have been formed.

HOLLANDER[1253] has pointed out that the *mechanical irritation* of the mucosa by an indwelling catheter may stimulate an abnormally high production of mucus, and he has designed a technique with which the catheter need only be in contact with the mucosa during the brief intervals when juice is removed for analysis[1254].

[1250] LIM, R. K. S., A. R. MATHESON, and W. SCHLAPP: An improved method for investigating the secretory function of the stomach and duodenum in the human subject. Quart. J. exp. Physiol. **13**, 333—345 (1923).

[1251] IHRE, B. J. E.: Human Gastric Function. Acta Med. Scandinav. Suppl. 95 (1938). Also published by Oxford Univ. Press 1939.

[1252] PAVLOV, I. P.: Die Arbeit der Verdauungsdrüsen. Wiesbaden 1898. The Work of the Digestive Glands. 2nd. Ed. London: Griffin 1910.

[1253] HOLLANDER, F.: The composition and mechanism of formation of gastric acid secretion. Science **110**, 57—63 (1949).

[1254] HOLLANDER, F., and G. R. COWGILL: Studies in gastric secretion I. Gastric juice of constant acidity. J. biol. Chem. **91**, 151—182 (1931).

ÖBRINK[1255] emphasized the problem of the *"dead space"* forming around an indwelling catheter, and THULL and REHM[1256] have recently shown that even the "dead space" of the fluid which is trapped in the mucosal folds and crypts may be considerable. The "dead space" gives rise to a "delay time" problem, similar to that encountered in renal physiology, and particularly invalidates observations on the volume rate-concentration relationship at rising or declining secretory flows. The dead space can be minimized by stomach washings, injection of air and continuous aspiration[1256], but these procedures are laborious and they may act as mechanical irritants to the mucosa. It is therefore a technical improvement that TEORELL[1257] and ÖBRINK[1255] have developed the constant intravenous histamine infusion technique. By changing the rate of histamine infusion, any desired constant secretion rate can be maintained for hours. The effect of the dead space is thus minimized due to the large total volumes, which can be recovered even at the critical low rates of secretion.

Pure gastric juice, obtained by one of the stated techniques, represents the composite of the secretory products of a number of different cell types, located in the gastric glands and on the mucosal surface. Histological and histochemical investigations and studies of comparative histology form the only basis for our present day knowledge of the secretory function of individual cells. The approach is open to criticism, but until better evidence is presented one has to accept the current hypothesis that the parietal (oxyntic) cell is the site of HCl formation and the chief (peptic) cell the site of pepsin formation, whereas the mucoid cell and the columnar surface epithelium secrete mucus.

Since it has not yet been possible to obtain the secretory product of one type of cell, uncontaminated by the secretion of other cells, knowledge about the volume and electrolyte composition of the component secretions can only be obtained indirectly. The main approach has been to study the composition of the mixed secretion under different conditions of stimulation and at varying rates of secretion. Such investigations require exacting experimental technique and the interpretation of the data is complicated by the fact that the gastric mucosa appears to be more or less permeable to all the secreted ions (p. 480), so that secondary alterations of the secreted juice may take place by diffusion of ions between the gastric contents and the plasma.

It is understandable that physiologists, forced to struggle with this hydra of variables, have not yet been able to reach final agreement on the problems concerning the secretory function of the individual cells in the gastric mucosa.

The presence of "fixed alkali" in gastric juice was first demonstrated by PROUT in 1824[1258]. In 1854 SCHMIDT[1259] found sodium as well as potassium in the secretion from a patient with a gastric fistula, and FROUIN[1260] verified the presence of both these alkali metals in the secretion from the fundic pouch of a dog. It is now well established that pure gastric juice is approximately isotonic with the plasma, that chloride is the chief anion, and that the secretion contains the

[1255] ÖBRINK, K. J.: Studies in the Kinetics of the Parietal Secretion of the Stomach. Acta physiol. scand. Suppl. 51 (1948):

[1256] THULL, N. B., and W. S. REHM: Composition and osmolarity of gastric juice as a function of plasma osmolarity. Amer. J. Physiol. **185**, 317—324 (1956).

[1257] TEORELL, T.: Untersuchungen über die Magensaftsekretion. Skand. Arch. Physiol. **66**, 225—317 (1933).

[1258] PROUT, W.: On the nature of the acid and saline matters usually existing in the stomach of animals. Phil. Trans. roy. Soc. London. Part I, 45—49 (1824).

[1259] SCHMIDT, C.: Über die Constitution des menschlichen Magensaftes. Liebigs Ann. Chem. **92**, 42—48 (1854).

[1260] FROUIN, A.: Sur l'acidité du suc gastrique. J. Physiol. Path. gén. **1**, 447—455 (1899).

cations: H^+, Na^+, K^+, and Ca^{++} in varying proportions depending upon the conditions of the experiment. There are perhaps also minor quantities of magnesium, sulphate and phosphate, but their concentrations are usually less than 1 meq/l. NH_4Cl is formed by the interaction between NH_3 and HCl in the stomach lumen and is not secreted by any cell. There appears to be convincing evidence that the "gastric urease" is of bacterial origin[1261].

In the following section the secretion of alkali metals by the gastric glands is discussed under the following headings:

1. Type of gland.
2. Rate of secretion.
3. Type of stimulus.
4. Duration of secretion.
5. Plasma concentration of the alkali metals (total osmolar concentration of plasma).
6. Mucosal blood flow and oxygen supply.
7. Gland temperature.
8. Salt depletion and adreno-cortical steroids.
9. Individual differences.
10. The secretion of lithium.
11. The alkali metals in the gastric mucosa.
12. Mechanism of alkali metal secretion.

Type of gland. The histology of the gastric glands differs regionally and individually. In most mammals the chief difference is related to the distribution of the parietal cells of which the glands of the corpus contain many, the glands of the fundus less and the glands of the pyloric antrum none or almost none. Further it appears, that the mucoid cells are particularly well developed in the pyloric glands. Accordingly studies of the "functional topography" of the gastric mucosa may represent one way of approaching the problem of individual cellular function (BABKIN[1262]).

HEIDENHAIN[1263] first examined the isolated secretion of the pyloric pouch of a dog. He found that the secretion was scanty, mucinous and rich in peptic activity. In confirmation, later workers have also found large concentrations of mucus[1264], strong peptic activity[1265, 1266, 1267] and low volume rates of secretion[1265, 1266, 1267, 1268, 1269, 1270]. Secretory rates vary between $1-2$[1265, 1267] and $4-6$[1264, 1270] ml/hr and appear to increase slightly during stimulation of the sympathetic nerves[1264], during weak stimulation of the vagi and by mechanical or chemical irritation of the mucosa. However, neither strong stimulation of the vagi nor pilocarpine affect the volume rate of secretion measurably[1270].

The relatively few analyses of the electrolyte content of pyloric juice are summarized in Table 33.

The secretion is approximately isotonic with the secretion of corpic pouches and with the plasma[1268, 1273] and it has a p_H approximately similar to that of the

[1261] KORNBERG, H. L., and R. E. DAVIES: Gastric urease. Physiol. Rev. **35**, 169—175 (1955).

[1262] BABKIN, B. P.: Some recent advances in the physiology of gastric secretion. Amer. J. Dig. Dis. **5**, 107—111 (1938).

[1263] HEIDENHAIN, R.: Über die Pepsinbildung in den Pylorusdrüsen. Pflügers Arch. ges. Physiol. **18**, 169—171 (1878).

[1264] BAXTER, S. G.: Sympathetic secretory innervation of the gastric mucosa. Amer. J. Dig. Dis. **1**, 36—39 (1934).

[1265] IVY, A. C., and Y. Oyama: Studies on the secretion of the pars pylorica gastrica. Amer. J. Physiol. **57**, 51—60 (1921).

[1266] TAKATA, M.: On the pyloric juice. J. Biochem. (Tokyo) **2**, 33—42 (1922).

[1267] LIM, K. S., and N. M. DOTT: Observations on the isolated pyloric segment and on its secretion. Quart. J. exp. Physiol. **13**, 159—177 (1923).

[1268] GAMBLE, J. L., and M. R. McIVER: The acid-base composition of the gastric secretions. J. exp. Med. **48**, 837—847 (1928)

[1269] COPE, O., H. BLATT, and M. R. BALL: Gastric secretion III. The absorption of heavy water from pouches of the body and antrum of the stomach of the dog. J. clin. Invest. **22**, 111—115 (1943).

[1270] IVY, J. S.: The effect of pilocarpine of mucus secretion by the pyloric mucosa. Gastroenterology **7**, 224—230 (1946).

Table 33. *Electrolyte composition of the pyloric secretion* (all data in meq/l)

Reference	Year	Species	pH	Cations				Anions		
				Na+	K+	Ca++	Total	Cl-	HCO₃-	Total
Ivy and Oyama[1265]	1921	dog	7.00—7.50	—	—	—	—	130—180	—	—
Takata[1266]	1922	dog	7.60—8.00	105	15.4	6.5	—	150	—	—
Lim and Doyt[1267]	1923	dog	"Alkaline"	—	—	—	—	—	—	—
Gamble and McIver[1268]	1928	cat	8.40	—	—	—	169	158	11	169
Baxter[1264]	1934	cat, dog	"Alkaline"	—	8.8	—	—	128—146	12—14	—
Wilhelmj et al.[1271]	1934	dog	—	—	—	—	—	107	40	147
Grant[1272]	1941	dog	—	—	—	4.9	—	—	—	—
Lifson et al.[1273]	1941	dog	—	100—120	—	—	—	—	—	—
Cope et al.[1269]	1943	dog	"Alkaline"	—	—	—	—	118—161	18—32	—
Ivy[1270]	1946	dog	—	—	—	—	—	—	—	—

plasma (the high values reported in Table 33 may be due to the fact that escape of CO_2 was not prevented[1268]). The high " bicarbonate" concentrations[1270, 1271] have obtained by titration of the non-dialysed pyloric secretion. The lower bicarbonate concentrations[1264, 1268] correspond to those reported for gastric mucus (p. 471).

Rate of secretion. The composition of the *pyloric secretion* has not been examined in relation to variations in secretory rate. Since the latter is low and varies within narrow limits it would probably also be an impracticable task to engage in such a study.

Ever since Heidenhain[1274] and Pavlov[1252] demonstrated the rate dependent variations in the acidity of *gastric juice from whole stomachs or corpic pouches* this problem has been studied by numerous investigators and it was soon found that — in general — does the concentration of "acid chloride" increase with secretory rate, whereas the concentration of "neutral chloride" varies inversely with the rate. In 1928 Gamble and McIver[1268] showed that sodium and potassium constitute the bulk of the "neutral chloride" of the earlier investigators. They demonstrated further, that the concentration of sodium varies inversely with rate and acidity, whereas the concentration of potassium remains relatively independent of these parameters. This finding was confirmed by Schairer[1275], Bliss[1276] and many later workers (for references see Table 34).

[1271] Wilhelmj, C. M., I. Neigus, and F. C. Hill: A comparison of intragastric and duodenal factors in lowering the acidity of gastric contents. Amer. J. Physiol. **107**, 490—507 (1934).

[1272] Grant, R.: The relation of calcium content to acidity and buffer value of gastric secretions. Amer. J. Physiol. **132**, 467—473 (1941).

[1273] Lifson, N., R. L. Varco, and M. B. Visscher: Relationship between osmotic activity and sodium content of gastric juice. Proc. Soc. exp. Biol. (N. Y.) **47**, 422—425 (1941).

[1274] Heidenhain, R.: Über die Absonderung der Fundusdrüsen des Magens. Pflügers Arch. ges. Physiol. **19**, 148—166 (1879).

However, very few investigators have examined the concentrations of H^+, Na^+, K^+ and Cl^+ simultaneously in samples of gastric juice obtained over a wide range of variation in secretory rates. Fig 22 illustrates 3 such experiments which are all performed on dogs with gastric pouches. TAKATA[1277] stimulated gastric secretion by the application of food to the main stomach, whereas GRAY and BUCHER[1278] used repetitive subcutaneous injections of histamine, and LINDE and ÖBRINK[1279] a continuous intravenous infusion of histamine.

Sodium. All three investigations clearly illustrate an inverse relationship between sodium concentration and secretory rate. However, there is some discrepancy about the absolute concentration of sodium at the very low rates. GRAY and BUCHER[1278] extrapolated a value of 154.5 meq/l from their data (compare Table 39), and LINDE and ÖBRINK[1279] actually found sodium concentrations of

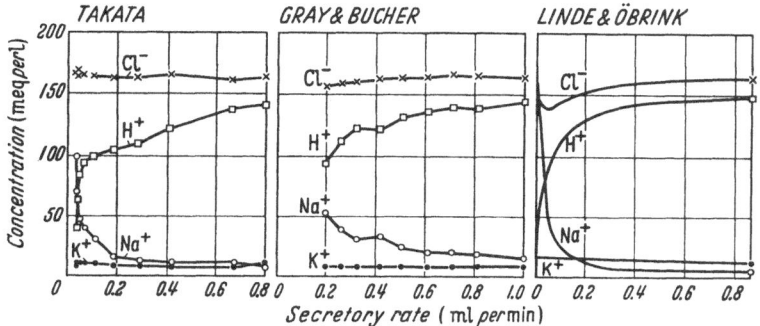

Fig. 22. Electrolytes of gastric juice in relation to secretory rate

about 160 meq/l at secretory rates below 0.1 ml/min. However, TAKATA[1277] only found sodium concentrations of about 100 meq/l at the lowest rates, but his results should probably be regarded with some reserve, since there appears to be an analytical error (H + Na + K does not equal Cl, particularly at the lower and lowest rates) and since a "delay time" effect cannot be excluded (see discussion on p. 466).

Potassium. The concentration of potassium is low relative to that of the other ions (mean values: 9.2[1277], 7.3[1278] and about 13[1279] meq/l) and does apparently not vary significantly with secretory rate. In LINDE and ÖBRINKS data there is perhaps a slight drop in potassium concentration with increasing rates (or with time?).

Table 34 summarizes the data on potassium concentration in gastric juice from 20 different investigations.

The data presented in Table 34 show considerably greater fluctuations in gastric juice K conc. than indicated by the results demonstrated in Fig. 22. Certainly, some of the data are open to criticism, since the results were obtained on human beings, in whom no measure was taken to prevent contamination with

[1275] SCHAIRER, E.: Beitrag zur Kenntnis der Ionenzusammensetzung des Mageninhalts. Klin. Wschr. 8, 1113—1115 (1929).

[1276] BLISS, T. L.: The acid-base composition of gastric juice during the secretory cycle. Ann. intern. Med. 3, 838—849 (1930).

[1277] TAKATA, C.: Über das Verhalten der Na und K Ionen im Magensafte und Blutserum des Hundes. Jap. J. Med. Sci. VIII (Intern. Med., Pediat. and Psychiat.) 3, 33—50 (1933).

[1278] GRAY, J. S., and G. R. BUCHER: The composition of gastric juice as a function of the rate of secretion. Amer. J. Physiol. 133, 542—550 (1941).

[1279] LINDE, S., and K. J. ÖBRINK: On the behavior of electrolytes in gastric juice induced by histamine. Acta physiol. scand. 21, 54—60 (1950).

Table 34. *Potassium in gastric juice* (all values in meq/l)

Reference	Year	mean	range	species	stimulus
SCHMIDT[1259]	1854	14.1		man	
FROUIN[1260]	1899	10.0		dog	sham-feeding
ROSEMANN[1280]	1907	9.5	7.9—11.1	dog	sham-feeding
GAMBLE and McIVER[1268]	1928	13.0	8.9—15.6	cat	sham-feeding
GRIMBERT and FLEURY[1281]	1929	16.0	14.5—17.5	man	histamine
SCHAIRER[1275]	1929	14.0	4—23	man	histamine
MAHLER[1282]	1930	7.6	1—23	man	fasting secretion
BLISS[1276]	1930		17—30	man	histamine
UMENO et al.[1283]	1930	8.7	3.6—16.4	man	alkohol test meal
AUSTIN and GAMMON[1284] .	1931		10—20	man	histamine
INGRAHAM and VISSCHER[1285]	1932	16.4	8.9—22.3	dog	histamine
TAKATA[1277]	1933	9.2	7.2—11.0	dog	sham-feeding
KOZAWA et al.[1286]	1933	10.2		man	fasting
		7.2		man	alkohol test meal
McCANCE[1136]	1938	17.3	15.9—18.5	man	histamine
GRAY and BUCHER[1278] . .	1941	7.3	7.0—7.4	dog	histamine
GUDIKSEN[1287]	1950		3.85—18.78	cat	histamine
			7.67—12.55	cat	pilocarpine
MARTIN[1288]	1950		15—20	man	fasting
			20—35	man	histamine
LINDE and ÖBRINK[1279] . .	1950		10—15	dog	histamine
BERNSTEIN[1289]	1952	13.0		man	histamine
THULL and REHM[1256] . . .	1956	10.9	9.5—12.4	dog	histamine

extragastric secretions[1281, 1275, 1276, 1286, 1280]. But even data obtained from animals with pouches show quite large ranges of variation in the hands of some investigators[1285, 1287]. The reasons for these variations cannot be stated. In contradistinction to BERNSTEIN[1289], MARTIN[1288] reported a temporary marked increase in gastric juice K following administration of histamine to humans, in whom swallowing of saliva was apparently prevented. Both COLCHER, JANOWITZ and HOLLANDER[1290] and THULL and REHM[1256] have noted a similar (but less pronounced) rise in gastric juice K following histamine stimulation of animals. It can thus not be excluded that there is a "potassium transient" phenomenon in the gastric mucosa like that

[1280] ROSEMANN, R.: Die Eigenschaften und die Zusammensetzung des durch Scheinfütterung gewonnenen Hundemagensaftes. Pflügers Arch. ges. Physiol. 118, 467—524 (1907).

[1281] GRIMBERT, L., and P. FLEURY: Contribution à la connaissance de la composition chimique des sucs gastriques chez l'homme. Bull. Soc. Chim. biol. 11, 1105—1121 (1929).

[1282] MAHLER, P.: Beiträge zur Chemie des menschlichen Magensaftes. Wien. Arch. inn. Med. 19, 413—450 (1930).

[1283] UMENO, M., K. KURIHARA, M. HORIUCHI, and C. TAKATA: Tokyo Ijishinshi. Nr. 2731. (1931); cit. from [1277].

[1284] AUSTIN, J. H., and G. D. GAMMON: Gastric secretion after histamine. Sodium and potassium content and peptic estimation. J. clin. Invest. 10, 287—307 (1931).

[1285] INGRAHAM, R. C., and M. B. VISSCHER: Inverse concentration ratios for sodium and potassium in gastric juice and blood plasma. Proc. Soc. exp. Biol. (N. Y.) 30, 464—466 (1932).

[1286] KOZAWA, S., K. FUKUSHIMA, M. UMENO, K. KURIHARA, C. TAKATA, and M. HORIUCHI: Über das Verhalten der Ionen im Magensaft bei verschiedenen Patienten. Jap. J. Med. Sci. VIII (Intern. Med.,Pediat. and Psychiat.) 3, 15—32 (1933).

[1287] GUDIKSEN, E.: Investigations on the Composition of Gastric Juice. C. R. Trav. Lab. Carlsberg s. Chim. 27, 145—261 (1950).

[1288] MARTIN, L.: The relationship of potassium to the electrolytes and to the proteins of the gastric juice of man. Gastroenterology 15, 326—340 (1950).

[1289] BERNSTEIN, R. E.: The potassium, sodium and calcium content of gastric juice. J. Lab. clin. Med. 40, 707—717 (1952).

[1290] COLCHER, H., H. D. JANOWITZ, and F. HOLLANDER: Potassium in gastric juice. Fed. Proc. 11, 26 (1952).

observed by BURGEN[1077] in the case of the salivary glands (p. 434). Studies of mucosal potassium balance have, however, not been performed. Apart from this initial increase in K conc. the best available data appear to indicate that the K conc. of the gastric juice remains relatively independent of secretory rate[1277, 1278, 1279, 1256, 1289]. This represents a parallel to the finding on those duct-possessing glands, which do not reabsorb sodium ions (Fig. 17). Time dependent variations in K conc. of gastric juice are discussed in a following section (p. 473).

Type of stimulus. The reader is referred to the monograph by BABKIN[1065] for details regarding the neural and humoral stimulation of gastric secretion.

Weak stimulation of the vagi[1291], stimulation of the splanchnic nerves[1264] and mechanical or chemical irritation of the mucosa[1292, 1293] provokes a secretion of mucus from the surface epithelium (and the mucoid cells?). This mucus is free from HCl and contains only small amounts of pepsin, desquamated epithelium and transsudate from the mucosa. The chemistry of gastric mucin has been extensively reviewed by GLASS[1294], but there are relatively few analyses of its electrolyte composition (Table 35).

Data on sodium and potassium concentrations are lacking, but with respect to p_H, Ca^{++}, Cl^- and HCO_3^- concentrations the gastric mucus appears closely similar to oesophageal mucus (p. 465), colonic mucus (p. 485) and pyloric secretion (Table 33, p. 468). The rate of secretion is low, possibly lower in the corpic region than in the pyloric region (BAXTER[1264]).

Conventional stimuli of gastric secretion in experimental and clinical work are:
1) Stimulation of the vagal nerve supply (animal work).
2) Insulin, which stimulates the vagal center via the induced hypoglycemia [replaces (1) in work on humans].
3) Cholinergic substances: Pilocarpine, metacholine.
4) Histamine or histaminase inhibitors.

It is generally assumed that the vagal and cholinergic stimuli act on the parietal cells as well as on the chief (peptic) cells and the mucus producing cells. In contrast, most workers regard histamine as a selective stimulant of parietal secretion.

Accordingly, it has been shown that "vagal juice" does always contain considerably more pepsin than histamine juice — even when the two juices are

Table 35. *Electrolyte composition of gastric mucus* (all data in meq/l)

Author	Year	Species	Stimulus	p_H	Ca^{++}	Cl^-	HCO_3^-
WEBSTER[1295]	1930	dog		—	—	132	16.8
VINEBERG[1291]	1931	dog	vagal	—	—	95—134	
BAXTER[1264]	1934	dog	splanchnic.	—	—	128—146	11.6—14.0
IHRE[1251]	1938	man	fasting	7.24—7.91	—	130—139	3.2—10.8
HOLLANDER[1292]	1946	dog	eugenol	—	5.0	—	—
HOLLANDER and LAUBER[1293]	1948	dog	eugenol	7.4—7.5	—	—	—

[1291] VINEBERG, A. M.: The activation of different elements of the gastric secretion by variation of vagal stimulation. Amer. J. Physiol. 96, 363 (1931).
[1292] HOLLANDER, F.: Calcium content of gastric mucus. Fed. Proc. 5, 49 (1946).
[1293] HOLLANDER, F., and F. V. LAUBER: The p_H of gastric mucus secretion after equilibration with alveolar air. Fed. Proc. 7, 56 (1948).
[1294] GLASS, G. B. J.: New physiological and clinical studies on the secretion of mucin in the human stomach. Rev. Gastroent. 16, 687—701 (1949).
[1295] WEBSTER, D. R.: The mucus of gastric juice and its variations. Trans. roy. Soc. Canada 24 Sect. 5, 199 (1930).

secreted at equal rates (cf. Table 36). The peptic activity of the histamine juice is generally assumed to be a "wash-out" phenomenon of preformed peptic cell secretion, which has been retained in the gastric gland tubules.

Data on possible variations in electrolyte concentrations with different stimuli are less clear cut than the enzyme studies.

Table 36. *Comparison of "Histamine Juice" and "Insulin Juice" From the data of* IHRE[1251]

	Histamine (0.6 mg)	Insulin (16 I.U.)
Volume (ml/60 min)	103	100
Chloride (meq/l)	151.4	156.4
Acidity (meq/l)	110.3	112.8
"neutral chloride" (meq/l)	41.1	43.6
Pepsin (units per ml)	36	100

HOLLANDER and COW-GILL[1254] found that the usual relationship between H^+ ion concentration and secretory rate was frequently eliminated in histamine experiments on dogs with gastric pouches. When the abundant flow of gastric juice had "washed out" the mucus from the gastric cavity, these workers obtained a secretion, which remained highly acid (H^+ ion conc.: 155—160 meq/l) despite considerable variations in the rate of secretion. GRAY and BUCHER[1278] and LINDE and ÖBRINK[1279] were not able to confirm this finding in their histamine experiments (cf. Fig. 22), and LINDE and ÖBRINK state that a delay time phenomenon may have masked the rate-concentration relationship in HOLLANDER and COWGILL's tests.

BABKIN[1065] cites some clinical data as indicating that a change of stimulus may cause rate-independent variations in the composition of gastric juice. Clinical data must, however, be regarded with some reserve since contamination with extragastric secretions is normally not prevented. Swallowing of saliva, which flows abundantly during cholinergic stimulation, may easily give the faulty impression of large gastric secretory rates combined with low acidities.

It is apparent from IHRE's data in Table 36, that the electrolyte concentrations of the histamine juice and the insulin juice are closely similar, despite the decided difference in peptic activity.

LINDE[1296] obtained a steady state secretion by a continuous intravenous infusion of histamine. The peptic activity of the gastric juice rose sharply when a vagal stimulus was superimposed on the histamine infusion, but secretory rate and electrolyte concentrations remained unchanged.

GUDIKSEN[1287] closely studied the relationship between stimulus and electrolyte composition of gastric juice. He used cats with gastric pouches, stimulated the secretion with histamine, pilocarpine and via the vagal nerve, collected the juice under careful control of the rate and analyzed the samples for all the chief ions present. His results are demonstrated in Table 37.

Table 37. *Electrolyte composition of "Histamine Juice", "Pilocarpine Juice" and "Vagal Juice". From the data of* GUDIKSEN[1207] (all values in meq/l)

Stimulus	Histamine	Pilocarpine	Vagal Stimulation
Dosage (mg)	0.25—0.75	0.4—2.0	—
Secretory rate (ml/15min) .	1.14—10.0	0.24—1.60	0.22—1.8
Cl⁻	162—191	155—179	165—177
$H^+(+NH_4^+)$	129—167 (1.2—8.9)	10—92 (4.3—15.5)	21—134 (3.4—9.1)
Na^+	3.9—17.2	38—138	13—136
K^+	10.2—18.8	7.7—14.9	4.0—13.4
Ca^{++}	0.07—2.3	—	—

[1296] LINDE, S.: Studies on the Stimulation Mechanism of Gastric Secretion. Acta physiol. Scand. Suppl. 74 (1950).

It appears from Table 37 that "pilocarpine juice" and "vagal juice" have lower acidities and higher sodium concentrations than "histamine juice". However, if the individual observations are represented in relation to secretory rate (Fig. 23) it becomes difficult to discern any difference between Gudiksen's data with different stimuli and data from experiments where only one type of stimulus has been used (Fig. 22). Further, it appears from Fig. 23 that there is no essential difference between the results of TAKATA, which are obtained in freeding experiments and the results of GRAY and BUCHER and LINDE and ÖBRINK which are obtained in histamine experiments.

According to the cited data of IHRE[1251], LINDE[1296], GUDIKSEN[1287], GRAY and BUCHER[1278] and LINDE and ÖBRINK[1279] it is thus hardly possible to distinguish the effect of stimulus from the effect of rate on the electrolyte composition of gastric juice. However, the results of pepsin analyses apparently preclude the simplest explanation for this phenomenon: That histamine excites the "non-parietal" cells to the same degree as do the vagal type stimuli.

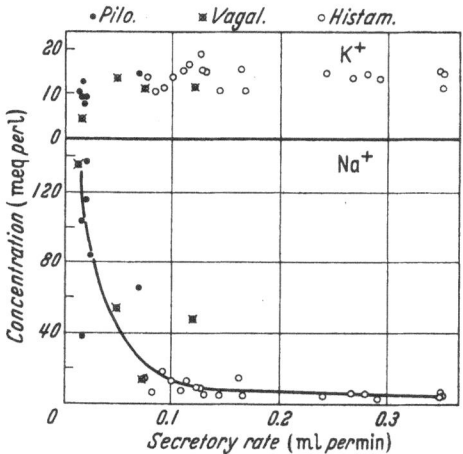

Fig. 23. Sodium and potassium in pilocarpine, vagal and histamine juice (from the data by GUDIKSEN)

The explanation is rather that *the volume of the "non-parietal" component is small and only little influenced by variations in the intensity of stimulation, whereas the volume of the parietal component is highly variable and represents the bulk of the gastric juice at most rates of secretory flow.* This conclusion is in accordance with the findings of TOBY[1297] and receives indirect support from the demonstration of the very low volume rates at which the entirely "non-parietal" pyloric juice is being secreted (p. 467).

Possible differences in electrolyte composition depending upon the type of stimulus will thus only show up at the very low rates of gastric secretion, in which range experimental error (delay time, exact determination of flow etc.) becomes large and reduces the statistical reliability of the observations.

Duration of secretion. THULL and REHM[1256] and LINDE and ÖBRINK[1279] both state that the concentration of potassium in gastric juice decreases slightly on long continued stimulation with histamine. In the course of 60 min of steady state secretory activity (in response to i.v. histamine) THULL and REHM thus found a decrease in K from 12.4 to 9.5 meq/l, whereas the concentrations of the other ions were not measurably affected. This latter finding agrees with old work on gastric secretion, stating that no change in the chloride concentration of the juice could be observed on long continued stimulation, unless severe chloride depletion was induced by deficient replacement of secretory losses (p. 476).

Plasma concentrations of Na and K (total osmolar concentration). GILMAN and COWGILL[1298, 1299] have demonstrated that variations in the total osmolar

[1297] TOBY, C. G.: Effect of different types of stimuli on the composition of gastric juice. Quart J. exp. Physiol. **26**, 45—51 (1936).

[1298] GILMAN, A., and G. R. COWGILL: The regulatory action of total blood electrolytes on the concentration of gastric chlorides. Amer. J. Physiol. **99**, 172—178 (1931—32).

[1299] GILMAN, A., and G. R. COWGILL: The osmotic relation of blood and gastric juice. Amer. J. Physiol. **103**, 143—152 (1933).

concentration of the plasma induced by the injection of hypertonic saline, resp. water are followed by almost parallel variations in the total osmolar concentration and chloride concentration of the gastric juice in dogs secreting in response to histamine. NOBLE and ROBERTSON[1300] confirmed this finding in histamine juice of cats receiving a rapid intravenous infusion of 30% NaCl. Both NOBLE and ROBERTSON[1300] and DAY and KOMAROV[1301] obtained a rise in the osmolar concentration of the gastric juice following intravenous injection of hypertonic glucose. This latter finding supports the conclusion of GILMAN and COWGILL that the effect of salt loading and water loading is chiefly (or exclusively?) due to alterations in the total osmolar concentration of the plasma and less (if at all) to a change in the concentration of individual electrolytes of the plasma. GILMAN and COWGILL[1299] found an inverse relationship between the secretory rate and the total osmolar concentration of the plasma. When the plasma was hypotonic secretory rate was increased over and above that of control experiments, whereas secretory rate always dropped markedly when the plasma became hypertonic. These findings are in accord with the results of similar experiments on the secretions of duct-possessing glands (p. 437), intestinal glands (p. 485) and the liver (p. 489).

THULL and REHM[1256] repeated GILMAN and COWGILL's experiments and arrived at closely similar conclusions. They studied the individual electrolytes of the gastric secretion and found an increase in sodium and a decrease in hydrogen ion concentrations when secretory rate dropped in response to hypertonic loading. During hypotonic loading (when secretory rate was increasing) sodium concentration remained low and hydrogen ion concentration remained high. Potassium concentration of the gastric juice was not significantly affected by variations in the osmolar concentration of the plasma.

CARONE and COOKE[1302] examined the gastric secretion of rats which were made K deficient by dietary K restriction supplemented with injections of DCA. Plasma K was reduced from 4.77 to 2.66 meq/l and there was a slight alkalosis (HCO$_3$ rose from 23 to 27.9 meq/l) with a parallel reduction in plasma chloride concentration. Gastric juice in the hypokalemic animals showed a reduced acidity, a slight decrease in Cl conc., a marked increase in Na conc. and a drop in K conc. from 8.6 to 4.9 meq/l. The authors conclude that the reduced plasma K conc. was responsible for the reduction of acid secretion. DELRUE[1303] first showed that omission of K from the medium of isolated frog mucosa caused a rapid decrease in the secretion of HCl.

Mucosal blood flow and oxygen supply. A detailed description of the *vascularization* of the stomach is given by BABKIN[1065]. BABKIN, ARMOUR and WEBSTER[1304] have shown that ligation of most arteries does not affect secretory rate nor acidity. This is an indication of the efficiency of the numerous anastomoses present.

[1300] NOBLE, R. L., and J. D. ROBERTSON: The effect of hypertonic solutions on gastric secretion and intraocular pressure. J. Physiol. **93**, 430—437 (1938).

[1301] DAY, J. J., and S. A. KOMAROV: Glucose and gastric secretion. Amer. J. Dig. Dis. **6**, 169—175 (1939).

[1302] CARONE, F. A., and R. E. COOKE: Effect of potassium deficiency on gastric secretion in the rat. Amer. J. Physiol **172**, 684—688 (1953).

[1303] DELRUE, G.: Etude de la sécrétion de l'estomac. II Sécrétion acide de la muqueuse isolée de l'estomac de grenouille. Action des ions. Arch. intern. Physiol. **36**, 129—135 (1933).

[1304] BABKIN, B. P., J. C. ARMOUR, and D. R. WEBSTER: Restoration of the functional capacity of the stomach when deprived of its main arterial blood supply. Canad. med. Ass. J. **48**, 1—10 (1943).

Gastric blood flow was measured by TEORELL[1257] in the cat. Average flow during stimulation was 10.3 ml/min, i.e. in considerable excess of secretory flow, which was 0.5—1.0 ml/min (compare data on blood flow versus secretory rate in salivary glands, p. 455). IVY and FARRELL[1305] showed that variations in blood flow affect the secretory response of the gastric pouch transplant. LIM, NECHELES and NI[1306] studied the isolated vivi-perfused stomach and concluded that gastric secretion can take place within wide limits independently of blood flow, although increased blood flow may increase secretion already in progress. HELLEBRANDT, BROGDON and HOOPES[1307] found a decrease in gastric secretory rate and acidity when untrained persons were subjected to heavy excercise. The depression was considered as being due to diversion of splanchnic blood flow and tended to disappear during adequate physical training[1307].

Mucosal oxygen consumption in vivo was measured by TEORELL[1257] in cats. Average oxygen consumption by the cat stomach was 0.54 ml O_2 per minute. Assuming that the mucosa of the stomach (like that of the intestine) utilizes 85% of the oxygen taken up by the entire viscus and dividing by the average mucosal weight of 12.1 g TEORELL arrived at the figure: 0.037 ($\pm$ 0.005) ml O_2 per gram mucosa per minute = 6.60 μeq of oxygen per gram mucosa per minute (1.65 μM are 6.60 μeq). This figure is slightly greater than the resting oxygen consumption of salivary and pancreatic glands (p. 435), but there was no sharp distinction between resting and secreting mucosae in TEORELL's experiments. The oxygen uptake of the isolated mucosa has been measured in relation to HCl secretion, but complete agreement upon the relation between oxygen uptake and HCl secretion rates has apparently not yet been reached. HELLEBRANDT, BROGDON and HOOPES[1308] did not find any significant depression of gastric secretion during severe anoxia in human beings.

TEORELL studied the mucosal a—v difference for CO_2 and found that the venous blood almost invariably contained less CO_2 than the arterial. It is known (p. 483) that the isolated frog gastric mucosa takes up one molecule of CO_2 from the nutrient medium for every H^+ ion secreted. TEORELL[1257] and BROWNE and VINEBERG[1309] showed that breathing of CO_2 enchances, whereas hyperventilation depresses gastric acid secretion. Introduction of CO_2 in the stomach lumen is followed by an increased flow of acid gastric juice (BABKIN[1065]). If external supplies of CO_2 are withdrawn from the medium of the isolated frog mucosa, the rate of acid secretion goes down and may become completely arrested (p. 483).

Gland temperature. The effect of variations in temperature on the secretion of the isolated mouse stomach has been studied by DAVENPORT and CHAVRÉ[1310]. A fall in temperature depressed the rate of acid secretion. The alkali metals were not studied.

Salt depletion and adreno-cortical steroids. CAHN[1311] found that severe chloride depletion induced by continuous removal of gastric secretion combined with

[1305] IVY, A. C., and J. I. FARRELL: Contributions to the physiology of gastric secretion. VIII. The proof of a humoral mechanism. Amer. J. Physiol. **74**, 639—649 (1925).

[1306] LIM, R. K. S., H. NECHELESS, and T. G. NI: Vasomotor reactions the vivi-perfused stomach. Chinese J. Physiol. **1**, 381—396 (1927).

[1307] HELLEBRANDT, F. A., E. BROGDON, and S. L. HOOPES: The disappearance of digestive inhibition with the repetition of exercise. Amer. J. Physiol. **112**, 442—450 (1935).

[1308] HELLEBRANDT, F. A., E. BROGDON, and S. L. HOOPES: The effect of acute anoxemia on hunger, digestive contractions and the secretion of hydrochloric acid in man. Amer. J. Physiol. **112**, 451—460 (1935).

[1309] BROWNE, J. S. L. and A. M. VINEBERG: The interdependence of gastric secretion and the CO_2 content of the blood. J. Physiol. **75**, 345—365 (1932).

[1310] DAVENPORT, H. W., and V. J. CHAVRÉ: Acid secretion and oxygen consumption by mouse stomachs in vitro. Amer. J. Physiol. **174**, 203—208 (1953).

NaCl restriction caused a depression of the volume rate and acidity of gastric juice in the dog. FROUIN[1312] verified this finding and demonstrated that administration of NaCl was followed by a normalization of the secretory response. McCANCE[1136] studied gastric secretion in human beings, who were sodium depleted by repeated periods of profuse sweating superimposed on a low sodium diet. McCANCE found the volume of secretion practically unchanged, a slight drop in acidity and chloride, a slight drop in sodium and a definite rise in potassium concentration (from 15.9— 18.5 meq/l before sodium depletion to 21.2—23.6 meq/l after sodium depletion). McCANCE does, however, point out that contamination with extragastric secretions may have taken place. ROSEMANN[1313] closely studied the relation between chloride depletion and gastric secretion. He showed that the gastric juice of dogs did not change in composition before severe chloride depletion (amounting to 50% of total body chloride) was induced and the animals were nearly dying. Shorter experiments with continuous removal of the gastric juice secreted in response to histamine demonstrate, that the volume and acidity remains unaffected by the duration of the secretion as well as by the moderate chloride depletion, which is induced[1314, 1315].

From these data it appears reasonable to conclude that the volume and composition of gastric juice is not affected by salt loss before a considerable depletion has developed and plasma chloride concentration is subnormal.

The problem concerning the effect of adrenal steroids on gastric secretion has received considerable attention in later years due to the frequency of peptic ulceration in patients treated with large doses of steroid for longer periods. The effect of adrenal steroids has mainly been studied in relation to acid secretion, whereas the effect on the alkali metals in the gastric juice has been little investigated Only a brief review is therefore given in this place. For more detailed information the reader is referred to the paper by GRAY[1316].

Patients with Addison's disease frequently have anacidity[1316] and a depression of acid secretion is also found in adrenalectomized animals[1317, 1318]. Administration of cortisone frequently normalises acid secretion in patients or animals with adrenal insufficiency[1316, 1317, 1318]. Normal dogs[1319] and normal man[1320] may show an increase in volume rate and acidity of gastric secretion following ACTH or cortisone without other stimulation being used. The effect of ACTH is abolished by adrenalectomy, but not by vagotomy[1319, 1320]. Stimulation of the anterior part of the hypothalamus is followed by marked gastric secretory activity, which is

[1311] CAHN, A.: Die Magenverdauung im Chlorhunger. Z. physiol. Chem. 10, 522—535 (1886).

[1312] FROUIN, A.: Action des chlorures de l'alimentation sur la sécrétion gastrique. Bull. Soc. Chim. biol. 4, 435—453 (1922).

[1313] ROSEMANN, R.: Die Magenverdauung bei Verminderung des Chlorvorrates des Körpers. Pflügers Arch. ges. Physiol. 142, 208—234 (1911).

[1314] ROTHLIN, E., and R. GUNDLACH: Etude expérimentale de l'influence de l'histamine sur la sécrétion gastrique. Arch. intern. Physiol. 17, 59—84 (1921—22).

[1315] LIM, R. K. S., and A. C. LIU: Ermüdung der Magensekretion. Pflügers Arch. ges. Physiol. 211, 647—662 (1926).

[1316] GRAY, J. S.: Relationship of the adrenal gland to peptic ulcer. Med. Clin. N. Amer. November 1957, 1471—1480.

[1317] TURKISCHER, E., and E. WERTHEIMER: Adrenalectomy and gastric secretion. J. Endocr. 4, 143—151 (1945).

[1318] MADDEN, R. J., and H. H. RAMSBERG: Gastric secretion in the adrenalectomized rat. Endocrinology 49, 82—85 (1951).

[1319] VILLARREAL, R., W. F. GANONG, and S. J. GRAY: Effect of adrenocorticotrophic hormone upon the gastric secretion of hydrochloric acid, pepsin and electrolytes in the dog. Amer. J. Physiol. 183, 485—494 (1955).

[1320] GRAY, S. J., C. RAMSEY, R. W. REIFENSTEIN, and J. A. BENSON: The significance of hormonal factors in the pathogenesis of peptic ulcer. Gastroenterology 25, 156—172 (1953).

abolished by vagotomy, whereas stimulation of the posterior hypothalamus causes secretory activity which is abolished by adrenalectomy, but not by vagotomy[1321]. The pathway for the latter stimulus to the adrenal gland remains unknown. Peptic activity appears to vary in parallel to acid secretion, indicating that the adrenal cortex is, somehow, of importance for the "non-parietal" as well as for the parietal secretion[1316, 1319, 1320].

The mechanism of the stimulating effect of adrenal cortical hormone is not clear. Histamine may provoke a normal acid secretion in adrenalectomized rats[1322]. If confirmed, this finding indicates that adrenocortical steroids do not excert their effect directly on the secretory cells, but that they may act via a change in normal stimulatory or inhibitory mechanisms.

VILLARREAL et al.[1319] found an increase in H^+ conc. and pepsin conc. and a decrease in Na^+ and K^+ of gastric juice following administration of adrenocorticotropin to dogs. It is however difficult to relate these changes to the simultaneous changes in rate. The depression of K^+ ion concentration is not in accord with the findings on other glandular secretions. The depression of Na^+ ion concentration may merely be secondary to the rise in secretory rate (cf. Fig. 22).

Individual differences. All workers agree that there are individual variations in the volume and the acidity of gastric juice secreted in response to a standard stimulus. Women produce gastric juice of a lower volume and acidity than men[1323, 1324, 1325] and the volume and acidity decreases with advancing age in both sexes[1326].

The secretion of lithium. GOOD[1206] and BERGER[1207] have shown that lithium is secreted into the gastric cavity. The kinetics of lithium secretion have not been studied.

The alkali metal content of the gastric mucosa. Several workers have determined the chloride content of gastric mucosa. ROSEMANN[1313] found 95.5 meq of chloride per kg of fresh mucosa before secretion and 75.5 meq of chloride per kg

Table 38. *Electrolyte composition of the gastric mucosa*

Author	Species (site)	Fresh tissue				Blood and fat free tissue			
		% water	meq/l of tissue water			% water	meq/l of tissue water		
			Na	K	Cl		Na	K	Cl
INGRAHAM and VISSCHER[1096]	dog	80.5	123	66	73	—	—	—	—
MANERY and HASTINGS[1096]	rat (fundus)	79.1	—	87.0	96.3	—	—	—	—
MANERY and HASTINGS[1096]	rabbit (pylorus)	84.9	34.4	—	76.8	85.3	34.1		77.9
MANERY and HASTINGS[138]	rabbit (fundus)	79.5	46.2	—	96.0	80.6	44.7		95.6

[1321] PORTER, R. W., H. J. MOVIUS, and J. D. FRENCH: Hypothalamic influences on hydrochloric acid secretion of the stomach. Surgery **33**, 875—880 (1953).

[1322] KULE, J., and R. B. WELBOURN: The influence of the adenohypophysis and the adrenal cortex on gastric secretion in the rat. Brit. J. Surg. **44**, 241—247 (1956).

[1323] POLLAND, W. S.: Histamine test meals. Arch. intern. Med. 51, 903—919 (1933).

[1324] BLOOMFIELD, A. L.: The mechanism of decrease of gastric secretion with advancing years. Amer. J. med. Sci. **190**, 325—330 (1935).

[1325] OSTERBERG, A. E., F. R. VANZANT, and A. V. ALVAREZ: Studies of gastric pepsin, methods of measurement and factors which influence it. J. clin. Invest. **12**, 551—556 (1933).

[1326] VANZANT, F. R., W. C. ALVAREZ, G. B. EUSTERMAN, H. L. DUNN, and J. BIRKSON: The normal range of gastric acidity from youth to old age. Arch. intern. Med. **49**, 345—359 (1932).

of fresh tissue after secretion. TEORELL[1257] found from $67-74$ meq/kg of fresh mucosa and could not demonstrate any difference between the resting and secreting state. The alkali metals of the gastric mucosa have been examined by INGRAHAM and VISSCHER[1056] and MANERY and HASTINGS[138]. INGRAHAM and VISSCHER did not find any difference between resting and stimulated mucosae. MANERY and HASTINGS do not specify whether their results have been obtained during secretory rest or during stimulation.

Mechanism of alkali metal secretion. Two different hypotheses have been forwarded to explain the rate dependent variations in electrolyte composition of gastric juice:

1) *The component theory*, stating that the variations are due to the mixing of (at least) two components of different composition.

2) *The diffusion theory*, stating that the chief reason for the variations is a partial equilibration between the secreted gastric juice and the plasma by diffusion of ions according to their concentration gradients.

These hypotheses have been extensively reviewed by HOLLANDER[1327, 1328, 1253], BABKIN[1065], TEORELL[1329], CONWAY[1330] and HEINZ and ÖBRINK[1331]. Only a brief outline is therefore presented in this place.

1) *The component theory.* This theory is based on the assumption that hydrochloric acid is secreted by the parietal cells in a constant (isotonic or slightly hypertonic) concentration[1252, 1254], but at widely varying secretory rates depending upon the intensity of the stimulus. Following discharge, the acid (parietal) component is neutralized and diluted by an alkaline component, which is secreted by the other cells of the gastric mucosa. The alkaline ("non-parietal") component is low in volume and its neutralizing effect therefore most pronounced at the low rates of gastric secretory flow.

The component theory was first proposed by PAVLOV[1252] and has received support from BABKIN[1332, 1333, 1065], HOLLANDER[1334, 1335, 1327, 1328, 1253] and several others (for references see Table 39). HOLLANDER clearly formulated the theory and stated the composition of the component secretions which best fitted his data on the variations in "neutral chloride" (i.e. total chloride minus hydrogen ion concentration) and "acid chloride" at different secretory rates. Unlike ROSEMANN[1280] and TAKATA[1277], but in confirmation of most other workers, HOLLANDER found that the chloride concentration of the gastric juice decreases with decreasing rates of secretion (see graphical representation of GRAY and BUCHER's data in Fig. 22).

[1327] HOLLANDER, F.: The chemistry and mechanics of hydrochloric acid formation in the stomach. Gastroenterology **1**, 410—430 (1943).

[1328] HOLLANDER, F.: Current views on the physiology of gastric secretion. Amer. J. Med. **13**, 453—464 (1952).

[1329] TEORELL, T.: Electrolyte diffusion in relation to the acidity regulation of the gastric juice. Gastroenterology **9**, 425—443 (1947).

[1330] CONWAY, E. J.: The Biochemistry of Gastric Acid Secretion. Springfield, Ill.: C. C. Thomas 1953.

[1331] HEINZ, E., and K. J. ÖBRINK: Acid formation and acidity control in the stomach. Physiol. Rev. **34**, 643—673 (1954).

[1332] BABKIN, B. P.: The physiological factors determining the acidity of the gastric juice and the gastric contents. Canad. med. Ass. J. **17**, 36—42 (1927).

[1333] BABKIN, B. P.: The factors regulating the composition of gastric juice. Canad. med. Ass. J. **25**, 134—139 (1931).

[1334] HOLLANDER, F.: Studies in gastric secretion. IV. Variations in chloride content of gastric juice and their significance. J. biol. Chem. **97**, 585—604 (1932).

[1335] HOLLANDER, F.: The components of the gastric secretion. Amer. J. Dig. Dis. **3**, 651 (1936).

Within a range of hydrogen ion concentrations from about 100 to about 160 meq/l HOLLANDER found a straight line relationship between the concentration of neutral chloride and the acidity. By extrapolation of this line to "zero neutral chloride" he arrived at the conclusion that the acid (parietal) component represented a 170 meq/l solution of HCl. Extrapolation to "zero acidity" gave a value of 100 meq/l of neutral chloride. HOLLANDER inferred from this finding that the remaining anion was buffer, probably bicarbonate, and stated that the alkaline ("non-parietal") component contained 100 meq of chloride and 70 meq of bicarbonate per liter without specifying the cations involved.

Broadly speaking similar views were taken by LIU, YUAN and LIM[1336], GRAY et al.[1337, 1338, 1278] and FISHER and HUNT[1339], although the different investigators are at slight variance regarding the H^+ ion concentration of the non-parietal component and the presence or absence of "neutral chloride" in the parietal component (see Table 39). Regarding the latter point most workers, who have actually determined the individual cations of the "neutral chloride", agree that the parietal

Table 39. *The composition of the component secretions.* Modified from HEINZ and ÖBRINK[395]. All values meq/l

Reference	Component	Cations					Anions		
		H^+	Na^+	K^+	Ca^{++}	Total	Cl^-	HCO_3^-	Total
HOLLANDER[1327] [1328]	Parietal	170		0		170	170	0	170
	Non-Parietal	0		170		170	100	70	170
LIU, YUAN and LIM[1336]	Parietal	176		0		176	176	0	176
	Non-Parietal 1	0		176		176	176	0	176
	Non-Parietal 2	0		176		176	0	176	176
GRAY[1338]	Parietal	158.6	0	7.4	0	166	166	0	166
	Non-Parietal	0	154.5	7.4	3.7	165.6	133	33	166
FISHER and HUNT[1339]	Parietal	160		10		170	170	0	170
	Non-Parietal	0		170		170	125	45	170

component contains small amounts of "neutral chloride" as KCl. Since K is the only ion of the gastric juice, which does not vary appreciably with the rate of secretion, it is presumably present in about equal concentration in both components (cf. Fig. 22).

It is inherent in the component theory that the interaction between the acid and the alkaline component results in the reaction: $HCl + NaHCO_3 = NaCl + H_2O + CO_2$ with a consequent reduction in the total osmolar concentration of the mixed gastric juice. According to the two-component hypothesis the reduction in osmolar concentration must be most pronounced at the intermediate secretory rates, whereas the osmolar concentration rises towards the high rates (where the gastric juice consists of almost unneutralized HCl) and towards the very low rates (where the gastric juice consists of almost unneutralized alkaline component).

[1336] LIU, A. C., I. C. YUAN, and R. K. S. LIM: Quantitative relationships between the oxyntic and other gastric component secretions. Chinese J. Physiol. 8, 1—36 (1934).

[1337] GRAY, J. S., G. R. BUCHER and N. M. HARMAN: The relationships between total acid and neutral chloride of gastric juice. Amer. J. Physiol. 132, 504—516 (1941).

[1338] GRAY, J. S.: The physiology of the parietal cell with special reference to the formation of acid. Gastroenterology 1, 390—400 (1943).

[1339] FISHER, R. B., and J. N. HUNT: The inorganic components of gastric secretion. J. Physiol. 111, 138—149 (1950).

The osmotic pressure relationships have been carefully studied by LIFSON, VARCO and VISSCHER[1340, 1341, 1273], who demonstrated that the gastric juice is isotonic (or slightly hypertonic) at the high rates, that the osmolar concentration drops to values about 30 mOsmol below plasma concentration at the intermediate secretory rates and rises again at the very low rates to reach approximate isotonicity. LIFSON et al. related these osmotic pressure variations to the sodium content and to the nitrogen content of the gastric juice, and in several experiments did they thus obtain results, which were at least not incompatible with a two-component hypothesis as suggested by HOLLANDER.

The two-component hypothesis requires that the isotonic gastric juice formed at low rates of secretion contains considerable quantities of bicarbonate (cf. Table 39). Analyses of gastric mucus (Table 35) and of pyloric secretion (Table 33) are however not in accord with this conclusion. Further, LINDE and ÖBRINK[1279] directly measured the variations in chloride concentration over a wide range of secretory rates and found, that the initial decline in chloride concentration with decreasing rates was followed by an increase to about 150 meq/l at the lowest rates of secretion (Fig. 22, p. 469). This finding, which was confirmed by IHRE[1251] clearly demonstrates the hazards of extrapolation procedures based on a limited sets of observations, but does not necessarily refute the essential validity of the component theory. The "non-parietal" component is elaborated by a number of different cells, and it is possible that the secretory product of the individual cells can vary in volume as well as in anionic composition. This possibility was actually suggested by LIU, YUAN and LIM (see Table 39) as well as by LIFSON, VARCO and VISSCHER[1341] in order to account for certain osmotic pressure variations, which could not be explained on the basis of a *two*-component mechanism. In later discussions of his component theory HOLLANDER[1328] has also suggested that the non-parietal component may comprise an alkaline solution as well as a solution of neutral saline.

2) *The diffusion theory.* This hypothesis was forwarded by TEORELL[1257] and has been reviewed by TEORELL[1329] and by HEINZ and ÖBRINK[1331]. It states that the chief reason for the rate dependent variations in the electrolyte composition of gastric juice is a diffusion of H^+ and Na^+ ions between the gastric lumen and the plasma according to their concentration gradients. It is an essential basis for the theory that the gastric mucosa has been shown to be a membrane with a definite, albeit low, permeability to H^+, Na^+ and Cl^-. This is apparent from evidence obtained by experiments on the intact stomachs of animals[1342,1343] and man[1251] as well as on the isolated gastric mucosa[1344, 1345, 1350]. A review of the permeability of the stomach mucosa to various substances has been made by KAREL[1346].

[1340] LIFSON, N., R. L. VARCO, and M. B. VISSCHER: Nitrogen content and total osmotic activity of gastric juice. Proc. Soc. exp. Biol. (N. Y.) **49**, 410—415 (1942).

[1341] LIFSON, N., R. L. VARCO, and M. B. VISSCHER: The relationship between the total osmotic pressure of gastric juice and its acidity. Gastroenterology **1**, 784—802 (1943).

[1342] TEORELL, T.: On the permeability of the stomach mucosa for acids and some other substances. J. gen. Physiol. **23**, 263—274 (1939).

[1343] COPE, O., W. E. COHN, and A. G. BRENIZER: Gastric secretion II. Absorption of radioactive sodium from pouches of the body and antrum of the stomach of the dog. J. clin. Invest. **22**, 103—115 (1943).

[1344] CRANE, E., and R. E. DAVIES: Transport of radioactive Na and K through the gastric mucosa. Biochem. J. **45**, 23—24 (1949).

[1345] HOGBEN, A. M.: The chloride transport system of the gastric mucosa. Proc. nat. Acad. Sci. (Wash.) **37**, 393—395 (1951).

[1346] KAREL, L.: Gastric absorption. Physiol. Rev. **28**, 433—450 (1948).

The diffusion theory apparently received great impetus when TEORELL[1257] and later LINDE, TEORELL and ÖBRINK[1347] claimed that the hydrogen ion concentration of the acid (parietal) component was not 160—170 meq/l (Table 39), but as high as 350 or perhaps even 464 meq/l. In experiments designed to test the validity of the diffusion theory, they attempted to reduce the hydrogen ion concentration of the secreted juice by introduction of a suitable buffer: glycine. When glycine was introduced in the stomach, the titrable acidity of the removed specimens of gastric juice rose to the levels just stated. If this were the true "primary acidity" the volume and buffer concentration of the alkaline component had to be excessively large in order to account for the "secondary acidity" normally observed. Since this was impossible, the only alternative explanation appeared to be, that the primary acidity was reduced mainly by diffusion and only to a very limited extent by intragastric neutralization. CONWAY[1330] and later HEINZ[1348] have, however, pointed out that the "primary acidities" measured with the glycine buffer were abnormally high, due to the artificial reduction in osmolar concentration and hydrogen ion concentration of the secreted juice. The interaction between the three ions: H^+, Cl^- and $CH_2(NH_3^+)COO^-$ gives the two ions: Cl^- and $CH_2(NH_3^+)COOH$. This means a *reduction in the osmolar concentration gradient* causing less water to be "secreted" along with the hydrochloric acid. The result is an increase in "primary acidity" and a decrease in volume (CONWAY[1330]). However TEORELL et al. did not find any change in volume, so possibly the explanation of HEINZ[1348] is better under the circumstances. HEINZ pointed out that the binding of H^+ to the buffer caused a *reduction in the H^+ ion concentration gradient* over the canalicular wall with the result that more H^+ ions were transferred into the stomach lumen with a resulting increase in acidity without change in volume. In their review HEINZ and ÖBRINK[1331] accordingly refuted the theory of the high "primary acidities" and stated that the HCl is secreted in approximate isotonicity.

Thus the chief argument for claiming that a diffusion mechanism had to be by far the most important factor in acidity reduction failed to stand up to critical revision. Nevertheless, one can by no means exclude, that a diffusion does occur and that it may even be an important factor under certain circumstances.

According to the approximation by GUGGENHEIM[1349] one can look upon the diffusion across a membrane separating say HCl and NaCl as occurring in ion pairs, not as individual ions. Due to the smaller molecular size of HCl the "HCl side" will become temporarily hypotonic to the "NaCl side" before complete equilibration has taken place. The validity of this view point was confirmed by TEORELL in model experiments using a membrane separating a small volume of isotonic HCl from a large volume of isotonic NaCl. The HCl reservoir represented the stomach and was replentished by the introduction of more isotonic HCl at varying rates ("secretion"). The large NaCl reservoir represented the plasma. In such model experiments, and in instillation experiments in stomachs, he found that the Cl concentration and the total osmolar activity decreased with decreasing "secretory rates" showing a rise to approximate isotonicity at the lowest rates. These osmotic relations are in complete accord with the measurements by LIFSON, VARCO and VISSCHER[1273, 1340, 1341]. Further, the alterations in ionic composition (notably in

---

[1347] LINDE, S., T. TEORELL, and K. J. ÖBRINK: Experiments on the primary acidity of gastric juice. Acta physiol. scand. 14, 220—232 (1947).

[1348] HEINZ, E.: Über die primäre Azidität der Magensäure. Biochim. biophys. Acta 6, 434—444 (1950—1951).

[1349] GUGGENHEIM, E. A.: A study of cells with liquid-liquid junctions. J. Amer. Chem. Soc. 52, 1315—1337 (1930).

chloride concentration), which were observed by TEORELL in his instillation experiments were similar to the rate dependant alterations observed by LINDE and ÖBRINK[1279] in gastric juice obtained in response to histamine (cf. Fig. 22). It should also be mentioned that TERNER[1350] has demonstrated that an equilibrium diffusion may take place across the secreting, isolated gastric mucosa, and in some experiments (but not in all) did he find this process to account quantitatively for the observed reductions in acidity. TERNER does, however, point out that the isolated mucosa represents a special system, which cannot necessarily be compared to the intact mucous membrane.

In conclusion it can be said that the component theory rests on a sound foundation of histological, histochemical and physiological observation. The question is, whether an exchange diffusion may also be involved and perhaps even play a decisive role under circumstances. LINDE and ÖBRINK[1279] claim that admixture of non-parietal components could be excluded in their histamine experiment (Fig. 22), since histamine does not stimulate other cells than the parietal. However, the difficulties in quantitating the admixture of non-parietal components following different stimuli has been pointed out in a previous section of this treatise (p. 473). It appears wise not to draw too definite conclusions from analyses of the gastric juice obtained at the very low secretory rates. Conceivably therefore, the solution of the problem as to which mechanism is the more important in "acidity reduction" must come from studies, in which other experimental approaches are attempted.

3) *The intimate mechanism of alkali metal secretion by the gastric mucosa.*

a) *Electrolyte transport. The parietal component.* The parietal component contains H^+, Cl^- and according to the opinion of most workers also small quantities of K^+. Considerable attention has been given to the problem of HCl secretion. This work has been reviewed by DAVIES[1351,1352], CONWAY[1330], DAVENPORT[1353,1354], REHM[1355], REHM and DENNIS[1356] and HEINZ and ÖBRINK[1331]. It appears clearly from these reviews that the mechanism by which HCl is secreted remains incompletely understood. There are, however, certain experimental findings upon which there seems to be no disagreement, and these findings shall briefly be recapitulated. It has long been known that there is a potential difference over the gastric wall. REHM showed that this potential is localized in the mucosa and that the secretory side is negative to the nutrient. The potential decreases when secretory activity is stimulated. HOGBEN[1345] has presented good evidence that there exists an active transport mechanism for chloride ions across the gastric mucosa, and his findings have been confirmed by other investigators. However, the source of the hydrogen ions in the parietal cells and the manner in which they are transported across the

[1350] TERNER, C.: The reduction of gastric acidity by back-diffusion of hydrogen ions through the mucosa. Biochem. J. **45**, 150—158 (1949).

[1351] DAVIES, R. E.: Gastric Secretion. Mechanism. In: Jones, F. A.: Modern Trends in Gastroenterology p. 272—286 New York: Hoeber 1952.

[1352] DAVIES, R. E.: Gastric hydrochloric acid production. The present position. In Q. R. MURPHY, Metabolic Aspects of Transport across Cell Membranes. P. 277—293. Univ. Wisconsin Press. 1957.

[1353] DAVENPORT, H. W.: The secretion of acid by the gastric mucosa. Gastroenterology 1, 383—389 (1943).

[1354] DAVENPORT, H. W.: Metabolic aspects of gastric secretion. In: Murphy, Q. R.: Metabolic Aspects of Transport across Cell Membranes. P. 295—302. Univ. Wisconsin Press 1957.

[1355] REHM, W. S.: A theory of the formation of HCl by the stomach. Gastroenterology 14, 401—417 (1950).

[1356] REHM, W. S., and W. H. DENNIS: A discussion of theories of hydrochloric acid formation in the light of electrophysiological findings. In Q. R. MURPHY, Metabolic Aspects of Transport across Cell Membranes. P. 303—330. Univ. Wisconsin Press 1957.

canalicular wall and into the secretion remains unknown, although certain facts about H⁺ ion secretion have been established. It is known that the gastric mucosa contains considerable quantities of carbonic anhydrase (DAVENPORT). This enzyme catalyzes the reaction: $CO_2 + H_2O \rightarrow H_2CO_3 (\rightarrow H^+ + HCO_3^-)$. DAVIES has demonstrated that the isolated mucosa for every H⁺ ion secreted takes up 1 mol of CO_2 from the nutrient medium and gives off 1 HCO_3^- ion to the nutrient medium. Omission of external supplies of CO_2 (DAVIES) or application of potent carbonic anhydrase inhibitors (DAVENPORT) arrests acid secretion by the isolated mucosa.

The non-parietal component concists chiefly of Na⁺ and Cl⁻ and smaller quantities of K⁺ and HCO_3^- in an approximately isotonic solution. Whether an active outward transport of chloride does also take place in the "non-parietal cells" is unknown. HOGBEN[1345] has stated that the movement of Na across the gastric mucosa approaches the behaviour of a passive ion. REHM[1355] has proposed a theory of gastric secretion according to which the Cl ions and the water are secreted by the parietal cells, whereas the H, Na and K ions are secreted by the surface epithelial cells. There are, however, several objections to such an hypothesis and the crucial experiments to prove or disprove its validity are still lacking.

b) Water transport. Blood pressure is not the driving force for the water transport across the gastric mucosa. This is evident from the histological structure of the mucosa and the organization of the blood supply as well as from the fact that the isolated mucosa can secrete (even against considerable hydrostatic pressure). As in the case of other secreting organs it must be assumed that water moves from the nutrient to the secretory side in passive sequence of active electrolyte transport, forming an isotonic or slightly hypertonic secretory product. This assumption is supported by the findings on the effect of variations in plasma osmolarity on the volume and composition of the gastric juice (cf. p. 473).

c) The intestinal mucosa

Comparatively pure intestinal secretions can be obtained from man by the use of special intubation methods (see i.a. OWLES[1357]). Most data on the composition of the intestinal secretions have, however, been obtained in acute or chronic experiments on animals with surgical isolation of parts of the intestine. A surgical procedure for isolation of the duodenum with restoration of normal drainage of bile and pancreatic juice has been described by FLOREY and HARDING[1358]. Segments of the jejunum or of the ileum are rather easily isolated as Thiry-Vella fistula, and a segment of the colon can be exposed in a similar manner.

Most analyses of intestinal secretions are concerned with enzyme activities, whereas there are surprisingly few data on the electrolyte concentrations. In evaluating electrolyte concentrations and volume rates of the succus entericus it is of importance to realize that these secretions are delivered into a viscus, which is readily permeable to most of the secreted ions and which moreover posesses mechanisms for active reabsorption of sodium ions (cf. section on intestinal absorption of electrolytes, p. 508).

Type of gland. *Duodenum.* The duodenal secretion is mucinous, highly viscous and waterclear. The volume rates from isolated duodenal segments of various animals range from about 1 to about 8 ml/hr, depending upon the size of the animal. Secretory rate increases slightly after a meal, slightly after injection of hista-

---

[1357] OWLES, W. H.: Investigations of the function of the small intestine in man by intestinal intubation. Clin. Sci. **3**, 1—36 (1937).

[1358] FLOREY, H. W., and H. E. HARDING: The nature of the hormone controlling Brunner's glands. Quart. J. exp. Physiol. **25**, 329—339 (1935).

mine[1359] or pilocarpine[1360] and to a somewhat larger extent following injection of secretin[1358],[1359].

The secretion is approximately isotonic with the plasma and has a p_H ranging from about 8 to about 9.3 in different species. The duodenal secretion of the rabbit is thus more alkaline than that of the dog[1361]. The entire buffer capacity of the duodenal secretion is due to the presence of bicarbonate. The mucus has almost no buffer capacity[1362]. The electrolyte composition has been examined by FUKUSHIMA[1363] and FLOREY and HARDING[1361]:

p_H	8.0— 9.3[1361]	(dog, rabbit)
Na meq/l	101 —130[1363]	(dog)
K meq/l	23.7— 20.5[1363]	(dog)
Cl meq/l	122 —130[1363]	(dog)
HCO_3 meq/l	40 — 86[1361]	(dog, rabbit)

The K concentration reported by FUKUSHIMA appears surprisingly large as compared to the K conc. in the other intestinal secretions.

Jejunum. Secretory rate is about 3—5 ml per hour in loops of 10—30. cm's length. The rate is only little affected by ingestion of food. The jejunal secretion is approximately isotonic with the plasma. Electrolyte concentrations have been examined by GAMBLE and McIVER[1220], DEBEER, JOHNSTON and WILSON[1364] and SCHRIFFIN and NASSET[1365]. Their results are shown in Table 40.

Table 40. *Electrolytes in jejunal secretion.* All data in meq/l

Reference	[1220]	[1364]	[1365]
Species	cat	dog	dog
p_H	—	6.80 (6.30—7.28)	—
Na		142 (131—152)	—
K	172 (157—194)*	6.45 (4.2—10.2)	—
Ca		3.4 (1.6—5.4)	—
Cl	130 (129—131)	148 (141—153)	130—150
HCO_3	—	19.2 (5.2—30.0)	10

     * Total "base"

Ileum. Secretory rate is slightly lower than in the jejunum[1365] and little, if at all, affected by the ingestion of food. Electrolyte concentrations have been determined by DEBEER, JOHNSTON and WILSON[1364] and SCHRIFFIN and NASSET[1365]. Their results are illustrated in Table 41.

[1359] FOGELSON, S. J., and W. H. BACHRACH: Response of Brunner's glands to secretin. Amer. J. Physiol. **128**, 121—123 (1939).

[1360] FLOREY, H. W., and H. E. HARDING: The functions of the Brunner's glands and the pyloric end of the stomach. J. Path. Bact. **37**, 431—453 (1933).

[1361] FLOREY, H. W., and H. E. HARDING: Further observations on the secretion of the Brunner glands. J. Path. Bact. **39**, 255—276 (1934).

[1362] HAVARD, R. E.: The buffering power of the duodenal mucin obtained in the secretion of the Brunner's glands. J. Path. Bact. **39**, 277—279 (1934).

[1363] FUKUSHIMA, K.: On the ion concentration of the digestive juices. Med. J. Osaka Univ. **2**, 583—586 (1951).

[1364] DEBEER, E. J., C. G. JOHNSTON and D. W. WILSON: The composition of the intestinal secretions. J. biol. Chem. **108**, 113—120 (1935).

[1365] SCHRIFFIN, M. J., and E. S. NASSET: The response of jejunum and ileum to food and enterocrinin. Amer. J. Physiol. **128**, 70—80 (1939).

Table 41. *Electrolytes in ileal secretion.* All data in meq/l

Reference	1364	1365
Species	dog	dog
p$_H$ . . .	7.61	—
Na. . . .	151 (146—156)	—
K	4.7	—
Ca . . .	5.5	—
Cl	78 (68—87)	96—101
HCO$_3$ . .	83 (69—97)	63—64

Table 42. *Electrolytes in colonic secretion.* All data in meq/l

Reference	1364	1366
Species	dog	cat
p$_H$ . . .	7.99 (7.94—8.03)	8.3—8.4
Na. . . .	147 (136—153)	—
K	7.2 (5.7—8.6)	—
Ca . . .	4.2 (3.2—5.0)	1
Cl	77 (59—88)	100
HCO$_3$ . .	90 (86—93)	—

Colon. The secretion of the colon is mucinous and viscous. WRIGHT, FLOREY and JENNINGS[1366] found no secretion from the unstimulated colonic mucosa of the cat. When pilocarpine or eserine were injected or when the nervi erigentes were electrically stimulated secretion rate was about 10 ml/hr from the entire viscus. Mucus was reabsorbed from the colon at the rate of 23 ml per 3 hr.

The electrolytes in the colonic secretion have been determined by DeBEER, JOHNSTON and WILSON[1364] and by WRIGHT, FLOREY and JENNINGS[1366]. The results are shown in Table 42.

Rate of secretion. The variations in secretory rate appear to be small, particularly in the small intestine. It is the impression of FUKUSHIMA[1363] as well as of SCHRIFFIN and NASSET[1365] that the electrolyte composition of duodenal, jejunal and ileal secretions is not influenced by the minor increases in secretory rate which follow ingestion of a meal.

Plasma concentration of the alkali metals (total osmolar concentration of the plasma). DeBEER, JOHNSTON and WILSON[1364] studied the effect of intravenous administration of hypertonic NaCl and Na$_2$CO$_3$ on the composition of the jejunal, ileal and colonic secretions of the dog. The results are presented in Tables 43 and 44.

It appears from Tables 43 and 44 that a variation in the total osmolar concentration of the plasma by hypertonic loading is followed by an almost parallel variation in the total osmolar concentration of the jejunal and the ileal contents. The colonic secretion is little affected, but the increase in plasma Cl was small in this experiment. Whether NaCl or Na$_2$CO$_3$ is used does not appear to make any difference with respect to the changes in Cl and HCO$_3$ concentration of the jejunal contents. It must be born in mind that the mucosa of the small intestine is readily permeable to water and electrolytes (cf. p. 508). The alterations observed in the

Table 43. *Effect of loading with hypertonic NaCl.* All data in meq/l.

	Jejunal secretion		Ileal secretion		Colonic secretion	
	before	after	before	after	before	after
Plasma Cl . .	110	160	114	160.9	117	128
Secretion p$_H$.	6.73	6.47	8.66	7.30	7.92	7.96
Na$^+$ . . .	136.4	163.8	155.2	180.4	149	150
K$^+$ . . .	6.6	5.4	6.8	10.2	5.0	5.5
Ca^{++} . .	2.7	3.0	5.0	4.9	1.5	1.5
Cl$^-$ . . .	147.6	184.6	80.1	112.7	90	88
HCO$_3$$^-$ . .	23.8	17.9	114.0	94.0	90.3	97

[1366] WRIGHT, R. D., H. W. FLOREY, and M. A. JENNINGS: The secretion of the colon of the cat. Quart. J. exp. Physiol. 28, 207—229 (1938).

jejunal and ileal contents during hypertonic loading may therefore be due to a secondary equilibration between the secreted juice and the plasma by diffusion through interstitial spaces or through cells other than those engaged in the secretory process. On the other hand it is worth remembering that a similar close correlation between plasma and secretion osmolarity has been found in a number of other secreting organs (cf. p. 437, 473 and 489).

Table 44. *Effect of loading with hypertonic* Na_2CO_3. *All data in meq/l.*

	Jejunal secretion	
	before	after
Plasma		
Cl . . .	107.6	97.2
HCO$_3$.	32.2	49.4
Secretion		
Na$^+$ . . .	148.4	158.6
K$^+$.	5.3	3.0
Ca^{++} . .	1.4	2.2
Cl$^-$ . . .	143.6	160.7
HCO$_3$$^-$	24.7	16.3

The alkali metals in the intestine. MANERY and HASTINGS[138] have determined the alkali metals in the intestine (mucosa, muscularis, serosa). The results are demonstrated in Table 45.

The mechanism of intestinal secretion. The mechanism of intestinal secretion remains unknown. In the small intestine there is hardly any potential difference across the mucosa, a finding which is in keeping with the fact that the mucosa of the small intestine is highly permeable to ions (cf. p. 509). In the large intestine there is a decided potential difference between the outside ("secretory side") and the inside ("nutrient side or blood side"), the latter being positive as compared to the outside. By his short-circuiting technique, USSING has shown that the large intestinal potential in the isolated mucosa is entirely due to active reabsorption of sodium ions (p. 137). In parallel to the frog skin (p. 118) one might have expected a small contribution to the potential by the secretory cells in the colon (active outward transport of chloride), but in the isolated mucosa this is either non-existing or too small to be resolved from the overwhelming influence of the active inward sodium transport.

Table 45. *Electrolyte composition of the intestine*

Species (site)	Fresh tissue				Blood and fat free tissue			
	% water	meq/l of tissue water			% water	meq/l of tissue water		
		Na	K	Cl		Na	K	Cl
rabbit (small intestine)	82.5	60.5	—	52.5	83.1	60.0	—	51.8
rabbit 1 (cocum)	87.1	46.9	—	28.2	87.3	46.9	—	28.3
rabbit 2 (coecum)	79.5	66.8	—	30.6	81.5	66.4	—	30.3
rabbit (colon)	74.8	74.9	—	58.7	78.3	74.8	—	58.6

C) The liver and the gall bladder

a) Hepatic bile

Collection of hepatic bile. Fractional collection of bile originating chiefly from the liver or chiefly from the gall bladder ("A, B, and C bile") can be performed by duodenal aspiration following instillation of magnesium sulfate or injection of cholecystokinin. The demarcation between the fractions is, however, not sharp and contamination with other duodenal secretions is inescapable. Most analyses of the composition of human bile have therefore been carried out on specimens obtained from patients with surgical drainage of the biliary tract. A great many of the older reports refer to the composition of bile flowing from cholecystostomies. These analyses must be regarded with considerable reserve, since the bile has been exposed for undetermined periods to the concentrating activity of the gall bladder. The total quantity of bile solids excreted is probably little affected by this circumstance, but the volume and the electrolyte concentrations have been altered to an unpredictable extent. Analyses of bile from a choledochal drainage in cholecystectomized patients are more reliable measures of the composition of hepatic bile provided that liver function is unimpaired. Normally it is, however, not possible to obtain an estimate of the total quantity of bile secreted, since a variable amount is flowing into the duodenum and leaking into the pericholedochal space. Only in work on animals is it possible to get a quantitative recovery of the total volume of bile secreted by the liver. A method for permanent sterile drainage of the common duct has been devised by Rous and McMaster[1367].

One problem is common to all methods of external bile drainage in man and in animals, i.e. the effect of the complete removal of the bile on the volume and composition of the hepatic secretion. There appears to be a species difference in the tolerance to the procedure, but the effect on all species is a gradual reduction in the rate of biliary secretion due to the interruption of the normal circulation of the bile acids. Ideally therefore, chronic fistula methods should involve a devise for the reintroduction into the intestine of the greater part of the harvested bile.

The electrolyte composition of hepatic bile. Analyses of the electrolyte composition of hepatic bile are listed in Table 46.

Table 46. *Electrolyte composition of hepatic bile.* All data in meq/l.

Reference	[1368]	[1369]	[1220]	[1370]	[1371]	[1372]	[1373]	[1374]
Species	man	man	cat	rabbit	dog	dog	dog	man
p_H	—	7.30	—	—	7.1—8.6	7.40	—	—
Na	133	—	172	151	174	174	221	—
K	8.7	4.9		5.7		6.6	6.08	4.5
Ca	0.4	5.0		4.8		8.8	—	—
Mg	—	1.5		0.5		3.6	—	—
Cl	117	96	120	75	55	64	—	—
HCO_3 ...	3	—	—	—	64.8	34	—	—

[1367] Rous, P., and P. D. McMaster: A method for the permanent sterile drainage of intraabdominal ducts as applied to the common duct. J. exp. Med. **37**, 11—20 (1923).

[1368] Hammarsen, O.: Zur Kenntnis der Lebergalle des Menschen. Nova Acta Soc. Scient. Uppsaliensis. **16**, Ser. III, 1—44 (1893).

[1369] Tschopp, E.: Rückresorption als biologisches Prinzip. Schweiz. med. Wschr. **57**, 1065—1067 (1927).

[1370] Stransky, E.: Pharmakologie der Gallensekretion. IV: Ausscheidung von Stoffen durch die Galle. Z. ges. exp. Med. **77**, 807—841 (1931).

[1371] Ravdin, J. S., C. G. Johnston, C. Riegel, and S. L. Wright: Studies on gall bladder function VII. The anion-cation content of hepatic bile and gall bladder bile. Amer. J. Physiol. **100**, 317—327 (1932).

[1372] Reinhold, J. G., and D. W. Wilson: Acid base composition of hepatic bile. Amer. J. Physiol. **107**, 378—405 (1934).

[1373] Cook, D. L., C. A. Lawler, L. D. Calvin, and D. M. Green: Mechanisms of bile formation. Amer. J. Physiol. **171**, 62—74 (1952).

[1374] Gilleland, J. L., J. H. Gast, and B. Halpert: Sodium and potassium concentration in bile from human gallbladders. Proc. Soc. exp. Biol. (N. Y.) **94**, 118—119 (1957).

The concentration of total solids in hepatic bile is usually about $2-4\%$[1368, 1375], but values up to 10% have been reported[1375]. The fluctuation in total solids may at, least in part be due to experimental conditions. Thus SCHMIDT et al.[1376] found an excretion of 1.2 to 1.6 g of bile acids per day in dogs if the bile drainage was not fed back to the animals. If the harvested bile was reintroduced in the intestine, the total quantity of bile acids ranged from 6.5 to 9.0 g with minor day to day fluctuations in the individual dog. It appears from Table 46 that the p_H, the sodium concentration and partly also the chloride concentration of the bile are quite variable. Most workers find p_H values between 7.00 and 7.60[1369, 1372, 1375, 1377]. The high p_H values (8 or above 8) which have been reported by some investigators are probably due to analytical error (escape of CO_2). REINHOLD and WILSON[1372] have presented evidence indicating that the fluctuations in bile acid concentration, p_H and sodium concentration are interrelated. They found the following relationship in the dog (only extreme values are presented):

Bile acids:	$37.8-101.5$	meq/l
Sodium:	$157\ \ -178$	meq/l
Chloride:	$69\ -\ 64$	meq/l
Bicarbonate:	$55.7-\ 22.7$	meq/l

According to these analyses an increase in bile acid concentration is followed by a marked decrease in bicarbonate, a small decrease in chloride and a pronounced increase in sodium concentration of the bile.

The high sodium concentrations which run parallel to high concentrations of bile acids do not cause an increase in the osmotic pressure of the hepatic bile. All workers agree that the total osmolar concentration of hepatic bile (as measured by freezing point depression) is very constant and approximately equal to that of the plasma (see i.a.[1233, 1372, 1375, 1378, 1379]). It must therefore be assumed that part of the sodium ions are held in an osmotically inactive form, probably by electrostatic forces in macromolecular complexes of bile salts, lipids and protein.

Rate of secretion. The total volume of bile secreted by the human liver cannot be stated exactly. Quantitative recovery is normally not possible in patients with choledochal drainage (cf. p. 487) and the secretory activity of the liver depends upon whether the collected bile is discarded or returned to the patients digestive tract. Most workers consider the daily production of hepatic bile to be about 700 to 1500 ml in man (see SOBOTKA[1375]).

The liver secretes continuously with certain fluctuations in the course of the day. BRAND[1378] thus found a maximum in the late afternoon and a minimum during night. BRAND states that the salt concentration of the bile is not affected by these spontaneous variations in the volume rate of secretion.

SCHIFF[1380] first demonstrated that the complete external drainage of bile leads to a reduction in the rate of bile formation and that the reintroduction of the

---

[1375] SOBOTKA, H.: Physiological Chemistry of the Bile. Baltimore: Williams & Wilkins 1937.

[1376] SCHMIDT, C. R., J. M. BEAGELL, A. L. BERMAN, A. C. IVY, and A. J. ATKINSON: Studies on the secretion of bile. Amer. J. Physiol. **126**, 120—135 (1939).

[1377] REINHOLD, J. G., and L. K. FERGUSON: Reaction of human bile and its relation to gall stone formation. J. exp. Med. **49**, 681—694 (1929).

[1378] BRAND, J.: Beitrag zur Kenntnis der menschlichen Galle. Pflügers Arch. ges. Physiol. **90**, 491—522 (1902).

[1379] STRAUSS, H.: Osmotischer Druck der menschlichen Galle. Berlin. klin. Wschr. **40**, 261—264 (1903).

[1380] SCHIFF, M.: Gallenbildung abhängig von der Aufsaugung der Gallenstoffe. Pflügers Arch. ges. Physiol. **3**, 598—613 (1870).

secreted bile into the intestinal tract restores normal rates. This finding has been confirmed by all later workers in the field, and it has been shown that there is a species difference in the tolerance to external drainage (cf. SOBOTKA[1375]).

Administration of *bile acids* (or salts of the bile acids) to man and animals has a stimulating effect on bile flow. A temporary increase in secretory rate of about 100—300% is not uncommonly seen. Apparently, the conjugated bile acids (glyco- or taurocholate) cause an increase in the volume as well as in the concentration of total solids in the bile ("choleretic effect"). The unconjugated cholic acid (or its less toxic derivates) promote bile flow, but not solid excretion and the concentration of total solids decreases ("hydrocholeretic effect"). For details the reader is referred to the papers by NEUBAUER[1381], ADLERSBERG and NEUBAUER[1382] and HOEHN and JOHNSON[1383] as well as to the monograph by SOBOTKA[1375].

The concentrations of the different electrolytes in the bile are not measurably affected by variations in the rate of bile production following administration of "hydrocholeretic" substances (COOK, LAWLER and GREEN[1384]).

Unconjugated and conjugated bile acids have hydrocholeretic resp. choleretic effect on the bile formation in isolated livers, which are perfused at a constant rate (BRAUER and PESSOLLI[1385]). BRAUER and PESSOLLI interprate this finding as indicating that the bile acid preparations act directly on the liver cells and not via a change in liver blood flow. The mechanism by which the bile acids stimulate bile flow remains unknown.

Secretin has a moderate "hydrocholeretic" effect on bile secretion in patients with choledochal drainage[1386]. *Cholinergic substances* and *atropine* do not measurably affect the volume rate of secretion[1376].

According to WESTPHAL et al.[1387] stimulation of the right vagal nerve causes a moderate increase in the flow of hepatic bile in the well-hydrated dog, but depresses bile flow in the thirsting dog.

Plasma concentration of the alkali metals (total osmolar concentration of the plasma). GILMAN and COWGILL[1233] have shown that extreme variations in the total osmolar concentration of the plasma, produced by the injection of hypertonic saline or water, results in parallel changes in the osmolar concentration of the hepatic bile in the dog. This finding corresponds closely to the results of similar studies on the gastric secretion (p. 473), the intestinal secretions (p. 485) and the pancreatic secretion (p. 462) The variations in the concentration of individual electrolytes in bile and plasma were not studied by GILMAN and COWGILL.

Hepatic blood flow and oxygen supply. The blood supply of the liver differs fundamentally from that of other secreting systems and the formation of bile represents only one out of many hepatic functions. The mechanism by which hepatic bile is formed remains unknown. An attempt at correlating blood flow,

[1381] NEUBAUER, E.: Dehydrocholsäure, ein wirksames ungiftiges Glied der Gallensäuregruppe. Klin. Wschr. 2, 1065—1067 (1923).

[1382] ADLERSBERG, D., and E. NEUBAUER: Einfluß von Dehydrocholsäure auf Galle, Blut und Harn. Z. exp. Med. 48, 291—305 (1926).

[1383] HOEHN, W. H., and R. JOHNSON: Toxicity of sodium 3.1.2 dihydroxy-7-cholanate and its influence on the bile flow in rats. J. Amer. Pharm. Ass. 35, 296—297 (1946).

[1384] COOK, D. L., C. A. LAWLER, and D. M. GREEN: Studies on the effect of hydrocholeretic agents on hepatic excretory mechanisms. J. Pharm. exp. Ther. 110, 293—299 (1954).

[1385] BRAUER, R. W., and R. L. PESSOLLI: Effect of choleretic and hydrocholeretic agents on bile flow and bile solids in the isolated perfused liver. Science 115, 142—143 (1952).

[1386] GROSMAN, M. I., H. D. JANOWITZ, H. RALSTON, and K. S. KIM: The effect of secretin on bile formation in man. Gastroenterology 12, 133—138 (1949).

[1387] WESTPHAL, K., F. GLEICHMANN, and G. SOIKA: Thierexperimentelle Untersuchungen über nervös bedingte Resorptionsschwankungen der Gallenblase mit teilweiser Berücksichtigung des Lebergallenflusses. Pflügers Arch. ges. Physiol. 227, 204—219 (1931).

oxygen uptake and electrolyte transport rates is therefore futile at the present time.

COOK, LAWLER, CALVIN and GREEN[1373] found that ligation of the hepatic arteries in the dog does neither affect bile flow nor the concentrations of sodium, potassium and chloride in the bile. POPPER, JEFFERSON, WULKAN and NECHELESS[1388] ligated the hepatic artery and the portal vein of dogs and found that the formation of bile proceeded at unaltered rates in the surviving animals. These workers conclude that the small amount of arterial blood which reaches the liver through the hepatic branches of the phrenic arteries and through filamentous arterial collaterals is sufficient to maintain bile production. Conflicting reports in the older litterature regarding the tolerance to hepatic arterial and portal vein ligation and its effect on bile secretion are probably due to individual variations in the development of this collateral cirvulation.

These findings indicate that the rate of bile secretion from the liver *in situ* is independent of large variations in blood supply. BRAUER, LEONG and HOLLOWAY[1389] obtained similar results on the *isolated* perfused rat liver. However, if the rate of blood perfusion was reduced below a certain critical limit bile flow fell off sharply. This critical perfusion rate increased, if the oxygen tension of the perfusate was lowered (BRAUER, ELROY, LEONG and HOLLOWAY[1390]).

Temperature. Local application of heat to the liver region has been advocated as having a choleretic effect on patients. Experimental results on animals are somewhat conflicting, but on the whole they have not confirmed the clinical impression. With constant perfusate pressure, but variable perfusate temperature, BRAUER et al. found maximal volumes of secretion between 38 and 40° C in the isolated rat liver. Above and below this temperature there was a rapid decline in secretory rate and irreversible damage to the secretory mechanism was noted if extremes of perfusate temperature were maintained for too long.

The excretion of lithium in the hepatic bile. COOK et al.[1373] have found that lithium is excreted in the bile following intraperitoneal injection of LiCl. The bile/plasma concentration ratio was not stated.

The mechanism of alkali metal excretion in the bile. The unique character of the hepatic secretion as an excretum and a digestive juice, the apparent high permeability of the bile capillaries to a number of substances, not normally appearing in other secretions, and the low pressures against which the flow of bile is completely arrested represent some of the more puzzling differences between bile and other secretory products. Processes of filtration, active secretion, passive backflow and active reabsorption have all been considered as essential to bile production, but the mechanism of bile formation and particularly the electrolyte secretion has not yet been clarified in detail.

On the basis of renal clearance techniques COOK et al.[1373] have suggested that a process of filtration by pressure difference is responsible for the outward transport of water and several bile solutes, including the chief electrolytes. According to this theory the hepatic cells only contribute to the bile such compounds, for which active secretory processes must be surmised (bilirubin, bromsulfalein, several antibiotics etc.).

The hypothesis by COOK et al.[1373] has been critisized by BRAUER and his collegues[1389]. Bile secretion can take place against pressures which exceed portal

[1388] POPPER, H. L., N. C. JEFFERSON, E. WULKAN, and H. NECHELES: Bile secretion and blood supply of the liver. Amer. J. Physiol. 181, 435—438 (1955).
[1389] BRAUER, R. W., G. F. LEONG, and R. J. HOLLOWAY: Mechanics of bile secretion. Effect of perfusion pressure and temperature on bile flow and bile secretion pressure. Amer. J. Physiol. 177, 103—112 (1954).
[1390] BRAUER, R. W., R. E. McELROY, G. F. LEONG and R. J. HOLLOWAY: Mechanism of bile formation. Role of oxygen supply. Fed. Proc. 14, 322 (1955).

vein pressure in the intact animal as well as in the isolated perfused liver preparation. BRAUER et al.[1389] further showed that the flow of bile from the isolated liver is independent of a wide range of variation in perfusate pressure. The drop in bile flow, which is noted at the lowest perfusate pressures, is presumably due to a decrease in blood flow (which may become unevenly distributed to different liver lobules) and not to the decrease in blood pressure. BRAUER et al. conclude that a filtration mechanism plays little (if any) role in the process of bile formation. They consider the secretion of bile to be dependent upon active secretory mechanisms in the hepatic cells. These secretory mechanisms can be specifically depressed or stimulated by procedures which involve no change in perfusion pressure or flow [cf. section on temperature effect on bile flow (p. 490) as well as the discussion of the action of hydrocholeretic and choleretic agents on the isolated liver preparation (p. 489)]. The findings of BRAUER et al.[1389] further indicate that the arrest of bile flow which occurs when the pressure in the biliary ducts exceeds a certain critical limit is due to a backflow of bile from the ducts and not to an arrest of bile production.

The demonstration by COOK et al.[1373] that inulin and certain other non-electrolytes such as glucose, appear in the bile in concentrations almost equal to those of the plasma does not necessarily mean that the hepatic bile is elaborated by a filtration process. The hepatic cells, and particularly the intercellular substance in the region of the bile ducts through which back flow of bile can occur may well be highly permeable structures. An equilibration by simple diffusion processes between the forming bile and the plasma is by no means a remote possibility. Inspection of the data by COOK et al.[1373] reveals considerable variations in the individual B/P ratios (inulin about $1/2$, glucose about $1/1$) indicating that the different substances do not equilibrate with the bile at equal rates. The standard deviations of the different B/P ratios are, however, so large that the figures do not permit a statistical study of the respective rates of transfer.

The intimate secretory mechanism of the hepatic cells is not understood. The statement by KELLER[1391] that the bile ducts are electrically negative as compared to the surrounding tissue is based on staining reactions. The actual potential difference over the walls of the bile ducts has not been directly measured. If the bile ducts are as readily permeable to ions as they appear to be to certain non-electrolytes[1373], it is quite possible that a measurable potential difference cannot be maintained between the lumen and the blood side, even in the case that an active outward net transport of anion or cation does occur (compare section on intestinal secretion, p. 486).

BRAND[1378] first suggested the possibility that the bile ducts (like the gall bladder) possess reabsorptive functions. BRAND comments on the inverse relationship between chloride concentration and the concentration of total solids and suggests that the bile is concentrated in the ducts by reabsorption of salt and water. With a number of substances which are concentrated in the bile (bilirubin, bromsulfalein, antibiotics etc.) it has however been shown that the B/P ratios and the clearance rates decrease with increasing plasma concentration (COOK et al.[1373]). This suggests an active outward secretion of these solutes rather than a concentration by reabsorption of water from a precursor secretion, which is in equilibrium with the plasma. The back flow of bile which has been demonstrated by BRAUER et al. does not occur unless bile pressure exceeds a certain critical limit and is probably dependent upon simple hydrostatic forces. At the present time there is thus no evidence to suggest that electrolytes and water are actively reabsorbed by the bile ducts.

[1391] KELLER, R.: Zur Elektrochemie der Leber und der Galle. Biochem. Z. **257**, 78—85 (1933).

b) Gall bladder bile

The secretion of bile from the liver is a continuous process, although certain spontaneous variations do occur. The outflow of bile into the duodenum is, however, a discontinuous process in such species as are in possession of a gall bladder and a choledocho-duodenal sphincter.

As long as the sphincter of Oddi is closed the continuous flow of bile from the liver causes the pressure in the choledochus to increase. The increase in pressure forces the bile to enter the gall bladder via the cystic duct. The cystic duct does not have a sphincter of its own, but it is possible that the valves of Heister subserve such function, since it has been suggested that they offer less resistance to flow from the common duct towards the gall bladder than in the reverse direction (LÖHNER[1392]). In response to humoral or nervous stimuli elicited from the duodenal mucosa the gall bladder contracts and the sphincter Oddii relaxes with the result that gall bladder contents are emptied into the duodenum.

The volume of the gall bladder is small as compared to the volume of bile produced by the liver, even within a limited period of time. The reservoir function of the bladder would thus be negligeable were it not for the fact that its reabsorptive capacity is considerable. In fact, the reabsorptive capacity is so large that it has been estimated that the gall bladder can hold in a concentrated from about $^1/_4$ to $^1/_2$ of the total daily bile production. Besides having a reabsorptive function the gall bladder mucosa adds to the bile a secretion of its own, probably consisting chiefly of mucus.

Most analyses of gall bladder bile have been performed on single specimens removed during surgery on man or animals. Naturally such data only give a static picture of the dynamic processes of reabsorption (and secretion) in the gall bladder.

The electrolyte composition of gall bladder bile. There are surprisingly few analyses of the electrolyte composition of gall bladder bile. Table 47 presents the data of GAMBLE and McIVER[1220], RAVDIN, JOHNSTON, RIEGEL and WRIGHT,[1371] GILLELAND, GAST and HALPERT[1374], TELFER[1393] and HERMAN, WILSON and KAZYALE [1397].

Table 47. *Electrolyte composition of gall bladder bile.* All data in meq/l

Reference	1374	1393	1220	1371	1397
Species	man*	man	cat	dog	guinea pig
pH	6.72 (±50)	—	—	6.3—7.5	—
Na	169 (±25)	—	} 261—318	} 287—325	—
K	27 (±11)	—			7.06 (6.1 - 7.7)
Ca	—	4—29			—
Cl	—	30—70	0—20	1.4—4.7	—
HCO/	—	—	—	—	—
bile acid . .	—	—	—	289—343	—

* post mortem

The concentration of solids in gall bladder bile is usually much higher than in the hepatic bile. According to different investigators the concentration of solids ranges from about 10 to about 35% (for references see SOBOTKA[1375]).

[1392] LÖHNER, L.: Zur Füllungs- und Entleerungsmechanik der Gallenblase und zur Funktion der Valvulae Heisteri. Pflügers Arch. ges. Physiol. **211**, 356—372 (1926).
[1393] TELFER, S. V.: Concentration of human bile constituents in human gall bladder. Glasgow med. J. **30**, 395—399 (1949).

The reaction of gall bladder bile is usually more acid than that of hepatic bile (see Table 48).

The osmotic pressure of gall bladder bile is almost identical to the osmotic pressure of the plasma. This was clearly demonstrated by BRAND[1378] and has been confirmed by all later investigators. It must thus be assumed that a considerable fraction of the sodium in gall bladder bile is held in an osmotically inactive form by binding to complexes of bile acids, cholesterol and protein. RAVDIN et al.[1371] thus found 287 to 325 meq of sodium in bladder bile (cf. Table 47), but the freezing point depression of the bile was only $0.563-0.576°$ C.

The reabsorptive functions of the gall bladder. The physiology of the gall bladder has been extensively reviewed by IVY[1398] in 1934.

The high concentration of solids in the gall bladder bile has been

Table 48. p_H of hepatic bile and gall bladder bile

Author	Species	p_H hepatic bile	p_H gall bladder bile
DRURY, MCMASTER and ROUS[1394]	dog	8.20	5.18—6.00
BARRY and LEVINE[1395]	man	7.2—7.8	5.6—7.2
TSCHOPP[1369]	man	7.3	6.2
STERN[1396]	man	6.9	6.0—7.0
REINHOLD and FERGUSON[1377]	man	6.86—7.39	6.78—7.15
RAVDIN, JOHNSTON, RIEGEL and WRIGHT[1371]	dog	7.1—8.6	6.3—7.5

known from an early date, and it has been assumed for a long time that the gall bladder exerts its concentrating function chiefly by reabsorption of water from the hepatic bile. The first clear suggestion of such an hypothesis was presented by BRAND[1378] who studied the relationship between the total solids of the bile and its concentration of chloride. BRAND found that the chloride concentration invariably decreases as the concentration of solids increases. He concluded that the gall bladder mucosa concentrates the hepatic bile by the reabsorption of an isotonic solution of sodium chloride.

This hypothesis has received experimental support from investigations on the reabsorption of salt solutions and of hepatic bile from cannulated or ligated gall bladders *in situ*. The classical work by ROUS and MCMASTER[1399, 1400] and the extensive studies by RAVDIN and collaborators[1401, 1371] represent the first attempts to clarify the dynamics of the reabsorptive process by such technique. In this place we shall consider first the fate of salt solutions which are introduced into the bile free, ligated gall bladder.

[1394] DRURY, D. R., P. D. MCMASTER, and P. ROUS: Observations on some causes of gall stone formation. J. exp. Med. **39**, 403—423 (1924).

[1395] BARRY, W. M., and V. E. LEVINE: The oxidation and reduction of bile pigments. J. biol. Chem. 59, LII (1924).

[1396] STERN, R.: Klinische Bedeutung des Cholesterins in der Galle. Naunyn-Schmiedebergs Arch. exp. Path. Pharmak. **131**, 221—232 (1926).

[1397] HERMAN, R. H., T. H. WILSON, and L. KAZYALE: Electrolyte migration across the guinea pig gall bladder. J. coll. comp. Physiol. **51**, 133—144 (1958).

[1398] IVY, A. C.: The physiology of the gall bladder. Physiol. Rev. 14, 1—102 (1934).

[1399] ROUS, P., and P. D. MCMASTER: The concentrating activity of the gall bladder. J. exp. Med. **34**, 47—73 (1921).

[1400] ROUS, P., and P. D. MCMASTER: Physiological causes for the varied character of stasis bile. J. exp. Med. **34**, 75—95 (1921).

[1401] RAVDIN, I. S., C. G. JOHNSTON, J. H. AUSTIN, and C. RIEGEL: Studies on gall bladder function. IV. The absorption of chloride from the bile free gall bladder. Amer. J. Physiol. **99**, 638—647 (1931—32).

a) *The reabsorption of salt solutions*. BILLARD and CAVALIÉ[1402] were apparently the first investigators who studied this problem. They showed that the bile free ligated gall bladder absorbed water at the rate of about 3 ml/hr, and that the rate of reabsorption was faster from isotonic than from hypertonic solutions. The first investigation in which the transfer of water and electrolytes was quantitated was performed by RAVDIN, JOHNSTON, AUSTIN and RIEGEL[1401]. RAVDIN et al. found that water flows out of the gall bladder at the rate of about 6 ml/hr when isotonic solutions of sodium chloride are introduced. It appears from their tables that outward salt transfer was slightly greater than the rate of water outflow, since the concentration of total anions in the bladder contents was consistently slightly lower at the end of an experiment than at the beginning. This finding indicates that the reabsorptive process operates on the salt and not on the water. A better indication of active salt reabsorption is, however, furnished by some experiments in which it was found, that a net outward transfer of chloride takes place against the concentration gradient from hypotonic solutions (68.4 mM).

GRIM and SMITH[1403] have recently studied the water fluxes across ligated gall bladders which were filled with iso- and anisotonic solutions of NaCl in D_2O. These workers found that a net outflux of water occurred at about equal rates from isotonic and hypotonic solutions. Net outflux was arrested when the sodium conc. of the introduced solutions exceeded 220 mEq/l. With isotonic solutions net outflux rates of the order of 200 to 260 μl/min could be observed, and according to GRIM and SMITH this net transfer is larger per unit surface area than that of the ileum.

If solutions of sodium chloride are left for a sufficient period of time in the gall bladder they are completely absorbed by the mucosa (HERMANN[1404]).

b) *The reabsorption of hepatic bile*. The reabsorptive functions of the gall bladder can be estimated by simultaneous analyses of hepatic bile and gall bladder bile. Determination of "total solids" indicates that the gall bladder bile is from 5 to 20 times more concentrated than the hepatic bile (for detailed references see IVY[1398]). The best reference substances to test the degree of concentration are apparently the bile pigments. Bile pigment is neither reabsorbed to any measurable degree, nor is it secreted by the bladder wall.

Single determinations of the bladder bile/hepatic bile concentration ratio for bile pigment can however at most give a measure of the maximal concentrating capacity of the gall bladder, but yields no information about the dynamics of the reabsorptive process. ROUS and McMASTER[1399] first studied the rate of reabsorption and found that a gall bladder, emptied at the beginning of an experiment and left to fill from the liver, concentrated 49.8 ml of bile reaching it in $22^1/_2$ hr to 4.6 ml or about 10 fold. The average concentration in a series of experiments of this type was 7.1 fold. However, if hepatic bile was introduced through the fundus and recovered from the cystic duct it was concentrated from 2.3 to 4.8 times *merely in its passage through the bladder*.

RAVDIN, JOHNSTON, RIEGEL and WRIGHT[1401] instilled measured quantities of hepatic bile in dog gall bladders by the same method as used in the experiments with salt solutions (see above). The composition of the hepatic bile, which was introduced was the following:

[1402] BILLARD, and CAVALIÉ: L'absorption par la vésicule biliaire. C. R. Soc. Biol. **52**, 780—783 (1900).

[1403] GRIM, E., and G. A. SMITH: Water fluxes across dog gallbladder wall. Amer. J. Physiol. **191**, 555—560 (1957).

[1404] HERMANN, H. E.: Tierexperimentelle Studien über Resorption und Ausstoßung des Gallenblaseninhaltes.

Total "base"	183	(174—192)	meq/l
Calcium	6.5	(3.4—9.9)	meq/l
Chloride	84.1	(55.0—107)	meq/l
Bicarbonate	48.0	(34.4—64.8)	meq/l
Bile salt	35.7	(28.1—45.9)	meq/l

After a short exposure to the absorptive functions of the gall bladder the bile was not uniform with respect to the alterations in electrolyte concentrations that had occurred. Chloride and bicarbonate generally decreased in concentration while p_H always decreased. Calcium always, and bile salt generally, tended to increase in concentration.

When the bile had remained in the gall bladder for about 20 hr and the average degree of concentration was 10 fold (5.3—12.5 fold) the composition was as follows:

Total "base"	245.8	(224—305)	meq/l
Calcium	27.3	(23.4—31.1)	meq/l
Chloride	9.0	(1.1—33.7)	meq/l
Bicarbonate	8.1	(0.9—16.9)	meq/l
Bile salt	233.3	(114—334)	meq/l

It appears from these data that the ionorganic anions were markedly reduced in concentration. The bile acids were increased but their concentration was slightly lower than was to be expected from the measured change in volume, indicating that small amounts of bile acids may have been reabsorbed. The sodium concentration exceeded the average concentration of sodium in the hepatic bile, but a considerable fraction must have been present in some osmotically inactive form, since the bile remained isotonic with the plasma during the process of reabsorption.

Thus the concentrating functions of the gall bladder are apparently arrested, when the inorganic anions have been almost completely reabsorbed. The relations between chloride concentration, bile acid concentration and the amount of possible macromolecular aggregations in the bile has, however, not been worked out sufficiently well to permit a decision as to whether these findings indicate, that the gall bladder concentrates the hepatic bile to a constant concentration rather than to a constant volume. It further complicates these considerations that a certain quantity of bile acids may become reabsorbed, although the amount is probably small (cf. Ivy[1398]).

c) *The intimate mechanism of reabsorption by the gall bladder mucosa.* Two possibilities are at hand. Either water is actively transported and electrolytes follow passively or electrolytes are actively reabsorbed and water flows passively. The data of RAVDIN et al.[1401] are strongly indicative of the latter possibility in showing, that a net outflux of chloride ions takes place even from hypotonic solutions of NaCl, which are introduced into the lumen of the gall bladder. Whether the hypothetical active electrolyte transport mechanism operates on the sodium ions or on the chloride ions cannot be stated. The following observations point to active transport of sodium: 1) There are some chloride ions left over even in maximally concentrated gall bladder bile. 2) It appears that other anions (cholates) are reabsorbed to a limited extent. 3) The potassium concentration of the bile rises during the process of reabsorption. This was clearly shown by HERMAN, WILSON and KAZYALE[1397], who found that the conc. of K of guinea pig hepatic bile, when exposed to the reabsorptive functions of the gall bladder, rose from 4.6 (4.0—5.3) to 7.1 (6.1—7.7) meq per liter of bile.

It is thus possible, that there is a parallel between the gall bladder mucosa and other structures engaged in the active transport of electrolyte from the morphological outside to the blood side (the frog skin, the tubular cells of the glomerular nefron, the striated ducts of the salivary glands) in that all these structures appear to transport Na. It must be assumed that the gall bladder mucosa is readily permeable to water and to chloride ions which are transferred from lumen to plasma due to the osmotic and electrostatic forces created by active sodium reabsorption. On the other hand the mucosa must be relatively impermeable to cholates and other larger anions, since the rate of reabsorption slows down and is eventually arrested, when the bile consists chiefly of sodium in combination with cholates or macromolecules.

The potentials and ion fluxes in the isolated gall bladder have apparently not been determined.

The secretory functions of the gall bladder. The gall bladder mucosa produces small amounts of mucus (about 10—20 ml per day). The electrolyte composition of this mucus remains unknown.

c) The alkali metals in hepatic tissue

Measurements of the electrolyte composition of hepatic tissue are presented in Table 49.

Table 49. *Electrolyte composition of liver tissue*

Reference	Species	% water	meq/l of tissue water		
			Na	K	Cl
FENN[1405]	dog	70.8	—	137	—
HEPPEL[1406]	rat	70.1—73.9	33.1—39.4	132—142	38.6—41.4
MANERY and HASTINGS[138] . .	rat	72.1	—	127	41.7
HOLLAND and AUDITORE[1407] . .	guinea pig	70.0	—	120	—
MANERY and HASTINGS[138] . .	rabbit	71.3—74.0	45—47.5	—	37—43.5

HOLLAND and AUDITORE[1407] and BERGER[1408] have studied the intracellular distribution of potassium in the liver and found that potassium is accumulated in the nuclei and in the mitochondria which retain the ion despite repeated washings in sucrose or NaCl. HOLLAND and AUDITORE estimated the intramitochondrial water to contain 192.5 meq of potassium per liter.

The chloride space of the liver has been measured to be 18.1% (FERRARI and HARKNESS[1409]), the sodium space is 20% (SCHWARTZ and OPIE[1410]).

Thus the liver is an organ with a very high intracellular concentration of potassium and with most of the sodium located extracellularly.

In relation to the mechanism of bile formation it is of interest that LEONG, HOLLOWAY and BRAUER[1411] after injection of ^{42}K found an initial rapid uptake in

[1405] FENN, W. O.: The fate of potassium liberated from muscles during activity. Amer. J. Physiol. **127**, 356—373 (1939).

[1406] HEPPEL, L. A.: The electrolytes of muscle and liver in potassium depleted rats. Amer. J. Physiol. **127**, 385—392 (1939).

[1407] HOLLAND, W. C., and G. V. AUDITORE: Distribution of potassium in liver kidney and brain of the rat and guinea pig. Amer. J. Physiol. **183**, 309—313 (1955).

[1408] BERGER, M.: Studies on the distribution of potassium in the rat liver cell and the mechanism of potassium accumulation. Biochim. biophys. Acta **23**, 504—509 (1957).

[1409] FERRARI, V., and R. D. HARCKNESS: Free amino acids in liver and blood after partial hepatectomy in normal and adrenalectomized rats. J. Physiol. **124**, 443—463 (1954).

[1410] SCHWARTZ, I. L., and E. L. OPIE: The osmotic activity of cells of mammalian tissues. J. clin. Invest. **33**, 964 (1954).

[1411] LEONG, G. F., R. J. HOLLOWAY, and R. W. BRAUER: Bile formation in the isolated liver. Transfer of ^{42}K from perfusate to bile. Fed. Proc. **13**, 379—380 (1954).

the isolated liver, followed by a phase of more gradual uptake. ^{42}K made its appearance in the bile 20 min after it had been added to the perfusion fluid.

D) The mammary gland

For details regarding the physiology of lactation and milk secretion the reader is referred to the treatises by PETERSEN[1412], ZARIBNICKY[1413] and ESPE and SMITH[1414].

The sodium and potassium concentrations of human milk are illustrated in Table 50.

The concentrations of sodium and of potassium are largest in the early stages of lactation and decrease as lactation proceeds. Sodium apparently decreases more than potassium and the Na/K ratio is depressed. At the end of the lactation period when the babies are weaned there is again a slight increase in Na/K. These relations are apparent from Table 51.

Table 50. *The alkali metals of human milk.*
All data in meq/l of milk

Reference	year	Na	K	Na/K
SCHLOSS[1415] . .	1910	8.2	13.6	0.60
HOLT, COURTNEY and FALES[1416]	1915	6.7	13.8	0.48
KUROSAWA[1417, 1418]	1937	—	—	0.61
MACY[1419]	1949	7.5	13.1	0.57

This relationship between the stage of lactation and the sodium (resp. chloride) content of the milk were confirmed in the studies by STEFFEN[1420]. The work of FRUNZ[1421] and VUK and VON SANDOR[1422] demonstrates that closely similar fluctuations occur also in other species.

Table 51. *The alkali metals of human milk during different stages of lactation.* All data in meq/l of milk

HOLT, COURTNEY and FALES[1416]				MACY[1419]			
Period	Na	K	Na/K	Period	Na	K	Na/K
1—12 days	19.7	24	0.82	1— 5 days	21.8	19.1	1.14
13—30 days	11.1	18.2	0.61	6—10 days	12.8	16.3	0.78
1— 4 months	6.7	13.8	0.48	$^{1}/_{2}$—15 months	7.5	13.1	0.57
4— 9 months	5.7	15.6	0.37				
10—20 months	8.5	14.7	0.53				

[1412] PETERSEN, W. E.: Lactation. Physiol. Rev. 24, 340—371 (1944).

[1413] ZARIBNICKY, F.: Die Frauenmilch, ihre Eigenschaften und Zusammensetzung. Ergebn. inn. Med. Kinderheilk. 64², 1217—1306 (1945).

[1414] ESPE, D., and V. R. SMITH: Secretion of Milk. Ames, Iowa: Iowa State College Press 1952.

[1415] SCHLOSS, E.: Die chemische Zusammensetzung der Frauenmilch auf Grund neuer Analysen. Mschr. Kinderheilk. 9, 636—640 (1910).

[1416] HOLT, L. E., A. M. COURTNEY, and H. L. FALES: A chemical study of woman's milk especially its inorganic constitutients. Amer. J. Dis. Child. 10, 229—248 (1915).

[1417] KUROSAWA, T.: The Arakawa reaction and the sodium content of human milk. Tôhoku J. exp. Med. 31, 81—94 (1937).

[1418] KUROSAWA, T.: The Arakawa reaction and the potassium content of human milk. Tôhoku J. exp. Med. 31, 106—123 (1937).

[1419] MACY, I. G.: Composition of human cholostrum and milk. Amer. J. Dis. Child. 78, 589—603 (1949).

[1420] STEFFEN, F.: Über den Salzgehalt von Milch, Cholostrum und Galle. Med. Wschr. 12, 204—205 (1931).

[1421] FRUNZ, A.: Über die mineralischen Bestandteile der Kuhmilch und ihre Schwankungen im Verlaufe einer Lactationsperiode. Z. physiol. Chem. 40, 263—320 (1903—1904).

[1422] VUK, M., and Z. VON SANDOR: Änderungen des Natriumgehaltes der Milch einiger Säugetiere während der Lactationsperiode. Z. Untersuch. Lebensmitt. 75, 312—316 (1938).

MILLER[1423] has shown that the chloride concentration of human milk is constantly larger in women with inadequate lactation than in women who have an ample yield of milk. It further appears that samples of milk taken before a breast feed have a lower chloride concentration than samples withdrawn immediately afterwards (KERMARCK and MILLER[1424]).

Despite the low concentrations of inorganic electrolytes woman's milk is isotonic with the plasma (for ref. see [1413]). JACKSON and ROTHERA[1425] examined milk from many different species and found that the osmotic pressure of the milk is invariably equal to that of the plasma. JACKSON and ROTHERA showed that milk sugar was the chief osmotically active substance in most milks, and they demonstrated an inverse correlation between the concentration of ash and the concentration of sugar in milk samples from different species.

Milk secretion goes on continuously between feedings and the milk is retained in the ducts and alveoles of the glands. This has been shown i.a. by post-mortem miling of excised glands when a cow was killed immediately before usual milking time[1412, 1426, 1427].

The maximal pressure against which milk can be secreted by the cow is 40 to 45 mm Hg (see [1414]). If the mammary gland is not emptied at normal feeding times the rate of milk secretion goes down. PETERSEN and RIGOR[1428] injected hypo- and hypertonic solutions in the udder of the cow and found a more marked depression in the rate of milk secretion with the hyper- (and iso-) tonic solutions than with hypotonic. Whether this phenomenon has a bearing on the mechanism of milk secretion as discussed below cannot be stated.

The different *hormonal factors* involved in normal mammary gland development are not to be discussed in this place. The reader is referred to the review by PETERSEN[1412]. Adrenalectomy causes a depression in the rate of milk secretion, which is not improved by administration of excess salt. Adrenal steroids restore normal secretion (COWIE[1429]). The composition of the milk with respect to alkali metal concentration following steroid administration and adrenalectomy has not been thoroughly investigated. BUNGE[1430] claimed that intake of excess salt caused the sodium concentration in milk to increase and the potassium to decrease. This finding has not been confirmed by later investigators, who found that the mineral content of milk was largely independent of intake (cf.[1414]). Acethylcholine has no effect on the rate of milk secretion[1431].

The *blood flow* through the mammary gland has been measured by different methods in the cow and is about 1—1.5 l/min. No good method has yet been developed for determinations of mammary blood flow in women[1432, 1433].

[1423] MILLER, R. A.: Electrical conductivity and chloride content of woman's milk. Part 3: Relation to adequacy of lactation. Arch. Dis. Childh. 26, 325—329 (1951).

[1424] KERMARCK, W. O., and R. A. MILLER: Electrical conductivity and chloride content of woman's milk. Part 2: The effect of factors relating to lactation. Arch. Dis. Child. 26, 320—324 (1951).

[1425] JACKSON, L. C., and A. C. ROTHERA: Milk, its sugar, conductivity and depression of freezing point. Biochem. J. 8, 1—27 (1914).

[1426] PETERSEN, W. E., L. S. PALMER and C. H. ECKLES: The synthesis and excretion of milk fat. I. The time of milk and fat secretion. Amer. J. Physiol. 90, 573—581 (1929).

[1427] SWETT, W. W., F. W. MILLER, and R. R. GRAVES: Quantity of milk obtained from amputated cow udders. J. Agr. Res. 45, 385—400 (1932).

[1428] PETERSEN, W. E., and T. V. RIGOR: Osmotic pressure and milk secretion. Proc. Soc. exp. Biol. (N. Y.) 30, 259—264 (1932).

[1429] COWIE, A. T.: Influence of replacement value of adrenal cortical steroids of dietary sodium. Endocrinology 51, 217—225 (1952).

[1430] BUNGE, G.: Der Kali, Natri und Chlorgehalt der Milch usw. Z. Biol. 21, 295—335 (1874).

[1431] EMERY, F. E., C. E. GOSSETT, W. C. YOUNG, and E. DODGE: Effects of acethylcholine on guinea pigs, rats and humans. Texas Rep. Biol. Med. 10, 493—495 (1952).

The *intimate mechanism of alkali metal secretion* remains unknown. It is quite obvious that all theories of a "pressure dialysis" have to be abandoned. Somehow the cells must actively transport electrolyte(s) and water from plasma to alveolar lumen. The nature of this electrolyte transport mechanism remains undetermined.

It has been shown that J[1434, 1435, 1436, 1437, 1438] and possibly also Br[1439] are concentrated in human milk. Certain salivary glands and the gastric glands similarly excrete such anions as J, Br, SCN etc. with high S/P ratios. This points to a certain functional similarity between the mammary gland alveoles and the secreting epithelia of the other glands, but does of course not warrant the conclusion that their outward electrolyte transport mechanisms are identical.

The finding that all milks are isotonic with the plasma and shown an inverse correlation between the concentration of Na(Cl) and the concentration of milk sugar is interesting. This fact may be explained if it is assumed, that water moves from plasma to alveolar lumen in passive sequence of the osmotic "pull" created by active outward electrolyte transport and by the excretion of milk sugar. The mammary epithelium must be so readily permeable to water that it offers no restriction to the establishment of approximate isotonicity between plasma and milk at all rates of secretion. On the other hand the epithelium must be relatively impermeable to the backdiffusion of milk sugar from alveolar lumen to plasma. Under these circumstances the low (and variable) sodium concentrations of milk may well be a characteristic of the "primary secretion" and one needs not assume, that reabsorption of Na does occur in the mammary gland ducts.

These relations are, however, still uncertain until the process of milk formation has been studied by more refined techniques. The work of FORBES, FORBES and NYELAND[1440], showning that there is a slight negative deflection of the galvanometer (about 1 mV) when the potential is measured between the outpouring milk and the skin on the anterior surface of the chest, is not conclusive as it stands.

E) Male organs of reproduction

Table 52 shows the electrolyte concentrations in *human semen, prostatic fluid and seminal vesicle fluid* according to the analyses by HUGGINS, SCOTT and HEINEN[1441]. The prostatic fluid and the seminal vesicle fluid were obtained by massage of the respective organs, the semen by ejaculation in a glass tube.

[1432] PICKLES, R. V.: An instrument for the study of the physiology and pathology of the human mammary gland. Quart. J. exp. Physiol. **35**, 219—231 (1949).

[1433] PICKLES, V. R.: Blood flow estimations as indices of mammary activity. J. Obstet. Gynec Brit. Emp. **60**, 301—311 (1953).

[1434] KOLDA, J.: Die Passage des substances médicamenteuses dans le lait. Lait **6**, 12—24 (1926).

[1435] HONOUR, A. J., N. B. MYANT, and E. N. ROWLANDS: Secretion of radioiodine in digestive juices and milk. Clin. Sci. **11**, 447—462 (1952).

[1436] MILLER, H., and R. S. WEETEH: Excretion of radioactive iodine. Lancet **269**, 1013 (1955).

[1437] BROWN-GRANT, K.: Gonadal function and thyroid activity. J. Physiol. **131**, 71—84 (1956).

[1438] BROWN-GRANT, K.: The iodide concentrating mechanism of the mammary gland. J. Physiol. **135**, 644—654 (1957).

[1439] YEUNG, G. T. C.: Skin eruption in new-born due to bromism derived from mothers milk. Brit. med. J. 1950; 769.

[1440] FORBES, A., A. P. FORBES, and NYELAND: Action potentials in human mammary gland. J. appl. Physiol. **7**, 675—682 (1954—55).

[1441] HUGGINS, C., W. S. SCOTT, and J. H. HEINEN: Chemical composition of human semen and of the secretion of the prostate and seminal vesicles. Amer. J. Physiol. **136**, 467—473 (1942).

Tabelle 52. *Electrolyte composition of human semen, prostatic fluid and seminal vesicle fluid* (from HUGGINS et al.[441]). All data in meq/l of fluid

	Semen		Prostatic fluid		Seminal vesicle fluid	
p_H	7.19	(6.9—7.36)	6.45	(6.33—6.6)	7.29	(7.26—7.32)
$H_2O^0/_{00}$	918	(891—944)	932	(927—936)	890	(880—900)
Na	117	(100—133)	153	(149—158)	103	
K	22.9	(17—27.4)	48.3	(28.7—61.4)	17.8	(14.3—21.2)
Ca	6.22	(5.3—7.15)	30.2	(28.6—32.7)	—	
CO_2	24	(19.2—33.2)	4.2	(3.1—5.4)	—	
Cl	42.8	(28.3—57.3)	38.1	(34.8—46.1)	—	

ROTSCHILD and BURNS[1442] found that the seminal plasma of the bull contains 112 meq of Na and 44 meq of K per liter, and MANN[1443] states a high K conc. in the seminal plasma of the pig. The low Na/K ratios of seminal plasma as compared to blood plasma are hardly due to escape of K from sperm cells in exchange for Na, since HOWARD and DEFEO[1444] have recently demonstrated that the ejaculate of a vasectomized man contains 130.5 meq of Na and 28.7 meq of K per liter of fluid.

Prostatic fluid has been obtained from dogs, in which the prostate gland and the urethra can be isolated surgically from the bladder and the epididymis closed by ligature. This prostatic fluid is only contaminated by minor quantities of secretion from the parurethral glands (amounting to about 2% of the total volume[1445]).

The composition of prostatic secretion has been examined with this technique by FARRELL[1446], but the only complete analyses are those by HUGGINS, MASINA, EICHELBERGER and WHARTON[1445], which are shown in Table 53.

Table 53. *Electrolyte composition of canine prostatic fluid* (from HUGGINS et al.[1445]). All data in meq/l of fluid

p_H	$H_2O^0/_{00}$	Na	K	Ca	Cl
5.29—6.16	981 (±3)	159 ($\pm2,6$)	5.1 (±0.2)	0,3	160 (±2.7)

Secretory rate in the unstimulated state is about 2—20 ml per day[1445] but increases markedly on stimulation of the nervi erigentes and by injection of pilocarpine[1445, 1446]. The volume following pilocarpine may reach 4—5 times resting levels. Secretory pressure following pilocarpine is about 143 cm of prostatic fluid. The secretion is isosmotic with the plasma[1446]. The p_H is 5.29—6.16 according to the analyses by HUGGINS et al., and 6.8 according to FARRELL.

The resting secretory rate is depressed after testectomy and returns to normal following substitution therapy with androgens. Thyroidectomy, parathyroid-

---

[1442] ROTSCHILD, L., and H. BURNS: Constituents of bull seminal plasma. J. exp. Biol. **31**, 561—572 (1954).

[1443] MANN, T.: The Biochemistry of Semen. London 1954.

[1444] HOWARD, E., and V. J. DE FEO: Potassium and sodium content of uterine and seminal vesicle secretions. Amer. J. Physiol. **196**, 65—67 (1959).

[1445] HUGGINS, C., M. H. MASINA, L. EICHELBERGER, and J. D. WHARTON: Quantitative studies of prostatic secretion I. Characteristics of the normal secretion. The influence of thyroid, suprarenal and testis extirpation and androgen substitution on the prostatic output. J. exp. Med. **70**, 543—556 (1939).

[1446] FARRELL, J. S.: The newer physiology of the prostate gland. J. Urol. **39**, 171—185 (1938).

ectomy and adrenalectomy have no measurable effect on the volume of secretion. None of the stated procedures affect the electrolyte concentrations of the secretion[1445].

The fluid in the *seminal vesicle* of the guinea pig has been examined by BREUER and WHITTAM[1447]. Their results are shown in Table 54.

HOWARD and DEFEO found a very high solid content in the seminal vesicle fluid of rats (25%). The concentrations of Na and K (expressed in meq/kg of water) were 33.6 and 1.10 respectively.

Table 54. *Electrolyte concentrations in seminal vesicle fluid and seminal vesicle mucosa of the guinea pig* (from BREUER and WHITTAM[1447])

	Na	K	Cl
Fluid (meq/l) . .	13.5 ($\pm$2.3)	1.6 ($\pm$0.8)	11.1 ($\pm$1.6)
Mucosa (meq/kg)	33.5 ($\pm$7.4)	102.5 ($\pm$9.4)	46.5 ($\pm$7.6)
Plasma	143	8	101

The osmolality of the seminal vesicle fluid is not on record.

Electrolyte transport in the isolated seminal vesicle has been discussed by USSING on page 107.

The reader is referred to the reviews by MANN and LUTWAK-MANN[1448] and by HUGGINS[1449] for further details on the physiology of the male accessory organs of reproduction.

Dogs *testis* contains 87% of water, 60 meq of Cl, 46 meq of Na, 91 meq of K, 1.7 meq of Ca and 10 meq of Mg per kg of fat-free tissue/according to the data of HUGGINS and EICHELBERGER[1450].

F) Female organs of reproduction

SHIH, KENNEDY and HUGGINS[1451] have examined the *uterine secretion* of rats, rabbits and dogs. The uterine secretion was obtained either by aspiration from the uterus after opening of the abdomen or it was collected from uterine fistula or segments of the uterus which were enclosed between ligatures. Table 55 shows the results.

WARREN[1452] has clearly demonstrated, that

Table 55. *Electrolyte composition of uterine fluid* (from SHIH et al.[1451]). All data in meq/l of fluid

Species	H_2O ($^0/_{00}$)	p_H	Na	K	Ca	Cl	CO_2
Dog	984	6.09	162	5.2	3.5	167	3.0
Rabbit	979	7.78	158	6.1	4.7	98	53.6
Rat	982	7.55	169	4.3	1.5	98	61.8

the volume of secretion formed by the uterine mucosa of the rat is under influence of the stage of the sexual cycle. WARREN found a 20-fold increase in secretory rate during prooestrus and oestrus as compared to the secretory rate during dioestrus. SHIH, KENNEDY and HUGGINS do not state the period during which their animals were examined. It is of considerable interest that HOWARD

[1447] BREUER. H. J., and R. WHITTAM: Ion movements in seminal vesicle mucosa. J. Physiol. **135**, 213—225 (1957).

[1448] MANN, T., and C. LUTWAK-MANN: Secretory function of male accessory organs of reproduction in mammals. Physiol. Rev. **31**, 27—55 (1951).

[1449] HUGGINS, C.: The physiology of the prostate gland. Physiol. Rev. **25**, 281—295 (1945).

[1450] HUGGINS, C., and L. EICHELBERGER: Water and electrolyte content of testicular tumors . . . etc. Cancer Res. **4**, 447—452 (1944).

[1451] SHIH, H. E., J. KENNEDY, and C. HUGGINS: Chemical composition of uterine secretions. Amer. J. Physiol. **130**, 287—291 (1940).

[1452] WARREN, M. R.: Observations on the uterine fluid of the rat. Amer. J. Physiol. **122**, 602—608 (1938).

and DeFeo[1444] found the following composition of the uterine secretion of rats during prooestrus (Table 56).

Table 56. *The sodium and potassium of uterine fluid in rats during prooestrus before and after copulation* (from Howard and De Feo[1444])

	Na meq/l	K meq/l	H_2O %	Na + K meq/ kg of water
Uterine fluid before copulation	115.3	37.4	98.5	155.0
Serum	139.1	4.18	92.5	154.9
Uterine fluid after copulation	102.3	37.5	97.1	143.9
Serum	133.5	3.83	92.2	149.0

The rat uterine fluid during prooestrus is thus apparently characterized by a considerable K concentration. The K conc. is not modified by copulation, indicating that rat semen, like the semen of man, bull and pig (see above), is also high in K. Howard and DeFeo draw attention to the high K conc. in egg white and in the sea water of the pre-Cambrian oceans and state that this electrolyte environment, which would be toxic to most other cells, must be the natural habitat of the earliest and most primitive stages of life.

G) The glands of the respiratory tract

The present writer was not able to find data on the electrolyte composition of the secretion from the *nasal mucous membrane*.

The nasal gland, glandula lateralis nasi, which was first described by Stensen (Nicolao Steno)[1453], exists only in an embryological stage in man and other mammals. However, in birds with a marine habitat the gland is well developed and appears to play a role in the homeostasis of these species (gull, albatros, pelican, penguin). The physiological performance of the gland was unknown until the recent studies by Schmidt-Nielsen and collaborators[1454, 1455]. These workers found that the gland was stimulated to secrete when marine birds were drinking sea water or when hypertonic solutions of NaCl or of glucose were injected intravenously. A brisk flow of a watery secretion was then discharged. In cormorants (phalocrocorax auritus) it had the composition shown in Table 57.

Table 57. *Electrolyte composition of the secretion from the avian salt gland* (from Schmidt-Nielsen et al.[1454]). All values in meq/l of secretion

	Na	K	Cl
Average . . .	529 (±84)	12.1 (±5)	517 (±67)
Range	392—687	5.0—25.5	390—648

During brisk secretory activity the elimination rates for the chief electrolytes were the following:

Elimination rate (μeq/min)

Na . .	40—114.5
K . .	0.7— 2.5
Cl . .	40—102.5

This means, that the entire NaCl of the body of a cormorant could be eliminated by the gland within 10 hours.

The composition of the secretion is apparently independent of secretory rate. The gland is stimulated by a branch of the facial nerve in response to hypertonic loading. Mecholyl provokes secretion. Atropine inhibits secretion.

[1453] Steno, N.: De musculi et glandulis. Thesis. Amsterdam 1664.

[1454] Schmidt-Nielsen, K., C. Barker-Jørgensen, and H. Osaki: Extrarenal salt excretion in birds. Amer. J. Physiol. **193**, 101—107 (1958).

[1455] Fänge, R., K. Schmidt-Nielsen, and M. Robinson: Control of secretion from the avian salt gland. Amer. J. Physiol. **195**, 321—326 (1958).

The gland is extremely interesting from a physiological point of view. It probably plays a role in the homeostasis of marine birds, when ingesting sea water, since the kidney is not able to excrete the salt load thus imposed. Furthermore, it is of considerable interest, that it is the only gland, hitherto desribed (apart from the kidney), which produces a strictly hypertonic secretion.

The secretion of *the bronchial glands* of different animals was examined by BOYD, JACKSON, MACLACHLAN, PALMER, STEVENS and WHITTAKER[1456], who found the following values for Na and Cl:

The very low concentrations of Na and Cl are surprising if compared to the values in the secretions of other mucinous glands (oesophageal, gastric, colo-

	rabbit	cat	dog
Cl (meq/l) . .	13.1 ($\pm$1.5)	18.8 ($\pm$1.3)	18.8 ($\pm$0.5)
Na (meq/l) . .	15.7 ($\pm$3.4)	18.2 ($\pm$2.0)	14.3 ($\pm$3.2)

nic). It can hardly be excluded, that the bronchial secretion was diluted by condensation of water from alveolar air or inhaled air (which was kept at 100% relative humidity).

H) Concluding remarks on glandular secretion

According to the work of HEIDENHAIN[1101], ANREP[1102], KOMAROV, LANGSTROTH and McRAE[1103] and others the process of secretion must be subdivided into the more or less continuous synthesis of enzymes and other specific substances by the gland cells and the intermittent glandular discharge of watery solutions in which the enzymes are dissolved and propelled to the exterior (p. 435). In this treatise we have not discussed in further detail the elaboration of enzymes by the gland cells, but their excretion is of interest to the current problems due to the fact, that these large molecular compounds can transgress in some way the membranes of cells, which are otherwise impermeable to ions and non-electrolytes of much smaller size[1457, 1458]. We do not know in which manner this transfer takes place. The terms "apocrine", "eccrine" and "holocrine" glands, forwarded by the old histologists, are still of little meaning to the physiologist, and the character of the socalled "secretory granula" in the cytoplasm of the glandular cells remains unknown.

Even when we limit our interest to the intermittent glandular discharge of electrolytes and water, a survey of the composition of the different secretory products represents at first glance a complex and bewildering picture. Most secretory products are about isotonic, a few are decidedly hypotonic (sweat and certain types of saliva) and at least one gland produces a strictly hypertonic secretion (the avian salt gland). Certain secretions vary in electrolyte composition with their volume rate of formation, whereas others have an unvaried electrolyte composition at all rates of flow. We are not able to account for these differences between secretions, nor do we fully understand the successive transfers of ions and water, which lead to the variations in the composition of one and the same secretory product at different rates of formation. Our current knowledge of these

---

[1456] BOYD, E. M., S. JACKSON, M. MACLACHLAN, B. PALMER, M. STEVENS and J. WHITTAKER: The lipid, sodium, chloride and nitrogen content of the respiratory tract fluid of normal animals. J. biol. Chem. **153**, 435—438 (1944).

[1457] THAYSEN, J. H., and I. L. SCHWARTZ: The permeability of human sweat glands to a series of sulfonamide compounds. J. exp. Med. **98**, 261—268 (1953).

[1458] KILLMANN, S. A., and J. H. THAYSEN: The permeability of the human parotid gland to a series of sulfonamide compounds, paraaminohippurate and inulin. Scand. J. clin. Lab. Invest. **7**, 86—91 (1955).

problems is limited, at least if the situation is compared to the advances, which have been made in the study of the glomerular nephron.

In the study of the glomerular nephron we have the advantage, that the "primary urine" — the glomerular filtrate — represents a solution of well defined composition and volume rate of formation. The subsequent modifications, which the filtrate undergoes during its passage of the tubules, can be quantitated by clearance techniques and have in part also been located to the different sections of the tubules by "stop-flow" experiments, tubular micropuncture and tissue analyses. Due to the morphological differences between the glomerular nephron and the glands these different methods cannot all be directly applied to a study of the manner in which the "primary secretions" are modified before reaching the site of collection, but the "stop-flow" studies of NITTA[1066] on the sweat glands and the micropuncture work of LUNDBERG[1073] on the salivary glands indicate, that the techniques of renal physiology might be applied to advantage on a larger scale, than has hitherto been the case. However, up until the present time attempts to locate the successive transfers of ions and water by direct methods are few, and most of our concepts of glandular electrolyte secretion are still based on indirect evidence obtained from examination of the final secretory products, as they can be collected from the opening of a glandular duct or aspirated from the lumen of a viscus. One approach has been to examine the effect on the final secretions of substances, which are supposed to enchance or depress specifically the function of one or the other cell type (cf. the stimulating effect of histamine versus metacholine on gastric secretion, p. 471, the stimulating effect of secretin versus metacholine on pancreatic secretion, p. 461, and the inhibitory action of ethionine versus alloxan on the pancreatic gland, p. 463).

Based on the results of such studies and on other evidence, which is admittedly also of an indirect nature, it seems to be the current concept, that any one histological cell type forms a secretion, which has an unvaried electrolyte composition at all rates of flow. This hypothesis, which was first advanced in the case of the parietal and the "non-parietal" cells of the gastric mucosa, is not incongruent with the fact, that little complex glandular structures — consisting mainly or exclusively of one type of cells — form secretions in which the concentrations of the different electrolytes are independent of the volume rate of secretory flow. The reader is referred to the sections on sublingual (p. 453), prostatic (p. 500) and mucinous (p. 465, 467, 471, 485) secretions.

As the secretory product from one type of cells flows down the ducts or spreads on the mucosal surface of glandular structures of greater histological differentiation, it may become modified in one or more of the following ways:

1. By addition of the secretory products from other cell types.

2. By diffusion of ions between the forming secretion and the plasma according to their concentration gradients.

3. By active reabsorption of electrolyte(s).

Singly or in combination these different processes may account for the occurrence of rate dependent variations in the electrolyte composition of the final secretory products, but conclusive evidence pertaining to the relative importance of the stated ionic transfers is lacking. Thus it is still under discussion, whether the rate dependent variations in the cationic composition of the gastric juice are due to the mixing of "acid" and "neutral" component secretions in variable proportion or to the partial equilibration between the forming secretion and the plasma by diffusion of hydrogen and sodium ions according to their concentration gradients. The reader is referred to the section on the "component theory" versus the "diffusion theory" of gastric secretion (p. 478). Similar considerations may be forwarded in the case of the rate dependent variations in the anionic composition of the pancreatic, parotid and submaxillary secretions, although a "component theory" appears at present to have the greater appeal in these instances (p. 430). With respect to the third possibility: Active reabsorption of electrolyte(s) we appear to stand on somewhat firmer ground, since the existance of such a mechanism in the sweat gland and in certain salivary glands has been suggested by the results of several and independent methods of investigation, but also here final proof of the mechanism and of which ion is actively reabsorbed is lacking (p. 431).

When we turn to the problem of the manner in which the individual cells "secrete" or "reabsorb" electrolytes and water our knowledge is also quite limited, although a few points are worthy of comment.

The volume and the electrolyte composition of a secretory product appears to be independent of the duration of glandular discharge (p. 442, 454, 461, 473), and it has been shown, that the variations in the quantity of water and electrolytes in discharging glands are negligeable in comparison to secretory losses (p. 434). These findings indicate, that the glands do not function as sponges, which are "squeezed" of their contents when stimulated by the secretory nerves and left to refill in intervals between periods of discharge. In fact, BURGEN[1077] has demonstrated that during the steady state of secretion there is a quantitative relationship between the amount of water and electrolytes carried to the salivary glands via the arteries on the one side and the amount appearing in the saliva and carried away via the venous effluent on the other (p. 435). There is thus little reason to doubt, that the water and the electrolytes of a secretory product are derived directly from the plasma perfusing the gland.

During periods of discharge the amount of plasma perfusing the glands goes up, roughly in parallel to the volume of secretion formed. The exact relationship between secretory flow and plasma flow has only been examined in some of the duct possessing glands, notably the salivary glands (p. 455). In these glands the ratio between secretory flow and plasma flow appears to be about 1 : 5, yielding a "secretion fraction" of about 20% at all rates of glandular discharge. It is not known why plasma flow goes up, when the glands are stimulated to discharge, but HILTON and LEWIS[1189] have presented evidence, that a vasodilator substance is released from the stimulated submaxillary gland.

It has been claimed, that blood pressure is the driving force for the transport of water and electrolytes from plasma to glandular lumen. According to this theory, the only work performed by the gland cells is the synthesis of enzymes and other specific substances, whereas variations in the electrolyte composition of different secretory products are merely due to a differential permeability of the various glandular epithelia. This concept of a "pressure dialysis" in the secretory process has to be abandoned not only from histological considerations (in particular the arrangement of glandular blood supply), but also on experimental grounds. It has thus been shown, that secretory pressure can exceed arterial blood pressure (p. 427), that secretion can continue for a certain period following complete occlusion of glandular blood supply (p. 443, 455), and that the isolated, non-perfused gastric mucosa can secrete, when suspended in an appropriate medium (p. 483). Similarly, the secretion of bile by the isolated perfused liver is independent of a wide range of variation in perfusate pressure (p. 491), but — despite constant perfusate pressure — appreciably affected by such factors as are known to interfere with normal cellular metabolism (p. 490, 491).

All these findings indicate, that the glandular discharge of water and electrolytes — like the synthesis of enzymes — must somehow depend upon cellular activity. It appears to be the current concept, that electrolytes are actively transported and that water follows passively due to the osmotic forces thus created (p. 429, 483). This assumption is in keeping with the current theories of electrolyte and water transport in other systems (the renal tubule, p. 241, the intestinal mucosa, p. 509) and is not incongruent with the variations in secretory electrolyte composition, which have been shown to follow alterations in plasma osmolarity (p. 443, 455, 462, 473, 485, 489.)

According to the concept of an active electrolyte transport and a passive transfer of water by osmosis *outward transport* ("secretion") must result in the formation of products, which are either isotonic or hypertonic, depending upon the permeability of the "secreting" epithelia to water. Similarly, *inward transport* ("reabsorption") must lead either to a reduction in volume or to a reduction in tonicity of the original secretory product, depending upon the resistance, which the reabsorbing structures offer to the transfer of water from glandular lumen to plasma. Apparently both types of "secreting" resp. "reabsorbing" epithelia are met with in the glandular systems, which have been discussed in this chapter. A strictly hypertonic secretion (containing 400—700 meq of Na per liter) is formed by the avian salt gland (p. 502), indicating a "secreting" epithelium of low permeability to water (we are here disregarding the possibility, that the avian salt gland is in possession of a loop system like that of the glomerular nephron). In contrast all other "secreting" epithelia form isotonic or slightly hypertonic products, indicating that these epithelia offer little resistance to water transfer (p. 427, 479, 483, 489, 498). Hypotonic secretions with total electrolyte concentrations considerably lower than those of the plasma are formed by the sweat gland and by certain salivary glands, indicating that primary secretions are modified by reabsorption of electrolytes through epithelia of restricted permeability to water (p. 431). In contrast, water flows out freely following electrolyte reabsorption in the gall bladder with the result, that the volume of bile is reduced without appreciable change in its original isotonicity (p. 493).

Hypothetically, the active electrolyte transport mechanisms in the glands may operate on anions (cations following passively), on cations (anions following passively) or on both. Since electrophysiological studies are still scanty, these problems are by no means finally settled. However, evidence has been presented, that the active outward transport mechanism ("secretion") operates on the chloride ion in the glands of the frog skin (Part I, p. 118), in the acini of the submaxillary and sublingual glands (p. 428) and in the gastric mucosa (p. 482). Furthermore, there are data suggesting, that active inward transport of electrolyte ("reabsorption") takes place in the ducts of the sweat gland and certain salivary glands (p. 431) as well as in the mucosa of the gall bladder (p. 495), and that this transport mechanism operates on the sodium ion. If experimentally verified this latter process represents a parallel to the course of events in other systems such as the frog skin (part I, p. 114), the tubule of the glomerular nephron (p. 241) and the intestinal mucosa (p. 509), where electrolyte transport from the morphological outside to the blood side has been demonstrated to depend on active transport of the sodium ion. Due to the paucity of experimental data it is, however, still uncertain, whether the generalization is warranted, that the organism operates with one mechanism in outward transport (chloride "secretion") and another in inward transport (sodium "reabsorption"). The reader is referred to the discussion by USSING in part I (p. 113).

The more or less continuous secretory activity of certain glands (e. g. the liver, p. 488) appears to proceed without the interaction of any known stimulus, but most other glands — which secrete intermittently — receive a signal to discharge via the secretory nerves. Since the isolated and non-perfused gastric mucosa is stimulated by acethylcholine and histamine, there is little doubt that the chemical transmitters, which are released at the nerve endings, act directly upon the glandular cells. The manner in which the chemical transmitters excite the glandular cells to initiate outward electrolyte transport ("secretion") remains undetermined however. It is only known, that the initial reaction to stimulation is a loss of K and an equivalent uptake of Na by the submaxillary gland cells (p. 434), and that similar electrolyte changes may well take place also in other glandular tissues (p. 428, 470). Whereas the release of a chemical transmitter is in some way or other necessary to initiate the process of secretion in most glands, it appears that inward electrolyte transport ("reabsorption") proceeds without the interaction of nervous stimuli. The reabsorption of Na by the duct cells of the sweat gland and of certain salivary glands occurs at a constant rate, independently of the rate at which the "primary secretions" are formed (p. 431). Similarly, no nervous stimuli have been demonstrated, which accelerate the rate of re-absorption by the gall bladder in situ. This course of events corresponds to the situation in other sodium reabsorbing structures (the frog skin, the renal tubule, the intestinal mucosa). At present we can only speculate on the reason for these apparent differences between outward and inward electrolyte transport in the glands. To answer the problems further knowledge is obviously needed about the permeability to ions of the inner and outer cellular membranes as well as about the location of the hypothetical mechanisms for active electrolyte transport.

The intimate mechanism by which electrolytes are actively transported across the gland cell membranes remains unknown. It is an intriguing fact, however, that the energy requirement for active electrolyte transport, as measured by the superbasal oxygen consumption, is about the same in the isolated frog skin (part I, p. 120), in the kidney (p. 261) and in the duct possessing glands (p. 435). In all these structures the ratio between active electrolyte transport and superbasal oxygen consumption is about 4—6 when both parameters are expressed in equivalents. Likewise, the glands respond to ischemia, to changes in temperature and to adreno-cortical steroids in a manner, which is not fundamentally different from that of other electrolyte transporting systems. These findings seem to indicate, that the basic mechanisms may well be the same in all systems. Nature possesses only a few mechanisms of electrolyte transport, but combines them in a multiplicity of ways to subserve the varied functions of highly complex organs and organisms.

VI. Intestinal absorption of alkali metal ions

By

P. KRUHØFFER and J. HESS THAYSEN

A. Introduction

Since many of the basic features of the intestinal absorption of alkali metal ions have been thoroughly dealt with in pp. 131 to 139 in Part I of this book, only certain aspects remain to be considered here.

As is well-known — and has been discussed in detail in the preceding section — alkali metal ions are lost from the body at appreciable rates with the secretions of the digestive tract. An estimate of the 24 hours outputs of a normal human subject by this route is given in Table 58. Obviously these figures are only approximations, and in the case of the secretions of the intestines they are no more than rough estimates, because the simultaneous occurrence in these organs of glandular secretion, active absorption, and diffusion precludes the separate measurement of outputs.

Table 58. *Approximate magnitude of the 24 hr outputs of Na, K and water in the digestive secretions of a normal human subject*

Type of secretion	Salivary	Gastric	Pancreatic	Biliary	Intestinal	Colonic	Total	Total as per cent of exchangeable body contents
Volume (ml/24 hr)	1000 to 1500	1500 to 2500	500 to 1000	500 to 1000	2500 to 3500	100 to 200	6100 to 9700	about 20
Na (meq/24 hr)	30—45	45—75	80 to 160	80 to 160	400 to 560	20—40	650 to 1040	about 30
K (meq/24 hr)	15—20	15—25	2—5	2—5	15—25	1—2	50—82	about 3

In the normal subject these losses are only transient, since the alkali metal ions secreted — and others contained in the food — are very efficiently absorbed, as evidenced by the fact that only minute fractions are lost with the faeces. E. g. the following 24 hours faecal losses were reported by DANOWSKI and GREENMAN[1459] on the basis of 23 analyses: 3.9 ± 4.5 meq Na/24 hours and 9.7 ± 4.8 meq K/24 hours. Further examples may be found in p. 517.

Only a rather limited number of investigations have been undertaken to determine the amounts of Na, K (and water) which, at a particular time, are located in the gastrointestinal tract. References may be found in a recent paper by GOTCH et al. [1460]. As one might expect considerable species differences exist. In rabbits as much as 12% of the total body water has been found to be located in this "extracorporal" position. In human subjects studies have only been performed (6—22 hours) post mortem; about 1.5% of the total body contents of

---

[1459] DANOWSKI, T. S., and L. GREENMAN: Changes in fecal and serum constituents during ingestion of cation and anion exchangers. Ann. N. Y. Acad. Sci. 57, 273—279 (1954).

[1460] GOTCH, F., J. NADELL, and J. S. EDELMAN: Gastrointestinal water and electrolytes. IV. The equilibrium of deuterium oxide (D_2O) in gastrointestinal contents and the proportion of the whole body water (T. B. W.) in the gastrointestinal tract. J. clin. Invest. 36, 289—296 (1957).

water and sodium were found in the digestive tract, but obviously these figures may be greatly different from those of a living subject in good condition. In the latter case the figures are probably appreciably higher and, of course, subject to considerable variation with the stage of digestion. Altogether it appears that the gastrointestinal contents of Na (which exchanges quite rapidly with that of the body) may be large enough to constitute a perceptible error in the determination of (intracorporal) exchangeable Na. It has even been suggested by SWEET et al.[1461] that a diminution of the gastrointestinal contents of Na, Cl and water should be the major source for a 34% expansion of the extracellular space (inulin space) which they observed in monkeys in the course of 5 days treatment with desoxy-corticosterone.

.. It is important to remember that, when the intestinal absorption is impaired in a variety of pathological conditions, severe losses of alkali metal ions (in particular Na) may be inflicted upon the subject, either by losses to the outside or by trapping inside the gastrointestinal tract. For details of such cases the reader is referred to several monographs and reviews listed elsewhere[1-15].

From the discussion in pp. 131 to 138 the following facts are apparent: (1) Active absorption of sodium takes place in all parts of the mammalian intestine, and the small intestine may also be capable of absorbing chloride actively, (2) Per unit length of intestine the capacity of the sodium absorbing mechanism is larger in the small intestine than in the large intestine (but not necessarily so per unit of epithelial surface area), (3) The passive permeability to Na^+ and Cl^- is much larger in the small intestine than in the large intestine, and consequently the small intestine is not capable of establishing nearly as high Na^+ (and Cl^-) concentration gradients across the epithelium as is the large intestine. The very recent studies by BERGER et al.[1462a] on the simultaneous fluxes of sodium into and out of intestinal loops of dogs have provided further support for these conclusions. Cf. also the review by DURBIN et al.[1462b].

Evidently then, the small intestine is built for bulk absorption of (salt + water), whereas the colon is suited for absorption of salt without proportional amounts of water, or in other words for reducing the sodium concentration in the intestinal contents to very low levels. As far as potassium is concerned it is apparently not yet clear whether this ion is subject to active intestinal absorption.

It might be expected from these facts that the sodium concentration of the intestinal contents would be rather high in the proximal parts and decline progressively through the distal parts of the intestinal tract. This has also been confirmed by analyses of intestinal contents from various levels, and further support has come from analyses of the cations bound to cation exchange resins removed from various levels of the intestinal tract. Since the use of cation exchange resins has also contributed some information on factors influencing the intestinal absorption of alkali metal ions, and has further received consideration as tools to retard the intestinal absorption of these ions, a short survey on these substances will be given here, before proceeding. For further details the reader is referred to several papers in the symposium edited by MINER[1463].

[1461] SWEET, A. Y., M. F. LEVITT and H. L. HODES: The effects of desoxycorticosterone acetate on water and electrolyte distribution. J. clin. Invest. **37**, 65—69 (1958).

[1462a] BERGER, E. Y., G. KANZAKI, M. A. HOMER, and I. M. STEEL: Simultaneous flux of sodium into and out of the dog intestine. Amer. J. Physiol. **196**, 74—82 (1959).

[1462b] DURBIN, R. P., P. F. CURRAN, and A. K. SOLOMON: Ion and water transport in stomach and intestine. In Advances in biological and medical physics. Vol. VI, p. 1—36. New York: Acad. Press 1959.

[1463] MINER, R. W. (Ed), Symposium: Ion exchange resins in medicine and biological research. Ann. N. Y. Acad. Sci. **57**, 61—324 (1954.)

B. Resins and intestinal absorption of alkali metal ions

Properties of ion exchange resins. Ion exchange resins are crosslinked polymers of "infinite" molecular size (and consequently generally insoluble) in which acidic or basic groups are attached to the hydrocarbon network.

In connection with the problems here to be considered only resins with acidic groups, i. e. cation exchangers, are of interest, and among these, those carrying carboxylic or sulfonic groups have received by far the greatest attention.

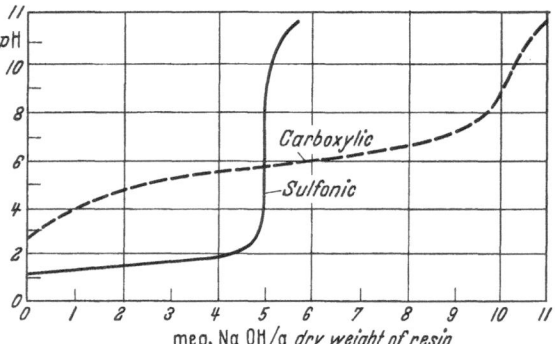

Fig. 24. *Titration curves for typical "high capacity" carboxylic and sulfonic resins.* From BREGMAN[1464]

At sufficiently high p_H values the acidic groups will dissociate leaving negatively charged groups on the resin. These will attract ("bind") other positively charged ions (among which Na^+ and K^+) if such are present in the surrounding solution.

The factors determining the number of, say, sodium ions, which will be "bound" per gram of resin are complex and mutually interrelated. Obviously, the inherent maximal capacity for cation binding is dependent upon the number of acidic groups per gram of resin. The fraction of these groups actually available for exchange depends on the p_H of the surrounding solution, and may be read from the resin titration curve. Examples of such curves for two typical resins, one of the carboxylic and one of the sulfonic type, are shown in Fig. 24. It is apparent that the sulfonic groups, being rather strong acids, are fully dissociated, and thus available for cation binding, already at p_H about 3. In the case of the carboxylic resin dissociation only begins at p_H values above this and continues up to p_H values around 10. It is apparent that for these two typical resins the maximal exchange capacity of the carboxylic resin is definitely superior to that of the sulfonic resin (10 meq/gram versus 5 meq/gram), but it is also evident that at p_H values around 5—6, i. e. the p_H encountered in the intestinal contents, the available capacities are of similar magnitude. It should be added that titration curves as those pictured are obtained with high concentrations of a neutral salt (NaCl) present in the surrounding solution, so that an excess of Na^+ is available to replace hydrogen ions dissociating from the resin (cf. BREGMAN[1464]); obviously sufficient time was allowed for equilibrium to be established. Less exchange will take place, of course, if the concentration of the exchanging cation in the solution is lowered below a certain level, or if less than a certain time is allowed for the exchange.

If various kinds of cations are present in the surrounding solution they will compete for attachment to the acidic groups. The amount of a particular cation then being bound will depend partly on its concentration relative to those of other cations in the solution and partly on the relative affinities of the resin for each of these cations. The latter property is expressed by ion selectivity coefficients, which, however, are not fixed values for a particular resin, but subject to some variation with the conditions, i. e. the ionic strength of the equilibrating solution

[1464] BREGMAN, J. I.: Cation exchange processes. Ann. N. Y. Acad. Sci. **57**, 125—143 (1954).

and the relative proportions of different cations dissolved in it, the temperature etc. Ingestion of cation exchange resins (generally as a mixture of the ammonium and potassium forms) was originally proposed as a remedy for sodium depleting therapy, the aim being to increase the faecal losses of sodium. In this respect the resins have fallen short of expectations, primarily because it has so far been impossible to produce resins with sufficiently high exchange capacities and with Na/K selectivity coefficients appreciably above unity.

The state of charging of resins present in the intestinal contents. The propulsion of the intestinal contents, especially in the colon, should be slow enough to allow a finely granulated resin passing along the intestine essentially to reach exchange equilibrium with the cations of the intestinal contents at each level. That this actually occurs was shown by SPENCER et al.[1465] who removed cation exchange resins from various levels of the intestinal tract of patients on a low sodium diet (in some cases post-mortally following sudden death). Sodium was found to make up a high fraction of the (Na + K) bound to the resin, when the latter was removed from the proximal parts of the intestinal tract, but only a small fraction when the resin was removed from the most distal parts. A similar observation was made by FIELD et al.[1466] in dogs with terminal ileal fistulae. When carboxyl resin was administered, resin removed through the fistulae had a much higher Na/K ratio than resin obtained from the faeces. It was apparent therefore that the cation exchange of the resin continues throughout the intestinal tract, and that sodium which is once bound in the proximal parts is again detached further distally, and in part replaced by potassium. Consequently the amounts of Na and K lost with a resin in the faeces will be solely determined by the ion composition of the contents of the most anal parts of the colon (as long as the intestinal passage is not unusually fast). Now, as mentioned above, sodium is very efficiently absorbed in these parts of the intestine, and the contents normally have an appreciably higher concentration of potassium than of sodium. It is therefore quite understandable that it has been a common experience (cf. e. q. SPENCER et al.[1465] for references) that cation exchange resins remove as much (or more) potassium as sodium when they are excreted in the stools, even when they have been fed to subjects on a normal diet (and irrespective of the kind of cation charging of the resin administered). Under such conditions the ingestion of resins — carboxylic and sulfonic alike — by normal subjects has generally been found to lead to faecal losses of some 1.5—2 meq of (Na + K) per gram of resin, with fairly equal amounts of the two cations. There is no great difference between the available carboxyl and sulfonic resins as regards ability to raise faecal losses of (Na + K), as might be expected from the titration curves and the existence of a p_H around 6—7 in the lower parts of the colon. It is also noteworthy that the (Na + K) bound represents only a fraction of the total available capacity of the resin at this p_H. McCHESNEY[1467] has shown that even when Ca and Mg are also considered only some 60% of the total available capacity of the (sulfonic) resin (some 5 meq/g) is "covered", the remainder probably being occupied by ammonium and hydrogen ions.

From the above discussion it is apparent that a daily intake of some 40—50 g of resin (which is about as much as a person can take because of the unpleasant

[1465] SPENCER, A. G., E. J. ROSS, and H. G. L. LLOYD-THOMAS: Cation exchange in the gastrointestinal tract. Brit. med. J. **1954** I, 603—606.

[1466] FIELD, H., JR., L. SWELL, R. E. DAILEY, E. C. TROUT, and R. S. BOYD: Electrolyte changes in ileal contents and in feces during restriction of dietary sodium with or without the administration of cation exchange resin. Circulation **12**, 625—629 (1955).

[1467] McCHESNEY, E. W.: *In vivo* uptake of cations by two types of exchange resins. Amer. J. Physiol. **168**, 44—54 (1952).

texture, poor palatability and the tendency to cause gastrointestinal distress) could at most produce a faecal loss of sodium of some 40—50 meq per day. Evidently, the use of cation exchange resins can be no more than an adjunct in sodium depleting therapy, and it could not allow one to dispense from a rather rigid restriction of the sodium intake. Actually the sodium depleting effect of resins is even smaller than this, because, as discussed below, body responses to sodium depletion make the resins less efficient as sodium removers.

C. Influence of corticoids on intestinal absorption of alkali metal ions

In dogs with chronic loops of ileum DENNIS and WOOD[1468] found that the rate of net absorption of sodium and chloride (and to a smaller extent, potassium) from the loops was appreciably reduced upon withdrawal of adrenal cortical extract treatment from adrenalectomized dogs maintained on a high sodium, low potassium diet. In some cases there occurred even a net movement of sodium into the intestine. A large depression of the rate of sodium and chloride absorption from the small intestine has also been observed in rats following adrenalectomy, and desoxycorticosterone administration was reported to normalize the rates (STEIN and WERTHEIMER[1469]). It is not possible, from these and similar findings, to say whether corticoids enchance the absorption of sodium in the small intestine by a direct effect upon the epithelium. Indirect effects, e. g. by way of changes in the blood circulation in the intestine, cannot be excluded.

Most other studies concerning the effect of corticoids on the intestinal absorption of alkali metal ions pertain to the absorption in the colon.

After the introduction of resin therapy it was soon recognized that the efficiency of resins as sodium removers varies considerably from one patient to another, and in the same patient under different conditions. It was also soon established that less sodium is removed under conditions of a low sodium diet than if the sodium intake is high. E. g. only 0.4—0.5 meq of Na were reported by McCHESNEY et al.[1470] to be removed per gram of resin in subjects on low Na intakes against 0.9—1.2 meq per gram during medium or high intakes. In similar vein it was observed by EMERSON et al.[1471] that during continued resin therapy (in subjects on a restricted Na intake) a gradual decline occurred in Na excretion in the stools, and that simultaneously there was a tendency for the K excretion to increase. These findings, and others indicating a reduced efficiency of resins as sodium removers in patients accumulating oedema (BERGER and STEEL[1472]), suggested that an enhanced absorption of sodium in the colon might be part of a general sodium saving reaction of the body in response to sodium depletion.

As discussed in the section on the kidney (cf p. 312 and 384) the secretion of aldosterone is increased under such conditions, and it is reasonable to assume that the low Na output in the stools results from stimulation of the absorption of Na in the colon by aldosterone. It is consonant with this view that BERGER

[1468] DENNIS, C., and E. H. WOOD: Intestinal absorption in the adrenalectomized dog. Amer. J. Physiol. **129**, 182—190 (1940).

[1469] STEIN, L., and E. WERTHEIMER: Effect of adrenalectomy on intestinal absorption involving osmotic work in rats. Proc. Soc. exp. Biol. (N. Y.) **46**, 172—174 (1941).

[1740] McCHESNEY, E. W., F. C. NACHOD, and M. L. TAINTER: Some aspects of cation exchange resins as therapeutic agents for sodium removal. Ann. N. Y. Acad. Sci. **57**, 252—259 (1954).

[1471] EMERSON, K., JR., S. S. KAHN, and D. JENKINS: The role of the gastrointestinal tract in the adaptation of the body to the prevention of sodium depletion by cation exchange resins. Ann. N. Y. Acad. Sci. **57**, 280—290 (1954).

[1472] BERGER, E. Y., and J. M. STEEL: Suppression of sodium excretion by the colon in congestive heart failure and cirrhosis of the liver demonstrated by the use of cation exchange resins. J. clin. Invest. **31**, 451—456 (1952).

et al.[1473] found that the amounts of sodium removed by resins could be greatly reduced in human subjects and in rats by administration of large doses of desoxy-corticosterone. Further support has come from studies in patients with adreno-cortical insufficiency. EMERSON et al.[1471] reported that desoxycorticosterone treatment of Addisonian patients greatly reduced the extra loss of Na in the stools which resulted from resin administration. The same authors also described a dramatic increase in faecal excretion of Na following the administration of 45 g of resin per day to a patient who had been subjected to bilateral adrenalectomy: 252 meq of Na were lost per day with the stools against 28—65 meq in the non-resin control period. This meant that the resin had induced a Na loss in the faeces some five fold as great as any induced by a similar amount of resin in a normal subject. This observation is not, however, very convincing as an argument for a specific action of the corticoids on the Na absorption in the colon since the faecal loss of sodium equalled, or rather exceeded, the total available cation binding capacity of the resin administered; it seems most likely that the large loss of Na was a consequence of a diarrhoea induced by the resin.

It deserves also to be mentioned that DAVIS and associates (cf. DAVIS et al.[1474]) have reported very low Na/K ratios in the stools of dogs (without resin treatment) in which experimental ascites had been produced by various procedures (con-strictive pericarditis, constriction of the thoracic inferior vena cava) and in which the urinary output of aldosterone was increased. Cf. also DUNCAN et al.[1475] for related findings in human subjects.

Glucocorticoids, on the other hand, do not seem to influence the absorption of sodium in the colon, since DANOWSKI and GREENMAN[1459] did not find any reduction in faecal Na losses during resin treatment when cortisone or ACTH was administered.

The studies of FIELD et al.[1466] provide some indication that the intestinal "sodium saving" in sodium deficiency may not be confined to the colon. These authors reported that, with or without administration of resins, serere restriction of the dietary sodium (to about 1 meq/day) was followed by a marked decrease in the concentration of Na in the intestinal contents removed via a fistula to the terminal ileum in dogs. In view of the findings in the above-mentioned studies on the effect of adrenocortical insufficiency and of desoxycorticosterone (cortin) on ileal absorption it is natural to think of aldosterone as responsible for this "sodium saving" in the upper intestinal tract, but evidently there is no proof that this is so.

The problem whether the intestinal absorption of alkali metal ions is (speci-fically) influenced by *other hormones* still remains largely unsettled. DAVIS et al.[1474] found that in normal dogs as well as in dogs with thoracic caval constriction hypophysectomy was generally followed by an increased excretion of both Na and K in the stools, the Na increase being more pronounced than the K increase. As discussed elsewhere (p. 311) hypophysectomy is generally held to produce only a moderate fall in the aldosterone secretion, a fact which makes it difficult

[1473] BERGER, E. Y., G. P. QUINN, and M. A. HOMER: Effect of desoxycorticosterone on the colon: Its relation to the action of cation exchange resins in man. Proc. Soc. exp. Biol. (N.Y.) **76**, 601—604 (1951).

[1474] DAVIS, J. O., W. C. BALL, JR., R. C. BAHN, and M. J. GOODKIND: Relationship of adrenocortical and anterior pituitary function to fecal excretion of sodium and potassium. Amer. J. Physiol. **196**, 149—152 (1959).

[1475] DUNCAN, L. E., JR., G. W. LIDDLE, and F. C. BARTTER: The effect of changes in body sodium on extracellular fluid volume and aldosterone and sodium excretion by normal and edematous men. J. clin. Invest. **35**, 1299—1305 (1956).

to ascribe the increased faecal cation losses to a reduced secretion of this hormone. In the dogs with caval constriction the authors did, however, observe a fall in the urinary excretion of this hormone following hypophysectomy. This, of course, does not prove that the aldosterone secretion was reduced; an impaired renal excretion might be an alternative explanation.

D. Use of resin therapy for potassium depletion

From the above discussion on resins it is apparent that ingestion of cation exchange resins induce not only a loss of Na, but also — and sometimes more so — a loss of K. Consequently the administration of resins charged exclusively with non-K cations will induce a net loss of K, and when the K intake is low a severe K depletion may occur with prolonged therapy. When resins were still given with the aim of producing Na depletion, such K losses constituted an undesirable side-effect, and to counteract them part of the resin was administered in the K-cycle, and some authors further advised an oral supplement of a potassium salt.

Since our present resins are too imperfect tools for sodium depletion therapy, these problems are no longer of importance. The observation that resins may induce faecal losses of K has, however, lead to some attemps to use them as K-depleting agents. For this purpose they have, of course, been administered in a non-K charged state, and generally this has been the ammoniated form. Such treatment has apparently been successful in the treatment of various cases of hyperkalaemia, in which a very quick and large K-depletion was not required (cf. Knowles and Kaplan[1476]; Evans et al.[1477]). The usefulness of resins for this purpose is, however, limited by the fact that renal failure is by far the most common cause of hyperkalaemia (K-intoxication). In such cases resins given in hydrogen or ammonium charged form are apt to precipitate an acidosis, because the ability of the kidneys to excrete hydrogen ion equivalents is often reduced along with the impairment of the potassium secretion capacity.

E. Intestinal lavage as a measure to correct electrolyte imbalances

Since the passage of Na and K across the intestinal epithelium is quite rapid in both directions, in particular in the small intestine, these cations may be added to or removed from the body at appreciable rates by perfusion of the intestinal lumen with solutions containing Na and K in suitable concentrations. Therapeutically this method has only been applied in a rather limited number of cases, mainly to remove potassium and water (and uraemic metabolites) in cases of renal failure. For details the reader is referred to a recent review by Schloerb[1478].

F. Intestinal absorption as a problem in ureterocolic anastomoses

Rather peculiar problems as regards intestinal absorption (and secretion) of electrolytes have presented themselves in those cases where anastomoses have been established between the ureters and the intestine as a surgical treatment of a variety of pelvic diseases.

[1476] Knowles, H. C., Jr., and S. A. Kaplan: Treatment of hyperkalaemia in acute renal failure using exchange resins. Arch. intern. Med. **92**, 189—194 (1953).

[1477] Evans, B. M., N. C. Hughes Jones, M. D. Milne, and H. Yellowlees: Ion exchange resins in the treatment of anuria. Lancet **1953 II**, 791 — 795.

[1478] Schloerb, P. R.: Peritoneal dialysis and newer methods of intestinal perfusion in renal failure. Arch. intern. Med. **102**, 914—921 (1958).

Anastomoses to the (upper parts of the) small intestine is not tolerated, since uremia develops from reabsorption of toxic components of the urine (HINMAN and BELT[1479]).

Anastomoses to the colon, generally to the sigmoideum, are, however, well tolerated, although disturbances in the body electrolytes develop in a considerable number of cases. Hyperchloraemic acidosis is the disturbance most commonly encountered (FERRIS and ODEL[1480], JACOBS and STIRLING[1481]), but hypokalaemia has also been reported in several cases.

In an attempt to clarify the genesis of these disturbances PERS[1482, 1483] has studied the electrolyte transfers to and from urine samples introduced into an isolated loop of colon in dogs. The *net* absorption of chloride was found to exceed that of sodium, and in particular when concentrated urine samples were introduced. Production of an intestinal secretion, containing high concentrations of sodium and bicarbonate, but little chloride, was offered as the most likely explanation. This state of affairs provides a satisfactory explanation for the hyperchloraemia, and since the loss of bicarbonate represents an addition of hydrogen ion equivalents to the body it also serves to account for the tendency towards acidosis. Intestinal absorption of hydrogen ions (as such, or masked as NH_4^+ by combination with ammonia) from the urine constitutes, however, another way of addition of hydrogen ion equivalents to the body, and a distinction between these possibilities is not feasible. As pointed out by PERS and others, supervention of an impaired renal secretion of hydrogen ions (from pyelonephritis) greatly favours the development of a hyperchloraemic acidosis in these cases.

A moderate net absorption of potassium was also a common finding in PERS' experiments, and he was inclined to think that the hypokalaemia occasionally found in patients with ureterocolic anastomoses is caused by increased renal losses induced by the acidosis, rather than being a consequence of a loss of potassium to the urine during its stay in the intestine.

[1479] HINMAN, F., and A. E. BELT: An experimental study of ureterosigmoidostomy. J. Amer. med. Ass. **79**, 1917—1924 (1922).

[1480] FERRIS, D. O., and H. M. ODEL: Electrolyte pattern of the blood after ureterosigmoidostomy. J. Amer. med. Ass. **142**, 634—641 (1950).

[1481] JACOBS, A., and W. B. STIRLING: The late results of ureterocolic anastomosis. Brit. J. Urol. **24**, 259—316 (1952).

[1482] PERS, M.: Reabsorption from urine in colon. Scand J. clin. Lab. Invest. **6**, 189—202 (1954).

[1483] PERS, M.: The influence of time on reabsorption from urine in colon. Scand. J. clin. Lab. Invest. **7**, 103—110 (1955).

VII. Intakes and general turnovers

By

NIELS A. THORN

A. Intakes

a) Contents in food components

For tables with the contents of sodium and potassium in various foods and diets the reader is referred to MATTICE[1484], MCCANCE and WIDDOWSON[1485] and the pamphlet on sodium-restricted diets issued by the U. S. National Research Council[1486]. The latter publication also has tables on the sodium content of public water supplies in a number of North American states.

b) Normal intakes

The normal intakes of sodium and potassium vary considerably according to food habits. Also, the amount of NaCl used for flavouring by different individuals varies considerably.

Sodium. Few analyses of the actual intake of sodium in normal persons are available. A recent study of a group of American adults (DAHL[1487]) showed a rough average (calculated from urinary excretion) of some 180 meq taken per day with variations from 70 to 450 meq. — This agrees well with the results of a study of urinary chloride excretion in a group of Americans (ASHE and MOSENTHAL[1488]). — There is an interesting sex difference in that among females there seem to be more "low-salt eaters" and among males more "high-salt eaters".

DAHL[1487] also discusses differences in sodium intake in various countries and communities.

Development of hypertension has been claimed to be more frequent in persons who ingest much salt (see also p. 520), and it has been recommended that the intake of salt by normal persons should be decreased below the level of 180 meq/day since salt appetite generally seems greatly to exceed salt requirements (DAHL[1487]). cf. sweating is not prominent. A sodium chloride content in the diet of 0.15 to 2.0% was considered by MENEELY and BALL[1489] to be optimal for rats.

Potassium. Normally the ratio of intake of potassium to that of sodium is $1/4$ to $1/1$, depending on the diet. (DAHL[1487]).

[1484] MATTICE, M. R.: Bridger's Food and Beverage Analyses. 3. ed. Philadelphia: Lea & Fibiger 1950.

[1485] MCCANCE, R. A., and E. M. WIDDOWSON: Chemical composition of foods. H. M. Stat. Office. London 1946.

[1486] Sodium-restricted diets. The rationale, complications, and practical aspects of their use. Nat. Acad. of Sciences-Nat. Research Council. Washington D. C. 1954.

[1487] DAHL, L. K.: Salt intake and salt need. New Engl. J. Med. 258, 1152—1157, 1205—1208 (1958).

[1488] ASHE, B. J., and H. O. MOSENTHAL: Protein, salt and fluid consumption of 1000. residents of New York. J. Amer. med. Ass. 108, 1160—1163, 1937

[1489] MENEELY, G. R., and C. O. T. BALL: Experimental epidemiology of chronic sodium chloride toxicity and the protective effect of potassium chloride. Amer. J. Med. 25, 713—725 (1958).

A recent study (DEMPSEY et al.[1490]) of 31 patients on a metabolic study regimen showed daily voluntary intakes from 40—194 meq.

c) Diets ensuring low intakes

Sodium-restricted diets have been used therapeutically in congestive heart failure, cirrhosis of the liver, essential hypertension and various other disease states. For a description of such diets (e. g. the Kempner rice diet and others) the reader is referred to the pamphlet issued by the U. S. National Research Council[1486]. Sodium-restricted diets comprise both foods naturally low in Na (e. g. rice) as well as such which have been deprived of part of their sodium content (e. g. dialyzed milk) and finally utilize the principle of keeping addition of sodium during the preparation of diets to a minimum. Recently bananas have been advocated as a major component of sodium-restricted diets (WACKER et al.[1491]). Several sodium-restricted diets are difficult to keep because of monotony. The pamphlet on sodium-restricted diets[1486] also contains a chapter on salt substitutes and on the complications and potential dangers of sodium-restricted diets. Such problems are furthermore treated in the clinical treatises listed in the introduction and in the paper by DANOWSKI et al.[1492].

Descriptions of diets low in Na used for experimental animals are found e. g. in the paper by MENEELY and BALL[1493]. Diets low in K are described in the papers by FRIEDMAN et al.[1493] and GARDNER et al.[1494].

B. Daily turnovers

For a person in a steady state obviously intake balances output. A daily intake and output of 180 meq (see p. 518) of sodium for a 70 kg man would mean a turnover of some 4% of the total body sodium (see p. 231). Similarly, a daily intake and output of some 115 meq of potassium (see p. 518) would mean a turnover of some 3% of total body potassium (see p. 231).

Discrepancies between intake and output are found in pregnancy and growth and a number of abnormal states.

For a discussion of salt appetite the reader is referred to STRAUSS[1495]. Given the choice of various sodium salts adrenalectomized rats showed a specific appetite for NaCl and gained weight only on this salt. LiCl can not function as a substitute for NaCl (FREGLY[1496]).

Losses of sodium normally mainly occur in the urine. For a discussion of the processes involved in the renal excretion the reader is referred to p. 233. The excretion in the stools is normally small and pretty constant (on daily intakes from some 2—200 meq only about 0.5 to 5 meq appeared in the stools (DOLE et al.[1497]). This figure agrees well with the average of 3.1 meq found by DEMPSEY et al.[1490].

[1490] DEMPSEY, E. F., E. L. CARROLL, F. ALBRIGHT, and P. H. HANEMAN: A study of factors determining fecal electrolyte excretion. Metabolism 7, 108—118 (1958).

[1491] WACKER, W. E. C., M. MARGOSHES, A. F. BARTHOLOMAY, and B. L. VALLEE: Bananas as a low-sodium dietary staple. New Engl. J. Med. 259, 901—904 (1958).

[1492] DANOWSKI, T. S., E. B. FERGUS, and F. M. MATEER: The low salt syndromes. Ann. intern. Med. 43, 643—657 (1955).

[1493] FRIEDMAN, M., R. H. ROSENMAN, and S. C. FREED: Depressor effect of potassium deprivation on the blood pressure of hypertonic rats. Amer. J. Physiol. 167, 457—461 (1951).

[1494] GARDNER, L. J., N. B. TALBOT, C. D. COOK, H. BERMAN and C. URIBE: The effect of potassium deficiency on carbohydrate metabolism. J. Lab. clin. Med. 35, 592—602 (1950).

[1495] STRAUSS, M. B.: Body water in man. London: Churchill 1951.

[1496] FREGLY, M. J.: Specificity of the sodium chloride appetite of adrenalectomized rats, substitution of lithium chloride for sodium chloride. Amer. J. Physiol. 195, 645—653 (1958).

[1497] DOLE, V. P., L. K. DAHL, G. C. COTZIAS, H. A. EDER, and M. E. KREBS: Dietary treatment of hypertension: clinical and metabolic studies of patients on rice-fruit diet. J. clin. Invest. 29, 1189—1206 (1950).

Minimal losses in the skin have been given as less than 1 meq per day (DAHL et al.[1498]). A detailed discussion of the consequences of losses in sweat are found on p. 447 and in [1499]. The various factors influencing excretion by the different routes have been discussed in the pertinent sections in this book. In contrast to what is the case for sodium, losses of K of some magnitude occur in the cells and bacteria of feces so that minimum fecal K loss exceeds that of sodium. The excretion of potassium in the feces seems to be pretty constant and little affected by intake. It was found by DEMPSEY et al.[1490] in 31 patients to be some 9 meq daily (range 3—21) on an intake of 40—194 meq. Losses of K in the sweat are normally small since the concentration of potassium in sweat is small (see p. 441). It was claimed by BASS et al.[1499] that a "relative" potassium deficiency may develop when persons taking 78 meq/man/day of potassium are exposed to heat. In a recent study[1500], however, physical performances in heat were carried out normally by a group of 15 normal males receiving 70—75 meq of potassium daily. Dietary supplementation to provide an intake of double as much K did not influence physical performances.

[1498] DAHL, L. K., B. C. STALL III, and G. C. COTZIAS: Metabolic effects of marked sodium restriction in hypertensive patients: skin electrolyte losses. J. clin. Invest. **34**, 462—470 (1955).

[1499] BASS, D. E., C. R. KLEEMAN, M. QUINN, A. HENSCHEL, and A. H. HEGNAUER: Mechanism of acclimatization to heat in man. Medicine **34**, 323—380 (1955).

[1500] FREGLY, M. J., and P. F. IAMPIETRO: Dietary potassium supplementation and performance in the desert. Metabolism **7**, 624—634 (1958).

VIII. Effects of excesses and deficits

By

NIELS A. THORN

A. Introduction (remarks on homeostasis)

Both for sodium and potassium, the average daily intake far exceeds minimum need. In spite of this and in spite of the considerable variations in intake the total body contents and distribution are normally rigidly maintained. This must involve signal systems for detection of changes in these parameters and very efficient effectors securing an adequate response to changes. Some of these mechanisms are fairly well known, e.g. the hypothalamicohypophyseal regulation of the osmolarity of the blood (water concentration) and thereby plasma sodium concentration (since sodium is the predominant cation). It seems now also, that considerable depots exist for Na and K. These have been described in the chapters on cartilage and bone (p. 208) and also on p. 202.

The function of these systems, however, only secures the regulation of concentrations in the extracellular phase, whereas the regulation of the capacity factor, total sodium and potassium mass is little known.

That the total volume of intra- and extracellular fluid is rigidly controlled is evident from the small magnitude of fluctuations in body weight. Such fluctuations are kept within ± 500 g. (LOWE[1501]). LOWE and coworkers (see LOWE[1502] for references) have studied factors influencing the volume of body fluids. The body must be considered as a fluid reservoir, an "open" system, with a continuous inflow and outflow of fluid. LOWE et al. have constructed a model on which the effects of changes in the variables of such a system could be studied.

The constancy of volume of intracellular fluid must be a reflection of the vivid regulation in each cell. The control of the active extrusion of sodium and the accumulation of potassium is discussed in part I, p. 65. Total potassium content is predominantly dependant on the number of negative counter-ions (proteins, phosphateesters etc.) present in the cells, but obviously also on the ion pumps of the cellular membranes ensuring that K is the predominant intracellular cation. For a discussion of the possible role of basic amino-acids substituting for K ions as intracellular cations the reader is referred to the papers by ECKEL et al.[1503, 1504].

The idea of a volume receptor sensitive to some volume of extra-cellular fluid (which contains the major part of body Na) (Arterial-tree volume, central venous

[1501] LOWE, T. E.: A model representing the control of body fluid volume in man. Australasian Ann. Med. **4**, 16—25 (1955).

[1502] LOWE, T. E.: Control of body fluid volume in man: Further observations on intake, outflow and volume of body fluid. Australasian Ann. Med. **5**, 42—48 (1956).

[1503] ECKEL, R. E., J. E. C. NORRIS, and C. E. POPE II: Basic amino acids as intracellular cations in K deficiency. Amer. J. Physiol. **193**, 644—652 (1958).

[1504] ECKEL, R. E., C. E. POPE II, and J. E. C. NORRIS: Influence of lysine and NH$_4$Cl feeding on the electrolytes of normal and K-deficient rats. Amer. J. Physiol. **193**, 653—656 (1958).

phase, total extracellular fluid or a small section of extravascular fluid) has been attracting great interest recently. This is discussed on p. 368.

a) Effects of sodium loading

Since this subject has been thoroughly treated in this handbook (Ergänzungs-werk volume 10) by EICHLER, the reader is referred to that volume. The present description will center on the literature which has appeared since that chapter was written.

B. Acute

Acute. Recently the effects of intake of large doses of isotonic sodium chloride (10% of the body weight by gastric tube during 21 hr) has been studied in man (MARKLEY et al.[1505]). The renal effects were an increase of 32% of glomerular fil-tration rate at the termination of the period, with no change in effective plasma flow. The body weights returned to baseline values within 3 hr after the termination of the load. — This study seems to show that man can excrete a large load of sodium chloride solution with a speed equivalent to that of a dog. This is in contrast to earlier findings by CRAWFORD and LUDEMAN[1506]. The differences may, however, be due to the fact that the doses and the rapidity of administra-tion differed widely in the studies cited. Mice tolerate i.v. infusions of isotonic saline in doses up to 250 ml/kg. After an average infusion of 345 ml/kg death occurred with the rate of injection employed (WINBERRY and CRITTENDEN[1507]). Strongly hypertonic sodium chloride solutions given to rabbits or dogs release an unidentified depressor substance, possibly related to adenosine, from the blood cells[1508].

b) Chronic

A daily load for 24 days of 50% of the total body content of sodium produced no toxic effects in rats (NICHOLS and NICHOLS[76]). The sodium content of plasma, muscle and liver was unchanged whereas there was a considerable increase in the sodium content of bone (see chapter II).

More prolonged increased intake of sodium chloride in rats, however, produces a state mimicing human essential hypertension (for references see DAHL[1487] and MENEELY and BALL[1489]). As an example it may be cited (MENEELY and BALL[1489]) that rats fed for 9 months with a diet containing 3—10% NaCl developed sustained arterial hypertension. Increased simultaneous intake of potassium prolonged the survival and lowered the blood pressure in the group receiving large supple-ments of NaCl.

Chronic sodium loading in rats in combination with K deficit causes con-siderable changes in body composition and a marked alkalosis (CHEEK and WEST[1509]).

[1505] MARKLEY, K., M. BOCANEGRA, G. MORALES, and M. CHIAPPORI: Oral sodium loading in normal individuals. J. clin. Invest. **36**, 303—308 (1957).

[1506] CRAWFORD, B., and H. LUDEMAN: The renal response to intravenous injection of sodium chloride solutions in man. J. clin. Invest. **30**, 1456—1462 (1952).

[1507] WINBERRY, M. M., and P. J. CRITTENDEN: Intravenous saline tolerance in mice. Proc. Soc. exp. Biol. (N. Y.) **69**, 220—221 (1948).

[1508] DEYRUP, I. J., and W. W. WALCOTT: Studies on the mechanism of the potentiation of circulatory effects of hypertonic solutions resulting from admixture of these solutions with homologous blood. Amer. J. Physiol. **160**, 509—518 (1950).

[1509] CHEEK, D. B., and C. D. WEST: Alterations in body composition with sodium loading and potassium restriction in the rat: the total body sodium, nitrogen, magnesium and calcium, J. clin. Invest. **35**, 763—774 (1956).

When humans were given about 20—30 g of sodium per day, there was an initial increase in extracellular fluid space and body weight as well as an increase in venous pressure (LADD and RAISZ[1510]). Later a balance was achieved between intake and output. McDONOUGH and WILHELMJ[1511] giving doses of 25—60 g of NaCl also saw an increased body weight and an elevation of blood pressure as well. These changes were normalized immediately on stopping the excessive intake. — The dog seems to have a more effective adaption to sodium loading[1510] WILHELMJ[1512] giving dogs 2.5 g/kg of NaCl daily for up to 205 days found an elevation of the systolic blood pressure which subsided on continuous administration. If the salt was suddenly withdrawn, a sudden fall of systolic and diastolic blood pressure occurred. — It has been claimed that excessive intake of sodium chloride aggravates dermatoses as urticaria and eczema[1513].

C. Effects of potassium loading

a) Acute

For a discussion of the clinical symptoms of potassium intoxication the reader is referred to the clinical treatises listed in the introduction and to the paper by FINCH et al.[1514]. The most striking clinical symptoms are: Numbness of the extremities, muscle weakness and paralysis. The ECG manifestations comprise: (as plasma K increases): Peaked T-waves of increased amplitude, auricular arrest, spreading of QRS, biphasic QRST, ventricular fibrillation. The latter usually occurs at plasma concentrations of some 12 meq/l.

The present section will be restricted to a discussion of the necessary doses for production of intoxication on loading.

It was shown already in 1871 (BUNGE[1515]) that a normal person can tolerate a rapid oral intake of 140 meq of K. The demonstration by KEITH et al.[1516] that doses of 2.5 meq/kg body weight elevates serum K considerably with ECG signs of toxic manifestations indicate that toxic effects are possible after oral intake. In 2 of 5 patients given this dose a 30% decrease in inulin and urea clearances occurred. — 5 meq per kg of potassium taken orally in 1—3 hr has been shown to cause profound muscular weakness and ataxia. — Increased tolerance can develop in the rat and dog after continued administration, however. (THATCHER and RADIKE[1517]). This phenomenon may last for 1 week or longer after stopping the K intake. The main cause is probably an increases efficiency in the renal elimination, possibly caused by adrenocortical stimulation.

After acute potassium loading the excess potassium is transiently stored outside the extracellular fluid and is normally excreted again within 1—3 hours (DRESCHER et al.[1526]).

[1510] LADD, M., and L. G. RAISZ: Response of the normal dog to dietary sodium chloride. Amer. J. Physiol. 159, 149—152 (1949).

[1511] McDONOUGH, J., and C. M. WILHELMJ: Effect of excess salt intake on human blood pressure. Amer. J. Dig. Dis. 21, 180—181 (1954).

[1512] WILHELMJ, C. M., E. B. WALDEMANN, and T. F. McGUIRE: Effect of prolonged high sodium chloride ingestion and withdraval upon blood pressure of dogs. Proc. Soc. exp. Biol. (N. Y.) 77, 379—382 (1951).

[1513] KEINING, E., and G. HOPF: Injurious effects of sodium chloride and their prevention. Arch. Derm. Syph. 32, 739—745 (1935).

[1514] FINCH, C. A., C. G. SAWYER, and J. M. FLYNN: Clinical syndrome of potassium intoxication. Amer. J. Med. 1, 337—352 (1946).

[1515] BUNGE, G.: Über·die physiologische Wirkung der Fleischbrühe und der Kalisalze. Arch. ges. Physiol. 4, 235—282 (1871).

[1516] KEITH, N. M., A. E. OSTERBERG, and H. B. BURCHELL: Some effects of potassium salts in man. Ann. intern. Med. 16, 879—892 (1942).

[1517] THATCHER, J. S., and A. W. RADIKE: Tolerance to potassium intoxication in albino rat. Amer. J. Physiol. 151, 138—146 (1947).

Growing animals tolerate much higher loads than starving young animals because of the deposition of K with protein and glycogen (see p. 533).

Tolerance is decreased in renal failure. Thus in a group of patients with renal failure 3 hr after administration of some 1 meq/kg of body weight, only 4—39% of the K had appeared in the urine (normal patients excreted 49—100%). Serum K in some cases rose to 8 or 9 meq/l for several hours[1525].

It has recently been shown (LARAGH and CAPECI[1518]), (ANDERSON and LARAGH[1519]) that Na depletion sensitizes the organism to the toxic effects of K-loading. This was interpreted to mean that in the Na-depleted animal there are limits to the capacity of the organism to remove K from the extracellular fluid. The renal excretion was not diminished after K-loading as compared to control values.

A high potassium content in mice sensitizes these animals to the toxic effects of histamine (MACMILLAN[1520]). Administration of glutathione decreases the toxic effects of potassium (ZWEMER et al.[1521]). Desoxycorticosterone acetate protects normal rats from KCl poisoning. Thyroid extract has the opposite effect (LOWENSTEIN and ZWEMER[1522]).

Infusion of KCl to dogs caused a lowering of the plasma p_H and bicarbonate (ROBERT et al.[1523]).

The potassium excretion after an increase in potassium intake is greatly diminished in K-deficient subjects (see p. 292, 531). In anaesthetized cats intrathecal injection of small amounts (0.1—0.2 ml of 1.15% or weaker solutions) of KCl produce an elevation of blood pressure, mydriasis and changes in the heart and respiratory rhythms. These effects may be neutralized with $CaCl_2$ (CALMA and WRIGHT[1524]).

The mechanism of the naturetic effect of potassium is discussed on p. 294.

b) Chronic

Doses as high as 5 meq/kg of potassium per day taken over prolonged periods by normal persons do not produce toxic symptoms (McQUARRIE et al.[1527], TALBOTT et al.[1528]. In this connection it is also of interest that persons who live largely on potatoes may have a daily intake of potassium of some 500 to 1000 meq

[1518] LARAGH, J. H., and N. E. CAPECI: Effect of administration of potassium chloride on serum sodium and potassium concentration. Amer. J. Physiol. **180**, 539—544 (1955).

[1519] ANDERSON, H. M., and J. H. LARAGH: Renal excretion of potassium in normal and sodium depleted dogs. J. clin. Invest. **37**, 323—331 (1958).

[1520] MACMILLAN, W. K.: Antagonism of depressed extracellular potassium levels against histamine toxicity in mice. Amer. J. Physiol. **191**, 583—586 (1957).

[1521] ZWEMER, R. L., E. P. VOLLMER, and M. M. CAREY: Glutathione protection against Potassium in mice. Amer. J. Physiol. **164**, 766—769 (1951).

[1522] LOWENSTEIN, B. E., and R. L. ZWEMER: Resistance of rats to potassium poisoning after administration of thyroid or of desoxycorticosterone acetate. Endocrinology **33**, 361 to 365 (1943).

[1523] ROBERTS, K. E., M. G. MAGIDA, and R. F. PITTS: Relationship between potassium and bicarbonate in blood and urine. Amer. J. Physiol. **172**, 47—59 (1953).

[1524] CALMA, I., and S. WRIGHT: Effects of intrathecal injection of KCl and other solutions in cats. Excitatory action of K ions on posterior nerve root fibers. J. Physiol. **106**, 211—235 (1947).

[1525] KEITH, N. M., and A. E. OSTERBERG: Tolerance for potassium in severe renal insufficiency: study of 10 cases. J. clin. Invest. **26**, 773—783 (1947).

[1526] DRESCHER, A. N., N. B. TALBOT, P. A. MEARA, M. TERRY, and J. D. CRAWFORD: A study of the effects of excessive potassium intake upon body potassium stores. J. clin. Invest. **37**, 1316—1322 (1958).

[1527] McQUARRIE, I., W. H. THOMPSON, and J. A. ANDERSON: Effects of excessive ingestion of sodium and potassium salts on carbohydrate metabolism and blood pressure in diabetic children. J. Nutr. **11**, 77—101 (1936).

[1528] TALBOTT, J. H., and R. S. SCHWAB: Recent advances in biochemistry and therapeutics of potassium salts. N. E. J. M. **222**, 585—590 (1940).

apparently without toxic symptoms. — Also intakes as high as 500 meq daily have been tolerated well by patients with myasthenia gravis[1528].

In the study of DRESCHER et al.[1526] rats were given loads of potassium which were increased stepwise from a normal intake of 1.6 to as much as 38.4 meq/100 g body weight per day. Not until the intake exceeded 25.6 meq/100 g were any toxic symptoms noted. Of those which were given more than 25.6 meq/100 g, one half died in K intoxication within 3 days after reaching intake levels of 28.8 to 38.4 meq/100 g. The surviving one half showed intoxication symptoms: roughening of coat, irritability, lethargy, weakness but no significant change in total carcass K content or concentration. (There was a decrease in cardiac intracellular K.) These findings compared with the fact that storing can transiently take place on acute loading suggested to the authors that the maintenance of cellular potassium levels is regulated by adrenocortical function. When the maximal capacity for storing K has been reached, accumulation of K in the extracellular fluid with severe intoxication ensues.

D. Effects of lithium loading.

A detailed discussion of lithium intoxication has recently been published by SCHOU[145]. — Toxic effects of lithium in man have been known for very long, but only recently has the role of the sodium intake in the development of lithium intoxication been clarified. — This was started when lithium salts were used as a sodium substitute for patients on a low sodium diet. In these patients severe intoxications and even deaths occurred (CORCORAN et al.[1529]). The mechanism of this potentiation of toxicity is discussed on p. 419. The use of lithium as a sodium chloride substitute in the diet has now been abandoned. The same is the case with its previous use in uric acid gout. The only rational use of lithium of present seems to be as a drug against protracted or frequently occurring phases of manio-depressive phychosis (CADE[1530], SCHOU et al.[148]). Unfortunately the therapeutic index is pretty low. — Few systematic studies have been done on the toxicity of lithium with simultanous control of sodium intake, so most statements of toxic doses must be treated critically. — Symptoms of lithium intoxication in man have been seen on a low sodium diet after as small a total intake as 5.2 g of lithium chloride. — LEUSEN and

Table 59. *Toxicity of LiCl (given orally) in dogs.* Modified from RADOMSKI et al.[146]

diet	daily dose mg/kg	number of dogs	number of deaths	survival time in days
normal (0.061 meqNa/g)	100	2	2	22—42
	50	2	0	150*
	20	2	0	150*
low-sodium (0.0072 meq/g)	50	2	2	12—18
	20	2	2	18—30

* After that, administration discontinued.

DESMEESTER[1531] saw symptoms similar to the ones following oral intake when they injected lithium intracisternally.

Toxic symptoms derive mainly from the gastrointestinal tract, the kidneys and the central nervous system. In acute poisoning death appears to ensue from toxic effects on the heart. The cause of death in subacute — chronic intoxication is

[1529] CORCORAN, A. C., R. D. TAYLOR, and I. PAGE: Lithium poisoning from the use of salt substitute. J. Amer. med. Ass. **139**, 685—688 (1949).

[1530] CADE, J. F. J.: Lithium salts in the treatment of psychotic excitement. Med. J. Aust. **2**, 349—352 (1949).

[1531] LEUSEN, I., and G. DEMEESTER: Au sujet de la toxicité du chlorure de lithium. Acta med. scand. **138**, 232—236 (1950).

held by some to be renal failure. — Generally, at serum concentrations below 0.7 meq/l no symptoms are found. From 0.7—1.1 meq/l gastrointestinal symptoms occur,whereas severe toxic symptoms are seen at concentrations between 3—4 meq/l. The lethal conc. in man seems to be approximately 5 meq/l.

Gastrointestinal tract. Symptoms occur in animals and man both after i. v. injection and oral intake. They are nausea, salivation, vomiting and diarrhoea, occasionally watery, hemorrhageous stools. — Hyperaemia of the gastrointestinal tract mucosa, sometimes with small ulcerations, seem to be the only pathological findings. — In animals atropin sulphate, (1—2 mg/kg of body weight) has alleviated these symptoms.

Muscular and nervous systems. Beginning symptoms of lithium intoxication are tremor of the hands, occasionally of the lips and mandible, later muscular weakness with ataxia, positive Romberg's symptoms, drowsiness, tinnitus, slurred speach and blurred vision. In some cases mental confusion has occurred. More severe symptoms are muscular hyperirritability, nystagmus, chorea-athetosis and Parkinson-like symptoms. In the most severe cases epileptic seizures and coma are found. For a detailed description of these and other symptoms see SCHOU[145]. EEG changes are mainly dominated by severe slow dysrhythmia with frequencies of 4—6 Hz and voltages to 150 mV. The same changes may be seen in patients treated with lithium, but showing no toxic symptoms. No pathological anatomical changes in the muscular and nervous systems have been reported. MORACCI[1532] applied lithium salts to the exposed motor area of dog's cortex. Tonic and clonic seizures were seen in the corresponding muscles — sometimes a more generalized reaction occurred. The rats studied by DAVENPORT[147] had lower seizure thresholds to electric stimuli than the control animals.

Circulation. A decreased heart rate is often seen in animals and man. Flattening of T waves, even inversion (after 25—50 meq/day) is seen in man, also after therapeutic doses, associated with no other signs of intoxication. The changes are reversible. Reports on effects on blood pressure seem conflicting. In more severe lithium intoxication the simultaneous elevations of serum K conc. may be responsible for part of the effect. Cardiac arrest may be seen.

Kidneys. Some authors consider renal failure with oliguria and azotemia the main cause of death in subchronic-chronic lithium-poisoning. — In the lighter intoxications a transient proteinuria or hematuria may be found. — Also after small doses a vasopressin-resistant diabetes insipidus may be found.

Recently SCHOU[1533] has published a careful study of lithium intoxication in rats after i.p. injection and with control of sodium intake. Rats kept on a low sodium intake (less than 0.5 meq/kg per day) tolerated well a lithium intake less than 3 meq/kg per day, and their excretion kept pace with the intake. The only symptoms were a certain lethargy and a reversible polyuria, resistant to vasopressin. — Intakes above 3 meq/kg per day produced irreversible intoxication. The serum concentration of lithium rose, first slowly, then rapidly. This condition was characterized by a comatose state with occasional convulsions. Serum potassium concentrations remained within a normal range, but a negative sodium balance occurred. The terminal states were characteristic of renal insufficiency. — Slight pathological changes (a moderate vacuolization) in the zona glomerulosa and fasciculata of the adrenals were found, but marked changes (acute degeneration) occurred in the proximal part of the nephron. (In the dog experiments of RA-DOMSKI et al.[146] the lesions were located to the distal part of the nephron.) When

---

[1532] MORACCI, E.: Azione di alcuni sali applicati direttamente sui centre corticali sensitivo-motori del cane. Arch. Fisiol. **29**, 487—492, 493—511 (1931).

[1533] SCHOU, M.: Lithium studies I. Toxicity. Acta pharmacol. (Kbh.) **15**, 70—84 (1958).

the sodium intake was increased to 5 meq/kg per day the rats tolerated up to 5 meq/kg of lithium per day.

Treatment of lithium intoxication. It seems well established that a high sodium intake is of prophylactic value against lithium intoxication, also that the administration of large amounts of NaCl may accelerate the excretion of lithium in cases of light intoxication. The question of a probable beneficial effect of sodium chloride in cases of severe intoxication is unsolved.

E. Effects of rubidium loading
a) Acute

In the acute toxicity of rubidium seen after infusions in dogs, symptoms from the heart are predominant. These symptoms on the whole resemble those produced by potassium intoxication. However, some differences are seen. — Kunin et al.[1534]* injected Rb^{86} labelled rubidium chloride solutions of 25—100 meq/l (made isotonic with NaCl or $NaHCO_3$) into dogs. The potassium concentration in the plasma rose, although no potassium was infused. At concentrations of Rb of 0.2—1.0 meq/l (Rb + K: 4—5 meq/l) a decrease in heart rate, peaking of T waves and increased S waves in the ECG occurred. Later the amplitude of T increased, S disappeared and R diminished. When Rb conc. reached 2.0—3.5 meq/l (Rb + K: 7—8 meq/l), P disappeared and varying degrees of A—V block and nodal or ventricular beats appeared. At Rb + K of 9.5—13.0 meq/l ventricular tachycardia developed. Control injections of KCl gave similar symptoms except extrasystoles. Tarail et al.[1535] found a somewhat similar picture. Although the actual lethal doses were not given in that study it was stated that the mean lethal dose of Rb was larger than that of K. The predominance of ventricular tachycardia — ventricular flutter in Rb intoxication was stressed. The LD_{50} for mice of Rb_2CO_3 was found by Zipser and Freedberg[1536] to be 0.65 mg/g body weight. Overdosage produced generalized paralysis leading to respiratory failure.

b) Chronic

Prolonged intake of Rb in experimental animals leads to symptoms from the nervous system, mainly increased irritability[153]. Although Rb causes acidosis[1537] there is some indication that the effects on the neuromuscular system are independent of those caused by the acidosis (Relman[153]). — The acidosis produced is mild. In the experiments of Relman et al.[1538] rats given daily 3 meq/kg RbCl for 6 days had a p_H in the plasma of 7.50 ± 0.04 and a plasma CO_2 of 22.5 ± 1.3 8mMol/l. The CO_2 of the control group was 26,2 ± 1.92 mMol/l. There is some indication of a decreased ammonia production in Rb loaded rats[1537]). Young rats receiving a K-deficient diet plus 0.85% KCl and 0.5% RbCl showed a poor growth and lesions of the myocardium[1536]. The profound changes in muscular composition after feeding Rb for a longer period (see p. 225) may explain the symptoms.

[1534] Kunin, A. S., E. H. Dearborn, and A. S. Relman: Electrocardiographic changes produced by rubidium infusions in the dog. Amer. J. Physiol. **183**, 636 (1955).

[1535] Tarail, R., T. E. Bennett, and W. K. Noell: A comparison of electrocardiographic, electroencephalographic, and chemical effects of rubidium and potassium in dogs. J. clin. Invest. **34**, 966—967 (1955).

[1536] Zipser, A., and A. Stone Freedberg: The distribution of administered radioactive rubidium (Rb^{86}) in normal and neoplastic tissues of mice and humans. Cancer Res. **12**, 867—870 (1952).

[1537] Lambie, A. T., A. M. Roy, A. S. Relman, B. A. Burrows, and W. B. Schwartz: On the mechanism of rubidium induced acidosis. Clin. Res. Proc. **4**, 128 (1956).

' * See also: Kunin, A. S., E. H. Dearborn, and A. S. Relman: Effect of infusion of rubidium chloride on plasma electrolytes and the electrocardiogram of the dog. Amer. J. Physiol. **197**, 231—235 (1959).

F. Effects of cesium loading
a) Acute

HAZARD et al.[1539] injected intravenously solutions of 350 meq/L of cesium at a rate of 9 ml/min to dogs with a weight of approximately 10 kg. The symptoms seen in the ECG were: inhibition of sinus activity, sinus arrythmia, sino-auricular block, ventricular tachycardia, ventricular fibrillation and death. The severe symptoms were usually seen when some 60 ml or 21 meq had been injected. LD_{50} after i.p. injection in rats were found by COCHRAN et al.[1540] to be as given in Table 60.

b) Chronic

FOLLIS[1541] gave a group of normal rats a K-deficient diet with a supplement of 0.5% CsCl and 0.85% KCl. These animals showed a fine growth for 3 weeks, then the growth stopped and a wt. loss occurred. At the same time they showed signs of hyperirritability, later developing into fits lasting 3—4 min, in which the animal, following auditory stimuli, trembled, ran wildly about, fell on one side with both legs extended and had spastic extremities with a fine, muscular tremor. — The profound changes caused in muscular composition (225) after feeding Cs or Rb for a longer period may explain the muscular symptoms.

c) Factors influencing the excretion of cesium.

Since cesium is one of the more important long-lived fission products, considerable interest is attached to the behaviour of this metal in the body. HOOD and COMAR[121] in a study of the metabolism of cesium[137] in rats and farm animals reported a total cesium[137] excretion by the rat of 70% of the dose in 7 days with 12 times more cesium in the urine than in the feces. The predominance of the renal route of excretion was confirmed by MRAZ et al.[1542]. — MRAZ et al.[1543, 1544] showed that dietary potassium increased the rate of excretion of cesium in rats. Sodium also increased the excretion, when the diet was adequate in K.

Table 60. LD_{50} for various cesium compounds given i.p. to rats. Modified from COCHRAN et al.[1540]

Compound	LD_{50} of compound mg/kg	LD_{50} of metal mg/kg
Cesium chloride . .	1500	1118
Cesium hydroxide .	100	89
Cesium bromide . .	1400	874
Cesium iodide . . .	1400	715

Various natural foodstuffs increased the excretion of cesium[134] in the feces, probably due to adsorption (MRAZ et al.[1545, 1546]). Parathyroid extract, large doses

[1538] RELMAN, A. S., A. M. ROY, and W. B. SCHWARTZ: The acidifying effect of rubidium in normal and potassium-deficient alkalotic rats. J. clin. Invest. **34**, 538—544 (1955).

[1539] HAZARD, R., J. R. BOISSUR, J. HAZARD, and P. MOUILLI: Action cardiovasculaire du cesium. Arch. int. Pharmacodyn. **110**, 203—221 (1957).

[1540] COCHRAN, K. W., J. DOULL, M. MAZUR, and K. P. DU BOIS: Acute toxicity of zirconium, columbium, strontium, lanthanum, cesium, tantalum and yttrium. Arch. Industr. Hygiene and Occupat. Medicine **1**, 637—650 (1950).

[1541] FOLLIS, R. H., jr.: Histological effects in rats resulting from adding rubidium or cesium to a diet deficient in potassium. Amer. J. Physiol. **138**, 246—250 (1943).

[1542] MRAZ, F., M. LeNOIR, J. PINAJIAN, and H. PATRICK: Influence of parathyroid extract, cortisone and dienestrol diacetate on metabolism of cesium in rats. Arch. Biochem. Biophys. **63**, 73—76 (1956).

[1543] MRAZ, F. R., and H. PATRICK: Factors influencing excretory patterns of cesium[134], potassium[42] and rubidium[86] in rats. Proc. Soc. exp. Biol. (N. Y.) **94**, 409—412 (1957).

[1544] MRAZ, F. R., M. LeNOIR, J. J. PINAJIAN, and H. PATRICK: Influence of potassium and sodium on uptake and retention of cesium[134] in rats. Arch. Biochem. Biophys. **66**, 177—182 (1957).

Table 61. *Influence of parathyroid extract, dienestrol diacetate and massive vitamin D₂ on the metabolism of Cesium-134* (mean % dose/g × 100, except blood which is mean % dose/ml × 100). Modified from WILLIAMS and PATRICK[581b]

	whole blood	muscle	liver	kidney	spleen
control	0.33	2.1	2.3	4.0	1.3
treated with PTH	0.44	2.9	3.2	4.0	2.1
treated with dienestrol diacetate . .	0.50	3.8	4.1	7.5	3.0
treated with massive doses of vitamin D₂	0.56	2.7	4.8	6.9	3.0

of vitamin D_2 and dienestrol diacetate caused a greater uptake or retention of Cs in the tissues studied following the administration of a single subcutaneous dose in rabbits[1547] (see Table 61).

G. Sodium depletion

a) Acute

One of the ways most often used in producing fairly rapid sodium depletion is the one employed by DARROW and YANNET[1548] consisting in injecting intraperitoneally large loads of isotonic glucose and withdrawing the sodium containing fluid after some time. This principle was also used in the recent studies of WOODBURY[77] and that of WHITE et al.[1549]. A rapid "pure" sodium depletion can be achieved by vivodialysis against a fluid only differing from plasma in its sodium concentration (NICHOLS and NICHOLS[75]).

The most striking features of sodium depletion are weakness, muscle cramps and decrease of the circulating blood volume with final circulatory failure. This, in man, occurs when some 1000 meq of sodium have been lost (ELKINTON and DANOWSKI[9]). For discussion of the clinical syndromes involved the reader is referred to clinical treatises listed in the introduction to this part, especially those by ELKINTON and DANOWSKI[9] and DANOWSKI et al.[1492] and also to p. 447 and [1499].

NICHOLS and NICHOLS[75] have published a careful study of the effects af acute sodium depletion on the composition of tissues in dogs. Approximately 23% of total body sodium was removed by dialysis. The extracellular phase contributed 70%, bone 25% and body cells only 5% of the sodium removed. Of the sodium which was lost from the extracellular phase, approximately 60% came from the skin and extracell phase of muscle, tendon and extracell water of bone yielded another 26%, plasma only 12%. — The rate of mobilization of sodium from bone decreased with time. — The distribution of the loss of Na from extracellular fluid, bone and cells is in fairly good agreement with earlier results found by BERGSTROM in rats[68]. — The clinical symptoms developing in the dogs were mainly hyperpnea and a metabolic acidosis. This in the cases where death occurred had become incompensated. In the animals which had some 100 meq of sodium removed, there was a compensated metabolic acidosis. These animals were

[1545] MRAZ, F. R., and H. PATRICK: Organic factors controlling the excretory pattern of potassium[42] and cesium[134] in rats. J. Nutr. **61**, 535—546 (1957).

[1546] MRAZ, F. R., and H. PATRICK: Some factors influencing the excretory pattern of cesium[134] in rats. Arch. Biochem. Biophys. **71**, 121—125 (1957).

[1547] WILLIAMS, L. G., and H. PATRICK: Metabolism of cesium[134] in rabbits. Arch. Biochem. Biophys. **70**, 464—468 (1957).

[1548] DARROW, D. C., and H. YANNET: Changes in distribution of body water accompanying increase and decrease in extracellular electrolyte. J. clin. Invest. **14**, 266—275 (1935).

very slow in recovering from the procedure, usually being lethargic and refusing food for 2—3 days.

WHITE et al.[1549] by intraperitoneal dialysis removed 30% of body sodium from adult rats. The sodium loss was mainly accounted for by loss from extracellular fluid, only small changes were found in the sodium content of bone. The discrepancies found in the litterature regarding concepts of mobilization of bone sodium and the nature of the stimulus for such mobilizations are discussed p. 213.

A detailed study of the changes in the composition of various tissues in acute hyponatremia was undertaken by WOODBURY[77] who stresses the individual differences in the changes in the tissues; e.g. brain actually gained sodium.

Renal responses to a diminution of total blood volume are discribed on p. 369.

b) Chronic

The sodium conserving power of the organism. From the studies of DAHL et al. (see DAHL[1487]) it seems that humans may exist for years on a diet as low in sodium content as some 5 meq per day without any signs of deficiency. Several reports are available on the effect of sodium restriction on body metabolism. Chronic restriction of sodium to some 5 meq daily causes a decrease in the plasma concentration of Na and a decrease in total exchangeable sodium (Na$_e$) (DAHL[1487]). A whole set of laboratory tests and tests of adrenocortical function were all normal in these patients. A weight loss of some 1.5% probably due to loss of extracellular fluid was found by THOMAS et al.[1550]. Other studies of the effects of sodium restriction are those of RENWICK et al.[1551]. One of the most predominant responses to sodium restriction is an activation of the production of aldosterone[1552], with ensuing effects on the sodium transport in the kidneys, the terminal ileum, salivary glands and sweat glands. The maximal response in these various organs does not result at the same time. After restricted sodium intake the kidneys adapt completely in hours, the sweat glands take 4—5 days and the salivary glands about 2 weeks. These responses are further discussed on p. 212.

The adaptation of the ileum (which takes approximately two weeks) is discussed also in the paper by FIELD et al.[1553]. — A discussion of the effects of aldosterone on fecal excretion of sodium and potassium is found in the paper by DAVIS et al.[1554a].

Due to the efficient conservation of sodium induced by aldosterone, severe experimental sodium depletion in man has mainly been studied in patients with

[1549] WHITE, H. L., M. AUDIA, and D. ROLF: Comparison of total body and tissue losses of sodium and chloride with losses from sucrose space in salt-depleted rats. Amer. J. Physiol. **196**, 54—58 (1959).

[1550] THOMAS, C. B., HOWARD and H. ISAACS: The effect of sodium withdrawal upon the body weight of normal young men. Bull. Johns Hopk. Hosp. **85**, 115—134 (1949).

[1551] RENWICK, R., J. S. ROBINSON, and C. P. STEWART: Observations upon the withdrawal of sodium chloride from the diet in hypertensive and normotensive individuals. J. clin. Invest. **34**, 1037—1043 (1955).

[1552] CRABBÉ, J., E. J. ROSS, and G. W. THORN: The significance of the secretion of aldosterone during dietary sodium deprivation in normal subjects. J. Clin. Endocr. **18**, 1159 to 1177 (1958).

[1553] FIELD, H., jr., R. E. DAILEY, R. S. BOYD, and L. SWELL: Effect of restriction of dietary sodium on electrolyte composition of the contents of the terminal ileum. Amer. J. Physiol. **179**, 477—480 (1954).

[1554a] DAVIS, J. O., W. C. BALL, JR., R. C. BAHN, and M. J. GOODKIND: Relationship of adrenocortical and anterior pituitary function to fecal excretion of sodium and potassium. Amer. J. Physiol. **196**, 149—152 (1959).

decreased adrenocortical function. From studies of adrenalectomized humans on a restricted sodium diet and receiving maintenance doses of cortisone LIPSETT and PEARSON[1554b] concluded that when sodium loss is gradual, a deficit of some 50% of total exchangeable sodium may be reached before the development of hyponatremia whereas a hyponatremia will be caused by a much smaller deficit if it occurs suddenly.

Because of the high content of sodium in the body an organism can survive a small negative balance of sodium for a considerable period, e. g. a negative balance of 3 meq/day of sodium in the course of 50 days would be equivalent to only the loss of the sodium in 1 l of extracellular fluid.

In a sodium-depleted animal potassium produces a hyperkaliemia (ANDERSON and LARAGH[1519]) which is not due to a deficient renal secretion, but most likely to a relative inability of the hyponatremic organism to store K within the cell. Young rats fed a diet containing 0.002% of sodium chloride in 19 weeks died with symptoms of retarded growth and ocular lesions. The serious symptoms started in the 14'th week (ORENT-KEILES et al.[1556]). — Rats fed on a diet deficient in NaCl for periods of 30—150 days developed decreased weight of thymus and spleen, but increased weight of the kidney, no changes in cardiac weight. There was an increased weight of the adrenals with a reduction of the ascorbic acid content (DANFORD and HERRING[1557]). This was interpreted as showing stimulation of mineralocorticoid (and glucocorticoid) secretion.

H. Potassium depletion

a) Acute

Potassium depletion can be rapidly produced by vivodialysis. A more gradual depletion occurs on a low-potassium diet with or without the additional administration of ionic-exchange resin.

For a detailed description of the clinical causes and symptoms of acute and chronic potassium depletion the reader is referred to the clinical treatises listed in the introduction and also to the papers by SURAWICZ et al.[1555], BROOKS et al.[1558] that of CONN and MACH[1559]. The main clinical symptoms are: Weakness, even paralysis of skeletal muscles, first in the extremities, then respiratory, mental function impairment, later atonia of smooth muscles. ECG changes comprise: (as the conc. of K in plasma decreases) decreased amplitude and broadening of T waves, sagging S—T segments, A—V block.

SURAWICZ et al. state that the only clinical abnormality in hypopotassemia showing some correlation with the degree of hypopotassemia was the decrease of the activity of the deep tendon reflexes.

The present chapter will be restricted to a discussion of recent reports on the structural and functional derangements seen in these conditions.

[1554b] LIPSETT, M. B., and O. H. PEARSON: Sodium depletion in adrenalectomized humans. J. clin. Invest. **37**, 1394—1402 (1958).

[1555] SURAWICZ, B., H. A. BRAUN, W. B. CRUM, R. L. KEMP, S. WAGNER, and S. BELLET: Clinical Manifestations of Hypopotassemia. Amer. J. med. Sci. **233**, 603—616 (1957).

[1556] ORENT-KEILES, E., and E. V. McCOLLUM: Mineral metabolism of rats on an extremely sodium-deficient diet. J. biol. Chem. **133**, 75—81 (1940).

[1557] DANFORD, H. G. and R. C. HERRING: Some physiological effects of salt restrictions in the rat. Amer. J. Physiol. 165, 128—134 (1951).

[1558] BROOKS, R. V., R. R. McSWINEY, F. T. G. PRUNTZ, and F. J. Y. WOOD: Potassium deficiency of renal and adrenal origin. Amer. J. Med. **23**, 391—407 (1957).

[1559] MACH, R.-S.: Les états de déplétion en potassium. Schw. Med. Wschr. 88, 1299—1305 (1958).

Vivodialysis in dogs (WELLER et al.[1560], HABIB et al.[1561]) and in man (GJØRUP and HESS THAYSEN[1562]) against a potassium-free fluid produces a rapid "pure" loss of potassium often in 2 phases, one partly from extracellular fluid, another from cellular sources, exclusively, with the conc. in the extracellular fluid remaining constant — These latter sources do not seem to include heart, liver or skeletal muscle. Their character is unknown. — It might be that the potassium of bone (see p. 214) functions as a (small) depot. The fact that no loss of K from muscle was found in these acute experiments is in contrast to the findings in chronic potassium depletion where muscular potassium is exchanged for sodium.

An acute increase of the extracellular fluid volume by 53% with a K-free solution causes mobilization of potassium so efficiently that only an insignificant decrease is seen in plasma potassium concentration (SCRIBNER et al.[1563]).

One of the most characteristic disturbances in potassium depletion is an extracellular alkalosis, presumably due to a loss of hydrogen ions by the kidney and from extracellular fluid into the cells (see chapter IV)*.

Changes in the cardiac function are reflected in ECG changes. The following changes in dogs were noted by WELLER et al.[1560]: Accelerated heart rate, increased P waves, increased A—V conduction time. The ventricular changes were: a widening of the QRS, broadening and rounding of the T wave and depression of ST. For detailed discussions of the myocardial changes the reader is referred to GOODOF and McBRYDE[1564] and KEY[1565]. The clinical cardiac manifestations were described by PERKINS et al.[1566].

FINKENSTAEDT et al.[1567] by hemodialysis rapidly depleted 8 normal dogs of up to 25% of their K content. The symptoms developing were profound muscular weakness and apathy, elevated pCO_2, but little change in bicarbonate content, and a decrease in inulin clearance to some 40—50%.

DARROW[1568] noted similarity of the symptoms of K deficiency and those of paralytic ileus and suggested that the intestinal paralysis might be caused by a decrease in plasma K. STREETEN and WILLIAMS[1569] in animal experiments showed that the depression of intestinal propulsion may be related causally to a reduction in cellular K. In the recent experiments of DANIEL and BASS[1570] potassium

---

* See also the paper by J. E. HUTH, R. D. SQUIRES, and J. E. ELKINTON: Experimental potassium depletion in normal human subjects II. Renal and hormonal factors in the development of extra cellular alkalosis during depletion. J. clin. Invest. 38, 1149—1165 (1959).

[1560] WELLER, J. M., B. LOWN, R. V. HOIGNE, N. F. WYATT, M. CRISCITIELLO, J. P. MERRILL, and S. A. LEVINE: Effects of acute removal of potassium from dogs. Changes in the electrocardiogram. Circulation 11, 44—52 (1955).

[1561] HABIB, Y. A., G. C. NICHOPOULOS, and R. R. OVERMAN: Effect of acute removal of potassium from the body on tissue electrolytes. Amer. J. Physiol. 193, 634—638 (1958).

[1562] GJØRUP, S., and J. H. THAYSEN: Distribution of potassium excess in oliguric patients Scand. J. clin. Lab. Invest. 10, 5—10 (1958).

[1563] SCRIBNER, B. H., H. KLEINBERG, and J. M. BURNELL: Failure of change in extracellular volume to alter plasma potassium concentration. Amer. J. Physiol. 195, 448—450 (1958).

[1564] GOODOF, J. I., and C. M. MACBRYDE: Heart failure in Addison's disease with myocardial changes of potassium deficiency. J. clin. Endocr. 4, 30—34 (1944).

[1565] KEYE, J. D.: Death in potassium deficiency; report of case including morphologic findings. Circulation 5, 766—770 (1952).

[1566] PERKINS, J. G., A. B. PETERSEN, and A. J. RILEY: Renal and cardiac lesions in potassium deficiency due to chronic diarrhoea. Amer. J. Med. 8, 115—123 (1950).

[1567] FINKENSTAEDT, J. T., A. RUIZ-GUINAZA, L. MOREAU, R. S. MORRISON and J. P. MERRILL: Experimental acute potassium depletion in dogs. Clin. Sci. 16, 171—179 (1957).

[1568] DARROW, D. C.: Medical progress; body-fluid physiology: role of potassium in clinical disturbances of body water and electrolyte. New Engl. J. Med. 242, 978—983 (1950).

[1569] STREETEN, D. H. P., and E. M. V. WILLIAMS: Loss of cellular potassium as a cause of intestinal paralysis in dogs. J. Physiol. 118, 149—170 (1952).

[1570] DANIEL, E. E., and P. BASS: Influence of sodium, potassium and adrenal hormones on gastrointestinal motility. Amer. J. Physiol. 187, 253—258 (1956).

deficiency decreased gastrointestinal motility only when associated with sodium depletion. The activation of mineralocorticoid activity caused by such states — with ensuing loss of K from the smooth muscle fibers — further strengthens the concept that the contraction of intestinal muscle depends critically on its K contents (see also p. 193 and 533).

b) Chronic

The potassium conserving power of the organism. Studies of the potassium conserving power of the organism have been hampered until recently by the difficulty in producing diets low in potassium. — Although the potassium conserving mechanism of the kidneys are able to work against procedures which usually increase the excretion of K (alkali intake, osmotic diuresis) (EVANS et al.[1571]), and although it has been reported that the daily losses of K by the kidneys may be restricted to values around 1 meq (WESTON et al.[1572]), the overall conservation by the body, does not reach the capacity of the sodium conservation (see also p. 293)*. Considerable amounts of K are lost with the feces (see p. 518). Unlike for Na there is no K-conserving mechanism in the colon. Activation of the Na-conserving mechanism causes increased loss of K[1553]. Other factors than the lack of K alone significantly influence the development of K deficiency symptoms. Among these factors are protein deficiency (CANNON et al.[1573]) a simultaneous high intake of Na, (CANNON et al.[1574]) or phosphate (SELYE and BAJUSZ[1575]). The role of cellular sodium intoxication in potassium deficiency has recently been discussed by SPATER et. al.[1576] A rapid repletion occurs in rats when potassium salts are injected (SCHWARTZ et al.[1577]).

Renal changes. Some of the most striking effects of potassium depletion are the structural and functional changes seen in the kidney. These have recently been thoroughly described in several reviews, among them those by RELMAN and SCHWARTZ[1578] and MILNE et al.[1579]. The syndrome has been produced experimentally, especially in rats (given a diet containing 0.07 meq K per 100 g) HOLLANDER et al.[1580] and has been seen in various clinical conditions, among them the recently

---

* See also the paper by R. D. SQUIRES and E. J. HUTH: Experimental potassium depletion in normal human subjects I. Relation of ionic intakes to the renal conservation of potassium. J. clin. Invest. **38**, 1134—1148 (1959).

[1571] EVANS, B. M., N. C. HUGHES JONES, M. D. MILNE, and S. STEINER: Electrolyte excretion during experimental potassium depletion in man. Clin. Sci. **13**, 305—316 (1954).

[1572] WESTON, R. E., J. GROSSMAN, E. R. BORUN, H. A. GUERIN, H. MARK, T. D. ULLMAN, M. WOLFMAN, and L. LEITER: Metabolic studies on the effects of ion exchange resins in edematous patients with cardiac and renal disease. Amer. J. Med. **14**, 404—424 (1953).

[1573] CANNON, P. R., L. E. FRAZIER, and R. H. HUGHES: Influence of potassium on tissue protein synthesis. Metabolism **1**, 49—57 (1952).

[1574] CANNON, P. R., L. E. FRAZIER, and R. H. HUGHES: Sodium as toxic ion in potassium deficiency. Metabolism. **2**, 297—312 (1953).

[1575] SELYE, H., and E. BAJUSZ: Provocation and prevention of potassium deficiency by various ions. Proc. Soc. exp. Biol. (N. Y.) **98**, 580—583 (1958).

[1576] SPATER, H., A. HUNT, R. TODD, P. MEARA, M. TERRY, J. D. CRAWFORD, and N. B. TALBOT: Development and therapy of cellular sodium intoxication in potassium deficiency. Metabolism **8**, 28—38 (1959).

[1577] SCHWARTZ, R., J. COHEN, and W. M. WALLACE: Distribution of injected potassium salts in tissues of the potassium-deficient rat. Amer. J. Physiol. **182**, 39—44 (1955).

[1578] RELMAN, A. S., and W. B. SCHWARTZ: The kidney in potassium depletion. Amer. J. Med. **24**, 764—773 (1958).

[1579] MILNE, M. D., R. C. MUERHCKE and B. E. HEAD: Potassium deficiency and the kidney. Brit. med. Bull. **13**, 15—18 (1957).

[1580] HOLLANDER, W., R. W. WINTERS, T. F. WILLIAMS, J. BRADELEY, J. OLIVER, and L. G. WELT: Defect in the renal tubular reabsorption of water associated with potassium depletion in rats. Amer. J. Physiol. **189**, 557—563 (1957).

discovered syndrome of primary hyperaldosteronism[16a]. — No information is available on the severity and minimum duration of the K-deficiency required to cause symptoms in man.

Structural changes. The most striking structural changes are an increase in kidney size. This occurs within few days in both man and the rat. — Microscopic lesions are found after 1 week. In man a vacuolization of the convoluted tubules is the characteristic change. In the rat the lesion is primarily located to the collecting tubules. (A hyperplastic obstructing lesion which secondarily leads to proximal dilatation and degeneration). For a detailed description see OLIVER et al.[1581] *. The changes seem to be reversible provided they have not persisted too long.

Functional changes. These involve all parts of the nephron, but the most characteristic feature seems to be a vasopressin-resistant diabetes insipidus. (Also a decreased response to a water load is found.) The effect of potassium depletion on the distal tubular electrolyte transport (enhanced sodium reabsorption enhanced ammonia excretion) has been discussed on p. 294. Glomerular filtration rate is reduced, and there seems to be an inhibition in the proximal tubular transport mechanism for PAH and phosphate. Several enzyme systems function in a deficient way (IACOBELLIS[1582]), but on the other hand glutaminase and carbonic anhydrase activity is increased. It is interesting that the normal diurnal cycle in potassium excretion (see p. 387) is abolished (EVANS et al.[1571]). — In potassium depletion there is often a sodium retention. The mechanism of this phenomenon is unknown. It might be due to the increased ammonia excretion.

Myocardial changes. It is very difficult to lower the potassium content of the myocardium of rats by restricted K intake (St. GEORGE et al.[1583]). Considerable pathological changes occur in the myocardium of man, however, in chronic potassium depletion[1584]. The essential finding is a myocardial fibrosis (McALLEN[1585]). In there studies a diminution of the K cone. of the myocardium was found.

Other changes. A diet low in potassium leads to partial exchange of muscular K for Na [see part I, chapter VII B (b)]. Severe K-deficiency in rats was associated with an inhibited tissue glycogenesis (GARDNER et al.[1494]).

The symptoms seen in dogs on a low-K diet are fairly similar to those seen in humans (MUNTWYLER et al.[1586], SMITH[1587]). The same is the case in rats. — Rats fed on a K-deficient diet (DANFORD and HERRING[1557]) had increased weight of the adrenals with lowered ascorbic acid content, decreased weight of the thymus and a

[1581] OLIVER, J., M. MacDOWELL, L. G. WELT, M. A. HOLLIDAY, W. HOLLANDER, R. W. WINTERS, T. F. WILLIAMS, and W. E. SEGAR: The renal lesions of electrolyte imbalance. I The structural alterations in potassium-depleted rats. J. exp. Med. 106, 563—574 (1957).

* See also M. A. HOLLIDAY, R. W. WINTERS, L. G. WELT, M. MACDOWELL and J. OLIVER: The renal lesions of electrolyte imbalance II. The combined effect on renal architecture of phosphate loading and potassium depletion. J. exp. Med. 110, 161—168 (1959).

[1582] IACOBELLIS, M., E. MUNTWYLER, and G. E. GRIFFIN: Enzyme concentration changes in the kidneys of protein-and/or potassium-deficient rats. Amer. J. Physiol. 178, 477—482 (1954).

[1583] ST. GEORGE, S., S. C. FREED, R. H. ROSENMAN, and S. WINDERMAN: Influence of potassium deprivation and adrenalectomy on potassium concentration of the myocardium. Amer. J. Physiol. 181, 550—552 (1955).

[1584] Human heart changes in prolonged potassium deficiency. Nutr. Rev. 14, 9—10 (1956).

[1585] McALLEN, P. M.: Myocardial changes occurring in potassium deficiency. Brit. Heart J. 17, 5—14 (1955).

[1586] MUNTWYLER, E., G. E. GRIFFIN, G. S. SAMUELSEN, and L. G. GRIFFITH: The relation of the electrolyte composition of plasma and skeletal muscle. J. biol. Chem. 185, 525—536 (1950).

[1587] SMITH, S. G.: Magnesium, — potassium antagonism as it affects respiration. Fed. Proc. 10, 394 (1951).

relative increase of kidney weight. There was also a lowering of the percentage of lymphocytes and eosinophils.

In rats made potassium deficient by a low K diet and injections of DCA a rise in the p_H of the gastric juice, a fall in titrable acidity and in the conc. of K and Cl in the gastric juice were noticed. The conc. of Na at the same time showed a considerable rise. (CARONE and COOK[1588].) Muscle and kidney of K-deficient rats have an increased content of free basic amino acids. Lysine may contribute significantly to the total cation content of muscle in K-deficiency[1504].

Potassium deficient rats have several features in common with adrenalectomized rats, thus a lowered blood pressure, and diminished blood pressure response to pressor substances (FREED and ROSENMAN[1589]). — Evidence against this being due to a suppression of the secretion of adrenocortical steroids was found in the experiments of ROSENMAN et al.[1590].

In potassium-deficient rats FREED et al.[1591] have found a decreased concentration of K in the aorta associated with a hypotension. Cortisone caused a fall in the sodium concentration of the aorta and restored the blood pressure to normal levels*.

It has recently been suggested by SPATER et al.[1576] that potassium depletion by itself may be a largely symptomless condition but that the functional and biochemical derangements usually associated with K-depletion become manifest when the normal metabolic functions of the cell are affected in the way that the sodium extrusion is hampered, cellular sodium intoxication ensuing.

Magnesium deficiency produces a secondary potassium depletion (MACINTYRE and DAVIDSON[133b]).

I. Function of rubidium and cesium in replacement of potassium

As regards general physiological effects K and Rb are often very nearly interchangeable, but Cs, although it resembles K more closely than Na or Li, is never a physiological substitute for K. The interchangeability of K, Rb and Cs was discussed by HÖBER[1592] (see also p. 230).

Rubidium and to certain extent Cs can replace K as an essential nutrient in rats (FOLLIS[617]). More than $1/_2$ of the total tissue K content was replaced by Rb when the latter was added to a low-K dient (HEPPEL and SMITH[1593]). It should be remembered, however, that organisms will not tolerate indefinite replacement of K with Rb or Cs because of their toxic effects.

LiCl cannot replace NaCl in the diet (FREGBY[1496]). These two salts apparently taste differently, and rats reject LiCl.

[1588] CARONE, F. A., and R. E. COOKE: Effect of potassium deficiency on gastric secretion in the rat. Amer. J. Physiol. 172, 684—688 (1953).

[1589] FREED, S. C., and R. H. ROSENMAN: Effect of potassium depletion upon vascular reactivity of the rats's mesoappendix. Amer. J. Physiol. 184, 183—187 (1956).

[1590] ROSENMAN, R. H., S. S. GEORGE, S. C. FREED, and M. K. SMITH: The effect of potassium deficiency upon adrenocortial secretion in the rat. J. clin. Invest. 34, 1726—1729 (1955).

[1591] FREED, S. C., S. ST. GEORGE, and R. H. ROSENMAN: Aorta electrolytes of hypotensive potassium-deficient rats. Amer. J. Physiol. 195, 445—447 (1958).

* A somewhat similar finding for rat myocardium has recently been reported by S. C. FREED and S. ST. GEORGE: Myocardial sodium and potassium content in relation to blood pressure. Amer. J. Physiol. 197, 214—216 (1959).

[1592] HÖBER, R.: Alkali- und Erdalkalimetalle, in Handbuch der Experimentellen Pharmakologie. Vol. III, Part 1, p. 254. Berlin: Springer 1927.

[1593] HEPPEL, L. A., and C. L. A. SCHMIDT: Studies on the potassium metabolism of the rat during pregnancy, lactation and growth. Univ. of Calif. Publ. in Physiol. 8, 189—205 (1938).

J. Influence of age on the efficiency of homeostasis

New-born mammals present very special problems in homeostasis (for a recent review see McCance and Widdowson[1594]). They are characterized by having low renal clearances of urea and sodium and chloride. However, the low urea clearances do not lead to any elevation of blood urea since the main part of the protein ingested is used for synthesis (growth) whereas a very low fraction of the calories of basal metabolism is derived from protein catabolism. — This balance between anabolism and catabolism may be more important than renal excretion for maintaining homeostasis for potassium. Thus the presence of growth allows an animal to tolerate much larger doses of potassium than when no growth occurs. This was demonstrated by McCance and Widdowson[1595] using new born piglets. Potassium chloride given in water led to a retention of 2.9 meq/kg starting weight, associated with paralysis and widespred signs of toxicity in 40 hr. The same amount of potassium given *in milk* was followed by a retention of 10.5 meq/kg which did not produce any toxic symptoms. The deposition of protein (and K) and the upkeep of tissue glycogen (and K) stores in the latter case, would explain this phenomenon. The low clearances of sodium and chloride have implications for sodium homeostasis. If the concentration of sodium in the food exceeds that of normal milk, sodium retention and oedema will ensue (McCance and Widdowson[1596]).

The high fraction of total body sodium exchangeable with labelled sodium in infants and its relation to the special composition of bone sodium in the young have been thoroughly discussed on p. 230.

[1594] McCance, R. A., and E. M. Widdowson: New thoughts on renal function in the early days of life. Brit. med. Bull. **13**, 3—6 (1957).

[1595] McCance, R. A., and E. M. Widdowson: The response of the new-born piglet to an excess of potassium. J. Physiol. **141**, 88—96 (1958).

[1596] McCance, R. A., and E. M. Widdowson: Hypertonic expansion of the extracellular fluids. Acta paediat. (Uppsala) **46**, 337—353 (1957).

IX. Internal shifts and displacements of alkali metal ions
By
NIELS A. THORN

A. Mobilization from or deposition in extracellular structures, especially bone

In the chapters on the sodium and potassium of connective tissues, cartilage and bone it is described how considerable amounts of sodium are found in these tissues partly as extracellular fluid, partly bound to polyelectrolytes, partly in a non-organic binding in bone. A considerable part of this sodium can be mobilized on appropriate stimuli. These involve hyponatremia, acidosis or administration of certain adrenocortical hormones. In addition to the references found on p. 213 it might be added that STREETEN and CONN[1597] have produced some evidence that aldosterone mobilizes sodium from bone. Whether hyponatremia *per se* an mobilize sodium from bone is discussed on p. 213. In the section on corium it is concluded that skin does not function as a depot for "dry" sodium chloride, but that large amounts of extracellular fluid can be mobilized or deposited here. — Although it seems that some of the potassium of bone may also be in a "depot" form, it is yet unclarified to which extent it might function as such. Further discussion of the sources for easily mobilized potassium is found in the section on potassium depletion p. 530.

B. Factors affecting the distribution of alkali metals between cells and extracellular fluid

Many aspects concerning these problems have been dealt with thoroughly in part I of this book. — Since they have also been treated thoroughly from the point of view of the intact organism in various recent reviews (see among others ELKINTON and DANOWSKI[9], EDELMAN and NADELL[1598], DARROW and HELLERSTEIN[14 a], they will only dealt with here in a sketchy way.

In the section on plasma it has been stressed how very small changes in the high intracellular/extracellular concentration ratio of potassium will lead to considerable changes in the concentration in plasma. Among the many causes of such disturbances it might be pertinent to stress the fact that any impairment of cellular metabolism causes a loss of potassium from the cells.

a) Hormones

Various hormones seem to be able to affect the distribution of alkali metals between cells and extracellular fluid.

Corticoids. SWINGLE et al.[1599] first suggested that corticoids control the distribution of water, Na and K between cells and their surroundings. This seemed

[1597] STREETEN, H. P., and J. W. CONN: Effects of primary aldosteronism on the slowly exchangeable component of body sodium. Clin. Res. 7, 253 (1959).

[1598] EDELMAN, I. S., and J. NADELL: Recent progress in the study of potassium metabolism. Stanford med. Bull. 13, 511—525 (1955).

[1599] SWINGLE, W. W., J. J. PFIFFNER, H. M. VARS, and W. M. PARKINS: The effect of fluid deprivation and fluid intake upon the revival of dogs from adrenal insufficiency. The relation between blood pressure, blood urea nitrogen and fluid balance of the adrenalectomized dog. Amer. J. Physiol. 108, 144—150 and 428—437 (1934).

to be confirmed in the studies of HILLS et al.[1600] who showed that cortisone, in patients with acute adrenocortical insufficiency, very quickly corrected the serum electrolyte abnormalities — long before any correction of the deficit in total amount had taken place. Quite recently SWINGLE et al.[1601] have resumed experiments along these lines using pure steroids and derivatives. Thus they have demonstrated that 2-methyl-9 α-fluorocortisol administered to dogs with adrenocortical insufficiency has a rapid effect on BP and serum electrolytes in the absence of exogenous sources of fluid, Na and Cl. In a recent paper[1602] they put forward the hypothesis that only glucocorticoids affect the distribution of Na and K between cells and extracellular fluid. — Several workers have noted changes in inulin space in humans given corticotropin or cortisol. — WOODBURY[1603] found that corticotropin given to fasted nephrectomized rats, produced a decrease in the concentration of K in the muscles. Other studies suggesting extrarenal effects of corticoids are those of GAUDINO and LEVITT[1604] and FLANAGAN et al.[79a] LEVITT and BADER[1605] and SWEET et al.[1606]. FREED et al.[1615] showed beneficial effects of cortisone on Na/K ratio in the aorta of K-deficient rats. In an evaluation of these studies, it must be kept in mind, that a considerable part, if not all of the effects, at least on sodium metabolism, can be explained by the effects of corticoids on the depots in bone. They may thus be mainly a redistribution *within* the extracellular phase, and not a redistribution over the cell boundaries. Due to their catabolic effect glucocorticoids or corticotrophin may cause appreciable losses of potassium from cells. Anabolic steroids and growth hormone have opposite effects. These facts complicate interpretations.

It seems that some of the best studies of the effects of adrenocortical hormones on the distribution of Na and K within the body are those performed in adrenalectomized, nephrectomized animals. — Such studies have been performed in acutely nephrectomized (previously adrenalectomized) rats by TOMPKINS et al.[1607] and in adrenalectomized, nephrectomized dogs maintained for up to 40 days by peritoneal lavage by GROLLMAN[1608]. The latter procedure has the advantage that such changes as occur have ample time to develop to a detectable degree. GROLLMAN found an increase in the sodium concentration, especially of skeletal muscle and liver and a decrease of potassium concentration in skeletal muscle

[1600] HILLS, A. G., T. M. CHALMERS, G. D. WEBSTER, and O. ROSENTHAL: Adrenal cortical regulation of the distribution of water and electrolytes in the human body. J. clin. Invest. **32**, 1236—1247 (1953).

[1601] SWINGLE, W. W., J. DaVANZO, E. FEDOR, H. C. CROSSFIELD, D. GLENISTER, M. OSBORNE and G. WAGLE: Plasma volume and electrolyte changes induced by 2-methyl-9-α fluorohydrocortisone in fasted adrenalectomized dogs. Proc. Soc. exp. Biol. (N. Y.) **97**, 416—419 (1958).

[1602] SWINGLE, W. W., J. P. DaVANZO, D. GLENISTER, H. C. CROSSFIELD and G. WAGLE: Role of gluco- and mineralocorticoids in salt and water metabolism of adrenalectomized dogs. Amer. J. Physiol. **196**, 283—286 (1959).

[1603] WOODBURY, D. M.: Extrarenal effects of desoxycorticosterone, adrenocortical extract and adrenocorticotrophic hormone on plasma and tissue electrolytes in fed and fasted rats. Amer. J. Physiol. **174**, 1—19 (1953).

[1604] GAUDINO, M., and M. F. LEVITT: Influence of the adrenal cortex on body water distribution and renal function. J. clin. Invest. **28**, 1487—1497 (1949).

[1605] LEVITT, M. F., and M. E. BADER: Effect of cortisone and ACTH on fluid and electrolyte distribution in man. Amer. J. Med. **11**, 715—723 (1951).

[1606] SWEET, A. Y., M. F. LEVITT, and H. L. HODES: The effect of desoxycorticosterone acetate on water and electrolyte distribution. J. clin. Invest. **37**, 65—69 (1958).

[1607] TOMPKINS, M. J., E. ECKMAN, and L. SHARE: Extrarenal action of the adrenal cortex on electrolyte metabolism in nephrectomized and nephrectomized-eviscerated rats. Amer. J. Physiol. **196**, 141—144 (1959).

[1608] GROLLMAN, A.: Water and electrolyte content of tissues of the adrenalectomized and adrenalectomized-nephrectomized dog. Amer. J. Physiol. **179**, 36—38 (1954).

and the gut. The discrepancy between these results and those of previous studies was suggested to be due to the fact that the previous studies had been done in acute adrenocortical insufficiency where contraction of extracellular fluid volume and hyponatremia and hyperkalemia dominate the picture. TOMPKINS et al. in adrenalectomized, eviscerated, nephrectomized rats found an increased concentration of potassium in the plasma. — Desoxycorticosterone reduced the plasma K concentration in these animals. HEPPS et al.[1609] found an increased uptake of K^{42} in the tissue of adrenalectomized rats after large doses of cortisone.

Both endogenous and exogenous histamine is capable of releasing large amounts of potassium from the cells (MACMILLAN[1610], SUDAK et al.[1611]).

Norepinephrine seems to release potassium from smooth muscle (TOBIAN and FOX[1612], see also MUIRHEAD[39a]). On the other hand RAGOFF[1613] found that infusion of epinephrine at a physiological rate caused hypokalemia. This latter paper contains a discussion of the discrepancies found in reports on effects of epinephrine on serum potassium level. It is suggested that they are due to differences in dosage or method or rate of administration.

A few reports have appeared on a decrease in inulin space after vasopressin. For a critical discussion see THORN[655].

Insulin induces deposition of potassium with glycogen when potassium supplies are available (FENN[1614], WILLEBRANDS et al.[1615], CALKINS et al.[1616], NICHOLS[133a] and DURY[1617]).

Glucagon is known to cause a transient marked hyperkalimia (WOLFSON and ELLIS[1618]) followed by a much larger, milder hypokalemia. This effect might be related to hepatic glycogenolysis.

It is common to all these effects of hormones that very little is known about the mechanism of action.

b) Excesses or deficits — primary changes in p_H

The effects of excesses and deficits of the various alkali metals on their distribution in the body have been dealt with in chapter VIII.

Considerable changes in the distribution of the alkali metals between cells and extracellular fluid are caused by changes in the acid-base metabolism of the body.

[1609] HEPPS, S. A., F. A. HARTMAN, and K. A. BROWNELL: Effect of cortisone and desoxycorticosterone on distribution of radioactive potassium in the adrenalectomized rat. Amer. J. Physiol. 196, 153—155 (1959).

[1610] MACMILLAN, W. H.: Exogenous and endogenous histamine-induced potassium release as modified by the antihistaminics. Amer. J. Physiol. 191, 587—590 (1957).

[1611] SUDAK, F. N., C. WYMAN, and G. P. FULTON: Effect of histamine on electrocardiograms and serum electrolytes of intact, cortisonetreated and adrenalectomized hamsters. Amer. J. Physiol. 194, 53—56 (1958).

[1612] TOBIAN, L., and A. FOX: The effect of nor-epinephrine on the electrolyte composition of arterial smooth muscle. J. clin. Invest. 35, 297—301 (1956).

[1613] ROGOFF, J. M., J. M. QUASHNOCK, E. NOLA NIXON, and A. W. ROSENBERG: Adrenal function and blood electrolytes. Proc. Soc. exp. Biol. (N. Y.) 73, 163—169 (1950).

[1614] FENN, W. O.: The deposition of potassium and phosphate with glycogen in rat livers. J. biol. Chem. 128, 297—307 (1939).

[1615] WILLEBRANDS, A. F., J. GROEN, CHR. E. KAMMENGA, and J. R. BLICKMAN: Quantitative aspects of the action of insulin on the glucose and potassium metabolism of the isolated rat diaphragm. Science 112, 277—278 (1950).

[1616] CALKINS, E., J. M. TAYLOR, and A. BAIRD HASTINGS: Potassium exchange in the isolated rat diaphragm; effect of anoxia and cold. Amer. J. Physiol. 177, 211—218 (1954).

[1617] DURY, A.: The effect of epinephrine and insulin on the plasma potassium level. Endocrinology 49, 663—670 (1951).

[1618] WOLFSON, S. K., and S. ELLIS: Effects of glucagon on plasma potassium Proc. Soc. exp. Biol. (N.Y.) 91, 226—228 (1956).

Usually shifts of sodium ions are most predominant in these in the way that hydrogen ions deficiencies or excesses are compensated by oppositie movements of sodium and (potassium) ions. — On the other hand, primary changes in the potassium content of the cells lead to secondary changes in the hydrogen ion distribution.

This can be caused by such effects on the renal tubular cells (see p. 296) and partly the other cells in the body.

Loading with potassium chloride produces a hyperkalemic acidosis (ROBERTS et al.[1523], FULLER and MACLEOD[1619]). On the other hand potassium deficiency seems to be an important factor in the development and maintenance of extracellular alkalosis and intracellular acidosis. It seems somewhat unclear, whether potassium deficiency alone can produce this syndrome or whether additional factors are required (ELKINTON and DANOWSKI[9] and MOORE et al.[1620]).

Since these shifts may be said to have mainly clinical interest and since the mechanisms and symptoms have very recently been thoroughly and competently surveyed by among others ELKINTON and DANOWSKI[9] and ELKINTON[1621] this subject will not be treated further here.

[1619] FULLER, G. R., and M. B. MACLEOD: Effect of potassium infusions on renal tubular reabsorption of bicarbonate. Fed. Proc. **13**, 49—50 (1954).

[1620] MOORE, F. D., E. A. BOLING, H. B. DITMORE, jr., A. SICULAR, J. E. TETERICK, A. E. ELLISON, S. J. HOYE, and M. R. BALL: Body sodium and potassium V. The relationship of alkalosis potassium deficiency and surgical stress to acute hypokalemia in man. Metabolism **4**, 379—402 (1955).

[1621] ELKINTON, J. R.: Whole body buffers in the regulation of acid-base equilibrium. Yale J. Biol. Med. **29**, 191—210 (1956).

Author Index

Page numbers in *italics* refer to the bibliography

Abbot, B. C., and D. Ballantine *126*
— R. *94*
Abele, W. A. see Welt, L. G. *402*
Abrahams, V. C., and M. Pickford *343*
Acheson, G. H. see Kahn jr., I. B. *80*
Ackermann, H. see Schwarzenbach, G. *5*
Adam, W. E. see Fleckenstein, A. *182*
Adams, M. see Wilder, R. M. *302*
Adamson, jr., K. see Dyke, H. B. *333, 343*
Addison, Thomas 303
Adler, F. H. *217*, 221
Adlersberg, D., and E. Neubauer *489*
Adolph, E. F. *447, 449*
Adrian, R. H. *145*
— see Keynes, R. D. *50*
Aebi, H. *25, 26, 66*
Agna, J. W., H. C. Knowles and G. Alverson *210*, 211
Ågren, G., and H. Lagerlöf *460, 463, 465*
— see Hammarsten, E. *463*
Aikawa, J. K. *231*
— and M. B. Rhyne *231*
Aitken, E. H. see Preedy, J. R. K. *339*, 340
Akeson, W. H. see Eichelberger, L. T. *208*
Akman, L. C. see Hwang, W. *374*
Albert, A. see Mattox, V. R. *308*
— see Sprague, R. G. *320*
Albrectsen, S. R., and J. H. Thaysen *432*, 438
Albright, F. see Dempsey, E. F. *517*
Albrink, M. J., P. M. Hald and E. B. Man 199, *200*
— — — and J. R. Peters 199, *200*
Albritton, E. C. *198*, 199
Alexander, D. P., D. A. Nixon, W. F. Widdas and F. X. Wohlzogen *218*
— G. V., R. E. Nusbaum and N. S. MacDonald *214*

Alexander, R. S. see Pitts, R. F. 252, 253, 297
Allers, W. D., and E. C. Kendall *301*
Alles, G. A., and R. C. Hawes *19*
Alonso, L. G. see Maren, T. H. *298*
Alvarez, A. V. see Osterberg, A. E. *477*
Alverson, G. see Agna, J. W. *210*, 211
Amatruda, T. T., and L. G. Welt *443, 448, 456*
Ambache, N. *193*
Amberson, W. R. *116*
— T. P. Nash, A. G. Mulder and D. Binns *237*
Amelung, D. see Hübener, H. J. *319*
Ames, A. *104*
— and A. B. Hastings *104*
— see Mudge, G. H. *400, 409*
Amoore, J. E., W. Bartley and R. van Heyningen *220*
Amson, K. see Mond, R. *86*
Andersen, B. *61*
— and H. H. Ussing 46, 53, *60*, 128
— see Ussing, H. H. *137*
— D. H. see Darling, R. C. *446*
— see Kessler, W. R. *446*
— R., and K. Lehmann *8*
Andersh, M. see Höber, R. *144, 151*
Anderson, C. E. see Bucher, G. R. *132*
— C. M., M. McCally and G. L. Farrell *369*
— E. *327*
— H. M., and J. H. Laragh 522, 529
— and G. H. Mudge *294*
— J. A. see McQuarrie, I. *522*
— J. S. see Emeleus, H. J. *2*
— W. A. D., and W. R. Bethea *390*
Andersson, B., and S. M. McCann 362, *364*
Ando, S. see Araki, Y. *432*
Anfinsen, C. B. see Hastings, A. B. *30*
Anner, G. see Wettstein, A. *305*, 308

Anrep, G. V. *435, 454, 503*
Ansell, J. S., and B. Zimmermann *230*
Anslow, W. P. see Wesson, L. G. *236, 239, 244, 245, 281, 282, 401*
— jr., L. G. Wesson jr., A. A. Bolomey and J. G. Taylor *345*
— see Wesson, L. G. jr. *266*, 270
Anthonisen, P., T. Hilden and Aa. C. Thomsen *364*
Antonowicz, I. see Metcoff, M. S. *300*
Appelmans, F. see Duve, C. de *22*
Araki, Y., and S. Ando *432*
Archibald, R. M. see Slyke, D. D. *254*
Arisz, W. H. *38*
Arlt, F. *464*
Arman, C. G. van *415*
— and H. R. Dettelbach *415*
— see Kagawa, C. M. *320, 418*
Armour, J. C. see Babkin, B. P. *474*
Armstrong, E. F., and H. E. Armstrong *18*
— see Armstrong, E. F. *18*
— see Scatchard, G. *9*
Arnett, V., and W. S. Wilde *102*
Arons, H. L. see Laidlaw, J. C. *320*
— W. L., R. J. Vanderlind and A. K. Solomon *228*
— see Robinson, C. V. *227*
— see Thorn, G. W. *304*
Arrington, T. M. see Kattus, A. *415*
Ashe, B. J., and H. O. Mosenthal *516*
Ashford, C. A., and K. C. Dixon 24, 28
Assali, N. S. see Dignam, W. S. *340*
Astwood, E. B. see Talbot, N. B. *194*
Atchley, D. W., R. F. Loeb, D. W. Richards jr., E. M. Benedict and M. E. Driscoll *281*
— see Ferrebee, J. W. *334*
— see Kuhlman, D. *323*

Atchley, D. W. see Loeb, R. F. *302*
— see Ragan, C. *334*
— see Stahl, J. *301*
Atherden, L. M. *338*
Atkins, E. L., and J. W. Pearce *371*
Atkinson, A. J. see Schmidt, C. R. *480*
Atwood, W. G. see Meigs, E. B. *85*
Audia, M. *207*
— see White, H. L. *528*
Auditore, G. V. see Holland, W. C. *229, 496*
— J. V. see Hartmann, R. C. *222*
Auerbach, T. see Fine, D. *312*
Austin, J. H., and G. D. Gammon *470*
— see Ravdin, I. S. *492, 493, 494, 495*
Axelrad, B. J. *307*
— B. B. Johnson and J. A. Luetscher *311*, 312
Axelrod, D. R., and R. F. Pitts *289, 407*, 408
— see Capps, J. N. *403*
— see Luetscher, J. A. jr. *311, 312*
Ayer, J. L. see Pitts, R. F. *238*
Ayres, P. J., J. Barlow, O. Garrod, A. E. Kellin, S. A. S. Tait, J. F. Tait and G. Walker *310*

Babkin, B. P. *425, 455, 464, 465, 467, 471, 472, 474, 475, 478*
— J. C. Armour and R. D. Webster *474*
— and W. W. Sawitsch *461*
Bach, R. O. *5*
Bachman, D. M., and W. B. Youmans *377*
Bachrach, E., and N. Guillot *185*
— and A. Reinberg *186*
— W. H. see Fogelson, S. J. *484*
Bacq, Z. M. *176*
— see Goffart, M. *166, 176*
— see Szent-Györgyi, A. *9, 172, 173,* 174, *190*
Baden, H. see Edelman, I. S. *210*, 211
Bader, M. E. see Levitt, M. F. *332, 536*
— R. A., J. W. Eliot and D. E. Bass *352*
Baetjer, A. M. *88, 177*
Bahn, R. C. see Davis, J. O. *513, 528*
Bailey, K. *173*

Baird, and Haldane, J. B. S. *349*
— S. L., G. Karreman, H. Mueller and A. Szent-Györgyi *9*
Bajusz, E. see Selye, H. *531*
Baker, C. see Swingle, W. W. *307, 322, 335*
Baldes and Smirk *349*
Baldwin, D., E. M. Kahana and R. W. Clarke *270*
Bale, W. F. see Manery, J. F. *210*
Balint, P., and A. Fekete *366*
— — and S. Szalay *370*
Ball, C. O. T. see Meneely, G. R. *516, 520*
— E. G. *461*, 462
— Helen F. Tucker, A. K. Solomon and Birgit Vennesland *430*
— M. R. see Cope, O. *467*, 468
— see Moore, F. D. *538*
— see Wilson, G. M. *213*
— W. C. see Davis J. O. *513*, 528
— jr. see Davis J. O. *310, 385*
Ballantine, D. see Abbot, B. C. *126*
Ballou, G. A. see Lineweaver, H. *19*
Bammer, H. *168*
— and K. E. Rothschuh *167*
Banga, J. *10*
Banks, R. C. see Farrell, G. L. *311*
Barber, D. E. see Visscher, M. B. *133*, 134, 135, 136
— J. K. see Bartter, F. C. *312*
Barclay, A. E. see Trueta, J. *358*
— J. A., W. T. Cooke, R. A. Kennedy and M. E. Nutt *387*
— R. A. Kennedy and M. E. Nutt *347*
— W. R., and R. H. Ebert *303*
Barcroft, I. *436*
Barfour, A., G. M. Bull, B. M. Evans, N. C. Hughes Iones and I. Logothetopoulos *352*
Ba ger, A. C. *379*
Barker, E. S., R. B. Singer, I. R. Elkinton and I. K, Clark *291*
— see Singer, R. B. *290*
Barker, M. H. see Lindberg, H. A. *390*
Barlow, G. see Swingle, W. W, *306, 307, 335*
— I. see Ayres, P. I. *310*
Barnafi, L. see Croxatto, H. *355*

Barnes, H. see Lord Rothschild *142*
— L. E. see Byrnes, W. W. *337*
— see Lyster, S. L. *337*
— see Stafford, R. O. *336*, 337
Barry, W. M., and V. E. Levine *493*
Bartholomay, A. F. see Wacker, W. E. C. *517*
Bartlay, W., and R. E. Davies *22, 37*
— — and H. A. Krebs *37*
— see Amoore, J. E. *220*
Bartram, E. A. *398*
— see Christian, H. A. *412*
Bartter, F. C. *314*
— G. W. Liddle, L. E. Duncan jr., J. K. Barber and C. Delea *312*
— see Duncan, L. E. jr. *513*
— see Leaf, A. *345, 348*
— see Liddle, G. W. *311, 322*
— see Schwartz, W. B. *364*
Bass, A. C. see Davis, A. K. *318*
— D. E. *352*
— C. R. Kleeman, M. Quinn, A. Henschel and A. H. Hegnauer *518*
— see Bader, R. A. *352*
— P. see Daniel, E. E. *530*
Bassett, S. H. see Blahd, W. H. *293*
— see Goldman, R. *381*
Bates, J. C. see Geyer, R. P. *31*
Battley, E. H., and J. M. Klotz *9*
Batts, A. A. see Stein, J. D. jr. *342*
Bauer, G. C. H. *214*
— W., M. W. Ropes and H. Waine *214*
— see Beckman, W. W. *297*
Baumann, E. J., and S. Kurland *301*
— see Marine, D. *301*
Baumberger, J. P., V. Suntzeff and E. V. Cowdry *207*
Bayliss, L. E., and E. Lundsgaard *266*
— W. M., and E. H. Starling *461*
Baxter, C. F. see Page, L. B. *357*
— H. *452, 453, 467, 468, 471*
Beadle, L. C. *143*
Beagell, J. M. see Schmidt, C. R. *488*
Beall, W. A. see Langley, L. L. *456*
Beams, H. W., T. N. Tahmisian, R. L. Devine and L. E. Roth *21*

Beccari, L. *185*
Beck, R. N. *285*
Becker, E. L. see Wasserman, K. *32*
— W. H. see Farber, S. J. *373, 374*
Becker-Christensen, P. *298*
Beckman, W. W., E. C. Rossmeisl, R. B. Pettengill and W. Bauer *297*
Beer, E. J. de, and D. W. Wilson *456*
Behrens, O. K. see Bromer, W. W. *354*
Beinert, H., D. F. Green, P. Hele, H. Hift, R. W. v. Korff and C. V. Ramakrishnan *15*
Bellet, S. *222*
— see Cooper, E. S. *215*
— see Surawicz, B. *529*
Belt, A. E. see Hinman, F. *515*
Ben, M. see Swingle, W. W. *307, 322, 335*
Benedict, E. M. see Atchley, D. W. *281*
— see Loeb, R. F. *294, 302*
Benesch, E. see Benesch, R. *408*
— R., and R. E. Benesch *408*
Benirschke, K. see Dingman, J. F. *311, 312, 313*
Bennett, A. L. see Still, E. U. *429*
— L. L. see Liddle, G. W. *295*
— see Stein, J. D. jr. *342*
— see Thorn, G. W. *330*
— see Whitney, J. E. *342*
— T. E. see Tarail, R. *525*
— W. A. see Cuxton, H. E. *323*
— W. see Schwartz, W. B. *364*
Benson, J. A. see Gray, S. J. *476*
Berdasco, G. A. see Weston, R. E. *293, 345, 348*
Bergenstal, D. M. see Landau, R. L. *339*
Berger, E. Y., M. Galdston and S. A. Horwitz *289*
— G. Kanzaki, M. A. Homer and I. M. Steel *509, 512*
— G. P. Quinn and M. A. Homer *513*
— J. *459, 477*
— M. *496*
Bergerard, J., and A. Reinberg *185*
Bergmann, F., S. Dickstein, J. Menczel and T. D. Ullmann *261*
Bergstrand, A. *280*
— H. see Lundegårdh, H. *223*

Bergstrom, W. H. *211, 212, 214*
— and W. M. Wallace *210*
Berliner, K. W. see Orloff, J. *2565*
— R. W. *239, 258, 287, 297, 298, 299, 300*
— and D. G. Davidson *244*
— and T. J. Kennedy *400*
— — and J. G. Hilton *399*
— — and J. Orloff *397, 408, 409, 422*
— — jr. *257*
— — and J. Orloff *239, 258, 287, 297, 298, 299, 300*
— N. G. Levinsky, D. G. Davidson and M. Eden *249*
— see Davidson, D. G. *240, 258*
— see Levinsky, N. G. *353, 423*
— see Orloff, J. *256*
Berman, A. L. see Schmidt, C. R. *488*
— H. see Gardner, L. I. *294, 517, 532*
— M. D. see Shanes, A. M. *96*
Bernard, Claude *356, 358*
Berne, R. M. *357*
— W. K. Hoffman jr., A. Kagan and M. N. Levy *360, 361*
— see Driscol, T. E. *385*
— and M. N. Levy *384*
— see Levy, M. N. *375*
Bernfeld, P. see Meyer, K. H. *57, 125*
Bernini, G. see Capraro, V. *128, 129*
Bernstein, J. *54, 57, 87, 144, 146, 151*
— R. *200, 470*
Berson, S., A. and R. S. Yalow *206*
Berthet, L. see Duve, C. de *22*
Bertrand, D. *77, 223*
— see Bertrand, G. *224, 225*
— G., and D. Bertrand *224, 225*
Best, C. see Sirek, O. V. *335, 336*
Bethe, A. *180*
— and F. Franke *176*
Bethea, W. R. see Anderson, W. A. D.
Bethune, J. E. see Ross, E. J. *418*
Bevier, G., and A. E. Shershy *328*
Beyer, K. H. *415, 416, 417*
Beyl, G. see Sheppard, C. W. *74, 76*
Bezeky, G. V. *141*

Bickford, R. G., and F. R. Winton *266*
Billard and Cavalié *494*
Billings, C. see Klein, R. *318*
Binger, M. W. see Keith, N. M. *392*
Binns, D. see Amberson, W. R. *237*
Birchard, W. H., J. D. Rosenbaum and M. B. Strauss *349*
— and M. B. Strauss *350*
Birkenfeld, L. W. see Edelmann, I. S. *200*
— see O'Meara, M. P. *229*
Birmingham, J. R. see Dancis, J. *352*
M. R. see Pearse, M. L. *375, 376*
Birnbaum, D., and F. Hollander *463*
Birnie, J. H. *333*
— W. J. Eversole, W. R. Boss, C. M. Osborn and R. Gaunt *333*
— see Gaunt, R. *327*
Bishop, G. H. *98*
Black, D. A. K. *196, 197*
— and E. W. Emery *258*
— and M. D. Milne *293*
— R. Platt and S. W. Stanbury *372*
— see McCance, R. A. *246*
— E. see Cope, C. L. *310*
— M. M. see Zweifach, B. W. *303*
— S. *16*
Blackmore, W. P. *355*
Blahd, W. H., and S. H. Bassett *293*
Blair, E. A. see Erlanger, J. *162*
Blake, W. D. *361, 387*
— R. Wegria, R. P. Keating and H. P. Ward *275*
— — H. P. Ward and C. W. Frank *270*
— see Bradley, S. E. *379*
— see Orloff, J. *371*
Bland, J. H. *197*
Blatt, H. see Cope, D. *467, 468*
Blickman, J. R. see Kamminga, C. E. *30*
— see Willebrands, A. F. *537*
Blinks, L. R. *109, 111*
Bliss, E. L., S. Rubin and T. Gilbert *361*
— T. L. *468, 469, 470*
Bloch, K. *16*
— see Johnston, R. B. *15*
— see Snoke, E. J. *15, 16*
Block, J. D. *200*
Blomhert, G. *349*

Blomhert, G., J. Gerbrandy, J. A. Molhuysen, L. A. de Vries and J. G. G. Borst 349
— see Borst, J. G. 338
Blomstrand, R. see Linder, E. 204
Bloomfield, A. L. 477
Bloor, W. R. see Fenn, W. O. 86
Blount, R. W. 110, 111
Blumgart, H. L., D. R. Gilligan, R. V. Levy, M. G. Brown and M. C. Volk 397, 411, 414
Bocanegra, M. see Markley, K. 270, 520
Bock, J. 256, 295, 410, 413
Bockris, J. O. M. 4
Bodo, R. C. de 352
— and K. F. Prescott 352
— I. L. Schwartz, J. Greenberg, M. Kurtz, D. P. Earle and S. J. Farber 341
— see Earle, D. P. jr. 341
— see Lane, N. 310, 315
Boehm, R. 184
Bohrer, B. B. see Robinson, S. 448, 449, 450
Boissur, J. R. see Hazard, R. 526
Bojesen, E. 267, 268, 269, 270, 272, 286
Boling, E. A. see Moore, F. D. 538
Bolomey, A. A. see Anslow, W. P. jr. 345
— see Wesson, L. G. jr. 266, 270, 349
Boné, G. J. 140
Booth, V. H. see Roughton, F. J. W. 296
Borden, C. see Cooper, J. A. D. 228
Borman, A., F. M. Singer and P. Numerof 337
— see Fried, J. 337, 419
Borrero, L. M. see Pappenheimer, J. R. 53, 54
Borst, J. G. G. 379, 384
— G. Blomhert, J. A. Molhuysen, J. Gerbrandy, K. P. Turner and L. A. de Vries 338
— see Blomhert, G. 349
— see Molhuysen, J. A. 338
Borth, R. see Mach, R. S. 317
Borun, E. R. see Grossman, J. 397, 402, 409
— see Weston, R. E. 293, 531
Bose, M. see Gupta, S. L. 6
Boss, W. R. see Birnie, J. H. 333
Bott, P. A. see Walker, A. M. 234, 242, 245, 247

Bott, P. A. see Wirz, H. 240
Bouckaert, J. J., J. P. Bouckaert and A. K. Noyons 185
— J. P. see Bouckaert, J. J. 185
Bowditch, H. P. 188
Bowen, E. H. see Hilton, J. G. 377, 378
— W. J., and T. D. Kerwin 18
Bowes, J. H., and M. M. Murray 214
Bowie, E. J. see Geyer, R. P. 31
— M. A. see Rosenthal, O. J. 210
Bowman, B. J. see Byrnes, W. W. 337
— see Stafford, R. O. 336, 337
Bowyer 69
Boyd, E. M., S. Jackson, M. MacLachlan, B. Palmer, M. Stevens and J. Whittaker 503
— E. S., and W. F. Neuman 209
— R. S. see Field, H. jr. 511, 513, 528
— T. E. see Zwikster, G. H. 185
Boyer, P. D. 11, 12
— H. A. Lardy and P. H. Phillips 11
— see Kachmar, J. F. 12
Boylan, J. W., E. P. Colbourn and R. A. McCance 218
Boyle, P. J., and E. J. Conway 20, 146, 165
Bradeley, J. see Hollander, W. 531
Bradley and H. O. Wheeler 258, 267
— G. P. see Bradley, S. E. 276
— L. B. see Kielly, W. W. 18
— S. E., and W. D. Blake 379
— and G. P. Bradley 276
— see Nickel, J. F. 257, 355, 360
— see Smythe, C. M. C. 360
Brady, A. J., and J. W. Woodbury 161, 164
— T. G. see Conway, E. J. 108
Braganza, B. de see Korey, S. R. 14
Brandfonbrenner, M. see Selkurt, E. E. 273, 274
Brauer, R. W., R. E. McElroy, G. F. Leong and R. J. Holloway 490, 491

Brauer, R. W., G. F. Leong and K. J. Holloway 490, 491
— and R. L. Pessolli 489
— see Leong, G. F. 496
Braun, H. A. see Surawicz, B. 529
Braveman, W. S. see Rubin, A. L. 351
Brazeau, P., and A. Gilman 238, 289, 290
Breed, E. S. see Maxwell, M. H. 243, 380
Bregman, J. I. 6, 510
— and Y. Murata 5
— see Gregor, H. P. 6
Breitoff, J. 182
Brenizer, A. G. see Cope, O. 480
Breuer, H. J., and R. Whittam 60, 107, 501
Brewer, F. M. see Sidgwick, N. V. 5
Bricker, N. S., W. R. Guild, J. P. Rearden and J. P. Merrill 360
Brickner, E. W. see Dowds, E. G. 290
Briggs, A. P., D. M. Fowell, W. F. Hamilton, J. W. Remington, N. C. Wheeler and J. H. Winslow 383
Brink, F., D. W. Bronk and M. G. Larrabee 166
Britton, S. W. see Silvette, H. 327
Brodie, T. B. 282
Brodsky, W. A., and H. N. Graubarth 391, 397
— see Rapoport, S. 367
Brøndsted 197
Brogdon, E. see Hellebrandt, F. A. 475
Bromer, W. W., L. G. Sinn, A. Staub and O. K. Behrens 354
Bronk, D. W. see Brink, F. 166
Brooke, L. see Wilson, G. M. 213
Brooks, C. McC., B. F. Hoffman, E. E. Suckling and O. Orias 65
— E. see Moore, F. D. 232
— L. see Edelman, I. S. 230
— R. V., R. R. McSwiney, F. T. G. Prunitz and F. J. Y. Wood 529
— S. C. 110
Bro-Rasmussen, F., S.-Å. Killmann and J. H. Thaysen 426
Brota, L. de see Pearcy, M. 443, 448

Brown, B. see Eichelberger, L. T. *208*
— D. E. S., and F. J. M. Sichel *178*
— see Shanes, A. M. *98*
— G. L., and U. S. von Euler *177*
— and W. Feldberg *193*
— and F. C. MacIntosh *166*
— H. see Lindsay, A. E. *416*
— J. B., and N. J. Klotz *453*
— M. G. see Blumgart, H. L. *397*, *411*, *414*
Brown-Grant, K. *499*
Browne, J. S. L., and A. M. Vineberg *475*
Brownell, K. A. *305*
— see Hepps, S. A. *537*
Brücke, E. Th. v. *182*
Brun, C., T. Hilden and F. Raaschou *399*
— E. O. E. Knudsen and F. Raaschou *350*
— see Zak, G. A. *246*
Brunn, F. *128*
Brunner, H., G. Kuschinsky, O. Münchow and G. Peters *353*
Buchanan, D. L., and A. Nakao *212*
— J. M., A. B. Hastings and F. B. Nesbett *29*, *30*
— see Hastings, A. B. *29*, *30*
— T. J. see McGillivray, I. *231*
Buchborn, E. see Wolff, H. P. *312*, *370*, *384*, *385*
Buchem, F. S. P. van, H. Doorenbos and H. S. Elings *316*
Bucher, G. R., C. E. Anderson and C. S. Robinson *132*
— see Gray, J. S. *469*
Bucht, H. see Werkö, L. *390*
Buchthal, F. *170*
— and J. Lindhard *170*
Budolfsen, S. E. *132*, *133*, *138*
Bülbring, E. *147*
Buie, R. M. see Lewis, J. M. jr. *375*
Bull, G. M. see Barfour, A. *352*
Bullock, T. H. *168*
Bulmer, M. G. *432*
— and G. D. Forwell *426*
Bundschuh, H. E. see Kuschinsky, G. *353*
Bunge, G. *295*, *392*, *498*, *521*
Bungenberg de Jong, H. G. see Teunissen, P. H. *5*
Burack, W. R. see Kellogg, R. H. *329*
Burch, G. E., C. T. Ray and S. A. Threefoot *206*

Burch, G. E., see Love, W. D. *77*
— see Ray, C. T. *422*
— see Threefoot, S. A. *230*, *423*
— P. R. J., and F. W. Spiers *227*
Burchell, H. B. see Keith, N. N. *521*
Bureau, V. *40*
Burgen, A. S. V. *427*, *428*, *433*, *434*, *435*, *441*, *456*, *459*, *471*, *505*
— and P. Seeman *438*
— and K. G. Terroux *65*, *147*
— — and E. Gouder *438*
— see Terroux, K. G. *436*, *455*
Burgess, W. W., A. M. Harvey and E. K. Marshall jr. *247*
Burn, G. P. see Harris, E. J. *55*, *87*, *89*, *93*, *94*
— see Burn, J. H. *352*
— J. H., L. H. Truelove and I. Burn *352*
Burnell, J. M. see Scribner, B. H. *203*, *204*, *530*
Burnett, A. F. see Weiner, I. M. *406*
— C. H. *327*
— B. A. Burrows, R. R. Commons and B. T. Towery *291*
— see Welt, L. G. *240*
— see Wilkins, R. W. *350*, *372*
— D. W. Seldin and M. Walser *327*
— see Ingbar, S. H. *332*
Burns, H. S., and M. B. Visscher *132*
— H. see Rothschild, L. *500*
Burrows, B. A. see Burnell, C. H. *44*
— see Ingbar, S. H. *332*
— see Lambie, A. T. *525*
— see Relman, A. S. *44*, *224*, *225*
— see Wilkins, R. W. *350*, *372*
Burston, R. A., and O. Garrod *328*, *330*, *334*
— see Garrod, O. *327*, *330*
Burt, A. S. see Moore, A. R. *36*
Bush, I. E. *309*
— see Simpson, S. A. *308*
Bushey, M. S. see Visscher, M. B. *133*, *134*, *135*, *136*
Butler, A. M. see Mackey, E. M. *295*, *392*
Byers, C. see Klein, R. *318*

Byrnes, W. W., L. E. Barnes, B. J. Bowman, W. E. Dubin, E. H. Morley and R. O. Stafford *337*
— see Lyster, S. L. *337*

Cade, J. F. J. *523*
Cafruny, E. J., and A. Farah *405*
Cahill jr., G. see Garrod, O. *330*, *331*
Cahn, A. *476*, *477*
Caldwell, P. C. *88*, 191
— and R. D. Keynes *60*
Cales, J. O. see Perlman, H. B. *218*
Calkins, E., J. M. Taylor and A. B. Hastings *60*, *89*, *95*, *537*
Calhoon, D. see Sartorius, O. W. *324*, *347*
Calma, I., and S. Wright *166*, *522*
Calvin, D. B., G. Decherd and G. Herrmann *397*, *411*
— see Cook, D. L. *487*, *489*, *490*, *491*
— M. C. see Martell, A. E. M. *4*
Camacha, E. see Kinsey, V. E. *217*
Camara, A., and F. Schemm *332*
Camazon, L. see Croxatto, H. *355*
Campanella, D. A. see Wazer, J. R. *8*
Canaga, B. L. see Scott, G. H. *225*
Cannon, P. R., L. E. Frazier and R. H. Hughes *531*
Canzanelli, A., G. Rogers and D. Rapport *24*
Capeci, N. E. see Laragh, J. H. *287*, *522*
Capps, J. N., W. S. Wiggins, D. R. Axelrod and R. F. Pitts *403*
Capraro, V., and G. Bernini *128*, *129*
Carey, M. J., and E. J. Conway *45*, *86*, *90*, *91*, *94*
— M. M. see Zwemer, R. L. *522*
Carlin, M. R., C. B. Mueller and H. L. White *387*
— see Mueller, C. B. *271*, *272*
Carlsen E. see Tosteson, D. *78*
— J. A. see Love, W. D. *78*
Carnes, W. H. see Ferrebee, J. W. *334*
Carone, F. A., and R. E. Cooke *474*, *532*
Carr, C. W., and L. Topol *9*

Carr, C. W. see Visscher, M. B. *132, 134, 135, 136*

Carroll, E. L. see Dempsey, E. F. *517*

Carruthers, C., and V. Suntzeff *220*

Carter, N. see Seldin, D. W. *322*

Carton, E. see Conway, E. J. *108*

Casper, A. G. T. see Liddle, G. W. *322*

Castillo, J. del, and B. Katz *168*

Catchpole, H. R., N. R. Joseph, and M. B. Engel *55*

Cavalié see Billard *494*

Cavanaugh, G. A. see Kinsey, *217*

Cella, J. A. see Kagawa, C. M. *418*

Chalfin, D. see Cooperstein, I. L. *136*

Chaikoff, I. L. see Montgommery, M. L. *463*

Chalmers, see Cox, L. W. *218, 219*

— see Hills, A. G. *536*

— T. M., M. G. Fitzgerald, A. H. James and H. Scarborough *316*

— and A. A. G. Lewis *330, 331*

— — and G. L. S. Pawan *347, 372*

Chambers, R. *36*

Chance, B., and G. R. Williams *61*

Chang, T. H., M. Shaffer and R. W. Gerard *25*

Chapman, M. see Martin, M. M. *227*

Charney, W. see Herzog, H. L. *336*

Chart, J. J., N. Hetzel and R. Gaunt *330*

— see Gaunt, R. C. *333*

— see Renzi, A. A. *330*

Chasis, H., H. A. Ranges, W. Goldring and H. W. Smith *413, 414, 415*

Chavré, V. J. see Davenport, H. W. *475*

Cheek, D. B. *365*

— and C. D. West *520*

— — and C. C. Golden *206, 210, 211*

Cheng, C. P. see Woodbury, D. M. *318*

Chetrick, A. see Goodyer, A. V. *370*

Chiappori, M. see Markley, K. *270, 520*

Child, C. M. *34*

Chinard, R. P. *271*

Christensen, H. N. *105*

— and T. R. Riggs *105*

— — and B. A. Coyne *105*

Christian, H. A., and E. A. Bartram *412*

Churney, L., and F. Moser *179*

Cicardo, V. H. *166*

Citterio, P. see Ranzi, S. *35*

Cizek, L. J., and K. C. Huang *328*

Clark, A. J. *184*

— see Daly de Burgh, I. *184, 186*

— H. E. see Davies, D. F. *446*

— I. see Opdyke, D. F. *203, 204*

— J. A., and R. A. MacLeod *13, 17*

— J. K. see Barker, E. S. *291*

— see Singer, R. B. *290*

Clarke, H. T. *46*

— R. W. see Baldwin, D. *270*

— see Talso, R. J. *223, 419, 420, 421*

Claude, A. *21*

Cluxton, H. E., W. A. Bennett, M. H. Power and E. J. Kepler *323*

Cobb, D. M. see Fenn, W. O. *85, 165*

— see Hegenauer, A. H. *26, 145, 175*

Cobbey, T. S. see Farah, A. *402, 406*

Cobet, R. *131*

Cochran, K. W., J. Doull, M. Mazur and K. P. Du Bois *526*

Cohen, E. M. *405*

— J. see Schwartz, R. *531*

Cohn, E. T. see Cohn, W. E. *71*

— M., and J. Monod *16*

— S. see Meyer, L. F. *295, 392*

— W. E., and E. T. Cohn *71*

— see Cope, D. *480*

Colbourn, E. P. see Boylan, J. W. *218*

Colcher, H., H. D. Janowitz and F. Hollander *470*

Cole, H. N. see Sollman, T. *396*

— K. S., and H. J. Curtis *101, 151, 152*

— see Curtis, H. J. *148, 149, 154, 165*

Collander, R. *36*

Collier, H. B. see Solvonuk, P. F. *12*

Collins, E. J. *311*

— E. see Swingle, W. W. *306*

Comar, C. L. see Hood, S. L. *43, 219, 220, 225, 526*

Comfort, M. W., and A. E. Osterberg *462*

Commons, R. R. see Burnett, C. H. *291*

Compère, E. L. *302*

Conan, N. J. see Farber, S. J. *199, 200*

Conly, S. S., J. O. Crider and J. E. Thomas *461*

Conn, J. W. *318, 323, 445*

— M. W. Johnston and L. H. Louis *445*

— and L. H. Louis *197, 312, 445*

— see Streeten, D. H. P. *312, 320, 535*

— Louis, M. W. Johnston and B. J. Johnson *445*

Consolazio, F. C. see Pitts, G. C. *448*

— see Johnson, R. E. *444*

— W. V. see Talbott, J. H. *328*

Constant, M. see Kinsey, V. E. *217*

Conway, E. J. *45, 68, 84, 91, 92, 108, 109, 165, 478*

— and T. G. Brady *108*

— — and E. Carton *108*

— and M. Downey *108*

— and E. O'Malley *108*

—, H. Ryan and E. Carton *108*

— see Boyle, P. J. *20, 146, 165*

— see Carey, M. J. *45, 86, 90, 91, 94*

Cook, C. D. see Corsa, L. jr. *228*

— see Gardner, L. J. *517*

— C. A. Lawler and D. M. Green *489*

— — L. D. Calvin and D. M. Green *487, 490, 491*

Cooke, R. E. see Carone, F. A. *474, 532*

— see Nyhan, W. L. *365*

— W. T. see Barclay, J. A. *387*

— see Flear, C. T. G. *227*

Coombs, J. S., J. C. Eccles and P. Fatt *160, 171*

Cooper, E. S., E. Lechner and S. Bellet *215*

— J. A. D., N. S. Radin and C. Borden *228*

Cooperstein, I. L., D. Chalfin and C. A. M. Hogben *136*

Cope, C. L., and E. Black *310*

— O., H. Blatt and M. R. Ball *467, 468*

— W. E. Cohn and A. G. Brenizer *480*

Copenhaver, J. H. see Rector, F. C. jr. *256*

— see Seldin, D. W. *322*

Coquin-Carnot, M. see Hanon, F. *218*
Corcoran, A. C., R. D. Taylor and I. Page *419, 523*
— see Schneckloth, R. *355*
Cordsen, M. see Gaunt, R. *361*
Cornec, A. see Hazard, R. *193*
Corner, G. W. see Csapo, A. *195*
Cornfield, J. see Liddle, G. W. *322*
Cori, G. T., and M. W. Slein *12*
Corsa, L. jr., D. Gribetz, C. D. Cook and N. B. Talbot *228*
Cort, J. H. *367, 372*
— see Seldin, D. W. *287*
— see Welt, L. G. *287*
Cotzias, G. C. see Dole, V. P. *517*
Counihan, T. B., B. M. Evans and M. D. Milne *298*
Courtney, A. M. see Holt, L. E. *497*
Cowan, S. L. *102, 148, 165*
Cowdry, E. V. see Baumberger, J. P. *207*
Cowgill, G. R. see Gilman, A. *462, 473, 474, 489*
— see Hollander, F. *465, 472*
Cowie, A. T. *498*
— D. B. see Flexner, L. B. *218, 219*
— see Roberts, R. B. *38*
Cox, L. W., and T. A. Chalmers *218, 219*
Coyne, B. A. see Christensen, H. N. *105*
Crabbé, J., E. J. Ross and G. W. Thorn *528*
— see Hernando, L. *311*
— see Renold, A. E. *418*
Crane, E., and R. E. Davies *480*
— M. M. *246*
Cranefield, P. F., J. A. E. Eyster and W. E. Gilson *164*
Crawford, B., and H. Ludeman *270, 520*
— J. D. see Drescher, A. N. *521, 522, 523*
— see Spater, H. *531, 533*
— M. A. see Milne, M. D. *256, 336*
Creese, R. *39, 86, 94, 95*
— M. W. Neil and G. Stephenson *90*
Crescitelli, F. *163*
— and T. A. Geismann *163*
— see Lipsett, M. N. *24*
Crider, J. O. see Conly, S. S. *461*
— see Thomas, J. E. *462*

Crititiello, M. see Weller, J. M. *530*
Crittenden, P. J. see Winberry, M. M. *520*
Croghan, P. C. *50*
Cross, R. J., and J. V. Taggart *32*
Crossfield, H. C. see Swingle, W. W. *304, 536*
Crowder jr., C. H. see Maxwell, M. H. *362*
Croxatto, H., L. Barnafi, L. Camazon and V. Parra *355*
Crum, W. B. see Surawicz *529*
Csapo, A. *194, 195*
— and G. W. Corner *195*
Culbertson, J. W. see Wilkins, R. W. *350, 372*
Curby, W. A. *451*
Curelop, S. see Schwartz, W. B. *364*
Curran, P. F., and A. K. Solomon *136, 137*
— see Durbin, R. F. *509*
Currie, D. J. see Webster, D. R. *193*
Curtis, G. M. *411*
— H. J., and K. S. Cole *148, 149, 154, 165*
— see Cole, K. S. *101, 151, 152*
Cushing *321, 323, 413*
Cushny, A. R. *410*
— and C. G. Lambie *413*
— see Wallace, G. B. *131*
Cutling, W. C. see Marshall, E. K. *297*

Dahl, B. C. Stall III and G. C. Cotzias *518*
— L. K. *516, 520, 528*
— see Dole, V. P. *517*
Dailey, R. E. see Field, H. jr. *511, 513, 528*
Dainty, J. see MacRobbie, E. A. C. *36, 111*
Dale, R. A., and P. H. Sanderson *397, 403*
Daly de Burgh, I., and A. J. Clark *184, 186*
— see Clark, A. J. *184, 196*
— W. J. see Robinson, S. *444, 449, 450*
Dancis, J., J. R. Birmingham and S. H. Leslie *352*
Danford, H. G., and R. C. Herring *529, 532*
Daniel, E. E. *222*
— and P. Bass *530*
— J., and F. Högler *347*
Danielli, J. F. *63, 68*
Danowski, T. S. *72, 196, 197, 293, 379*
— E. B. Fergus and F. M. Mateer *517, 527*

Danowski, T. S. and L. Greenman *507, 527*
— see Elkinton, J. R. *196, 197, 198*
Darling, P. A. di Sant'Agnese, G. A. Perera and D. H. Anderson *446*
— R. C. *446*
— see Sant'Agnese, P. A. *446*
Darrach, J. H. see Welt, L. G. *402*
Darrow, D. C. *138, 193, 291, 530*
— and S. Hellerstein *197, 203, 206, 220, 535*
— and H. Yannet *288, 527*
— see Harrison, H. E. *178, 206, 328, 329*
— see Miller, H. C. *86*
Da Vanzo, J. see Swingle, W. W. *304, 536*
Davenport, V. D. *223, 224, 482, 483, 524*
— and V. J. Chavré *475*
— and A. E. Wilhelmi *240*
Davidson, D. D. see Levinsky, N. G. *353*
— D. G., N. G. Levinsky and R. W. Berliner *240, 258*
— see Berliner, R. W. *244, 249*
Davidsson, O. see MacIntyre, J. *221, 533*
Davies, B. M. A., and J. Yudkin *255*
— D. F., and H. E. Clark *446*
— H. W., J. B. S. Haldane and E. L. Kennaway *289*
— J. T. *4*
— R. E. *50, 430, 482, 483*
— and A. W. Galston *106*
— H. L. Kornberg and G. M. Wilson *232*
— see Bartlay, W. *22, 37*
— see Crane, E. *480*
— see Kornberg, H. L. *467*
— see Whittam, R. *60, 106*
— S. A. see Garrod, O. *330, 331*
Davis, A. K., A. C. Bass and R. R. Overman *318*
— see Flanagan, J. B. *213, 536*
— D. M. see Marshall, E. K. *328*
— J. O., W. C. Ball jr., R. C. Bahn and M. J. Goodkind *513, 528*
— and D. S. Howell *331, 333*
— — and R. E. Hyatt *385*
— B. Kliman, N. A. Yankopoulos and R. E. Peterson *375*
— A. E. Lindsay and J. L. Southworth *384*

Davis, A. K., M. M. Pechet, W. C. Ball jr. and M. J. Goodkind *310, 385*
— and N. W. Schock *411, 413, 414*
— see Howell, D. S. *324*
— R. K. see Rosenbaum, J. D. *329, 344, 376, 387*
— see Strauss, M. B. *349, 371*
Davson, H. *72, 75, 79, 207, 215, 221*
Day, J. J., and S. A. Komarov *474*
— T. D. *206*
Dayton, A. B. see Goldschmidt, S. *131, 132*
Dean, R. B. *57, 92*
— and O. Gatty *114*
— see Visscher, M. B. *132, 134, 135, 136*
Deane, H. W., J. H. Shaw and R. O. Greep *315*
Dearborn, E. H. see Kunin, A. S. *525*
De Beer, E. J., C. G. Johnston and D. W. Wilson *484, 485*
Decherd, G. see Calvin, D. B. *397, 411*
Deitrick, J. E. see Hanlon, L. W. *419*
Delea, C. see Bartter, F. C. *312*
Delrue, G. *474*
Delvaux, P. *187*
Demarret, J. C., E. Engel and R. S. Mach *231*
Demeester, G. see Leusen, I. *523*
Deming, Q. B., and J. A. Luetscher *384*
Demunbrun, T. W., A. D. Keller, A H Levkoff and R. M. Purser jr. *354*
— see Levkoff, A. H. *354*
Dempsey, E. F. *518*
— E. L. Carroll, F. Albright and P. H. Haneman *517*
Dennis, C. *132, 136*
— and M. B. Visscher *133*
— and E. H. Wood *138, 512*
— W. H. see Rehm, W. S. *482, 483*
Denton, D. A. *451, 457*
— I. R. Donald, J. Munro and W. Williams *257*
— M. Maxwell, I. R. McDonald, J. Munro and W. Williams *290*
— see Goding J. R. *457*
Desaulles, P., W. Schuler and R. Meier *318*
— J. Tripod and W. Schuler *321, 322*
— see Schuler, W. *316, 317*

Desmedt, J. E. *88*, 164
D'Esopo, L. M. see Lavieties, P. H. *347*
Dessert, A. M. see Miller, W. H. *297*
Dettelbach, H. R. see Arman, C. G. van *415*
Deucher, F. *40*
Devine, R. L. see Beams, H. W. *21*
Deyrup, I. J. *66*
— and H. H. Ussing *32*
— and W. W. Walcott *520*
Dhyse, F. G. see Hertz, R. *418*
Diamond, J. S., and S. A. Siegel *460, 463*
Dickens, F., and G. D. Greville *24*
Dicker, S. E. *354*
— and H. Heller *354*
Dignam, W. S., J. Voskian and N. S. Assali *340*
Dill, D. B. *448*
— F. G. Hall and H. T. Edwards *444*
Dimiek, D. F. see Landau, R. L. *339*
Dingman, J. F. *331, 349*
— K. Benirschke and G. W. Thorn *311, 312, 313*
— see Laidlaw, J. C. *320*
— see Thorn, G. W. *304*
Ditmore, H. B. jr. see Moore, F. D. *538*
Dixon, K. C. *104*
— see Ashford, C. A. *24, 28*
Dobson, A. *130*
— and A. T. Phillipson *130*
Dodge, E. see Emery, F. E. *498*
Dole, V. P., L. K. Dahl, G. C. Cotzias, H. A. Eder and M. E. Krebs *517*
— B. G. Stall and I. L. Schwartz *445*
— and J. H. Thaysen *439, 440, 441*
— see Schwartz, I. L. *432, 434, 443*
Donald, I. R. see Denton, D. A. *257*
Doorenbos, H. see Buchem, F. S. *316*
Dorfman, R. I. *306*
— see Rosenfeld, G. *314*
Dorman, P. J., W. J. Sullivan and R. F. Pitts *238, 290*
Dorrance, S. S. see Lewis, R. A. *289*
Dosekun, F. O., and D. Mendel *221*
Dott, N. M. see Lillie, R. S. *467, 468*

Doull, J. see Cochran, K. W. *526*
Dowds, E. G., E. W. Brickner and E. E. Selkurt *290*
Downey, M. see Conway, E. J. *108*
Draper, M. H., and S. Weidmann *147, 164, 186*
Dray, S. see Sollner, K. *56*
Dreiling, D. A. *460*
— and F. Hollander *460, 462, 463*
— H. Janowitz and M. Halpern *463*
Dreizen, S., W. Niedermeier, A. I. Reed and T. D. Spies *457*
Drenckhahn, F. O. see Ullrich, K. J. *248*
Drescher, A. N., N. B. Talbot, P. A. Meara, M. Terry and J. D. Crawford *521, 522, 523*
Dreyer, N. B., and E. B. Verney *269*
Drill, V. A. see Saunders, F. J. *340*
Driscol, T. E., M. M. Maultsby, G. L. Farrell and R. M. Berne *385*
Driscoll, M. E. see Atchley, D. W. *281*
— see Loeb, R. F. *294*
Drury, A. N. see Lewis, T. *186*
— D. R., P. D. McMaster and P. Rous *493*
— J. P. Henry and J. Goodman *351*
Dso, L. see Winter, H. A. *193*
Dube, A. H. see Streeten, D. H. P. *312*
Dubin, W. E. see Byrnes, W. W. *337*
Du Bois, K. P. see Cochran, K. W. *526*
Du Bois Reymond, E. *114*
Dubuisson, M. *40*
Duckert, A. see Mach, R. S. *317*
Ducommun, P. see Mach, R. S. *317*
Duggan, J. J., and R. F. Pitts *397, 404, 406*
— see Pitts, R. F. *397, 400, 401, 406*
Dumm, M. E. see Orti, E. *313*
Duncan, L. E. jr., G. W. Liddle and F. C. Bartter *513*
— D. H. Solomon, M. P. Nichols and E. Rosenberg *361*
— see Bartter, F. C. *312*
— see Liddle, G. W. *311*
Dunham, E. T. *61*

Dunham, E. T. see Tosteson, D. 78
— see Love, W. D. 78
Dunker, E. 216
— and H. Passow 78, 79
Durant, T. M. see Lasche, E. C. 384
Durbin, R. P., P. F. Curran and A. K. Solomon 509
— H. Frank and A. K. Solomon 54
Dury, A. 537
Duve, C. de, J. Berthet, L. Berthet and F. Appelmans 22
Dyke, H. B. van, K. Adamson jr., and S. L. Engel 333, 343
— and A. B. Hastings 193

Earle, D. P. see Bodo de, R. C. 341
— see Farber, S. J. 199, 200
— jr., R. C. de Bodo, I. L. Schwartz, S. J. Farber, M. Kurtz and J. Greenberg 341
— S. J. Farber, R. C. de Bodo, M. Kurtz and M. W. Sinkoff 341
Ebbecke, U. 151
Ebert, R. H. see Barclay, W. R. 303
Eccles, J. C. 160
— and W. V. MacFarlane 168
— see Coombs, J. S. 160, 171
Eckel, R. E. 79
— C. E. Pope II and J. E. C. Norris 519
Eckles, C. H. see Petersen, W. E. 498
Eckman, E. see Tompkins, M. J. 536
Eddleman, E. E. see Lombardo, T. A. 369, 370
Edelman, I. S., A. H. James, H. Baden and F. D. Moore 210, 211
— — L. Brooks and F. D. Moore 230
— J. Leibman, M. P. O'Meara and. L. W. Birkenfeld 200
— and J. Nadell 196, 197, 535
— J. M. Olney, A. H. James, L. Brooks and F. D. Moore 227
— see Gotch, F. 507
— see James, A. H. 228
— see Moore, F. D. 232
— see O'Meara, M. P. 229
— see Weston, R. E. 293, 399, 400, 401
Eden, M. see Berliner, R. W. 249

Eder, H. A., H. D. Lauson, R. P. Chinard, R. L. Greif, G. C. Cotzias and D. D. van Slyke 271
— see Dole, V. P. 517
Edlund, T., and H. Linderholm 398
Edsall, D. L. 450
Edward, B. see Thomas, C. 528
Edwards, C., and E. J. Harris 147
— C. J. see Hinkle, L. E. jr. 352
— J. G. 399
— H. T. see Dill, D. B. 444
Eggleston, L. V. see Krebs, H. A. 70, 103, 106
— see Stern, J. R. 65
Eggleton, L. V. see Terner, G. 25, 106
— M. G. 352
— J. R. Pappenheimer and F. R. Winton 269, 273
Eichelberger, L. and M. Roma 202, 207, 220
— see Huggins, C. 500, 501
— W. H. Akeson and M. Roma 208
— L. T., B. Brown and M. Roma 208, 209
Eichler, O. 2, 520
Eichna, L. W. see Farber, S. J. 373, 374
Eiseman, B. see Vivion, C. G. 423
Eisenberg, S. see Lombardo, T. A. 369, 370
— see Viar, W. N. 376, 377
Eisenstein, A. B. see Hartroft, P. M. 315
— B. see Frieden, J. 373
Eisler, M. see Swingle, W. W. 322
Ek, J. 389, 411, 414, 415
Eldridge, J. S. see Tyor, M. P. 43
Elings, H. S. see Buchem, F. S. 316
Eliot, J. W. see Bader, R. A. 352
Elisberg, E. I. see Frieden, J. 372, 373
Elkinton, J. R. 387, 527, 535, 538
— and T. S. Danowski 196, 197, 198
— and A. W. Winkler 287
— see Barker, E. S. 291
— see Singer, R. B. 290
Ellinger, A. 414
— P. 238
Elliott, K. A. C. see McLennan, H. 29

Ellis, S. see Wolfson, S. K. 537
Ellison, A. E. see Moore, F. D. 538
Elmadjian, F., J. M. Hope and G. Pencus 338
Elrick, H., E. R. Hoffman, C. J. Hlad jr., N. Whipple and A. Staub 355
— see Hlad, C. J. jr. 229
— see Staub, A. 355
Elsom, K. A. see Walker, A. M. 413, 414
Embden, G. and H. Lange 26
Emeleus, H. J., and J. S. Anderson 2
Emerson, K. see Marshall, E. K. 297
— see Renold, A. E. 418
— K. jr., S. S. Kahn and D. Jenkins 512, 513
— see Forsham, P. H. 323
Emery, E. W. see Black, D. A. K. 258
— F. E., C. E. Gossett, W. C. Young and E. Dodge 498
Emmelin, N. 455
— and W. Feldberg 193
Engbaek, L., and T. Hoshiko 122
— see Hoshiko, T. 122
Engel, E. see Demarret, J. C. 231
— F. L. see Teabeaut, R. 323
— L. L. see Thorn, G. W. 318, 319, 339, 340
— M. B. see Catchpole, H. R. 55
— S. L. see Dyke, H. B. 333, 343
Engström, A. 212
— W. W., and A. Liebman 364
Enns, L. H. see Rothstein, A. 108
Eppstein, F. H. 251
— see Hendrik, A. 251
Epstein, E. 38
— F. H. 38, 352, 373, 377
— A. V. N. Goodyer, F. D. Lawrason and A. S. Relman 375
— R. S. Post and M. McDowell 272
— see Lamdin, E. 352
Erdös, T. 9
Ericson, D. see Visscher, M. B. 132, 134, 135, 136
Erlanger, J., and E. A. Blair 162
Escher, D. J. W. see Weston, R. E. 293, 399, 400, 401, 407, 409
Espe, D., and V. R. Smith 497

Essellier, A. F. see Jeanneret, P *325*
Ethridge, C. B., D. W. Myers and M. N. Fulton *407*
Etsten, B. see Relman, A. S. *238, 290,* 294
Euler v., U. S. see Brown, G. L. *177*
Euw, J. v. see Reichstein, T. *307*
— see Simpson, S. A. *308*
Evans, B. M., N. C. Hughes Jones, M. D. Milne and S. Steiner 300, *531, 532*
— — — and H. Yellowlees 300, *514*
— see Counihan, T. B. *298*
— see Barfour, A. *352*
— see Milne, M. D. *292, 336*
— J. see Koch, H. J. *142*
— W. J., and S. Smiles *5*, 300
Eversole, W. J., F. A. Giere and M. H. Rock *361, 362*
— see Gaunt, R. *327*
Eyring, Henry see Frank H. Johnson *49*
Eyster, J. A. E. see Cranefield *164*
Eyzaguirre, C., and S. W. Kuffler *161*

Fabre, J. see Mach, R. S. *317*
Fänge, R., K. Schmidt-Nielsen and M. Robinson *502*
Fajans, S. S. see Streeten, D. H. P. *312*
Falbriard, A., A. F. Muller, R. Neher and R. S. Mach *313*
Fales, H. L. see Holt, L. E. *497*
Falkenheim, M. see Ranzi, S. *34*
Farah, A., T. S. Cobbey jr. and W. Mook 402, *406*
— and G. Maresh *396*, 401
— see Cafruny, E. J. *405*
Farber, S. J., W. H. Becker and L. W. Eichna *373*, 374
— E. D. Pellegrino, N. J. Conan and D. P. Earle *199*, 200
— see Bodo de, R. C. *341*
— see Earle, D. P. jr. *341*
— S., and M. Schubert 205, 209
Farrell, G. *314*
— G. L., R. C. Banks and S. Koletshy *311*
— E. W. Rauschkolb, P. C. Royce *307*
— — — and H. Hirschmann *307, 309,* 311
— and J. B. Richards *308*, 321

Farell, G., R. S. Rosnagle and E. W. Rauschkolb *312*, 370
— see Driscol, T. E. *385*
— see Newman, A. E. *313*
— see Rauschkolb, E. W. *313*
— see Rosnagle, R. S. *314*
— see Sweat, M. L. *309*
— S. I. see Ivy, A. C. *475*
— J. S. *500*
Fasman, G. D., and C. Niemann 19
Fatt, P. *169*
— and B. Katz 161, *163, 169,* 170
— see Coombs, J. S. *160, 171*
Fedor, E. see Swingle, W. W. *306, 307, 335, 536*
Feigen, G. A. *172,* 191
Fekete, A. see Balint, P. *366*
Feldberg, W., and S. L. Sherwood *216*
— see Brown, G. L. *193*
— see Emmelin, N. *193*
Feng, T. B., and Y. M. Liu *148, 162, 163*
— L. Y. Lee, C. W. Meng and S. C. Wang *177*
Fenn, W. O. *26, 84, 86, 174, 177, 496, 537*
— and D. M. Cobb *85, 165*
— J. F. Manery and W. R. Bloor *86*
— and R. Gershman *98*
— see Hegenauer, A. H. *26,* 145, 175
— see Mullins, L. J. *71*
— see Noonan, T. R. *39*
Feode, V. J. *500, 501, 502*
Fergus, E. B. see Danowski, T. S. *517,* 527
Ferguson, B. C. see Rosenbaum, J. D. *344, 387*
— F. P., and D. C. Smith 289
— L. K. see Reinhold, J. G. *488*
— M. H. see Hildes, J. A. *451, 452,* 459
Fernandez, C. see Tasaki, I. *141*
Fernelius, W. C. *2*
Ferrari, V., and R. D. Harckness *496*
Ferrebee, J. W., D. Parker, W. H. Carnes, M. K. Gerity, D. W. Atchley and R. F. Loeb *334*
— see Kuhlman, D. *323*
— see Ragan, C. *334*
Ferris, D. O., and H. M. Odel *515*
Fetcher, E. S. see Visscher, M. B. *133, 134, 135, 136*
Feyel, P., and R. Vieillefosse *259*

Field, H. jr., R. E. Dailey, R. S. Boyd and L. Swell *528*
— L. Swell, R. E. Dailey, E. C. Trout and R. S. Boyd *511*, 513
Finberg, L. see Harrison, H. E. *351*
Finch, C. A., C. G. Sawyer and J. M. Flynn *512*
Findley, T. jr. see Walker, A. M. *235, 236,* 247
Fine, D., L. E. Meiselas and T. Auerbach *312*
Finkenstaedt, J. T., A. Ruiz-Guinaza, L. Moreau, R. S. Morrison and J. P. Merrill *530*
— see Laidlaw, J. C. *320*
Fischer, S. see White, H. L. *375*
Fishel, L. see Newman, W. *381*
Fisher, R. B. *134,* 136
— and J. N. Hunt *479*
Fishman, A. P. see Puck, T. T. *31*
— see Wasserman, K. *32*
— R. A. *377*
Fitzgerald, M. G., and P. Fourman *294*
— see Chalmers, T. M. *316*
Fitzhugh, A. J. see Freeman, O. W. *387*
— F. W. see Freeman, O. W. *387*
Flanagan, J. B., A. K. Davis and R. R. Overman *213*, 536
Flear, C. T. G., R. Cawley, W. T. Cooke and A. Quinton *227*
— — A. Quinton and W. T. Cooke *227*
Fleckenstein, A. *175,* 179, 180
— and H. Hertel *181*
— H. Hille and W. E. Adam *182*
— E. Wagner and K. H. Göggel *181*
— see Hardt, A. *175*
Fleischman, E. see Harrison, H. E. *351*
Fletcher, H. M. see Langley, J. N. *452, 453, 455, 456*
— W. M. see Loewi, O. *412,* 413
Fleury, P. see Grimbert, L. *470*
Flexner, L. B. *215*
— B. D. Cowie and G. J. Vosburgh *218,* 219
— and A. Gellhorn *218,* 219
— see Gellhorn, A. *219, 220*

Flexner, L. B. see Pohl, H. A. *220*

Flink, E. B., A. B. Hastings and J. K. Lowry *60*

— E. see Forsham, P. H. *323*

— see Thorn, G. W. *330*

Florey, H. W., and H. E. Harding *483, 484*

— see Wright, R. D. *484*

Flynn, F., and M. Maizels *78*

— J. M. see Finch, C. A. *521*

Füldi, M. see Kovách, A. G. *306*

Fogelson, S. J., and W. H. Bachrach *484*

Folk, B. P., K. L. Zierler and J. L. Lilienthal jr. *202, 203*

Follis, R. H. jr. *526, 533*

Fomon, S. J. see Kaplan, S. A. *357, 358*

— see West, C. D. *261*, 290

Forbes, A., A. P. Forbes and Nyeland *499*

— A. P. see Forbes A. 499

— G. B. *210*, 211, 226

— and A. M. Lewis 220

— G. L. Mizner and A. Lewis *210, 211*

— and A. Perley *231*

- R. B. Tobian and H. Lewis *213*

Forsham, P. H., E. Flink, K. Emerson jr. and G. W. Thorn 323

— see Frawley, T. F. *457*

— see Liddle, G. W. *295*

— see Thorn, G. W. *330*

Forster, R. P., and J. V. Taggart *31*

Forsyth, B. T. *321*

Fortunato, J. see Klein, R. *318*

Forwell, G. D. see Bulmer, M. G. *426*

Foulks, J., G. H. Mudge and A. Gilman 223, *419, 420, 421, 422*

— see Mudge, G. H. 257, *281*, 397, *400, 409*

Fourman, P. 293, 340

— and P. Leeson *364*

— see Fitzgerald, M. G. *294*

Fowell, D. M., J. A. Winslow, V. P. Sydenstricker and N. C. Wheeler *411*

Fox, A. see Tobian, L. *537*

Francis, W. L. *117*

Franck, J., and J. E. Mayer *69*

Franglen, G. T., E. McGarry and A. G. Spencer *291*

Frank, C. W. see Blake, W. D. *270*

— H. see Durbin, R. P. *54*

Franke, F. see Bethe, A. *176*

Frankenhaeuser, B., and A.L. Hodgkin *158*, 160

Fraser, A. M. *353*

Frawley, T. F., and P. H. Forsham *457*

Frayser, R. see Hickam, J. B. *203*

Frazier, L. E. see Cannon, P. R. *531*

Freed, S. C., S. St. George and R. H. Rosenman *533*, 536

— and R. H. Rosenman *533*, 536

— — S. St. George and M. K. Smith *304*, 536

— see Friedman, M. *517*

— see Rosenman, R. H. *304*, 533

— see St. George, S. *532*

Freedberg, A. Stone see Zipser, A. *525*

— S. see Zipser, A. *224*

Freeman, O. W., G. W. Mitchell, J. S. Wilson, F. W. Fitzhugh and A. J. Fitzhugh *387*

Fregly, M. J., and P. F. Lampietro *517, 518*, 533

Fremont-Smith, F. see Merritt, H. H. *215*

— K. see Scribner, B. H. *203*

French, J. D. see Porter, R. W. *477*

Frenkel, M. see Pelser, H. E. *338*

Freygang, W. see Shanes, A. M. *158*

Friberg, O. *352*

Fricker, R. see Knowlton, K. *340*

Fried, J., and A. Borman *337, 419*

— and E. F. Sabo *337*

Frieden, J., L. Rice and E. I. Elisberg *372*

— — — B. Eisenstein and L. N. Katz *373*

Friedman, C. L. see Friedman, S. M. *374*

— M., R. H. Rosenman and S. C. Freed *517*

— S. M., M. Nakashima and C. L. Friedman *374*

— see Sréter, F. A. *200*

Friess, E. T. *18*

Fritz, I., and R. Levine *303*

Frouin, A. *466, 470, 476*

Fruhman, G. J. see Gaunt, R. *317*

Frunz, A. *497*

Fuhrman, F. A., and H. H. Ussing *127*, 128

Fukushima, K. *484, 485*

— see Kozana, S. *470*

Fuller, G. R., and M. B. MacLeod *294, 538*

Fulton, G. P. see Sudak, F. N. *537*

— see Wyman, L. C. *303*

— M. N. see Ethridge, C. B. *407*

Futcher, P. H. see Kriss, J. P. *356*

— see Slyke, D. D. *254*

Fuyat, H. N. see Radomski, J. L. 223, *419*, 420, 523, 524

Gabrilove, J. L. see Soffer, L. J. *321, 334*

Gaddum, J. H. *362*

Gaillard, L. M. *328*

Galdstonand, M. see Berger, E. Y. *289*

Gale, E. F. *38*

Galeotti, G. *114*, 120, 246

Galston, A. W. see Davies, R. E. *106*

Gamble, J. L. 196, *197*

— and M. A. McIver *461, 467, 468, 470, 484, 492*

— see McIver, M. A. *461, 467, 468, 470, 484, 492*

Gammel, J. A. see Sollman, T. *396*

Gammon, G. D. see Austin, J. H. *470*

Ganong, W. F. see Villarreal, R. *476*, 477

— and P. J. Mulrow *326*

Gamstorp, I., M. Hauge, H.F. Helweg-Larsen, H. Mjösnes and U. Sagild *197*

Gantier, E. see Prader, A. *452, 458, 499*

— R. see Prader, A. *452, 458, 499*

Garb, S. *186*

Garby, L. *53, 218, 219, 264*

Gardner, L. I., E. A. Mac Lachlan and H. Berman *294, 532*

— N. B. Talbot, C. D. Cook, H. Berman and C. Uribe *517*

Gárdos, G. *80*

Garrod, O., and R. A. Burston *327, 330*

— S. A. Davies and G. Cahill jr. *330, 331*

— see Ayres, P. J. *310*

— see Burston, R. A. *328, 330, 334*

Gasser, H. S. *175*

Gassman, F. K. see Lewy, F. H. *367*

Gast, J. H. see Gilleland, J.L. *487, 492*

Gatty, O. see Dean, R. B. *114*

Gaudino, M., and M. F. Levitt 328, 536
Gauer, O. H., J. P. Henry, H. O. Sieker and W. E. Wendt 351
— see Henry, J. P. 351
— see Sieker, H. O. 351
Gaunt, R. 335, 646
— J. H. Birnie and W. J. Eversole 327
— A. S. Gordon, A. A. Renzi, J. Padawer, G. J. Fruhman and M. Gilman 317
— M. Liling and M. Cordsen 361
— W. Lloyd and J. J. Chart 333
— J. W. Remington and M. Schweizer 334
— see Birnie, J. H. 333
— see Chart, J. J. 330
— see Renzi, A. A. 330
Gehrsitz, L. B. see Harris, J. E. 221
Geisman, T. A. see Crescitelli, F. 163
Geller, H. M. see Selkurt, E. E. 273, 274
— J. see Soffer, L. J. 334
Gellhorn, A., L. B. Flexner and L. M. Hellman 219
— — and H. A. Pohl 220
— M. Merrill and R. M. Rankin 229
— see Flexner, L. B. 218, 219
— see Pohl, H. A. 220
— E. 176
Gemzell, C. A. see Luft, R. 314
Genest, J. see Kattus, A. A. 375, 387
George, S. S. see Rosenman, R. H. 533
Gerard, R. W. 98
— see Chang, T. H. 25
— see Jenerick, H. P. 166, 167
— see Ling, G. 145, 146
Gerbrandy, J. see Blomhert, G. 349
— see Borst, J. G. 338
— see Molhuysen, J. A. 338
Gergely, J., M. A. Gouvea and D. Karibian 18
Gerity, M. K. see Ferrebee, J. W. 334
Gerking, S. D., and S. Robinson 447
— S. G. see Robinson, S. 442
Gersh, I. 40
Gershman, R. see Fenn, W. O. 98
Gershou, S. see Treutner, E. M. 224

Geyer, R. P., E. J. Bowie and J. C. Bates 31
— M. F. Meadows, L. D. Marshall and M. S. Gongaware 31
Giardini, A., and J. R. E. Roberts 464
Giarman, N. J. see Green, J. P. 187
Giebisch, G. 239
Giere, F. A. see Eversole, W. J. 361, 362
Gilbert, T. see Bliss, E. L. 361
Gill, T. J. see Solomon, A. K. 80
Gilleland, J. L., J. H. Gast and B. Halpert 487, 492
Gilligan, D. R. see Blumgart, H. L. 397, 411, 414
Gilman, A., and G. R. Cowgill 462, 473, 474, 489
— see Brazeau, P. 238, 289, 290
— see Foulks J. 223 419, 420, 421, 422
— see Mudge, G. H. 257, 281, 397, 400, 409
— M. see Gaunt, R. 317
Gilroy, F. J. see Hanlon, L. W. 419
Gilson, W. E. see Cranefield, P. F. 164
Ginetzinsky, A. G. 243
Ginsburg, J. M., and W. S. Wilde 229
Girerd, R. J., C. L. Rassaert, G. di Pasquale and R. L. Krog 338
— see Green, D. M. 213, 214
Gitths, R. D. see Streeten, D. H. P. 312
Gjørup, S., and J. H. Thaysen 530
Glass, G. B. J. 471
Glatzel, H., and W. Mecke 288, 295, 392
Gleichmann, F. see Westphal, K. 489
Glenister, D. see Swingle, W. W. 304, 536
Glenn, W. W. L. see Goodyer, A. V. N. 278, 282
Glick, D. 19
Glynn, I. M. 64, 72, 74, 75, 77, 78, 80, 326
Goding, J. R., and D. A. Denton 457
Göggel, K. H. see Fleckenstein, A. 181
Goetz, F. C. see Thorn, G. W. 304
Goffart, M., and Z. M. Bacq 166, 176
— and W. L. M. Perry 65
— see Bacq, Z. M. 166, 176

Goffart, M. see Szent-Györgyi, A. 9, 172, 173, 174, 176, 190
Gold, G. L., and A. K. Solomon 77
— see Solomon, A. K. 80
Goldacre, R. J., and I. J. Lorch 68
Goldberg, H. see Stamler, J. 374
Golden, C. C. see Cheek, D. B. 206
Goldfien, A., J. C. Laidlaw, N. A. Haydar, A. E. Renold and G. W. Thorn 337
Goldinger, J. M. see Perlman, H. B. 218
Goldman, D. E. 48, 56, 146
— M. L. see Kriss, J. P. 356
— R., and S. H. Bassett 381
Goldner, F. see Gordon, G. L. 364
Goldring, W. see Chasis, H. 413, 414, 415
Goldschmidt, S., and A. B. Dayton 131, 132
Goldstein, M. S., E. R. Ramey and R. Levine 303
— see Ramey, E. R. 303
Golup, J. R. see Hilton, J. G. 377, 378
Gongaware, M. S. see Geyer, R. P. 31
Good, C. A. 459, 477
Goodkind, M. J., see Davis, J. O. 310, 385, 513, 528
Goodman, H. C. sée Sellers, A. L. 355
— J. see Drury, D. R. 351
— L. S. see Woodbury, D. M. 318
Goodof, J. I., and C. M. MacBryde 530
Goodyer, A. V., L. R. Mattie and A. Chetrick 370
— A. V. N., and W. W. L. Glenn 278, 282
— E. R. Peterson and A. S. Relman 270
— see Epstein, F. H. 375
— see Tarail, R. 286
— see Welt, L. G. 402
Gook, H. van 429
Gordillo, G. see Metcoff, M. S. 300
Gordon, A. S. see Gaunt, R. 317
— see Stamler, J. 374
— F. H. see Oncley, J. L. 9
— G. L., and F. Goldner 364
Gossett, C. E. see Emery, F. E. 498
Gotch, F. A. see O'Meara, M. P. 229

Gotch, F., J. Nadell and J. S. Edelman 507

Goth, A. see Muirhead, E. E. 203

Gottschalk, C. W., and M. Mylle 249, 264, 265, 266, 268, 284

Gottstein, U. see Taugner, R. 174

Gouder, E. see Burgen, A. S. V. 438

Gould, R. G. see Hastings, A. B. 30

Gourea, M. A. see Gergely, J. 18

Gourley, D. R. H., and H. Jonas 39

Govaerts, P. 398

Grad, B. 457, 459

Grant, R. 468

—, W. M. see Kinsey, V. E. 216

Graubarth, H. N. see Brodsky, W. A. 391, 397

Graves, R. R. see Swett, W. W. 498

Grawford, J. H., and J. F. McIntosh 397

Gray, J. S. 476, 479

— and G. R. Bucher 469

— — and N. M. Harman 470, 472, 473, 478, 479

— M. J., and A. A. Plentl 231

— S. J., C. Ramsey, R. W. Reifenstein and J. A. Benson 476

— see Villarreal, R. 476, 477

Greco, F. del see Schneckloth, R. 355

Green, D. F. see Beinert, H. 15

— D. M., T. B. Reynolds and R. J. Girerd 213, 214, 221

— see Cook, D. L. 487, 489, 490, 491

— H. D. see Nichols, J. 315

— I. see Mommaerts, W. F. H. M. 18

— J. P., N. J. Giarman and W. T. Salter 187

— J. W., and A. K. Parpart 78

Greenberg, J. see Bodo de, R. C. 341

— see Earle, D. P. jr. 341

Greenman, L. see Danowski, T. S. 507, 527

Greep, R. O., and others 210

— see Deane, H. W. 315

— see Knobil, E. 203

Gregersen, M. I., and E. N. Ingalls 453, 454

Gregor, H. P. 6

— and J. I. Bregman 6

Gregor, H. P. see Visscher, M. B. 133, 134, 135, 136

Greif, R. L. see Eder, H. A. 271

Greig, M. E., and W. C. Holland 79

— see Lindvig, P. E. 79

Greven, K. 115

Greville, G. D. see Dickens, F. 24

Gribetz, D. see Corsa, L. jr. 228

Griffin, G. E. see Iacobellis, M. 532

— see Muntwyler, E. 532

Griffith, L. G. see Muntwyler, E. 532

Grim, E., and G. A. Smith 494

— see Sollner, K. 56

Grimbert, L., and P. Fleury 470

Grob, D., A. Liljestrand and R. J. Johns 200, 201

Groen, J. see Kamminga, C. E. 30

— see Pelser, H. E. 338

— see Willebrands, A. F. 537

Grollman, A. 536

Grosman, M. I., H. D. Janowitz, H. Ralston and K. S. Kim 489

Gross, F. 314

Grossman, J., R. E. Weston, E. R. Borun and L. Leiter 397, 402, 409

— — R. A. Lehman, J. P. Halperin, T. D. Ullman and L. Leiter 405, 409

— see Weston, R. E. 293, 345, 348, 352, 399, 400, 401, 407, 531

— and A. C. Ivy 463

— see Kalser, M. H. 463

Grundfest, H. 98, 152, 159, 171

— see Shanes, A. M. 158

Grundy, H. M., S. A. Simpson and J. F. Tait 308

— — — and M. Woodford 308

— see Tait, J. F. 308

Gudiksen, E. 470, 472, 473

Guerin, H. A. see Weston, R. E. 293, 531

Guggenheim, E. A. 481

Guild, W. R. see Bricker, W. R. 360

Guillot, N. see Bachrach, E. 185

Gukelberger, M., and H. Tschumi 266

Gundlach, R. see Rothlin, E. 476

Gunthorpe, C. H. see Langley, L. L. 456

Gupta, S. L., M. Bose and S. K. Mukherjee 6

Gurd, F. R. N. 9

— see Oncley, J. L. 9

— R. S. see Kessler, R. H. 403

Gustafson, T. see Runnström, J. 33

Gustavson, K. H. 206

Gutman, A. see Soffer, L. J. 334

Guttman, R. 150

Gydell, K. see Skanse, B. 316, 518

Habib, Y. A., G. C. Nichopoulos and R. R. Overman 530

Hacker, E. S. see Tarail, R. 199, 202

Hadidan, Z., and N. W. Pirie 19

Haege, L. see Mullins, L. J. 71

Hagiwara, S. see Tasaki, I. 161

Hahn, L., and G. Hevesy 71

— see Hevesy, G. 71

Hajdu, S. 188, 189, 190, 191

— and A. Szent-Györgyi 173, 188, 189, 190, 195

Hald, P. M. see Albrink, M. J. 199, 200

— P. T. 184, 185

Haldane, J. B. S. see Baird 349

— see Davies, H. W. 289

— see Hancock, W. 440, 441

Hall, A. D. see Luetscher, J. A. jr. 271

— F. G. see Dill, D. B. 444

— P. W. see Selkurt, E. E. 275

— III, P. W., and E. E. Selkurt 275

Hallman, L. F. see Hertz, R. 418

Halperin, J. P. see Grossman, J. 405, 409

— M. H. see Judson, W. E. 373

Halpern, M. see Dreiling, D. A. 463

Halpert, B. see Gilleland, J. L. 487, 492

Hamilton, J. G. 225

— P. B. see Slyke D. D. van 254

Hammarsen, O. 487

Hammarsten, E. 8

— G. Ågren and H. Lagerlöf 463

— and E. Jorpes 429

Hammarsten, J. E. see Jacobson, W. E. 359
Hancock, W., A. G. R. Whitehouse and J. S. Haldane 440, 441
Handler, P. see Kamin, H. 254
Handley, C. A., and J. H. Moyer 361
— J. Telford and M. Laforge 400
— T. see Platts, M. M. 415
Haneman, P. H. see Dempsey, E. F. 517
Hanenson, I. B. see Weston, R. E. 293, 345, 348, 352
Hanlon, L. W., M. Romaine, F. J. Gilroy and J. E. Deitrick 419
Hannon, J. P., A. M. Larson and D. W. Young 203
Hanon, F., M. Coquin-Carnot and P. Pignard 218
Hanzon, V. see Sjöstrand, F. S. 21
Harckness, R. D. see Ferrari, V. 496
Harding, H. E. see Florey, H. W. 483, 484
Hardt, A., and A. Fleckenstein 175
Hare, K. see Hare, R. S. 244, 347
— see Hickey, R. 349
— R. S., K. Hare and D. M. Phillips 244, 347
Hardin, B. see Mudge, G. H. 407, 408
Hargitay, B., and W. Kuhn 247, 249
— see Wirz, H. 247
Harman, N. M. see Gray, J. S. 470, 472, 473, 478, 479
Harned, H. S., and B. B. Owen 2
Harper, A. A., and H. S. Raper 461
Harreveld, A. van 98
Harris, E. J. 39, 42, 56, 62, 72, 74, 75, 82, 84, 87, 89, 90, 92, 93, 94
— and G. P. Burn 55, 87, 89, 93, 94
— and H. McLennan 55
— and M. Maizels 76, 77, 78
— and T. A. J. Prankerd 80
— and H. B. Steinbach 39, 44
— see Edwards, C. 147
— see Niedergerke, R. 188
— E. S. see Osterhout, W. J. V. 146
— J. E., and L. B. Gehrsitz 221
— J. D. Hauschildt and L. T. Nordquist 221

Harris, E. J. see Heinricks, D. J. 221
— R. see McGavack, T. H. 321, 328
Harrison, H. C. see Harrison, H. E. 416
— H. E., and D. E. Darrow 178, 328, 329
— — and H. Yannet 206, 210
— L. Finberg and E. Fleischman 351
— and H. C. Harrison 416
— see Lavieties, P. H. 347
— R. I. see Silva, J. L. de 219, 220
— T. R. see Lewis, J. M. jr. 375
— see Lombardo, T. A. 369, 370
— see Lusk, J. A. 376, 377
— see Viar, W. N. 376, 377
Harrop, G. A., L. J. Soffer, W. M. Nicholson and M. Strauss 301, 302
— A. Weinstein, L. J. Soffer and J. H. Trescher 302
Hart, W. M., and J. E. Thomas 461
Hartman, F. A., and K. A. Brownell 305
— — and W. E. Hartman 305
— see Hepps, S. A. 537
— W. E. see Hartman, F. A. 305
Hartmann, R. C., J. V. Auditore and D. P. Jackson 222
Hartroft, P. M., and A. B. Eisenstein 315
Hartott, P. M. see Pitcock, J. A. 314
Harvey, A. M. see Burgess, W. W. 247
— R. B. see Simmons, D. H. 326
Hashida, K. 114
Hashish, S. E. E. 39
Hasselbach, W. 18
Hastings, A. B., and J. M. Buchanan 29, 30
— and E. L. Compère 302
— A. K. Solomon, C. B. Anfinsen, R. G. Gould and J. M. Rosenberg 30
— C. T. Teng, F. B. Nesbett and F. M. Sinex 30
— see Ames, A. 104
— see Buchanan, J. M. 29, 30
— see Calkins, E. 60, 89, 95
— see Dyke, H. B. van 193
— see Flink, E. B. 60
— see Manery, J. F. 222, 477, 478, 486
— see Raker, J. W. 73, 74, 76, 78
— see Taylor, I. M. 79

Hatcher, J. D. see Judson, W. E. 373
Haugaard, N. see Stadie, W. C. 27, 31
Hauge, M. see Gamstorp, I. 197
Haurowitz, F. see Rona, P. 202
Hauschildt, J. D. see Harris, J. E. 221
Havard, R. E. 484
Havill, W. H., J. A. Lichty and G. H. Whipple 406
Hawes, R. C. see Alles, G. A. 19
Hayashi, T., and R. Rosenblueth 173
Haydar, N. A. see Goldfien, A. 337
Hays, D. R. see Hilton, J. G. 377, 378
Hayward, H. R. see Scott, G. T. 109
Hazard, J. see Hazard, R. 526
— R., J. R. Boissur, J. Hazard and P. Mouilli 526
— and A. Cornec 193
— and A. Quinquaud 195
Head, B. E. see Milne, M. D. 531
Hecht, H. H. 221
Hechter, O., and G. Pincus 305, 309, 319
— A. Zaffaroni, R. P. Jacobsen, H. Lery, R. W. Jeanloz, V. Schenker and G. Pinkus 307
— see Kass, E. H. 309
Hegnauer, A. H., W. O. Fenn and D. M. Cobb 26, 145, 175
— see Bass, D. E. 518
Heide, R. M. van der see Pelser, H. E. 338
Heidenhain, R. 131, 435, 452, 453, 454, 455, 467, 468, 503
Heilbrunn, L. V. 179
Heinbecker, P. see White, H. L. 341
Heinen, J. H. see Huggins, C. 499, 500
Heinricks, D. J., and J. E. Harris 221
Heinz, E. 481
— and K. J. Öbrink 478, 480, 481, 482
Hele, P. see Beinert, H. 15
Hellebrandt, F. A., E. Brogdon and S. L. Hoopes 475
Heller, B. I. see Jacobson, W. E. 359
— H. 128, 333
— see Dicker, S. E. 354

Hellerstein, S. see Darrow, D. C. *197*, 203, 206
Hellman, L. M. see Gellhorn, A. *219*
— see Weston, R. E. 293, *399*, 400, 401
Helmsworth, J. A. *215*
Helweg-Larsen, H. F. see Gamstorp, I. *197*
Hempling, H. G. *103*, *105*, 106
Hems, R. see Stern, J. R. 65
Hench, P. S. see Sprague, R. G. *320*
Henderson, V. E. see Loewi, O. *412*, 413
Henrikson, W. H. see Webster, D. R. *193*
Henry, J. P. see Gauer, O. H. *351*
— see Sieker, H. O. *351*
Hepler, O. E. see Simonds, J. P. *399*
Heppel, L. A. *86*, 87, *496*
— and C. L. A. Schmidt *533*
Hepps, S. A., F. A. Hartman and K. A. Brownell *537*
Hendrikx, A., and F. H. Eppstein *251*
Henle 244, 249, 251, 259, 260, 265, 326, 399, 401, 402
Henriques, V., and S. L. Ørskov *71*
Henry, J. P., O. H. Gauer and J. L. Reeves *351*
— and J. W. Pearce *351*
— see Drury, D. R. *351*
Henschel, A. see Bass, D. E. *518*
Herbst, A. L. see Yates, F. E. *277*
— C. *32*
Hering, H. E. *184*
Herman, F. G., and F. R. Winton *276*
— R. H., T. H. Wilson and L. Kazyale 492, *493*, 494, 495
Hermann, H. E. *494*
Hernando-Avendano, L. see Renold, A. E. *418*
Hernando, L., J. Crabbé, E. J. Ross, W. J. Reddy, A. E. Renold, D. H. Nelson and G. W. Thorn *311*
Herring, R. C. see Danford, H. G. *529*, 532
Herrmann, G. see Calvin, D. B. *397*, 411
Hers, H. *13*
Hershberg, E. B. see Herzog, H. L. *336*
Hertel, H. see Fleckenstein, A. *181*
Hertz, H. *165*

Hertz, R., W. W. Tullner, J. A. Schricker, F. G. Dhyse and L. F. Hallman *418*
Herzog, H. L., A. Nabile, S. Tolksdorf, W. Charney, E. B. Hershberg, P. L. Perlman and M. M. Peshet *336*
Hess Thaysen 113
Hestrin, S. see Nachmansohn, D. *14*
Hetzel, N. see Chart, J. J. *330*
Heuverswyn, J. van *151*
Hevesy, G. see Hahn, L. *71*
Heyningen, R. E. van, and J. S. Weiner 442, 443, 444
— see Amoore, J. E. *220*
— see Weiner, J. S. 442, *443*
Hiatt, E. P. *237*
Hickam, J. B., W. P. Wilson and R. Frayser *203*
Hickey, R., and K. Hare *349*
Hierholzer, K. see Kessler, R. H. *403*
Hift, H. see Beinert, H. *15*
Hild, W., and G. Zetler *343*
Hilden, T. see Anthonisen, P. *364*
— see Brun, C. *399*
Hildes, J. A., and M. H. Ferguson *451*, 452, 459
Hilger, H. H., J. D. Klümper and K. J. Ullrich *260*
— see Klümper, J. D. *260*
Hill, A., and P. S. Kupalov *42*
— A. V. *179*
— and L. Macpherson *174*
— F. C. see Wilhelmj, C. M. *468*
— F. S. *196*, 197
Hille, H. see Fleckenstein, A. *182*
Hiller, A. see Slyke, D. D. *254*
Hills, A. G. *197*
— T. M. Chalmers, G. D. Webster and O. Rosenthal *536*
Hilton, J. G. *408*
— D. M. Kanter, D. R. Hays, E. H. Bowen, J. R. Golup, J. H. Keating and R. Wegria 377, *378*
— S. M., and G. P. Lewis 455, 505
— see Berliner, R. W. *399*
Hines, C. R. see McKeever, W. P. *415*
Hinkle, L. E. jr., C. J. Edwards and S. Wolf *352*
Hinman, F., and A. E. Belt *515*
Hlad, C. J. jr., E. R. Huffman and H. Elrick *229*

Hlad, R. Nelson and J. H. Holmes *423*
— see Elrick, H. *355*
— see Vivion, C. G. *423*
Hoagland, H. see Rosenblueth, A. *182*
Hodes, H. L. see Sweet, A. Y. *509*, 536
Hodgkin, A. L. *72*, 84, *95*, 97, 102, 164
— and P. Horowitz *146*
— and A. F. Huxley 99, *100*, 101, 102, *151*, *152*, *154*, 155, 157, 158, 159, 160, 164, 166
— — and B. Katz *153*, 154
— and B. Katz *56*, 146, 149, 150, *152*, 153, 154, 162
— and R. D. Keynes 40, *42*, 51, *60*, 62, 78, *92*, 95, 96, 97, 98, 99, 100, 101, 158, 159
— see Frankenhaeuser, B. *158*, 160
— see Nastuk, W. L. *150*, 163, 164
Höber, J. see Höber, R. *144*, 151
— R. *1*, *45*, *131*, 138, *144*, 146, 150, 151, *152*, 533
— M. Andersh, J. Höber and B. Nebel *144*, 151
— and H. Strohe *150*
Högler, F. see Daniel, J. *347*
Hoehn, W. H., and R. Johnson *489*
Høhnson, C. G. see Walker, A. M. *413*, 414
Hökfelt, B. see Skanse, B. *197*, 518
Hoel, J. *334*
Hoeltzenbein, J. see Surtshin, A. *357*
Hörstadius, S. *34*
Hoff, H. E. see Winter, H. A. *193*
Hoffman, B. F. see Brooks, C. McC. *65*
— E. R. see Elrick, H. *355*
— J. F. see Parpart, A. K. *72*, 79
— jr., W. K. see Berne, R. M. *360*, 361
Hogben, A. *138*
— A. M. *480*, 482
— C. A. M. *113*, *138*
— see Cooperstein, I. L. *136*
Hogeboom, G. H., W. C. Schneider and G. E. Pallade *22*
Hogg, J. A., F. H. Lincoln, R. W. Jackson and W. P. Schneider *337*
Hoigne, R. V. see Weller, J. M. *530*

Holland, B. C., and E. A. Stead jr. *376*
— W. C., and C. V. Auditore *229*, *496*
— see Greig, M. E. *79*
Hollander, F. *465*, *471*, *478*, *479*, *480*
— and G. R. Cowgill *465*, *472*
— and F. V. Lauber *471*
— see Birnbaum, D. *463*
— see Colcher, H. *470*
— see Dreiling, D. A. *460*, *462*, *463*
— W., R. W. Winters, T. F. Williams, J. Bradeley, J. Oliver and L. G. Welt *531*
— see Judson, W. E. *373*
— see Oliver, J. *532*
Hollenberg, G. J. *110*
Holley, H. L. see Shaw, C. W. *215*
Holliday, M. A. see Oliver, J. *532*
Holloway, R. E. see Brauer, R. W. *490*, 491
— R. J. see Leong, G. F. *496*
Holman, Mollie E. *148*
Holm-Jensen, I. *143*
— A. Krogh and V. Wartiovaara *36*
Holmes, H. J. *281*, 328
— J. H. see Hlad, C. J. jr. *423*
Holt, L. E., A. M. Courtney and H. L. Fales *497*
Holtmeier, H. J. see Jeanneret, P. *325*
Homer, M. A. see Berger E. Y. *509, 513*
Honour, A. J., N. B. Myant and E. N. Rowlands *499*
Hood, M. see Roberts, K. E. *293*, 296
— S. L., and C. L. Comar *43*, 219, *220*, 225, 526
Hoopes, S. L. see Hellebrandt, F. A. *475*
Hope, J. M. see Elmadjian, F. *338*
Hopf, G. see Keining, E. *521*
Hopkins, W. S. see Shanes, A. M. *25*, 148
Horiuchi, M. see Kozawa, S. *470*
Horowitz, H. B. see Weston, R. E. *293*, *352*
— P. see Hodgkin, A. L. *146*
Horvath, B. *194*
Horwitz, S. A. see Berger, E. Y. *289*
Hoshiko, T., and Lise Engbaek *122*
— see Simmons, D. H. *326*
Howard, E., and V. J. de Feo *500*, 501, 502

Howarth, S., J. McMichael and E. P. Sharpey-Schafer *411*
Howell, D. S., and J. O. Davis *324*
— see Davis, J. O. *331*, 333
Hoye, S. J. see Moore, F. D. *538*
Hoyle, G. *162*
Huang, K. C. see Cizek, L. J. *328*
Hudson, C. L. see Walker, A. M. *235*, 236, 247
— P. B., A. Mittelman and M. Podberezec *338*
Hübener, H. J. *305*
— and D. Amelung *319*
Huf, E. G. *114*, *115*, 119, 129, 139
— and J. Wills *120*
Huffman, E. R. see Hlad, C. J. jr. *229*
Huggins, C., W. S. Scott and J. H. Heinen *499*, 500
— and L. Eichelberger *501*
— M. H. Masina, L. Eichelberger and J. D. Wharton *500*
— see Shih, H. E. *501*
Hughes, R. H. see Cannon, P. R. *531*
Hughes-Jones, N. C., G. W. Pickering, P. H. Sanderson, H. Scarborough and J. Vandenbroucke *355*
— see Barfour, A. *352*
— see Evans, B. M. 300, *531*, 532
Hulet, W. H., and G. A. Perera *355*
Hunt, A. see Spater, H. *531*, 533
— J. N. see Fisher, R. B. *479*
Hunter, C. B. see Hutchinson, D. L. *218*
— see Neslen, E. D. 218, *219*
Hurwitz, J. see Muntz, J. A. *14*
Hutchinson, D. L., C. B. Hunter, E. D. Neslen and A. Plentl *218*
Huxley, A. F. *40*, 41, *157*, 179
— and R. Stämpfli *148*, *149*, 150, 153, 154, 162, 165
— and R. E. Taylor *179*
— see Hodgkin, A. L. *99*, *100*, *101*, *102*, *151*, *152*, 154, 155, *157*, 159, 160, 164, 166
Hwang, W., L. C. Akman, A. J. Miller, E. N. Silber, J. Stamler and L. N. Katz *374*
Hyatt, R. E. see Davis, J. O. *385*

Hydén, S. see Sperber, I. *129*, 130
Iacobellis, M., E. Muntwyler and G. E. Griffin *532*
Ihre, B. J. E. *465*, *471*, *472*, 473
Ikkos, D., H. Ljunggren and R. Luft *342*
— R. Luft and B. Sjögren *342*
— — and H. Olivecrona *334*
— see Ljunggren, H. *228*
— see Luft, R. *213*, *314*, *319*, 320, 321, 323
Ingalls, E. N. see Gregersen, M. I. *453*, 454
Ingbar, S. H., E. H. Kass, C. H. Burnett, A. S. Relman, B. A. Burrows and J. H. Sisson *332*
Ingle, D. J. *303*
— R. Sheppard, E. A. Oberle and M. H. Kuizenga *320*
Ingraham, R. C., H. C. Peters and M. B. Visscher *69*
— and M. B. Visscher 131, *132*, 134, *138*, *470*, 477
Ingram, W. R. see Winter, C. A. 333, 335
Iob, V., and W. W. Swanson *210*
Isaacs, H. see Thomas, C. *528*
Ishikawa, Y. see Sollman, T. *192*
Ivy, A. C. *493*, *494*
— and J. I. Farrell *475*
— and Y. Oyama *467*, 468
— see Grossman, M. I. *463*
— see Schmidt, C. R. *488*
— J. S. *467*, 468
Jackson, D. P. see Hartmann, R. C. *222*
— L. C., and A. C. Rothera *498*
— R. W. see Hogg, J. A. *337*
— S. see Boyd, E. M. *503*
Jacobs, A., and W. B. Stirling *515*
— M. see Soffer, L. J. *321*
— M. D. see Soffer, L. J. *321*
— M. H. *53*
Jacobsen, R. P. see Hechter, O. *307*
Jacobson, H. N., and R. H. Kellogg *353*
— W. E., J. E. Hammarsten and B. I. Heller *359*
Jacox, R. F., M. K. Johnson and R. Koontz *214*
Jacques, A. G. *110*
Jaffe, L. see Moehlig, R. C. *335*
James, A. H., L. Brooks, I. S. Edelman, J. M. Olney and F. D. Moore *228*

James, A. H. see Chalmers, T. M. *316*
— see Edelman, I. S. *210*, 211, *227, 230*
— see Moore, F. D. *232*
— M. B. see Metcoff, M. S. *300*
Janecek, J. see Tobian, L. *314*
Janowitz, H. D. see Colcher, H. *470*
— see Dreiling, D. A. *463*
— see Grosman, M. I. *489*
Jarausch, K. H., and K. J. Ullrich *260*
— see Ullrich, K. J. *248*
Jeanloz, R. W. see Hechter, O. *307*
Jeanneret, P. *275, 276*
— A. F. Essellier and H. J. Holtmeier *325*
Jefferson, N. C. see Popper, H. L. *490*
Jenerick, H. P., and R. W. Gerard *166*, 167
Jenkins, D. see Emerson, K. jr. *512*, 513
— see Thorn, G. W. *304*
Jennings, M. A. see Wright, R. D. *484*
Jensen, R. L. see Schwartz, W. B. *255*, 286
Jessen, J. *282*
Jewell, P. A. *348*
Jiminez-Diaz, C. *324*
Jørgensen, C. B. *128*
Johansson, S. see Skanse, B. *316*, *518*
John, H. M. see Nachmansohn, D. *14*
Johns, R. J. see Grob, D. 200, 201
Johnson, B. B., A. H. Lieberman and P. J. Mulrow *313*
— see Axelrad, B. J. *311*, 312
— B. J. see Conn, J. W. *445*
— Frank H., Eyring, Henry and Milton J. Polissar *49*
— J. A. *64*, 89, 90
— J. see Tosteson, D. *83*
— M. K. see Jacox, R. F. *214*
— R. see Hoehn, W. H. *489*
— R. D. see Streeten, D. H. P. *312*
— R. E., G. C. Pitts and F. G. Consolazio *444*
Johnsson, R. E. see Pitts, G. C. *448*
Johnston, C. G. see De Beer, E. J. *484, 485*
— see Ravdin, I. S. *487*, 492, 493, 494, 495
— M. W. see Conn, J. W. *445*
— R. B. and K. Bloch *15*
Johnstone, B. M. see Shaw, F. H. *42*

Jonas, H. see Gourley, D. R. H. *39*
Jones, H. S. see Locke, W. *440*, 442
— I. C., and A. Wright *334*
— J. see Muirhead, E. E. *203*
— N. C. H. see Milne, M. D. *292*, 336
Jong, J. C. de see Molhuysen, J. A. *338*
Jorpes, E. see Hammarsten, E. *429*
Joseph, N. R. see Catchpole, H. R. *55*
Joyce, C. R. B., and M. Weatherall *80*
Judson, W. E., J. D. Hatcher, W. Hollander, M. H. Halperin and R. W. Wilkins *373*
— see Wilkins, R. W. *350*, 372
Juel-Nielsen, N. see Schou, M. *224*
Jungmann, P. *366*
— and E. Meyer *365*

Kachmar, J. F., and P. D. Boyer *12*
Kagan, A. see Berne, R. M. *360*, 361
Kagawa, C. M., and C. G. van Arman *320*
— J. A. Cella and C. G. van Arman *418*
Kahana, E. M. see Baldwin, D. *270*
Kahn, A. J. see Sandow, A. *174*, 178, 179
— jr., J. B., and G. H. Acheson *80*
— S. S. see Emerson, K. jr. *512*, 513
Kahnt, F. W., and A. Wettstein *319*
Kalckar, H. M. see Kielly, W. W. *18*
Kalser, M. H., and M. I. Grossman *463*
Kamin, H., and P. Handler *254*
Kammenga, E. see Willebrands, A. F. *537*
Kamminga, C. E., A. F. Willebrands, J. Groen and J. R. Blickman *30*
Kampitsch, E. see Schwarzenbach, G. *5*
Kanter, D. M. see Hilton, J. G. *377*, 378
Kaplan, S. A., S. J. Fomon and S. Rapoport *357, 358*
— and S. Rapoport *356*, 358
— C. D. West and S. J. Fomon *357, 358*

Kaplan, see Knowles, H. C. jr. *514*
— see West, C. D. *261*, 290
Karel, L. *480*
Karibian, D. see Gergely, J. *18*
Karreman, G. see Baird, S. L. *9*
Kascht, M. E. see Landau, R. L. *339*
Kass, E. H., O. Hechter, I. A. Macchi and T. W. Mou *309*
— see Ingbar, S. H. *332*
Kato, G. *162*
Kattus, A., T. M. Arrington and E. V. Newman *415*
— A. A., B. Sinclair-Smith, J. Genest and E. V. Newman *375*, 387
Katz, B. *161*, *162, 177*
— see Castillo, J. del *168*
— see Fatt, P. *161*, *163, 169*, 170
— see Hodgkin, A. L. *56*, 146, 149, 150, 152, *153, 154*, 162
— L. N. see Frieden, J. *373*
— see Hwang, W. *374*
— see Stamler, J. *374*
Katzenellenbogen, M. *131*, 138
Katzin, L. J. *115*
Katzman, R., and P. H. Leiderman *229*
Kawahata, A., and H. Sakamoto *446*
— see Tanaka, M. *446*
Kawata, N. see Steinbach, H. B. *150*
Kaye, M. *300*
Kazyale, L. see Herman, R. H. 492, 493, 494, 495
Keating, J. H. see Hilton, J. G. *377, 378*
— R. P. see Blake, W. D. *275*
Keele, D. see Klein, R. *318*
Keilholz, A. *223*
Keilin, D. see Mann, T. *296*
Keining, E., and G. Hopf *521*
Keith, N. M., and M. W. Binger *392*
— H. E. King and A. E. Osterberg *257*
— and A. E. Osterberg *522*
— — and H. B. Burchell *521*
Keller, A. D. see Demunbrun, T. W. *354*
— R. *491*
Kellin, A. E. see Ayres, P. J. *310*
Kellogg, R. H., and W. R. Burack *329*
— see Jacobson, H. N. *353*

Kelsey, W. M. see Little, J. M. *333, 341*

Kemp, R. L. see Surawicz, B. *529*

Kendall, A. E. see Walker, A. M. *413*, 414

— E. C. see Allers, W. D. *301*

— see Sprague, R. G. *320*

— see Wilder, R. M. *302*

Kennaway, E. L. see Davies, H. W. *289*

Kennedy, J. see Shih, H. E. *501*

— E. P., and A. L. Lehninger *21*

— see Lehninger, A. L. *23*

— R. A. see Barclay, J. A. *347, 387*

— T. J. see Berliner, R. W. *397, 400*, 408, 409, *422*

— T. J. jr. see Berliner, R. W. *257*

Kenyon, A. T. see Knowlton, K. *340*

Kepler, E. F. see Robinson, F. J. *327*

— E. J. see Cluxton, H. E. *323*

— see Wilder, R. M. *302*

Kermarck, W. D., and R. A. Miller *498*

Kerpel-Fronius, E. *281*

Kerwin, T. O. see Bowen, W. J. *18*

Kessler, R. H., K. Hierholzer, R. S. Gurd and R. F. Pitts *403*

— R. Lozano and R. F. Pitts *406*

— W. R., and D. H. Andersen *446*

Kesztyus, L., and J. Martin *455*

Keye, J. D. *530*

Keynes, R. D. *64, 87, 89, 90*, 91, 93, *94*, 95, *96*, 100, 102, 162, *171*

— and R. H. Adrian *50*

— and G. W. Maisel *26, 60*, 62, 88, 92

— see Caldwell, P. C. *60*

— see Hodgkin, A. L. 40, 42, *51, 60*, 62, 78, 92, 95, 96, 97, 98, 100, 101, 158, 159

— and P. R. Lewis *96*

— see Swan, R. C. *50*

Keys, A. see Mickelsen, O. *444*

Kiel, F. *278*

Kielly, W. W., H. M. Kalckar and L. B. Bradley *18*

Killmann, S. A., and J. H. Thaysen 452, *503*

— see Bro-Rasmussen, F. *426*

Kilpatrick, R., H. E. Renschler, D. S. Munro and G. M. Wilson *43*, 230

Kim, K. S. see Grosman, M. I. *489*

Kimura, K. K. see Randall, W. C. *439*, 445

Kincaid, R. K. see Robinson, S. 442, *444*, 449, 450

King, A. L. see Robinson, S. *448*, 449, 450

— C. V. *396*

— E. J. see Wottom, I. D. P. *199*

— H. E. see Keith, N. M. *257*

Kinsey, V. E. 216, *217*

— E. Camacha, G. A. Cavanaugh, M. Constant and D. A. McGinty *217*

— and W. M. Grant *216*

— see Cavanaugh, G. A. *217*

Kinter, W. B., and J. R. Pappenheimer *268*

— see Pappenheimer, J. R. *267*, 414

Kirkwood, J. G. *52*

Kirschner *81*

— L. B. *118*, 122, 127

Kitayama, K. see Rosenberg, H. *165*

Kitchener, J. A. see Kressman, T. R. E. *3*

Kitching, J. A. *37*

Kittsteiner, C. 440, 442

Kleeman, C. R. see Bass, D. E. *518*

— see Lamdin, E. *352*

Klein, R., P. Taylor, C. Papadatos, Z. Laron, D. Keele, J. Fortunato, C. Byers and C. Billings *318*

Kleinberg, H. see Scribner, B. H. *530*

Kleinzeller, A. *26*

Kliman, B. see Davis, J. O. *375*

Klotz, J. M. *8*

— see Battley, E. H. *9*

— N. J. see Brown, J. B. *453*

Klümper, J. D., K. J. Ullrich and H. H. Hilger *260*

— see Hilger, H. H. *260*

Knafel-Lenz, E., and S. Nogaki *132*

Knobil, E., and R. O. Greep *203*

Knowles, H. C. see Agna, J. W. *210*, 211

— jr., and S. A. Kaplan *514*

Knowlton, A. I. see Plotz, C. M. *323*

— F. P. *269*

— K., A. T. Kenyon, I. Sanddiford, G. Lotwin and R. Fricker *340*

Knudsen, E. O. E. see Brun, C. *350*

Kobinger, W., and F. J. Lund *416*

Koch, H. *62, 142, 143*

— H. J., and J. Evans *142*

— — and E. Schicks *142*

— and A. Krogh *143*

Koczorek, Kh. R. see Wolff, H. P. *312*, 370, 384, *385*

Koefoed-Johnsen, V. *126*

— H. Levi and H. H. Ussing *116*

— and H. H. Ussing 46, 53, *78, 123*, 124, 128, *243*

— — and K. Zerahn *113*

Koepf, G. F. see Lewis, R. A. *289*

Kolda, J. *499*

Koletshy, S. see Farrell, G. L. *311*

Kolls, A. C. see Marshall, E. K. jr. *356*

Kolm, R., and E. P. Pick *185*

Koltay, E. see Kovách, A. G. *366*

Komarov, S. A., G. O. Langstroth and D. R. McRae 435, 461, *503*

— see Day, J. J. *474*

— see Langstroth, G. O. *435*

— see Vineberg, A. M. *464*

Koontz, R. see Jacox, R. F. *214*

Kopaczewski, M. W. *19*

Korey, S. R., B. de Braganza and D. Nachmansohn *14*

Korff, R. W. v. *15*

— see Beinert, H. *15*

Kornberg, H. L., and R. E. Davies *467*

— see Davies, R. E. *232*

Kovách, A. G., B. M. Földi, N. Papp, P. S. Roheim and E. Koltay *366*

Kozawa, S., K. Fukushima, M. Umeno, K. Kurihara, C. Takata and M. Horiuchi *470*

Kraus, S. D. *338, 339*

Krebs, H. A., L. V. Eggleston and C. Terner 70, *103*, 106

— see Bartley, W. *37*

— see Stern, J. R. *65*

— see Terner, C. 25, 106

— M. E. see Dole, V. P. *517*

Kremer, V. L. see Luetscher, J. A. jr. *271*

Kressman, T. R. E., and J. A. Kitchener *3*

— see Kitchener, J. A. *3*

Kreutman, E. H. see Waterhouse, C. *328*

Krjevic, K. *95, 163*

Krimsky, I. see Racker, E. *17*

Kriss, J. P., P. H. Futcher and M. L. Goldman *356*
Krog, R. L. see Girerd, R. J. *338*
Krogh, A. *46*, 57, 84, 87, *115*, 129, *142*
— A. L. Lindberg and B. Schmidt-Nielsen *191*
— C. G. Lund and K. Pedersen-Bjergaard *464*
— see Holm-Jensen, I. *36*
— see Koch, H. J. *143*
Kronenberg, G., and H. Ocklitz *361*, *362*
Kroop, I. G. see Sirota, J. H. *257*
Kruhøffer, P. *236*, *237*, *238*, 246, *255*, 257, 266, 277, 281, 288, 291, 414
Kuffler, S. W. *168*, *170*, *175*, *176*
— and E. M. Vaughan Williams 90, 163, *177*
— see Eyzaguirre, C. *161*
Kuhlman, D., C. Ragan, J. W. Ferrebee, D. W. Atchley and R. F. Loeb *323*
Kuhn, W. see Hargitay, B. *247*, 249
— see Wirz, H. *247*
Kuizenga, M. H. see Ingle, D. J. *320*
Kule, J., and R. B. Welbourn *477*
Kulonen, E. see Mäkinen, P. *215*
Kunin, A. S., E. H. Dearborn and A. S. Relman *525*
Kunitz, M. see Northrop, J. H. *9*
Kuno, Y. 433, 439, *439*, 441, 449, 450
Kupalov, P. S. see Hill, A. *42*
Kupfer, S., D. D. Thompson and R. F. Pitts 398, 400, *412*
Kurihara, K. see Kozawa, S. *470*
Kurland, S. see Baumann, E. J. *301*
Kurosawa, T. *497*
Kurtz, M. see Bodo de, R. C. *341*
— see Earle, D. P. jr. *341*
— see White, A. G. *352*
Kuschinsky, G., and H. E. Bundschuh *353*
— see Brunner, H. *353*

Ladd, M. 347, *349*, *371*, *403*
— and L. G. Raisz *521*
— see Wesson, L. G. jr. *266*, 270, *349*
Ladell, W. S. S. *442*, *443*, 445, *446*, *448*, 449, 450

Laehr, H. *387*
LaForge, M. see Handley, C. A. *400*
Lagerlöf, H. O. *460*, 462, 463
— H. see Ågren, G. *460*
— see Hammarsten, E. *463*
Laidlaw, J. C., J. F. Dingman, W. L. Arons, J. T. Finkenstaedt and G. W. Thorn *320*
— see Goldfien, A. *337*
— see Thorn, G. W. *304*
Lajta, A. *10*
Laken, B. see Orti, E. *313*
Lallier, R. 35
Lambie, A. T., A. M. Roy, A. S. Relman, B. A. Burrows and W. B. Schwartz *525*
— see Relman, A. S. *44*, 224, 255
— C. G. see Cushny, A. R. *413*
Lamdin, E., C. R. Kleeman, M. Rubini and F. H. Epstein *352*
Lamm, O., and H. Malmgren *8*
Lampietro, P. F. see Fregly, M. J. *517*, *518*, *533*
Lamy, H., and A. Mayer *280*
Landau, R. L., D. M. Bergenstal, K. Lugibihl and M. E. Kascht *339*
— K. Lugibihl and D. F. Dimiek *339*
Lane, N., and R. C. de Bodo *310*, 315
Lange, H. see Embden, G. *26*
Langham, M. E. *216*
Langley, J. N., and H. M. Fletcher 452, 453, 455, 456
— L. L., C. H. Gunthorpe and W. A. Beall 456
Langstroth, G. O., D. R. McRae and S. A. Komarov *435*
— D. R. McRae and G. W. Stavraky *427*, 433, *435*, 453, 454
— see Komarov, S. A. *435*, 461, 503
Laporte, Y. see Walker, S. M. *170*
Laragh, J. H. *379*
— and N. E. Capeci *287*, *522*
— and H. C. Stoerk *313*
— see Anderson, H. M. *522*, 529
Lardy, H. A. *11*
— and J. A. Ziegler *11*
— see Boyer, P. D. *11*
— see Pressman, B. C. *23*
Laron, Z. see Klein, R. *318*

Larrabee, M. G. see Brink, F. *166*
Larramendi, L. M. H., R. Lorente de Nó and F. Vidal *161*
— see Lorente de Nó, R. *161*
Larsen, E. E. see Weir, J. F. *346*
Larson, A. M. see Hannon, J. P. *203*
Lasche, E. C., W. H. Perloff and T. M. Durant *384*
Lashley, K. S. *451*
Lasnitzki, A. *28*
— and O. Rosenthal *28*
Latimer, W. M. *2*
Latorre, G. see Surtshin, A. *272*
Lauber, F. V. see Hollander, F. *471*
Lauson, H. D. see Eder, H. A. *271*
— H. O. *348*
Lavender, A. R., and T. N. Pullman *417*
Lavieties, P. H., L. M. D'Esopo and H. E. Harrison *347*
Lawler, C. A. see Cook, D. L. *487*, *489*, *490*, *491*
Lawrason, F. D. see Epstein, F. H. *375*
Leaf, A. *66*, 68, 120, *130*
— F. C. Bartter, R. F. Santos and O. Wrong *345*, 348
— and A. R. Mamby *350*
— — H. Rasmussen and J. P. Marasco *335*
— and A. Renshaw *61*, *120*
— W. B. Schwartz and A. S. Relman *298*
Le Brie, S. J. see Swingle, W. W. *322*
Lechner, E. see Cooper, E. S. *215*
Lee, D. H. K. 449
— L. Y. see Feng, T. P. *177*
Leeson, P. see Fourman, P. *364*
Lehman, R. A. see Grossman, J. *405*, 409
Lehmann, F. E. *33*
— J. E. *166*
— K. see Andersen, R. *8*
Lehninger, A. L. *2*
— and E. P. Kennedy *23*
— see Kennedy, E. P. *21*
Leibman, J. see Edelman, I. S. *200*
Leiderman, P. H. see Katzman, R. *229*
Leifer, E. see Nickel, J. F. *257*
Leiter, L. see Grossman, J. *397*, 402, *405*, 409
— see Mokotoff, R. *277*

Leiter, see Weston, R. E. 293, 352, 397, 399, 400, 401, 407, 409, 531
— see White, A. G. 347
Leland, J. see Loeb, R. F. 302
Le Noir, M. see Mraz, F. R. 526, 527
Lenstra, J. B. see Molhuysen, J. A. 338
Leonard, E., and J. Orloff 256
Leong, G. F., R. J. Holloway and R. W. Brauer 496
— see Brauer, R. W. 490, 491
Leopold, J. H. see Smolens, J. 464
Le Page, G. A. 17
Leslie, S. H. see Dancis, J. 352
Lesnick, G. see Soffer, L. J. 321
Leusen, I. 216
— and G. Demeester 523
Levi, H., and H. H. Ussing 50, 62, 87, 89, 91, 92, 139
— see Koefoed-Johnsen, V. 116
Levin, L. K. see Schneyer, L. H. 451
Levine and others 303
— H. C. see Somerville, W. 304
— R. see Fritz, I. 303
— see Goldstein, M. S. 303
— see Ramey, E. R. 303
— S. A. see Weller, J. M. 530
— V. E. see Barry, W. M. 493
Levinsky, N. G., and R. W. Berliner 423
— D. D. Davidson and R. W. Berliner 353
— see Berliner, R. W. 249, 303, 345
— see Davidson, D. G. 240, 258
Levitt, M. F., and M. E. Bader 332, 536
— L. B. Turner and A. Y. Sweet 372
— — — and D. Pandiri 211, 214
— see Gaudino, M. 328, 536
— see Sweet, A. Y. 509, 536
Levkoff, A. H. see Demunbrun, T. W. 354
Levy, M., and G. Nora 191, 192
— M. N., and R. M. Berne 375
— see Berne, R. M. 360, 361
— see Blumgart, H. L. 397, 411, 414
— H. see Hechter, O. 307
Lewis, A. see Forbes, G. B. 210, 211, 220

Lewis, A. A. G. see Chalmers, T. M. 330, 331
— G. P. see Hilton, S. M. 455, 505
— H. see Forbes, G. B. 213
— J. M. jr., R. M. Buie, S. M. Sevier and T. R. Harrison 375
— P. R. see Keynes, R. D. 96
— R. A., G. W. Thorn, G. F. Koepf and S. S. Dorrance 289
— see Thorn, G. W. 318, 319
— T. 186
— and A. N. Drury 186
Lewy, F. H., and F. K. Gassmann 367
Li, C. H. see Stein, J. D. jr. 342
— see Whitney, J. E. 342
— M. C. see MacLean, J. P. 311
Lichty, J. A. see Havill, W. H. 406
Liddle, C. M. 418
— G. W. 418
— L. L. Bennett and P. H. Forsham 295
— J. Cornfield, A. G. T. Casper and F. C. Bartter 322
— L. E. Duncan and F. C. Bartter 311
— J. E. Richard and G. M. Tomkins 337
— see Bartter, F. C. 312
— see Duncan, L. E. 513
Lieberman, A. H. 379
— see Johnson, B. B. 313
Liebman, A. see Engström, W. W. 364
Lifson, N., R. L. Varco and M. B. Visscher 480, 481
— see Visscher, M. B. 132, 134, 135, 136
Lilienthal, J. L. see Zierler, K. L. 321
— jr. see Folk, B. P. 202, 203
Liling, M. see Gaunt, R. 361
Liljestrand, A. see Grob, D. 200, 201
— see Grob, D. 200, 201
Lillie, R. S. 151
Lim, K. S., and N. M. Dott 467, 468
— R. K. S., and A. C. Liu 476
— A. R. Matheson and W. Schlapp 465
— H. Necheless and T. G. Ni 475
— see Liu A. C. 479, 480
Lincoln, F. H. see Hogg, J. A. 337
Lindahl, P. E. 34
— and L. O. Öhman 34

Lindberg, A. L. see Krogh, A. 191
— H. A., M. H. Wald and M. H. Barker 390
Linde, S. 472
— and K. J. Öbrink 469, 470, 472, 473, 480, 482
— T. Teorell and K. J. Öbrink 481
Linder, E., and R. Blomstrand 204
Linderholm, H. 48, 49, 57, 114, 122
— see Edlund, T. 398
Lindhard, J. see Buchthal, F. 170
Lindsay, A. E., and H. Brown 416
— see Davis, J. O. 384
Lindvig, P. E., M. E. Greig and S. W. Peterson 79
Lineweaver, H., and G. A. Ballou 19
Ling, G. 42, 44
— and R. W. Gerard 145, 146
Lipmann, R. W. 406
Lipschitz, W. L., and E. Stokey 415
Lipsett, M. B., and O. H. Pearson 529
— C. D. West, J. P. MacLean and O. H. Pearson 320
— see MacLean, J. P. 311
— M. N., and F. Crecitelli 24
Little, J. M., W. M. Kelsey and E. H. Yount jr. 333, 341
Liu, A. C., I. C. Yuan and R. K. S. Lim 479, 480
— see Lim, R. K. S. 476
— Y. M. see Feng, T. B. 148, 162, 163
Ljungberg, E. 248, 259
Ljunggren, H., D. Ikkos and R. Luft 228
— see Luft, R. 213, 319, 320, 321, 323
— see Ikkos, D. 342
Lloyd, W. see Gaunt, R. C. 333
Lloyd-Thomas, H. G. see Spencer, A. G. 415, 511
Lobitz, W. C., and A. E. Osterberg 439
— and H. L. Mason 439
Locke, F. S. 169
— W., N. B. Talbot, H. S. Jones and J. Worcester 440, 442
Lockett, M. F. 333
Loeb, R. F. 301, 302
— D. W. Atchley, E. M. Benedict and J. Leland 302
— — D. W. Richards, E. M. Benedict and M. E. Driscoll 294

Loeb, and J. Stahl *302*
— see Atchley, D. W. *281*
— see Ferrebee, J. W. *334*
— see Kuhlman, D. *323*
— see Ragan, C. *334*
— see Stahl, J. *301*
Löhner, L. *492*
Loewi, O. *237, 413*
— W. M. Fletcher and V. E. Henderson *412, 413*
Logan, M. A. *214*
Logothetopoulos, J. see Barfour, A. *352*
Lojkin, M. E. see Mulinos, M. G. *334*
Lombardo, T. A. *377*
— S. Eisenberg, B. B. Oliver, W. N. Viar, E. E. Eddleman and T. R. Harrison *369, 370*
— see Viar, W. N. *376, 377*
Longuevalle, S. see Parrot, J. L. *65*
Lontie, R. A. see Oncley, J. L. *9*
Loosjes, R. see Schuffelen, A. C. *112*
Lorch, I. J. see Goldacre, R. J. *68*
Lorente de Nó, R. *161, 162, 163, 166*
— F. Vidal and L. M. H. Larramendi *161*
— see Larramendi, L. M. H. *161*
Lotspeich, W. D. *313, 329*
— and R. F. Pitts *254*
— see Pitts, R. F. *238, 254*
Lotwin, G. see Knowlton, K. *340*
Louis, L. H. see Conn, J. W. *197, 312, 445*
— see Streeten, D. H. P. *312*
Love, W. D., and G. E. Burch *77*
— J. A. Carlsen and E. T. Dunham *78*
— R. B. Romney and G. E. Burch *43*
Lowe, K. G. *293*
— T. E. *519*
Lowenstein, B. E., and R. L. Zwemer *522*
Lown, B. see Weller, J. M. *530*
Lowrance, P. B. see Nickel, J. F. *257*
Lowry, J. K. see Flink, E. B. *60*
— O. H. see Smith, C. A. *141, 217*
— see Talbot, N. B. *194*
Lozaityte, I. see Mathews, M. B. *209*

Ludeman, H. see Crawford, B. *270, 520*
Ludwig, C. *241, 272, 274, 427*
— and R. H. Curtis *384, 385*
— see Axelrad, B. J. *311, 312*
— see Deming, Q. B. *384*
— jr., and B. J. Axelrad *311, 312*
— A. D. Hall and V. L. Kremer *271*
Lüttgau, H. C. see Niedergerke, R. *188*
Luft, R., D. Ikkos and C. A. Gemzell *314*
— B. Sjögren, D. Ikkos, H. Ljunggren and H. Tarukaski *213, 319, 320, 321, 323*
— see Ikkos, D. *228, 342*
Lugibihl, K., see Landau, R. L. *339*
Lund, F. J. see Kobinger, W. *416*
— G. H. see Lyster, S. L. *337*
— E. J., and P. Stapp *117*
Lund, A. *423*
— C. G. see Krogh, A. *464*
— E. J. *115*
Lundberg, A. *426, 427, 428, 429, 430, 433, 437, 452, 454, 455, 504*
Lundegardh, H. *61, 68, 112*
— and H. Bergstrand *223*
Lundsgaard, E. see Bayliss, L. E. *266*
Lusk, J. A., M. N. Viar and T. R. Harrison *376, 377*
Lutwak-Mann, C. see Mann, T. *501*
Lyster, S. L., L. E. Barnes, G. H. Lund, M. M. Meinzinger and W. W. Byrnes *337*

MacArthur, J. W. *34*
Macaulay, D. see McCrory, W. W. *365*
MacBryde, C. M. see Goodof, J. I. *530*
Macchi, I. A. see Kass, E. H. *309*
MacDonald, N. S. see Alexánder, G. V. *214*
MacDougal, E. J., and F. Verzar *132, 133*
— M. see Oliver, J. *532*
MacDowell, M. C. see Walker, A. M. *234, 242, 245, 247*
MacFarlane, W. V. see Eccles, J. C. *168*
Mach, R. S. *529*
— J. Fabre, A. Duckert, R. Borth and P. Ducommun *317*
— see Demarret, J. C. *231*

Machado, A. L. see Nachmansohn, D. *14*
MacIntosh, F. C. see Brown, G. L. *166*
MacIntyre, J., and O. Davidsson, *221, 533*
MacKay, E. M. see Smith, F. M. *346, 347, 348*
— G., C. P. Stewart and J. D. Robertson *220*
MacKey, E. M. and A. M. Butler *295, 392*
MacLachlan, A., see Gardner, L. I. *294, 532*
— M. see Boyd, E. M. *503*
MacLean, J. P., M. B. Lipsett, M. C. Li, C. D. West and O. H. Pearson *311*
— see Lipsett, M. B. *320*
MacLeod, M. B. see Fuller, G. R. *294, 538*
— R. A. see Clark, J. A. *13, 17*
MacMillan, W. H. *537*
MacMillan, W. K. *522*
Macollum, A. B. *36*
Macpherson, L. see Hill, A. V. *174*
MacRobbie, E. A. C. *111*
— and J. Dainty *36, 111*
Macy, I. G. *497*
Madden, R. J., and H. H. Ramsberg *476*
Madinaveitia, J., and T. H. H. Quibell *19*
Mäkinen, P., and E. Kulonen *215*
Magaard, H. *463*
Magida, M. G. see Roberts, K. E. *291, 294, 522, 538*
Magnus Caryl, J. see Moore, F. D. *227*
Magnus, R. *269, 280*
Mahler, P. *470*
Main, E. R. see Neuman, W. F. *212*
Maisel, G. W. see Keynes, R. D. *26, 60, 62, 88, 92*
Maitland, A. I. L. *393*
Maizels, M. *60, 72, 73, 77, 78, 81, 82, 83*
— M. Remington and R. Truscoe *105*
— see Flynn, F. *78*
— see Harris, E. J. *76, 77, 78*
Maletich, W. S. see Robinson, S. *448, 449, 450*
Malmgren, H. see Lamm, O. *8*
Malvin, R. L., W. S. Wilde and L. P. Sullivan *239, 260*
— — A. J. Vander and L. P. Sullivan *241*
Mamby, A. R. see Leaf, A. *335, 350*

Man, E. B. see Albrink, M. J. 199, *200*

Manchester, R. C. *348*

Mandel, H. *179*

— see Sandow, A. *179*

Manery, J. F. *84*, 201, *202, 204, 206, 208, 210, 211,* 220

— and W. F. Bale *210*

— and A. B. Hastings *222,* 477, 478, 486

— see Fenn, W. O. *86*

— see Wilson, D. L. *103*

Mann, P. J. G., M. Tennenbaum and J. H. Quastel *28*

— T. *500*

— and C. Lutwak-Mann *501*

— and D. Keilin *296*

Manning see Muller, A. F. *376*

Marasco, J. P. see Leaf, A. *335*

Maren, T. H. *298,* 300

— B. C. Wadsworth, E. K. Yale and L. G. Alonso *298*

Maresch, G. see Farah, A. *396,* 401

Margoshes, M. see Wacker, W. E. C. *517*

Marine, D., and E. J. Baumann *301*

Marinelli, L. D. see Miller, C. E. *227*

Mark, H. see Weston, R. E. *293, 531*

Markley, K., M. Bocanegra, G. Morales and M. Chiappori 270, *520*

Marmorston, J. see Sellers, A. L. *355*

Marnay, A. see Nachmansohn, D. *175*

Maroney, W. H. see Welt, L. G. *402*

Marriott, H. L. 191, *192*

Marshall, E. K., W. C. Cutling and K. Emerson *297*

— and D. M. Davis *328*

— jr. *389*

— and A. C. Kolls *356*

— L. D. see Geyer, R. P. *31*

— see Burgess, W. W. *247*

Martell, A. E. M., and M. C. Calvin *4*

Martin, E. G. *184,* 185

— J. see Kesztyus, L. *455*

— L. *470*

— M. M., and G. Walker *227*

— — and M. Chapman *227*

— W. R. see Sheppard, C. W. *73, 74,* 76

Masina, M. H. see Huggins, C. *500*

Mason, H. L. see Lobitz, W. C. *439*

— see Mattox, V. R. *308*

— see Sprague, R. G. *320*

Massart, J. *464*

Mateer, F. M. see Danowski, T. S. *517, 527*

Matheson, A. R. see Lim, R. K. S. *465*

Mathews, M. B. *209*

— and I. Lozaityte *209*

Mathiesen, D. R. see Sprague, R. G. *320*

Mathis, H. *459*

Mathison, G. C. *184,* 193

Matthies, H. *67*

Mattice, M. R. *516*

Mattie, L. R. see Goodyer, A. V. *370*

Mattox, V. R., H. L. Mason and A. Albert *308*

— see Salassa, R. M. *419*

Maultsby, M. M. see Driscoll, T. E. *385*

Maurice, D. M. *208, 217*

Maxwell, M. see Denton, D. A. *290*

— M. H. and E. S. Breed *243*

— — and I. L. Schwartz *380*

— P. Morales and C. H. Crowder jr. *362*

— R. see Swingle, W. W. *307, 335*

— S. S. *128*

Mayer, A. see Lamy, H. *280*

— J. E. see Franck, J. *69*

Mazia, D. *179*

Mazur, M. see Cochran, K. W. *526*

McAllen, P. M. *532*

McCance, R. A. *444, 446,* 470, 476

— and E. M. Widdowson *257, 289, 291, 328, 516, 533, 534*

— W. F. Young and D. A. K. Black *246*

— see Boylan, J. W. *218*

— see Widdowson, E. M. *226*

— see Wilkinson, B. M. *328*

McCann, S. M. see Andersson, B. *362, 364*

McChesney, E. W. *511*

— F. C. Nachod and M. L. Tainter *512*

McClean, D. *20*

McClure see Randall, W. C. *441*

McCollum, E. V. see Orent-Keiles, E. *293, 529*

McCracken, B. H. see Thorn, G. W. *304*

McCrory, W. W., and D. Macaulay *365*

McDonald, I. R. see Denton, D. A. *290*

— R. K., and J. H. Miller *399*

McDonough, J., and C. M. Wilhelmj *521*

McDowall, R. J. S., and A. A. I. Soliman *192*

— and A. F. Zayat 187, *188*

McDowell, M. see Epstein, F. H. *272*

McElroy, R. E. see Brauer, R. W. *490,* 491

McGarry, E. see Franglen, G. T. *291*

McGavack, T. H., A. Saccone, M. Vogel and R. Harris *321, 328*

McGillivray, I., and T. J. Buchanan *231*

McGinty, D. A. see Kinsey, V. E. *217*

McGuire, T. F. see Wilhelmj, C. M. *521*

McIntosh, J. F. see Grawford, J. H. *397*

McIver, M. A. see Gamble, J. L. *461, 467, 468, 470, 484,* 492

McKeever, W. P., C. R. Hines and I. C. Winter *415*

McLean, F. C., and M. R. Urist *210*

— see Slyke, D. D. van *201*

McLennan, H. *63*

— and K. A. C. Elliott *29*

— see Harris, E. J. *55*

McMaster, P. D. see Drury, D. R. *493*

— see Rous, P. *487, 493, 494*

McMichael, J. see Howarth, S. *411*

McMurrey, J. D. see Moore, F. D. *227*

McQuarrie, I., W. H. Thompson and J. A. Anderson *522*

McQueen-Williams, M., and K. W. Thompson *340*

McRae, D. R. see Langstroth, G. O. *427, 433, 435, 453,* 454

— see Komarov, S. A. *435,* 461, 503

McSwiney, R. R. see Brooks, R. V. *529*

Meadows, M. F. see Geyer, R. P. *31*

Meara, P. A. see Drescher, A. N. *521, 522, 523*

— P. see Spater, H. *531, 533*

Meares, P., and H. H. Ussing *53*

Mecke, W. see Glatzel, H. *288, 295, 392*

Meier, R. see Desaulles, P. 318
— see Schuler, W. 316, 317
Meigs, E. B., and W. G. Atwood 85
Meinzinger, M. M. see Lyster, S. L. 337
— see Stafford, R. O. 336, 337
Meisel, E. see Wachstein, M. 399, 405
Meiselas, L. E. see Fine, D. 312
Melchior, N. C. 7
Mellanby, J. 462
Melville, R. S. see Talbott, J. H. 328
Menczel, J. see Bergmann, F. 261
Mendel, B., D. Mundell and F. Strelitz 19
— D. see Dosekun, F. O. 221
Meneely, G. R., and C. O. T. Ball 516, 520
Meng, C. W. see Feng, T. P. 177
Mercier, F., and J. Mercier 193
— J. see Mercier, F. 193
Merkel, F. 424, 425, 430, 434
Merrill, A. J. 378, 382
— J. A. see Warren, J. V. 381
— J. P. see Bricker, N. S. 360
— see Finkenstaedt, J. T. 530
— see Weller, J. M. 530
— M. see Gellhorn, A. 229
Merritt, H. H., and F. Fremont-Smith 215
Metcalf, W. 370
Metcoff, M. S., M. B. James, G. Gordillo and I. Antonowicz 300
Meyer, E. see Jungmann, P. 365
— K. 19
— K. H., and P. Bernfeld 57, 125
— and M. M. Rapport 19
— and J. F. Sievers 56, 57
— L. F., and S. Cohn 295, 392
Meyerhof, O., and J. R. Wilson 17
Meyler, F. L. 185
Mickelsen, O., and A. Keys 444
Millar, F. K. see Steward, F. C. 38
Miller, A. J. see Hwang, W. 374
— C. E., and L. D. Marinelli 227
— F. W. see Swett, W. W. 498
— D. I. see Pearcy, M. 443, 448
Miller, G. E. 379

Miller, H., D. S. Munro and G. M. Wilson 213
— and R. S. Weetch 499
— and G. M. Wilson 216, 227
— H. C., and D. C. Darrow 86
— H. G. 295, 392
— J. H. see McDonald, R. K. 399
— R. A. 498
— see Kermarck, W. O. 498
— W. H., A. M. Dessert and R. O. Roblin 297
Milne, M. D., N. C. H. Jones and B. M. Evans 292, 336
— R. C. Muerheke and B. E. Head 531
— B. H. Schreiner and M. A. Crawford 256, 336
— see Black, D. A. K. 293
— see Counihan, T. B. 298
— see Evans, B. M. 300, 531, 532
Miner, R. W. 5, 205, 509
Mitchell, G. W. see Freeman, O. W. 387
— P. 38
Mittelman, A. see Hudson, P. B. 338
Miyamoto, S., and C. L. A. Schmidt 9
Mizner, G. L. see Forbes, G. B. 210, 211
Mjösnes, H. see Gamstorp, I. 197
Modell, W. 388, 410
Moehlig, R. C., and L. Jaffe 335
Möller, F. see Skanse, B. 316, 518
Møller, K. O. 393, 397, 398, 411
Mokotoff, R., and G. Ross 384
— — and L. Leiter 277
Molhuysen, J. A., J. Gerbrandy, L. A. de Vries, J. C. de Jong, J. B. Lenstra, K. P. Turner and J. G. G. Borst 338
— see Blomhert, G. 349
— see Borst, J. G. 338
Mommaerts, W. F. H. M. 172
— and I. Green 18
Mond, R., and K. Amson 86
— and H. Netter 86
Monod, J. see Cohn, M. 16
Montgomery, H., and J. A. Pierce 238, 252
Montgomery, M. L., G. E. Sheline and I. L. Chaikoff 463
Montigel, C. 9
Mook, W. see Farah, A. 402, 406
Moore, A. R., and A. S. Burt 36

Moore, F. D. 197
— I. S. Edelman, J. M. Olney, A. H. James, E. Brooks and G. M. Wilson 232
— E. A. Boling, H. B. Ditmore jr., A. Sicular, J. E. Teterick, A. E. Ellison, S. J. Hoye and M. R. Ball 538
— J. D. McMurrey, H. V. Parker and J. Caryl Magnus 227
— see Edelman, I. S. 210, 211, 227, 230
— see James, A. H. 228
— see Wilson, G. M. 213
Moracci, E. 524
Morales, G. see Markley, K. 270, 520
— P. see Maxwell, M. H. 362
Morel, F. 258, 330
Morison, R, S. see Rosenblueth, A. 177
Morley, E. H. see Byrnes, W. W. 337
Morris, R. see Treutner, E. M. 224
Morrison, R. S. see Finkenstaedt, J. T. 530
Moser, F. see Churney, L. 179
Motokawa, K. 114, 115
Mou, T. W. see Kass, E. H. 309
Mouilli, P. see Hazard, R. 526
Moulin, M., and W. Wilbrandt 191
Moustgaard, J. 266
Movius, H. J. see Porter, R. W. 477
Moyer, J. H. see Handley, C. A. 361
Mraz, F. R., and H. Patrick 526, 527
— M. Le Noir, J. Pinajian and H. Patrick 526
Mudge, G. H. 60, 66, 106, 107
— A. Ames, J. Foulks and A. Gilman 400, 409
— J. Foulks and A. Gilman 257, 281, 397
— and B. Hardin 407, 408
— and J. V. Taggart 197
— and K. Vislocky 291
— and I. M. Weiner 396, 408
— see Anderson, H. M. 294
— see Foulks, J. 223, 419, 420, 421, 422
— see Stanbury, S. W. 22, 39
Mueller, B. see Surtshin, A. 357
— C. B., A. Surtshin, M. R. Carlin and H. L. White 271, 272
— see Carlin, M. R. 387

Mueller, H. see Baird, S. L. *9*
Münchow, O. see Brunner, H. *353*
Muerheke, R. C. see Milne, M. D. *531*
Muirhead, E. E., A. Goth and J. Jones *203*, *537*
Mukherjee, S. K. see Gupta, S. L. *6*
Mulder, A. G. see Amberson, W. R. *237*
Mulinos, M. G., C. L. Spingarn and M. E. Lojkin *334*
Muller, A. F., and C. M. O'Connor *314*, 376
— see Falbriard, A. *313*
— Manning and Riondel 376
Mullins, L. J. *54*
— W. D. Fenn, T. R. Noonan and L. Haege *71*
Mulrow, P. J. see Ganong, W. F. *326*
— see Johnson, B. B. *313*
Munck, O. *261*, *268*
Mundell, D. see Mendel B. *19*
Munro, D. S., R. S. Satoskar and G. M. Wilson *210*, *213*
— see Denton, D. A. *257*, *290*
— see Kilpatrick, R. *43*, *230*
— see Miller, H. *213*
Muntwyler, E., G. E. Griffin, G. S. Samuelsen and L. G. Griffith *532*
— see Iacobellis, M. *532*
Muntz, J. A. *13*, *14*
— and J. Hurwitz *14*
Murata, Y. see Bregman, J. I. *5*
Murphy, R. J. F. *347*
Murray, M. M. see Bowes, J. H. *214*
Mustakallio, K. K., and A. Telkkä *399*
Muylder, de *356*, *359*
Myant, N. B. see Honour, A. J. *499*
Myers, D. W. see Ethridge, C. B. *407*
Mylle, M. see Gottschalk, C. W. *249*, *264*, *265*, *266*, *268*, *284*
Myrden, J. A. see Wilson, G. *213*
— M. R. see Wilson, G. M. *213*

Nabatoff, R. A. see Sirota, J. H. *276*
Nabile, A. see Herzog, H. L. *336*
Nachmansohn, D. *19*, *168*
— S. Hestrin and H. Voripaieff *14*
— and H. M. John *14*
— and A. L. Machado *14*

Nachmansohn, J. Wajzer and A. Marnay *175*
— and I. B. Wilson *168*
— see Korey, S. R. *14*
— see Wilson, I. B. *65*
Nachod, F. C. see McChesney, E. W. *512*
Nadell, J. see Edelman, I. S. *196*, *197*, *507*, *535*
Näj, D. see Prader, A. *452*, *458*, *499*
Nakao, A. see Buchanan, D. L. *212*
Nakashima, M. see Friedman, S. M. *374*
Nash, T. P. see Amberson, W. R. *237*
Nasset, E. S. see Schriffin, M. J. *484*, *485*
Nastuk, W. L., and A. L. Hodgkin *150*, *163*, *164*
Nebel, B. see Höber, R. *144*, *151*
Necheless, H. see Lim, R. K. S. *475*
— see Olson, W. H. *393*
— see Popper, H. L. *490*
Needham, D. M. *172*
— J. *33*
— see Peters, J. P. *366*
— J. W. see Sims, E. A. H. *351*
Neher, R. see Simpson, S. A. *308*
Neigus, I. see Wilhelmj, C. M. *468*
Neihof, R. see Sollner, K. *56*
Neil, M. W. see Creese, R. *90*
Nelson, A. A., and G. Woodard *315*
— see Radomski, J. L. *223*, *419*, *420*, *523*, *524*
— D. H. see Hernando, L. *311*
— see Renold, A. E. *418*
— K. R. see Thorn, G. W. *339*
— R. see Hlad, C. J. jr. *423*
— W. P., and L. G. Welt *347*, *367*
— III., W. P. see Rosenbaum, J. D. *329*, *376*
Nesbett, F. B. see Buchanan, J. M. *29*, *30*
— see Hastings, A. B. *30*
Neslen, E. D., C. B. Hunter and A. A. Plentl *218*, *219*
— see Hutchinson, D. L. *218*
Netravisesh, V. *375*, *376*, *377*
— and H. L. White *369*, *370*
Netter, H. *86*, *151*
— see Mond, R. *86*
Neubauer, E. *489*
— see Adlersberg, D. *489*
Neuman, M. W. see Neuman, W. F. *210*, *212*

Neuman, W. F., and M. W. Neuman *210*, *212*
— — E. R. Main, J. O'Leary and F. A. Smith *212*
— see Boyd, E. S. *209*
— see Stoll, W. R. *211*
Newburgh, L. H. *449*
Newman, A. E., E. S. Redgate and G. L. Farrell *313*
— E. V. *379*
— see Kattus, A. *375*, *387*, *415*
— see Pearce, M. L. *375*, *376*
— W., and L. Fishel *381*
Ni, T. G. see Lim, R. K. S. *475*
Nichols, G. jr., and N. Nichols *207*, *213*, *520*, *527*
— see Nichols, N. *212*, *213*
— and H. D. Green *315*
— and H. L. Sheehan *315*
— M. P. see Duncan jr., L. E. *361*
— N. *221*, *537*
— and G. Nichols jr. *212*, *213*
— see Nichols, G. jr. *207*, *212*
Nicholson, W. M. see Harrop, G. A. *301*, *302*
Nichopoulos, G. C. see Habib, Y. A. *530*
Nickel, J. F., P. B. Lowrance, E. Leifer and S. E. Bradley *257*
— C. McC. Smythe, E. M. Papper and S. E. Bradley *355*, *360*
— see Smythe, C. McC. *360*
Nicolas, J. R. see Robinson, S. *444*, *449*, *450*
Niedergerke, R. *191*
— H. C. Lüttgau and E. J. Harris *188*
Niedermeier, W. see Dreizen, S. *457*
Niemann, C. see Fasman, G. D. *19*
Nistler, L. *136*
Nitta, H. *426*, *504*
Nixon, D. A. see Alexander, D. P. *218*
— Nola, E. see Rogoff, J. M. *537*
Noack, C. H. see Treutner, E. M. *224*
Noble, R. L., and J. D. Robertson *474*
— and N. B. G. Taylor *350*
Noell, W. K. see Tarail, R. *525*
Nogaki, S. see Knafel-Lenz, E. *132*
Noonan, T. R., W. O. Fenn and L. Haege *39*
— see Mullins, L. J. *71*

Nora, G. see Levy, M. 191, 192
Nordquist, L. T. see Harris, E. J. 221
Norris, J. E. C. see Eckel, R. E. 519
Northrop, J. H., and M. Kunitz 9
Novelli, A. 128
Noyons, A. K. see Bouckaert, J. P. 185
Numerof, P. see Borman, A. 337
Nussbaum, R. E. see Alexander, G. V. 214
— see Alexánder, G. V. 214
Nutt, M. E. see Barclay, J. A. 347, 387
Nyeland see Forbes, A. 499
Nyhan, W. L., and R. E. Cooke 365

Oberle, E. A. see Ingle, D. J. 320
O'Brien, J. M., and W. S. Wilde 182
— see Wilde, W. S. 182
Ochoa, S. see Ohlmeyer, P. 11
— see Stern, J. R. 15
Ochwadt, B. 289
Ocklitz, H. see Kronenberg, G. 361, 362
O'Connor, C. M. see Muller, A. F. 314, 376
— see Wolstenholme, G. 215
— E. W. see Wolstenholme, G. 215
— W. J. 352, 358
Odel, H. M. see Ferris, D. O. 515
Odenthal, I. 316
Öbrink, K. J. 454, 466
— see Heinz, E. 478, 480, 481, 482
— see Linde, S. 469, 470, 472, 473, 480, 481, 482
Öhman, L. O. see Lindahl, P. E. 34
Oehme, C. 288
Orskov, S. L. see Henriques, V. 71
Oettingen van, W. F. see Sollman, T. 192
Offenbacher, R. 398
Ohara, K. 435
Ohlmeyer, P., and S. Ochoa 11
Okkels, H. 258, 259
O'Leary, J. see Neuman, W. F. 212
Olivecrona, H. see Ikkos, D. 334
Oliveira, H. L. de 256
Oliver, B. B. see Lombardo, T. A. 369, 370

Oliver, see Viar, W. N. 376, 377
— J., M. MacDowell, L. G. Welt, M. A. Holliday, W. Hollander, R. W. Winters, T. F. Williams and W. E. Segar 532
— see Hollander, F. 531
— see Walker, A. M. 234, 242, 245, 247
Olney, J. M. see Edelman, I. S. 227
— see James, A. H. 228
— see Moore, F. D. 232
— see Wilson, G. M. 213
Olsen, N. S., and G. G. Rudolph 215, 216
— see Rudolph, G. G. 215
Olson, W. H., and H. Necheles 393
O'Malley, E. see Conway, E. J. 108
O'Meara, M. P., L. W. Birkenfeld, F. A. Gotch and I. S. Edelman 229
— see Edelman, I. S. 200
Opdyke, D. F., and I. Clark 203, 204
Opie, E. L. 66
— see Schwartz, I. L. 496
Oncley, J. L., F. H. Gordon, F. R. N. Gurd and R. A. Lontie 9
Onsager, L. 51
Orbeli, L. A. 114
Orent-Keiles, E., and E. V. McCollum 293, 529
Orias, O. see Brooks, C. McC. 65
Orloff, J. 291
— and R. W. Berliner 256
— and W. D. Blake 371
— L. G. Welt and L. Stowe 271
— see Berliner, R. W. 239, 258, 287, 297, 298, 299, 300, 397, 408, 409, 422
— see Leonard, E. 256
— see Peters, J. P. 366
— see Sims, E. A. H. 351
— see Stevenson, J. A. F. 364
— see Welt, L. G. 270, 350
Orti, E., E. P. Ralli, B. Laken and M. E. Dumm 313
Osborn, C. M. see Birnie, J. H. 333
— M. see Swingle, W. W. 536
Osterberg, A. E., F. R. Vanzant and A. V. Alvarez 477
— see Comfort, M. W. 462
— see Keith, M. N. 257, 521, 522
— see Lobitz, W. C. 439
Osterhout, W. J. V. 5
— and E. S. Harris 146

Ostwald, W. 144
Ottoson, D., F. Sjöstrand, S. Stenström and G. Swaetichin 122
Overman, R. R. 196, 197
— see Davis, A. K. 318
— see Flanagan, J. B. 213, 536
— Habib, Y. A. 530
Overton, E. 162, 174, 175
Owen, B. B. see Harned, H. S. 2
Owles, W. H. 483
Oyama, Y. see Ivy, A. C. 467, 468

Packer, D. M. see Scott, G. H. 41
Padawer, J. see Gaunt, R. 317
Page, I. H. 355
— see Schneckloth, R. 355
— I. see Corcoran, A. C. 419, 523
— L. B., C. F. Baxter, G. H. Reem, J. C. Scott-Baker and H. W. Smith 357
Palade, A. E. 21
Pallade, G. E. see Hogeboom, G. H. 22
Palmer, B. see Boyd, E. M. 503
— L. S. see Petersen, W. E. 498
Pandiri, D. see Levitt, M. F. 214
Panikkar, N. K. 143
Papadatos, C. see Klein, R. 318
Papp, N. see Kovách, A. G. 366
Pappenheimer, J. R. 262, 264, 265, 267
— and W. B. Kinter 267, 414
— E. M. Renkin and L. M. Borrero 53, 54
— see Eggleton, M. G. 269, 273
— see Kinter W. B. 268
Papper, E. M. see Nickel, J. F. 355, 360
Parker, D. see Ferrebee, J. W. 334
— H. V. see Moore, F. D. 227
— J. see Smolens, J. 464
Parkins, W. M. see Swingle, W. W. 535
Parpart, A. K., and J. F. Hoffman 72, 79
— see Green, J. W. 78
Parra, V. see Croxatto, H. 355
Parrot, J. L., J. Thouvenot and S. Longuevalle 65
Parthasarathy, D., and A. T. Phillipson 130

Pasquale di, G. see Girerd, R. J. *338*
Passow, H. see Dunker, E. *78, 79*
Patrick, H. see Mraz, F. R. *526, 527*
— see Williams, L. G. *527*
Paudiri, D. see Levitt, M. F. 211, *214*
Pauling, L. 3
Pavlov, I. P. *465*, 468, 478
Pawan, G. L. S. see Chalmers, T. M. *347, 372*
Pearce, J. W. see Atkins, E. L. *371*
— see Henry, J. P. *351*
— M. L., E. V. Newman and M. R. Birmingham *375, 376*
Pearcy, M., S. Robinson, D. I. Miller, J. T. Thomas jr. and L. de Brota *443, 448*
— see Robinson, S. *444, 449, 450*
Pearson, O. H. see MacLean, J. P. *311*
— see Lipsett, M. B. *320, 529*
Pechet, M. M. see Davis, J. O. *310, 385*
Pecora, L. H. see Talbott, J. H. *328*
Pedersen-Bjergaard, K. *464*
Pellegrino, E. D. see Farber, S. J. *199*, 200
Pelser, H. E., A. F. Willebrands, M. Frenkel, R. M. van der Heide and J. Groen *338*
Pencus, G. see Elmadjian, F. *338*
Perera, G. A. *323*
— see Darling, R. C. *446*
— see Hulet, W. H. *355*
— see Sant'Agnese, P. A. di *446*
Perkins, J. G., A. B. Petersen and A.˙J. Riley *530*
Perley, A. see Forbes, G. B. *231*
Perlman, H. B., J. M. Goldinger and J. O. Cales *218*
— P. L. see Herzog, H. L. *336*
Perlmutter, M. see Stadie, W. C. 27, 31
Perloff, W. H. see Lasche, E. C. *384*
Perry, W. L. M. see Goffart, M. *65*
Pers, M. *515*
Peschel, E., and G. J. Race *315*, 316
Peshet, M. M. see Herzog, H. L. *336*
Pessoli, R. L. see Brauer, R. W. *489*

Peter, K. *246*
Peters, G. see Brunner, H. *353*
— H. C. see Ingraham, R. C. *69*
— J. P. *368, 379*
— L. G. Welt, E. A. H. Sims, J. Orloff and J. Needham *366*
— see Albrink, M. J. 199, *200*
Petersdorf, R. G., and L. G. Welt *270*
Petersen, A. B. see Perkins, J. G. *530*
— W. E. *497*, 498
— L. S. Palmer and C. H. Eckles *498*
— and T. V. Rigor *498*
Peterson, E. R. see Goodyer, A. V. N. *270*
— R. E. *310*
— and J. B. Wyngaarden *309*
— see Davis, J. O. *375*
— S. W. see Lindvig, P. E. *79*
Petow, H. see Rona, P. *202*
Pettengill, R. B. see Beckmann, W. W. *297*
Pfiffner, J. J. see Swingle, W. W. *535*
Pfyfe, P. see Ragan, C. *334*
Phillips, D. M. see Hare, R. S. *244, 347*
— P. H. see Boyer, P. D. *11*
— R. A. see Slyke, D. D. van *254*
Phillipson, A. T. see Dobson, A. *130*
— see Parthasarathy, D. *130*
Pick, E. P. see Kolm, R. *185*
Pickering, G. W., and M. Prinzmetal *355*
— see Hughes-Jones, N. C. *355*
Pickford, M. see Abrahams *343*
Pickles, V. R. *499*
Pierce, J. A. see Montgomery, H. *238, 252*
Pignard, P. see Hanon, F. *218*
Pinajian, J. see Mraz, F. R. *526, 527*
Pincus, G. see Hechter, O. *305, 307, 309, 319*
Pinto, H. B. see Zipser, A. *224*
Pirie, A., and R. van Heyningen *221*
— N. W. see Hadidan, Z. *19*
Pitcock, J. A., and P. M. Hartrott *314*
Pitts, G. C., R. E. Johnsson and F. C. Consolazio *448*
— see Johnson, R. E. *444*
— R. F. *253*, 388, 396, 398, 406, 417

Pitts, and R. S. Alexander *252, 253, 297*
— J. L. Ayer and W. A. Schiess *238*
— and J. J. Duggan *397, 400, 401, 406*
— and W. D. Lotspeich *238, 254*
— R. S. Wilde and L. P. Sullivan *260*
— see Axelrod, D. R. *289, 407, 408*
— see Capps, J. N. *403*
— see Dorman, P. J. *238, 290*
— see Duggan, J. J. *397, 404, 406*
— see Kessler, R. H. *403, 406*
— see Kupfer, S. *398, 400, 412*
— see Lotspeich, W. D. *254*
— see Magida, M. G. *291, 294, 522, 538*
— see Roberts, K. E. *322*
— see Roemmelt, J. C. *325, 327, 346*
— see Sartorius, O. W. *255, 388, 393, 394, 404, 405*
— see Thompson, D. D. *271, 272*
Plant, O. H. see Richards, A. N. *412*
Platt, R. see Black, D. A. K. *372*
Platts, M. M., and T. Handley *415*
Plentl, A. A. 218, *219*
— see Neslen, E. D. 218, *219*
— see Gray, M. J. *231*
— see Hutchinson, D. L. *218*
Plotka, C. *193*
Plotz, C. M., A. I. Knowlton and C. Ragan *323*
Podberczec, M. see Hudson, P. B. *338*
Pohl, H. A., L. B. Flexner and A. Gellhorn *220*
— see Gellhorn, A. *220*
Polissar, J. Milton, see Johnson, Frank H. *49*
Polland, W. S. *477*
Polley, H. F. see Sprague, R. G. *320*
Ponder, E. 38, 39, 43, *78, 79*
Pont, M. E. see Streeten, D. H. P. *320*
Pope II, C. E. *519*
Popper, H. L., N. C. Jefferson, E. Wulkan and H. Necheles *490*
Porter, R. W., H. J. Movius and J. W. French *477*
Portzehl, H. see Weber, H. H. *172*
Post, R. S. see Selkurt, E. E. *277*

Potor, A. *242*

Potter, V. R. *23*

— and R. O. Recknagel *22*

Power, M. H. see Cluxton, H. E. *323*

— see Robinson, F. J. *327*

— see Salassa, R. M. *419*

— see Sprague, R. G. *320*

Prader, A., E. Gantier, R. Gantier, D. Näj, J. S. Semer and E. J. Rotschild *452, 458, 499*

Prankerd, T. A. J. see Harris, E. J. *80*

Preedy, J. R. K., and E. H. Aitken *339,* 340

Prescott, D. M., and E. Zeuthen *54*

— K. F. see Bodo, R. C. de *352*

Pressman, B. C., and H. A. Lardy *23*

Prinzmetal, M. see Pickering, G. W. *355*

Prout, W. *466*

Prunitz, F. T. G. see Brooks, R. V. *529*

Puck, T. T., K. Wasserman and A. P. Fishman *31*

Pullman, T. N. see Lavender, A. R. *417*

Pulver, R., and F. Verzar *103, 108*

Purser jr., R. M. see Demunbrun, T. W. *354*

Quashnock, J. M. see Rogoff, J. M. *537*

Quastel, J. H. see Mann, P. J. G. *28*

Quibell, T. H. H. see Madinaveitia, J. *19*

Quinn, G. P. see Berger, E. Y. *513*

— M. see Bass, D. E. *518*

Quinquaud, A. see Hazard, R. *195*

Quinton, A. see Flear, C. T. G. *227*

Raaschou, F. see Brun, C. *399*

Rabinowitch, J. *132,* 133

Race, G. J. see Peschel, E. *315,* 316

Racker, E., and I. Krimsky *17*

Radike, A. W. see Thatcher, J. S. *521*

Radin, N. S. see Cooper, J. A. D. *228*

Radomski, J. L., H. N. Fuyat, A. A. Nelson and P. K. Smith *223, 419,* 420, *523,* 524

Ragan, C., J. W. Ferrebee, P. Pfyfe, D. W. Atchley and R. F. Loeb *334*

— see Kuhlman, D. *323*

— see Plotz, C. M. *323*

Raisz, L. G. see Ladd, M. *521*

— see Wesson, L. G. jr. *266,* 270, *349*

Raker, J. W., I. M. Taylor, J. M. Weller and A. B. Hastings 73, 74, 76, *78*

Ralli, E. P. see Orti, E. *313*

Ralston, H. see Grosman, M. I. *489*

Ramage, H. see Sheldon, J. H. *224*

Ramakrishnan, C. V. *15*

Ramey, E. R., M. S. Goldstein and R. Levine *303*

Ramsay, J. A. *140*

Ramsberg, H. H. see Madden, R. J. *476*

Ramsey, C. see Gray, S. J. *476*

Randall, H. T. see Roberts, K. E. *293,* 296, *320,* 324

— W. C. *439, 441, 443*

— and McClure *441*

— and K. K. Kimura *439,445*

Ranges, H. A. see Chasis, H. *413,* 414, 415

Rankin, R. M. see Gellhorn, A. *229*

Ranzi, S., and P. Citterio *35*

— and M. Falkenheim *34*

Raper, H. S. see Harper, A. A. *461*

Rapoport, S., C. D. West and W. A. Brodsky *367*

— see Kaplan, S. A. *356, 357,* 358

— see West, C. D. *261, 285,* 290

Rapport, D. see Canzanelli, A. *24*

— M. M. see Meyer, K. H. *19*

Rashbass, C., and W. A. H. Rushton *163*

Rasmussen, H. see Leaf, A. *335*

Rassaert, C. L. see Girerd, R. J. *338*

Rauschkolb, E. W., and G. L. Farrell *313*

— see Farrell, G. L. *307, 312,* 370

— J. E. see Sollman, T. *396*

Ravdin, I. S., C. G. Johnston, J. H. Austin and C. Riegel *492, 493,* 494, 495

— J. S., C. G. Johnston, C. Riegel and S. L. Wright *487*

Raven, C. P. *33*

Rawson, A. J. see Starr, I. *381*

Ray, C. T., S. A. Threefoot and G. E. Burch *422*

— see Burch, G. E. *206*

— see Threefoot, S. A. *230, 423*

Rearden, J. P. see Bricker, N. S. *360*

Reaser, P. see Threefoot, S. A. *230*

Recknagel, R. O. see Potter, W. R. *22*

Rector, F. C. jr., D. W. Seldin, A. D. Roberts jr. and J. H. Copenhaver *256*

— see Seldin, D. W. *322*

Reddy, W. J. see Hernando, L. *311*

Redgate, E. S. see Newman, A. E. *313*

Reed, A. I. see Dreizen, S. *457*

Reem, G. H. see Page, L. B. *357*

Reeves, J. L. see Henry, J. P. *351*

Rehberg, P. B. *236*

Rehm, W. S. *482,* 483

— and W. H. Dennis *482*

— see Thull, N. B. *466,* 470, 473, 474

Reichstein, T. *309*

— and J. v. Euw *307*

— and C. W. Shoppee *304*

— see Simpson, S. A. *308*

Reid, E. W. *128*

Reifenstein, R. W. see Gray, S. J. *476*

Reinberg, A. *185*

— see Bachrach, E. *186*

— see Bergerard, J. *185*

Reinhold, J. G., and L. K. Ferguson *488*

— and D. W. Wilson *487,* 488

Reiss, R. S. see Thorn, G. W. *330*

Relman, A. S. *43, 224, 422*

— B. Etsten and W. B. Schwartz *238, 290, 294*

— A. T. Lambie, A. M. Roy and B. A. Burrows *44, 224,* 225

— A. M. Roy and W. B. Schwartz *526*

— and W. B. Schwartz *531*

— see Epstein, F. H. *375*

— see Goodyer, A. V. N. *270*

— see Ingbar, S. H. *332*

— see Kunin, A. S. *525*

— see Lambie, A. T. *525*

— see Leaf, A. *298*

— see Schwartz, W. B. *255, 256, 286, 298*

Remington, J. W. see Gaunt, R. *334*

Remington, see Swingle, W. W. 302, *303*
— M. see Maizels, M. *105*
Renkin, E. M. see Pappenheimer, J. R. 53, 54
Rennick, B. R. see Weiner, I. M. *406*
Renold, A. E., J. Crabbé, L. Hernando-Avendano, D. H. Nelson, E. J. Ross, K. Emerson and G. H. Thorn *418*
— see Goldfien, A. *337*
— see Hernando, L. *311*
Renschler, H. E. see Kilpatric, R. *43, 230*
Renshaw, A. see Leaf, A. *61*, 120
Renwick, R. J., S. Robinson and C. P. Stewart 213, *528*
Renzi, A. A., M. Renzi, J. J. Chart and R. Gaunt *330*
— see Gaunt, R. *317*
Reynolds, S. R. M. *194*
— T. B. see Green, D. M. 213, *214*, 221
Rhamy, R. K. see Robinson, S. *444*, 449, 450
Rhyne, M. B. see Aikawa, J. K. *231*
Rice, L. see Frieden, J. 372, *373*
Richard, J. E. see Liddle, G. W. *337*
Richards, A. N. 235, *238*
— and O. H. Plant *412*
— see Walker, A. M. 235, 236, 247
— D. W. see Atchley, D. W. *281*
— J. B. see Farrell, G. L. 308, *321*
— see Loeb, R. F. *294*
Richterich, R. *416*
Richter-Quittner, M. *202*
Ridley, F. *464*
Riegel, C. see Ravdin, I. S. *487*, 492, 493, 494, 495
Riemer, A. D. *332*
Riesser, O. *175*
Riggs, T. R. see Christensen, H. N. *105*
Rigor, T. V. see Petersen, W. E. *498*
Riley, A. J. see Perkins, J. G. *530*
Ringer, S. *183*, 269
Riondell see Manning 376
Robert, F. *347*
Roberts jr., A. D. see Rector, F. C. jr. *256*
— I. Z. see Roberts, R. B. 38
— J. R. E. see Giardini, A. *464*

Roberts, K. E., M. G. Magida and R. F. Pitts *291, 294, 522*, 538
— and R. F. Pitts *322*
— and H. T. Randall *320, 324*
— — H. L. Sanders and M. Hood *293*, 296
— K. see Sartorius, O. W. *346*
— R. B., and I. Z. Roberts 38
— — and D. B. Cowie 38
— S., and C. M. Szego *194*
Robertson, J. D. *143*
— see Mackay, G. 220
— see Noble, R. L. *474*
— J. S. see Tosteson, D. C. 60, 73, 83
Robinson, A. H. see Robinson, S. *438*, 440, 441, 442
— C. S. see Bucher, G. R. *132*
— C. V., W. L. Arons and A. K. Solomon 227
— F. J., M. H. Power and E. F. Kepler *327*
— J. R. 66
— M. see Fänge, R. *502*
— S., S. G. Gerking, E. S. Turrell and R. K. Kincaid *442*
— R. K. Kincaid and R. K. Rhamy *444*, 449, 450
— R. T. Maletich, W. S. Robinson, B. B. Bohrer and A. L. King *448*, 449, 450
— J. R. Nicolas, J. H. Smith, W. J. Daly and M. Pearcy *444*, 449, 450
— and A. H. Robinson *438, 440*, 441, 442
— see Gerking, S. D. *447*
— see Pearcy, M. *443*, 448
Roblin, R. D. see Miller, W. H. 297
Robson, J. S. see Renwick, R. 213, *528*
Roche, M. see Thorn, G. W. *330*
Rock, M. H. *361*, 362
Roemmelt, J. C., O. W. Sartorius and R. F. Pitts *325*, 327, 346
— see Sartorius, O. W. 255, *393, 394*
Roepke, R. R. see Visscher, M. B. *132*, 134, 135, 136
Rogers, G. see Canzanelli, A. 24
Rogoff, J. M., and G. N. Stewart *301*
— J. M. Quashnock, E. Nola Nixon and A. W. Rosenberg *537*
Roheim, P. S. see Kovách, A. G. *366*

Rolf, D. see White, H. L. *324, 341, 528*
Roller, D., and G. Wiedemann *414*
Roma, P., F. Haurowitz and H. Petow *202*
— M. see Eichelberger, L. T. *208*
Romaine, M. see Hanlon, L. W. *419*
Romney, R. B. see Love, W. D. *43*
Ropes, M. W. see Bauer, W. *214*
Rosemann, R. *470, 476*, 477
Rosemberg, E. see Rosenfeld, G. *314*
Rosen, I. T. see White, H. L. *375*
Rosenbaum, J. D., R. K. Davis and B. C. Ferguson *344*
— B. C. Ferguson, R. K. Davis and E. C. Rossmeisl *387*
— W. P. Nelson III, M. B. Strauss, R. K. Davis and E. Rossmeissl *329*, 376
— see Birchard, W. H. *349*
— see Strauss, M. B. *349, 371*
Rosenberg, A. W. see Rogoff, J. M. *537*
— E. see Duncan, L. E. jr. *361*
— H., and K. Kitayama *165*
— J. M. see Hastings, A. B. 30
— T. *4*, 46
Rosenblueth, A., and R. S. Morison *177*
— J. W. Wille and H. Hoagland *182*
— see Hayashi, T. *173*
Rosenfeld, G., E. Rosemberg, F. Ungar and R. I. Dorfman *314*
Rosenman, R. H., S. C. Freed and M. K. Smith *304*
— S. S. George, C. Freed and M. K. Smith *533*
— see Freed, S. C. *517, 533*, 536
— see St. George, S. *532*
Rosenthal, H. O. see Ashe, B. J. *516*
— O. J., M. A. Bowie and G. Wagoner *210*
— O. see Hills, A. G. *536*
— see Lasnitzki, A. 28
Rosnagle, R. S., and G. L. Farrell *314*
— see Farrell, G. L. *312*, 370
Ross, E. J., and J. E. Bethune *418*
— see Crabbé, J. *528*
— see Hernando, L. *311*
— see Renold, A. E. *418*

Ross, see Spencer, A. G. *511*
— G. see Mokotoff, R. *384*
Rossmeisl, E. C. see Beckman, W. W. *297*
— see Rosenbaum, J. D. *387*
— see Strauss, M. B. *349, 371*
Rossmeissl, E. see Rosenbaum, J. D. *329, 376*
Roth, L. E. see Beams, H. W. *21*
Rothenberg, M. A. *96*
Rothera, A. C. see Jackson, L. C. *498*
Rothlin, E. and R. Gundlach *476*
Rothschild, Lord, and H. Barnes *142*
Rothschuh, K. E. *168*
— see Bammer, H. *167*
Rothstein, A., and L. H. Enns *108*
Rotschild, G. *202*
— J. see Prader, A. *452, 458, 459*
— L., and H. Burns *500*
Roughton, F. J. W., and V. H. Booth *296*
Rourke, G. M. see Stewart, J. D. *389*
Rous, P., and P. D. McMaster *487, 493, 494*
— see Drury, D. R. *493*
Rowlands, E. N. see Honour, A. J. *499*
Rowntree, L. G. see Weir, J. F. *346*
Roy, A. M. see Lambie, A. T. *525*
— see Relman, A. S. *44, 224, 225, 526*
Royce, P. C. see Farrell, G. L. *397, 309, 311*
Rubin, A. L., and W. S. Braveman *351*
— G. see White, A. G. *347, 352*
— S. see Bliss, E. L. *361*
Rubini, M. see Lamdin, E. *352*
Rudolph, G. G., and N. S. Olsen *215*
— see Olsen, N. S. *215, 216*
Ruiz-Guinaza, A. see Finkenstaedt, J. T. *530*
Rundo, J., and U. Sagild *227*
Runels, E. A. see Salter, W. T. *186*
Runnström, J. *34, 35*
— and T. Gustafson *33*
Rushton, W. A. H. see Rashbass, C. *163*
Ryan, H. see Conway, E. J. *108*
Ryberg, C. *255*
Rynearson, E. H. see Wilder, R. M. *302*

Ryssing, F. *199*

Sabo, E. F. see Fried, J. *337*
Saccone, A. see McGavack, T. H. *321, 328*
Sagild, U. *197, 228*
— see Gamstorp, I. *197*
— see Rundo, J. *227*
Sakai, T. *183, 184*
Sakamoto, H. see Kawahata, A. *446*
Salassa, R. M., V. R. Mattox and M. H. Power *419*
Salit, P. W. *220*
Salter, W. T., and E. A. Runels *186*
— see Green, J. P. *187*
Samuelsen, G. S. see Muntwyler, E. *532*
Sand, H. F. *429*, 458
Sanddiford, I. see Knowlton, K. *340*
Sanders, H. L. see Roberts, K. E. *293, 296*
Sanderson, P. H. *328*
— see Dale, R. A. *397, 403*
— see Hughes-Jones, N. C. *355*
Sandor, Z. von see Vuk, M. *497*
Sandow, A. *175, 179, 182*
— and A. J. Kahn *174, 178, 179*
— and H. Mandel *179*
Sant'Agnese, P. A. di *446, 447*
— R. C. Darling, G. A. Perera and E. Shea *446*
— see Darling, R. C. *446*
Santos, R. F. see Leaf, A. *345, 348*
Sartorius, O. W., D. Calhoon R. F. Pitts *324, 347*
— and K. Roberts *346*
— J. C. Roemmelt and R. F. Pitts *255, 393, 394*
— O. W. see Roemmelt, J. C. *325, 327, 346*
Sass-Kortsák, A., F. C. Wang and F. Verzár *317*
Satoskar, R. S. see Munro, D. S. *210, 213*
Saugman, B. *237, 259, 403*
Saunders, F. J., and V. A. Drill *340*
Sawitsch, W. W. see Babkin, B. P. *461*
Sawyer, C. G. see Fineh, C. A. *521*
— W. H. *128, 353*
Sayers, G. see Woodbury, D. M. *318*
Scarborough, H. see Chalmers, T. M. *316*
— see Hughes-Jones, N. C. *355*

Scatchard, G. *56*
— J. H. Scheinberg and S. H. Armstrong *9*
Schairer, E. *468, 469, 470*
Schatzmann, H. J. *79, 80*
Scheinberg, J. H. see Scatchard, G. *9*
Schemm, F. R. *389*
— F. see Camara, A. *332*
Schenker, V. see Hechter, O. *307*
Schicks, E. see Koch, H. J. *142*
Schiess, W. A. see Pitts, R. F. *238*
Schiff, M. *488*
Schindler, O. see Simpson, S. A. *308*
Schlapp, W. see Lim, R. K. S. *465*
Schloerb, P. R. *514*
Schloss, E. *497*
Schmidt, A. *340*
— C. *461, 466, 470*
— C. F. see Walker, A. M. *413, 414*
— C. L. A. see Heppel, L. A. *533*
— see Miyamoto, S. *9*
— C. R., J. M. Beagell, A. L. Berman, A. C. Ivy and A. J. Atkinson *488*
— E. *413*
Schmidt-Nielsen, B. *242*
— see Krogh, A. *191*
— see Schmidt-Nielsen, K. *247*
— K. *502*
— and B. Schmidt-Nielsen *247*
— see Fänge, R. *502*
Schmitz, H. L. *414*
Schneckloth, R., I. H. Page, F. del Greco and A. C. Corcoran *355*
Schneider, W. C. see Hogeboom, G. H. *22*
— W. P. see Hogg, J. A. *337*
Schneyer, L. H. *451*
— and L. K. Levin *451*
Schock, N. W. see Davis, J. O. *411, 413, 414*
Schoffeniels, E. *118*
Schou, M. *109, 223, 281, 419, 420, 421, 524*
— N. Juel-Nielsen, E. Strömgren and H. Voldby *224*
— P. B. *237*
Schreibner, N. E. see Solman, T. *396*
Schreiner, B. H. see Milne, M. D. *256, 336*
Schricker, J. A. see Hertz, R. *418*

Schriffin, M. J., and E. S. Nasset *484*, 485
Schubert, M. see Farber, S. *205*, 209
Schuffelen, A. C. and R. Loosjes *112*
Schuler, W., P. Desaulles and R. Meier 316, *317*
— see Desaulles, P. *318*
Schumm, O. *460*
Schwab, R. S. see Talbott, J. H. *522*
Schwartz 451
— I. L., and E. L. Opie *496*
— and J. H. Thaysen *426*, 441
— — and V. P. Dole *432*, 434, 443
— see Bodo de, R. C. *341*
— see Dole, V. P. *445*
— see Earle, D. P. jr. *341*
— see Maxwell, M. N. *380*
— see Thaysen, J. H. *426*, 427, 431, 433, 441, 447, 453, 454, *503*
— see Thorn, I. L. 456, *457*
— R., J. Cohen and W. M. Wallace *531*
— W. B. *197*
— W. Bennett, S. Curelop and F. C. Bartter *364*
— R. L. Jensen and A. S. Relman 255, *286*
— and A. S. Relman *298*
— and W. M. Wallace *409*
— see Lambie, A. T. *525*
— see Leaf, A. *298*
— see Relman, A. S. *238*, 290, 294, 526, *531*
Schwarzenbach, G., and H. Ackermann *5*
— E. Kampitsch and R. Steiner *5*
— A. Willi and R. O. Bach *5*
Schweizer, M. see Gaunt, R. *334*
Scott, G. H., and B. L. Canaga *225*
— and D. M. Packer *41*
— G. T., and H. R. Hayward *109*
— V. B. see Still, E. U. *429*
— W. S. see Huggins, C. 499, *500*
Scott-Baker, J. C. see Page, L. B. *357*
Scott Russel, R. *111*
Scribner, B. H., and J. M. Burnell 203, *204*
— K. Fremont-Smith and J. M. Burnell *203*
— H. Kleinberg and J. M. Burnell *530*
Seeman, P. see Burgen, A. S. V. *438*

Segar, W. E. see Oliver, J. *532*
Seitzer, H. S. see Streeten, D. H. P. *312*
Sekelj, P. see Terroux, K. G. 436, *455*
Seldin, D. W., F. C. Rector jr., N. Carter and J. Copenhaver *322*
— L. G. Welt and J. H. Cort *287*
— and R. Tarail *282*
— see Burnett, C. H. *327*
— see Rector, F. C. jr. *256*
— see Tarail, R. *286*
— see Welt, L. G. 287, *367*
— see Wilson, J. D. 322, *324*
Selkurt, E. E. 196, *197*, 271, 277, 278, 279, 280, *290*
— M. Brandfonbrener and H. M. Geller 273, *274*
— P. W. Hall and M. P. Spencer *275*
— and R. S. Post *277*
— see Dowds, E. G. *290*
— see Hall III, P. W. *275*
Sellers, A. L., S. Smith III, H. C. Goodman and J. Marmorston *355*
Selye, H., and E. Bajusz *531*
Semer, J. S. see Prader, A. 452, 458, *499*
Serby, A. M. *397*
Sevier, S. M. see Lewis, J. M. jr. *375*
Shaffer, M. see Chang, T. H. *25*
Shanes, A. M. 63, 95, *96*, 97, 98, 99, *102*, 158
— and M. D. Berman *96*
— and D. E. S. Brown *98*
— H. Grundfest and W. Freygang *158*
— and H. S. Hopkins 25, 148
Shannon, J. A. *344*, 345, 348
Shapiro, B. see Stern J. R. *15*
Share, L. *273*
— see Tompkins, M. J. *536*
Sharpey-Schafer, E. P. see Howarth, S. *411*
Shaw, C. W., and H. L. Holley *215*
— F. H., and S. E. Simon 42, 45
— — and B. M. Johnstone *42*
— J. H. see Deane, H. W. *315*
Shea, E. see Sant'Agnese, P. A. di *446*
Sheehan, H. L. see Nichols, J. *315*
Sheeten, H. P., and J. W. Conn *535*
Sheldon, J. H., and H. Ramage *224*

Sheline, G. E. see Montgommery *763*
Sheppard, C. W. 72, 77
— and W. R. Martin 73
— — and G. Beyl *74*, 76
— R. see Ingle, D. J. *320*
Sherwood, S. L. see Feldberg, W. *216*
Shevshy, A. E. see Bevier, G. *328*
Shih, H. E., J. Kennedy and C. Huggins *501*
Shipley, R. E., and R. S. Study *272*
Shohl, A. T. *226*
Shoppee, C. W. *305*
— see Reichstein, T. *304*
Shorr, E. see Zweifach, B. W. *303*
Shulman, M. H. see Wyman, L. C. *303*
Sichel, F. J. M. see Brown, D. E. S. *178*
Sicular, A. see Moore, F. D. *538*
Sidgwick, N. V., and F. M. Brewer *5*
Siebert, G. see Taugner, R. *174*
Siegel, S. A. see Diamond, J. S. *460*, 463
Sieker, H. O., O. H. Gauer and J. P. Henry *351*
— see Gauer, O. H. *351*
Sievers, J. F. see Meyer, K. H. *56*, 57
Silber, E. N. see Hwang, W. *374*
Silva, J. L. de, and R. I. Harrison 219, *220*
Silverman, L. see Taggart, J. V. *27*
Silvette, H., and S. W. Britton *327*
Simmons, D. H., R. B. Harvey and T. Hoshiko *326*
Simms, H. S. *9*
Simon, S. E. see Shaw, F. H. 42, 45
Simonds, J. P., and O. E. Hepler *399*
Simpson, S. A., and J. F. Tait *308*, 321
— — and I. E. Bush *308*
— — A. Wettstein, R. Neher, J. von Euw and T. Reichstein *308*
— — — — — O. Schindler and T. Reichstein *308*
— see Grundy, H. M. *308*
— see Speirs, R. S. *317*
— see Tait, J. F. *308*
— S. L. *327*

Sims, E. A. H., L. G. Welt, J. Orloff and J. W. Needham *351*
— see Peters, J. P. *366*
Sinclair-Smith, B. *375, 387*
Sinex, F. M. see Hastings, A. B. *30*
Singer, F. M. see Borman, A. *337*
— R. B., J. R. Elkinton, E. S. Barker and J. K. Clark *290*
— see Barker E. S. *291*
Sinkoff, M. W. see Earle, D.P. *341*
Sinn, L. G. see Bromer, W.W. *354*
Sirek, O. V., and C. H. Best *335, 336*
Sirota, J. H., and I. G. Kroop *257*
— and R. A. Nabatoff *276*
Sisson, J. H. see Ingbar, S.H. *332*
Sjögren, B. see Luft, R. *213, 319,* 320, 321, 323, *342*
Sjöstrand, F. S., and V. Hanzon *21*
— see Ottoson, D. *122*
Skanse, B., and B. Hökfelt *197, 518*
— F. Möller, K. Gydell, S. Johansson and H. B. Wulff *316, 518*
Skou, J. C. *17*
Slein, M. W. see Cori, G. T. *12*
Slessor, A. see Thorn, G. W. *330*
— H. *328*
Slocumb, C. H. see Sprague, R. G. *320*
Slyke, D. D. van, R. A. Phillips, P. B. Hamilton, R. M. Archibald, P. H. Futcher and A. Hiller *254*
— H. Wu and F. C. McLean *201*
— see Eder, H. A. *221*
Smiles, S. see Evans, W. J. *5*
Smirk see Baldes *349*
Smith *252*
— C. A., M. Wu and O. H. Lowry *141, 217*
— C. G., and D. Y. Solandt *26*
— D. C. see Ferguson, F. P. *289*
— F. A. see Neuman, W. F. *212*
— F. M., and E. M. MacKay *346, 347,* 348
— G. A. see Grim, E. *494*
— H. W. *236, 247,* 349, *378*
— see Page, L. B. *357*
— see Zak, G. A. *246*

Smith, see Chasis, H. *413,* 414, 415
— J. H. see Robinson, S. *444,* 449, 450
— M. K. see Rosenman, R. H. *304, 533*
— P. K. see Radomski, J. L. *223, 419,* 420, *523, 524*
— S. G. *532*
— V. R. see Espe, D. *497*
— III, S. see Sellers, A. L. *355*
Smolens, J., J. H. Leopold and J. Parker *464*
Smyth, D. H., and C. B. Taylor *134*
Smythe, C. McC., J. F. Nickel and S. E. Bradley *360*
— see Nickel, J. F. *355, 360*
Snell, A. M. see Wilder, R. M. *302*
— F. M. *7*
Snoke, E. J., and K. Bloch *15,* 16
Sobieranski, W. v. *413*
Sobotka, H. *488, 489, 492*
— H. H. see Soffer, L. J. *321*
Soffer, L. J., J. L. Gabrilove and M. D. Jacobs *321*
— A. Gutman, J. Geller and J. L. Gabrilove *334*
— G. Lesnick, S. Z. Sorkin, H. H. Sobotka and M. Jacobs *321*
— see Harrop, G. A. *301, 302*
Soika, G. see Westphal, K. *489*
Solandt, D. Y. *26,* 175
— see Smith, C. G. *26*
Soliman, A. A. I. see McDowall, R. J. S. *192*
Sollman, T. *237*
— W. F. van Oettingen and Y. Ishikawa *192*
— N. E. Schreibner, H. N. Cole, J. A. Gammel and J. E. Rauschkolb *396*
Sollner, K. *56*
— S. Dray, E. Grim and R. Neihof *56*
Solomon, A. K. *63, 64, 72, 73,* 75, 76, 77, 78, 81
— see Arons, W. L. *228*
— see Ball, E. G. *430*
— see Curran, P. F. *136,* 137
— see Durbin, R. P. *54, 509*
— see Gold, G. L. *77*
— see Hastings, A. B. *30*
— see Robinson, C. V. *227*
— see Streeten, D. H. P. *73,* 74, *80*
— D. H. see Duncan, L. E. *361*
— S. *139, 237,* 259

Solomon, T. J. Gill and G. L. Gold *80*
Solvonuk, P. F., and H. B. Collier *12*
Somerville, W., H. C. Levine and G. W. Thorn *304*
— see Thorn, G. W. *330*
Sorkin, S. Z. see Soffer, L. J. *321*
Southworth, H. see Strauss, M. B. *296*
— J. L. see Davis, J. O. *384*
Spater, H., A. Hunt, R. Todd, P. Meara, M. Terry, J. D. Crawford and N. B. Talbot *531, 533*
Spealman, C. R. *186,* 187
Spector, W. G. *22*
Speirs, R. S., S. A. Simpson and J. F. Tait *317*
Spek, J. *34*
Spencer, A. G., and H. G. Lloyd-Thomas *415*
— E. J. Ross and H. G. L. Lloyd-Thomas *511*
— see Franglen, G. T. *291*
— M. P. see Selkurt, E. E. *275*
Sperber, I., and S. Hydén *129,* 130
Spiegelman, S. see Steinbach, H. B. *95,* 150
Spiers, F. W. see Burch, P. R. J. *227*
Spies, T. D. see Dreizen, S. *457*
Spingarn, C. L. see Mulinos, M. G. *334*
Sprague, R. G., M. H. Power, H. L. Mason, A. Albert, D. R. Mathiesen, P. S. Hench, E. C. Kendall, C. H. Slocumb and H. F. Polley *320*
Spray, C. M. see Widdowson, E. M. *226*
Springs, V. see Staub, A. *355*
Sréter, F. A., and S. M. Friedman *200*
Stadie, W. C., N. Haugaard and M. Perlmutter *27,* 31
— and J. A. Zapp jr. *30*
Stadtman, E. R. *15*
— see Stern, J. R. *15*
Stämpfli, R. *148*
— see Huxley, A. F. *148, 149,* 150, 153, 154, 162, 165
Stafford, R. O., L. E. Barnes, B. J. Borman and M. M. Meinzinger *336,* 337
— R. O. see Byrnes, W. W. *337*
Stahl, J., D. W. Atchley and R. F. Loeb *301*
— see Loeb, R. F. *302*

Stall III, B. C. see Dahl, L. K. *518*
— B. G. see Dole, V. P. *445*
Stamler, J., H. Goldberg, A. Gordon, M. Weinsel and L. N. Katz *374*
— J. see Hwang, W. *374*
Stanbury, S. W., and G. H. Mudge *22, 39*
— and A. E. Thomson *289*
— see Black, D. A. K. *372*
Stapp, P. *117*
— see Lund E. J. *115, 117*
Starling, E. H. see Bayliss, W. M. *461*
Starr, I. *380*
— and A. J. Rawson *381*
Staub, A., V. Springs, F. Stoll and H. Elrich *355*
— see Bromer, W. W. *354*
— A. see Elrick, H. *355*
Stavraky, G. W. see Langstroth, G. O. *427, 433, 435, 453, 454*
Stead, E. A. jr. *379*
— see Holland, B. C. *376*
— see Warren, J. V. *381*
Steel, I. M. see Berger, E. Y. *509, 512*
Steffen, F.
Stehle, R. L. *348, 395*
Stein, J. D. jr., L. Leslie Bennett, A. A. Batts and C. H. Li *342*
— K. E. see Thorn, G. W. *346, 347*
— L., and E. Wertheimer *512*
Steinbach, H. B. *40, 62, 78, 86, 87, 88, 146, 148*, 165
— and S. Spiegelman *95*
— — and N. Kawata *150*
— see Harris, E. J. *39, 44*
Steiner, R. see Schwarzenbach, G. *5*
— S. see Evans, B. M. *300, 531, 532*
Sten-Knudsen, O. *183*
Steno, N. *502*
Stephenson, G. see Creese, R. *90*
Stern, J. R., L. V. Eggleston, R. Hems and H. A. Krebs *65*
— B. Shapiro, E. R. Stadtman and S. Ochoa *15*
— L. *216*
— R. *419, 493*
Stevens, M. see Boyd, E. M. *503*
Stevenson, J. A. F., L. G. Welt and J. Orloff *364*
Steward, F. C., and F. K. Millar *38*

Stewart, G. N. see Rogoff, J. M. *301*
— C. P. see Mackay, G. *220*
— see Renwick, R. *215, 528*
— J. D. and G. M. Rourke *389*
St. George, S., S. C. Freed, R. H. Rosenman and S. Winderman *532*
— see Freed, S. C. *304, 533, 536*
Still, E. U., A. L. Bennett and V. B. Scott *429*
Stirling, W. B. see Jacobs, A. *515*
Stoerk, H. C. see Laragh, J. H. *313*
Stokey, E. see Lipschitz, W. L. *415*
Stoll, F. see Staub, A. *355*
— W. R., and W. F. Neuman *211*
Stowe, L. see Orloff, J. *271*
Stransky, E. *487*
Straub, F. B. *80, 81*
Strauss, H. *488*
— M. B. *387, 517*
— R. K. Davis, J. D. Rosenbaum and E. C. Rossmeisl *349, 371*
— see Rosenbaum, J. D. *329, 376*
— and H. Southworth *296*
— see Birchard, W. H. *349*
— M. see Harrop, G. A. *301, 302*
Streeten, D. H. P. *191*
— J. W. Conn, L. H. Louis, S. S. Fajans, H. S. Seitzer, R. D. Johnson, R. D. Gitths and A. H. Dube *312*
— see Thorn, G. W. *304*
— M. E. Pont and J. W. Conn *320*
— and A. K. Solomon *73, 74, 80*
— and E. M. V. Williams *530*
Strelitz, F. see Mendel, B. *19*
Strömgren, E. see Schou, M. *224*
Strohe, H. see Höber R. *150*
Study, R. S. see Shipley, R. E. *272*
Suckling, E. E. see Brooks, C. McC. *65*
Sudak, F. N., C. Wyman and G. P. Fulton *537*
Sullivan, L. P. see Malvin, R. L. *239, 241, 260*
— see Pitts, R. F. *260*
— W. J. see Dorman, P. J. *238, 290*
Sundin, T. *376*
Suntzeff, V. see Baumberger, J. P. *207*

Suntzefl, see Carruthers, C. *220*
Surawicz, B., H. A. Braun, W. B. Crum, R. L. Kemp, S. Wagner and S. Bellet *529*
Surtshin, A., and J. Hoeltzenbein *357*
— and G. Latorre *272*
— B. Mueller and H. L. White *357*
— see Mueller, C. B. *271, 272*
Sutcliffe, J. F. *111*
Swaetichin, G. see Ottoson, D. *122*
Swan, R. C., and R. D. Keynes *50*
Swanson, W. W. see Iob, V. *210*
Sweat, M. L., and G. L. Farrell *309*
Swell, L. see Field, H. jr. *511, 513, 528*
Sweet, A. Y., M. F. Levitt and H. L. Hodes *509, 536*
— see Levitt, M. F. *211, 214, 372*
Swett, W. W., F. W. Miller and R. R. Graves *498*
Swingle, W. W. *305*
— M. Ben, R. Maxwell, C. Baker, E. Fedor and G. Barlow *307*
— E. Collins, G. Barlow and E. J. Feder *306*
— J. Da Vanzo, E. Fedor, H. C. Crossfield, D. Glenister, M. Osborne and G. Wagle *536*
— — D. Glenister, H. C. Crossfield and G. Wagle *536*
— — — H. C. Crossfield and G. Wagle *304*
— E. J. Fedor, M. Ben, R. Maxwell, C. Baker and G. Barlow *332*
— R. Maxwell, M. Ben, C. Baker, S. J. Le Brie and M. Eisler *323*
— J. J. Pfiffner, H. M. Vars and W. M. Parkins *535*
— and J. W. Remington *302, 303*
Sydenstricker, V. P. *411*
Szalay, S. see Balint, P. *370*
Szego, C. M. see Roberts, S. *194*
Szent-Györgyi, A. *9, 172, 173, 174, 190*
— Z. M. Bacq and M. Goffart *176*
— see Baird, S. L. *9*
— see Hajdu, S. *173, 188, 189, 190, 195*

Taggart, J. V. *396*, 416
— L. Silverman and E. M. Trayner 27
— see Cross, R. J. *32*
— see Forster, R. P. *31*
— see Mudge, G. H. *197*
Tahmisian, T. N. see Beams, H. W. *21*
Tainter, M. L. see McChesney, E. W. *512*
Tait, J. F., S. A. Simpson and H. M. Grundy 308
— S. A. S. see Ayres, P. J. *310*
— see Grundy, H. M. *308*
— see Simpson, S. A. *308*, 321
— J. F. see Speirs, R. S. *317*
Takata, C. *469*
— see Korawa, S. *470*
— M. *467*, 468, 470, 473, 478
Talbot, N. B., O. H. Lowry and E. B. Astwood *194*
— see Corsa, L. jr. *228*
— see Drescher, A. N. 521, *522*, 523
— see Gardner, L. J. *517*
— see Locke, W. *440*, 442
— see Spater, H. *531*, 533
Talbott, J. H., L. H. Pecora, R. S. Melville and W. V. Consolazio 328
— and R. S. Schwab 522
Talso, P. J., and R. W. Clarke *223*, *419*, 420, 421
Tammann, G. *8*
Tanaka, M. *446*
— and A. Kawahata *446*
Tarail, R., T. E. Bennett and W. K. Noell 525
— E. S. Hacker and R. Taymor *199*, 202
— D. W. Seldin and A. V. N. Goodyer 286
— see Seldin, D. W. *282*
Tarukaski, H. see Luft, H. *213*, *319*, 320, 321, 323
Tasaki, I., and C. Fernandez *141*
— and S. Hagiwara *161*
Taugner, R., G. Siebert and U. Gottstein *174*
Taylor, C. B. see Smyth, D. H. *134*
— H. see Teabeaut, R. *323*
— I. M., J. M. Weller and A. B. Hastings 79
— see Calkins, E. *60*, 89, 95
— see Raker, J. W. *73*, 74, 76, 78
— J. G. see Anslow, W. P. jr. *345*
— N. B. G. see Noble, R. L. *350*
— P. see Klein, R. *318*

Taylor, R. D. see Corcoran, A. C. *419*, 523
— R. E. see Huxley, A. F. *179*
Taymor, R. see Tarail, R. *199*, 202
Teabeaut, R., F. L. Engel and H. Taylor 323
Teitel, P. *67*
Telfer, S. V. *492*
Telford, J. see Handley, C. A. *400*
Telkkä, A. see Mustakallio, K. K. *399*
Teloh, H. A. *199*
Teng, C. T. see Hastings, A. B. *30*
Tenennbaum, M. see Mann, P. J. G. *28*
Teorell, T. *48*, 56, 57, *100*, *466*, 475, *478*, 480, 481, 482
— and Linderholm 49
— see Linde, S. *481*
Terner, C. *482*
— L. V. Eggleton and H. A. Krebs *25*, 106
— see Krebs, H. A. *70*, *103*, 106
Terroux, K. G., P. Sekelj and A. S. V. Burgen *436*, 455
— see Burgen, A. S. V. *65*, *147*
Terry, M. see Drescher, A. N. 521, *522*, 523
— see Spater, H. *531*, 533
Teterick, J. E. see Moore, F. D. *538*
Teunissen, P. H., and H. G. Bungenberg de Jong *5*
Thatcher, J. S., and A. W. Radike 521
Thaysen, J. H. 424, *426*, 428, 434, 440
— and I. L. Schwartz 447, 503
— and N. A. Thorn 426, 427, 432, 441, 464
— — and I. L. Schwartz 426, 427, 431, 433, 441, 453, 454
— see Albretsen, S. R. *432*, 438
— see Bro-Rasmussen, F. *426*
— see Dole, V. P. *439*, 440, 441
— see Gjørup, S. *530*
— see Killmann, S. A. *432*, 503
— see Schwartz, I. L. *426*, 432, 434, 443
— see Thorn, G. W. 456, 457
Thomas, C., B. Edward and H. Isaacs 528
— J. E. *460*
— and J. O. Crider *462*

Thomas, see Conly, S. S. *461*
— see Hart, W. M. *461*
— J. T. see Pearcy, M. *443*, 448
Thompson, D. D., and R. F. Pitts 271, *272*
— see Kupfer, S. *398*, 400, *412*
— J. see Tobian, L. *314*
— K. W. see McQueen-Williams, M. *340*
— W. H. see McQuarrie, I. *522*
Thomsen, Aa. C. *364*
Thomson, A. E. see Stanbury, S. W. *289*
Thorn, D. W. see Thorn, G. W. *339*
— G. W., and L. L. Engel *339*, 340
— — and R. A. Lewis 318, *319*
— P. H. Forsham, L. L. Bennett, M. Roche, R. S. Reiss, A. Slessor, E. B. Flink and W. Somerville 330
— D. Jenkins, J. C. Laidlaw, F. C. Goetz, J. F. Dingman, W. L. Arons, D. H. P. Streeten and B. H. McCracken 304
— K. R. Nelson and D. W. Thorn 339
— and K. E. Stein 346, *347*
— see Crabbé, J. *528*
— see Dingman, J. F. *311*, 312, 313
— see Forsham, P. H. *323*
— see Goldfien, A. *337*
— see Hernando, L. *311*
— see Laidlaw, J. C. *320*
— see Lewis, R. A. *289*
— see Renold, A. E. *418*
— see Somerville, W. *304*
— I. L. Schwartz and J. H. Thaysen 456, *457*
— N. A. *244*, 348, 386, 451, 537
— see Thaysen, J. H. *426*, 427, 431, 432, 433, 441, 453, 454, 464
Thorup, O. A. jr. see Welt, L. G. *240*
— see Womersley, R. *325*
Thouvenot, J. see Parrot, J. L. *65*
Threefoot, S. A., G. E. Burch and C. T. Ray 423
— — and P. Reaser 230
— C. T. Ray and G. E. Burch 230
— see Burch G. E. *206*
— see Ray, C. T. *422*

Thull, N. B., and W. S. Rehm
  466, 470, 473, 474
Tinsley, C. M. see Wilkins,
  R. W. *350, 372*
Tobian, L., and A. Fox *537*
— J. Thompson, R. Twedt
  and J. Janecek *314*
— R. B. see Forbes, G. B. *213*
Toby, C. G. *473*
Todd, R. see Spater, H. *531,
  533*
— W. R. see West, E. S. *197*
Tolksdorf, S. see Herzog, H. L.
  336
Tomkins, G. M. see Liddle,
  G. W. *337*
Tompkins, M. J., E. Eckman
  and L. Share *536*
Topol, L. see Carr, C. W. *9*
Tosteson, D. C. *7, 50, 67, 72,
  74, 75, 78*
— E. Carlsen and E. T. Dun-
  ham *78*
— and E. T. Dunham *77*
— and J. Johnson *83*
— and J. S. Robertson *60,
  73, 83*
Toth, L. A. *361*
Towery, B. T. see Burnett,
  C. H. *291*
Trayner, E. M. see Taggart,
  J. V. *27*
Treherne, J. E. *143*
Trescher, J. H. see Harrop,
  G. A. *302*
Treutner, E. M., R. Morris,
  C. H. Noack and S. Ger-
  shou *224*
Tripod, J. see Desaulles, P.
  321, 322
Trout, E. C. see Field, H. jr.
  511, 513
Truelove, L. H. see Burn, J. H.
  352
Trueta, J., A. E. Barclay, P.
  M. Daniel, K. J. Franklin
  and M. M. L. Prichard *358*
Truscoe, R. see Maizels, M.
  105
Tscherning, R. *398*
Tschopp, E. *487*
Tschumi, H. see Gukelberger,
  M. *266*
Tucker, Helen F. see Ball, E.
  G. *430*
Tullar, P. E. *451*
Tullner, W. W. see Hertz, R.
  418
Turkirscher, E., and E. Wert-
  heimer *476*
Turner, K. P. see Borst, J. G.
  338
— see Molhuysen, J. A. *338*
— L. B. see Levitt, M. F. 211,
  214, 372

Turolt, M. *194*
Turrell, E. S. see Robinson, S.
  442
Twedt, R. see Tobian, L. *314*
Tyor, M. P., and J. S. Eldridge
  43, 422

Uhlenbrock, P. *114*
Ullmann, T. D. see Bergmann,
  F. *261*
— see Grossman, J. *405, 409*
— see Weston, R. E. *293, 531*
Ullrich, K. J. *433*
— F. O. Drenckhahn and K.
  H. Jarausch *248*
— H. H. Hilger and J. D.
  Klümper *260, 279, 286*
— see Hilger, H. H. *260*
— see Jarausch, K. H. *260*
— see Klümper, J. D. *260*
Umeno, M. see Kozawa, S.
  470
Ungar, F. see Rosenfeld, G.
  314
Uribe, C. see Gardner, L. J.
  517
Urisz, M. R. see McLean, F. C.
  210
Urquhart, J. see Yates, F. E.
  277
Ussing, H. H. *46, 49, 50, 53,
  74, 84, 97, 114, 115, 116,
  118, 119, 120*
— and B. Andersen *137*
— and K. Zerahn *116*, 117,
  121
— see Andersen, B. *46, 53, 60*,
  128
— see Deyrup, I. J. *32*
— see Fuhrman, F. A. *127*,
  128
— see Koefoed-Johnsen, V.
  46, 53, 78, 113, 123, 124,
  128, 243
— see Levi, H. *50, 62, 87, 89*,
  91, 92, 139
— see Meares, P. *53*
Utter, M. F. *11*, 17
Umeno, M., K. Kurihara, M.
  Horiuchi and C. Takata
  470
Unna, K., and L. Walterskirchen *348*
Vallee, B. L. see Wacker, W.
  E. C. *517*
Vandenbroueke, J. see Hu-
  ghes-Jones, N. C. *355*
Vander, A. J., R. L. Malvin,
  W. S. Wilde and L. P. Sullivan *403, 417*
— — — J. Lapides, L. P. Sullivan and V. M. McMurray
  326
— see Malvin, R. L. *241*

Vanderling, R. J. see Arons,
  W. L. *228*
Vanzant, F. R., W. C. Alva-
  rez, G. B. Eusterman, H.
  L. Dunn and J. Birkson
  477
— see Osterberg, A. E. *477*
Varco, R. H. see Visscher, M.
  B. *132, 134, 135, 136*
— R. L. see Lifson, N. *480,
  481*
Varnauskas, E. see Werkö, L.
  390
Vaugham Williams, E. M. see
  Kuffler, S. W. *90, 163, 177*
Veal, N., H. J. Fisher, J. C.
  M. Brown and J. E. S.
  Bradley *228*
Veis, A. *8*
Verney, E. B. *348*
— and F. R. Winton *412, 413*
— see Dreyer, N. B. *269*
Verzár, F. see MacDougal, E.
  J. *132, 133*
— see Pulver, R. *103, 108*
— see Sass-Kortsák, A. *317*
— see Wang, F. C. *317*
Vesin, P., and R. Cattan *332*
Vennesland, Birgit see Ball,
  E. G. *430*
Venning, E. H., J. Dysen-
  furth and J. C. Beek *311*
— A. Carballeira and I. Dy-
  renfurth *312*
Viar, W. N., B. B. Oliver, S.
  Eisenberg, T. A. Lombar-
  do, K. Willis and T. R.
  Harrison *376, 377*
— see Lombardo, T. A. *369,
  370*
— see Lusk, J. A. *376, 377*
Vidal, F. see Larramendi, L.
  M. H. *161*
Vieillefosse, R. see Feyel, P.
  259
Vigneaud, V. du *343*
Villarreal, R., W. F. Ganong
  and S. J. Gray *476, 477*
Villee, C. A. *30*
Vineberg, A. M. *471*
— and S. A. Komarov *464*
— see Browne, J. S. L. *475*
Vislocky, K. see Mudge, G. H.
  291
Visscher, M. B., E. S. Fetcher,
  C. W. Carr, H. P. Gregor,
  M. S. Bushey and D. E.
  Barber *133, 134, 135, 136*
— R. R. Roepke and N. Lif-
  son *132, 134, 135, 136*
— R. H. Varco, C. W. Carr,
  R. B. Dean and D. Eric-
  son *132, 134, 135, 136*
— see Burns, H. S. *132*
— see Dennis, C. *133*

Visscher, see Ingraham, R. C. *69*, 131, *132*, 134, *138*, *470*, 477
— see Lifson, N. *480*, 481
Vivion, C. G., C. J. Hlad and B. Eiseman *423*
Vogel, M. see McGavack, T. H. *321*, *328*
Vogl, A. *388*
Voldby, H. see Schou, M. *224*
Volk, M. C. see Blumgart, H. L. *397*, *411*, 414
Vollmer, E. P. see Zwemer, R. L. *522*
Voripaieff, H. see Nachmansohn, D. *14*
Vosburgh, D. J. see Flexner, L. B. *218*, 219
Voskian, J. see Dignam, W. S. *340*
Vries de, L. A. see Blomhert, G. *349*
— see Borst, J. G. *338*
— see Molhuysen, J. A. *338*
Vuk, M., and Z. von Sandor *497*

Wachstein, M., and E. Meisel *399*, 405
Wacker, W. E. C., M. Margoshes, A. F. Bartholomay and B. L. Vallee *517*
Wadsworth, B. C. see Maren, T. H. *298*
Wagle, G. see Swingle, W. W. *304*, 536
Wagner, E. see Fleckenstein, A. *181*
— S. see Surawicz, B. *529*
Wagoner, G. see Rosenthal, O. J. *210*
Waine, H. see Bauer, W. *214*
Wajzer, J. see Nachmansohn, D. *175*
Walcott, W. W. see Deyrup, I. J. *520*
Wald, M. H. see Lindberg, H. A. *390*
Waldemann, E. B. see Wilhelmj, C. M. *521*
Waldron, A. M. *419*
Walker, A. M., P. A. Bott, J. Oliver and M. C. MacDowell 234, *242*, 245, 247
— and C. L. Hudson 235, 247
— — T. Findley jr. and A. N. Richards 235, 236, 247
— C. F. Schmidt, K. A. Elsom, A. E. Kendall and C. G. Høhnson *413*, 414
— G. see Ayres, P. J. *310*
— see Martin, M. M. *227*
— S. M. *177*, 178
— and Y. Laporte *170*

Wallace, G. B., and A. R. Cushny *131*
— W. M. see Bergstrom, W. H. *210*
— see Schwartz, W. B. *409*, 531
Wallenius and Garby 264
Waller, D. S. see Wiley, F. H. *288*
Walser, M. see Burnett, C. H. *327*
Walt, de J. L. see Winthers, R. W. 212, 213
Wang, F. C., and F. Verzár *317*
— see Sass-Kortsák, A. *317*
— S. C. see Feng, T. P. *177*
Ward, H. P. see Blake, W. D. 270, 275
Warren, J. V., J. A. Merrill and E. A. Stead jr. *381*
— and E. A. Stead jr. *381*
— M. R. *501*
Wartiovaara, V. see Holm-Jensen, I. *36*
Wasserman, K., E. L. Becker and A. P. Fishman *32*
— see Puck, T. T. *31*
Waterhouse, C., and E. H. Kreutmann *328*
Waters, L. see Winternitz, M. C. *341*
Watman, R. N. 460, 463
Wazer, J. R. van, and D. A. Campanella *8*
Weatherall, M. see Joyce, C. R. B. *80*
Weber, A. *173*
— H. H., and H. Portzehl *172*
— and H. H. Weber *173*
— see Weber, A. *173*
Webster, D. R. *471*
— W. H. Henrikson and D. J. Currie *193*
— see Babkin, B. P.*474*
— G. D. see Hills, A. G. *536*
Webb, D. A. *143*
— and J. Z. Young *162*
Weeteh, R. S. see Miller, H. *499*
Wegria, R. see Blake, W. D. 270, 275
— see Hilton, J. G. *377*, *378*
Weidmann, S. *65*, *158*, 160, *164*, 167
— see Draper, M. H. *174*, 164, 186
Weil-Malherbe, H. *25*
Weiner, I. M., A. F. Burnett and B. R. Rennick *406*
— J. S., and R. E. van Heyningen *442*, *443*
— see Heyningen, R. E. van *442*, *443*, 444
— see Mudge, G. H. *396*, 408

Weinsel, M. see Stamler, J. *374*
Weinstein, A. see Harrop, G. A. *302*
Weir, J. F., E. E. Larsen and L. G. Rowntree *346*
Weiss, O. *464*
Welbourn, R. B. see Kule, J. *477*
Weller, J. M., B. Lown, R. V. Hoigne, N. F. Wyatt, M. Cricitiello, J. P. Merrill and S. A. Levine *530*
— see Raker, J. W. *73*, 74, 76, 78
— see Taylor, I. M. *79*
Welt, L. G. 196, *197*, 349
— A. V. Goodyer, J. H. Darrach, W. A. Abele and W. H. Maroney *402*
— and J. Orloff 270, *350*
— D. W. Seldin and J. H. Cort *287*
— — W. P. Nelson *367*
— D. T. Young, O. A. Thorup jr. and C. H. Burnett *240*
— see Amatruda, T. T. *443*, 448, 456
— see Hollander, W. *531*
— see Nelson, W. P. *347*
— see Oliver, J. *532*
— see Peters, J. P. *366*
— see Petersdorf, R. G. 270
— see Seldin, D. W. *287*
— see Sims, E. A. H. *351*
— see Stevenson, J. A. F. *364*
— see Winthers, R. W. 212, 213
— see Womersley, R. *325*
·Wendt, H. *393*
— W. E. see Gauer, O. H. *351*
Werkö, L., J. Ek, H. Bucht and E. Varnauskas *390*
Wertheimer, E. *129*
— see Stein, L. *512*
Werther, M. *425*, 434, 452
Wesson, L. G. *233*, 388
— and W. P. Anslow *236*, *239*, *244*, 245, *281*, *282*, 401
— jr., W. P. Anslow jr., L. G. Raisz, A. A. Bolomey and M. Ladd 266, 270, *349*
— see Anslow, W. P. 345
West, C. D., S. A. Kaplan, S. J. Fomon and S. Rapoport *261*, 290
— and S. Rapoport *285*, 290
— see Cheek, D. B. *206*, 520
— see Kaplan, S. A. *357*, 358
— see Lipsett, M. B. *320*
— see MacLean, J. P. *311*
— see Rapoport, S. *285* 367
— E. S., and W.R. Todd, *197*

Weston, R. E., J. Grossman, E. R. Borum, H. A. Guerin, H. Mark, T. D. Ullman, M. Wolfman and L. Leiter 293, *531*
— — I. S. Edelman, D. J. W. Escher, L. Leiter and L. Hellman 293, *399*, *400*, *401*
— — and L. Leiter 293, *397*
— D. J. W. Escher, J. Grossman and L. Leiter 293, *407*, *409*
— I. B. Hanenson, J. Grossman, G. A. Berdasco and M. Wolfman 293, *345*, *348*
— H. B. Horowitz, J. Grossman, I. B. Hanenson and L. Leiter 293, *352*
— see Grossman, J. *397*, *402*, *409*
Westphal, K., F. Gleichmann and G. Soika *489*
Wettstein, A. *305*, *310*, *313*, *316*, *319*
— and G. Anner *305*, *308*
— see Kahnt, F. W. *319*
— see Simpson, S. A. *308*
Wharton, J. D. see Huggins, C. *500*
Wheeler, H. O. see Bradley, S. E. *267*
— N. C. see Fowell, D. M. *411*
Whelan, M. *295*
Whipple, G. H. see Havill, W. H. *406*
— N. see Elrick, H. *355*
White, A. G., M. Kurtz and G. Rubin *352*
— G. Rubin and L. Leiter *347*
— H. L. *341*
— M. Audia and D. Rolf *528*
— P. Heinbecker and D. Rolf *341*
— and D. Rolf *324*
— I. T. Rosen, S. Fischer and G. H. Wood *375*
— see Carlin, M. R. *387*
— see Mueller, C. B. *271*, *272*
— see Netravisesh, V. *369*, *370*
— see Surtshin, A. *357*
Whitehead, R. W. *192*
Whitehouse, A. G. R. *440*, *441*
Whitlock, R. T. see Winthers, R. W. *212*, *213*
Whitney, J. E., L. L. Bennett and C. H. Li *342*
Whittaker, J. see Boyd, E. M. *503*
Whittam, R. *80*, *106*
— and R. E. Davies *60*, *106*
— see Breuer, H. J. *60*, *107*
Widdas, W. F. see Alexander, D. P. *218*

Widdowson, E. M., R. A. McCance and C. M. Spray *226*
— see McCance, R. A. *257*, *289*, *291*, *328*, *516*, *533*, *534*
Wiedemann, G. see Roller, D. *414*
Wiggers, C. J. *186*
Wiggins, W. S. see Capps, J. N. *403*
Wilbrandt, W. *78*, *79*, *151*
— see Moulin, M. *191*
Wilde, R. S. see Pitts, R. F. *260*
— W. S. *84*
— and J. M. O'Brien *182*
— see Arnett, V. *102*
— see Ginsburg, J. M. *229*
— see Malvin, R. L. *239*, *241*, *260*
— see O'Brien, J. M. *182*
Wilder, R. M., A. M. Snell, E. J. Kepler, E. H. Rynearson, M. Adams and E. C. Kendall *302*
Wiley, F. H., L. L. Wiley and D. S. Waller *288*
— L. L. see Wiley, F. H. *288*
Wilhelmi, A. E. see Davenport, H. W. *240*
Wilhelmj, C. M., I. Neigus and F. C. Hill *468*
— E. B. Waldemann and T. F. McGuire *521*
— see McDonough, J. *521*
Wilkins, R. W., C. M. Tinsley, J. W. Culbertson, B. A. Burrows, W. E. Judson and C. H. Burnett *350*, *372*
— see Judson, W. E. *373*
Wilkinson, B. M., and R. A. McCance *328*
Wille, J. H. see Rosenblueth, A. *182*
Willebrands, A. F., J. Groen, Chr. E. Kammenga and J. R. Blichman *537*
— see Kamminga, C. E. *30*
— see Pelser, H. E. *338*
Willi, A. see Schwarzenbach, G. *5*
Williams, E. M. see Streeten, D. H. P. *530*
— G. R. see Chance, B. *61*
— L. G., and H. Patrick *527*
— T. F. see Oliver, J. *532*
— Vaughan, E. M. see Kuffler, S. W. *90*, *163*, *177*
— W. see Denton, D. A. *257*, *290*
Willis, K. see Viar, W. N. *376*, *377*
Wills, J. see Huf, E. G. *120*
— J. H. *429*, 455

Wilson, D. L., and J. F. Manery *103*
— D. W. see Beer de, E. J. *456*, *484*, *485*
— see Reinhold, J. S. *487*, *488*
— G. M., J. M. Olney, L. Brooke, J. A. Myrden, M. R. Ball and F. D. Moore *213*
— see Davies, R. E. *232*
— see Kilpatric, R. *43*
— see Miller, H. *213*, *216*
— see Moore, F. D. *232*
— see Munro, D. S. *210*, *213*
— I. B., and D. Nachmansohn *65*
— see Nachmansohn, D. *168*
— J. D., and D. W. Seldin *322*, *324*
— J. R. see Meyerhof, O. *17*
— J. S. see Freeman, O. W. *387*
— T. H. *66*
— see Herman, R. H. *492*, *493*, *494*, *495*
— W. P. see Hickam, J. B. *203*
Winberry, M. M., and P. J. Crittenden *520*
Winderman, S. see St. George, S. *532*
Winkler, A. W. see Elkinton, J. R. *287*
Winslow, J. A. see Fowell, D. M. *411*
Winter, C. A. *335*, *336*
— and W. R. Ingram *333*, *335*
— H. A., H. E. Hoff and L. Dso *193*
— I. C. see McKeever, W. P. *415*
Winternitz, M. C., and L. L. Waters *341*
Winters, R. W. see Oliver, J. *532*
Winthers, R. W., R. T. Whitlock, J. L. de Walt and L. G. Welt *212*, *213*
Winton, F. R. see Bickford, R. G. *266*
— see Eggleton M. G. *269*, *273*
— see Herman, F. G. *276*
Wirz, H. *247*, *249*, *257*, *264*, *325*
— and P. A. Bott *240*
— B. Hargitary and W. Kuhn *247*
Wise, B. L. *368*
Wohlgemuth, J. *461*
Wohlzogen, F. X. see Alexander, D. P. *218*
Woinar, A. O. *461*

Wolf, A. V. *287, 294, 295, 371, 389, 392*
— S. see Hinkle, L. E. jr. *352*
Wolff, H. P., Kh. R. Koczorek and E. Buchborn *312, 370, 384, 385*
Wolfman, M. see Weston, R. E. 293, *345*, 348
Wolfson, S. K., and S. Ellis *537*
Wolstenholme, G. E. W., and C. M. O'Connor *215*
Womersley, R., O. A. Thorup jr. and L. G. Welt *325*
Wood, F. H. see Dennis, C. *138, 512*
— F. J. Y. see Brooks, R. V. *529*
— G. H. see White, H. L. *375*
Woodard, G. see Nelson, A. A. *315*
Woodbury, D. M. *207, 213, 525, 536*
— C. P. Cheng, G. Sayers and L. S. Goodman *318*
— J. W. see Brady, A. J. *161*, 164
Woodford, M. see Grundy, H. M. *308*
Woodward, K. F. *281*
Worcester, J. see Locke, W. *440*, 442
Woronzow, D. S. *166*
Wottom, I. D. P., and E. J. King *199*
Wright, A. see Jones, I. C. *334*
— R. D., H. W. Florey and M. A. Jennings *484*
— S. see Calma, I. *166*
— S. L. see Ravdin, J. S. *487*
Wrong, O. *344*
— see Leaf, A. *345*, 348
Wu, H. see Slyke, D. D. van *201*

Wu, M. see Smith, C. A. *141, 217*
Wulff, H. B. see Skanse, B. *316*, 518
Wulkan, E. see Popper, H. L. *490*
Wyatt, N. F. see Weller, J. M. *530*
Wyman, C. see Sudak, F. N. *537*
— L. C., G. P. Fulton and M. H. Shulman *303*
Wyngaarden, J. B. see Peterson, R. E. *309*

Yale, E. K. see Maren T. H. *298*
Yalow, A. see Berson, S. *206*
— R. S. see Berson, S. *206*
Yankopoulos, N. A. see Davis, J. O. *375*
Yannet, H. see Darrow, D. C. *288, 527*
— see Harrison, H. E. *206*, 210
Yates, F. E. *277*
— J. Urquhart and A. L. Herbst *277*
Yellowlees, H. see Evans, B. M. 300, *514*
Yeung, G. T. C. *499*
Yoffey, J. M. *315*
Youmans, W. B. *379*
— see Bachman, D. M. *377*
Young, A. C. *102*
— D. W. see Hannon, J. P. *203*
— D. T. see Welt, L. G. *240*
— J. Z. see Webb, D. A. *162*
— W. C. see Emery, F. E. *498*
— W. F. see McCance, R. A. *246*
Yount jr., E. H. see Little, J. M. *333, 341*

Yuan, I. C. see Liu, A. C. *479*, 480
Yudkin, J. see Davies, B. M. A. *255*

Zaffaroni, A. 307
— see Hechter, O. *307*
Zak, G. A., C. Brun and H. W. Smith *246*
Zapp jr., J. A. see Stadie, W. C. *30*
Zaribnicky, F. *497*
Zayat, A. F. see McDowal *187, 188*
Zebrowski, v. *451*
Zerahn, K. 28, *60, 61*, 68, 69, *118*, 120, 121, *436*
— see Koefoed-Johnsen, V. *113*
— see Ussing, H. H. *116*, 117, 121
Zetler, G. see Hild, W. *343*
Zeuthen, E. see Prescott, D. M. *54*
Ziegler, J. A. see Lardy, H. A. *11*
Zierler, K. L., and J. L. Lilienthal *321*
— see Folk, B. P. 202, *203*
Zimmermann, B. see Ansell, J. S. *230*
Zipser, A., H. B. Pinto and S. Freedberg *224*
— and A. Stone Freedberg *525*
Zwaardemaker, H. *185*
Zweifach, B. W. *112*
— E. Shorr and M. M. Black *303*
Zwemer, R. L., E. P. Vollmer and M. M. Carey *522*
— see Lowenstein, B. E. *522*
Zwikster, G. H., and T. E. Boyd *185*

Subject Index

Page numbers followed by "*T*" refer to tables. Numbers followed by "*F*" refer to footnotes. The use of names of experimental animals as keywords is restricted to the first section, such animals being of relatively little interest in the second part.

Acclimatization to cold,
  effect on plasma K and Na
    203
Acetamide,
  neurohypophyseal hormones and permeability
    of frog skin towards
    128
Acetate-activating enzyme,
  effects on 14
Acetazoleamide see carbonic
  anhydrase inhibitors
Acetylation of Coenzyme A,
  activation by K, Rb 14, 15
  inhibition by Li 15
Acetylcholine,
  benadryl as antagonist of
    193
  effect on heart "potassium-
    paradox" 185
  — — hemolysis 79
  — — influx of Na and K
    into red cells 79
  effects on release 170
  — — synthesis 28, 29
  electromotive action at
    motor end-plate 169^F
  heart muscle and 168, 185
  ionic permeability and 55,
    64, 171
Acid polysaccharides,
  binding of K and Na by 8
  interaction with alkali me-
    tal ions in enzymatic
    processes 8
Acidification,
  of urine 240, 252, 285–301
Acidosis
  in adrenocortical insuffi-
    ciency 323
  renal effects 288–292,
    393–395
ACTH see corticotropin
Actin
  in non-living models 172
Action potential,
  effect of alkali metal ions
    on 152
  — — Li on nerve 154
  of heart false tendons 167
  — isometric contraction,
    effect of K on 178

Action potential
  of Loligo giant nerve
    162^F
  — squid giant axon 151
  relation of external Na to
    nerve 153
  — — K to nerve 154
  sodium hypothesis and
    151, 153
Activance 16, 20
Activation analysis,
  determination of K in
    muscle by 94
Active extrusion
  of Na, coupling with K up-
    take 77
Active state of nerve and
  muscle 151
Active transport
  as a "forced exchange" 57
  concept 46
  effects of drugs and hor-
    mones on 63
  inhibition by scillaren and
    digitoxin in erythro-
    cytes 80
  mechanism 67, 81
  of alkali metal ions 45, 57
  — Cl, in frog skin glands
    113, 118, 130
  — —, in frog small inte-
    stine 138
  — K, in the formation of
    bull seminal plas-
    ma 142
  — Na, caloric efficiency
    in muscle 92
  — —, coulomb efficiency
    92
  — —, electromotive force
    in frog skin 122
  — —, energy require-
    ment in frog
    muscle 91
  — —, in muscle 87
  — —, inhibitors in am-
    phibian skin
    125
  — —, relation to frog skin
    potenti-
    al 114

Active transport
  of Na, relatio to intestinal
    poten-
    tials 136
  — —, — — water trans-
    port a-
    cross
    frog skin
    128
  — —, work performed in
    frog skin 120
  quantitative relationship
    between oxygen con-
    sumption and 61
  relation to metabolism 60,
    78
  stoichiometric efficiency 62
Activity,
  K and Na shifts during
    nerve 102
Actomyosin 172
  resting potential and 190
Addison's disease (see also
    adreno-cortical insuffi-
    ciency) 302, 303, 320, 327
Adenohypophysis,
  renal effects 340
Adenosine diphosphate 11
Adenosine triphosphatase
    (ATP-ase) from brain and
    crab nerve 11
Adenosine triphosphate,
  binding of K and Na by 7
  effect on actomyosin 172
  fructokinase and 13
  pyruvic phosphoferase
    and 11
ADH see vasopressin
Adrenal cortical steroids see
    corticosteroids
Adrenalectomy (see also adre-
    nocortical insufficiency),
  effect on gastric secretion
    477
  — — intestinal absorp-
    tion 138
  — — milk secretion 498
  — — prostatic secretion
    501
  — — salivary secretion
    457
Adrenalin see epinephrine

Adrenocortical hormones see corticosteroids
Adrenocortical insufficiency, effects of 301–304, 324, 327
Adrenocorticotropic hormone see corticotropin
Aedes,
Malpighian tubules 140ᵀ
reabsorption of K and Na by rectum 141
African tortoise 83
After-hyperpolarization of motoneurons 161
Age,
influence on homeostasis 533
— — K in serum 198
— — Na in bone 210
— — — — cartilage 208
Albumin (serum),
renal salt excretion and 270
Aldehyde dehydrogenase, effects on 16
Aldosterone,
blood loss and secretion 370
control of secretion 310–314, 369
effect on renal electrolyte excretion 321–326
— — salivary secretion 458
— — sweat secretion 445
identification and synthesis 308
in pregnancy 339
mineralocorticoid activity 308, 318, 321
rate of secretion 307, 309, 370, 375, 384
sodium retaining activity 308, 318, 321
volume receptors and secretion 369
Aldosteronism,
primary, 316, 323, 419
Alkaline earth metal ions,
K-effect on nerve and 150
Alkalosis,
renal effects 288–292
resulting from aldosteronism 323
— — desoxycorticosterone 323
— — potassium deficiency 293, 323
serum K and 203
All-or-none reaction
of heart to stimuli 185
All-or-none response 155
Amino acid accumulation
in mouse ascites carcinoma, effects on 105
p-Aminohippurate,
effects on accumulation in kidney slices 23, 27ᵀ

p-Aminohippurate,
respiration of kidney slices and transport of 32
tubular excretion 27ᶠ
p-Aminohippurate clearance 382
Aminometramide and Aminometradine 415
6-Aminouracil 415
Ammonia,
excretion in urine 255, 260, 324, 394
formation in kidney 254, 260
Ammonium salts,
effects on enzymatic processes 10ᵀ
— — renal electrolyte excretion 393
Amniotic fluid,
K and Na in 218
Amphenone B 417
Amphibian skin (see also frog skin) 114–129
inhibitors of active Na transport in 125, 126ᵀ
stimulants of active Na transport in 127ᵀ
work performed by active Na transport in 120
Anaerobiosis,
effect on active ion transport in toad nerve 98
— — K content of liver slices 106
Anaesthesia,
effects on renal electrolyte excretion 357
Anal papillae,
absorption of K and Na in mosquito larvae through 143
Androgens,
anabolic effects 340
electrolyte metabolism and 340
in adrenal cortex 305
Animalizing substances,
viscosity of fibrillar protein solutions and 35
Anionenatmung, definition 61
Anodal polarization,
block of nerve conduction and 166
Anoxia,
active Na extrusion from yeast and 108
ionic movement in nerve and 98
kidney cortex slices and 106
Antialdosterones,
renal effects 417

Anticholinesterases,
active Na transport and 125, 143
Antidiuresis (vasopressin), 264, 270, 343
resulting from barbiturates 352
— — emotional stress, 352
— — morphine 352
— — nicotine 352
Antidiuretic hormone see vasopressin
Antidididiuretic substances
in adrenocortical insufficiency 333
Antikaliuresis,
resulting from adrenocortical insufficiency 302, 323
— — androgens 340
— — growth hormone 342
— — increased ureteral pressure 273
— — mercurial diuretics 299, 409
— — potassium deficiency 292
— — respiratory acidosis 290
Antinatriuresis,
resulting from aldosterone 321–326
— — anaesthesia 357
— — androgens 340
— — assumption of upright posture 375
— — blood loss 369
— — circulatory failure 378–386
— — desoxycorticosterone 317, 319, 321, 326
— — exercise 387
— — glucocorticoids 320
— — growth hormone 342
— — hyperoncotic serum albumin 270
— — hypertensin (in man) 355
— — increased extrarenal pressure 276
— — — renal venous pressure 275
— — — ureteral pressure 273
— — licorice extract 338
— — lowered renal arterial pressure 271

Antinatriuresis
    resulting from oestrogens
        239
— — peripheral venous
        congestion 372
— — respiratory acidosis
        290
— — serotonin 355
— — stress 358
— — surgery 357
— — sympathomimetic
        amines 359
— — vasopressin 346
Appetite for "salt" 517
Apyrase 17
Aqueous humour 216
Arabic acid,
    binding of K and Na by 8
Argentophilic cells (renal tu-
    bular) 259
Arsenic,
    permeability of intestinal
        walls to sulfate and 134
Arsenite,
    inhibition of Na transport
        in frog skin 126^T
Artemia salina,
    exchange of Na and K 50
Arthropods,
    active K and Na uptake
        143
Ascites carcinoma cells,
    cardiac glycosides and ac-
        tive ion transport in
        mouse 64
    transport of electrolytes
        and amino acids in 105
Aspartate,
    effect on seminal vesicle
        mucosa 107
— — squid axon mem-
        brane potential
        159
"Asymmetrically collapsing
    lattice" theory,
    mechanism proposed for
        active transport 69
ATP see adenosine triphos-
    phate
ATP-ase see adenosine tri-
    phosphatase
Atrial receptors
    left, controlling vasopres-
        sin secretion 358
    right, controlling aldoste-
        rone secretion 369
Atrium,
    effect of K on 183
Atropine,
    effect on active Na trans-
        port in amphi-
        bian skin 127^T
— — heart "potassium-
        paradox" 185

Autoregulation (renal vascu-
    lar) 271, 274, 359
"Availability"
    of K in bone 216
— — — cartilage 208
— Na in bone 212
— — — cartilage 209
Avian salt gland 502
Axoplasm,
    Na activity in 153
Azide,
    effect on cephalopod giant
        axons 99
— — erythrocytes 79
— — frog skin 126^T
— — kidney cortex sli-
        ces 106
— — sea urchin larvae
        34
— — yeast 108

Bacterial hexokinase,
    effects on 13
BAL,
    active Na transport in
        amphibian skin and
        127^T
    antimercurial action 299,
        396, 402, 405
Barium chloride,
    effect on frog nerve 150
Barley roots 112
Benadryl,
    effect on gut as antagonist
        of acetylcholine 193
Benemid,
    kidney cortex slices and
        106
Bernstein hypothesis 87,
    144^F, 145
    muscle experiments not in
        accord with 146
    Nernst equation and 146
Bicarbonate,
    secretion by colon 515
Bicarbonate, tubular
    reabsorption 239, 252
    effects of acid-base status
        of body on
        288–292
— — carbonic anhydr-
        ase inhibitors
        on 296–300
— — potassium on
        294–296
Bile,
    gall bladder bile 492–496
    hepatic bile 486–491
    K in 486–496
    Li in 490
    mechanism of reabsorp-
        tion in gall
        bladder 493
— — secretion by liver 490
    Na in 486–496

Bile acids 489
Bioelectric phenomena,
    relation of alkali metal
        ions to 144–172
Bioelectric potential,
    ionic permeability and the
        development of 56
Bird red cells,
    transport of K and Na in 82
Block of conduction
    in frog ventricle strip due
        to K 167
— nerve due to K 166
Blood volume,
    effects of changes in
        distribution 372
— on renal electrolyte
        excretion 369
Bone,
    K in 210
    Na in 210
Boyle-Conway hypothesis 146
Brain adenosinetriphospha-
    tase 17
Brain slices,
    cation transport system
        104
    effects on oxygen con-
        sumption 24, 25
    exchange of cellular K 103
    glycolysis 28
Brine shrimp,
    exchange of K and Na 50
Bromide,
    active Na transport in
        amphibian skin and
        127^T
Bronchial mucosa 503
Bronchial secretion 503
Bufo bufo,
    inhibitors of Na transport
        in skin of 126^T
    stimulants of active Na
        transport in skin of
        127^T
    urinary bladder 130
Bufo marinus,
    K level in muscle 45
Bull-frog,
    Cl and Na transport in
        small intestine 138
Bull seminal plasma,
    active K transport in the
        formation of 142

Calcium chloride,
    effect on frog nerve 150
Caloric efficiency of Na
        transport in muscle 92
Carbon dioxide,
    Na transport in amphi-
        bian skin and 126^T
Carbon monoxide,
    active ion transport in
        erythrocytes and 79

Carbonic anhydrase inhibitors,
active ion transport in erythrocytes and 79
— Na transport in frog skin and 125
increasing renal excretion of Na, 296–300, 416
— tubular secretion of K 139, 296–300, 416
intraocular pressure and 217
lowering renal citrate excretion 416
— tubular bicarbonate reabsorption 239, 252, 296
— — hydrogen ion secretion 139, 239, 252, 296
renal effects 139, 239, 296–301, 416
resistance to 300
Carcinus maenas,
effect of Na on nerve 162
K and Na in nerves 95^T
— — — movements in unmyelinated nerves 101^T
— — — uptake through gills 143
— loss of nerve during stimulation 102
Cardiac failure,
renal excretion and 378–386
venous pressure in 380
— tone in 380
Cardiac glycosides,
effect on active transport mechanism 64
— — ion transport in erythrocytes 79, 80
— — Na flux in mouse ascites carcinoma 106
Cardiac potentials,
measurement using intracellular electrodes 147^F
Carrier molecules,
exchange diffusion and 51
required for ion transport through cell membranes 50, 67, 68
Cartilage,
K and Na in 208
Casein,
binding of alkali metal ions by 9

Cat,
K and Na in erythrocytes 82^T
— — — — nerves 95^T
— — — — serum 199^T
resting potential of auricle effect of K on 147
Cation exchange processes,
distal tubular 252
proximal tubular 240
Cation exchange resins 5, 510
Cation fluxes in nerve,
effect of temperature on 98
Cation pump 67, 106
Cell sap,
ionic composition of giant algal 110^T
Cell separation hypothesis (renal) 267, 270
Cellular accumulation of various substances,
effects on 31
Cellular volume – see volume of living cells
Central nervous system,
effects on renal sodium excretion 362–368
— — water excretion 362–368
— — — intake 362–365
Cephalopod giant axons,
active Na transport in 60^F, 97, 99
Cerebral salt wasting 366
Cerebrospinal fluid,
K and Na in 215
Cesium,
affinity for β-galactosidase 16
complex formation with protein 38
Cs^{131}, Cs^{134}, Cs^{137}, 3
distribution after administration 43, 225
— of naturally occurring 225
effect of loading, acute 526
— — — chronic 526
— on acetylcholine synthesis 29
— — aldehyde dehydrogenase 16
— — bacterial hexokinase 13
— — enzymatic reactions 10^T, 20
— — mitochondria preparations 23

Cesium,
effect on oxygen consumption of brain slices 24
— — — resting potential of muscle and nerve 151
fecal excretion 526
function of in replacement of K 159, 533
ionic radius 3^T
metabolic effects on tissue slices 24
permeability of cell surfaces to 47
— — sepia nerve to 159
radioactive 3
renal excretion 423, 526
state in living cells 43
transport in human erythrocytes 77
Characeans 36, 111
Chelates 4
Chelydra serpentina 164
Chloride,
active transport of 113, 118, 130, 138
concentration in renal tissue 248
distal tubular reabsorption 258
flux ratio in frog skin 116
movement in intestinal mucosa 133
proximal tubular reabsorption 237
renal handling 234–238, 242–254
Chlormerodrin – see mercurial diuretics
Chlorothiazide,
renal effect 416
Chloruresis (see also natriuresis) 417
Choleretic effect 489
Choline
as substitute for Na 100, 153, 163
permeability of frog skin to 118
Choline acetylase,
effects on 14
Cholinergic substances,
gastric secretion and 471
Cholinesterase,
effect of esters split by 79
— on sub-synaptic membrane 171
Cholinesterase,
sensitivity towards alkali metal ions 19
Chondroitin sulphate,
binding of K and Na by 8, 205, 209

Circulatory failure
   in adrenocortical insuf-
     ficiency 302–304
   renal electrolyte excre-
     tion, effect on 378–386
Coecum,
   active Na transport in
     guinea-pig 133, 136
   potential difference in
     guinea-pig 136
Coenzyme A,
   acetylation 14, 15
   binding of K and Na by 7
Collagen,
   binding of K and Na by 206
Colloid osmotic pressure see
   pressure, oncotic
Colon,
   active transport of NaCl
     in 133
   Na-flux in dog 134, 135^r
   potential difference in 138
Colonic mucosa 485
Colonic secretion 485
Common shore crab,
   uptake of K and Na
     through gills 143
Compartmentalization of
   cellular K 45
Complex formation 6, 50
Component theory,
   gastric secretion and 478,
     504
   pancreatic secretion and
     430, 462, 504
   salivary secretion and 430,
     504
Concentrating mechanism,
   renal 244–251
   corticoids, effects on 326
   urea, effects on 251
Concentration ratio
   of K in nerve 97
Conduction,
   effects of external Na on,
     162–164
   — — K on 165–168
Conduction block
   caused by K 167, 168
   — — Na deficiency 162
Conductivity
   of heart muscle 183
Congenital adrenal hyper-
   plasia 318, 339
Connective tissue,
   mobility of K and Na in
     symphyseal 55
Conn's Syndrome see
   aldosteronism, primary
Constant field theory of
   Goldman 48^F, 146
Contractibility,
   effect of K on 177, 194
Contractibility of heart 183
   relation to irritability 186

Contracture 176, 177, 189
Conway's hypothesis 92
Copper,
   effect on frog skin 118,
     119^r
   — — kidney cortex
       slices 106
   — — potential of inte-
       stinal mucosa
       137
   — — uptake of K and
       Na in Daphnia
       magna 143
Corium, K and Na in 207
Cornea, K and Na in 207
Cortex, adrenal 301–338
Corticoids see corticosteroids
Corticosteroids (see also
   glucocorticoids and mine-
   ralocortocoids) 301–337
   antagonistic effects 318
   bioassay 305, 307
   biosynthesis, inhibition of
     417
   chemical nature 304–308
   competition 318
   control of secretion
     310–314
   depression of secretion
     315, 417
   derivatives of 336
   effect on gastric secretion
     475
   — — ion transport in
       erythrocytes 80
   — — milk secretion 498
   — — Na in bone 213
   — — renal electrolyte
       excretion 316–334
   — — renal water ex-
       cretion
       326–334
   — — salivary secretion
       457
   — — sweat secretion 445
   — — vascular tone 303
   effects of insufficient pro-
     duction 301–304
   epinephrine and produc-
     tion 351
   inactivation in liver 277,
     375
   — inhibited by licorice
     extract 338
   polyuria induced by
     334–336
   rates of secretion 309
   sites of production
     314–316
   transformations 319
Corticotropin,
   effects on renal electrolyte
     excretion 320
Cortisol and cortisone see
   glucocorticoids

Coulomb efficiency,
   definition 92
Countercurrent arrangements
   in renal medulla 247–251
Coupled Na – K pump 58
   evidence for existence 70
   in mouse ascites carci-
     noma cells 105
Coupling
   between K influx and Na
     outflux 99
   — — uptake and active
       Na extrusion 77
Crab muscle,
   inapplicability of sodium
     theory to 161
   measurements using intra-
     cellular glass elec-
     trodes 88
Crab nerve,
   effect of K on respiration
     25
   reversible inexcitability
     165, 166
Cricket,
   effects on dorsal blood
     vessel 185
Critical potential,
   for propagated impulses
     in frog muscle 167
Crustacean muscle,
   effects on action potential
     163
Crystal radii,
   determination 3
   of alkali metal ions 3^r
Curare,
   active Na transport in
     amphibian skin and
     127^r
   reduction of end-plate
     potential by 170
Curarine 177
Curarized fibres
   effect of Na on end-plate
     potential in 170
Cushing's Syndrome 321,
   323, 445
Cyanide,
   effect on active fluxes
     of K and Na in cephalo-
     pod nerve 98
   — — — ion transport
         in ascites
         carcinoma
         106
   — — — Na extrusion of
         yeast 108
   — — — — transport in
         frog skin
         116,
         126^r,
         129

Cyanide,
  effect on cephalopod
              giant axons 99
  — — ion transport in
              erythrocytes 79
  — — kidney cortex
              slices 106
  — — Na outflux 88, 99
  — — transport of water
              across frog skin
              129
Cytidine triphosphate,
  bindung of K and Na by 7

Daphnia magna 143
DDD 315
Dead space errors (urinary
  tract) 268
Debye-Hückel theory,
  activity coefficients of
              phosphates and 8
"Delay time" phenomon,
  gastric secretion, in 466
  salivary secretion, in 453
Depletion
  of K, acute 529
  — —, chronic 531
  — Na, acute 527
  — —, chronic 528
Depolarization 151
  produced by adding KCl
              to muscle and nerve
              149
  rise in K permeability,
              caused by 101
Derivatives of corticosteroids
  336
Desheathed nerves,
  effect of K on 148
  properties 163
11-Desoxycorticosterone,
  effect on intracellular K
              level 189
  — — staircase pheno-
              menon 188
  effects on renal electrolyte
              excretion 316, 319,
              321–326
  glucocorticoid activity 317
  mineralocorticoid activity
              318
  question of adrenal secre-
              tion 305, 307
Diabetes insipidus 242
Diabetes mellitus,
  effect on urinary electro-
              lyte excretion 354, 395
Diamox see carbonic an-
  hydrase inhibitors
Diaphragm,
  glycogen formation by rat
              30
Dichloro-2,2-bis(p-chlorophenyl)-ethane (DDD) 315

Diencephalon,
  controlling aldosterone
              secretion 313, 365
Diethylmalonate,
  active Na transport in
              frog skin and 126ᵀ
Diffusion potential
  of K and Na in frog skin
              123
Diffusion resistance of interspaces 55
Diffusion theory of gland
  secretion 480, 504
Digestive tract,
  contents of K and Na
              508
  secretory output of K and
              Na 508
Digitalis,
  effect on intracellular
              K level 189
Digitalis glucosides,
  effect on staircase phe-
              nomenon 188
Digitoxigenin,
  effect on ion transport
              in erythrocytes 79
Digitoxin,
  ion flux in ascites carci-
              noma and
              106
  — — — erythrocytes
              and 80
Diisopropylfluorophosphate
  143
Dilution diuresis 269
2,3-Dimercaptopropanol
  (BAL),
  active Na transport in
              amphibian skin and
              127ᵀ
  antimercurial action 299,
              396, 402, 405
4,6-Dinitro-o-cresol,
  effect on Ulva lactuca 109
Dinitrophenol,
  effect on cephalopod giant
              axons 99
  — — energy-rich phos-
              phate bonds
              106
  — — erythrocytes 79
  — — frog skin 125, 126ᵀ
  — — intestinal prepa-
              rations 137
  — — kidney cortex slices
              106
  — — mitochondria 22
  — — muscle 88
  — — nerve 98, 99, 100
  — — yeast 108, 109
Dioestrus 501
Distal tubular system 242, 261
  acidification of urine 252

Distal tubular system
  alkali metal ion transport
              by 242–259
  ammonia secretion by 254
  cation exchange in 252
  chloride reabsorption by
              258
  effects of mineralocorti-
              coids 321–326
  K secretion by 256
  water transport by
              242–251
Distal tubules see distal
  tubular system
Distribution
  of alkali metal ions be-
              tween cells and their
              surroundings 36
  — Cs, after administra-
              tion 43, 225
  — — naturally occur-
              ring 225
  — Li, after administra-
              tion 223
  — —, naturally occur-
              ring 223
  — Rb, after administra-
              tion 43, 224
  — —, naturally occur-
              ring 224
Distribution kinetics of K
  and Na 229
Diuregan see mercurial diuretics
Diuresis,
  "conduction" 388
  "propulsion" 388
  "tubular salt rejection"
              389
  water 242, 388
Diuretic agents 388–419
  acidifying 393
  antialdosterones 417
  carbonic anhydrase inhibi-
              tors 416
  chlorothiazide 416
  mercurials 395
  "osmotic" 390
  purines and pyrimidines
              415
  salts 391
  water 389
  xanthine 410
Dixippus, Malpighian tubules,
  140ᵀ
DOC and DOCA see desoxy-
  corticosterone
Donnan ratios see Gibbs-
  Donnan ratios
Drinking centers (hypothalamic) 362
Duodenal secretion 483—484
Duodenum 133, 483—484

Dynamic haematocrit 267
Dytiscus, Malpighian tubules, 140^T

Ehrlich breast carcinoma 105
Elasmobranchs 84
Electric activity (see also relation of alkali metal ions to)
"sodium theory" 151, 160
Electric organs 171
effect of neurohormones on 161
Electric potential difference of red cells 72
Electrochemical potential 47, 100
Electromotive force,
methods of estimating in frog skin 122^T
of active Na transport 122
Electroneutral ion pump 57
Electron-linked carrier transport,
theory of active ion transport 68
Electroosmosis 53, 69
Electrophorus 171, 172
Electroplaques,
properties of and arrangement in electric organs 171
Emys orbicularis,
effect of K on heart 187
Endolymph,
K and Na in 141^T, 217
potential difference between perilymph and 141
Endothelium,
intercellular diffusion 112
End-plate,
effects of K and Na on 169, 170
End-plate potential 169, 170
Energy requirement of active Na transport in frog muscle 91
Energy-rich phosphate bonds, 2,4-dinitrophenol and 106
ion transport in red cells and consumption of 81
Enzymatic reactions,
effect of alkali metal ions on 10
Ephedrine,
effects on renal electrolyte excretion 362
Epinephrine,
effect of K on release 195
— on active Cl transport in frog skin glands 113, 118, 130
effects on corticoid production 361

Epinephrine,
effects on electrolyte excretion 359, 362
— — ionic permeability 65
— — Na-flux and short-circuit current 118, 119^T, 130
— — renal circulation 359, 362
Epineurium,
permeability to inorganic ions 148
properties of frog nerve 162^F
Epithelial cells, salt transport in 59
Epithelial membranes,
transport through 112
Eriocheir sinensis,
ion uptake by gills 142
oxygen consumption and ion transport 62
Erythrocyte ghosts,
ion transport by 80, 81
Erythrocyte membrane,
nature of diffusion of alkali metal ions through 81
Erythrocytes 71–84, 105, 222
coupling between active Na extrusion and K uptake 77
energy-rich phosphate bonds and ion transport 81
equations for influx of K and Na 75
— — outflux of K and Na 75, 76
K and Na in 82^T, 222
Li in human 77
phytic acid in bird 83
relation of ion transport to metabolism 78
saturation kinetics of K in human 74
state of K in 43
transport of ions in bird 82
— — — human 73, 75, 77
Eserin,
effect on active Na transport in frog skin 125, 126^T
— — Na uptake in Eriocheir sinensis 143
Estradiol
electrolyte pattern of cells and 63, 64
K retention in rat uterus, caused by 194
"Estrogen withdrawal" 195

"Excess", Na
in bone 212
— cartilage 210
Exchange
of muscle K against Na caused by low K diets 86
transcapillary of Na 229
Exchange diffusion,
mechanism 50
nature of carrier 51
of Na in amphibian skin 63
— — — erythrocytes 63
— — — frog muscle 92
— — — kidney mitochondria 50
— — — nerve 63, 102
Exchange resins 5, 6, 510
Exchangeability
of K, in liver mitochondria 39
— , — muscle 39^F, 95
— , — various organs 229
— Na, in bone 212
— —, — cartilage 210
— —, — erythrocytes 71
Excitability,
effect of alkali metal ions on heart 183
— — K on muscle 177
— — — nerve 166
Excitation,
effects of external Na on 162–164
— — K on 165–168
"sodium" theory of 151
Excretion of alkali metal ions, renal 233, 423
Excretion, fecal
cesium 526
potassium 518
sodium 517
Exercise,
effect on renal Na excretion 387
Exocrine glands (see resp. glands)
Exocrine secretions (see resp. secretions)
Expansion, extracellular
urine excretion, effects on 270, 371
Extracellular Na 90
Extracellular space,
relation to Na-space 205
Extracellular volume,
expansion from intestinal sources 509
renal electrolyte excretion, effects on 270, 371
— Na-excretion in regulation of 368

Extragastrulation,
  produced by Li 33
Extrarenal pressure,
  effects on urine excretion
    276

False tendon,
  effects on resting poten-
    tial 150, 167
Fast muscle fibres,
  properties of 54, 90, 163
Fatty acid metabolism,
  effects on 31
Fatty acid oxidation com-
  plex 22
Fecal excretion
  of Cs 526
  — K 518
  — Na 517
Feedback mechanisms 368
Female organs of reproduc-
  tion 501, 502
Ferricyanate,
  renal effect 237, 280
Filtration coefficient (glome-
  rular), 264
Filtration rate see glomerular
  filtration rate
Fistula (arterio-venous),
  renal Na excretion and
    272, 378
Fixed charge hypothesis,
  alternative to sodium
    pump theory 44, 87
  analysis and criticism of
    45
Fleckenstein hypothesis 179
Flexner-Jobling tar carci-
  noma
  effect of K on glycolysis 28
Flounder,
  isolation of renal tubules
    of 31
Fluid circuit mechanisms 69
Fluoride,
  effect on anoxic ion shifts
    in nerve 98
    — ion transport in
      red cells 78, 83
    — — K contents of liver
      slices 106
    — — Na transport in
      frog skin 126^T
    — — seminal vesicle
      mucosa 107
  shrinkage of erythrocytes,
    produced by 79
Fluoroacetate,
  effect on Na transport in
    frog skin 126^T
Flux ratio 49
  membrane structure and
    74
  of Cl, in amphibian skin
    116

Flux ratio
  of K, in cephalopod
    nerve 100
  — Na, in intestinal mu-
    cosa 135
Forced exchange 57
Formoguanamine 415
Francium 2
Free water clearance,
  negative 245, 251
  positive 245, 251
Frog large intestine,
  active Na transport 133
  potential difference 136
Frog muscle,
  effect of external K on
    membrane po-
      tential 166
    — — Na on excitability
      174
  energy requirements of
    active Na transport 91
  K diffusion coefficient 55
  — equilibrium concen-
    tration in perfused
      85, 86
  — exchange 90, 94
  — flux 93
  Na diffusion coefficient 55
  — flux across membrane
    89
  Q_{10} for active Na trans-
    port 62, 63^T
Frog nerve,
  effect of K on sciatic nerve
    165, 166
    — — Na on excitation
      and conduction
        162
    — — quaternary am-
      monium ions on
        161, 162
  properties of epineurium
    162^F
Frog skin,
  effect of cardiac glycosides
    on 64
    — — pH on Na trans-
      port 125
  effects of neurohypophy-
    seal hormones on
      128
  — on oxygen consump-
    tion of isolated 27
  electromotive force of ac-
    tive Na transport 122
  inhibitors of active Na
    transport 125, 126^T
  measurements using iodine
    coulometer 117^F
  potentials 114, 123
  relationship between
    transport of Na and
      water across 128

Frog skin,
  stimulants of active Na
    transport 126, 127^T
Frog skin glands,
  active Cl transport in 113,
    118, 130
Frog ventricle,
  effects on 164, 168
Fructokinase,
  antagonism between K
    group and Na group 20
  effects on 12
  important ions for action
    27
Fructose,
  energizing of cation trans-
    port by 78
  seminal vesicle mucosa,
    effect on 107
Fructose-1,6-diphosphate,
  binding of K and Na by
    7

β-Galactosidase,
  effects on 16, 20
Gall bladder 492, 496
  reabsorption in 493
  secretion by 496
Gall bladder bile 492
Gastric mucosa 465, 483
  alkali metal ions in 477
  electrophysiology of 482
  mechanism of secretion by
    478, 483
Gastric mucus 471
Gastric secretion 465, 483
  effect of cholinergic sub-
    stances on 471
  — — corticosteroids on
    475
  — — duration of secre-
    tion on 473
  — — glandular blood
    flow on 474
  — — histamine on 471
  — — insulin on 471
  — — K depletion on 474
  — — Na depletion on
    474
  — — plasma conc. of Na
    and K on 473
  — — rate of secretion on
    469
  — — temperature on 475
  individual variations in
    477
  Li in 477
  mechanism of formation of
    478
  type of gland 467
  — — stimulation 471
Gastrointestinal atonia 192
Gastrointestinal tract see digestive tract

Gelatin,
  binding of alkali metal ions
    by 9
Genitals see male, resp. female
    organs of reproduction
Giant algal cells,
  ionic compositions of cell
    sap and potential of
    110^r
Giant axon,
  active K and Na transport
    in cephalopod 60^F, 97
Giant nerve,
  effect of cardiac glycosides
    on 64
Gibbs-Donnan distribution
    of H in Carcinus muscle
    191
  — K in living cells 37, 70
Gibbs-Donnan equilibrium,
  exchange resins and 6
Gibbs-Donnan ratios,
  K and Na in plasma 201,
    202^r
Gizzard slices,
  K—Na distribution in pi-
    geon 70
Glands, exocrine see different
    glands
γ-Globulin,
  binding of alkali metal
    ions by 9
Glomerular capillary pressure
    262, 273, 332
Glomerular factors,
  salt and water excretion
    and 261–272
Glomerular filtration rate,
  decrease by cardiac failure
    382
  — — hypophysectomy
    341
  — — neurophyseal de-
    struction 354
  increase by extracellular
    expansion 270
  — — glucocorticoids 330
  — — oxytocin 354
Glomerular membrane,
  resistance in 261
Glomerular propulsive pres-
    sure 261
  antinatriuresis from lower-
    ing of 271, 358, 359,
    383, 387
  natriuresis from elevation
    of 271, 355, 358, 359,
    413
Glomerular ultrafiltration 261
Glucagon,
  renal electrolyte excretion
    and 354
Glucocorticoids 307, 309, 315,
    316, 319–320

Glucocorticoids
  effects on filtration rate
    330
  — — proximal fluid re-
    absorption 331
  — — renal blood flow
    330
  — — — electrolyte ex-
    cretion
    319–334
  in treatment of cardiac
    oedema 332
Glucose, active transport in
    small intestine 134
  as osmotic diuretic 281,
    391, 395
  ascites carcinoma cells and
    105
  brain slices and 25
  energizing of cation trans-
    port by 78
  seminal vesicle mucosa
    and 107
  yeast cells and 108
Glucose-1-phosphate 7
Glucose-6-phosphate 7
Glutamate,
  brain slices and 25, 103
  isolated retina and 104
  seminal vesicle mucosa
    and 107
  squid axon membrane po-
    tential and 159
Glutaminase activity (renal)
    256
  in adrenocortical insuffi-
    ciency 324
  — K deficiency 294
Glutamine,
  isolated retina and 104
  renal ammonia formation
    and 254, 260
  seminal vesicle mucosa
    and 107
Glutathione synthesizing en-
    zyme system,
  effects on 15
Glycerophosphate 7
Glycine,
  accumulation by ascites
    carcinoma cells 105
Glycogen formation
  by various organs 27, 30
  effects on 29, 31
Glycogenolysis 29
Glycolysis,
  active ion transport and 60
  effects on 28
  energizing of cation pump
    in ascites carcinoma
    cells by 106
  relation to K and Na in
    nerve 98
Glycyrrhetinic acid see licori-
    ce extract

Glycyrrhizine (-inic acid) see
    licorice extraxt
Goldman equation 48, 49, 56,
    146
Gras snake
  cation transport in red
    cells of 83
Growth hormone,
  renal effects 314, 342
Guiacol,
  complex formation with K
    5
Guanidinium,
  restoration of Na deficient
    frog nerve by 161
Guanosine triphosphate 7
Guinea-pig
  brain slices 103
  coecum 133, 136
  K in serum 199^r
  kidney cortex slices 66,
    107
  liver slices 70
  seminal vesicle mucosa 60,
    107
  symphyseal connective
    tissue 55

Haematocrit,
  dynamic (renal) 267
Haemorrhage,
  effect on renal electrolyte
    excretion 369
Half-life,
  in plasma, Na^{22} 203
  of radioactive alkali metal
    ions 2, 3
Halicystis 36, 57, 109
Halicystis ovalis,
  active Na transport in 110
  ionic composition of cell
    sap 110^r
Hajdu hypothesis 188
Halogenated corticoids 318,
    336
Head organizer,
  morphogenetic effect of Li
    on 33
Heart muscle 147, 164,
    183–191
  all-or-none reaction to sti-
    muli 185
  diminution of intracellular
    K level 189
  effect of cardiac glycosides
    on active trans-
    port mecha-
    nism in 64
  — — K on development
    of ten-
    sion 189
  — — — excitation
    and con-
    duction
    167

Heart muscle
    factors influencing mecha-
        nical response 186
    ionic antagonism in 184
    K contracture 175, 189
    — release during contrac-
        tion 182
    temperature and ionic ef-
        fects on 185
    voltage clamp 164
Heart rate,
    effects on 186
Heavy metals (see also Cu,
        Hg, Pb),
    osmotic regulation in
        Daphnia magna and 143
Heavy water 46^r, 53
Helodes 143
Hemerythrin,
    binding of alkali metal
        ions by 9
Hemoglobin,
    binding of alkali metal
        ions by 9
Hen red cells 82, 83
Heparin,
    binding of alkali metal
        ions by 8
Hepatic bile 486–491
    effect of blood flow on 489,
        490
    — — plasma conc. of K
            and Na on 489
    lithium in 490
    mechanism of formation
        of 490
    rate of secretion 488
Hepatic tissue 496
Heterogeneity of intracellular
        K in muscle 90
Higher plants,
    accumulation of cations by
        111
Histaminase inhibitors,
    gastric secretion and 471
Histamine,
    active Na transport in am-
        phibian skin and 127
    gastric secretion and 471
    release of K from intesti-
        nal muscle, caused by 65
Hodgkin-Huxley-Goldman
        equation 124
Hodgkin theory of electric ac-
        tivity 102, 151, 164
Hormones,
    extrarenal effects on K,
        Na 535
    plasma conc. of K, Na, ef-
        fect on 203
    renal effects 301–355
    transport of alkali metal
        ions and 63
Hyaluronic acid 8, 19, 205
Hyaluronidase 19, 20

Hydrated radii of alkali metal
        ions 3^r
Hydrocholeretic effect 489
Hydrocyanic acid,
    permeability of intestinal
        walls to sulfate and 134
Hydrodynamics of the
        nephron 261, 268, 279, 282
Hydrogen ions, renal excre-
        tion, osmotic diuresis and
        285
Hydrogen ions, tubular secre-
        tion 239, 252
    effects of acid-base status
        of body on
            288–292
    — — carbonic anhydrase
            inhibitors on
            296–300
    — — potassium on
            294–296
17-Hydroxycorticoids see glu-
        cocorticoids
Hypercapnia see respiratory
        acidosis
Hyperchloraemia (see also hy-
        pernatraemia)
    resulting from paroptic
        ganglion destruction 367
Hyperkalaemia 203
    resulting from adrenocor-
        tical insufficiency 301,
        323
Hypernatraemia 203
    resulting from aldostero-
        nism 323
    — — diabetes insipidus
            363
    — — neurogenic oligo-
            dipsia 363, 364
Hyperpolarization 101, 161
Hypertensin,
    effects on renal electrolyte
        excretion 355
Hypertonia
    of body fluids see hyperna-
        traemia
    — urine 243–251
Hyperventilation see respira-
        tory alkalosis
Hypocapnia see respiratory
        alkalosis
Hypokalaemia 203
    resulting from aldostero-
        nism 323
    — — desoxycortico-
            sterone 323
    — — neurogenic oligo-
            dipsia 364
Hyponatraemia 203
    — resulting from adreno-
        cortical insuf-
        ficiency 301

Hyponatraemia
    resulting from
    — — cardiac failure 386
    — — cerebral disorders
            366
    — — neurogenic poly-
            dipsia 363
    — — spinal cord trans-
            section 366
    — — unbridled secre-
            tion of ADH 363,
            364
β-Hypophamine see vaso-
        pressin
Hypophysectomy,
    defective water diuresis
        after 334
    effects on aldosterone ex-
        cretion 311,
        513, 514
    — — salt metabolism
        310, 341
    reduced glomerular fil-
        tration from 341
    — renal blood flow from
        341
Hypotonia
    of body fluids see hypo-
        natraemia
    — urine 242–251
Hypoventilation see respi-
        ratory acidosis

Ileal secretion 484, 485^r
Ileum 484
    Na fluxes 133, 134, 135^r
Inactivation of membrane
        elements,
    permeable to K, Na 157, 158
Indoleacetate,
    effect on amino acid and
        ion uptake 105
Influx
    of K and Na in red cells
        75, 76
Inhibitors of active ion trans-
        port 82, 125, 126^r
Injury potential 144, 145
Inner ear,
    composition of endolymph
        and perilymph in ver-
        tebrate 141
Inosine triphosphate,
    binding of K and Na by 7
Insects,
    Malpighian tubules of 59,
        140
Insulin 354
    gastric secretion and 471
Intercellular cements,
    permeability of 55
Interspaces,
    diffusion resistance of 55
Interstitial tissue fluid,
    K, Na in 204

Intestinal absorption of K and Na 508–515
effects of corticoids on 512
— hypophysectomy on 513
— — resins on 510
in ureterocolic anastomoses 514
Intestinal lavage,
use in electrolyte imbalances 514
Intestinal mucosa,
factors influencing Na transport in 133, 137
net transport of Na 131
secretion by 483–486
unidirectional Na flux 134
Intestinal muscle,
effect of K on 192
— — Na on 191
K release by histamine 65
Intestinal potentials,
relation to active Na transport 136
Intestinal wall,
permeability towards sulfate 134
transport of K across 138
Intestine (see also large and small intestine)
alkali metal ion absorption in 134, 508–515
Intestine contents,
K and Na conc. in 139, 509, 511
potential difference between blood and 136
Intracellular electrodes (see also micro-electrodes),
measurements using 147, 148
Intracellular glass electrodes,
measurement of intracellular pH using 88, 191
Inulin 104
Inulin clearance see glomerular filtration rate
Inulin space 104, 194
Iodine coulometer 117^F
Iodoacetate,
effect on active Na transport in frog skin 126^T
— — anoxic ion shifts in nerve 98
— — ion transport in ascites carcinoma cells 106
— — — — in muscle 88
— — — — in red cells 78
— — — — in Valonia 110

Iodoacetic acid,
effect on erythrocytes 72
— — muscle 175
Ion-exchange resins,
binding of alkali metal ions by 5
intestinal absorption of alkali metal ions and 510
Ionic antagonism
in enzymatic action 20
— heart 184
Ionic concentrations
of endolymph and perilymph 141^T
Ionic diameter,
solvent drag and 53
Ionic permeability,
bioelectric potentials and 56
Ionic potential,
complex formation and 4
Ionic radii,
determination 3
of alkali metal ions 3^T
selectivity of exchange resins and 6
Irritability
of heart muscle 186
Ischaemic cationshifts 84
Isethionate 7
Isotopes of alkali metal ions 2, 3

Jejunal secretion 484
Jejunum 484
Na flux in dog 134, 135^T
transport of NaCl and water 133
Jensen sarcoma,
effects on glycolysis of 28
Juxta-glomerular apparatus 314, 359

Kaliuresis,
resulting from acidosis 295, 394
— — aldosterone 321–326
— — ammonium chloride 394
— — carbonic anhydrase inhibition 296–300
— — desoxycorticosterone 324
— — diabetes mellitus 395
— — glucagon 354
— — licorice extract 338
— — lithium intake 421
— — mercurial diuretics 286, 409
— — natriuresis 286

Kaliuresis,
resulting from non-respiratory alkalosis 291
— — osmotic diuresis 285
— — oxytocin 353
— — respiratory alkalosis 289
— — serotonin 355
K_e (total exchangeable K) 227
Ketoglutarate,
effect on brain slices 25
— — kidney cortex slices 106, 107
Kidney (see also renal)
blood flow see renal blood flow
handling of alkali metal ions by 233–423
oxygen consumption 260
Kidney cortex slices 106
accumulation of sulfate by 32
swelling associated with metabolic inhibition 66
Kidney medulla slices,
accumulation of sulfate by 32
Kidney mitochondria,
exchange diffusion of Na in 50
Kidney slices,
accumulation of p-aminohippurate by 27^T, 32
effects of alkali metal ions on fatty acid metabolism of 31
— on oxygen consumption of 27
exchangeable K in 39
Kidney tubules 139
isolation of flounder 31
reabsorption of NaCl in 62
transport of phenol red in 31

Lacrymal gland 463–464
mechanism of secretion of 424–438
Lacrymal secretion, alkali metals in 463–464
effect of duration of secretion on 464
— — plasma conc. of K and Na on 464
— — rate of secretion on 464
Lactate,
effects on erythrocytes 78, 82
Lactose,
ionic effects on enzymatic hydrolysis of 16

Large intestine,
active Na transport in frog 133, 136
— — — — toad 133, 136
— — —, relation to intestinal potentials 136
factors influencing Na transport in 133
"one-sidedness" of Na transport in 134, 136
potentials 136

Latency relaxation,
effect of K on 178

Latent period
of isometric contraction, effect of K on 178

Lead,
effect on ion uptake in Daphnia magna 143
— — K conc. of red cells 71

Lens,
K and Na in 220

Leucocytes 103
K and Na in 103^T, 222

Libinia emarginata 99

Limnaea embryos,
morphogenetic effect of Li on 33

Limnaea stagnalis,
extragastrulation caused by Li treatment of 33

Limulus leg nerve,
effect of stimulation on K content 102^F

Lipaemia,
plasma Na and 199

Liquid junction potential for water/axoplasm 149

Lithium,
affinity for exchange resins 6
— — β-galactosidase 16
biology and pharmacology of 109^F
chemical properties 3
competition with Na transport mechanism in yeast 109
conc. in blood 77, 223
distribution after administration 223
— of naturally occurring 77, 223
effect on acetate activating enzyme 15
— — action potential 154
— — aldehyde dehydrogenase 16

Lithium,
effect on enzymatic reactions 10^T, 16, 20
— — fatty acid matabolism 31
— — frog skin potential 114
— — heart muscle contraction 188
— — mitochondria preparations 23
— — nerve excitability 162
— — octanoate metabolism of kidney 31
— — oxygen consumption of brain slices 25
— — phosphotransacetylase 15
— — pyruvic phosphoferase 12
— — respiratory enzymes 35
— — resting potential 150, 151
— — skeletal muscle 162^F, 174
— — staircase 190
— — uptake of K and Na by Eriocheir sinensis 142
in gastric secretion 477
— hepatic bile 490
— saliva 459
— salivary gland 460
ionic radius 3^T
kaliuretic effect 421
loading 523
metabolic effects 24
morphogenetic effects 32
— —, mechanism 34
natriuretic effect 421
permeability of cell surfaces to 47
— — frog skin epithelium to 159
— — sepia nerve to 159
radioactive 2
renal excretion 419–422
transport in frog skin 118, 120
— — human erythrocytes 77
—, passive 47
— through epithelial membranes 113
uptake by Eriocheir sinensis 142
— — sea urchin embryo 34

Liver 496

Liver slices 106
factors influencing fatty acid metabolism of 31
— — oxygen consumption of 25
glycogen formation in rat 30

Liver mitochondria,
K metabolism of 39

Lizzard muscle 170

Locusta,
Malpighian tubules of 140^T

Loligo axons,
resting potential of 149

Loligo forbesi,
K and Na in nerves of 95
— — — — movements in unmyelinated nerves of 101^T

Loligo giant axons,
active ion transport in 60^F 99
effect of Na on 162

Loligo pealii,
K and Na in nerves of 95^T
— — movements in unmyelinated nerves of 101^T

Loop of Henle
function in urinary concentration 246–251

Loop of Thiry-Vella see Thiry-Vella loops

Lymph,
K and Na in 203

Macromolecules, in interstitial spaces,
binding to 205

Magnesium chloride,
absorption of NaCl by intestinal mucosa and 131

Maia nerve 102^F

Maintained potentials,
relation of alkali metal ions to 144

Malapterurus 172

Male organs of reproduction 499–501

Malonate,
effect on brain slices 25
— — erythrocytes 79

Malpighian tubules of insects 59, 140

Mammalian muscle,
K fluxes of 95
temperature and K exchangeability in 39

Mammalian nerve,
effect of K on 166

Mammalian red cells,
    alkali metal ion transport
        in 82
Mammary gland, 497–499
    blood flow in 498
    electrophysiology of 499
    hormonal effects on 498
    mechanism of secretion of
        499
Mammary secretion 497–499
    effect of adrenalectomy on
        498
    — — corticosteroids on
        498
    — — sodium loading on
        498
    — — stage of lactation
        497
Mannitol,
    absorption of NaCl in in-
        testinal mucosa and
        131
    as osmotic diuretic 281
Mannose,
    energizing of cation trans-
        port by 78
Mechanical response,
    effects of K on 177
    factors influencing heart
        186
Medullary shunt (renal vascu-
    lar) 358
Membrane current,
    contribution of K and Na
        to squid axons 154
Membrane potential,
    dependency on K conc.
        145, 149, 166
    estimation from ion conc.
        56
    measurement using micro-
        electrodes 145, 147
Membrane structure,
    change in permeable state
        54
    passive permeability and
        54
Membrane theory 85
Mercurial diuretics 395–410
    effects on free water
        clearances 402
    — — Na and Cl reabsorp-
        tion 401
    — — renal electrolyte
        excretion 286,
        299, 395–410
    extrarenal effects 397
    factors influencing re-
        sponse to 406–408
    mechanisms of action
        397–406
    renal excretion 405
    site of action 399, 405

Mercury,
    effect on ion uptake in
        Daphnia magna
        143
    — — kidney cortex
        slices 106
Mercury chloride,
    permeability of intestinal
        walls to sulfate and
        134
Mersalyl,
    active Na transport in
        amphibian skin and
        127^T
Metabolic acidosis, alkalosis
    see non-respiratory
Metabolic inhibitors,
    effect on liver slices 106
Metabolism,
    relation of active and
        passive
        transport to
        78
    — — — transport to
        60, 81
Metacholine,
    gastric secretion and 471
Methylated corticoids 336
Michaelis constants 12, 16
Micro-catheterization of
    collecting tubules 260
Micro-electrodes,
    measurement of end-plate
        potential using 169
    — — frog skin potential
        using 122
    — — intracellular poten-
        tials using 149
    — — membrane poten-
        tials using 145,
        147, 148
    use of "double-barrelled"
        160
Micro-glass electrodes,
    measurement of intra-
        cellular pH using 88,
        191
Micro-injection technique 159
Micro-puncture of renal tubu-
    les 235, 247, 249
Milk see mammary secretion
Mineralocorticoids (see also
    aldosterone and desoxy-
    corticosterone)
    control of secretion
        310–314
    mineralocorticoid activity
        318
    rate of secretion 307, 309
    renal electrolyte excretion
        and 316, 319, 321–326
    urinary excretion 312
Mitochondria 21
    accumulation of ions in
        22, 37

Mitochondria
    exchange diffusion of Na
        in kidney 50
    exchangeability of K in
        liver 39
    isolation of functional 22
Monobromacetate,
    active Na transport in frog
        skin and 125
Monofluoroacetate,
    active Na transport in
        frog skin and 125, 126^T
Monoiodoacetate see iodo-
    acetate
Monoiodoacetic acid see iodo-
    acetic acid
Mosquito larvae,
    exchange of K and Na in
        140^F
    osmotic regulation in 140^F
    salt absorption by anal
        papillae 143
Motoneurons,
    after-hyperpolarization of
        161
    applicability pf "sodium
        theory" on mamma-
        lian 160
Motor endplates
    effect of neurohormones
        on 161
Mouse ascites carcinoma cells
    105
    cardiac glycosides and
        active transport in 64,
        106
Mucosa,
    alkali metal ions in gastric
        477
    — — — — intestinal
        486
    — — — — uterine
        194^T,
        222
    secretion of bronchial 503
    — — gastric 465–483
    — — intestinal 483–486
    — — oesophageal
        464–465
    — — pyloric 467—468
    — — uterine 501–502
Mucous membrane see mucosa
Mucus,
    bronchial 503
    colonic 485
    gastric 471
    oesophageal 464
    pyloric 467
Mucoviscoidosis 446
Muscle,
    deviation from Bernstein
        hypothesis in
        146

Muscle,
deviation from Donnan distribution in 44
effect of cardiac glycosides on active transport in 64
— — Cs on resting potential 151
— — K on excitation and conduction 166, 167
— — — — heart 147, 175, 189
— — — — intestinal 192
— — — — mechanical response 177
— — — — resting potential 144, 147
— — — — skeletal 174
— — — — smooth 148, 175
— — — — uterus 193
— — — — vascular 195
— — Li on resting potential 151
— — Na on electric activity in 164
— — — — excitation and conduction 163, 164
— — — — heart 164
— — — — intestinal 191
— — — — resting potential 150
— — — — skeletal 174
— — — — striated 163
— — — — uterus 192
— — Rb on resting potential 151
effects on heart 183
— — mechanical responses of 177, 186
— — oxygen consumption of 26
electric activity of 151
energy requirement of active Na transport in frog 91
fast fibres 54, 90, 163
K conc. in toad 45
— contracture 175, 181, 181, 189
— diffusion coefficient for frog sartorius 55
— displacement by Cs in 43, 44^r
— equilibrium conc. in perfused frog 85, 86

Muscle,
K exchange in frog toe 94
— fluxes of frog 93
— — — mammalian 95
measurement of intracellular pH 88, 191
Na diffusion coefficient for frog-sartorius 55
— flux across membrane 89
net transport of K and Na 88
Q_{10} for Na transport in 62, 63^r
slow fibres 90, 163, 177, 181
twich fibres 177, 181
Muscular activity,
alkali metal ion shifts in relation to 95
Muscular contraction,
role of alkali metal ions in 172
Muscular exercise,
effect on plasma K 200
Muscular tissues,
K and Na in 221
Myelinated nerve fibres,
effect of K on action potential 165
— — — — resting potential 149
— — Li on resting potential 150
Myosin 9, 172
Myosin ATP-ase 18

Na$_e$ (total exchangeable Na) 227
Nasal gland see avian salt gland
Nasal mucosa 502
Nasal secretion 502
Natriuresis
resulting from acidosis 394–395
— — adrenocortical insufficiency 302
— — antialdosterones 417
— — blood volume expansion 370
— — carbonic anhydrase inhibitors 296, 416
— — chlorothiazide 416
— — desoxycorticosterone 321
— — fall in plasma oncotic pressure 269

Natriuresis
resulting from glucagon 354
— — glucocorticoids 320
— — hypernatraemia of carotid blood 366
— — hypertensin 355
— — increase in plasma Na-conc. 277
— — — — renal arterial pressure 272
— — lithium intake 421
— — mercurial diuretics 395
— — neck compression 377
— — non-identified steroids 318
— — osmotic diuresis 280, 390
— — oxytocin 353
— — potassium excess 295, 392
— — progesterone 339
— — renal denervation 357
— — renin 355
— — respiratory alkalosis 289
— — sodium chloride intake 280
— — stimulation of brain stem 368
— — sympathomimetic amines 359
— — vasopressin (ADH) 345, 347
— — xanthine diuretics 410
Natriuretics see diuretic agents
Necturus,
cardiac glycosides and reabsorption of Na in kidney proximal tubules 64
Negative staircase
in uterus muscle 194
Nephron,
fluid transport in 261–269
hydrodynamic resistance in 261–267
Nephrosis 271
Nernst equation 93, 146
Nerve,
depolarization produced by adding KCl to 149, 151
effect of Cs on resting potential 151

Nerve,
    effect of K on excitation
        and con-
        duction
        165
    — — — — resting po-
        tential
        148, 149
    — — Li on action poten-
        tial 154
    — — — — resting po-
        tential
        150, 151
    — — Na on excitation
        and con-
        duction
        162
    — — — — resting po-
        tential
        150
    — — quarternary am-
        monium com-
        pounds on 161,
        162
    — — Rb on resting po-
        tential 151
    — — temperature on cat-
        ion fluxes in 98
    effects on oxygen con-
        sumption of peripheral
        25
    electric activity of 151
    gain of Na per impulse for
        isolated 101[r], 103
    ion transport in peripheral
        95
    K and Na in 95[r]
    — concentration ratio in
        97
    — effect, ionic dependen-
        cy 150
    — movement in resting
        96
    Na movement in resting 96
    net loss of K per impulse
        in 101[r], 103
    relation of K to action po-
        tential 154
    — — Na to action poten-
        tial 153
    resting potential 148
Nerve activity,
    K and Na shifts during 102
Nerve conduction,
    effect of alkali metal ions
        on 102, 152, 162, 165
Nerve endings 169
Nerve sheath,
    as a diffusion barrier 162
    effect on ion diffusion 96,
        165
Neurogenic salt wasting 363,
    365–367
Neurohormones,
    potential effects 161

Neurohypophyseal extract,
    effects on frog skin 119[r]
    — — toad urinary blad-
        der 130
Neurohypophyseal hormones
    65, 342
    effects on frog skin 65, 118,
        119[r], 127, 128
    — — intestinal mucosa
        137
Neuromuscular block 170
Neuromuscular junctions,
    relation of alkali metal
        ions to electric activity
        of 168
Neuromuscular transmission
    169
Nitella 57
Nitellopsis 36, 111
Nitrate,
    renal effects 237, 280
    — handling 237
o-Nitrophenol-β-(D)-galacto-
    pyranoside 16
4-Nitro-salicylaldehyde 105
Non-hydrated radii of alkali
    metal ions 3
Non-living models
    for muscular contraction
        172
Non-propagated impulses
    voltage clamp and 158
Non-respiratory acidosis,
    effect on urinary K excre-
        tion 292
    — — — Na excretion
        394
Non-respiratory alkalosis,
    urinary K excretion and
        291
Noradrenalin see norepine-
    phrine
Norepinephrine,
    effect on renal circulation
        359–362
    — — — electrolyte ex-
        cretion
        359–362
Normal passive behaviour of
    ions,
    relationship for deviations
        from 49
Novasurol see mercurial diu-
    retics
Nucleic acids,
    binding of alkali metal
        ions by 8

Octanoate breakdown 31
Oedema,
    cardiac, genesis of 378–386
    —, treated by glucocorti-
        coids 342
    in nephrosis 271
    pre-menstrual 339

Oesophageal mucus 464–465
Oestrogens,
    effects on hyaluronic acid
        340
    — — renal electrolyte
        excretion 339
    in adrenal cortex 305
Oestrus 501–502
Oligodipsia,
    neurogenic 364
Organ of Corti 141
Osmolar conc. of plasma,
    relation to conc. of Na 200
Osmoreceptors 348
Osmosis,
    intestinal absorption and
        137
Osmotic barrier,
    renal 246
Osmotic diuresis 236, 265
    effect on renal K and Na
        excretion 280–285, 390
    mechanism of 281
Osmotic gradient,
    transfer of water across
        frog skin and 128
Osmotic regulation 65
Outflux
    of K and Na from red cells
        75, 76
Ovaries,
    K and Na in 223
Overshoot of potential 152
Oxygen consumption,
    brain slices 24
    exocrine glands, basal 435,
        475
    — —, in relation to Na
        transport
        435–436, 507
    isolated frog skin 27
    — — —, in relation to Na
        transport 120
    kidney slices 27
    liver slices 25
    muscle 26
    peripheral nerve 25
    relation between active
        ion transport and 61
    renal, relation to Na trans-
        port 261
Oxytocin 127[r], 346, 353

Pace-maker regions 167
PAH see p-aminohippurate
Palaemonetes varians 143
Pancreas slices,
    K-Na distribution in pi-
        geon 70
Pancreatic gland 460–463
    alkali metal ions in 434
    mechanism of secretion by
        424–438

Pancreatic secretion 460–463
  effect of duration of secretion on 461
  — — plasma conc. of K and Na on 463
  — — rate of secretion on 461
  — — type of stimulation on 461
Pancreatitis,
  alloxan induced 463
  ethionine induced 463
Pancreozymine 461
Panhypopituitarism 310
  defective water diuresis in 334
Paralytic ileus
  correlation between plasma NaCl and 191
Paraventricular neurones 348
Parotid gland 451–452
  mechanism of secretion by 424–438
Parotid secretion 451–452
Passive permeability,
  acetylcholine and 64
  membrane structure and 54
Passive transport,
  effect of drugs and hormones on 63
  of alkali metal ions 45, 47
  — K in nerve during current flow 101
  — — through cephalopod giant axon membrane 100
  — Na through giant fibre membrane 101
  relation to metabolism 78
Pectic acid 19
Pectinesterases 19
Perfused frog muscle,
  K equilibrium conc. in 86
Perilymph,
  K and Na in 141^r, 217
  potential difference between endolymph and 141
Perineurium
  as diffusion barrier 150
Periodate,
  active Na transport in amphibian skin and 127^r
Peripheral nerve 95–103
  effects on oxygen consumption of 25
Permanganate,
  active Na transport in amphibian skin and 127^r
Permeability,
  bioelectric potentials and 56
  membrane structure and 54

Permeability,
  of intercellular cements 55
  — intestinal walls to sulfate 134
pH,
  effect on intestinal NaCl absorption 133
  — — Na transport in frog skin 125
  measurement of intracellular 88, 88^r, 191
Phenol red,
  transport in flounder renal tubules 31
Phenylacetate,
  effect on amino acid and ion transport 105
Phenylurethane,
  effect on Ulva lactuca 109
  — — Valonia 110
Phlorhizin,
  intestinal effects 134
Phosphate esters,
  binding of alkali metal ions by 6
Phosphocreatin 175
Phosphofructokinase,
  effects on 13
  purification and properties of brain 14
2-Phosphopyruvate 11
Phosphotransacetylase,
  effects on 15
Phytic acid
  in bird red cells 83
Pieris,
  Malpighian tubules of 140^r
Pilocarpine,
  active Na transport in amphibian skin and 127
  gastric secretion and 471
Pineal gland,
  relation to aldosterone secretion 313
Pinocytosis,
  theory of active ion transport 69
Pitocin see oxytocin
Pitressin see vasopressin
Pituitrin (see also vasopressin and oxytocin) 193
Placenta,
  transport of K and Na over 219
Placenta slices,
  glycogen formation by human 30
Plant cells,
  active Na transport in 57
Plant roots,
  oxygen consumption and ion uptake by 61

Plasma,
  K and Na in 198, 199^r
Polydipsia,
  primary neurogenic 364
  psychogenic 364
Polyelectrolyte,
  binding of K and Na by 205
Polymetaphosphate 8
Polyphosphates 6
Polyposia 364
Polyuria,
  from corticoid treatment 334
  — potassium deficiency 336
  — thyroxin 335
  — vasopressin insufficiency 243, 343, 364
  secondary to excessive drinking 364
Porous membranes 51, 56, 136
Positive staircase 194
Posture,
  influence on aldosterone excretion 377
  — — (nor) epinephrine excretion 376
  — — renal electrolyte excretion 375–378
Potassium,
  compartmentalization of cellular 45
  complex formation 5
  coupling between active Na extrusion and uptake of 77
  — — Na-outflux and K-influx 99
  determination by activation analysis 94
  diffusion potential 123
  distal tubular secretion 256, 286
  Donnan distribution 37
  effect on development of muscle tension 189
  — — enzymatic reactions 10^r
  — — resting potential 144–150
  — — staircase phenomenon 84, 173, 189, 195
  exchange between brain and cerebrospinal fluid 222
  — — — — plasma 222
  — diffusion in duck red cells 92

Potassium,
    exchangeability in mam-
        malian muscle 39, 95
    fluxes of frog muscle 93
    — — mammalian muscle
        95
    heterogeneity of intracel-
        lular 90
    in amniotic fluid 218
    — aqueous humour 216
    — ascites carcinoma cells
        105
    — bone 210
    — cartilage 208
    — cerebrospinal fluid 215
    — colon contents 139
    — corium 207
    — cornea 207
    — endolymph 141^T, 217
    — epidermis 220
    — erythrocytes 82^T, 222
    — food components 516
    — gastric juice 470^T
    — interstitial fluid 204
    — lens 220
    — leucocytes 222
    — lymph 203
    — muscular tissues 221
    — nerves 95^T
    — ovaries 222^T, 223
    — perilymph 141^T, 217
    — plasma 198
    — — and serum of labo-
        ratory animals
        199^T
    — secretions of exocrine
        glands see resp. se-
        cretions
    — serum 198
    — synovial fluid 214
    — tendon 206
    — testes 222^T, 223
    — thrombocytes 222
    — uterus 194^T, 222
    — vitreous humour 217
    ionic radius 3^T
    K^{40}, K^{42}, K^{45} 2, 3
    natriuretic effect 295, 392
    net loss in stimulated ner-
        ve fibres 101^T, 103
    passive movement through
        cephalopod giant
        axon membrane
        100
    — transport during cur-
        rent flow in nerve
        101
    proximal tubular reab-
        sorption 240
    release by histamine 65
    renal clearance 257
    — excretion see renal ex-
        cretion, kaliuresis,
        antikaliuresis
    restricted diets 86, 517

Potassium,
    state in living cells 37
    total exchangeable 227,
        231^T
    "transient" 427, 434, 470
    transport across the inte-
        stinal wall 138
    — in human erythrocytes
        73
    — — muscle 88, 93, 95
    — over placenta 219
Potassium contracture,
    175, 181, 184, 189
Potassium deficiency
    from corticoids 333
    renal effects of 336, 531
    vasopressin resistant poly-
        uria from 336
Potassium depletion see de-
    pletion
Potassium-free medium,
    effect on active extrusion
        of Na 105
Potassium intake,
    normal 516
Potassium loading,
    acute 521
    chronic 522
    renal effects 294
"Potassium paradox" 185
Potassium-restricted diets 86,
    517
Potassium selectivity
    of membranes 152
Potential (see also action and
        resting potential),
    cardiac 147^F, 150, 164
    endolymph 141^T
    frog skin, isolated 123, 139
    gastric 482
    giant algal cells 110^T
    mammary 499
    perilymph 141^T
    relation of alkali metal
        ions to maintained 144
    sublingual 428, 433
    submaxillary 428, 433
Potential difference
    between blood and colon
        lumen 138
    — endolymph and peri-
        lymph 141
    equation for 56
Potential "overshoot" 152
Prednisone and prednisolone
    (see also glucocorticoids)
    336
Pressure
    extrarenal, effect on urine
        excretion 276
    in renal tubules 264, 266,
        284
    intrarenal 268

Pressure
    oncotic, of plasma, effect
        on urine excretion 267,
        269
    renal arterial, effect on uri-
        ne excretion 271
    — venous, effect on urine
        excretion 274
    ureteral, effect on urine ex-
        cretion 272
    venous, in cardiac failure
        380
Progesterone
    competition with aldoste-
        rone 339
    effects on ion transport 63
    — — intracellular K le-
        vel 189
    — — renal electrolyte
        excretion 339
    — — uterus 194
    in adrenal cortex 305
Propagated impulses 158
Propelled carrier transport,
    hypothesis of active ion
        transport 68
Propulsion diuresis 388
Protein binding,
    plasma K and Na 201
Proximal tubules (renal),
    alkali metal ion transport
        by 234—242
    effects of adenohypophysis
        on 341
    — — glucocorticoids on
        330
    hydrogen ion secretion by
        240
    reabsorption of bicarbona-
        te by 238
    — — chloride by 234—242
    — — potassium by 240
    — — sodium by 231,
        234—242
    — — water by 234—242
Prussic acid,
    effect on permeability of
        intestinal walls 134
Purkinje fibres,
    resting potential 147, 150,
        164
Pyloric secretion,
    electrolyte composition
        468^T
Pyridoxal,
    effect on amino acid and
        ion transport 105
Pyrophosphate 7
Pyruvate,
    cation transport and 78
    formation 11
    — of carbohydrates from
        29, 30
Pyruvic phosphoferase,
    effects on 11

Pyruvic transphosphorylase,
    antagonistic effect of K
    and Na 20
    important ions for action
        of 27

Q_{10} for Na exchange 63
Quarternary ammonium com-
    pounds,
    effects on frog nerve 161,
        162, 163

Rabbit
    kidney slices 27, 32
    leucocytes 103
    plasma and serum 199^T
    red cells 82^T
    temperature and ionic
        effects on heart of 185
Radioactive alkali metal ions
    2, 3
Rana esculenta,
    effects on nerve potentials
        149
    inhibitors of Na transport
        in skin 126^T
    K-contracture in m. rectus
        abdominis 181
    stimulants of active Na
        transport in skin 127^T
Rana fusca,
    morphogenetic effect of Li
        on 33
Rana pipiens,
    inhibitors of Na transport
        in skin 126^T
    stimulants of active Na
        transport in skin 127^T
Rana temporaria,
    effect of Na on action
        potentials 163
    inhibitors of Na transport
        in skin 126^T
    stimulants of active Na
        transport in skin 127^T
Rat cerebral cortex slices 66
Rat diaphragm,
    effect of K on amino acid
        accumulation
        in 105
    — — Na on excitability
        174
    glycogen formation in 30
    K fluxes in 39^F, 95
Rat erythrocytes 82^T
Rat heart slices,
    glycogen formation in
        27^F
Rat kidney slices 27, 31, 32
Rat liver slices 30, 32, 66
Rat muscle,
    K-Na exchange in 86
    Q_{10} for Na exchange in 63
Rat plasma, serum 199^T
Rate of conduction 167

Rays,
    reactions in electric organ
        172
Reabsorption, tubular see
    tubular transport
Rectus abdominis of frog,
    K-contracture 181
Red cells see erythrocytes
Red cell "ghosts",
    ion transport in 80
Redistribution
    of K and Na in blood
        samples 200
Reissner membrane 141
Renal arterial pressure,
    effect on urine excretion
        271
Renal artery,
    effects of partial occlusion
        272
Renal blood flow,
    effects of cardiac failure
        on 382
    — — corticoids on 330,
        332
    — — hypertensin on
        355
    — — hypophysectomy
        on 341
    — — neurohypophyseal
        destruction on
        354
    — — oxytocin on 354
    — — renal nerves on
        356–359
    — — "stress" on 358
    — — symphathomi-
        metic amines
        on 359–362
    extracellular expansion,
        increase by 270
Renal denervation,
    effects on electrolyte ex-
        cretion 356
Renal excretion of alkali
    metal ions 233–423
    effects of physical factors
        on 268–277
Renal excretion of Cs 423, 526
Renal excretion of K (see
    also kaliuresis and anti-
    kaliuresis) 234, 285–301
    diurnal variations 387
    effects of sympathomi-
        metic amines on
        359–362
    relation to acid-base
        status of body
        288–292
    — — urinary acidifica-
        tion
        285–301
    — — — — Na excretion
        286

Renal excretion of Li
    419–422
    relation to Na load 421
    — — — plasma conc. 420
Renal excretion of Na (see
    also natriuresis and anti-
    natriuresis)
    diurnal variations 387
    effects of central nervous
        system on
        362–368
    — — corticoids on
        319–334
    — — extracellular
        volume expan-
        sion on 371
    — — extrarenal pres-
        sure on 276
    — — osmotic diuresis on
        280
    — — physical factors on
        268–277
    — — plasma oncotic
        pressure on
        269
    — — — sodium con-
        centration on
        277–280
    — — renal arterial pres-
        sure on 271
    — — — nerves on
        356–359
    — — — sympatho-
        mimetic
        amines on
        359–362
    — — — vascular tone
        on 356–362
    — — — venous pres-
        sure on 274
    — — ureteral pressure
        on 272
Renal excretion of Rb 422
Renal nerves,
    effects on electrolyte ex-
        cretion 356–359, 384
Renal venous pressure,
    effect on urine excretion
        274
Renin,
    effects on renal electrolyte
        excretion 355
Reproduction, organs of see
    male, resp. female organs
    of reproduction
Resins, cation exchange
    properties of 5, 510
    state of charging in inte-
        stine 511
    use in K depleting therapy
        514
    cation exchange
        use in Na depleting
        therapy 511

Resistances in nephrons 262, 279, 282, 332
Respiration,
    energizing of cation pump in ascites carcinoma by 106
    ion transport in lower vertebrates and 83, 84
Respiratory acidosis,
    effect on renal K excretion 290
    — — — Na excretion 290
    — — tubular bicarbonate reabsorption 290
    — — — hydrogen ion secretion 290
Respiratory alkalosis,
    effect on renal K excretion 288
    — — — Na excretion 288
    — — tubular bicarbonate reabsorption 288
    — — — hydrogen ion secretion 288
Respiratory enzymes,
    effect of Li on 35
Respiratory tract,
    glands of 502–503
Resting nerve,
    movements of K and Na in 96
Resting potential,
    effect of K on 144–150, 170
    — — Na on 150
    — — non-biological alkali metal ions on 151
    equation 146
Reticulo-rumen sack of sheep 130
Retina,
    isolated 103, 104^T, 221
Rhodnius,
    Malpighian tubules of 140^{TF}
Robinson-Power-Kepler water test 327
Root potential 112^F
Rubidium,
    affinity for ß-galactosidase 16
    distribution after administration 43^F, 224
Rubidium,
    distribution of naturally occurring 224

effect of loading, acute 525
— — — chronic 525
— on acetylcholine formation 29
— — aldehyde dehydrogenase 16
— — bacterial hoxokinase 13
— — enzymatic reactions 10^T, 20
— — K-contracture 176
— — membrane potential 159
— — oxygen consumption of brain slices 24
— — pyruvic phosphoferase 12
— — respiration of liver mitochondria 23
— — resting potential 151
function of in replacement of K 533
ionic radius 3^T, 20
metabolic effects on tissue slices 24
permeability of cell surfaces to 47, 159
Rb^{81}, Rb^{82}, Rb^{86}, Rb^{87} 2, 3
renal excretion 422
state in living cells 43, 44
transport in human erythrocytes 77
tubular secretion 422
Rumen,
    ion shifts in goat 129^T
    of ruminants 129
Rythmicity
    of heart 183

Saliva 450–459
    effect of corticosteroids on 457
    — — duration of secretion on 454
    — — glandular blood flow on 455
    — — plasma conc. of K and Na on 455
    — — sodium depletion on 456
    — — — loading on 456
    individual variations in composition of 459
    lithium in 459
    oxygen consumption and production of 435
    rate of secretion 454
    temperature effect on secretion of 454
Saliva
    type of gland 451
    — — stimulation 455

Salivary glands (see also individual glands) 450–459
    lithium in 460
    mechanism of secretion of 424–438
    potassium in 434
    sodium in 434
"Salt craving" and "salt hunger" 295, 365
Salt depletion see sodium depletion
Salt gland, avian see avian salt gland
Salt losing sweat glands (mucoviscoidosis) 446
Salt transport
    in epithelial cells 59
Saluresis see natriuresis, kaliuresis
Saluretics see diuretic agents
Salyrgan see mercurial diuretics
"Salzstich", chloruresis from 366
Saturation kinetics
    of K in human red cells 74
Schwann cells 159
Sciatic nerve,
    effect of injected KCl 166
Scillaren,
    action on red cells 80
Sea urchin embryos,
    morphogenetic effect of Li on 32, 34
Secretin,
    effect on duodenal mucosa 484
    — — liver 489
    — — pancreas 461
Secretion (see also resp. secretions and ions)
    apocrine 503
    eccrine 503
    exocrine glands see various glands
    holocrine 503
Secretory work
    performed in frog muscle 91
Selectivity coefficients of resins 510
Semen 499–501
Seminal vesicle 501
Seminal vesicle mucosa 107
    ion movements in 60, 107
Sensitizers to K 176
Sepia axons,
    active cation transport in 99
    effect of external Na on 162
    temperature coefficients for ion fluxes in 62, 63^T, 99

Sepia officinalis,
  K and Na in nerves of 95ᵀ
  — — — movements in
      stimulated
      nerves of
      101
Serotonin,
  effects on renal electrolyte
      excretion 355
Serum,
  K and Na in 198, 199ᵀ,
      215ᵀ
Sex hormones,
  effects on active and pas-
      sive ion transport 63
Shifts
  of alkali metals, internal
      535
Shore crab 102
Short-circuit current,
  frog skin 63, 117, 118ᵀ,
      119ᵀ, 120
  · toad large intestine 137ᵀ
  — urinary bladder 130
Short-circuiting device 117
Short-circuiting technique 117
Shrinkage of tubular cells
      279, 282
Silver,
  effect on active Na trans-
      port in amphibian skin
      127ᵀ
Simple membrane-carrier
      transport, theory of active
      ion transport 67
"Simple osmotic theory" 136
Simple passive transport 47
"Single file" movement of K
      51, 101, 160
  — Na 102
Sinus, ·
  effect of K on heart 183
Skeletal muscle,
  composed of twitch and
      slow fibres 177
  effects of cardiac glyco-
      sides on 64
  — — K on 144, 174–183
  — — Na on 174
  state of Cs and Rb in 43
Skin elasticity 192
Slow muscle fibres
  in m. rectus abdominis 181
  properties 90, 163, 177
Small intestine,
  effects of pH on absorp-
      tion in 133
  — — phlorhizin on 134
  — on ion transport in
      133, 134
Small intestine,
  exchange of intestine K
      for blood Na in 134
  NaCl transport in bull-
      frog 137, 138

Smooth muscle,
  effect of K on 148, 192
  — — Na on 191
  electric properties 147
  K-contracture in 175
Snail,
  temperature and ionic
      effects on ventricle of
      185
Snapping turtle,
  cation transport in red
      cells of 83
  effect of Na on heart 164
Sodium,
  active extrusion me-
      chanism of yeast 108
  balance see antinatriure-
      sis and natriuresis
  diffusion potential 123
  effect on enzymatic reac-
      tions 10ᵀ
  — — intestinal muscle
      191
  — — skeletal muscle 194
  — — staircase phenome-
      non 190
  — — uterus muscle 192
  energy requirement for
      active transport of 91
  excess, primary neuro-
      genic 363, 368
  extracellular 89, 90
  extrusion 88, 108
  flux across frog muscle
      fibre membrane 89
  — values and short-
      circuit current for
      toad intestine 137ᵀ
  in amniotic fluid 218
  — aqueous humour 216
  — ascites carcinoma
      cells 105
  — bone 210
  — cartilage 208
  — cerebrospinal fluid 215
  — corium 207
  — cornea 207
  — drinking water 516
  — endolymph 141ᵀ, 217
  — epidermis 220
  — erythrocytes 82ᵀ, 222
  — food components 516
  — interstitial tissue fluid
      204
  — lens 220
  — leucocytes 222
  — lymph 203
  — muscular tissues 221
  — nerves 95ᵀ
  — ovaries 223
Sodium,
  in perilymph 141ᵀ, 217
  — plasma 198
  — — and serum of labo-
      ratory animals 199ᵀ

Sodium,
  — secretions of exocrine
      glands see various
      secretions
  — serum 198
  — synovial fluid 214
  — tendon 206
  — testes 223
  — thrombocytes 222
  — uterus 194ᵀ, 222
  — vitreous humour 217
  inhibitors of active trans-
      port of 125
  intake, normal 516
  ionic radius 3ᵀ
  K uptake coupled with
      active extrusion of 77
  loading, acute and chronic
      520
  loss (renal) see natriuresis
  Na²², Na²⁴, experiments
      using
      71, 89, 134,
      137, 203, 213,
      216, 217, 218,
      219, 227, 228,
      229, 230, 231,
      232
  — — half lives 2
  net gain per impulse in
      nerve 101ᵀ, 103
  relation between active
      transport and
      frog skin poten-
      tial 114
  — — oxygen consump-
      tion and active
      transport of
      120
  renal excretion see renal
      excretion
  restricted diets 517
  retention see antinatriure-
      sis and oedema
  space 205
  state in living cells 44
  stimulants of active trans-
      port of 126
  total exchangeable 227,
      231ᵀ
  turnover, daily 517
Sodium chloride,
  effect of pH on intestinal
      absorption of 133
  — on renal Na excretion
      277, 282
  method of effecting deple-
      tion 192
Sodium deficiency (see also
      depletion and natriuresis),
  effect on colonic Na ab-
      sorption 512
  — — renal Na conser-
      vation 372

Sodium deficiency
    from adrenocortical in-
        sufficiency 301
    — cerebral disorders 363,
        366
Sodium depletion see deple-
    tion
Sodium depletion, chronic,
    effect on gastric secretion
        475
    — — salivary secretion
        456
    — — sweat secretion
        444, 449, 450
Sodium exchange
    between brain and cere-
        brospinal
        fluid 222
    — — — plasma 222
    in muscle 89
Sodium fluoride,
    effect on intestinal mucosa
        131, 134
"Sodium" hypothesis 153
Sodium loading, acute,
    effect on gastric secretion
        473, 474
    — — hepatic secretion
        489
    — — intestinal secre-
        tion 485
    — — salivary secretion
        455, 456
    — — sweat secretion 443
Sodium/oxygen ratio 61
Sodium-potassium pump 70,
    105, 141
Sodium potential 156
"Sodium pump" 37, 57–59,
    85–88
    temperature dependency
        of the 62
Sodium-retaining steroids see
    mineralocorticoids, aldo-
    sterone and desoxycorti-
    costerone
Sodium selectivity 152
Sodium space,
    relation to extracellular
        space 205
Sodium sulphate
    as osmotic diuretic 281^T
    effect on intestinal ab-
        sorption of NaCl 131
    permeability of intestinal
        walls to 134
Sodium theory of electric
    activity,
    applicability and limita-
        tions of 160
"Sodium" theory of excitation
    151, 155
Sodium transport (see also
    active, passive transport)
    effect of p_H on 76, 125

Sodium transport
    in human erythrocytes 75
    — intestinal mucosa 131
    — muscle 88
    over placenta 219
    through giant fibre mem-
        brane 101
Solute diuresis 388
Solvent drag 49, 51–54
    force arising from 52
    intestinal transport and
        69
    ionic diameter and 53
Somatotropin,
    renal effects 314, 342
Spider crab nerve 102, 150
Spinal roots 150, 151
Spirolactones,
    renal effects 418
Squid axon 149, 165, 166
Squid giant axon 148^F, 151
Staircase phenomenon 188
    effect of Na on 190
    of heart muscle 84, 173,
        188, 189, 195
    — uterus muscle 84, 194
Steroid hormones (see also
    corticosteroids)
    effects on active and pas-
        sive transport 63
Stimulants
    of active Na transport 126
Stoichiometric efficiency
    of ion transport 62
Stop flow analysis (renal) 241,
    260, 403, 417
Stratum germinativum 127
Striated muscle 144, 163, 166
Strontium chloride,
    effects on frog nerve 150
Strophantidin,
    effect on ion transport in
        erythrocytes 79
G-Strophantin,
    effect on ion transport in
        amphibian
        skin 64, 126
    — — Na transport in
        mouse ascites
        carcinoma 106
Strophantins,
    effects on ion transport in
        erythrocytes 79
Sublingual gland 426, 428,
    433, 452
    electrophysiology of 428,
        433
    mechanism of secretion of
        424–438
    potassium in 434
    sodium in 434
Sublingual secretion 452
Submaxillary gland,
    electrophysiology of 428,
        433

Submaxillary gland,
    mechanism of secretion of
        424–438
    potassium in 434
    sodium in 434
Submaxillary secretion 452
Sub-synaptic membrane 161,
    170
Succinate,
    effect on brain slices 25
Succinic dehydrogenase
    (renal)
    mercurials, effects on 399,
        404
Sucrose,
    renal effects 390
Sulfhydryl groups (renal)
    mercurials, effects of 405
Sulphanilamide,
    inhibition of Na transport
        in frog skin 126^T
Sulphate 131, 134, 281^T
    renal effect 280, 393
Sulphonamides see carbonic
    anhydrase inhibitors
Supraoptic neurones 348, 352,
    362, 365
Surgery,
    effects on renal electrolyte
        excretion 357
Sweat 438–450
    effect of corticosteroids on
        445
    — — duration of secre-
        tion on 442
    — — glandular blood
        flow on 443
    — — plasma conc. of
        alkali metals
        on 443
    — — rate of secretion on
        440
    — — sodium depletion
        on 444, 449,
        450
    — — — loading on 444
    individual variation in
        composition of 445
    temperature and secretion
        of 442
    type of gland 439
    — — stimulation 443
Sweat glands,
    mechanism of secretion of
        424–438
Sweating,
    effect on homeostasis
        447–450
Swelling,
    metabolic inhibition in
        tissue slices arising
        from 66
Sympathomimetic amines,
    renal effects 359–362

Synapses,
relation of alkali metal ions to electric activity of 168
Synovial fluid 20, 214

Taenia coli,
effects on muscular potentials of 147
Tail organizer,
morphogenetic effect of Li on 33
Tears (see also lacrymal gland) 463–464
Teleosts,
ion transport in red cells of 84
Temperature,
effect on cation fluxes in nerve 98
— — gastric secretion 475
— — hepatic secretion 490
— — ion transport in red cells 76
— — salivary secretion 454
— — sweat secretion 442
relation to ionic effects on heart 185
Temperature coefficients,
estimation from isotopic exchange 62
for ion transport in mouse ascites carcinoma 106
— — — — Sepia axons 99
— Na transport in tissues 62, 63^T
Tendomucoid,
binding of K and Na by 206
Tendon,
K and Na in 206
Tenebrio,
Malpighian tubules of 140^T
Testes,
K and Na in 223
Tetrabutylammonium,
effect on crustacean muscle 161
Tetraethylammonium,
effect on crustacean muscle 163
— — frog nerve 161, 162
— — spinal roots 151
— — squid nerve 161
Tetraethylfluorophosphate,
effect on Eriocheir sinensis 143

Tetraethylpyrophosphate,
effect on active Na transport in frog skin 125, 126^T
Tetramethylammonium-Ringer 163
Thallium,
renal excretion 423
Theophylline,
effects on kidney cortex slices 106
Thiocyanate,
renal effects 237
— excretion 259
sensitizing effect towards K 176
Thiomerin see mercurial diuretics
Thionin,
effect on Eriocheir sinensis 143
Thiosulphate,
renal effects 280
Thiourea,
permeability of frog skin towards 128
"Third compartment",
location of Na in 45
Thirst center (hypothalamic) 362
Thiry-Vella loops 134, 138
Threshold for electrical stimulation,
effect of K on 167
Thrombocytes,
K and Na in 222
Thymonucleic acid 8
Thyroxin,
diuretic effect 335, 352
Tissue slices,
metabolic effects on 23
Toad large intestine 133, 136
Toad muscle,
K in 45
Toad myelinated nerve fibres 96
Toad nerves,
K and Na in 95^T
Toad urinary bladder 130
p-Toluenesulfonamide,
effect on Na transport in frog skin 126^T
Tolypellopsis,
K and Na in sap and cytoplasm 36
Tonicity,
body fluid, effect on vasopressin secretion 348
of renal tissue 248
— urine 242–251
plasma see osmolar conc.
Torpedo,
properties of cholinesterases, isolated from 19

Torpedo,
reactions in electric organ 172
voltage 171
Total body contents
of K 226
Na 226
relation to K_e, Na_e 231
— — serum conc. 232
Total exchangeable contents
of K 227
— Na 227
relation to total body contents 231
Toxin from diniflagellate,
effects on frog 126
Tracer experiments,
determination of flux ratios using 49
Transcellular transport of Na 58
Transfer, tubular see tubular transport
Transmitter substance,
effects on sub-synaptic membrane 171
Transport
between cells and their surroundings 70
of ions through porous membranes 51
— water across frog skin, relation to active Na transport 128
Transport, tubular see tubular transport
Triphosphopyridine nucleotide (TPN),
binding of K and Na by 7
Triton alpestris,
morphogenetic effect of Li on 33
Tubocurarine,
effect on Eriocheir sinensis 143
Tubular excretion
of p-aminohippurate 27^F
Tubular factors
and renal salt water excretion 261–272
Tubular fluid,
analysis of 235, 247, 249
pH of 239
Tubular secretion
of hydrogen ions 239, 252, 288, 296, 322
— potassium 256, 286, 299, 322
— water 261
Tubular transport (renal)
effects of glucocorticoids on 319, 329
— — mineralcorticoids on 322

Tubular transport
  of alkali metal ions
      244–261
  — ammonia 254
  — anions 237
  — chloride 234, 238,
      242–254
  — water 234–261
  suppression 266
Tubules (renal)
  intraluminal pressures
      264–266, 284
  isolation of flounder 31
  micropuncture 235, 247,
      249
  permeability, change by
      vasopressin 243, 343
  resistances in 264–266, 284
Turtle heart,
  effects of K and acetylcho-
              line on
          187
  — — — — temperatu-
          re on
          185
  K release during contrac-
      tion 182
Twitch muscle fibres,
  properties 177, 181
Twitch tension of isometric
  contraction,
  effect of K on 178

Ulva 57
Ulva lactuca 109
"Unexchangeable" Na 213
Unmyelinated nerve fibres,
  movements of K and Na
      in stimulated 101^T
Urea
  as osmotic diuretic 280,
      281^T, 391
  effect on renal concentrat-
      ing mechanism 251
Urease 18
Ureteral pressure,
  effect on urine excretion
      272
Ureterocolic anastomosis and
  intestinal ion transfer 514
Uridine triphosphate 7
Urinary bladder,
  ion transport by isolated
      toad 130
Urinary bladder wall,
  ion transfer across 423
Urine,
  acidification of 252
  ammonia in 254
  formation of hypertonic
      242–251
  — — hypotonic 242–251

Uterine mucosa 501
Uterine secretion 501
Uterus muscle,
  effect of K on 193
  — — Na on 192
  K and Na in 194^T, 222
  staircase phenomenon 84,
      194

Valonia 36, 109
Valonia macrophysa 110
Vascular muscle,
  effect of K on 195
Vasopressin 343–353
  control of secretion
      348–352
  effect on active Na trans-
              port in amphi-
              bian skin 127^T
  — — sweat glands 448
  — — tubular water
              transfer
      243–251, 265,
      343
  effects on renal electrolyte
      excretion 344
  resistance towards 336,
      352, 421
  role in adrenocortical
              insufficiency
          333
  — — cardiac oedema
          386
Vegetalizing substances 35
Ventricle,
  effect of K on 184
Veratrine,
  effects on skeletal muscle
      176
Versene,
  activation of myosin
      ATP-ase by 18
  complex formation with
      Na 5
Vitreous humour,
  K and Na in 217
Voltage clamp,
  K^{42} outflux and membrane
      current in Sepia axons
      during 101
  membrane current in
      squid axons under 155
  of heart muscle 164, 167
  relation to spike of im-
      pulses 158
Voltage clamp current,
  separation into K and Na
      components 156, 157
Voltage clamp method,
  advantages of 155
  principle of 154

Volume of living cells,
  role of alkali metal ion
      transport in regulation
      of 65

Water,
  natriuretic effect 389
  renal handling of 234–251
Water deficiency,
  primary neurogenic 363,
      364
Water diuresis 242, 388
  reduced in adrenocortical
      insufficiency 327
  resulting from alcohol 352
  — — carbon dioxide 352
  — — cold 352
  — — corticoids 334
  — — epinephrine 352
  — — hyperthyroidism
          352
  — — potassium defi-
          ciency 336, 352
Water excess,
  primary neurogenic 363,
      364
Water intoxication 365
Water test 327
Woolhanded crab 142
Work performed
  by active Na transport
      mechanism 120

Xanthine diuretics 410–415
  diuretics chemically
      related to 415
  effects on glomerular fil-
      tration rate 414
  — — renal blood flow
          413
  — — — electrolyte
              excretion
          411
  extrarenal effects 411
  mechanism of action 411
Xanthines,
  effect on ion transport in
      frog skin 125

Yeast 108
  active transport of K and
              H in 38
  — — — Na in 57
  competition between Na
      and Li in active trans-
      port 109
  Na extrusion mechanism
      of 108

Z-membrane 179
"Zuckerstich",
  chloruresis from 365